DNA REPLICATION - CURRENT ADVANCES

Edited by **Hervé Seligmann**

DNA Replication - Current Advances
Edited by Hervé Seligmann

Published by InTech

Janeza Trdine 9, 51000 Rijeka, Croatia

Publishing Process Manager Ana Pantar

Technical Editor Teodora Smiljanic

Cover Designer InTech Design Team

Additional hard copies can be obtained from orders@intechopen.com

DNA Replication - Current Advances, Edited by Hervé Seligmann
p. cm.
ISBN 978-953-307-593-8

For EU product safety concerns:
IN TECH d.o.o., Prolaz Marije Krucifikse Kozulić 3, 51000 Rijeka, Croatia,
info@intechopen.com or visit our website at intechopen.com.

Meet the editor

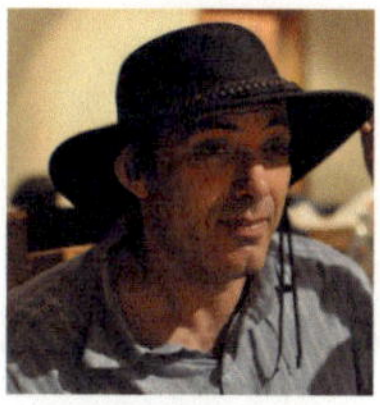

Dr. Hervé Seligmann has been a research associate of the National Collections of Natural History at the Hebrew University of Jerusalem since 2010. Following his research studies there at the Department of Botany (M. Sc. in plant physiology) he gained his Ph.D. there at the Department of Evolution, Systematics and Ecology in 2003 in vertebrate comparative ecomorphology. He was a visiting researcher at the Victoria University of Wellington, New Zealand, associate researcher at the University of Chicago, the Louisiana State University and the University of Oslo. He made major contributions to numerous international scientific journals in the disciplines of developmental physiology of plants, behavioural vertebrate ecomorphology, and molecular biology and evolution, notably on parallel/overlapping genetic codes. Current research interests develop explicit adaptive models of molecular mechanisms linking molecular phenomena and whole organism properties. He has co-authored more than 45 scientific publications and currently looks for a payed position.

Contents

Preface XIII

Part 1 DNA Structure 1

Chapter 1 **DNA Structure: Alphabet Soup for the Cellular Soul 3**
P. Shing Ho and Megan Carter

Chapter 2 **Replication Demands an Amendment of the Double Helix 29**
You Cheng Xu

Chapter 3 **Phosphorothioation: An Unusual Post-Replicative Modification on the DNA Backbone 57**
Lianrong Wang, Shi Chen and Zixin Deng

Chapter 4 **Mitosis and DNA Replication and Life Origination Hydrate Hypotheses: Common Physical and Chemical Grounds 75**
Ostrovskii Victor E. and Kadyshevich Elena A.

Part 2 Mutations 115

Chapter 5 **Strand-specific Composition Bias in Bacterial Genomes 117**
Feng-Biao Guo and Lu-Wen Ning

Chapter 6 **Mutation Patterns Due to Converging Mitochondrial Replication and Transcription Increase Lifespan, and Cause Growth Rate-Longevity Tradeoffs 137**
Hervé Seligmann

Chapter 7 **Mitochondrial DNA Replication in Health and Disease 167**
Nadezda Apostolova and Juan V. Esplugues

Chapter 8 **Damage and Replication Stress Responses 183**
Haiying Wang, Ping Shen and Wei-Guo Zhu

Part 3 Replication Origins, Forks, Chromatine Organization 201

Chapter 9 **Relationship between Fork Progression and Initiation of Chromosome Replication in *E. coli* 203**
Elena C. Guzmán, Israel Salguero, Carmen Mata Martín, Elena López Acedo, Estrella Guarino, Mª Antonia Sánchez-Romero, Vic Norris and Alfonso Jiménez-Sánchez

Chapter 10 **Replication Origin Selection and Pre-Replication Complex Assembly 221**
Kusic-Tisma Jelena and Stefanovic Dragana

Chapter 11 **The Coordination between DNA Replication Initiation and Other Cell Cycle Events 233**
Shijiao Huang and Chuanmao Zhang

Chapter 12 **The Organisation of Replisomes 253**
Anna Ligasová and Karel Koberna

Chapter 13 **Eukaryotic Replication Barriers: How, Why and Where Forks Stall 269**
Jacob Z. Dalgaard, Emma L. Godfrey and Ramsay J. MacFarlane

Chapter 14 **Control of Telomeric DNA Replication: Genetics, Molecular Biology, and Physiology 305**
Akira Matsuura and Aiko Matsui

Chapter 15 **Telomere Maintenance in Organisms without Telomerase 323**
James M. Mason, Hemakumar M. Reddy and Radmila Capkova Frydrychova

Chapter 16 **Eukaryote DNA Replication and Recombination: an Intimate Association 347**
Ramsay J. McFarlane, Khalid Al-Zeer and Jacob Z. Dalgaard

Part 4 The Cell Cycle and Replication 389

Chapter 17 **Cell Cycle Regulation of DNA Replication in *S. cerevisiae* 391**
Jorrit M. Enserink

Chapter 18 **Free Histones and the Cell Cycle 409**
Douglas Maya, Macarena Morillo-Huesca, Sebastián Chávez and Mari-Cruz Muñoz-Centeno

Chapter 19 **Involvement of Linker Histones in the Regulation of Replication Timing 427**
Christophe Thiriet, Gwenola Auda-Boucher and Yvonnick Chéraud

Chapter 20 **Replication Timing: Evolution, Nuclear Organization and Relevance for Human Disease 437**
Megan Lynne Wright and Frank Grützner

Chapter 21 **The Silencing Face of DNA Replication: Gene Repression Mediated by DNA Replication Factors 467**
Patricia Chisamore-Robert, Daniel Jeffery and Krassimir Yankulov

Part 5 Proteins in Replication 485

Chapter 22 **Faithful DNA Replication Requires Regulation of CDK Activity by Checkpoint Kinases 487**
Claus Storgaard Sørensen, Halfdan Beck, Viola Nähse-Kumpf and Randi G. Syljuåsen

Chapter 23 **Regulation of the G1/S Transition in Adult Liver: Expression and Activation of the Cyclin Dependent Kinase Cdk1 in Differentiated Hepatocytes is Controlled by Extracellular Signals and is Crucial for Commitment to DNA Replication 511**
Loyer Pascal and Corlu Anne

Chapter 24 **Binding of Human MCM-BP with MCM2-7 Proteins 549**
Ryoko Kon, Shunsuke Kusunoki, Naohito Nozaki and Yukio Ishimi

Chapter 25 **DNA Replication in Animal Systems Lacking Thioredoxin Reductase I 565**
Edward E. Schmidt

Part 6 Replication and Diseases 585

Chapter 26 **Prevalence of Reactivation of Hepatitis B Virus DNA Replication in Rheumatoid Arthritis Patients 587**
Yukitomo Urata, Ryoko Uesato and Dai Tanaka

Chapter 27 **Oncogenic Aspects of HPV Infections of the Female Genital Tract 595**
Josko Zekan, Maja Sirotkovic-Skerlev and Mihael Skerlev

Chapter 28 **The Role of E2 Proteins in Papillomavirus DNA Replication 613**
Reet Kurg

Chapter 29 **Topoisomerase I and II Expression in Recurrent Colorectal Cancer Cells: A Dubious Matter 639**
Panagiotis Gouveris, Elias Skopelitis and Nicolas Tsavaris

Chapter 30 **Bacterial Genetics of Large Mammalian DNA Viruses: Bacterial Artificial Chromosomes as a Prerequisite for Efficiently Studying Viral DNA Replication and Functions 669**
Felix Wussow, Tanja Spieckermann, Anne Brunnemann, Linda Hüske, Tuna Toptan and Helmut Fickenscher

Preface

This book includes a selection of authoritative reviews and contributions in the general field of DNA replication. One of the characteristics of this collection is that it touches a number of diverse domains, from the stereochemistry of DNA (chapters by Ostrovskii and Kadyshevich, Xu, Ho and Carter, Wang et al.), its physicochemical properties as determining the dynamics of mutations (chapters by Guo and Ning, Seligmann), the epidemiology of some replication-associated diseases (chapters by Kurg, Urata et al., Zekan et al., Gouveris et al.), and interactions with various protein complexes responsible for its replication and regulation of that process (most other chapters). Nevertheless, some subjects can be felt as missing or relatively neglected. For example, the functional protein family of DNA polymerases, given its central role in DNA replication, is fairly little mentioned, and only the famous DNA polymerase is given some attention (chapter by Apostolova and Esplugues). An analysis of fidelities of DNA polymerases would have been an adequate chapter subject in the scope of this book, especially if integrated with other, non-enzymatic processes leading to mutations, but current interests of the contributors did not focus on this. Similarly, viral DNA replication is relatively underrepresented in this volume, as compared to and despite its crucial contribution to the study of DNA replication in general (Wussow et al.). The book's contents therefore reflect mainly current trends on the subject of DNA replication.

Some chapters describe very surprising analyses, in the sense that they touch fundamental properties of DNA. One could have believed that basic DNA fundamentals are assessed and do not include major undiscovered or unresolved points after more than half a century of intensive study and exploration by the scientific community. Especially because this community currently happens to be the largest of its kind human history has ever known, and that the study of DNA involves major discoveries in terms of technical importance, outcompeted in importance only by discoveries such as that of fire, the number zero, the conceptualization of cause-effect relations or metallurgy .

Among these "new" DNA properties, for example, Wang et al. show in their chapter that the phosphate DNA backbone sometimes includes sulphur atoms, instead of oxygen, which is probably frequently used as a processing signal. Another major, perhaps controversial, issue is that of the orientation of the DNA's double helix (chapter by Xu) in which the author suggests that the double helix might be occasionally left-handed. The issue of left-handed DNA as a way of reducing physical tension in DNA molecules is in a way predicted by a number of other known phenomena, such as the inverse association between replication rates and distances between replication forks mentioned in the chapter by Guzmán et al. As amply explained in the chapter by Xu, this potential discovery, though contradicting commonly accepted concepts on DNA structure, does not revolutionize our understanding of DNA. It rather is a useful amendment to the model of DNA structure and function. Despite this, its publication necessitated a major, multidecennial effort on behalf of the author. This reflects more the theological-aristotelian origins of the modern scientific process of expansion of human knowledge through authority and sometimes censorship by a few rather than the current, ideally transparent, open (=published) evaluation and discussion of evidence and its interpretation, available to and by each one interested. The fact that some other chapters report no less or even more revolutionary findings on DNA, underlines the need to keep an open mind attitude, even towards commonly "accepted truths" on presumably well-known subjects. The deep conviction that no human knowledge is perfect, but only perfectible, should function as a fair safeguard in this respect. It is, in my opinion, a simple but effective way to prevent as much as possible the unavoidable psychological barriers that impede on the advancement of our understanding of natural phenomena through open discussion.

But perhaps the most astonishing and challenging novelty in this book is the approach of DNA structure and chemical dynamics by focusing on its interactions with its natural solvent, the water molecules, and the changes in water concentrations through the cell's life cycle (chapter by Ostrovskii and Kadyshevich). This most interesting hypothesis develops a concept that escapes conceptions established through the force of habit, which frequently result in dominant, yet unproven intuitive truths. This hypothesis will doubtlessly produce new, deep insights into every level of DNA-associated processes, and probably also general cell physiology, if given the deserved consideration and further developed. The approach in that chapter integrates processes associated with DNA and its structure with more basic physical properties at a lower scale of natural phenomena, namely the multimolecular dynamical structure of water. DNA properties can also be integrated with higher-scale phenomena: Seligmann suggests how whole-organism characteristics associate with details of DNA replication. Both chapters touch the issue of regulation of DNA replication and transcription, DNA versus RNA synthesis, the two main processes involving DNA molecules. The issue of integrating DNA and RNA synthesis is at least mentioned if not extensively explored by a large number of chapters (i.e Chisamore-Rob et al., Huang and Zhang). This suggests that the matter of coregulating DNA and RNA syntheses is very likely to be developed further by future activities in various subdisciplines dealing with DNA replication.

I chose to relatively neglect in this preface the mentioning of studies of the more complex organisation of eukaryotic chromosomes and their complex replication because this is the topic of the larger portion of this book's chapters (Matsuura and Matsui, Schmidt, Maya et al., McFarlane et al., Sørensen et al., Loyer and Corlu, Kon et al., Enserink). Several chapters deal with detection and regulation of eukaryotic replication origins (Grutzner and Wright, Kusic-Tisma and Stefanovic, Dalgaard et al., Ligasová and Koberna, Thiriet et al.), a matter not well established even in presumably simpler genomes (Guzman et al.), without forgetting the matter of DNA-associated DNA repair (i.e. Wang, Shen and Zhu). As shown by several chapters in this book, I do not think that it is an overstatement to assume that the study of DNA will continue for a while to be a leading front of scientific activities.

Luxemburg, 06 VII 2011

Hervé Seligmann,
Herpetological Collection National Natural History Collections (NNHC),
The Hebrew University of Jerusalem,
Israel

Center for Ecological and Evolutionary Synthesis,
University of Oslo,
Norway

Department of Life Sciences,
Ben Gurion University,
Israel

Part 1

DNA Structure

1

DNA Structure: Alphabet Soup for the Cellular Soul

P. Shing Ho and Megan Carter
Department of Biochemistry and Molecular Biology,
Colorado State University
USA

1. Introduction

The story of DNA structure is as varied as it is interesting, the most famous tale being the "discovery" of B-DNA by Watson and Crick. For many biologists, this simple, but elegant structure is all that is needed for a basic, albeit superficial understanding of cellular genetics. A deeper appreciation for how DNA functions comes from the recognition that this is a highly malleable molecule, providing the cell with a plethora of conformations to exploit in replication and transcription. Some of these conformations can give rise to mistakes, while others help to repair those mistakes in the genetic code. In this chapter, we dive into the cellular pot and find a literal alphabet soup of DNA structures. We start our journey by presenting the fundamental principles that serve as the vocabulary to analyze and describe the features of nucleic acid structures. We will explore the conformational variations that lead from double-helices to complexes composed of three or four strands, then consider how conformations interconvert through various intermediates. Although B-DNA is the standard form in the cell, we suggest that this dance away from the norm is essential for cellular function, giving the cell life and, hence, its genetic soul.

Replication is the process by which the cell creates an exact copy of the genetic information encoded in DNA—it is thus intuitive that we would be interested in the actual structure of DNA as a molecule. One would think that, for replication, we need only be concerned with the DNA duplex at the beginning, the single-stranded intermediate state, and the final duplex, since these structures generally tell us how the information is stored and read, and what the resulting product is. However, it is becoming clear that although the general structure of DNA is important in the overall mechanism of replication (Watson & Crick, 1953a), the conformational details are important for understanding how proteins recognize their cognate DNA sequence, and how mutations may be introduced and are repaired. Thus, we must explore and dissect the details in terms of variations that define the particular sequence dependent shape of DNA.

We will not attempt the impossible task of covering every aspect of DNA structure, only those that may be relevant to replication. Also, as crystallographers, we will have a bias towards studies derived from X-ray diffraction and other physical methods, although we will always attempt to relate these back to the biology of replication. In the process, we will explore the details of DNA structure that help elucidate structural principles that contribute to our understanding of the mechanism and fidelity of the replicative process.

2. A brief history of DNA structure

DNA structure has had over 55 years of history and, in that time, has undergone periods of discovery that have pushed the field forward in spurts. The evidence that DNA is the genetic molecule in the cell came from the studies of Avery, MacLeod, and McCarty (Avery *et al.*, 1944), and confirmed by Hershey and Chase (Hershey and Chase, 1952). The seminal experiments of Meselsen and Stahl (Meselson and Stahl, 1958) using heavy atom labeled DNA demonstrated that replication is semiconservative, with each newly replicated daughter strand being paired with one of the two parental strands. These classic studies from the 1940's and 1950's set the stage for a race to determine the molecular structure of DNA, a now familiar story that helps to bring perspective to the discussions in this chapter.

2.1 The race for the structure of DNA: X-ray fiber diffraction studies.

The key element in the race towards the structure of DNA was the availability of X-ray diffraction photographs of DNA fibers, the best of which came from the work of Franklin and Gosling in the lab of John Randall. It was clear at the time that DNA could adopt two different forms, an A-form under low humidity and a B-form at higher humidity. The A-DNA form gave the highest resolution data (Franklin and Gosling, 1953a), but, it was the lower resolution photograph of the "wetter" B-form (Franklin and Gosling, 1953b) (Fig. 1) that was more readily interpretable. From this photograph, DNA was clearly seen to be a helical structure (showing the characteristic "helical-X" in the diffraction pattern), with a repeat of 10 units (reflected in the pattern converging after 10 layer lines), and with a distance between repeating units of 3.4 Å (from the *d*-spacing of 10th layer line). What was not evident was the number of strands in the helix (indeed, Linus Pauling had initially proposed a three-stranded structure (Pauling and Corey, 1953)), whether it is left- or right-handed, and how the information is read and properly replicated. The interpretation of this data by Watson and Crick (Watson and Crick, 1953b) lead to the iconic right-handed, antiparallel, double-helical model of DNA that we all recognize.

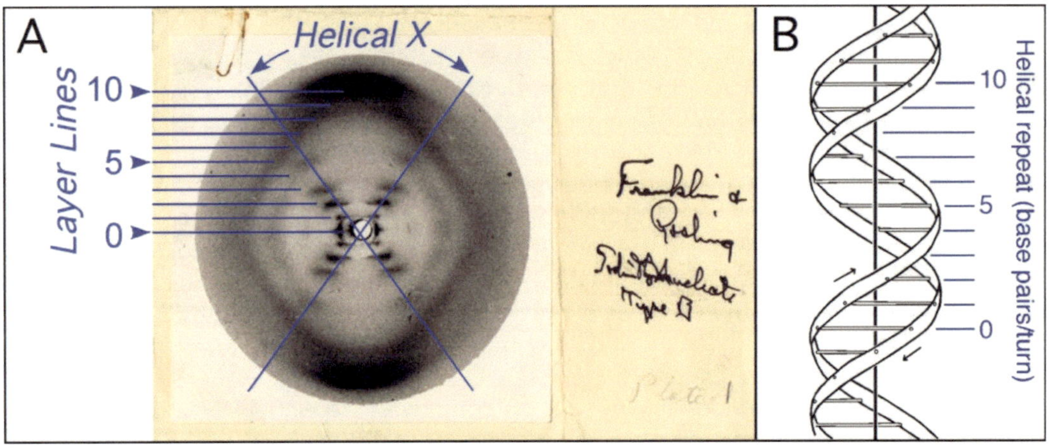

Fig. 1. Structure of B-DNA. A. Photograph 51 of B-DNA. X-ray diffraction photograph of a DNA fiber at high humidity (Franklin and Gosling, 1953b). Interpretation of the helical-X and layer lines added in blue. B. Watson-Crick model of B-DNA, adopted from (Watson and Crick, 1953b), with the helical repeat associated with the layer lines labeled.

Often missing from this story is that the Watson-Crick model depended not only on the large amount of biochemical and X-ray diffraction data being generated at the time, but also on a proper understanding of the chemical properties of DNA. One of the most important aspects of the Watson-Crick model was the proposal that guanines paired with cytosines and adenines with thymines. For this to occur, however, the nucleotide bases must be drawn in their proper tautomeric forms; however, up to that point, it was not clear, even to the organic chemists, what those forms should be. The initial assignment of guanine and thymine bases in their enol forms had lead to an early parallel model for DNA (Watson, 1968). It was not until the proper tautomers for the common nucleotides were assigned that the now familiar base pairs of G to C and A to T made sense, and, thus, provide a rationale for the well understood Chargaff rules for the complementary composition of nucleotides in the DNA of higher organisms (Chargaff, 1950) and a mechanism by which exact copies of the sequence information along a strand of DNA could result in an exact copy of a duplex through semiconservative replication (Watson and Crick, 1953a).

2.2 The single-crystal structures of DNA oligonucleotides

At this point, it should be stressed that Watson and Crick did not "discover" or "solve" the structure of DNA, but had presented a plausible and, basically, correct model that made important predictions that, in the end, led to the birth of modern molecular biology. However, several decades will pass before high resolution single crystals structures of synthetic DNAs emerge to support the essential elements of this model. For example, it was not immediately obvious that the Watson-Crick scheme, particularly for A=T base pairs, was correct—at the time the single-crystal structures of adenine bases paired with thymine or uracil bases showed geometries of Hoogsteen-type base pairs (this will be defined in Section 3). It was not until the crystal structure of the RNA dinucleotide phosphate ApU was determined to a remarkable 0.89 Å resolution (in crystallography, lower numbers refer to higher resolution) by Alexander Rich's group (Rosenberg *et al.*, 1973) that the Watson-Crick form of the A=U (and, thus, the analogous A=T) base pairs were confirmed. The concurrent structure of GpC also confirmed the Watson-Crick form of the G•C base pair (Day *et al.*, 1973) and, together, demonstrated for the first time that nucleotide double-helices (in this case, RNA dinucleotides) were antiparallel and had a right-handed twist.

In the late 1970's, it became possible to chemically synthesize "long" stretches of a defined DNA sequence for crystallographic studies. In 1979, Rich's group (Wang *et al.*, 1979) determined the single crystal structure of the DNA sequence CGCGCG (we write only one strand and drop the "p" for the phosphates for the sake of efficiency, even for double-helical structures). This structure showed DNA to be an antiparallel double-helix with Watson-Crick type base pairs, consistent with the 1953 model. However, it came with a new twist—this double-helix was left-handed and was called Z-DNA (for the zig-zagged backbone). It was not until 1981, with the single-crystal structure of the sequence CGCGTATACGCG (known as the Drew-Dickerson dodecamer (Drew *et al.*, 1981)), that the Watson-Crick structure for B-DNA was finally "proven" to be correct.

So, what of the dehydrated A-DNA form that Franklin had worked so hard on and struggled with? Soon after the Watson and Crick model of B-DNA, Franklin and Gosling published the structure of the fiber A-DNA form (Franklin and Gosling, 1953a), with a large number of single-crystals of A-DNA being determined and published in the 1980's and 1990's (the "heydays" of DNA crystallography (Mirkin, 2008)). The A-form was subsequently shown to be the native form of RNA duplexes, while DNA/RNA hybrids (primers for replication initiation) can interchange between the A- and B-forms.

Although it is well accepted that the B-DNA form is the most prevalent form in solution and in the cell, there is now a myriad of single-crystal DNA structures, including those assembled as double-, triple-, quadruple-, and even hexa- and octa-stranded complexes. There are hairpins from single-strands, structures with overhangs, etc., and a plethora of forms seen in complexes with proteins. We will discuss some of these in greater detail in Section 4 along with their relevant cellular functions, focusing on replication and the associated processes. First, we must delve into the detailed vocabulary used to describe DNA structure and provide a common language for the remainder of the chapter.

3. A vocabulary lesson for DNA structure

As with any description of a biopolymer, we will start the discussion of DNA structure at the simplest unit (the nucleotide building block), then develop the concepts of structure with increasing size and complexity. In order to reach this stage of complexity, we must first define terms that will be used in discussing DNA structure at all levels.

3.1 General principles

Almost every student today knows that DNA is composed of four basic building blocks, each defined by the unique chemical structure of the aromatic base, and each base attached to a phosphodeoxyribose backbone. The four common deoxyribonucleotides are categorized as the purine (deoxyadenosine, dA, and deoxyguanosine, dG) or pyrimidine (deoxythymidine, dT, and deoxycytosine, dC) nucleotides. The atoms of sugars are distinguished from those of the bases by a "prime" added to the atom name, so that the sugar carbons are C1′, C2′, C3′, C4′, C5′ (Fig. 2), starting with the carbon at the glycosidic bond that attaches the base to the sugar, and so forth around the ring. The deoxynucleotides of DNA lack a O2′ oxygen, which distinguishes them from ribonucleotides (RNA). For simplicity, we will simply assume the deoxyform and drop the "deoxy" and "d" prefixes from this point on (Hendrickson *et al.*, 1988).

3.2 What defines a stable DNA structure?

DNA in its functional form is not the isolated nucleotides, but a polymer built from the mononucleotides (G, C, A, T). A DNA polymer is constructed through condensation to form a phosphodiester linkage that bridges the O3′ and O5′ oxygens of sequential nucleotides (Fig. 2A). The primary structure, or sequence, of a DNA polymer strand is written in the direction that they are synthesized in the cell, starting at the free O5′ oxygen (5′-end) and progresses to the free O3′-end. Two complementary strands are brought together in a sequence specific manner to form an antiparallel double-strand, aligning one strand in the 5′ to 3′ direction and the complement 3′ to 5′. Nearly all functional secondary structures of DNA are multi-stranded, most commonly double-stranded. As the sequence of one strand dictates that of its complement, double-stranded DNA is often considered as a single biological molecule, even though the strands are not covalently linked.

3.2.1 Base pairing

Unlike proteins and RNA, the functional forms of DNA are typically complexes comprised of two or more strands, which are stabilized by base pairing, base stacking, and solvent interactions. Of these, base pairing is best understood for its important role in specifying the

sequence of newly synthesized DNA during replication and in general sequence recognition, but is perhaps the most misunderstood for its contribution to DNA stability.
The most commonly recognized form of DNA, B-DNA, is the double-stranded duplex stabilized by Watson-Crick base pairing (Fig. 2B). In standard Watson-Crick G•C and A•T base pairs, hydrogen bonds are formed between the respective donor and acceptor functional groups along what is called the "Watson-Crick" edges of the bases. The geometries of both purine-pyrimidine base pairs are similar in the relative positions of their bases and, consequently, the width of the resulting major and minor groove—the similarity in the geometries of correctly paired bases contributes to the fidelity of the replication polymerases [(Kool, 2001)]. The G•C base pair, however, is stabilized by three hydrogen bonds as opposed to the two that stabilize A•T base pairs; thus, G•C rich sequences tend to have higher stabilization energies and melting temperatures. With only two hydrogen bonds, A•T base pairs offer less resistance to deformations, including twisting of the individual bases from a common plane (called propeller twist, see below). Although the standard Watson-Crick base paired duplex DNA is most universally recognized, it is clear that DNA structures with non-standard pairing of bases are more prevalent and biologically significant than previously thought [(Neidle, 1999)].

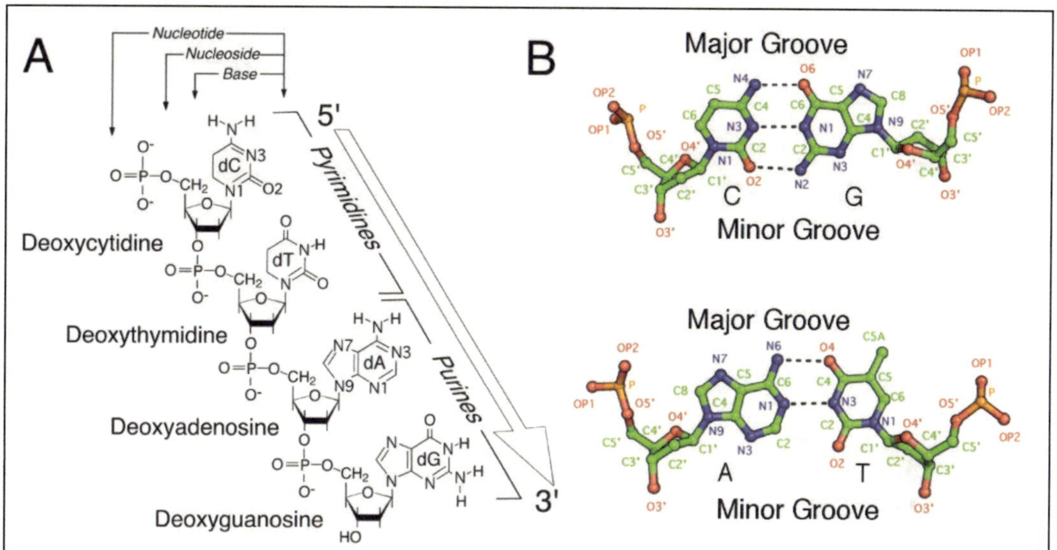

Fig. 2. Components of DNA. A. The four common deoxyribonucleotides are connected by phosphodiester bonds to form a single-strand, 5′ to 3′. B. Watson and Crick C•G and A•T base pairs with the major and minor grooves labeled.

Non-standard base pairs play critical roles in the varied structures observed in DNA and RNA. Wobble, mismatched, and reverse base pairs still use the Watson-Crick edges for hydrogen bonding. Reverse Watson-Crick base pairs are found in parallel duplexes, but are not immediately relevant to DNA replication. Wobble base pairing (Fig. 3A) is seen in mismatches between G•T and G•U base pairs incorporated into DNA and DNA:RNA complexes and play essential roles in the fidelity of DNA replication and transcription. Such mismatches can lead to genome mutations if not accurately detected and corrected by the

proof reading activity of DNA polymerase during replication, or post-replicative repair systems. Studies suggest that G•T and A⁺•C are the most frequent mismatches that cause point mutations in cells (Neidle, 1999). The energies of hydrogen bonding in proper and mismatched bases, relative to base stacking and steric effects, however, appear to have little influence on polymerase fidelity (Kool, 2001).
Hoogsteen base pairs take advantage of the Hoogsteen edge of a purine base, which is orthogonal to and, thus, can be accessed without disrupting the Watson-Crick base pairing edge (Fig. 3B). Consequently, Hoogsteen interactions allow the assembly of multi-stranded DNA complexes, including triplet helixes and G-quadruplexes.

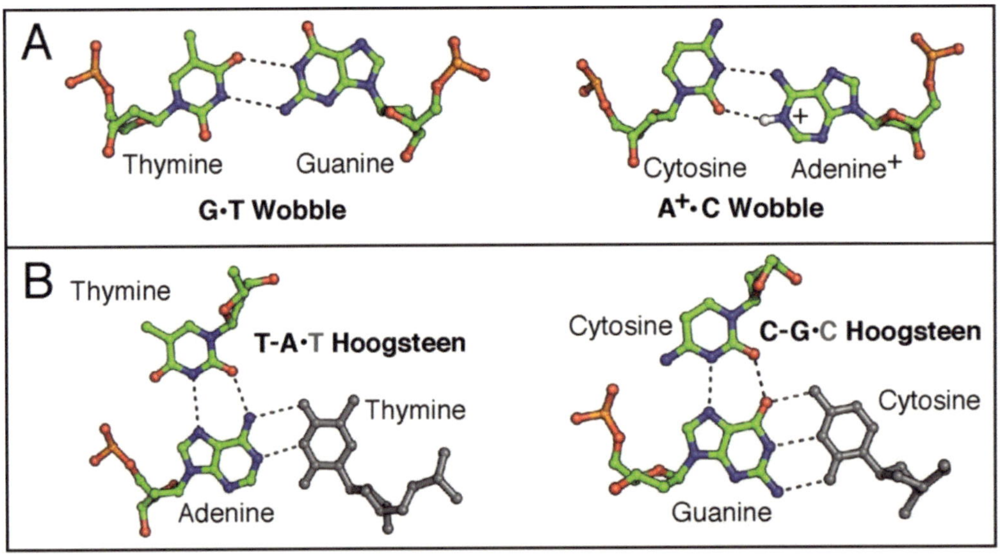

Fig. 3. Non-Watson Crick base pairs. A. G•T wobble and A^{+}•C wobble base pairs. B. Thymine Hoogsteen paired to A•T WC base pair, cytosine Hoogsteen paired to G•C WC base pair as observed in triplex strand formation.

3.2.2 Base stacking

Although not as intuitive, the stacking of bases into a column is as or more critical to the stability of multistranded DNAs (duplexes, triplexes, tetraplexes, etc) as base pairing. It is estimated that base stacking contributes as much as half of the total stabilizing free energy of a base pair in duplex DNA (Kool, 2001). Van der Waals interactions, electrostatic interactions, and solvent effects define the geometry and associated energies of stacked bases. Van der Waals forces drive bases to stack in a way that best complements their surface topologies. In addition, individual atoms carry permanent partial charges that contribute to either Coulombic attraction or repulsion between bases. This can be modeled as interactions between permanent dipoles, and it is this dipolar interaction, in conjunction with shape complementarities that helps to define the orientation of the stacked bases. The specific orientation of stacked base pairs contributes to the conformational stability of a DNA duplex. Likewise, deformations associated with specific base stacking geometries contribute to the mechanism of indirect sequence specific binding and recognition by proteins. Finally, since the nucleotide bases are aromatic and, therefore, primarily hydrophobic, stacking minimizes the solvent exposure of the base surfaces, thus, leading to the familiar face-to-face stacking of bases and base pairs. It is not surprising, therefore, that DNA conformations that increase exposure of bases are stabilized by organic solvents.

3.2.3 The phosphodeoxyribose backbone

The functional form of DNA links nucleotides together by phosphodiester bonds to form a continuous DNA strand. Phosphodiesters are highly acidic (*pKa'* ~1.5); thus, at neutral *pH*, the phosphate group is a monoanion with a formal -1 charge distributed among all four oxygens, with the two non-ester oxygens (OP1, OP2) carrying about twice the charge as the ester bonded oxygens (O5', O3'). As a consequence, the DNA phosphoribose backbone is overall negative and provides an opposing force to the base pairing and stacking interactions that hold a DNA duplex together. Indeed, if the backbone were uncharged, it would be much more difficult to unzip or displace a DNA strand and, consequently, it would take more energy to unwind a duplex to allow replication to start and to proceed.

The overall charge of DNA in solution is not simply a sum of -1 for each nucleotide—the backbone charges are counterbalanced by positive cations that accumulate around the DNA. These counterions are simple ions (monovalent Na^+ and K^+, or divalent Mg^{+2} and Ca^{+2} being the most prevalent in a cell), but include cationic polyamines (spermine and spermidine), drugs (ethidium or *cis*-platin), or proteins (*e.g.*, the histone proteins of nucleosomes). In general, DNA in solution is less negatively charged than expected—as a polyelectrolyte, each phosphate of a DNA duplex carries an "effective" charge of approximately -0.6, or that ~40% of the charge is counterbalanced by simple cations (Manning, 1977). The remaining net charge, however, acts to destabilize the double-helix. Consequently, structures with closely spaced phosphates are stabilized by increased concentrations of counter cations.

When a protein, such as DNA polymerase, binds to DNA, it must competitively displace the counterions associated with the DNA backbone. For example, nucleosome formation, which helps compact DNA in eukaryotes, is primarily driven by nonspecific interactions of the positive histones with the negative DNA backbone. In order to replicate or transcribe the information of the DNA, the respective polymerase and all of its associated proteins must compete against these non-specific interactions. Thus, the negative charge of the backbone is a platform for sequence independent electrostatic interactions with proteins in the cell (Rohs, et al., 2009).

3.2.4 Solvent effects

As with any biological molecule, solvent interactions directly influence DNA structure and function. Base pairing and stacking are in part stabilized by the hydrophobic effect. We have already seen how solvent (considered to consist primarily of water and salts) induces base pairs to stack and defines the effective charge of the phosphoribose backbone. Even base pairing is affected by solvent interactions. In forming a base pair, the hydrogen bond donor and acceptor groups of each base must break hydrogen bonds with water molecules first. If the enthalpy of any single hydrogen bond from one base to another base is essentially the same as they are from the base to water, why then do bases pair and exclude water (at 55.5 M concentration)? The primary answer is that sequestering hydrogen-bonding groups from the competing interactions of water increase the hydrogen bonding potential (Klotz, 1962). One can see from this why base stacking is so important in stabilizing double-, triple, and other multistranded DNA forms that are assembled through hydrogen bonding.

Water, however, is not entirely excluded from, but plays an important role in the structure of DNA. Even in a fully base paired duplex, numerous hydrogen bond donor and acceptor groups of the backbone and bases must be hydrated. There are classes of waters that can, in fact, be considered integral components of a DNA's structure. In a G•T wobble base pair, for example, the number of hydrogen bonds between the bases is reduced by one; however, bridging water molecules help to compensate for this loss (Ho *et al.*, 1985). Similarly, there are well-defined waters lining the minor groove of B-DNA duplexes (the so-called "spine of hydration") (Drew *et al.*, 1981) that exchange slowly with the bulk solvent (Liepinsh *et al.*, 1992) and, therefore, are considered to be integral parts of DNA. Thus, water promotes base stacking, which provides an environment for more stable hydrogen bonds within base pairs. Waters solvate the surfaces of the major groove and form well defined hydrogen bonded networks that bridge the two strands across the minor groove. In order to minimize the opposing repulsion between the phosphates of the DNA strands, cations help to mitigate the negative charges of the phosphoribose backbone (Hamelberg *et al.*, 2001). It is evident, therefore, just how important solvent really is for DNA structure and stability.

Finally, we must briefly discuss how solvent plays a role in DNA function. DNA is a hydrated molecule, until it is bound to a protein, at which point the DNA becomes dehydrated—*i.e.*, a protein must compete against water in order to bind to the DNA. The basic concept of direct read-out of DNA base pairs is a prime example of this. Direct read-out requires a protein to essentially stick its hydrogen bonding side-chain fingers into places where they would not normally belong, the major groove of a DNA duplex, for example. Both the proteins side chains and the DNA surface that they are trying to read would prefer to remain solvated; however, in order to form a strong complex with DNA, the protein must expel water from both surfaces and, as a result, the complex will become more stable than the sum of the individual parts. This, again, requires a balance between the stability of hydrogen bonds, the resulting decrease in conformational entropy of the protein side chains, and an increase in entropy of the water molecules as they return to the bulk solvent.

3.3 Conformations of the deoxyribose sugar

In addition to charge effects, the phosphoribose backbone helps to define the conformation of DNA *via* the conformation of the deoxyribose sugar. The detailed conformation of any polymer is defined by the rotations about each freely rotating chemical bond (Fig. 4A). We can define three categories of bonds: those of the phosphodiester holding two nucleotides together, those within the five-membered ring of the deoxyribose sugar, and the bond holding the nucleotide base to the sugar. The angles around the bonds that hold two nucleotides together start at the oxygen that links phosphate to the C5'-carbon of the ribose ring. Rotation about the P-O5' bond is the α-torsion angle, which is followed by the β-angle for the O5'-C5' bond, and so forth until we get to the ζ-angle that links the O3'-oxygen to the phosphate of the next nucleotide. These bonds adopt angles that help to minimize the repulsion of the negatively charged phosphates within and between DNA strands.

The bonds in the furanose ring are distinguished from those that flow linearly from one nucleotide to the next, and are designated as ν_1 for the C1'-C2' bond, ν_2 for the C2'-C3' bond, and so forth (Fig. 4A). The reader would recognize that the ν_3 angle within the ring coincides with the δ-angle along the chain. The ring is non-planar, and it is how particular atoms are placed either above or below a reference plane (the "sugar pucker") that facilitates formation of various conformational forms of DNA. The torsion angles are correlated to maintain reasonable bond lengths and angles within the ring, and are described by a single *pseudorotation angle* Ψ, which defines the sugar pucker (Saenger, 1984). Sugars with atoms puckered above the reference plane (on the same side as the base) are in an *endo*-form (C2'-

endo pucker has the C2′-carbon pointed up and towards the base), while a pucker that places an atom below this plane is in its *exo*-form (Fig. 5). The two general classes of sugar conformations commonly seen in DNA are the C2′-*endo* and C3′-*endo* puckers—the interconversion between these forms will be discussed in detail in section 5. The two conformations have profound effects on the overall DNA conformation in that they specify different phosphate-phosphate distances along each strand (~7 Å for C2′-*endo* and ~6 Å for C3′-*endo*). Thus, conformations constructed with C3′-*endo* sugars will require higher concentrations of salts to counter balance the shorter distance between the negatively charged phosphates.

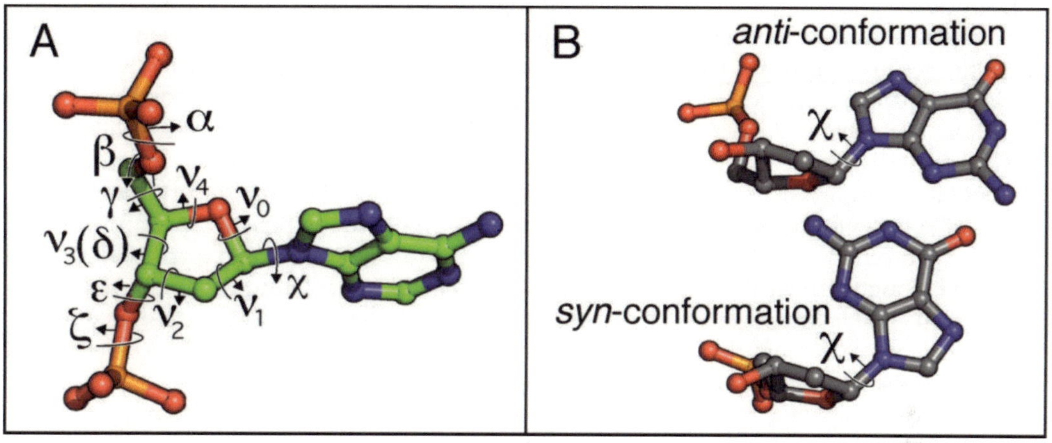

Fig. 4. Torsion angles of nucleic acids. A. Torsion angles along the backbone (α to ζ), within the sugar ring (ν_0 to ν_4), and the rotation of the nucleobase relative to the sugar. B. Rotation about the glycosidic bond defines χ-angles for the *anti*- and *syn*-conformations of the bases.

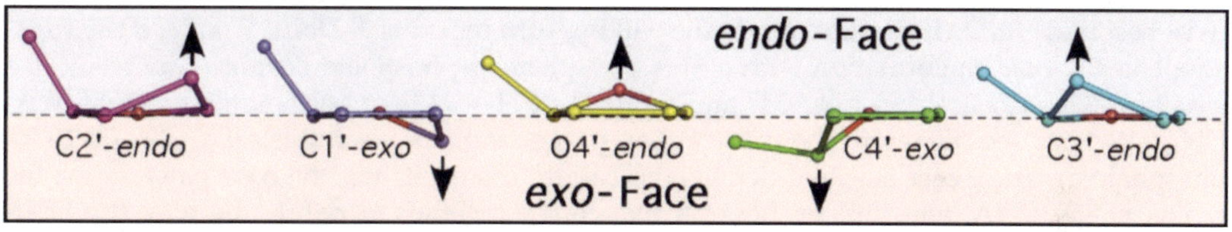

Fig. 5. Sugar pucker. Shown are the *endo* (above) and *exo* (below) faces of the 5-membered furanose sugar with the nucleotide base extended above the reference plane. Sugars are shown in order of transformation from C2′-*endo* to C3′-*endo*. Arrows indicate the atom that is puckered, and the direction of puckering.

The base of each nucleotide is attached *via* the glycosidic bond from the N1 nitrogen of pyrimidines or the N9 nitrogen of purines to the C1′-carbon of the deoxyribose sugar. The rotation about the glycosidic bond, the χ-angle, defines two general conformational classes: the *anti* conformation (+90° ≤ χ ≤ +180°), with the base extended away from the sugar, and the *syn* conformation (-90° ≤ χ ≤ +90°), with the base essentially lying on top of the sugar ring (Fig. 4B). The more compact *syn*-conformation is more susceptible to steric clashes than the extended *anti*-form. Although purine rings are generally larger, it has the smaller five-membered ring, as opposed to the six-membered ring of pyrimidines, attached directly to the sugar. Thus, purines will more readily adopt the compact *syn*-conformation than pyrimidines, because of reduced steric collisions. Similarly, the *syn* conformation is less sterically hindered when the sugar is puckered as C3′-*endo* than C2′-*endo*. From this, we can now start to appreciate how the interplay between sugar puckers and χ-rotations can have profound effects on the structures of DNA and the sequence dependence for their formation.

3.4 Helical parameters

Now that we have assembled well-defined helical structures, how do we describe these structures? We can certainly do this in a very descriptive and qualitative manner, using the classical A- and B-forms as examples. For instance, we can characterize the standard B-form of DNA as a right-handed double-helix held together by Watson-Crick type base pairs that stack directly along a helical axis, resulting in two well defined grooves. However, this raises numerous questions, for example, at which point does a distortion to the Watson-Crick base pair become a wobble base pair, how far off the helix axis is allowed in this definition, and what if the helix axis is not straight? To address these and other questions, a set of quantitative measures called the "helical parameters" were developed to characterize the regular secondary structures of nucleic acids (both DNA and RNA) (Lavery, 1998).

The most commonly recognized parameters for DNA include the helical repeat (number of base pairs in one complete turn) and the helical rise (distance between nucleotides when measured along the helical axis). The repeat defines the angle relating each base pair along the helix axis (the helical twist = 360°/repeat), while the product of repeat and rise is the pitch (distance between one complete turn) of the DNA. These parameters restrict the geometries of the DNA. Indeed, if we consider only the closest physical approach between base pairs (the rise = 3.4 Å, as defined by the thickness of a base), the maximum phosphate-phosphate distance along a strand (measured at ~7.5 Å by single-molecule stretching (Allemand *et al.*, 1998)), and the effective diameter of a duplex (9.5 Å), we see that the largest twist angle between stacked base pairs is ~42°, resulting in a smallest theoretical repeat of 8.5 base pairs per turn. This would be the most tightly or over-wound form of a DNA double-helix. If the phosphate-to-phosphate distance is relaxed to ~7 Å (for a C2′-*endo* sugar pucker), the helical twist becomes ~36°, which translates to the ~10 bp/turn repeat of B-DNA. Finally, if the sugar adopts a C3′-*endo* conformation with a ~6Å phosphate-to-phosphate distance, the result is a structure with a helical twist of ~31° and a repeat of 11 - 12 base pairs, similar to that of A-DNA. We can see, therefore, how the sugar pucker defines the intrastrand phosphate-to-phosphate distance, base stacking defines the base-to-base distance, the base pairs define the radius of the DNA, and, finally, how all this comes together to define the way the DNA double-helix twists into a specific conformation. Of course, these are only very rough approximations of DNA structures—the detailed descriptions require a complete set of helical parameters in addition to the two described so far.

The helical parameters can be categorized into two general classes to describe the absolute and relative conformations in nucleic acids (Fig. 6); base-pair parameters (for single base pairs) and base step parameters (for adjacent base pairs). We note that these classes are not mutually exclusive, but are interrelated. Twist and rise are clearly base step parameters, since they describe the relative angle and distance between two adjacent stacked base pairs. The other base-step parameters that are generally considered relevant include slide, roll, tilt, and shift. It is easy to see that slide can effectively increase the diameter of a DNA duplex and, consequently affect the helical twist and repeat. A-DNA, for example, shows a large slide between base pairs, while B-DNAs have small slides, placing the base pairs essentially stacked on top of each other. Not surprisingly, therefore, A-DNA has a larger overall diameter and, in fact, appears to have a hole down the middle when viewed down its helical axis.

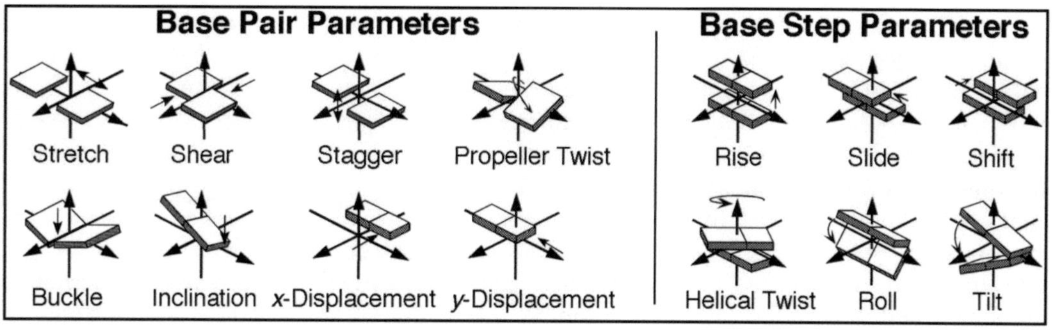

Fig. 6. Base Pair and Base Step Parameters. *Base Pair Parameters*: Translational and rotational relationships of bases within each base pair. *Base Step Parameters*: Translational and rotational relationsips between two stacked base pairs.

A conundrum in A-DNA is that it has a rise of ~2.5 Å, which would appear to violate the closest approach between stacked base pairs. In this case, the inclination associated with the roll and tilt of the base pairs, in conjunction with the helical twist result in a shortening of the vertical distance between base pairs along the helical axis, even though the stacking distance remains 3.4 Å. Indeed, A-like DNAs that have little or no roll and tilt have helical rises that are ~3.4 Å, as expected (Ng *et al.*, 2000; Vargason *et al.*, 2001).

Base pair parameters include those that relate the position or orientation of the base pair relative to the helical axis (inclination, *x*-displacement, and *y*-displacement), or the orientation and positions of the two bases in a pair (propeller twist, shear, stagger, stretch, buckle). It should be obvious that the inclination of a base pair will strongly influence the roll and tilt between base pairs, while slide defines the displacement perpendicular to the base pair (*x*) and along the base pair (*y*). Within the base pair itself, the large propeller twist seen in A•T base pairs has been attributed to the flexibility of two hydrogen bonds relative to three observed in G•C base pairs. At the extreme, this results in bifurcated hydrogen bonds, which are considered to be shared between adjacent A•T base pairs (Coll *et al.*, 1987).

Each of these base pair and base step parameters are defined relative to the helical axis that runs down the center of DNA. However, it should be recognized that defining this axis is not entirely straight forward, particularly if the DNA trajectory is bent or curved. There are two approaches to defining helical axes: the global axis and the local axis. The global axis is essentially the continuous curve that best runs down the center of all base pairs in a structure, while the local axis is the best line that defines the center of any two adjacent base pairs (local axes need not be continuous). Thus, helical parameters are analyzed in the context of global or local axes, and are not interchangeable and may be very different.

Two distinguishing features of double-helical DNAs are the grooves. The widths of the major and minor grooves are measured as the phosphate-to-phosphate distance across the two strands in a direction perpendicular to the trajectory of the strands. These groove widths provide an important means for proteins to interact with the base pairs of the DNA. The wide major groove of B-DNA allows direct read-out of the bases, while the narrow major groove of A-DNA does not—there is, however, an advantage to A-DNA having a wider minor groove, which we will discuss in the next section. It should be immediately obvious from the earlier discussion that the base pair and base step parameters described above conspire to define the groove widths for each form of DNA.

Finally, we can see how a parameter such as twist has such a strong effect on the overall behavior of genomic DNAs. DNA when confined in the cell or the cell's nucleus must be packaged into a compacted supercoiled form and, in the process, this induces stress that will perturb its secondary structure. For simplicity a set of terms have been defined for supercoiled DNA in the context of closed-circular double-stranded DNA such as those found in plasmids, bacterial chromosomes, and viral genomes. These terms can also be applied to linear eukaryotic DNAs that are spatially anchored and stressed through protein binding, DNA unwinding, and DNA compaction. In double-stranded DNA, the number of times the strands wrap around each other along the helical axis is defined as the twist (*Tw*), with positive *Tw* associated with right-handed and negative *Tw* for left-handed duplexes, and unwound duplexes (*e.g.*, melted domains) as *Tw* = 0. In closed-circular DNA, the ends are joined and not free to turn in accommodating a change in *Tw*; therefore, a change in twist has additional global effects (Fig. 7), resulting in supercoiling, or writhing (*Wr*), of the double-helix as it wraps around itself.

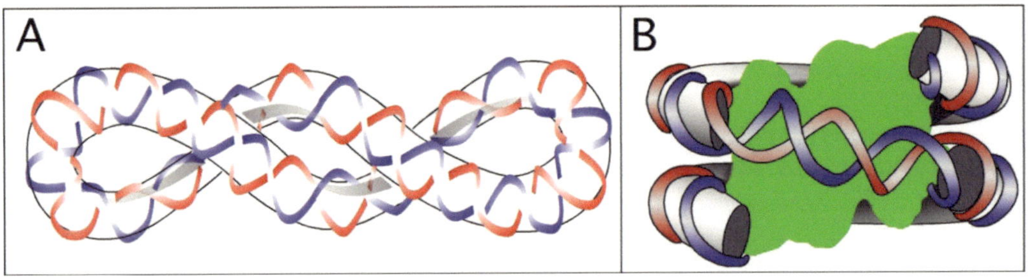

Fig. 7. Supercoiled DNA. A. Two negative supercoils are manifest as right-handed cross-overs in closed circular DNA. B. Similarly the DNA found in the nucleosome structure is wrapped ~twice around the histone core proteins (green) to form two negative supercoils (adapted from (Luger, *et al.*, 1997)).

Together, the twist and writhe define the topological properties of DNA. In truly closed-circular DNA that is unconstrained, twist and writhe are entirely correlated through the linking number (*Lk*) according to the equation $Lk = Tw + Wr$. Thus, if we unwind (reduce *Tw*) in closed circular DNA, the resulting strain must be relieved by increasing *Wr* (supercoiling). The only way to change *Lk* is by breaking the bonds of the backbone of one or both of the DNA strands, a process carried out by topoisomerases in the cells. How does all of this play out during replication? Consider the closed circular genome of a bacterium, or a domain of a eukaryotic genome that is locally constrained by nucleosomes and/or matrix attachment regions (MARs). As a DNA helicase plows through the DNA, it will locally unwind and melt the duplex (reduce *Tw*) for synthesis of the daughter strand. In doing so, the DNA in front of the polymerase will be positively supercoiled, while negative supercoils accumulate in its wake, both energetically unfavorable conditions. To relieve the strain, topoisomerases must relax the supercoils both in front of and behind the replisome.

4. The alphabet soup of DNA structures

DNA is highly polymorphic and, at least at the level of the helical structures, more variable than either proteins or RNA. The various forms of DNA have traditionally been named using the letters of the English alphabet and, from a survey of the literature, it was found that all but four letters have been assigned to at least one unique structural form (Ghosh and Bansal, 2003). We will, in this section, briefly describe a subset of DNA conformations that have been structurally characterized (Fig. 8 and 9) and the sequence propensities of these structures, starting with B-DNA and working our way through the variations on the double-helix and various multi-stranded conformations. Along the way, we will discuss their potential biological functions, particularly in DNA replication, as appropriate.

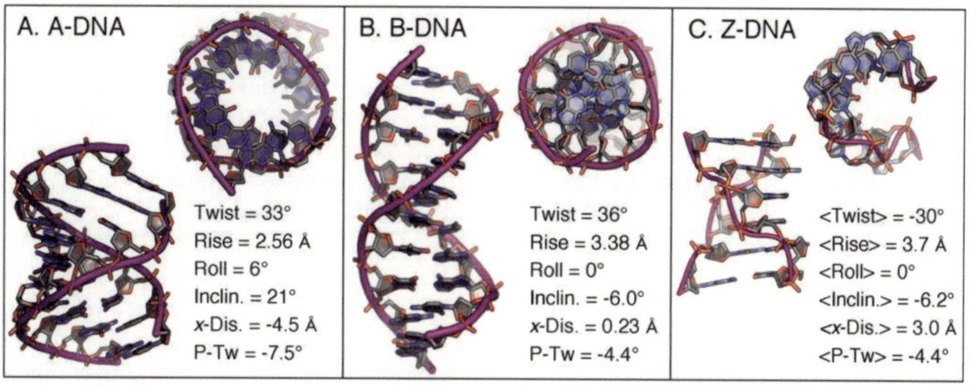

Fig. 8. Representatiive double-helical structures of DNA. Structures of A-DNA (Hays *et al.*, 2005), B-DNA (Privé *et al.*, 1991), and Z-DNA (Wang *et al.*, 1979). Abbreviations: Incl. = inclination, *x*-Disp. = *x*-displacment, P-Tw = propeller twist. For Z-DNA, the helical parameters are given as averages of the alternating dinucleotide steps.

4.1 B-DNA: The standard form

B-form DNA is the most recognized and common structural form of DNA in the cell, being considered the conformation adopted by nearly all sequences within a genome. Interestingly, while B-DNA has a distinguishing set of structural properties, it is now understood to be highly variable and malleable. B-DNA is a right-handed, antiparallel double-helix in which the Watson-Crick base pairs are stacked directly along and perpendicular to the helical axis, giving rise to major and minor grooves that are similar in depth. The bases are all in the *anti*-conformation with a majority of deoxyribose sugars in the C2′-*endo* form, although the sugar puckers are more variable than in many other conformations (Dickerson, 1999). The highly accessible major groove allows for direct readout of the polynucleotide sequence by proteins through patterns of hydrogen bond donors and acceptors that are complementary between the amino-acid side chains and each individual base pair. The more narrow minor groove, on the other hand, is characterized by a series of strongly coordinated waters and ions.

Although these properties are general for B-DNA, the structure is highly variable from one sequence to the next and for the same sequence under different conditions. The concept of *sequence-based differential deformability* recognizes that the B-form of a single sequence can adopt multiple conformations in response to the environment which can affect protein recognition. Therefore, the effect of sequence is important not in terms of any one structure, but instead in its malleability—the ability of that sequence to be deformed and molded as necessary for a particular function. For example, A•T base pairs and long stretches of A/T sequences (A-tract DNAs) seem to deviate significantly from the standard B-structure, showing larger propeller twists, along with narrower and more variable minor groove widths. Narrow minor grooves are shown to have preferential binding by arginine side chains of multiple DNA-binding protein families (Rohs *et al.*, 2009), and represent a specific example of protein recognition based on sequence perturbations to standard B-DNA. A-tract DNA sequences are also associated with large rolls and tilts of their base steps, resulting in rigid bending of the B-DNA duplex (Neidle, 1999). An extreme example of these perturbations is seen with the structure induced in gene promoter sequences by the TATA-binding protein in transcription (called TATA-DNA), which shows a significant tilt and roll of the base pairs, unwinding of the duplex, and widening of the minor groove in a manner similar to that seen with A-DNA (Burley, 1996).

Variations of the B-form have been primarily elucidated by detailed structural studies, particularly X-ray diffraction and NMR, on short oligonucleotides. The question that is often raised is whether these short lengths of DNA may in fact not be relevant (and, in the case of crystals, be otherwise distorted (Dickerson *et al.*, 1994)) relative to sequences embedded in a genomic context. Studies by Tullius' group using hydroxyl-radical foot printing (Greenbaum *et al.*, 2007), have shown significant sequence dependent variation in the solvent accessibility and, thus, the helical structure of protein-free genomic DNA. These structural variations at the genomic level are highly correlated with variations in helical parameters measured in DNA crystal structures (unpublished results) derived from a self-consistent data set (Hays *et al.*, 2005). In conclusion, there is growing recognition that even B-DNA is a highly variable structural form of the DNA double-helix, and that sequence dependent structural variations play a critical role in protein recognition and binding.

4.2 A-DNA: Underwinding for replication fidelity

A-form DNA is also a right-handed antiparallel helical duplex, but is characterized as an underwound structure that is more compact along the helix axis and broader overall across the helix relative to B-DNA. The nucleotide bases, all *anti*, are shifted by large x-displacements towards the minor groove, creating a shallow, wide minor groove and a channel associated with a deep, narrow major groove. The deoxyribose sugars are consistently C3'-*endo*, which minimizes the potential steric clashes as the sugar is pushed towards the phosphate to accommodate the sliding of the base (Dickerson, 1999).

A-DNA is involved in insuring the fidelity of DNA replication. An analysis of the structure of the *Bacillus* DNA polymerase in complex with duplex DNA showed a conformational switch from the B- to underwound A-form starting at the site of nucleotide incorporation and extending to four bases upstream (Kiefer *et al.*, 1998). Why is A-DNA induced by the polymerase? There are several perspectives on this answer, from an evolutionary view (the emergence of DNA polymerase from the primoidial RNA world where RNA polymerase reigned) to a functional view. We will discuss the latter in slightly greater detail. The direct read-out mechanism involves sticking amino acid side-chains into the DNA's major groove to read the unique pattern of hydrogen bonding donors and acceptors that specify a particular sequence. One would think that this would be a fairly straight forward way for a polymerase to insure the fidelity of the newly synthesized daughter strand and, thus would want the double-helix to adopt the standard B-form with its wide and accessible major groove. However, DNA polymerases are not sequence specific (*i.e.*, they will synthesize from any template sequence), so the enzyme must distinguish a proper Watson-Crick base pair from various mismatches without knowing what the base pair should be. The characteristic feature of mismatched bases (as in a wobble) is that the structure of the minor groove becomes perturbed (Kool, 2001); thus, by inducing the A-form, the polymerase exploits the structural features of the highly accessible minor-groove to insure that the correct base has been added relative to the template sequence.

4.3 Z-DNA: The left-handed duplex

Z-form DNA is noteworthy as the only characterized left-handed form of the double-helix. The zig-zagged backbone, its namesake, results from the alternation between *syn-* and *anti-* conformations, and the respective C3'-*endo* and C2'-*endo* sugar puckers. This alternating conformation imposes a sequence preference for alternating purine-pyrimidines, since purines adopt the *syn*-conformation more readily than do pyrimidines. Thus, the repeating unit is the dinucleotide rather than a single base pair, as in B-DNA. The major groove in Z-DNA is not so much a groove but more a convex outer surface, while the minor groove becomes a deep, narrow and largely inaccessible crevice (Wang *et al.*, 1979).

The biological function of Z-DNA has been widely debated and underappreciated; however, several cellular functions for the Z-form are now supported by experimental evidence (Rich and Zhang, 2003). Z-DNA was initially characterized as a structure induced by high salt conditions (3 M NaCl) (Pohl and Jovin, 1972), leading many to wonder whether it could exist in a cell. Subsequently, it has been shown that cytosine methylation, and other cations such as spermine and spermidine at millimolar concentrations also stabilize Z-DNA (Rich and Zhang, 2003). Most importantly, as a left-handed structure, Z-DNA is the most underwound form of the double-helix and, consequently, serves as a sink for the torsional tension in negatively supercoiled DNA (Rich and Zhang, 2003). This expands the range of cellular situations that could support the formation, at least transiently, of Z-DNA. In one model, RNA polymerase, as it transcribes through a gene, would generate negative supercoils in its wake (Liu and Wang, 1987) and, on the process drive Z-DNA formation upstream of the transcribing gene. A detailed study of the promoter for human CSF-1 gene showed that up-regulation by the chromatin remodeling BAF protein involves a Z-DNA element (Liu *et al.*, 2001). The authors suggested that Z-DNA upstream of the nuclear factor-1 binding site helped to maintain the gene in its activated, nucleosome-free state (nucleosomes do not bind to the very rigid Z-DNA form (Ausio *et al.*, 1987)). In support of its potential role in the regulation of eukaryotic genes, we have found that Z-forming sequences accumulate near the transcription start site of genes in humans and other eukaryotes (Khuu *et al.*, 2007; Schroth *et al.*, 1992), and that ~80% of the genes in human chromosome 22 have at least one Z-DNA sequence in the vicinity of their transcription start sites (Champ *et al.*, 2004).

The discovery of protein domains having very high specificity for Z-DNA (Rich and Zhang, 2003), in some cases with nanomolar K_D's, have suggested additional functions that include, for example, RNA editing and gene transactivation. Z-DNA sequences have also been implicated in genomic instability, that results in large scale breaks and rearrangements (Kha *et al.*, 2010). Thus, in addition to serving as a sink for superhelical tension, there are several potential functions for Z-DNA that may be either beneficial or deleterious to the cell.

4.4 H-DNA: Three's a crowd

When a single DNA strand invades the major groove of a DNA duplex, a triple helical structure is generated (Fig. 9). In order for the duplex to accommodate this third strand, it must unwind to broaden the major groove; thus, such triple-stranded helices are favored in negatively supercoiled DNA (Mirkin, 2008). The invading third strand can be intermolecular or intramolecular.

The interaction between strands involve the Hoogsteen edge of the Watson-Crick base pairs (Fig. 3) of the duplex to form base triplets, leading to the name H-DNA for such triplex structures. H-DNA is formed primarily in mirror repeat sequences (sequences that have dyad symmetry within a strand, as in ...AGAGGGnnnGGGAGA..., defined by the sequence preference to form base triplets). Mirror-repeats occur randomly in prokaryotes, but are three to six times more frequent in eukaryotic genomes (Schroth and Ho, 1995). Specific H-DNA forming sequences have been identified in multiple promoter regions with documented effects on gene expression of several disease related genes, including c-myc (Kinniburgh, 1989) and c-Ki-ras (Pestov *et al.*, 1991). As with Z-DNA, the repeating sequence motif of H-DNA appears to be a source of genetic instability resulting from double-strand breaks. Wang and Vasquez (2004) reported a ~20 fold increase in mutation frequency upon incorporation of an H-DNA forming sequence found in the c-myc promoter region into mammalian cells. These results suggest that naturally occurring DNA sequences can cause increased mutagenesis via non-standard DNA structure formation.

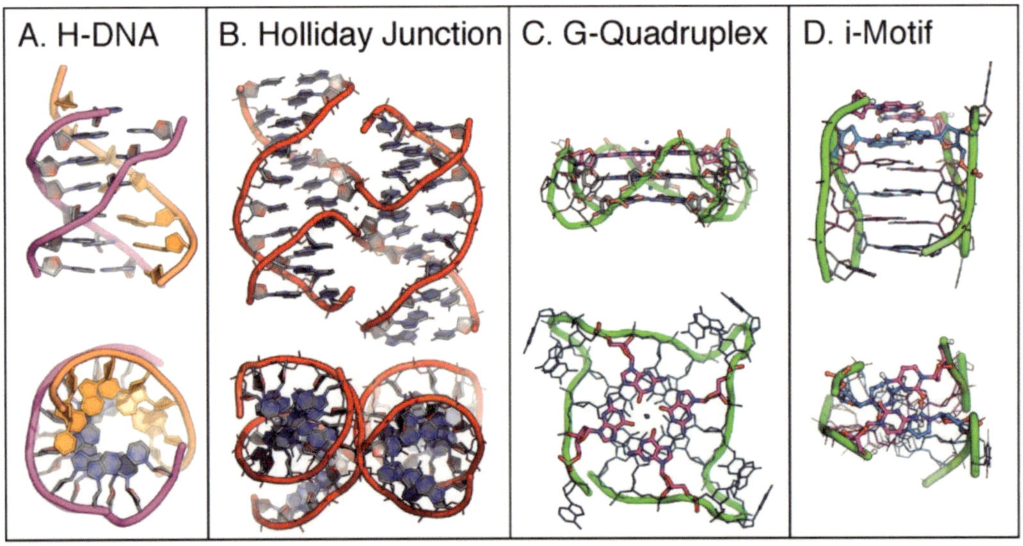

Fig. 9. Three- and four-stranded structures of DNA. The structures of triplex H-DNA (Radhakrishnan and Patel, 1993), the Holliday junction (Eichman et al, 2002), human telomeric G-quartet (Parkinson et al., 2002), and the i-motif (Weil et al., 1999), are viewed along (top) and down (bottom) their helical axes.

4.5 HJ, G, and I: The four-stranded DNAs

There are several conformations of DNA that can be assembled from four strands. The three structures discussed here show very different and unique helical forms, starting with a conformation that is most similar to standard B-DNA, and leading through forms that differ dramatically from the original Watson-Crick model (Fig. 9).

4.5.1 The four-stranded Holliday junction

Robin Holliday proposed in 1964 that a four-stranded junction would be involved as an intermediate to allow reciprocal exchange of genetic information through recombination across two homologous DNA duplexes (Holliday, 1964). These intermediates, now referred to as Holliday junctions, are essential to several cellular processes including recombination dependent DNA lesion repair, viral integration, restarting of stalled replication forks, and proper segregation of homologous chromosomes during meiosis *(Cox et al.*, 2000; Declais *et al.*, 2003; Dickman *et al.*, 2002; Haber and Heyer, 2001; Nunes-Duby *et al.*, 1987;

Subramaniam *et al.*, 2003). The structure of the Holliday junction has been the focus of intense biophysical studies for several decades (Lilley, 1999). Through a set of clever studies in which immobilized junctions are specifically cut by restriction enzymes or probed with fluorescent dyes, DNA junctions were shown to adopt either an extended open-X form under low-salt conditions or a more compact stacked-X conformation as the negatively charged phosphate backbone becomes shielded under high-salt conditions. In the stacked-X form, two continuous DNA strands are connected by two crossover strands, each forming a tight U-turn at the cross-over point, which restricts the migration of the junction. Single molecule studies have shown that migration requires a transition to the open-X structure (McKinney *et al.*, 2003), and that this is fairly rapid. As a result, enzymes that catalyze cellular processes that require junction migration (for example, during recombination dependent DNA repair by the RuvABC complex (Dickman *et al.*, 2002)) will recognize and bind the extended and topologically unrestrained open-X structure, while those that do not require junction migration (such as many resolving enzymes in recombination, including the resolvases from T4 and T7 (Biertumpfel *et al.*, 2007; Hadden *et al.*, 2007)) have active sites that bind to the topologically restrained stacked-X type structure.

Around the end of the 20th century, two groups almost simultaneously solved the single-crystal structures of the DNA Holliday junction (Ortiz-Lombardía *et al.*, 1999; Eichman *et al.*, 2000). Both structures strongly resembled the model derived from the solution studies (McKinney *et al.*, 2003), showing the junction to be essentially two B-DNA double-helices, with standard Watson-Crick type base pairs, linked by two crossing strands that connect the duplexes. A unique set of hydrogen bonds helps to stabilize the tight U-turns at the cross-over points (Eichman *et al.*, 2002), and impose a strong sequence dependence in the formation of Holliday junctions, with the inverted repeats GGTACC > GGCGCC > (GATATC = GGGCCC) in their stability as four-stranded stacked-X junctions (Hays *et al.*, 2005). In addition, the interactions define an ~40° angle relating the two linked duplexes—the structure of an asymmetric junction showed no interactions at the junction center, and an interduplex angle of ~60° (Khuu and Ho, 2009), similar to that determined in solution for analogous constructs (McKinney *et al.*, 2003). The structure of the junction has now been determined with the drug psoralen (Eichman *et al.*, 2001), methylated cytosines (Vargason and Ho, 2002), and various types of cations (Thorpe *et al.*, 2003), all showing effects on the detailed geometry of this four-stranded intermediate (Watson *et al.*, 2004). The effect of sequence on the formation and geometry of junctions lead to a model in which even non-sequence specific resolvases may show sequence preference, not as a result of any specific recognition motif between the protein and the DNA, but from the thermodynamic propensity of certain sequences to promote formation of the junction (Khuu, 2006).

In replication, Holliday junctions are essential intermediates in double-strand break repair (Cox *et al.*, 2000) in which RecA facilitates invasion of a single-strand into a homologous double-strand sequence, followed by junction migration and resolution by RuvABC (RecG). Homologous recombination also plays a crucial role in rescuing replication forks that stall because of DNA damage. Recombination proteins repair double-strand ends produced when a replication fork encounters a single-strand interruption and help reset replication at stalled forks by converting blocked replication forks into Holliday junctions. Thus, DNA junctions are involved in the repair of damaged DNAs both during and after replication.

4.5.2 G-Quadruplexes

The four-stranded structures assembled from guanine-rich sequences are called G-quadruplexes or G-quartets. Such sequences are found primarily in telomeric DNA repeats

(3′-overhangs at chromosome ends (Patel *et al.*, 2007)), but have recently been identified in various other central regions of the genome, including centrometric sequences (Brooks *et al.*, 2010) and in the immunoglobulin switch region. The strands are held together by pairing the Watson-Crick edge of each guanine with the Hoogsteen edge of an adjacent guanine, creating a cyclic arrangement of four guanines into G-tetrads. These tetrads are stacked with a right-handed helical twist, and are stabilized by monovalent cations (Na^+ or K^+) coordinated to the O2 oxygens of the guanines, and sandwiched between the base stacks.

G-quartets can be formed from the association of one, two, or four G-rich DNA strands with various topologies (Mirkin, 2008). Of these, the topologies that can be adopted by single-strands are perhaps most important for G-rich sequences at the 3′-ends (telomeric ends) of chromosomes (characterized as a single–stranded overhang of a guanine-rich sequence that assembles into a nucleo-protein structure). Such sequences have been shown to form G-quadruplex structures, from the DNA in the marconucleus of a ciliate (Mergny *et al.*, 2002) to the exceptionally stable G-quartet formed under physiological conditions by the human telomeric repeats ($(GGGTTA)_3GGG$) (Parkinson *et al.*, 2002). The telomer ends are replicated through the reverse transcriptase function of telomerase, which is itself a protein-RNA complex (Zakian, 2009). The precise length of each telomere controls the cell's ability to replicate, suggesting a regulatory role for their G-quadruplex structures. In normal cells, the length of the telomeric region is reduced during each round of replication until the Hayflick limit is reached, at which point the cell enters apoptosis (Zakian, 2009). The misregulation of telomerase activity can lead to immortality of cells and associated tumorogensis.

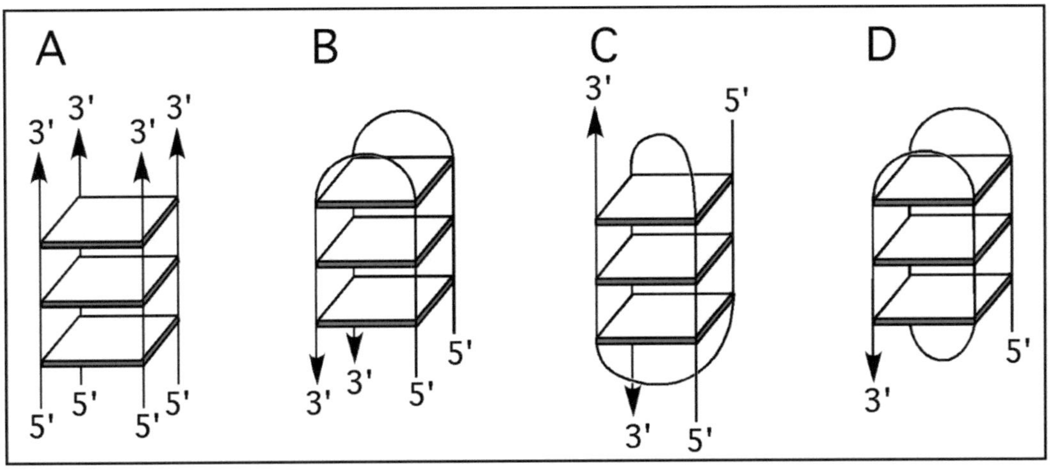

Fig. 10. Possible topologies for G-quartet structures. Topologies constructed from four parallel strands (A), from two strands that are non-crossing (B) or cross-over (C), and from a single strand (D).

Although it is easy to envision formation of a G-quartet structure at the single-stranded end of a chromosome, G-rich repeating sequences with the potential ability to form G-quadruplexes have also been identified at internal sites within genomes (Brooks *et al.*, 2010). Indeed, a recent study by Sarkies, *et al.* (Sarkies *et al.*, 2010) indicates that the specialized DNA polymerase Rev 1 is involved in replication through G-rich sequences and, when the polymerase is absent, DNA replication and histone recycling becomes uncoupled, leading to the assembly of nucleosomes with newly synthesized histones and, consequently, loss of epigenetic makers at or near these sites. Thus, internal G-quadruplex sequences are crucial for passing on to daughter cells genetic information beyond that of the linear sequence.

4.5.3 I-motifs

In order for a double-stranded G-rich region to extrude into a G-quartet structure, the complementary C-rich strand must also be extruded. The structure that is now associated with C-rich sequences is the four-stranded, intercalated i-motif. The i-motif, or I-form DNA, is fashioned from two parallel C-strands intercalated in a head-to-tail fashion [(Mills *et al.*, 2002). The two duplexes of poly(dC) are stabilized by base pairing the Watson-Crick edges of two cytosines to form hemi-protonated C•C+ pairs.

5. Getting from here to there: Structural transitions in DNA

B-DNA is recognized as the "standard" form in the cell; however, if everything remains standard and static, then life would not be as rich, nor might it exist at all. DNA is thus not only polymorphic, it is also dynamic. In this section, we will explore the mechanisms that drive DNA from the norm as B DNA, focusing on two transitions that present interesting and important insights into how DNA transforms between structural forms.

5.1 Going from B to A

As we have seen, A-type DNA plays an important role in replication as the induced form in the active site of DNA polymerase, allowing the non-sequence specific recognition of base mispairs in the template/daughter duplex. The transition from B- to A-DNA was one of the earliest characterized, with dehydration of DNA fibers showing a distinct shortening in the helical rise, unwinding of the helical twist, and broadening in the diameter (Franklin and Gosling, 1953a). The transition is also induced in solution by alcohol (a dehydrant), as well as methylation of cytosines (which affects the water structure around the base pairs). The question is, what are the structural and energetic steps involved in this transition? Although this is basically a transition from one right-handed antiparallel double-helix to another, several dramatic structural rearrangments must take place, including a conversion of the sugar pucker, along with large sliding and inclination of base pairs. The details of this conformational shift were observed crystallogaphically at the atomic level on the short DNA sequence GGCGCC (Vargason *et al.*, 2001), which was primarily in the B-form, but, upon cytosine methylation or bromination, adopts a number of conformational states, including true A-DNA forms and a set of logical intermediates between the B- and A-forms (Fig. 11). This study generates a structural map for how the sugar conformation works its way around the ring (Fig. 5), the order of translational and rotational distortions to the stacked base pairs, and the direction of propagation of a structural transition once initiated.

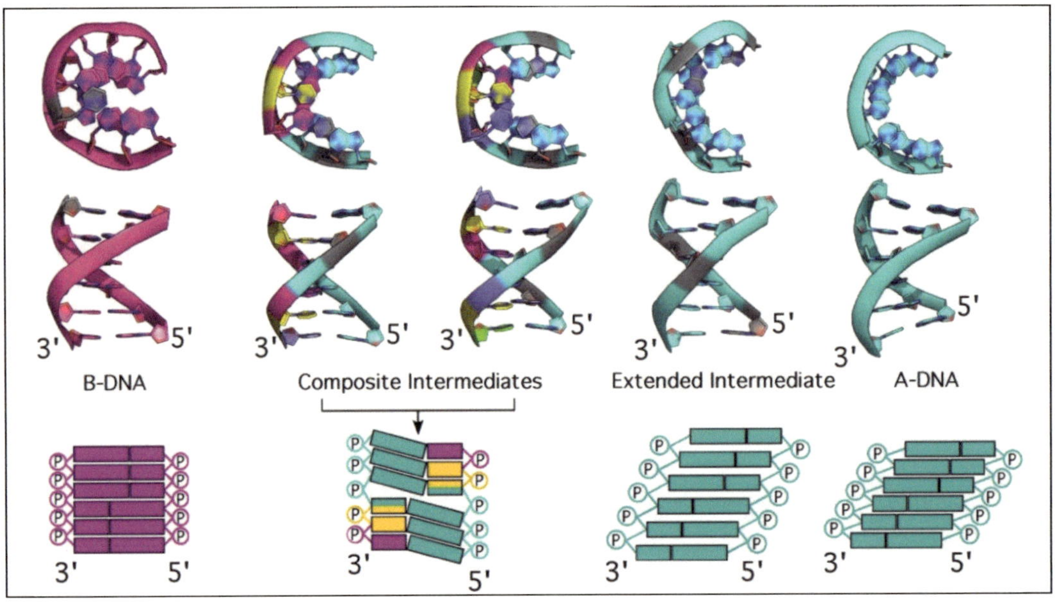

Fig. 11. B- to A-DNA transition. The structures of GGCGCC and methylated or brominated variants viewed down (top) and along (bottom) the helix axis. The series of structures show a transition from B-DNA, through a chimeric A-B intermediate and an extended intermediate, and leading finally to A-DNA. Nucleotides are colored according to their sugar puckers, as presented in Fig. 5.

The transition involves conversion of the sugar from the B-DNA C2′-*endo* pucker to C1′-*exo*, then O4′-*endo*, followed by C4′-*exo*, and finally to the C3′-*endo* pucker of A-DNA (Fig. 5) (Vargason *et al.*, 2001). Applying *ab initio* calculations on models of the deoxyribose derived from this study, we found that there is an ~4 kcal/mol energy barrier (primarily bonding energy) at the O4′-*endo* intermediate step. This is lower than the ~5-6 kcal/mol estimated for planar intermediates required for a direct conversion from C2′- to C3′-*endo*, and is similar to estimates from experimental (Olson and Sussman, 1982) and other *ab initio* calculations (Foloppe *et al.*, 2001) on the barrier (although about 2-fold higher than molecular dynamics estimates (Arora and Schlick, 2003; Harvey and Prabhakaran, 1986)).

Associated with the changes in sugar pucker are perturbations to the base stacking. As the sugars go through a transition from B- towards A-type sugars, the B-A chimeric intermediate (which is half B- and half A-type along each strand) induces a large buckle in the base pairs at the point of transition, which partially unstacks one of the two bases of the pair. The unstacking becomes complete when the sugars assume the full A-type pucker, resulting in an ~10% extension of the spacing between bases, or a rise of ~3.7 Å (Vargason *et al.*, 2000), thereby allowing the large slide and subsequent displacement of the base pairs away from the helical axis that is characteristic of A-DNA. Thus, large shifts between base pairs are predicated on breaking the base stacking interactions, as one would expect. In addition, it shows the transition to A-DNA propagating back towards the 5′-end of each strand. The tilt and roll that causes the inclination and resulting shortened rise of A-DNA are the final steps. The B- to A-DNA transition is unique in that specific intermediates have been trapped to provide an atomic level map for the transition—this is perhaps the most detailed description of a complete structural transition of any biological macromolecule.

5.2 Switching hands: The B- to Z-DNA transition

A more dramatic transition is from the right-handed B- to left-handed Z-DNA (Fig. 12), which has been studied extensively in solution and in plasmids. The B-Z transition, however, does not simply twist a right-handed double-helix in the opposite direction. The sugar for alternating nucleotides along a strand change from C2'-*endo* to C3'-*endo* puckers, concommitant with rotation of the base from the *anti*- to the *syn*-conformations. More significantly, the "sense" of the duplex must change—*i.e.,* the direction of the major and minor grooves are swapped (Dickerson, 1992).

In order to accommodate all of these radical changes, there is a junction with an overall zero twist (the B-Z junction) that serves to splice the right- and left-handed twisted duplexes (Peck and Wang, 1983). The structure of this junction was determined in a clever way using a Z-DNA binding protein to stabilize half the DNA in the left-handed form, while allowing the other half to remain in its relaxed B-form (Ha *et al.,* 2005). The structure shows that the bases at the B-Z junction itself have flipped out, which would allow for transition of the sugar pucker and rotation of the bases. It also allows the bases, when they pair again, to change the direction of the grooves sense, while maintaining stacking between the left- and right-handed columns. The B-Z transition, therefore, can be thought of as initiating with a melting of two base pairs (two B-Z junctions, with a nucleation energy of ~10 kcal/mol (Peck and Wang, 1983)), with each junction subsequently migrating in opposite directions to allow the propagation of the left-handed DNA between them (the propagation energy per base pair being sequence dependent and lowest in alternating GC dinucleotides (Ellison *et al.,* 1985)).

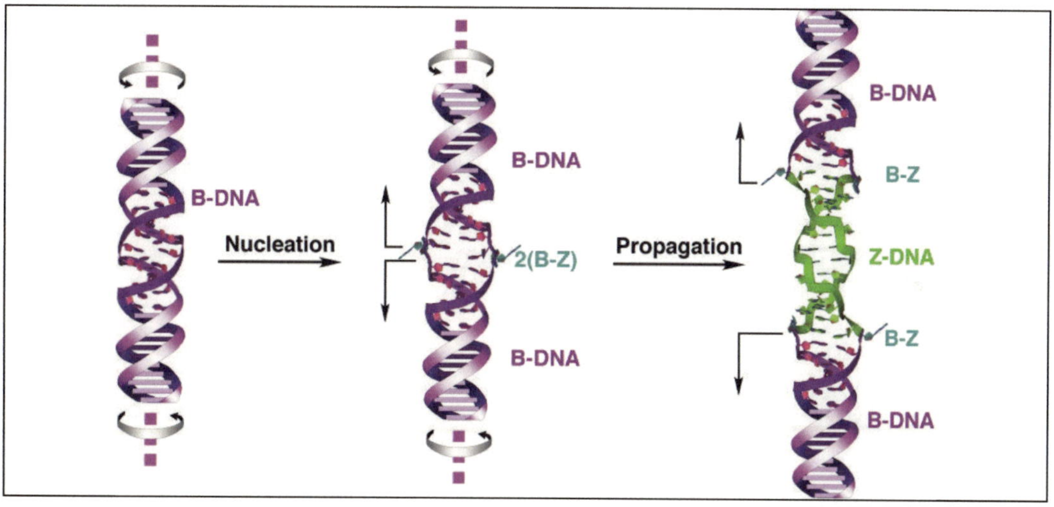

Fig. 12. B- to Z-DNA transition. B-DNA, when unwound by negative supercoiling, will first extrude two flipped out base pairs (serving as two B-Z junctions). Further unwinding results in the formation of left-handed Z-DNA between the two junctions as they migrate in opposite directions.

6. Conclusion

In this review, we have discussed a plethora of structures that come from physical biochemical studies, and show how these structures are defined by sequence and how they transform. Through its history, there has always been a nagging question of "Is this structure relevant?" Clearly, the B-DNA double-helix is relevant, not only to replication, but also to nearly all genetic processes. However, a clearer understanding for the biological roles of the non-B-type DNAs will require a detailed mapping of such structures (Ho, 2009), either experimentally or computationally, across genomes from various organisms.

7. References

Allemand, J.F., Bensimon, D., Lavery, R., & Croquette, V. (1998). Stretched and overwound DNA forms a Pauling-like structure with exposed bases. *Proc Natl Acad Sci, USA* 95: 14152-14157.

Arora, K., & Schlick, T. (2003). Deoxyadenosine sugar puckering pathway simulated by the stochastic difference equation algorithm. *Chem Phys Lett* 378: 1-8.

Ausio, J., Zhou, G., & van Holde, K. (1987). A reexamination of the reported B----Z DNA transition in nucleosomes reconstituted with poly(dG-m5dC).poly(dG-m5dC). *Biochemistry* 26: 5595-5599.

Avery, O.T., Macleod, C.M., & McCarty, M. (1944). Studies on the chemical nature of the substance inducing transformation of pneumococcal types: Induction of transformation by a desoxyribonucleic acid fraction isolated from pneumococcus Type Iii. *J Exp Med* 79: 137-158.

Biertumpfel, C., Yang, W., & Suck, D. (2007). Crystal structure of T4 endonuclease VII resolving a Holliday junction. *Nature* 449: 616-620.

Brooks, T.A., Kendrick, S., & Hurley, L. Making sense of G-quadruplex and i-motif functions in oncogene promoters. *FEBS J* 277: 3459-3469.

Burley, S.K. (1996). X-ray crystallographic studies of eukaryotic transcription initiation factors. *Philos Trans R Soc Lond B Biol Sci* 351: 483-489.

Champ, P.C., Maurice, S., Vargason, J.M., Camp, T., & Ho, P.S. (2004). Distributions of Z-DNA and nuclear factor I in human chromosome 22: a model for coupled transcriptional regulation. *Nucleic Acids Res* 32: 6501-6510.

Chargaff, E. (1950). Chemical specificity of nucleic acids and mechanism of their enzymatic degradation. *Experientia* 6: 201-209.

Coll, M., Frederick, C.A., Wang, A.H., & Rich, A. (1987). A bifurcated hydrogen-bonded conformation in the d(A.T) base pairs of the DNA dodecamer d(CGCAAATTTGCG) and its complex with distamycin. *Proc Natl Acad Sci, USA* 84: 8385-8389.

Cox, M.M., Goodman, M.F., Kreuzer, K.N., Sherratt, D.J., Sandler, S.J., & Marians, K.J. (2000). The importance of repairing stalled replication forks. *Nature* 404: 37-41.

Day, R.O., Seeman, N.C., Rosenberg, J.M., & Rich, A. (1973). A crystalline fragment of the double helix: the structure of the dinucleoside phosphate guanylyl-3',5'-cytidine. *Proc Natl Acad Sci U S A* 70: 849-853.

Declais, A.C., Fogg, J.M., Freeman, A.D., Coste, F., Hadden, J.M., Phillips, S.E., & Lilley, D.M. (2003). The complex between a four-way DNA junction and T7 endonuclease I. *EMBO J* 22: 1398-1409.

Dickerson, R.E. (1992). DNA structure from A to Z. *Methods Enzymol* 211: 67-111.

Dickerson, R.E. (1999). Helix structure and molecular recognition by B-DNA. In *Oxford Handbook of Nucleic Acid Structure*, S. Neidle, ed. (New York, Oxford University Press), pp. 145-197.

Dickerson, R.E., Goodsell, D.S., & Neidle, S. (1994). "...the tyranny of the lattice...". *Proc Natl Acad Sci, USA* 91: 3579-3583.

Dickman, M.J., Ingleston, S.M., Sedelnikova, S.E., Rafferty, J.B., Lloyd, R.G., Grasby, J.A., & Hornby, D.P. (2002). The RuvABC resolvasome. *Eur J Biochem* 269: 5492-5501.

Drew, H.R., Wing, R.M., Takano, T., Broka, C., Tanaka, S., Itakura, K., & Dickerson, R.E. (1981). Structure of a B-DNA dodecamer: conformation and dynamics. *Proc Natl Acad Sci USA* 78: 2179-2183.

Eichman, B.F., Mooers, B.H.M., Alberti, M., Hearst, J.E., & Ho, P.S. (2001). The crystal structures of psoralen cross-linked DNAs: drug dependent formation of Holliday junctions. *J Mol Biol* 301: 15-26.

Eichman, B.F., Ortiz-Lombardia, M., Aymami, J., Coll, M., & Ho, P.S. (2002). The inherent properties of DNA four-way junctions: comparing the crystal structures of holliday junctions. *J Mol Biol* 320: 1037-1051.

Eichman, B.F., Vargason, J.M., Mooers, B.H.M., & Ho, P.S. (2000). The Holliday junction in an inverted repeat sequence: sequence effects on the structure of four-way junctions. *Proc Natl Acad Sci, USA* 97: 3971-3976.

Ellison, M.J., Kelleher, R.J., 3rd, Wang, A.H., Habener, J.F., & Rich, A. (1985). Sequence-dependent energetics of the B-Z transition in supercoiled DNA containing nonalternating purine-pyrimidine sequences. *Proc Natl Acad Sci, USA* 82: 8320-8324.

Foloppe, N., Nilsson, L., & MacKerell, A.D., Jr. (2001). Ab initio conformational analysis of nucleic acid components: intrinsic energetic contributions to nucleic acid structure and dynamics. *Biopolymers* 61: 61-76.

Franklin, R.E., & Gosling, R.G. (1953a). Evidence for 2-chain helix in crystalline structure of sodium deoxyribonucleate. *Nature* 172: 156-157.

Franklin, R.E., & Gosling, R.G. (1953b). Molecular Configuration in Sodium Thymonucleate. *Nature (London)* 171: 740-741.

Ghosh, A., & Bansal, M. (2003). A glossary of DNA structures from A to Z. *Acta Crystallogr D Biol Crystallogr* 59: 620-626.

Greenbaum, J.A., Pang, B., & Tullius, T.D. (2007). Construction of a genome-scale structural map at single-nucleotide resolution. *Genome Res* 17: 947-953.

Ha, S.C., Lowenhaupt, K., Rich, A., Kim, Y.G., & Kim, K.K. (2005). Crystal structure of a junction between B-DNA and Z-DNA reveals two extruded bases. *Nature* 437: 1183-1186.

Haber, J.E., & Heyer, W.D. (2001). The fuss about Mus81. *Cell* 107: 551-554.

Hadden, J.M., Declais, A.C., Carr, S.B., Lilley, D.M., & Phillips, S.E. (2007). The structural basis of Holliday junction resolution by T7 endonuclease I. *Nature* 449: 621-624.

Hamelberg, D., Williams, L.D., & Wilson, W.D. (2001). Influence of the dynamic positions of cations on the structure of the DNA minor groove: sequence-dependent effects. *J Am Chem Soc* 123: 7745-7755.

Harvey, S.C., & Prabhakaran, M. (1986). Ribose Puckering: Structure, Dynamics, Energetics, and the Pseudorotation Cycle. *J Amer Chem Soc* 108: 6128-6136

Hays, F.A., Teegarden, A., Jones, Z.J., Harms, M., Raup, D., Watson, J., Cavaliere, E., & Ho, P.S. (2005). How sequence defines structure: a crystallographic map of DNA structure and conformation. *Proc Natl Acad Sci, USA* 102: 7157-7162.

Hendrickson, W.A., Smith, J.L., Phizackerley, R.P., & Merritt, E.A. (1988). Crystallographic structure analysis of lamprey hemoglobin from anomalous dispersion of synchrotron radiation. *Proteins* 4: 77-88.

Hershey, A.D., & Chase, M. (1952). Independent functions of viral protein and nucleic acid in growth of bacteriophage. *J Gen Physiol* 36: 39-56.

Ho, P.S. (2009). Thermogenomics: thermodynamic-based approaches to genomic analyses of DNA structure. *Methods* 47: 159-167.

Ho, P.S., Frederick, C.A., Quigley, G.J., van der Marel, G.A., van Boom, J.H., Wang, A.H., & Rich, A. (1985). G.T wobble base-pairing in Z-DNA at 1.0 A atomic resolution: the crystal structure of d(CGCGTG). *EMBO J* 4: 3617-3623.

Holliday, R. (1964). A mechanism for gene conversion in fungi. *Genet Res* 5: 282-304.

Kha, D.T., Wang, G., Natrajan, N., Harrison, L., & Vasquez, K.M. Pathways for double-strand break repair in genetically unstable Z-DNA-forming sequences. *J Mol Biol* 398: 471-480.

Khuu, P., & Ho, P.S. (2009). A rare nucleotide tautomer in the structure of an asymmetric DNA junction. *Biochemistry* 48: 7824-7832.

Khuu, P., Sandor, M., DeYoung, J., & Ho, P.S. (2007). Phylogenomic analysis of the emergence of GC-rich transcription elements. *Proc Natl Acad Sci, USA* 104: 16528-16533.

Khuu, P.A., Voth, A. R., Hays, F. A. and Ho, P. S. (2006). The stacked-X DNA Holliday junction and protein recognition. *J Mol Recognit* 19: 1-9.

Kiefer, J.R., Mao, C., Braman, J.C., & Beese, L.S. (1998). Visualizing DNA replication in a catalytically active Bacillus DNA polymerase crystal. *Nature* 391: 304-307.

Kinniburgh, A.J. (1989). A cis-acting transcription element of the c-myc gene can assume an H-DNA conformation. *Nucleic Acids Res* 17: 7771-7778.

Klotz, I.M. & Franzen, J.S. (1962). Hydrogen bonds between model peptide groups in solution. *J Am Chem Soc* 84: 3461-3466.

Kool, E.T. (2001). Hydrogen bonding, base stacking, and steric effects in dna replication. *Annu Rev Biophys Biomol Struct* 30: 1-22.

Lavery, R., & Zakrzewska, K (1998) in *Oxford Handbook of Nucleic Acid Structure*, S. Neidle, ed. (New York, Oxford University Press), pp39-76.

Liepinsh, E., Otting, G., & Wüthrich, K. (1992). NMR observation of individual molecules of hydration water bound to DNA duplexes: direct evidence for a spine of hydration water present in aqueous solution. *Nucleic Acids Res* 20: 6549-6553.

Lilley, D.M.J. (1999). Structures and interactions of helical junctions in nucleic acids. In *Oxford Handbook of Nucleic Acid Structure*, S. Neidle, ed. (New York, Oxford University Press), pp. 471-498.

Liu, L.F., & Wang, J.C. (1987). Supercoiling of the DNA template during transcription. *Proc Proc Natl Acad Sci, USA* 84: 7024-7027.

Liu, R., Liu, H., Chen, X., Kirby, M., Brown, P.O., & Zhao, K. (2001). Regulation of CSF1 promoter by the SWI/SNF-like BAF complex. *Cell* 106: 309-318.

Luger, K., Mader, A.W., Richmond, R.K., Sargent, D.F., & Richmond, T.J. (1997). Crystal structure of the nucleosome core particle at 2.8 A resolution. *Nature* 389: 251-260.

Manning, G.S. (1977). Limiting laws and counterion condensation in polyelectrolyte solutions. IV. The approach to the limit and the extraordinary stability of the charge fraction. *Biophys Chem* 7: 95-102.

McKinney, S.A., Declais, A.C., Lilley, D.M., & Ha, T. (2003). Structural dynamics of individual Holliday junctions. *Nat Struct Biol* 10: 93-97.

Mergny, J.L., Riou, J.F., Mailliet, P., Teulade-Fichou, M.P., & Gilson, E. (2002). Natural and pharmacological regulation of telomerase. *Nucleic Acids Res* 30: 839-865.

Meselson, M., & Stahl, F.W. (1958). The replication of DNA in Escherichia coli. *Proc Natl Acad Sci, USA* 44: 671-682.

Mills, M., Lacroix, L., Arimondo, P.B., Leroy, J.L., Francois, J.C., Klump, H., & Mergny, J.L. (2002). Unusual DNA conformations: implications for telomeres. *Curr Med Chem Anticancer Agents* 2: 627-644.

Mirkin, S.M. (2008). Discovery of alternative DNA structures: a heroic decade (1979-1989). *Front Biosci* 13: 1064-1071.

Neidle, S. (1999). Oxford Handbook of Nucleic Acid Structure (Oxford, Oxford Press).

Ng, H.L., Kopka, M.L., & Dickerson, R.E. (2000). The structure of a stable intermediate in the A <--> B DNA helix transition. *Proc Natl Acad Sci, USA* 97: 2035-2039.

Nunes-Duby, S.E., Matsumoto, L., & Landy, A. (1987). Site-specific recombination intermediates trapped with suicide substrates. *Cell* 50: 779-788.

Olson, W.K., & Sussman, J.L. (1982). How flexible is the furanose ring? 1. A comparison of experimental and theoretical studies. *J Am Chem Soc*: 270-278.

Ortiz-Lombardía, M., González, A., Eritja, R., Aymamí, J., Azorín, F., & Coll, M. (1999). Crystal structure of a DNA Holliday junction. *Nat Struct Biol* 6: 913-917.

Parkinson, G.N., Lee, M.P., & Neidle, S. (2002). Crystal structure of parallel quadruplexes from human telomeric DNA. *Nature* 417: 876-880.

Patel, D.J., Phan, A.T., & Kuryavyi, V. (2007). Human telomere, oncogenic promoter and 5'-UTR G-quadruplexes: diverse higher order DNA and RNA targets for cancer therapeutics. *Nucleic Acids Res* 35: 7429-7455.

Pauling, L., & Corey, R.B. (1953). A proposed structure for the nucleic acids. *Proc Natl Acad Sci, USA* 39: 84-97.

Peck, L.J., & Wang, J.C. (1983). Energetics of B-to-Z transition in DNA. *Proc Natl Acad Sci, USA* 80: 6206-6210.

Pestov, D.G., Dayn, A., Siyanova, E., George, D.L., & Mirkin, S.M. (1991). H-DNA and Z-DNA in the mouse c-Ki-ras promoter. *Nucleic Acids Res* 19: 6527-6532.

Pohl, F.M., & Jovin, T.M. (1972). Salt-induced co-operative conformational change of a synthetic DNA: equilibrium and kinetic studies with poly (dG-dC). *J Mol Biol* 67: 375-396.

Privé, G.G., Yanagi, K., & Dickerson, R.E. (1991). Structure of the B-DNA decamer C-C-A-A-C-G-T-T-G-G and comparison with isomorphous decamers C-C-A-A-G-A-T-T-G-G and C-C-A-G-G-C-C-T-G-G. *J Mol Biol* 217: 177-199.

Radhakrishnan, I., & Patel, D.J. (1993). Solution structure of a purine.purine.pyrimidine DNA triplex containing G.GC and T.AT triples. *Structure* 1: 135-152.

Rich, A., & Zhang, S. (2003). Timeline: Z-DNA: the long road to biological function. *Nat Rev Genet* 4: 566-572.

Rohs, R., West, S.M., Sosinsky, A., Liu, P., Mann, R.S., & Honig, B. (2009). The role of DNA shape in protein-DNA recognition. *Nature* 461: 1248-1253.

Rosenberg, J.M., Seeman, N.C., Kim, J.J., Suddath, F.L., Nicholas, H.B., & Rich, A. (1973). Double helix at atomic resolution. *Nature* 243: 150-154.

Saenger, W. (1984) *Principles of Nucleic Acid Structure*, Spinger-Verlag, New York

Sarkies, P., Reams, C., Simpson, L.J., & Sale, J.E. Epigenetic instability due to defective replication of structured DNA. *Mol Cell* 40: 703-713.

Schroth, G.P., Chou, P.J., & Ho, P.S. (1992). Mapping Z-DNA in the human genome. Computer-aided mapping reveals a nonrandom distribution of potential Z-DNA-forming sequences in human genes. *J Biol Chem* 267: 11846-11855.

Schroth, G.P., & Ho, P.S. (1995). Occurrence of potential cruciform and H-DNA forming sequences in genomic DNA. *Nucleic Acids Res* 23: 1977-1983.

Subramaniam, S., Tewari, A.K., Nunes-Duby, S.E., & Foster, M.P. (2003). Dynamics and DNA substrate recognition by the catalytic domain of lambda integrase. *J Mol Biol* 329: 423-439.

Thorpe, J.H., Gale, B.C., Teixeira, S.C., & Cardin, C.J. (2003). Conformational and hydration effects of site-selective sodium, calcium and strontium ion binding to the DNA Holliday junction structure d(TCGGTACCGA)(4). *J Mol Biol* 327: 97-109.

Vargason, J.M., Eichman, B.F., & Ho, P.S. (2000). The extended and eccentric E-DNA structure induced by cytosine methylation or bromination. *Nat Struct Biol* 7: 758-761.

Vargason, J.M., Henderson, K., & Ho, P.S. (2001). A crystallographic map of the transition from B-DNA to A-DNA. *Proc Natl Acad Sci, USA* 98: 7265-7270.

Vargason, J.M., & Ho, P.S. (2002). The effect of cytosine methylation on the structure and geometry of the Holliday junction: the structure of d(CCGGTACm5CGG) at 1.5 A resolution. *J Biol Chem* 277: 21041-21049.

Wang, A.H., Quigley, G.J., Kolpak, F.J., Crawford, J.L., van Boom, J.H., van der Marel, G., & Rich, A. (1979). Molecular structure of a left-handed double helical DNA fragment at atomic resolution. *Nature* 282: 680-686.

Wang, G., & Vasquez, K.M. (2004). Naturally occurring H-DNA-forming sequences are mutagenic in mammalian cells. *Proc Natl Acad Sci, USA* 101: 13448-13453.

Watson, J., Hays, F.A., & Ho, P.S. (2004). Definitions and analysis of DNA Holliday junction geometry. *Nucleic Acids Res* 32: 3017-3027.

Watson, J.D. (1968). The Double Helix: A Personal Account of the Discovery of the Structure of DNA (Atheneum).

Watson, J.D., & Crick, F.H. (1953a). Genetical implications of the structure of deoxyribonucleic acid. *Nature* 171: 964-967.

Watson, J.D., & Crick, F.H. (1953b). Molecular structure of nucleic acids; a structure for deoxyribose nucleic acid. *Nature* 171: 737-738.

Weil, J., Min, T., Yang, C., Wang, S., Sutherland, C., Sinha, N., & Kang, C. (1999). Stabilization of the i-motif by intramolecular adenine-adenine-thymine base triple in the structure of d(ACCCT). *Acta Crystallogr D Biol Crystallogr* 55: 422-429.

Zakian, V.A. (2009). The ends have arrived. *Cell* 139: 1038-1040.

2

Replication Demands an Amendment of the Double Helix

You Cheng Xu
UT Southwestern Medical Center at Dallas
USA

1. Introduction

DNA is a very important macromolecule in biology. It carries the genetic code for every living creature.

The finding of the double helix is undoubtedly one of the most significant discoveries in the twentieth century (Watson & Crick 1953a). It inspired many important discoveries in biology and medicine. Now, the double helix has become an icon of molecular biology (Olby, 2003).

Presently, DNA is widely accepted as a right-handed double helix taught in almost all textbooks of biochemistry and molecular biology. The knowledge of DNA is widely applied in scientific research, industry, agriculture and medicine. The information of DNA has been successfully used in many fields previously unimaginable: archaeology, drug design, forensic science, nanometer technology, etc.

After more than 50 years of intensive investigation, the basic idea of the Watson- Crick Model is still considered to be correct (Crick et al. 1979; Arnott 2006). Innumerable sequencing data proved that the two anti-parallel strands of the DNA are held by hydrogen bonds between A•T and G•C base pairs. The secondary structure of it was additionally supported by the X-ray crystallography from the double stranded oligo-deoxyribonucleotides. Ironically, prior to the right-handed B-DNA, the detailed molecular structure of main atoms in a left-handed Z-DNA was determined by X-ray crystallography (Wang, et al., 1979). Nevertheless, Z-DNA is generally assumed as a special form and seldom found in native DNA, since its presence needs alternative purine-pyrimidine sequence and some special conditions.

The helical nature of the double helix involves a topological problem for its replication. Watson and Crick (1953 b) were aware of the problem right after their discovery. They stated: "Since the two chains in our model are intertwined, it is essential for them to untwist if they are to separate.... Although it is difficult at the moment to see how these processes occur without everything getting tangled, we do not feel that this objection will be insuperable."

To avoid this objection, many side-by-side models were proposed. (Cyriax & Gäth, 1978; Rodley et al., 1976; Sasisekharan & Pattahireman 1978). Unfortunately, no substantial evidence was available for solving the puzzle of double helix (Yagil, 1991; Schvartzman & Stasiak, 2004).

2. The accumulated facts against the right-handed double helix

In 1958, Meselson and Stahl reported their classic experiment which convincingly proved that the two parental strands of *E.coli* were completely separated after each round of replication. That kind of semi-conservative mechanism becomes a basic rule in molecular biology. However, according to the Watson-Crick Model, there are 10 base pair per turn which raises a serious problem from the purely right-handed DNA duplex.

Let's focus our attention on the replication of DNA in *E.coli* which is the best known prokaryotic cell. It is well known that the DNA replication in *E.coli* is a very fast process. In rich medium, the doubling time of *E.coli* is only 20 minutes at 37°C. Each of the replication fork advances at 1 kb per second. According to the classical double helix model, the two parental strands have to untwist at the speed of 100 rounds per second or 6000 rounds per minute. The question is how can such a quick unwinding movement of the double helix proceed in the viscous cytosol where the friction is expected to be very high?

At first, the findings of the gyrase and other topoisomerases lead many scientists to believe that untwisting of DNA is no more a problem. Further investigation revealed that the only two enzymes responsible for untwisting DNA during *E.coli* replication are gyrase and topoisomerase IV. The reaction mechanisms of both enzymes are very complicated (Berger, et al 1996); and they catalyze an inter- or intra-molecular strand passing reaction respectively. And only 2 linking numbers were changed in each reaction.

Gyrase is the main operator for unwinding the DNA duplex, and its reaction rate is only 6 times per minute (Ullsperger & Cozzarelli, 1996). Whereas, topoisomerase IV is responsible for the separation of two mature chromosomal DNA molecules generated at the end of replication. Both enzymes were vital for the survival of *E.coli.*

The chromosomal DNA of *E.coli* is very long and circular. The base pair number in one of the sequenced *E.coli* DNA is 4,639,221 (Blattner et al. 1997). Hence, the linking number of *E.coli* chromosomal DNA should be around 4 X 10^5. The replication requires the two strands to be completely separated and distributed into two daughter cells. That means that the gyrase has to reduce the linking number from 4X 10^5 to exactly zero within a very short period of time (40 minutes in a fast growing *E.coli* cell). The slow reaction rate of gyrase definitely makes it unable to accomplish this task.

Digging deeper, more problems would be encountered: a) It is generally assumed that the DNA duplex can transfer the supercoiling from one region to another region like a car speedometer cable. In a rapidly growing *E.coli*, there are more than 6 replication forks (Skarstad et al. 1986). The positive supercoiling generated during the synthesis of new DNA is very difficult to transfer to the terminal along the highly twisted chromosomal DNA confined in the nucleoid (Zimmerman, 2004). b) At the same time, many tRNAs, ribosomal RNAs and mRNAs were being actively transcribed from the same chromosomal DNA. Hence many sites of the chromosomal DNA were occupied by various enzymes and nucleic acids. These macromolecules attached to the chromosomal DNA would physically block the advancement of DNA replication. In addition, the positive supercoiling generated in front of several replication forks and many transcription sites are also very difficult to pass through these regions. c) Each gyrase binds to around 150 base pairs, a toposite, on the chromosomal DNA (Bates & Maxwell, 1989; Condemine & Smith, 1990). Only the gyrase located in front of the replication fork is effective for the separation of parent strands. The effective toposites would be less and less as the bi-directional replication forks advance to their unique terminal. The rate of DNA replication would greatly slow down due to the less available toposites and consequently less effective gyrase. This imaginative effect has never been found. d) The structure of chromosome itself can cause additional trouble in DNA replication. Inside the bacteria, the chromosomal DNA is composed of many supercoiled domains; each of them containing abundant amounts of proteins, (Travers & Muskhelishvili, 2007). Although the detailed structure of these domains is not clear, they are topologically independent of each other. Besides, the binding of chromosomal DNA to the cell membrane may prevent the rotation of speedometer cable-like-DNA (Bravo et al. 2005).

In brief, these theoretical considerations or arguments are almost no use for solving the problem in reality. They just provide something for us to remember while investigating the mechanisms of DNA replication or RNA transcription.

From the view point of topology, how the linking number drops from $4x10^5$ to zero is an unavoidable and difficult question for any biochemist.

Scientists are not easily to be swayed by eloquence. To solve these topological problems, solid evidence is badly needed.

3. The disproof of the classical double helix

The topological problem involved in DNA replication is evident to many scientists. It greatly agitates the curiosity and interest of many scientists. Common sense tells us that the high speed unwinding is unlikely the answer for the quick DNA replication. It is our understanding that all biochemical processes can be deciphered by chemistry and physics. The complicated process of DNA replication should not violate the basic laws of chemistry and physics.

After the initial literature searching and inspired by the results of experimental exploration, a hypothesis was proposed that the two strands may not wind as strictly as announced in the Watson-Crick Model (Xu et al. 1982; Xu & Qian, 1983).

However, the evidence in these papers was unable to convince many scientists to believe that the native DNA may differ from the classical double helix model. Some experts in the field did not think the suggested idea worthy following. It is true that inspiration or intuition cannot be judged by logic reasoning for arguments in science. The author has to find some other concrete evidence to support this new hypothesis. An effective way is to find the illegitimacy of the assumption—"**All DNA duplex is right-handed double helix**", an assumption that is deeply rooted in the minds of many scientists.

When trying to argue with a prevalently accepted scientific doctrine, such as the idea of the Watson-Crick Model, disproof may be the only way of choice. Just as psychologist Csikszentmihalyi (1996) once stated: "What I try to do is to disprove certain widespread assumptions. The advantage of disproof over proof in science is that whereas a single case can disprove a generalization, even all the cases in the world are not enough for a conclusive positive proof. If I could find just one white raven that would be enough to disprove the statement: ‹**All ravens are black.**›"

Fortunately, such disproof was found after many years of investigation. The finding of a zero linking number topoisomer is similar to the finding of Achilles' heel. Except in Z-DNA, the presence of a zero linking number topoisomer is unexplained by the classical double helix model.

3.1 Finding of a zero linking number topoisomer

The most straight forward test is to measure the linking number of a set of pure topoisomers by electro-microscopy. The method was found serendipitously from relaxed plasmids (Xu, 2009).

pBR322, a head to tail dimer circular double stranded DNA containing 2 X 4361 base pairs, was chosen in this experiment (Watson, N. 1988). According to the double helix model, 10 base pair per turn, the linking number of this plasmid is estimated to be around L ≈ 2 X 4361/10 = 872.

In solution, the double helix is in B-DNA form, and the helical repeat is 10.4 base pair per turn. (Wang, 1979; Rhodes & Klug, 1980). So, the adjusted linking number of dimer pBR322 should be around L ≈ 2 X 4361/10.4 = 838.

Supercoiled DNA was prepared from an *E.coli* strain HB101 harboring the dimer pBR322. The pure plasmid was converted into relaxed form. Each relaxed DNA topoisomer was collected from a preparative agarose gel with great precaution. Each relaxed DNA was carefully denatured by glyoxal which effectively prevents the formation of hydrogen bonds between the complementary strands. After appropriate EM procedurals, the paired SSC DNAs of the individual topoisomer can be visualized by EM as shown in Figure 1. These EM pictures are just enlarged images of the tiny DNA molecules projected on a two dimensional plan.

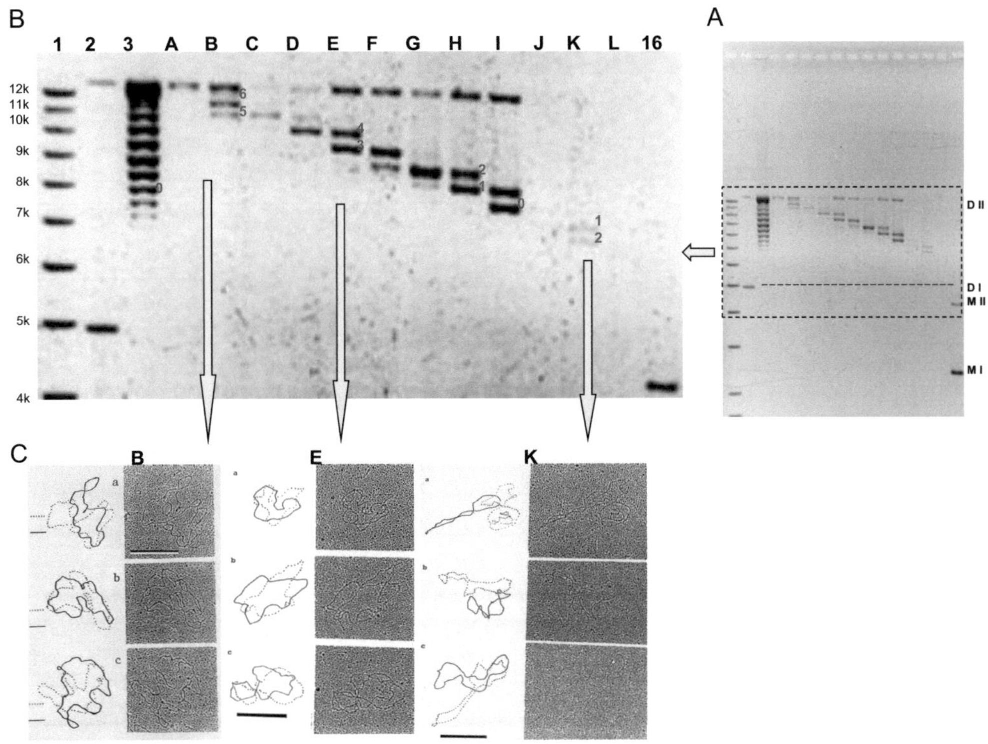

Fig. 1. The AGE purified pBR322 topoisomers were denatured and examined by EM. A) Relaxed pBR322 DNA dimers were purified by AGE and checked again on AGE. The electrophoresis buffer containing 1 μg chloroquine/ml. B) Lane 1, 1 kb DNA marker; Lane 2, supercoiled dimer; Lane 3, relaxed dimer; Lane A, B, C, D, E, F, G, H, I, J, K, L, are purified fractions; Lane 16, supercoiled monomer. (Only the nicked monomer appears in this picture). C) The fractions B, E, K were denatured by glyoxal and checked by EM. The bar represents 0.5μm. The red numbers represent absolute topological number, | Lk | (Xu, 2009).

Under optimal conditions, each linkage of the two rings generates two crossings on their two dimensional projection. The linking number of the denatured topoisomer molecule can be obtained by counting the crossing number of the two SSC DNAs on EM picture and divide it by two.

Surprisingly, the observed linking number greatly deviated from the value expected from the Watson-Crick Model.

Many reasons indicate that this result is not an artifact or an occasional occurance. Two of the cardinal reasons are that each topoisomer has the same measured linking number and that all the data is consistent with the established notion that the linking number differs by one between neighboring bands on the agarose gel (Crick et al. 1979). The individual EM pictures were thus fused into cohesive evidence.

The tricky part is that the zero linking number topoisomer itself could not be convincingly proved by checking the image of this denatured topoisomer. The reason is that an image of SSC DNA found under the EM may either come from a denatured zero linking number topoisomer or from the dissociated nicked DNA.

However, a zero linking number topoisomer can be definitely located on the agarose gel from the measured linking numbers of three different topoisomers.

A reasonable deduction is that the absolute linking number of supercoiled DNA is higher than that of relaxed DNA. This deduced result is remarkably different from the contemporary theory of DNA supercoiling.

An additional test was carried out to compare the EM pictures of supercoiled and relaxed monomer pBR322 DNA in their denatured form. Figure 2 clearly indicates that the absolute linking number of supercoiled DNA is higher than that of relaxed DNA. On the EM picture, the two SSC DNAs of relaxed pBR322 in relief exclude the possible overlapping of two independent SSC DNAs. Since the relaxed DNA samples were prepared from monomer pBR322 which is pure without any dimer as shown in figure 1 A and B, it excludes the presence of any catenated double stranded DNA.

It should be noted that similar EM pictures of denatured supercoiled PM2 DNA molecules were first published in 1975 (Brack et al.). Although the authors of the paper did not give their explanation to this phenomenon, their finding should be considered as extra evidence supporting the above results. PM2 DNA comes from a big bacterial virus carrying 10079 base pairs. Although its linking number cannot be clearly obtained from their EM pictures, its crossing number is estimated to be much less than $2\text{x } 10079/10.4 \approx 1938$.

With the observations from dimer or monomer pBR322 and PM2 DNA, it is appropriate to say that the linking numbers of covalently closed circular DNA are much less than that expected from the Watson - Crick Model.

Seeing is believing. Although the detailed winding direction of the two strands in the double helix was unable to be seen, the combination of EM and topological knowledge of circular DNA helps us to know that they could not always winding in one direction. That can be assumed as a disproof of the assertion that all DNA is right-handed double helix.

3.2 Annealing of two complementary SSC DNAs

The EM evidence has often worried some scientists who were not confident in the results obtained from this method. Further evidence is required to make sure that this eccentric idea is worth considering. To find out if the zero linking number topoisomer can be assembled by two independent complementary SSC DNAs, an experiment was performed as shown in Figure 3.

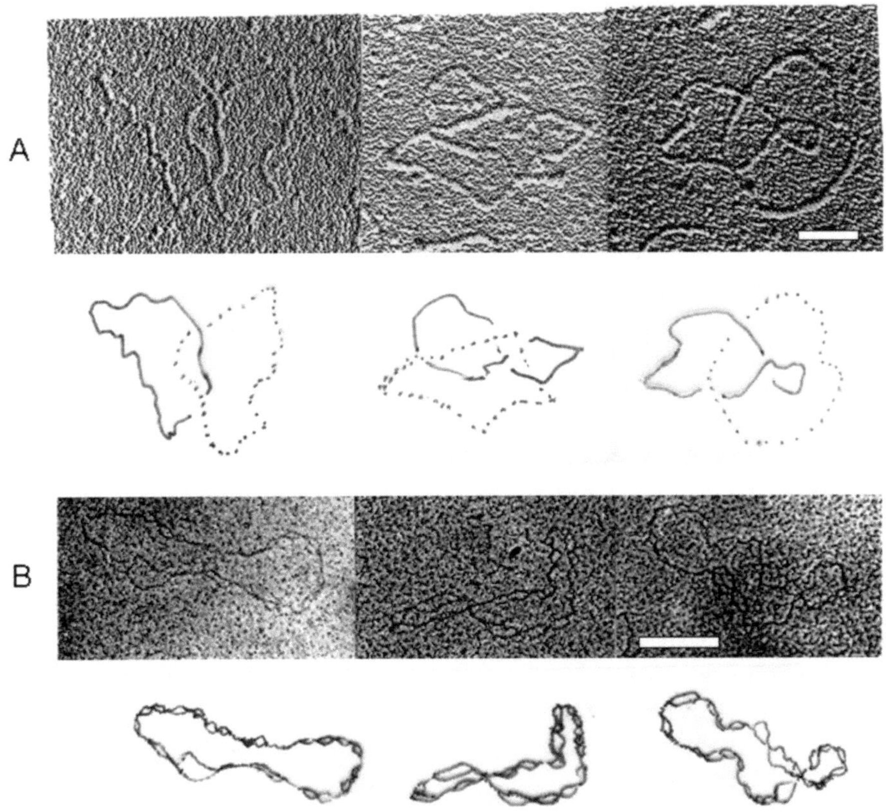

Fig. 2. EM pictures of pBR322 DNA molecules denatured by glyoxal. The bar represents 0.5μm. A) Relaxed DNA in relief, the EM samples were additionally shadowed in one direction. (B) Supercoiled DNA.

After singly nicked pBluescript DNA was obtained, a mixture of SSC DNA can be collected from alkaline sucrose gradient centrifugation. Under appropriate conditions, the annealing product of this SSC DNA was examined by a two dimensional AGE. A special topoisomer band appeared on the agarose gel, which is neither DNA II, DNA III nor DNA V (Stettler et al., 1979), but similar to one of the native topoisomers. According to topology, it strongly indicates that the linking number of this annealing product is zero, since the annealing solution contains nothing but the two complementary SSC DNAs together with a few chemical reagents.

Thus, the zero linking number topoisomer was proved to be the case by two different ways, i.e., disassembling and assembling with EM and AGE respectively.

Biegeleisen (2002) mentioned an interesting story about the assembling of complementary SSC DNA test conducted by Dr. Robert Chambers: "After becoming aware of the publication of the Stettler paper, Chambers retired his painstakingly isolated preparation of complementary single-stranded circular DNA to the refrigerator. Three months later, a significant portion of it had turned into Form I. Chambers, a staunch 'traditionalist' was unwilling to challenge the Watson-Crick theory, and, perhaps because he was unable to

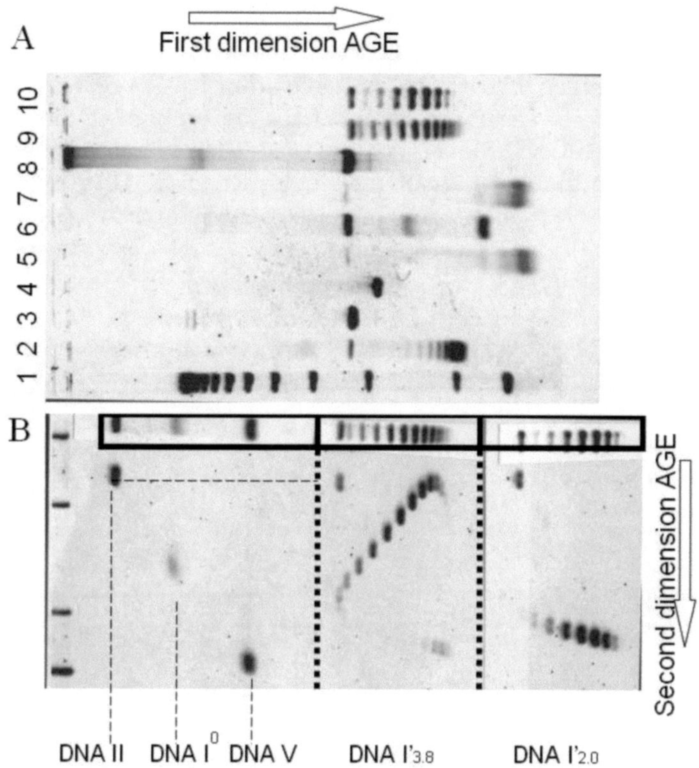

Fig. 3. The assembling products of pBluescript SSC-DNA. A) First dimension AGE in TBE buffer containing 1 µg chloroquine / ml. Lane 1, 1 kb molecular marker; Lane 2, supercoiled DNA; Lane 3, singly nicked DNA; Lane 4, linear DNA; Lane 5, SSC DNA; Lane 6, annealed SSC DNA; Lane 7, SSL DNA; Lane 8, annealed SSL DNA; Lane 9, DNA relaxed in the presence of 3.8 µg EthBr/ml; Lane 10, DNA relaxed in the presence of 2.0 µg EthBr/ml. B) Second dimension AGE in the TBE buffer containing 5µg EthBr/ml. Three slides of the sample in the first dimension were turned 90° for second dimension AGE. In the 3 square boxes, the 3 samples were electrophoresised in first dimension only and pasted in the way that keeps the nicked DNA alined with the corresponding nicked DNA in second dimension gel (Xu, 2009).

provide a satisfactory explanation for his discovery in terms of 'traditional' theory, he chose not to publish it (R.W. Chambers, personal communication, 1978)."
The finding of the zero linking number topoisomer is directly against the rule of DNA topology written in most textbooks. It is also a disproof of the idea that the two strands of DNA are always winding plectonemically in the right-handed direction.

3.3 Figure eight test

DNA structure is such an important molecule; that when trying to make even a slight modification one should be very careful and cautious. However, the finding of zero linking number questions the validity of the traditional double helix model. Advised by Wang, (A Mallinckrodt Professor of the department of Biochemistry and Molecular Biology at Harvard University), a figure eight test is designed to check whether DNA is really a right-handed duplex.

A 2 kb fragment of Hind III cleaved λDNA (from 23100 to 25157) was inserted into M13mp19 in opposite directions. The two SSC DNAs, each containing a 2 kb fragment complementary to the other one, can be prepared from two kinds of phage separately. It would be interesting to see the shape of the annealing product of these two SSC DNAs. According to the Watson-Crick Model, the annealed 2 kb fragment should have 200 right turns, that would force the rest part of the single stranded M13 turning 200 times left-handedly or turn the whole molecule into highly supercoiled form, so as to keep the linking number unchanged, i.e., $T_{right\text{-}handed} + T_{left\text{-}handed} + Wr = 0$. The experimental result is quite unexpected as shown in Figure 4.

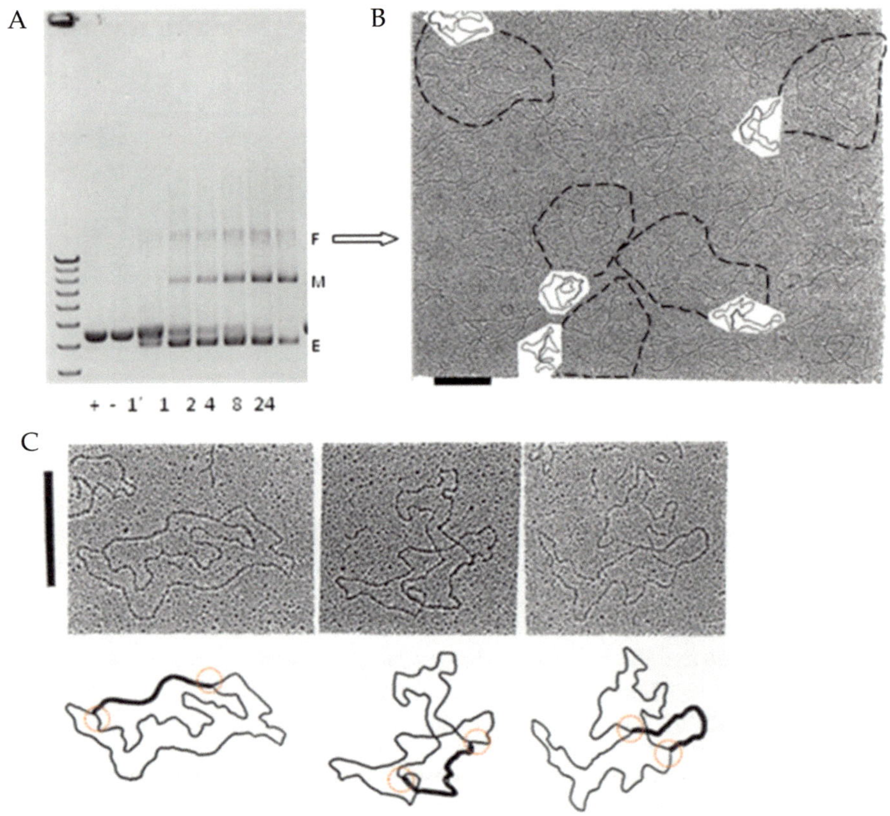

Fig. 4. Figure eight structures obtained from two SSC-DNAs with a 2 kb fragment inserted in opposite orientation. A) AGE of annealing products at different times. Lane 1, 1 kb DNA marker; Lane 2, SSC DNA+; Lane 3, SSC DNA–; Lane 4, 5, 6, 7, 8, 9, annealing of the two SSC DNA after 1 minute, 1, 2, 4, 8, 24 hours. B) The EM of annealing product from fraction F. A half sized image is pasted at the vicinity of each figure eight molecule. The bar represents 0.5μm. C) The three typical figure 8 molecules under EM. The bar represents 0.5μm (Xu, 2009).

The annealing product is just like figure Θ with two forks connecting the double stranded DNA with single-stranded DNA. Whereas, no product was found that resembles anything that could be expected from the double helix model.

The test clearly indicated that the 2 kb fragment of λHind III contains both right-handed and left-handed DNA. Due to the cancellation of the opposite twists, its net twist is close to zero. This result is consistent with other experimental findings showing that in native DNA, the two strands may wind in both directions. It constitutes one more piece of disproof of the right-handed double helix.

3.4 Denaturing singly nicked DNA

A much simpler experiment is also helpful to the understanding of the double helix. When singly nicked plasmid was denatured with alkaline, the fast denaturation process reflects the two strands of pBR322 DNA are unlikely winding 431 times. As shown in Figure 5, the singly nicked DNA can be denatured quickly within 10 minutes, one minute and even 1 second respectively.

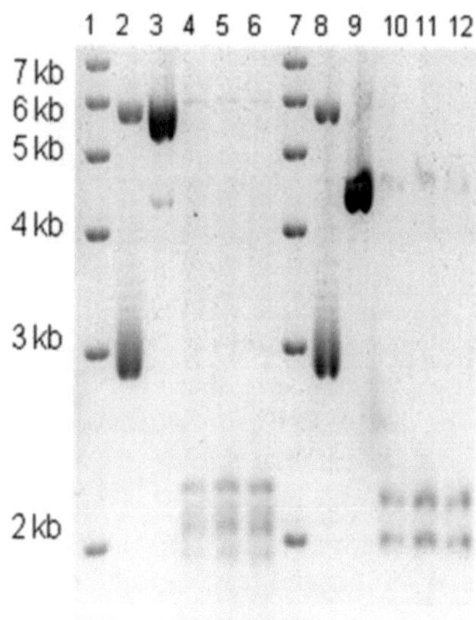

Fig. 5. AGE of pBR322 DNA II and DNA III denatured by NaOH. Lane 1 and 7, 1 kb DNA marker; Lane 2 and 8, supercoiled DNA; Lane 3, 0.5 µg of singly nicked DNA; Lane 4, 5, 6, 0.5 µg singly nicked DNA denatured by equal volume of 0.5 N NaOH after 10, 1 minute and 1 second; Lane 9, 0.5 µg linear DNA; Lane 10, 11, 12, 0.5 µg linear DNA denatured by equal volume of 0.5 N NaOH after 10, 1 minute and 1 second (Xu, 2009).

The powerful AGE separates the two kinds of SSC DNA and SSL DNA into 4 bands. It takes more thinking to figure out the denaturing process of this singly nicked DNA. In solution, the nicked DNA is moving in a three dimensional solution. Alkaline is supposed to destroy the hydrogen bond instantly that makes the SSL DNA departing from its complementary SSC DNA. According to the double helix model, a quick unwinding of the SSL DNA is required, that means that the two ends of the SSL DNA have to rotate in opposite directions. The question is that the rotating strand would cause tangling or knotting, which prevents the quick separation of the SSL DNA from SSC DNA. Besides, the SSC DNA is not always expanded at its extreme waiting for the two ends of SSL DNA to pass through. For better understanding of the process, a simplified cartoon is shown in Figure 6.

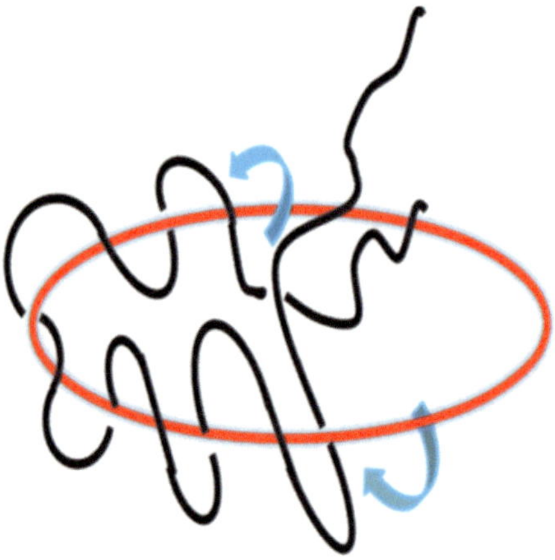

Fig. 6. The two ends of SSL DNA unwinding from SSC DNA in a nicked DNA

The observed phenomenon reflects that the twist number of singly nicked pBR322 DNA is probably very low, so that the two strands can be separated quickly without much topological impediment. However, this explanation is inconsistent with the right-handed double helix.

It is a real challenge to our wisdom as we have to explore the detailed winding directions of the two strands inside the double helix. There is no available protocol to follow. The present few tests were obtained after 30 years of trial-and-error experimentation. Here, only routine biochemical methods were used, combined with the topological knowledge of circular DNA duplex, a set of consistent evidences were obtained. They are supposed to provide a significant supplementary to the double helix model. Some of the tests are rather simple, but these experimental results need open-minded thinking.

3.5 Mobility of denatured topoisomers varies with their supercoiling

An additional test is useful in revealing the topological properties of the plasmid as shown in Figure 7.

Equal amounts of various pBR322 DNA samples, differing in their supercoiling, were denatured by alkaline first. The denatured products were examined by AGE. The mobility of denatured relaxed DNA moves the fastest. This phenomenon is difficult to explain by the Watson-Crick Model that assumes that the linking number of all these plasmids should be very big (from 430 of relaxed DNA to approximately 350 of highly supercoiled DNA); evidently these differences are relatively small and should not cause much difference in their denatured form.

On the other hand, suppose the linking number of relaxed pBR322 DNA is close to zero, after alkaline treatment, its two SSC DNAs should have more freedom to move in the alkaline solution. As soon as entering into the agarose gel under the electric force, they will renature instantly. A rigid entity is thus formed due to the formation of many illegitimate inter and intra-strand base pairs. The entity is so tight that it moves faster than the undenatured supercoiled DNA. Whereas, after denaturing, the mobility of those highly supercoiled DNA displays differently. This reflects that their linking number is higher; and the two strands are more topologically constrained and have much less freedom in alkaline solution. After entering the gel, they should have more chance, though not always, to find

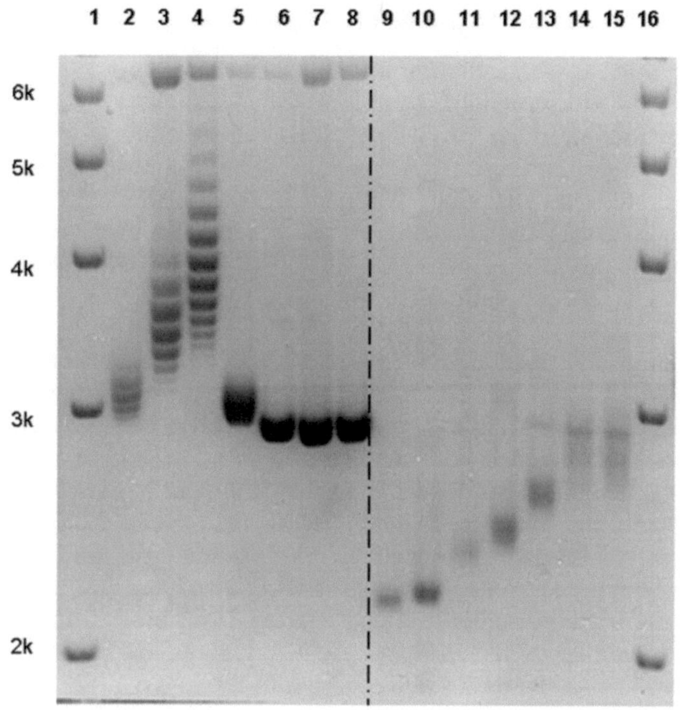

Fig. 7. Comparison of the pBR322 DNA with different supercoiling before and after alkaline denaturation. The electrophoresis buffer containing 2µg chloroquine/ml. Lane 1 & 16, 1 kb ladder; Lane 2, DNA I'_0; Lane 3, DNA $I'_{0.4}$; Lane 4, DNA I; Lane 5, DNA I'_3; Lane 6, DNA I'_5; Lane 7, DNA I'_{10}; Lane 8, DNA I'_{20}; Lane 9−15, same as 2−8 together with (1v/1v) 0.5 N NaOH.

their partners. Just as the thin band, seen in figure 7, moving with the same mobility as those untreated supercoiled DNA. However, most of them were renatured differently from those renatured relaxed counterparts due to their higher topological constrain.

All of these experiments afore-mentioned were designed to test a hypothesis that the two strands of the double helix are not restricted to wind right-handedly. Each experiment was conducted with a purely objective attitude, i.e., with no prejudgment. Just let the observed phenomena reflect the feature of DNA itself. The observed phenomena were explained independently of the prevailing theory. In order to assure the experimental results were reproducible, pure plasmids were used and the experiments were carried out under well defined conditions.

Although the five experiments have been independently carried out, the results were amazingly consistent with each other. Hence their combination makes a chain of evidence indicating that the two strands in the double helix cannot always wind right-handedly.

The provided evidence was designed on a hypothesis that is different from the canonical double helix model. It is by no means a challenge to anybody. It is not the intension of the author to commit blasphemy against authorities or leading scientists. The argument is totally in the field of science; hence no personal conflict is involved. However, our view point has to be declared for the sake of truth.

4. The ambidextrous model of the double helix

DNA generally presents as a uniform double helix, it can also adopt various different forms, such as left-handed Z-DNA, cruciform structures, three-stranded H-DNA, four stranded G-quartets or another four stranded PX DNA with reciprocal strand exchange (Mirkin, 2008; Wang, X. et al., 2010). Each of these DNA structures is important in its respective biological function. They are still rare structures that can seldom be found in native DNA. Even though their presence greatly expands our knowledge on DNA structure, they won't affect our understanding of the double helix. On the other hand, this ambidextrous model is different. It carries a conceptually different idea that may lead to some profound implications.

All our experiments, described above are consistent with each other and cannot be explained by the canonical double helix model. These results suggest that the two strands in native DNA must be wound bi-directionally. In other words, the two strands of DNA are winding ambidextrously, rather than plectonemically.

The meaning of this ambidextrous model is somehow similar to side-by-side DNA, which may cause some confusion and perplexity. Whereas, ambidextrous DNA implies that the two strands are mainly winding right-handedly or left-handedly at the same time in a native DNA duplex, which is an amendment to the classical double helix model.

The zero linking number topoisomer found in relaxed DNA indicates that there is a lot of left-handed DNA coexisting with right-handed DNA. It should be pointed out that the left-handed DNA found in these native DNAs is unlikely to be Z-DNA, because Z-DNA requires an alternative purine and pyrimidine sequence. It is plausible that Z-DNA is just a member of the left-handed DNA family.

An interesting finding is that the absolute linking number of relaxed DNA is less than that of supercoiled DNA which is contrary to the concept of traditional DNA topology.

Most native plasmids are negatively supercoiled DNA. The superhelical density of different plasmids has been measured to be similar, i.e., $\sigma \approx -0.05$. In a plasmid with N base pairs, its supercoiling is generally supposed to be around $Wr \approx \sigma N/10.4$, and the linking number should be $L_{w\text{-}c} \approx N/10.4$. Whereas, according to the ambidextrous model, the total twist number $T \approx 0$, so $L_{amb} = T + Wr \approx Wr$. It means that the two strands of native plasmid are still topologically inseparable. Hence, the ratio of $L_{w\text{-}c} / L_{amb} = 20$. It implies the linking number of a plasmid should be about 20 times less than the estimated value based on Watson-Crick Model.

An additional deduction is that the absolute linking number of positively supercoiled DNA is also higher than that of relaxed DNA. It further leads to the recognition that positively supercoiled DNA contains more left-handed DNA than right-handed DNA. This deduction has a significant implication on the understanding of heat resistance of DNA in hyperthermophilic strains.

5. The consequences of the amendment

Since the Watson - Crick Model is so widely accepted by the science community, it is likely that many scientists are unaware that some of their experimental phenomena may have alternative explanations.

The suggested ambidextrous double helix model is topologically different from the Watson-Crick Model. Consequently, many experimental results published previously could be explained differently with the ambidextrous DNA model. A few examples are presented here that may be of interest to the authors and other scientists.

5.1 The two strands of λDNA can be progressively separated by SS-DNA binding protein

Dalius et al. (1972) published an interesting picture of λDNA, which was completely denatured by SS-binding protein gene 32 as cited here (Figure 8).
The gene 32 binds the SSDNA in a cooperative way, and each gene 32 protein binds to 10 nucleotides.
Considering the dynamic nature of long λDNA in solution, the two strands of the DNA not only move together constantly, but also have transient impairing or "breathing" at some regions, especially at those AT rich regions and at two single stranded terminals. These SS

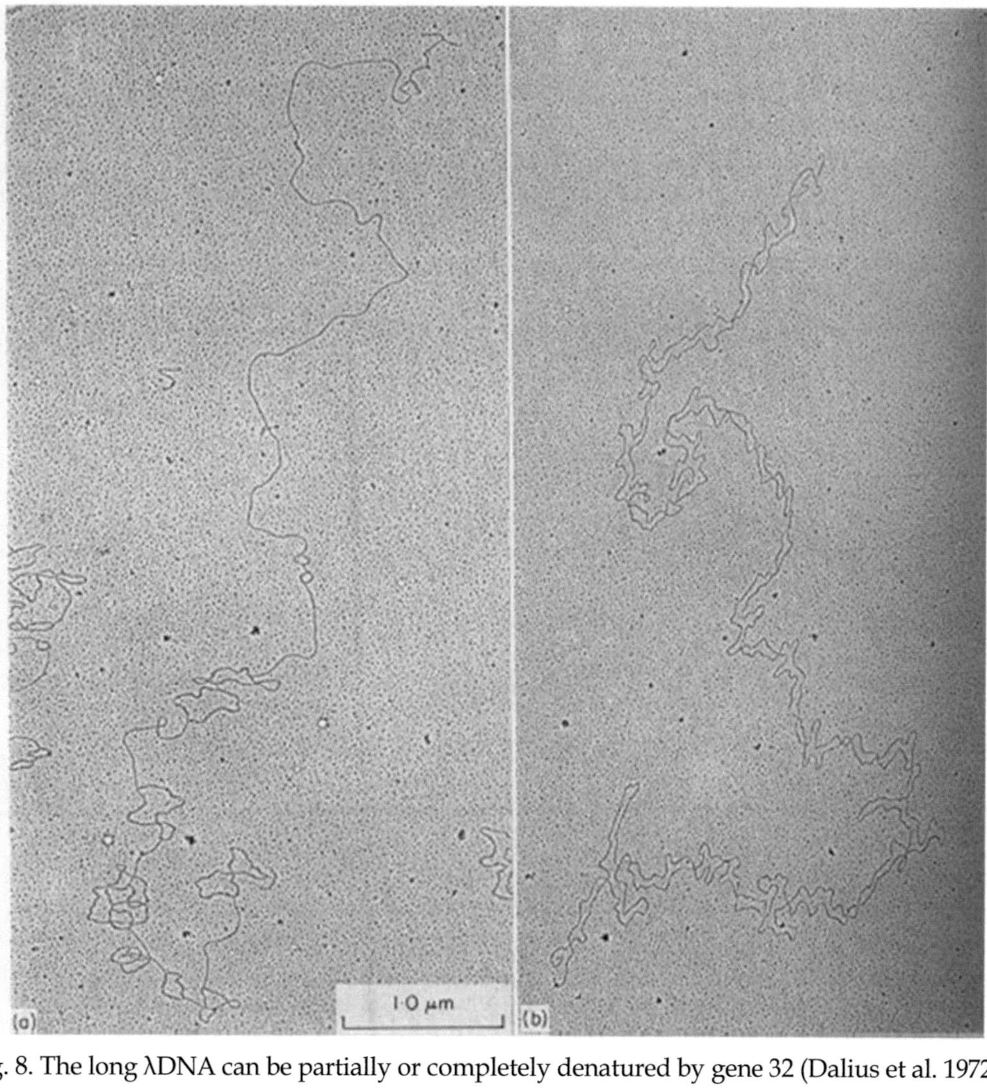

Fig. 8. The long λDNA can be partially or completely denatured by gene 32 (Dalius et al. 1972).

DNA regions were supposed to be preferentially occupied by gene 32 which has a molecular weight of 35,000Da. The gene 32 cooperatively occupied regions would be very clumsy and lumbering which would prevent their rotation in solutions as required by the Watson-Crick Model. As seen in Figure 8, the two strands of long λDNA were almost parallel as two side-by-side threads with no tangling. The complete separation implies that the two strands were not tightly winding in right-handed direction. Hence, the rotation of the gene 32 bound DNA is unlikely to happen.

5.2 The λDNA can be stretched to twice its normal size

Bensimon et al. (1995) proved that the λDNA can be stretched to twice its normal length. Lebrun and Lavery (1996) gave an instructive drawing as shown in Figure 9.

Only suppose the twist angle close to zero (θ= 0), it would be possible letting the two strands of λDNA to be stretched to almost parallel. It is well known that R = 3.4 Å (double helix pitch) and L = 7Å (supposed average distance between two adjacent phosphate atoms in stretched ss-DNA). The arithmetic tells us that the limit of a λDNA molecule could be stretched before rupture is let all the phosphate atoms line straight, i.e. let R ≈ L. The meaning of this experiment is much easier to be explained by the ambidextrous model, i.e., the net twist number in λDNA is close to zero.

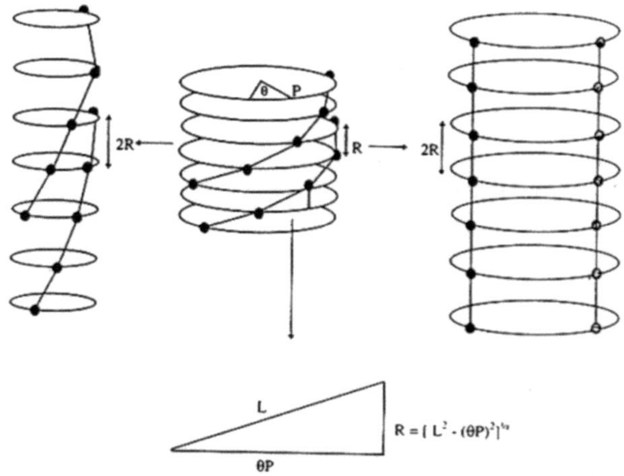

Fig. 9. Schematic model of DNA stretching: maintaining a constant inter-phosphate distance L within each strand of duplex, stretching to twice the normal rise R can be achieved by reducing the twist angle or by reducing the radius P of the duplex (Lebrun and Lavery 1996).

5.3 Sedimentation coefficient indicates the complete separation of T7 DNA

Freifelder & Davidson (1968) found the sedimentation coefficient of the denatured T7 DNA drops sharply at 54 °C as shown in Figure 10.

Freifelder and Davidson explained their observation this way: "We therefore interpret the change as a halving of the molecular weight of the DNA resulting from the physical separation of the strands." However, how could the two strands be physically separated?

T7 DNA is a long linear DNA duplex with 39936 base pairs. According to the canonical double helix model, the two strands should twist almost 4000 times. In solution, after the treatment of formaldehyde, the two ss DNA strands should be detached but still tangled with each other. Since the long strands of DNAs are very thin and curved, they are unlikely able to unwind quickly in solution. It would be almost impossible for the two strands of T7 DNA, highly tangled with each other as the classical double helix required, having such a dramatic change. Whereas, this observed phenomenon can be easily explained by the ambidextrous model.

Many other sedimentation experiments provided similar evidences indicating that the two strands are not tightly tangled with each other (Freifelder, 1983).

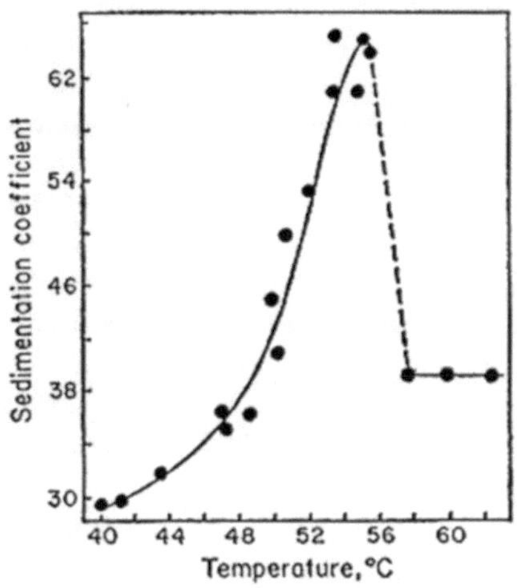

Fig. 10. Sedimentation coefficient of the sharp boundary of T7 DNA fully or partly denatured by heating for 10 minutes at the indicated temperatures in 12% HCHO, 0.1 M phosphate, pH 7.8 (Freifelder & Davidson 1968)

5.4 Point mutation shows the PCR reaction can be conducted on a plasmid

Point mutation is a clever method used in molecular biology. Stratagene Co. has successfully developed the method and a kit is ready for any users. In this method, DNA synthesis was started from two primers, differ in one specific site, on a supercoiled plasmid with Taq enzyme. The two new DNA were synthesized in opposite directions along the two strands of the same plasmid. It would be difficult for the two enzyme molecules to finish their job since two bulky enzymes would inevitably meet on their way and stop there. Whereas, if the two strands were not tightly wound, there would be enough space for both of them to pass through. This simplified explanation is based on an old idea explaining DNA synthesis. According to the presently accepted idea, the huge DNA polymerase is static, the template DNA moves in and the new DNA moves out like a movie projector. Nevertheless, it is still much easier to explain this phenomenon by the ambidextrous model.

5.5 The heat resistance of DNA in hyperthermophilic strains is difficult to explain

Hyperthermophilic strains live stably at high temperatures. An amazing strain even can duplicate at autoclaving temperature. The doubling time of strain 121 is 7 hr or 24 hr at 115°C or 115°C respectively (Kashefi & Lovley 2003). The strain is still alive after staying at 115°C for 2 hrs.

How can the double stranded DNA in an hyperthermophilic strain resist the high temperature without any damage or denaturation? It is suspected that both positive supercoiling and reverse gyrase are protecting DNA against high temperatures (Forterre & Elie, 1993; Kikuchi, 1990).
When the unique single gene of reverse gyrase was removed from a hyperthermophilic strain, the strain is still viable at high temperatures (Atomi et al. 2004). It strongly indicates that positive supercoiling is responsible for the heat resistance of double helix.
How does DNA gets positive supercoiling in the hyperthermophilic strain without reverse gyrase?
Several scientists revealed that the two strands of DNA are regularly turning left-handedly with elevated temperatures. They found the double helix unwinding angle for each base pair is Ω = -0.01° / °C/ bp. (Depew & Wang, 1975; Duguel, 1993). Hence at high temperatures, the chromosomal DNA of hyperthermophilic strain would turn left-handedly. As mentioned before, this left-handed chromosomal DNA would stay in positively supercoiled form which is supposed to be more stable at high temperatures. It is plausible that the positively supercoiled DNA is stable at high temperatures just as the negatively supercoiled DNA can. It is well known that negatively supercoiled DNA is stable at boiling temperatures, since a routine plasmid preparation protocols is the "boiling method".
Our finding of the relationship between left-handed DNA and positive supercoiling is critical for the understanding of the heat resistance of DNA at high temperatures. However, this connection can not be derived from the canonical double helix model.

5.6 The catabolite gene active protein (CAP) binds to left-handed DNA

McKay & Steitz (1981) determined the structure of catabolite gene activator protein (CAP) at 2.9 Å resolution by x-ray crystallography. They found this protein fitting quite well with the left-handed DNA rather than right-handed DNA as shown in Figure 11. Although no direct evidence of the left-handed B-DNA is obtained by their model building method, its significance in understanding the double helix should not be neglected.

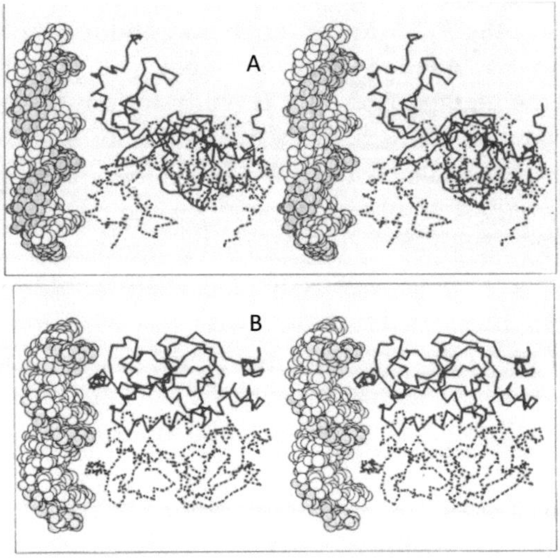

Fig. 11. Stereo drawing of the α–carbon backbone of the CAP dimer interacting with two kinds of DNA. One CAP subunit is drawn with dashed lines, the other subunit with solid lines. A) Right handed B-DNA; B) left-handed B-DNA (McKay & Steitz 1981).

All these evidences found in other labs imply that the two strands in the double helix are inconsistent to the right-handed B-DNA

Nowadays, nobody has the time or energy to read all the papers related to DNA. The listed six cases were just randomly found by the author. It is very likely that more interesting cases are hiding in the literature which may be explained differently. As seen in the above examples, except the last one, these papers did not suggest anything about the left-handed DNA. The hidden meaning on the shown facts has to be figured out after scrutinizing each paper.

Armed with the most advanced technique and instruments, the detailed information inside the native double helix is still unable to clearly figure out. The x-ray crystallography can only deal with short DNA fragments; the AEM can see some parts of DNA, but the image is not clear enough (Kato et al., 2009).

A special property of DNA is in its self-replicating function. Theoretically, the structure of this molecule enables its self- reproduction. It seems mysterious and inexplicable that after more than 50 years of research by many talented scientists, the topological problem is still unanswered.

6. The ambidextrous DNA model may be useful for understanding important biological mechanisms

Since the proposal of the central dogma (Crick 1970), great progress has been achieved; the framework of molecular biology was filled with abundant knowledge and evidence. It made modern biochemistry a reliable and valuable source of knowledge for young students. At the top of the central dogma, DNA plays a leading role in molecular biology. Any amendment of the double helix would have great implications in many aspects of molecular biology.

6.1 The mechanisms of DNA replication

Great progress accumulated over many years helps us gain a much better understanding of the mechanism of DNA replication. Nowadays, almost all elements involved in replication have been discovered and evaluated at the molecular level. Their individual function in the complicated replication process is known (Alberts, et al 2002). However, the topological problem involved in DNA replication is still largely unanswered.

Most of the knowledge on DNA replication is obtained from simple systems, i.e., in plasmids and prokaryotes, especially in *E. coli.* In principle, such knowledge is applicable to eukaryotes.

DNA replication needs a lot of proteins including DNA polymerase, helicase, ligase, primase, gyrase, single strand DNA binding proteins, etc. The huge DNA replicating machine which executes synthesizing DNA is called the replisome. It is believed that the replisome keeps stationary at the replication fork. The parental DNA rolled into the replisome; after processing, two new daughter DNAs were rolled out. The *in vitro* DNA synthesis system was proved to be valuable in elucidating the detailed replication process. The replication of leading strand and lagging strand was beautifully explained by the trombone model (Chastain et al. 2003). Now a simplified animation video of the DNA replication is available on internet. Albeit it does not mean we know the mechanism completely, especially how the double helix was untwisted. As mentioned above, the slow reaction rate of gyrase can not catch up the fast pace of DNA replication.

It should be noted that helicase, an active enzyme in DNA replication, can quickly open the double helix but is unable to cut and rebind DNA. It separates the energetically stable duplex DNA with the energy from NTP hydrolysis (Tuteja and Tuteja, 2004). The presence of this ubiquitous molecular motor protein implies that the two strands in the DNA duplex could not wind tightly as in the classical double helix model. According to the ambidextrous model, the function of helicase is reasonable and rational. The occasionally appeared topological problems would be easily solved by gyrase. However, if the DNA is really in the Watson-Crick Model, the accumulated positive supercoiling in front of the replication fork would be a big obstacle, because, the positive supercoiling is unable to be removed quickly by gyrase or to be transferred to the terminal.

The replication of DNA in eukaryotes is more complicated due to the presence of nucleosome structure and perhaps some other unknown problems. Anyone trying to uncover the mechanism of their DNA replication would encounter more topological problems. It is believed that the ambidextrous model may relieve that burden.

6.2 The mechanisms of RNA transcription

Accumulated evidence indicates that the DNA dependent RNA polymerase (RNAP) can read the information from the template strand through a relatively small "transcription bubble". At first, the finding of highly positively supercoiled pBR322 from a novobiocin treated *E.coli* strain (Lockshon & Morris, 1983) was unexpected. Later, a clever twin-supercoiled domain model was proposed, which nicely solved a difficult topological problem involved in transcription (Liu & Wang, 1987). In brief, the positive supercoiling generated in front of the RNAP is removed by gyrase, and the negative supercoiling behind the RNAP is removed by DNA topoisomerases I. When the activity of gyrase was inhibited by novobiocin or other inhibitors, the positive supercoiling were accumulated, which causes the yield of highly positively supercoiled DNA. It also explains why in a topoisomerase I mutant, the negatively supercoiled pBR322 is so unusually high (Pruss, 1985). The model was further proved by many excellent experiments (Wu et al. 1988; Tsao et al., 1989)

On the other hand, in a small extra-chromosomal DNA, the local positive supercoiling can be cancelled by the negative supercoiling concomitantly generated behind the RNAP through the speedometer like DNA. The question is how fast the diffusion of opposite supercoiling waves along the DNA could be within a topologically closed domain.

The devil is in the details.

Taking pBR322 as an example, the plasmid has 5 genes as shown in Figure 12. For simplicity, let's consider the two main genes first. According to the Watson - Crick Model, about 1182 /10.4 = 114 positive supercoilings should be generated from the transcription of tetracycline resistance (Tet) gene (86-1268), and 788/10.4 =76 positive supercoilings from β-lactamase gene (4084-3296),. Their transcriptions are oriented in opposite directions. If each gene initiated only once, their positive supercoilings generated should be additive, i.e., 76+114 = 190, which is much higher than that found in experiment. According to the result of Lockshon and Morris (1983), the positive supercoiling is estimated to be around +25, which is comparable to that of negative supercoiling (-25). The additional transcriptions from Rop and RNA II would make the situation even worse. Considering the transcriptions in a real pBR322 DNA, two successive positive supercoiling waves generated from β-lactamase and RNA II genes in one direction would clash with the other two successive positive supercoiling waves generated from Tet and Rop genes. The RNA I gene is relatively small; its contribution should be relatively small. What is the result of the clashing waves on pBR332 in a novobiocin treated living *E.coli* strain? The positive supercoiling should be more than that found experimentally.

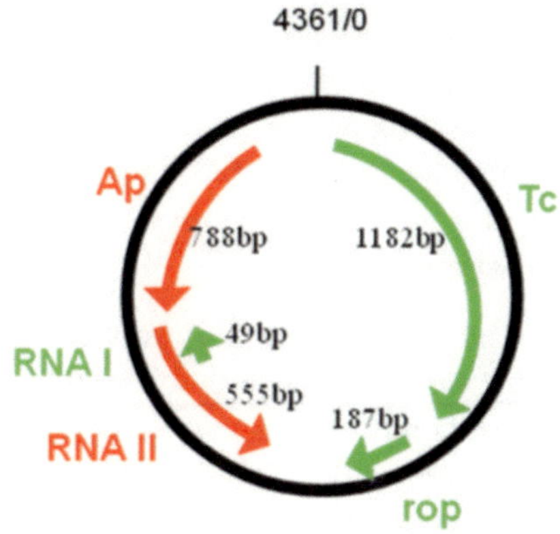

Fig. 12. The transcription orientations of 5 genes in pBR322 DNA

This remarkable discrepancy is favorable to the ambidextrous double helix model. Since the twist number is not necessarily proportional to the length of each gene, the positive or negative supercoiling generated in front of the RNAP should be much less than the expected value based on classical double helix model. It would greatly reduce the gap between experimental results and theoretical expectation. Thus, the mechanism of transcription can be understood more easily with less topological trouble.

In principle, the rules of transcription found from plasmids are applicable to the chromosomal DNA. As mentioned above, in the transcription of many genes from the chromosomal DNA, the positive supercoiling actually would not to cause any problem if the two strands are winding ambidextrously.

Transcription in eukaryotes is more complicated. However, the ambidextrous model would provide a good reason to believe that there is no topological problem during RNA transcription.

7. More problems waiting for answers

The suggested ambidextrous model seems to overcome a major topological obstacle in understanding the mechanism of DNA replication. However, it is still a hypothesis based on several topological evidences. We are not sure whether the left-handed DNA is determined or related to its sequence or not. The real nature of the two strands inside the double helix is largely unknown. Although the junction between B-DNA and Z-DNA in a 15 mer oligonucleotides was found by X-ray crystallography, in which two bases were extruded, it does not mean that similar junction could always be found in native DNA (Ha, et al., 2005).

Each restriction enzyme is sensitive to specific DNA sequence. This fact implies that secondary structure may not affect the activity of restriction enzymes. However, it is not clear that if the special sequence determines the secondary structure, and hence the activity of restriction enzymes is also affected. This is a question for future scientists to answer.

Crick et al. (1979) once stated: "DNA is such an important molecule that it is almost impossible to learn too much about it." Presently, our knowledge about the double helix has advanced much better than fifty years ago. However, many new findings remind us that probably there are still some secrets hidden in the double helix. For example: a) In dilute DNA solutions, some kind of short double stranded DNA can generate electromagnetic signal and the DNA can communicate with other DNA (Montagnier et al.2009) ; b) Concentrated solution of oligo- deoxyribonucleotide DNA duplex behave the character of both right-handed and left-handed DNA (Zanchetta et al. 2010); c) Alberts (2010) pointed out that the frontier of science is endless and "a total of about two-third of our genetic information –'our dark genome'- is needed for processes whose nature mostly remains a mystery".

8. It is time to make a conceptual change

In the history of discovery, similar stories incredibly repeated again and again. The garden pea experiment of Mendel was ignored by his contemporary scientists for 35 years; proteins were assumed to be the carriers of heredity for a very long period of time; the long stories in discovering Krebs cycle, transposon, prion, ribozyme happened in different scenarios (Grinnell, 2011). Almost all of these cases occurred due to an analogous reason — old minds die hard. The prevalently accepted dogma is always believed to be true and correct, and the new concept is believed to be bizarre and weird. The famous notion of "chance favors the prepared mind" is routinely displayed in an alternative way: "novel new concept is always being neglected, rejected or even hated by unprepared mind".

The basic idea of the Watson - Crick Model is correct and was proved by numerous experimental findings afterwards. Its contribution to molecular biology is highly evaluated. However, in native DNA, the winding direction of the two strands inside the double helix is very difficult to detect. Available evidence is scarce, obscure and questionable. The only source comes from the x-ray analysis of DNA fiber, which could not rule out the presence of left-handed DNA.

Currently, most people take the double helix as a scientific doctrine, but in 1953 it was merely an untested hypothesis as Watson and Crick recognized themselves. Even in a textbook of 1958, the double helix model was described as "an ingenious speculation". (Fruton & Simmonds, 1958)

Epistemology tells us that no theory is perfect. Even a theory as sound as Newtonian physics, is not unassailable. No matter how a theory survived the most rigorous tests, it does not mean it can pass all future tests.

The experimental results mentioned above strongly support another hypothesis that the two strands in native DNA are winding ambidextrously rather than plectonemically, a hypothesis which differs from the old hypothesis.

This amendment has been demanded for years by many facts found by various investigators. The author just weaves these findings together. The double helix is now inspected from a new viewpoint, i.e. the topological viewpoint and a new facet of the double helix is appeared.

It seems critical that while handling the problems of a long DNA molecule, we have to take it as a three dimensional structure. The negligence of the topology would lead to misinterpretation of the facts. An evident example is the extremely high unwinding rate of DNA derived from the classical double helix. The unwinding rate was assessed to be $12X10^7$ molecular weight per second at 37 °C (Freifeleder, 1983). It is equivalent to $1.8x\ 10^5$ base pair per second, or $1.08\ X\ 10^7$ rpm. It is plausible that a calculation based on a wrong premise could not tell the truth.

It is well known that DNA in solution is highly hydrated. The water content was 0.339g H_2O/g ds-DNA and 0.434g H_2O/g ss-DNA that is equivalent to 20 water molecules per base pair in ds-DNA and 7.8 water molecules per nucleotide in ss-DNA (Bastos et al 2004). These hydrated water molecules are closely contacting with more water molecules nearby. It makes the DNA strands very sluggish. While denaturing a stretch of pure DNA duplex in solution, once the unwinding of the double helix starts, the two SSL DNAs would have to unwind in opposite directions. The questions are: a) Where does the energy for the rotation of DNA strands come from; b) How can the rotation rate of delicate thin SSL DNA in solution reach the assessed value? According to our common sense, this value is intuitively unacceptable. As we know that when a car is running at its top speed, the rotation rate of its engine seldom reaches 6,000 rpm, which is made from steel and rotating in air. Although nobody can see how the two strands inside the double helix untwist while the hydrogen bonds were abruptly destroyed chemically or physically, it is unlikely that the delicate thin strands of DNA can rotate at 10 million rounds per minute in solution.

The suggested amendment is actually a minor change on the winding direction of the two strands inside the double helix. However, the concept of ambidextrous winding of the two strands is difficult for many scientists to accept. Just as everybody has a blind spot in one's vision, the conceptual blind spot of the double helix appears in some scientists' minds.

Perhaps the extreme success of the double helix in teaching and mentoring young scientists prevents them from thinking differently. According to psychology, the first impression makes a deep mark in the mind of everybody. And this impression is very difficult to be changed in an adult. It is possible that there were a few students who were skeptical on the accuracy or correctness of the double helix. However, their discrete voices were unable to be noticed by the science community.

Things are not always as they seem. It is well known that scientific knowledge is universal, objective and provisional. Except in the field of mathematics, all scientific knowledge has to be modified or improved by new findings or discoveries.

In exploring scientific truth, not artifact or illogical reasoning, but the incomplete fact or partially correct notion confuses people the most. All our knowledge about the double helix is gained from evidence achieved by many scientists and experts in the field. The various experimental phenomena provide the basis for us to have the vision below the surface, to figure out how the two strands should be. However, each scientist makes his/her own conclusion or assumption upon one's knowledge, skill, experience, wisdom, imagination and vision. Even the same evidence can lead to different conclusions or assumptions by different scientists. That is why further exploration is often necessary to verify the validity of various conclusions. Just like a jigsaw puzzle, the picture will never be perfect if some parts were missing or misplaced. However, there is no standard answer to an appropriate question asked either by a curious pupil or a scientist who is trying to know the reason of a phenomenon. In the objective world, each scientific result has to fit into the pre-existing framework, or on rare occasions modifies the theoretical framework. Scientists are not completely free of explaining their results.

As mentioned in section 3 and 5, many observed phenomena and new experimental findings found in different laboratories strongly suggest that the native DNA cannot always be a right-handed double helix. The function of DNA in replication especially demands an amendment of the double helix. Now it is the right time for making a conceptual change. Perhaps more time is needed for more people to realize this.

Through discussion, debate, refutation, re-examination, etc, our scientific knowledge gains momentum. In the arena of science, there is no discrimination of gender, race, ethnicity, age, social class, nationality, disability, political beliefs, religion, sexual orientation or other personal characteristics to any player. Nobody can act as a judge since nobody is perfect and nobody knows everything. Hence democracy is not applicable in determining which conclusion is correct. Perhaps only time can make the final verdict. Although the present peer reviewing system normally works well for the science community, it should be noted that it is by no means a best system for the promotion of science.

Different from material wealth, scientific truth is extremely precious and priceless. It is the mental product of many people who dare to explore the secrets of nature. It has no smell, no shape, no weight, and can not be physically felt. Once it is produced, it can be banned, neglected, rejected or even hated, but it can never be dismantled, burned or destroyed which is somehow different from some kind of art work. One valuable trait of scientific truth is that it can correctly predict something never happened before (under appropriate conditions) that is also the test of the correctness of any theory.

9. A double helix conjecture and some other predictions

Based on the hypothesis of the ambidextrous double helix model, it is reasonable to predict that a zero linking number topoisomer should be found among a mixture of relaxed topoisomers.

An idealized test is suggested for the validity of the ambidextrous DNA model as shown in Figure 13. This suggested experiment may be assumed as a test of double helix conjecture.

The test seems to be very simple — by manipulating a set of pure relaxed topoisomers and letting the zero linking number topoisomer disappear.

According to topology, the two complementary SSC DNAs of all topoisomers can not be completely separated except the zero linking number topoisomer. Hence, after the appropriate denaturing and renaturing treatment, all those non-zero linking number topoisomers should reappear, acting as ideal internal controls and only the zero linking number topoisomer is expected to be invisible on the agarose gel after AGE.

If such an expected experimental result could be obtained, that would be very strong evidence to prove the presence of a zero linking number topoisomer. It could be easily understood even by people with no knowledge of DNA topology. However, up to now, nobody has succeeded such an experimental demonstration. Therefore, the expected result is temporarily just a conjecture and must be verified.

The author believes this conjecture is feasible and attainable. It is hoped that readers of this paper will find the way to prove this conjecture.

Actually, as many conjectures, this conjecture will be very difficult to verify. One reason is that when destroying all the hydrogen bonds between the complementary strands of suitable topoisomer preparations, the long back bone of the plasmid is prone to be broken. Even if only a single nick occurred in a plasmid, the topological properties of the plasmid would be greatly changed and no meaningful information could be collected.

A conjecture is generally used in mathematics for a statement which is probably wise and true but has not been proven yet. According to Karl Popper's opinion, all scientific theories are provisional conjectures and subject to re-examination. Therefore, the new discoveries, the refutation of old theory and the proper conjectures or hypotheses presented at the right time and right place are helpful for the advancement of science.

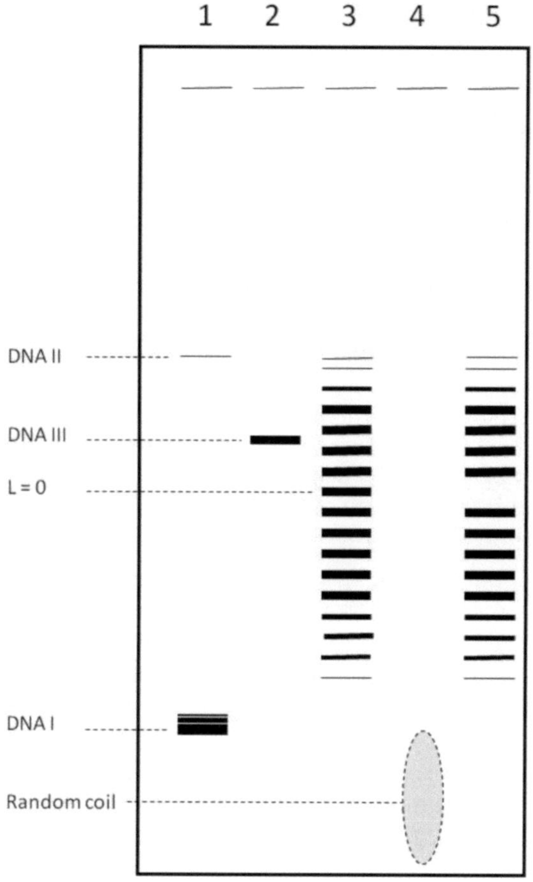

Fig. 13. The expected result of the double helix conjecture. Lane 1. Supercoiled DNA; Lane 2, Linear DNA; Lane 3, Relaxed DNA; Lane 4, Denatured relaxed DNA; Lane 5, Annealing product of samples from lane 4.

The proof of the famous Fermat conjecture took more than 300 years. (Now named as Fermat's last theorem: If an integer n is greater than 2, then the equation $a^n + b^n = c^n$ has no solutions in non-zero integers a, b and c). However, the quick advancement of modern biochemistry can not wait such a long period of time for the verification of this conjecture.

It is possible that when this conjecture is proven, the study of DNA and its various functions would be a new hot spot in biochemistry and molecular biology.

In addition to the double helix conjecture, according to the ambidextrous DNA model, the following assumptions or predictions are not difficult to be derived. It is also believed that they can be proven experimentally.

a. There is no quick rotation of the double helix during replication.
b. In any plasmid, the melting temperature of a zero linking number topoisomer should be very close to that of nicked DNA.

c. It is possible to make highly positively supercoiled DNA with superhelical density $\sigma >$ +0.1.

10. Conclusion

Is DNA really a double helix? The question has been asked by some scientists for many years. There is no doubt about the two anti-parallel strands and base pairing. The only question is about the winding direction of the two strands inside the double helix.

In his book 〈**What mad pursuit**〉, Crick (1988) wrote: "The double-helical structure of DNA was thus finally confirmed only in the early 1980s. It took over twenty-five years for our model of DNA to go from being rather plausible, to being very plausible (as a result of the detailed work on DNA fibers), and from there to being virtually certainly correct." Presently, most people believe that there are no problems in the double-helical structure of DNA.

There is no doubt that the structures of oligonucleotides determined by x-ray crystallography are correct and important. However, selectively choosing evidences favorable to right-handed DNA is not the best way in preventing imperfect conclusions. Besides, extrapolating the results obtained from short DNA fragments to long native DNA leaves room for error.

Instead of providing thousands of evidence favorable to the Watson-Crick Model, this chapter shows just a few examples that cannot be explained by that prevalently accepted theory. Based on topological evidence and many supporting facts, it is plausible that the two strands are winding ambidextrously, rather than plectonemically. This conceptually different idea can reasonably explain many experimental results that the classical double helix cannot.

The tough topological problems involved in clarifying the mechanisms of DNA replication and RNA transcription may be dissolved in the ambidextrous double helix model.

Surely, the DNA cannot speak for itself. Limited by personal knowledge, vision and time, our present hypothesis for the observed phenomena may be imperfect. As Horrobin (1975) pointed out: "Many and probably most of the hypotheses published in the journal will turn out in some way to be wrong. But if they stimulate determined experimental testing, progress is inevitable whether they are wrong or right. The history has repeatedly shown that when hypotheses are proposed it is impossible to predict which will turn out to be revolutionary and which ridiculous. The only safe approach is to let all see the light and to let all be discussed, experimented upon, vindicated or destroyed." It is hopeful that more investigation would help us understand the double helix deeper and better.

Perhaps the publication of this chapter would cause furious argument and refutation, because the subject is just at the center of molecular biology. It is evident that every scientist has his/her own experience and idea on the double helix. Only one thing the author can guarantee is that all his experimental results were reproducible. The author is responsible for every sentence written in this paper.

11. Acknowledgement

The author is grateful to the advice, support and help of Dr. J.C. Wang, H. Bremer, D. Lang, and T. Lance. Thanks to Drs. Z. X. Shen, A. Lazinica and Ms. V. Poffenberger for their careful examining of the manuscript. I am indebted to publishers of Nature and Elsevier for allowing me to cite the figures published in their journals. I owe special thanks to Dr. X.Y. Liu at the Shanghai Institute of Biochemistry and Cell Biology for allowing me working in his laboratory.

12. References

Alberts, et al. (2002) *Molecular biology of the cell*, 5 Th. Edition, Garland science.

Alberts, B. (2010). Is the frontier really endless? *Science*, 330, 1587.

Arnott. S. (2006). Historical article: DNA polymorphism and the early history of the double helix. *Trends Biochem. Sci.* 31, 349-354.

Atomi,H.; Matsumi, R. & Imanaka, T. (2004). Reverse gyrase is not a prerequisite for hyperthermophilic life. *J. Bacteriology*, 186 , 4829-4833.

Bates, A.D. & Maxwell, A. (1989). DNA gyrase can supercoil DNA circles as small as 174 base pairs. *EMBO*, 8, 1861-1866.

Bastos M et al. (2004) Hydration of ds-DNA and ss-DNA by neutron quasielastic scattering. Biophysical Journal 86, 3822-3827

Bensimon, D. et al. (1995). Stretching DNA with a receiding meniscus: Experiments and results. *Phys. Rev. Lett.* 74, 4754-4757.

Berger,J.M. et al. (1996). Structure and mechanism of DNA topoisomerases II. *Nature*.379, 225-232.

Biegeleisen, K. (2002). Topologically non-linked circular duplex DNA. *Bull. Math. Biol.* 64, 589-609.

Blattner et al., (1997). The complete genome sequence of *Escherichia coli* K-12, *Science*, 277, 1453-1562.

Brack, C; Bickle, T.A. & Yuan, B. (1975). The relation of single-stranded regions in bacteriophage PM2 supercoiled DNA to the early melting sequences. *J. Mol. Biol.* 96, 693-702.

Bravo, A.; Serrano-Heras, G. & Salas, M. (2005) Compartmentalization of prokaryotic DNA replication. *FEMS Microbiology Reviews* 29, 25-47.

Chastain, P.D. et al. (2003). Architecture of the replication complex and DNA loops at the fork generated by the bacteriophage T4 proteins. *J. Biol. Chem.* 278, 21276-21285.

Condemine, G. & Smith, C.L. (1990). Transcription regulates oxolinic acid-induced DNA gyrase cleavage at specific sites on the *E.coli* chromosome. *Nucleic acids Res.*18, 7389-7396.

Crick, F.H.C. (1970). Central dogma of molecular biology, *Nature*, 227, 161-163.

Crick, F.H.C. (1988). *What mad pursuit, A personal view of scientific discovery*, New York Basic Books.

Crick, F.H.C; Wang, J.C. & Bauer, W.R. (1979). Is DNA really a double helix? *J. Mol. Biol.* 129, 449-461

Csikszentmihalyi, M. (1996). *Creativity*, Harper Collins publishers.

Cyriax , B, & Gäth R(1978). The conformation of double-stranded DNA. *Naturwissenschaften* 65, 106-108

Dalius, H., Mantell, N.J. & Alberts, B. (1972) Characterization by electron microscopy of the complex formed between T4 bacteriophage gene 32-protein and DNA. *J. Mol. Biol.*, 67, 341-350.

Depew,D.E. & Wang, J.C. (1975) Conformation fluctuations of DNA helix. *Proc. Natl. Acad. Sci. USA*,72, 4275-4279.

Duguet, M. (1993). The helical repeat of DNA at high temperature. *Nucleic Acids Res.* 21, 463-468.

Forterre, P & Elie, C. (1993) Chromosome structure, DNA topoisomerases and DNA polymerases in archaebacteria. In Kates, M. Kushnes, D. & Matheson, A. (Eds) *The biochemistry of archaea.* 26, 325-361. Elsevier Science Publisher.

Ha, S.C. et al., Crystal structure of a junction between B-DNA and Z-DNA reveals two extruded bases. *Nature*,437, 1183-1186.

Kates, M. Kushnes,D. & Matheson, A. (Eds) *The biochemistry of archaea.* 26, 325-361.

Freifelder, D. & Davidson, P.F. (1963). Physicochemical studies on the reaction between formaldehyde and DNA. *Biophysical J.* 3, 49-63.

Freifelder, D. (1983). *Molecular biology.* p.117, Science books International.

Fruton, J.S. and Simmonds, S. (1958) *General Biochemistry*, p.200, Wiley.

Grinell, F. (2011). Book excerpt from Everyday practice of science. *The scientist,* 25, 76-77.

Ha. S.c. et al., (2005). Crystal structure of a junction between B-DNA and Z-DNA reveals two extruded bases. *Nature*,437, 1183-1186.

Horrobin, D.F. (1975). Ideas in biomedical science: reasons for the foundation of Medical Hypotheses. *Medical Hypothesis*, 1, 1-2.

Kashefi, K & Lovley, D.R.(2003). Extending the upper temperature limit for life. *Science* 301, 934.

Kato t. et al. (2009) High resolution structural analysis of a DNA nanostructure by cryoEM. *Nano Lett*, 9, 2747-2750.

Kikuchi, K. (1990) Reverse gyrase and other Archaebacterial topoisomerases. In N.R.Cozzarelli & J.C. Wang (eds) *DNA topology and its biological effects,* Cold spring Harbor Laboratory Press, NY. 285—298.

Lebrun and Lavery (1996). Modelling extreme stretching of DNA. *Nucleic Acids Res.* 24, 2260-2267

Liu, L.F. & Wang, J.C. (1987). Supercoiling of the DNA template during transcription. *Proc. Natl. Acad. Sci. USA*, 84, 7024-7027.

Lockshon, D. & Morris, D.R. (1983). Positively supercoiled DNA is produced by treatment of *Escherichia coli* with DNA gyrase inhibitor. *Nucleic Acids Res.* 11,2999-3017.

McKay, D.B. & Steitz, T.A. (1981). Structure of catabolite gene activator protein at 2.9A resolution suggests binding to left-handed B-DNA. *Nature*, 290, 744-749.

Mirkin, S.M. (2008). Discovery of alternative DNA structure: a heroic decade. (1979—1989). *Front Biosci.* 13, 1064—1071.

Meselson, M. & Stahl, F.W. (1958). The replication of DNA in *Escherichia coli. Proc. Natl. Acad. Sci, U.S.A.*44, 671-.682.

Montagnier, L. et al. (2009). Electromagmetic signals are produced by aqueous nanostructures derived from bacterial DNA sequences. *Interdiscip. Sci. Comput life Sci.*1, 81-90. DOI: 10.1007/s12539-009-0036-7

Olby, R. (2003). Quiet debut for the double helix. *Nature*, 421, 401-405.

Pruss, G.J. (1985). DNA topoisomerase I mutants. Increased heterogeneity inn linking number and other replicon-dependent changes in DNA supercoiling. *J. Mol. Biol.* 185, 51-63.

Sasisekharan V, & Pattahireman N (1978). Some implications of an alternative structure of DNA. *Proc. Natl. Acad. Sci. USA*, 75: 4092-4096

Schvartzman, J.B. & Stasiak, A. (2004). A topological view of the replicon. *EMBO reports*. 5, 256-261.

Skarstad, K; Boye, S & Steen, H.B. (1986). Timing of initiation of chromosome replication in individual *Escherchia coli* cells. *EMBO journal*, 5, 1711-1717.

Stettler,U. H. et al., (1979). Preparation and characterization of DNA V, the duplex DNA resulting from association of complementary circular single-stranded DNA. *店*131, 21-40.

Rhodes, D. & Klug, A. (1980). Helical periodicity of DNA determined by enzyme digestion. *Nature*. 286, 573-578.

Rodley G.A. et al. (1976). A possible conformation for double stranded polynucleotides. *Proc. Natl. Acad. Sci. USA*, 73, 2959-2963

Travers, A. & Muskhelishvili, G. (2007) A common topology for bacterial and eukaryotic transcription initiation? *EMBO reports*, 8, 147151.

Tsao, Y.P; Wu, H.Y. & Liu, L.F. (1989). Transcription-driven supercoiling of DNA: direct biochemical evidence from in vitro studies. *Cell*, 56, 111-118.

Tuteja, N & Tuteja R, (2004) Unraveling DNA helicases. *Eur. J. Biochem.* 271, 1849-1863.

Ullsperger, C & Cozzarelli, N.R. (1996). Contrasting enzymatic activities of topoisomerases IV and gyrase from *Escherichia coli*. *J. Biol. Chem.*, 271, 31549-31555.

Wang, A.H.J. et al., (1979) Molecular structure of a left-handed double helical DNA fragment at atomic resolution., *Nature*, 282, 680-686.

Wang, J.C. (1979). Helical repeat in solution. *Proc. Natl. Acad. Sci, U.S.A.*76, 200-203.

Wang, X. et al. (2010). Double-stranded DNA homology produces a physical signature. *Proc. Natl. Acad. Sci, U.S.A.107*, 12547-12552..

Watson, N. (1988). A new revision of the sequence of plasmid pBR322. *Gene*, 70, 399-403.

Watson, J.D. & Crick, F.H.C. (1953a). A structure for deoxyribose nucleic acids. *Nature*. 171, 737-738.

Watson, J.D. & Crick, F.H.C. (1953b). Genetical implications of the deoxyribonucleic acid. *Nature*. 171, 964-967.

Wu, H.Y. Shyy, S. Wang, J. C. & Liu, L. F. (1988). Transcription generates positively and negatively supercoiled domains in the template. *Cell*, 53, 433-440.

Xu, Y.C.; Li Qian &Tao, Z.J. (1982). A hypothesis of DNA structure.—Inspiration from the topological transformation of supercoiled DNA. *Scientia Sinica*. 25B, 827-836.

Xu, Y.C. & Li Qian (1983). Determination of linking number of pBR322 DNA. *Scientia Sinica*. 26B, 602-613

Xu, Y.C. (2009). Finding of a zero linking number topoisomer. *B.B.A.* 1790, 126-133

Yagil, G. (1991). Paranamic structure of DNA and their in DNA unwinding. *Critical review in Biochem. and Mol. Biol.* 26, 475-559.

Zanchetta, G. et al. (2010). Right-handed double-helix ultreshort DNA yields chiral nematic phases with both right- and left-handed director twist. *Proc. Natl. Acad. Sci, U.S.A.*107, 17492-17502.

Zimmerman, S.B. (2004). Studies on the compaction of isolated nucleoids from *Escherichia coli. J. structural Biol.*147, 145-158

3

Phosphorothioation: An Unusual Post-Replicative Modification on the DNA Backbone

Lianrong Wang[1,2], Shi Chen[1,2] and Zixin Deng[1,2]
[1]*State Key Laboratory of Microbial Metabolism, and School of Life Sciences & Biotechnology, Shanghai Jiaotong University, Shanghai*
[2]*Key Laboratory of Combinatorial Biosynthesis and Drug Discovery, Ministry of Education, and Wuhan University School of Pharmaceutical Sciences, Wuhan*
China

1. Introduction

DNA molecules are polymers composed of basic repeating subunits of deoxyribonucleotides, which consist of the deoxyribose sugar, phosphate groups, and a nitrogenous base. They appear to fulfill all requirements necessary to maintain the genetic function of DNA. The five elements of nitrogen, phosphorus, carbon, hydrogen, and oxygen had been regarded as the canonical composition of DNA until the discovery of phosphorothioation, with a sixth element, sulfur, identified as an additional naturally occurring constituent on the DNA backbone, as a sequence-selective, stereospecific post-replicative modification governed by the *dnd* gene cluster. Unlike any other DNA or RNA modification system, DNA phosphorothioation is the first-described physiological modification of the DNA sugar-phosphate backbone [1].

The physiological phosphorothioate modification is widespread in bacteria and occurs in diverse sequence contexts and frequencies in different bacterial genomes, implying a significant impact on bacteria [2]. Recently, a counterpart phosphorothioate-dependent restriction system capable of protection against the invasion of unmodified foreign DNA was discovered to maintain the genetic stability of the phosphorothioate modified host [3]. Another type IV endonuclease, ScoA3McrA, was found to be capable of specifically recognizing as well as cleaving phosphorothioate modified DNA [4]. Interestingly, the gene *sco4631*, which code for ScoA3McrA, is unable to coexist with the *dnd* gene cluster in the same host, causing immediate cell death [4]. Here we summarize the discovery of this first reported physiological modification on the DNA backbone, and provide insights and perspectives into the biological functions of the phosphorothioate modification in prokaryotic physiology.

2. Discovery of phosphorothioation as an unusual post-replicative modification on the DNA backbone

The study of the physiological DNA phosphorothioation originated from an observation that an unusual DNA modification in *Streptomyces lividans* renders DNA susceptible to *in vitro* Tris-dependent double strand cleavage, resulting in a DNA degradation (Dnd) phenotype during conventional and pulsed-field gel electrophoresis [5]. Zhou *et al.* demonstrated that such a Dnd phenotype was not due to nuclease contamination or improper *in vitro* genetic manipulation, but instead, an unusual DNA modification [5]. The modification sites are not randomly distributed in DNA. For instance, both plasmid pIJ101 and pIJ303 from Dnd^+ *S. lividans* underwent site-specific cleavage during electrophoresis, giving particular fragment profiles [5, 6]. Ray *et al.* then verified that the Dnd phenotype depends on the cleavage activity of an oxidative Tris derivative generated in the electrophoretic buffer adjacent to the anode [7]. In other words, the DNA isolated from *S. lividans* is intact, and the degradation only occurs during electrophoresis in the presence of oxidative Tris. Thiourea can react with the Tris derivative and thus inhibits the DNA scission. Alternatively, non-degradative electrophoresis of the DNA could also be achieved in a different buffer such as Hepes [7]. Based on these observations, it was proposed that the DNA degradation was the consequence of a site-specific modification, which suffered cleavage by oxidative Tris resulting in degradation during electrophoresis [5, 7].

Dyson and Liang *et al.* later revealed that the modification required a conserved consensus sequence, as well as flanking sequences with potential for secondary structure(s) (section 3) [8, 9]. Meanwhile, no Tris-mediated scission was detected in single-stranded plasmid replication intermediates, supporting the post-replicative mechanism. The modifying reagents most probably acted post-replicatively on unmodified double-stranded DNA substrates [8].

The chemical nature of this unusual DNA modification is an intriguing question. Based on the information that two genes involved in this modification are related to sulfur transfer (section 2), Zhou *et al.* were prompted to conduct the ^{35}S labeling experiment. Dnd^+ strains of *S. lividans*, *Streptomyces avermitilis* NRRL8165, and *Pseudomonas fluorescens* Pf0-1 were selected to propagate in media containing $^{35}SO4^{2-}$. Total genomic DNAs were prepared and analyzed on agarose gel followed by Southern blotting. ^{35}S signals were detected in the DNA from three Dnd^+ strains, but not in Dnd^- mutant ZX1 or *Streptomyces coelicolor*. This feeding experiment set up a link between the unusual DNA modification and sulfur [10].

The chemical nature of this unusual DNA modification was eventually found to be a phosphorothioate modification of the DNA backbone by Wang *et al.* In this modification, the non-bridging oxygen of the backbone phosphate group is replaced by sulfur [1]. Sequence specific phosphorothioate $d(G_{PS}A)$ and $d(G_{PS}G)$ were first detected in *E. coli* B7A and *S. lividans*, respectively. The discovery was based on the inability of nuclease P1 to cleave the phosphorothioate bond. Wang *et al.* fed Dnd^+ *E. coli* B7A with L-[^{35}S]-cysteine to label the DNA [1]. Enzymatic hydrolyzed and dephosphorylated nucleosides were resolved by liquid chromatography followed by scintillation counting to locate the ^{35}S containing molecules. Mass spectrometric analysis of the ^{35}S containing molecules revealed characteristic *m/z* of 597 accompanied by 446, 348, 152 and 136 fragments (Figure 1). 152 and 136 are characteristic *m/z* of guanine and adenine in positive mode, respectively. This suggests the presence of a G- and A-containing dinucleotide structure for the *m/z* of 597 molecular ion, with loss of guanine yielding the ion at *m/z* of 446. The 16-mass-unit increase over a canonical dG-dA dinucleotide (*m/z* 581) is the exact mass difference between a sulfur and an oxygen atom. The putative dinucleotide species can survive the enzymatic digestion to single nucleosides, indicating nuclease resistance. These features suggested phosphorothioate-containing species shown in Figure 1. Enzymatic digestion with nuclease P1 followed by dephosphorylation with alkaline phosphatase yields phosphorothioate modified dinucleotides and canonical nucleosides. Wang *et al.* eventually corroborated the phosphorothioate structure in *E. coli* B7A as d($G_{PS}A$) in R_P configuration by using synthetic d($G_{PS}A$) R_P and d($G_{PS}A$) S_P as references [1].

Remarkably, the phosphorothioate modification in *S. lividans* displayed different sequence selectivity as d($G_{PS}G$) R_P. To date, a repertoire of phosphorothioate-containing sequences, including d($C_{PS}C$), d($G_{PS}T$), d($A_{PS}C$), and d($T_{PS}C$), have been discovered in diverse bacterial species [2]. The substitution of sulfur creates a chiral center on the phosphate, resulting in two diastereoisomers, known as the R_P and S_P isomers. However, the physiological phosphorothioate modifications found in bacteria are all in the R_P configuration. DNA phosphorothioation thus represents a sequence-selective and stereo-specific physiological modification of the DNA backbone.

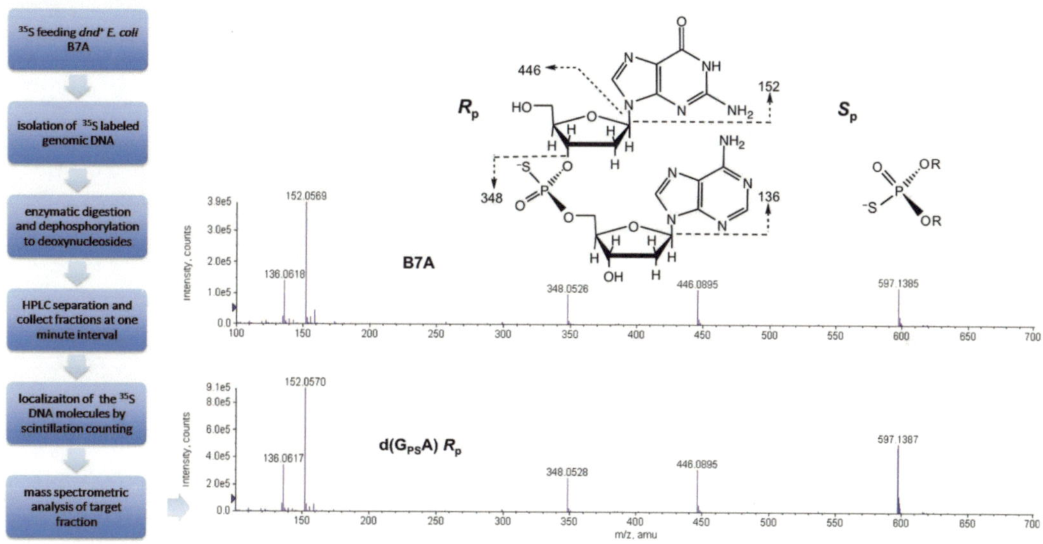

Fig. 1. The flowchart of the localization of phosphorothioate d($G_{PS}A$) R_P and mass spectra of isolated and synthetic d($G_{PS}A$) R_P. The fragmentation of d($G_{PS}A$) R_P is shown in the structural inset, with the [M+H] at *m/z* 597 in positive mode [1].

When phosphorothioate linked d($G_{PS}A$) R_P from *E. coli* B7A was treated with activated Tris buffer *in vitro*, the cleavage of the phosphorothioate bond was detected with the observation of dG and dA, whereas regular d(GA) without phosphorothioate bond remained intact. Therefore, the phosphorothioate modification was verified as the molecular basis for the Dnd phenotype during electrophoresis [1].

3. The *dnd* gene cluster is responsible for phosphorothioation

Evidence for a genetic link responsible for phosphorothioation came from the isolation of a mutant of *S. lividans*, ZX1, obtained by NTG ((*N*-methyl-*N*-nitro-*N*-nitrosoguanidine) mutagenesis [10]. In comparison to the wild-type, ZX1 has a ca. 90 kb chromosomal deletion and loses the Dnd phenotype, suggesting that the endogenous genes related to the unusual DNA modification are located in this 90 kb fragment.

A set of 13 overlapping cosmids covering the 90 kb region deleted in ZX1 but present in the wild-type were constructed and aligned as shown in Figure 2. When transformed into ZX1, cosmid 16C3 (ZX1::16C3) could restore the Dnd phenotype of mutant ZX1, indicating that 16C3 harbored genes associated with the DNA modification. By subsequent sub-cloning and Dnd phenotypic tests, a 6,665 bp *dnd* locus containing five *dnd* genes was precisely localized on cosmid 16C3 [11].

A.

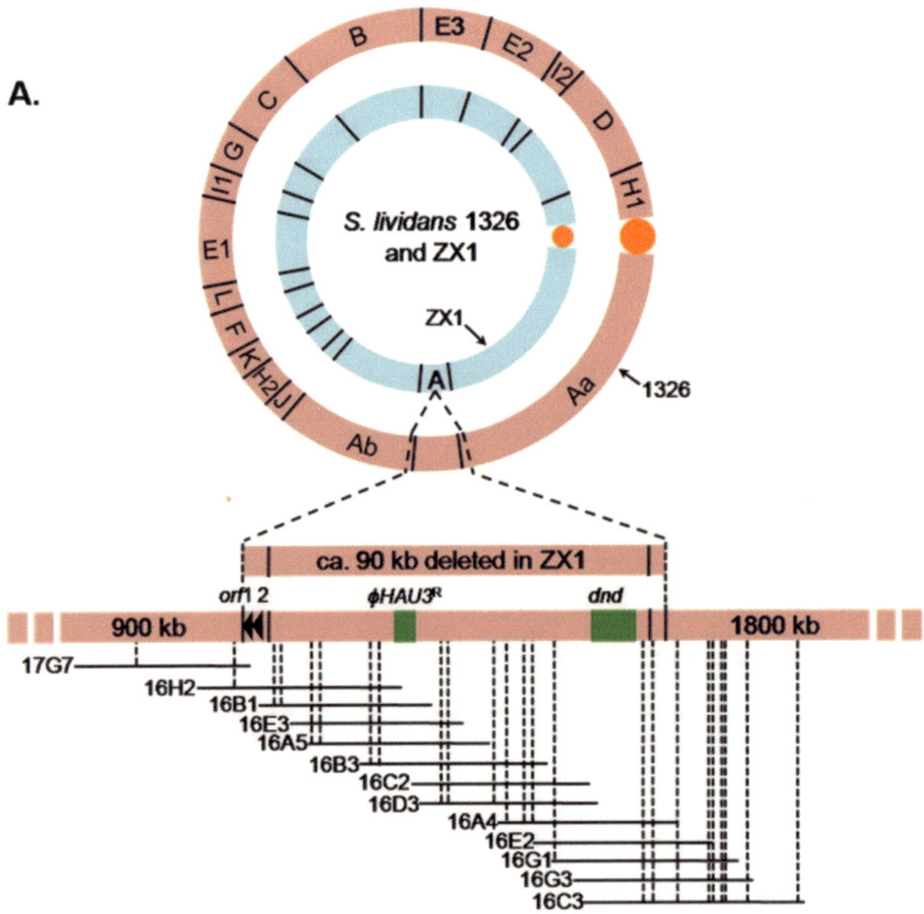

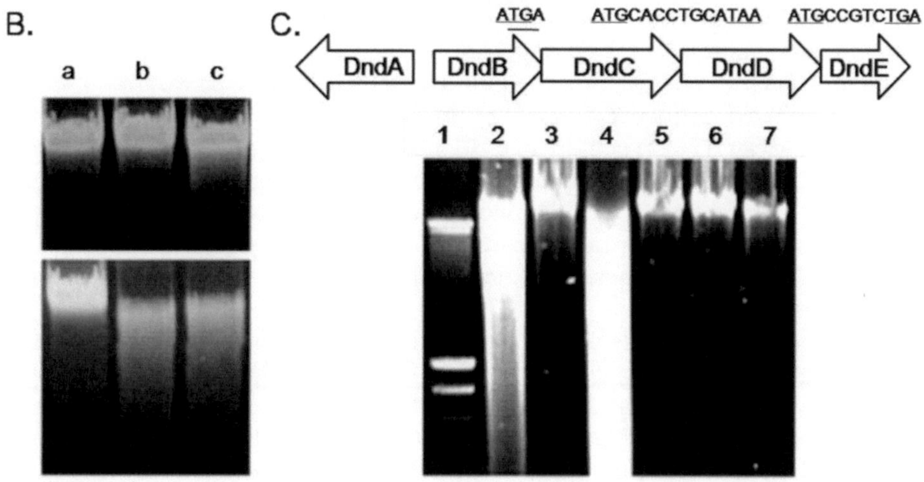

Fig. 2. (A) Physical maps of *S. lividans* 1326 and mutant ZX1. The ca. 90 kb region present in strain 1326 but not in ZX1 is enlarged to show 13 overlapping cosmids [11]. The *dnd* gene cluster and phage ΦHAU3 resistance gene, *ΦHAU3*^{R}, are shown in green boxes. The positions of two genes immediately flanking the left deletion junction, *orf1* (a P4-like integrase) and *orf2* (a putative transposase) are indicated by black triangles. (B) (top) Thiourea in the electrophoresis buffer can inhibit DNA degradation. (bottom) The Dnd phenotype of ZX1 can be complemented by cosmid 16C3 (lane b) but not 17G7(lane a). Wildtype *S. lividans* 1326 (lane c) is used as a positive control [10]. (C) (top) The five genes *dndABCDE* involved in the DNA phosphorothioate modification in *S. lividans* . (bottom) The disruption of *dndA* (lane 3), *dndC* (lane 5), *dndD* (lane 6) and *dndE* (lane 7) can abolish the Dnd phenotype, whereas the mutation of *dndB* (lane 4) aggravates the degradation. Wildtype *S. lividans* 1326 is used as control (lane 2). Lane 1 is a DNA marker [12]. Figure adapted from [11, 12].

The *dnd* gene cluster in *S. lividans* consists of five genes, *dndABCDE*. *dndBCDE* constitute an operon, which is divergently transcribed from the *dndA* gene (Figure 2C) [12]. The individual disruption of *dndA*, *dndC*, *dndD* or *dndE* abolishes phosphorothioation [10, 12]. *dndA* is predicted to encode a protein of 380 amino acids and homologous to cysteine desulfurase of IscS and NifS proteins in *E. coli.* Purified DndA protein is a pyridoxyl 5′-phosphate dependent homodimer and capable of catalyzing L-cysteine to produce elemental S and L-alanine. Cys327 in the C-terminal region of DndA is confirmed to be the active enzymatic center and surrounded by a consensus sequence of ATGSACTS [13]. The mobilized elemental sulfur by DndA could subsequently involve the assembly of a [4Fe-4S] cluster in the DndC protein. DndC possesses ATP pyrophosphatase activity, catalyzing hydrolysis of ATP to AMP and pyrophosphate, and is predicted to have phosphoadenyl sulphate reductase activity [13]. Meanwhile, DndC shares a unique adenylation specific P-loop motif of SGGKDS with SGGFDS in ThiI, an enzyme involved in the formation of 4-thiouridine in tRNAs.

DndD is homologous to the ATP-binding cassette (ABC) ATP-binding proteins and also shares extensive sequence similarity to the Structural Maintenance of Chromosomes (SMC) family of proteins associated with ATPase and DNA nicking activity. In addition, DndD possesses an ATP/GTP-binding Walker A motif (35-GLNGCGKT-42) and an ABC transporter family signature (556-LSAGERQLLAISLLW-570) [10]. Yao *et al.* located an *spfBCDE* gene cluster in Dnd-phenotypic *P. fluorescens* Pf0-1, which has an organization identical to that of *dndBCDE* in *S. lividans* 1326. The *spfBCDE* cluster is essential for the Dnd phenotype in *P. fluorescens* Pf0-1, and the putative SpfBCDE proteins exhibit 51%, 49%, 31% and 39% amino acid sequence homology to DndBCDE, respectively. SpfD, a DndD homolog, possesses an ATPase activity of 6.201 ± 0.695 units/mg and is proposed to provide the energy required in DNA phosphorothioation by hydrolyzing ATP [14].

DndE consists of merely 126 amino acids and shows 46% identity to a phosphoribosylaminoimidazole carboxylase (NCAIR synthetase) from *Anabaena variabilis* ATCC 29413 [10]. NCAIR synthetase is known to act at a condensing carboxylation step in purine biosynthesis [15].

Distinct from the others, the disruption of *dndB* does not abolish the Dnd phenotype, but instead it aggravates DNA degradation (Figure 2C). DndB shows 25% identity and 38% similarity to the ABC transporter ATPase from *Sphingomonas* sp. SKA58, and 26% similarity to a DNA gyrase (GyrB) from *Mycoplasma putrefaciens*. It also shows significant amino acid sequence homology to a group of putative transcriptional regulators. A run of 152 residues is 24% identical and 36% similar to the substrate-binding protein of an ABC transporter of *Streptococcus pneumoniae* TIGE4. In addition, it is noticeable that the predicted DndB is likely to be a basic protein (pI: 8.79) under physiological conditions and would conceivably bind nucleic acids to mediate the modification frequency [9].

In the tRNA sulfur modification system, IscS converts L-cysteine to L-alanine and sulfane sulfur in the form of a cysteine persulfide in its active site. The generated sulfane sulfur is sequentially transferred to ThiI to continue catalyzing the biosynthesis of 4-thiouridine [16]. Assembled by five Dnd proteins, the DNA phosphorothioation system appears to be more complicated than the tRNA sulfur modification system in accomplishing the sequence selective and stereo-specific sulfur substitution.

4. Widespread existence of phosphorothioation in bacteria

Homologous *dnd* clusters are found in phylogenetically diverse bacterial species including *Bacillus, Klebsiella, Enterobacter, Mycobacterium, Pseudomonas, Pseudoalteromonas, Roseobacter, Mesorhizobium, Serratia, Acinetobacter, Clostridium,* as well as certain archaea, etc. [12]. Moreover, *dnd* gene homologues are also detected in oceanic metagenomes, including the Sargasso Sea, Roca Redonda, the gulf of Mexico, etc. [2]. In some cases, *dndA* is not found adjacent to clustered *dndBCDE*. DndA is homologous to IscS, which usually has more than one copy in a genome. Therefore, an iscS homologue could be elsewhere in genomes and the cognate proteins may have served as functional homologues of DndA.

Apart from bacteria with a sequenced *dnd* cluster, a large part of bacteria not previously known to possess *dnd* clusters display the Dnd phenotype during electrophoresis. A survey on 74 actinomycetal strains from ecologically differentiated regions identified 5 Dnd$^+$ strains [17]. Genomic DNAs from 50% of the total of 69 tested *Mycobacterium abscessus* isolates degraded during pulse-field gel electrophoresis [18].

To investigate the phosphorothioate modification in diverse bacteria, Wang *et al.* developed a highly sensitive liquid chromatography-coupled electrospray ionization tandem quadrupole mass spectrometry technique (LC-MS/MS) that identifies phosphorothioate modifications at dinucleotide level [2]. Due to the specific resistance of the phosphorothioate bond (R_P) to nuclease P1, DNA harboring phosphorothioate sites generates nucleosides and phosphorothioate-linked dinucleotides upon digestion by nuclease P1 followed by dephosphorylation. As shown in Figure 3, quantification of phosphorothioate dinucleotides can be achieved using the non-physiological S_P stereoisomer of d(G_{PS}A) as an internal standard. This analytical approach makes it feasible to quantitatively screen all 16 phosphorothioate dinucleotides in DNA samples.

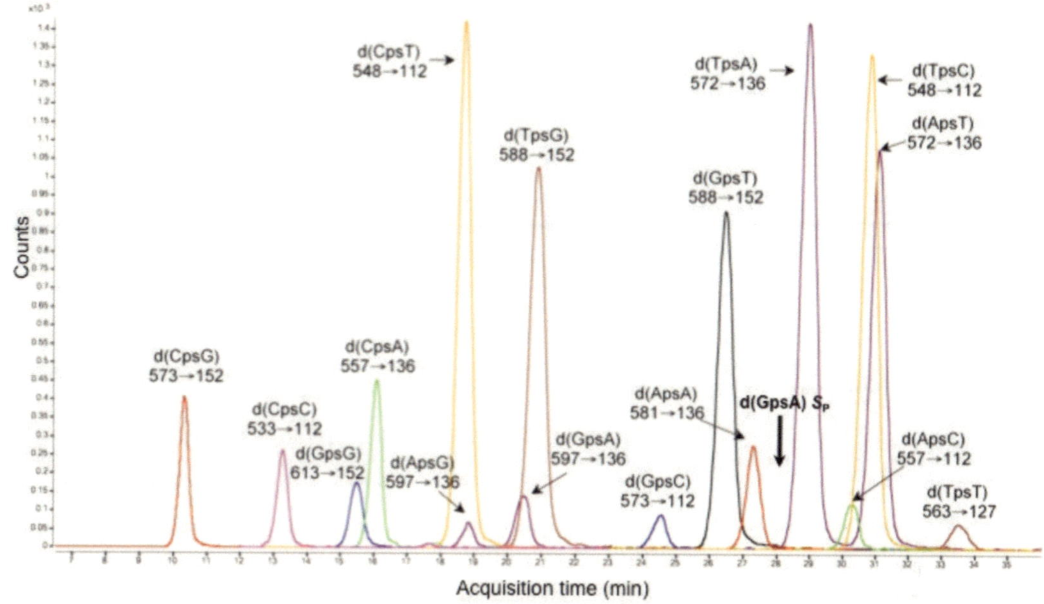

Fig. 3. The LC-MS/MS approach accounting for all 16 phosphorothioate linked dinucleotides in R_P configuration. All of the 16 possible phosphorothioate-linked dinucleotides were resolved by reversed-phase HPLC followed by MS/MS detection in multiple reaction monitoring mode. The ion transitions are labeled under each dinucleotide. Bold arrow indicates the internal standard of d(G_{PS}A) S_P for quantification [2]. Figure adapted from [2].

An extensive study of a collection of bacteria of variable origins and diverse habitats, including marine microbes *Shewanella pealeana* ATCC700345, *Bermanella marisrubri* RED65 and *Hahella chejuensis* KCTC2396, anaerobic *Geobacter uraniumreducens* Rf4, enterotoxigenic *E. coli* B7A and *Salmonella enterica* serovar Cerro 87, and one of the smallest known free-living bacteria *Candidatus* Pelagibacter ubique strain HTCC1002, reveals the common possession of DNA phosphorothioate modifications in these taxonomically unrelated bacterial strains (Table 1). It is conceivable that the *dnd*-associated DNA phosphorothioation is ubiquitous in prokaryotes [2].

The study of representative strains from various habitats, environmental DNA samples and 63 *Vibrio* strains reveals that the phosphorothioate modification occurs in a characteristic manner. In *S. enterica* 87, *E. coli* B7A and *Vibrio* 1F267, the phosphorothioate modification occurs in d(G_{PS}T) and d(G_{PS}A) at the ratio of 1:1. The marine bacteria *B. marisrubri* RED65 and *H. chejuensis* KCTC2396 possess d(G_{PS}A) accompanied by barely detectable d(G_{PS}T). A pair of d(G_{PS}T) and d(G_{PS}G) are simultaneously present in *G. uraniumreducens* Rf4 and *S. lividans* 1326, etc., but at levels that differed by two orders of magnitude. Three phosphorothioate contexts of d(C_{PS}C), d(A_{PS}C) and d(T_{PS}C) occur in *Vibrio* 1C-10, ZF264,

ZF29 and FF75, while the level of total phosphorothioation is almost 10 fold higher than that in other strains (Table 1) [2].

Bacterial strain	Total phosphorothioate (per 10^6 nt)	Phosphorothioate contexts (R_P)	Ratio	Putative 4 bp core sequence
E. coli B7A	768 ± 27	d(G$_{PS}$A), d(G$_{PS}$T)	1:1	5′-G$_{PS}$AAC-3′ 3′-CTT$_{PS}$G-5′
S. enterica 87	732 ± 20			
Vibrio 1F267	576 ± 34			
DH10B(pJTU1980)	1078 ± 109			
DH10B(pJTU1238)	1505 ± 103			
P. fluorescens Pf0-1	451 ± 9	d(G$_{PS}$G)	-	5′-G$_{PS}$GCC-3′ 3′-CCG$_{PS}$G-5′
S. lividans 1326	474 ± 39	d(G$_{PS}$G), d(G$_{PS}$T)	221:1	5′-G$_{PS}$GCC-3′ 3′-CCG$_{PS}$G-5′
G. uraniumreducens Rf4	520 ± 13		181:1	
Vibrio ZS139	581 ± 19		26:1	
Vibrio 1F230	400 ± 5		126:1	
B. marisrubri RED65	440 ± 23	d(G$_{PS}$A), d(G$_{PS}$T)	165:1	5′-G$_{PS}$ATC-3′ 3′-CTA$_{PS}$G-5′
H. chejuensis KCTC2396	286 ± 9		-	
S. pealeana ATCC700345	489 ± 11	d(G$_{PS}$A), d(G$_{PS}$T)	2:1	5′-G$_{PS}$AAC-3′ 3′-CTT$_{PS}$G-5′ or 5′-G$_{PS}$ATC-3′ 3′-CTA$_{PS}$G-5′
Virbrio 1C-10	3110 ± 71	d(C$_{PS}$C), d(A$_{PS}$C), d(T$_{PS}$C)	-	5′-C$_{PS}$CGG-3′ 3′-GGC$_{PS}$C-5′ or 5′-G$_{PS}$GCC-3′ 3′-CCG$_{PS}$G-5′
Virbrio ZF264	2270 ± 19			
Virbrio ZF29	2242 ± 57			
Virbrio FF75	2626 ± 22			

d(G$_{PS}$G) is the only phosphorothioate modification detected in *P. fluorescens* Pf0-1; dash indicates that the low frequency of d(G$_{PS}$T) in *H. chejuensis* KCTC2396, as well as of d(A$_{PS}$C) and d(T$_{PS}$C) in *Vibrio* 1C-10, ZF264, ZF29 and FF75 are far less than the major d(G$_{PS}$A) and d(C$_{PS}$C), respectively.

Table 1. Characteristic phosphorothioate modifications in diverse bacterial strains [2].

Wang *et al.* also analyzed the phosphorothioate modification in the environmental seawater from the Sargasso Sea and Oregon coast, leading to the discovery of phosphorothioate modifications of d(G_{PS}A), d(G_{PS}T), d(G_{PS}G) and d(C_{PS}C) in these metagenomes [2]. The Sargasso Sea is a low nutrient, low productivity, subtropical ocean gyre [19]. The oceanic water DNA samples represent microbial communities, including uncultured microbes. Interestingly, phosphorothioates d(C_{PS}C) and d(G_{PS}A) were found throughout the water columns off the Oregon coast (5–40 m) and in the Sargasso Sea (0–200 m), while d(G_{PS}G) was found only in deeper zones of the water column in both locations. More phosphorothioate sequence contexts and frequencies might be explored in the future.

5. Recognition sequences of the phosphorothioate modification

Authentic phosphorothioate modification in *S. lividans* requires not only a conserved consensus sequence but also a considerable flanking sequence with the potential to form secondary structures [8]. The investigations by two laboratories have demonstrated that phosphorothioate site selection requires recognition sequences. Dyson *et al.* and Liang *et al.* performed primer extension and cloning assays on the basis of Tris mediated DNA breakage, respectively, to localize the modification sites in *S. lividans*. At that time, the modification sites were proposed to be on closely opposed guanines on either strand of a stringently conserved 4 bp panlindromic core sequence of 5'-GGCC-3' in a region of 5'-c-cGGCCgccg-3' [8, 9]. It is clear now that the modification sites are actually phosphorothioation between two guanosines on both strands in *S. lividans*. Moreover, both groups confirmed that the phosphorothioate modification in *S. lividans* required a substantial portion of DNA sequences containing three 13 bp direct repeats. The central repeat contains the core sequence, while the left-hand and right-hand copies overlap two potential stem–loop structures (Figure 4). Deletion of either the left or right-hand repeat structures abolishes or alters modification within the core sequence [8].

Quantitative characterization of phosphorothioation in bacterial genomes provides an alternative way to predict the 4 bp core sequence for modification (Table 1). The predominant d(G_{PS}G) in *P. fluorescens* Pf0-1, *G. uraniumreducens* Rf4, *Vibrio* ZS139 and *Vibrio* 1F230 suggests a conserved palindromic 5'-G_{PS}GCC-3' core sequence as it does in *S. lividans*. The 1:1 ratio of d(G_{PS}A) and d(G_{PS}T) in *E. coli* B7A, *S. enterica* 87 and *Vibrio* 1F267 suggests the asymmetric complementary 5'-G_{PS}AAC-3' and 5'-G_{PS}TTC-3' core sequence. d(G_{PS}A) is the major phosphorothioation in *B. marisrubri* RED65 and *H. chejuensis* KCTC2396, indicating the 5'-G_{PS}ATC-3' core sequence.

The quantification shows that the d(G_{PS}G) modification of *S. lividans* occurs at the frequency of 474 ± 39 every 10^6 nt, whereas there are 1.1×10^5 d(GG) available on the chromosome (the genomic sequence of *S. lividans* is not available and the statistical calculation of d(GG) is based on *S. coelicolor*) [2]. Further statistical analysis revealed that even 4 nt 5'-GGCC-3' sequences still occur at too high frequency to serve as the consensus sequence. A 6 nt 5'-cGGCCg-3' with 2 bp extension, however, is more consistent with the phosphorothioate frequency on chromosomes. *E. coli* B7A, *P. fluorescens* Pf0-1, *Vibrio* ZS139 and *B. marisrubri* RED65, etc., have phosphorothioate frequencies close to that of *S. lividans*, indicating the consensus sequence in these bacteria is longer than the proposed 4 bp [2, 8].

Another pattern of phosphorothioate modification is represented by d(C_{PS}C) in *Vibrio* 1C-10, ZF264, ZF29 and FF75. It leads to the proposal of 5'-C_{PS}CGG-3' or 5'-G_{PS}GCC-3' as core sequences. The frequency in genomic DNA, 1 site per 333-500 nt, agrees well with a 4 bp consensus sequence which has the theoretical frequency of once every 256 bp (4^4). Thus, the four *Vibrio* strains might have recognition mechanisms that are distinct from the former group [2, 8].

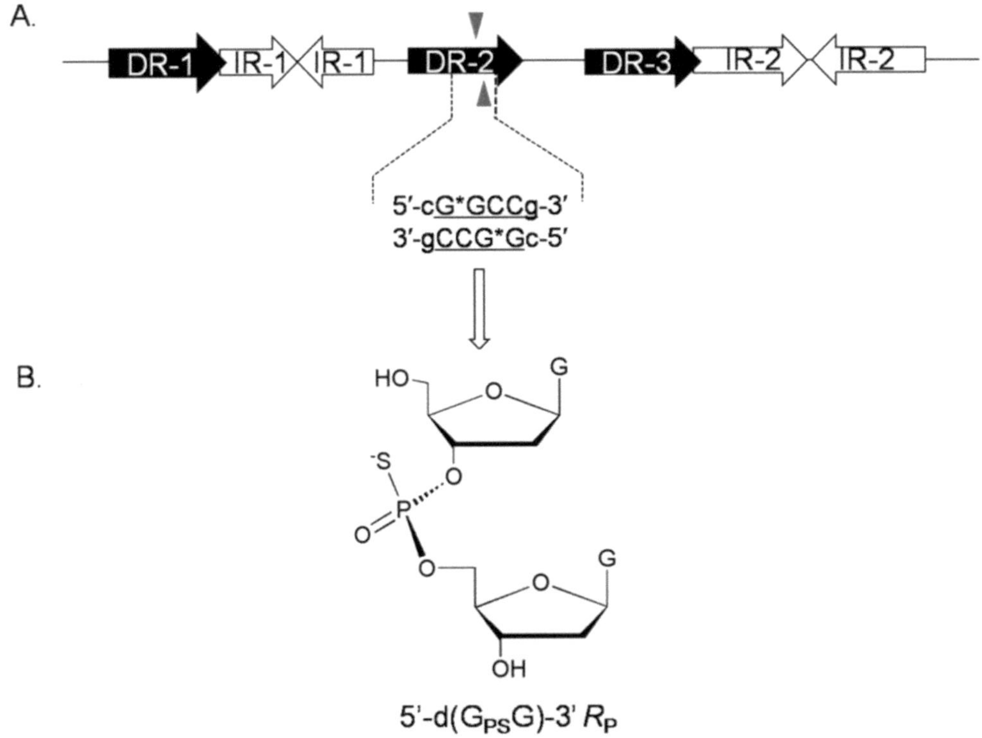

Fig. 4. (A) DNA phosphorothioate modification occurs within a highly conserved 4 bp core sequence, 5'-G_{PS}GCC-3' in *S. lividans*. In plasmid pIJ101, the modification sequence lies in the middle (DR-2) of the three direct repeats (DR1–3). The two inverted repeats (IR-1 and IR-2), overlapping direct repeat sequences of DR-1 and DR-3, have the potential to form stem-loop structures. (B) The chemical structure of d(G_{PS}G) R_P in *S. lividans* [9, 20]. Figure adapted from [20].

Apart from d(C_{PS}C), phosphorothioate modified d(A_{PS}C) and d(T_{PS}C) co-occur in the four *Vibrio* strains at low frequencies of 1-6 per 10^6 nt (Table 1). A similar situation holds for *S. lividans*, *G. uraniumreducens* Rf4 and *B. marisrubri* RED65, etc., in which low levels of d(G_{PS}T) are detected. To explain the low phosphorothioate frequencies, the *dnd* cluster from *S. enterica* 87 was inserted to a low- and high-copy vector of pACYC184 and pBluescript SK+, respectively, generating pJTU1980 and pJTU1238. Both plasmids still confer host *E. coli* DH10B with d(G_{PS}T) and d(G_{PS}A) modifications in a close 1:1 ratio. Moreover, the total phosphorothioate frequencies on chromosomes of DH10B(pJTU1980) and DH10B (pJTU1238) increased 1.5- and 2-fold in comparison to that of the original host *S. enterica* 87. Remarkably, three more phosphorothioate modifications of d(C_{PS}A), d(T_{PS}A), and d(A_{PS}A) at low levels appeared due to the increased expression of the *dnd* cluster. The low-frequency phosphorothioate modifications might result from relaxed DNA target recognition by Dnd proteins [2].

6. Phosphorothioation dependent restriction-modification system

After unveiling the chemical nature of the DNA phosphorothioate modification, an immediate question is what role this novel post-replicative DNA backbone modification plays. In bacteria, site-specific DNA modifications are often, but not always, associated with a sequence-specific endonuclease. The endonuclease is capable of making subtle distinctions between DNA molecules to prevent the invasion of foreign DNA from phage and plasmids that lack the specific DNA modification. For example, DNA methylation has been regarded as the classic restriction modification system. Because of the known resistance of phosphorothioate linkages to a variety of nuclease activities, as well as the post-replicative and site-specific nature of the modification, phosphorothioation of DNA could possibly function as a type of host defense mechanism, akin to restriction and modification systems [1].

Soon after the chemical nature of the Dnd modification was addressed, the *dnd* cluster was found to constitute a host-specific phosphorothioation-restriction system along with an adjacent *dptFGH* cluster in *S. enterica* 87 [3]. A 15 kb DNA fragment from *S. enterica* 87 conferred both host-specific phosphorothioation (*dptBCDE*) and restriction (d*ptFGH*) in *E. coli*. The two clusters are divergently transcribed. In addition to four phosphorothioation-related genes, three genes are responsible for restriction activity in this DNA fragment, confirmed by gene deletion experiments. With at least 7 genes, phosphorothioation-restriction components seem to form a large complex. The *dptFGH* restricts the invasion of non-phosphorothioate-modified pUC18 but not pUC18 with phosphorothioation. When transformed by pUC18 plasmid, *S. enterica* 87 reproducibly yielded about 100 times fewer colonies with non-phosphorothioate pUC18 than with phosphorothioate pUC18. Plasmids from *E. coli* that had escaped restriction were no longer restricted in *S. enterica* 87 [3]. This observation is similar to the phenomenon leading to the discovery of restriction and modification systems in 1950s [21]. Interestingly, once the modification cluster *dptBCDE* is disrupted, *dptFGH* loses the restriction function. The restriction genes *dptFGH* require the phosphorothioation genes *dptBCDE* to confer the restriction activity of *S. enterica* 87 to ensure that the attack on invasive DNA occurs only when the host DNA is already protected by phosphorothioation [3].

On the basis of subunit composition, sequence recognition and cofactor requirement, the DNA phosphorothioate modification is close to Type I restriction modification systems but far more complicated. Homologous phosphorothioation-restriction genes were identified in 19 diverse bacteria strains (Figure 5), including phosphorothioate tested *E. coli* B7A, *S. pealeana* ATCC700345, *B. marisrubri* RED65, *H. chejuensis* KCTC2396, as well as *E. cereus* E33L, *Vibrio cholera* MZO-2, etc. *E. coli* B7A was confirmed to possess a similar phosphorothioation-restriction system by transformation experiments. Plasmids from *dnd*⁻ XTG102 transformed *E. coli* B7A with 100-fold lower efficiency than phosphorothioate modified plasmid DNA from wild-type *S. enterica* 87. However, which restriction genes are responsible for DNA cleavage site selection and DNA sequence specificity is not clear. Many bacteria possess only the homologous *dnd* cluster without simultaneous *dptFGH* across their genomes, suggesting that the phosphorothioate modification may act not only as a sort of protective system against infection by bacteriophages, but also as an epigenetic signal for new biological function(s) that need to be explored [3].

The quantification of phosphorothioation is also supportive for a restriction-modification system. Analysis of the quantitative data revealed that the levels of phosphorothioation were classified into three distinct levels: 2-3 per 10^3 nt, 3-8 per 10^4 nt, and 1-6 per 10^6 nt [2]. Along with defined sequence contexts, the first two frequency ranges are consistent with a restriction-modification system with a 4-nt or 5-6 nt consensus sequence, respectively [22].

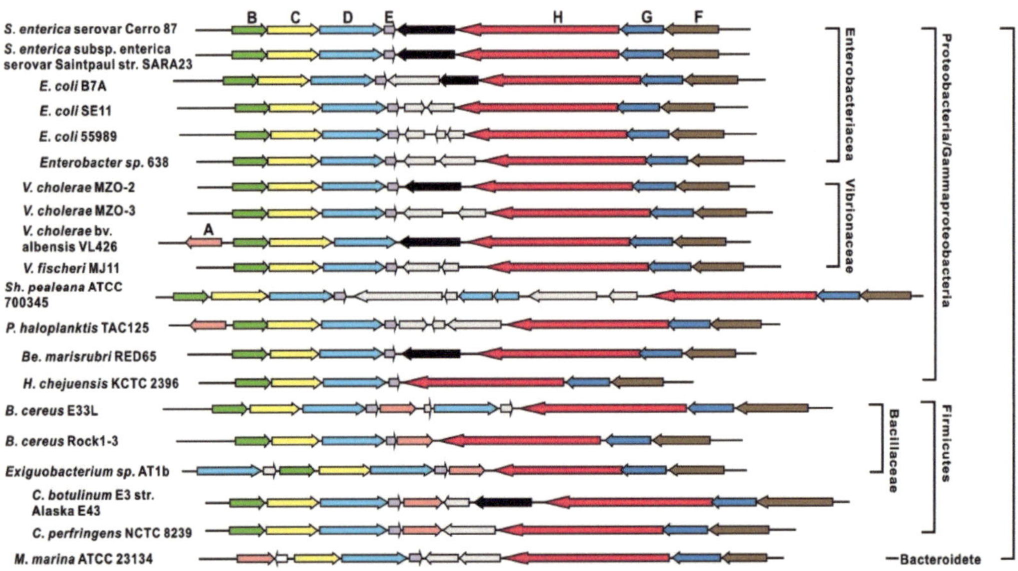

Fig. 5. Alignment of phosphorothioate modification (*dptABCDE*) and restriction (*dptFGH*) gene clusters from 20 bacterial strains. Colored arrows indicate homologous ORFs. Light gray arrows represent diverse ORFs without predicted functions that are not homologous to each other [3]. Figure adapted from [3].

7. Cleavage of phosphorothioate DNA by type IV restriction endonuclease ScoMcrA

When the bi-functional plasmid pIJ699 was isolated from *S. lividans* and *E. coli*, only pIJ699 from *S. lividans* degraded during electrophoresis, indicating that the Dnd phenotype selectively occurred in certain bacteria [2]. This is consistent with the observation that *dnd* is not present in *S. coelicolor* but is in *S. lividans*, although chromosomes of the two strains share an almost identical DNA banding pattern upon enzymatic digestion [5, 6]. Most of the *S. coelicolor* and *S. lividans* DNA sequenced is similar or even identical. Interestingly, a type IV restriction endonuclease (ScoA3McrA) coded by gene *sco4631* in *S. coelicolor* cuts foreign DNA containing phosphorothioates. The search for a phosphorothioate-cutting enzyme in *S. coelicolor* originated from the restriction to the *dnd* gene cluster. Liu *et al.* tried to introduce the *dnd* gene cluster from *S. lividans* into its close relative *S. coelicolor*. However, they unexpectedly failed, while the same gene cluster with a single base insertion for a frame-shift mutation in *dndE* gene generated exoconjugants [4]. This implied restriction towards phosphorothioate modification by *S. coelicolor*.

Comparison between the genome sequence of *S. coelicolor* and the *dnd*+ of *S. avermitilis*, revealed an endonuclease ScoA3McrA in *S. coelicolor* that is absent in *S. avermitilis*. *S. coelicolor* lost its restriction to the *dnd* gene cluster after disruption of ScoA3McrA. After integration of a vector containing ScoA3McrA into the genome, a *dnd* mutant *S. lividans* HXY6 confers restriction toward the *dnd* gene cluster. These knock-out and knock-in experiments confirmed the role of ScoA3McrA as the determinant of restriction of phosphorothioate in *S. coelicolor.* Moreover, *in vitro* in presence of Mn^{2+} and Co^{2+}, the purified ScoA3McrA protein cleaved *in vivo* phosphorothioated DNA as well as a synthesized 118 bp double strand DNA oligonucleotide bearing one phosphorothioate on each strand. ScoA3McrA specifically cleaves both the top and the bottom strand, and on both sides of the S-modification at multiple cleavage sites 16-28 nt away from the phosphorothioate sites. Liu *et al.* proposed that expression of the *dndA-E* gene cluster in *S. coelicolor* resulted in phosphorothioation of the host DNA. ScoA3McrA would then cleave the phosphorothioated host DNA near the modified sites and result in cell death as a cell suicide process. Purified ScoMcrA also cleaved Dcm-methylated DNA or Dcm-containing oligos 12-16 bp away from a C5mCWGG Dcm methylation site [4]. ScoA3McrA thus builds an interesting link between phosphorothioation and methylation.

8. Phylogenetic relationship and evolutionary path of *dnd* genes

The phylogeny of Dnd from 12 bacteria shows strong correlation between phosphorothioate modifications and four Dnd proteins (Figure 6). With the exception of *Candidatus* Pelagibacter ubique, the other 11 strains are well classified based on DNA phosphorothioate sequence contexts and frequencies. Results suggest the diversification of DNA phosphorothioate modifications depends on Dnd protein sequence but not on the phylogenetic descent of the bacteria strains. Furthermore, using phylogenetic analysis based on Dnd proteins and 16S rRNA, Wang *et al.* found the Dnd phylogenies do not follow their corresponding species tree. This is clearly seen in three *Vibrio* isolates (ZS139, 1F230, and 1F267) which are phylogenetically incoherent in all four DndBCDE proteins. The phylogenetic differentiation of the *Vibrio* isolates suggests horizontal gene transfer of *dnd* clusters facilitated by genomic islands in evolution [2, 17].

Sequence analysis reveals that the ca. 90 kb fragment containing the *dnd* cluster in *S. lividans* is indeed a genomic island with precise length of 92,770 bp [17]. The G+C content of the genomic island is 67.8%, lower than the average for *S. coelicolor* of 72.1%, indicating the *dnd* system may have originated from elsewhere. Genomic islands are discrete DNA segments, which differ among closely related strains. It explains why the *dnd* cluster occurs in *S. lividans* and *S. avermitilis*, but not in *S. coelicolor*, a close relative of *S. lividans* even at genomic sequence level. Genomic islands play a role in the evolution, diversification and adaption of microbes as they are involved in the dissemination of variable genes, including antibiotic resistance and virulence genes, as well as catabolic genes [23].

Active genomic island transfer has been reported in some cases. For instance, the PAPI-1 pathogenicity island in *P. aeruginosa* was shown to transfer from a donor strain into *P. aeruginosa* strains [24]. ICE*Hin1056*, an integrative and conjugative element from *Haemophilus influenzae*, proceeds conjugative transfer between two *H. influenzae* strains. Moreover, ICE*clc* of *Pseudomonas* sp. strain B13 can self-transfer to *P. putida*, *Cupriviadus necator* or *P. aeruginosa* at similar frequencies [25]. He *et al.* demonstrated that the 93 kb genomic island in *S. lividans* was capable of spontaneous excision from the chromosome at a level of 0.016%-0.027%. However, exposure to MNNG (*N*-methyL-*N'*-nitro-*N*-nitrosoguanidine) can increase the excision frequency by at least five fold. The excised island loses its capabilities of inter and even intra-species transmission between *Streptomyces* strains. This genomic island may have lost genes required for its transfer during evolution in order to maintain a relatively stable inheritance with the host [17].

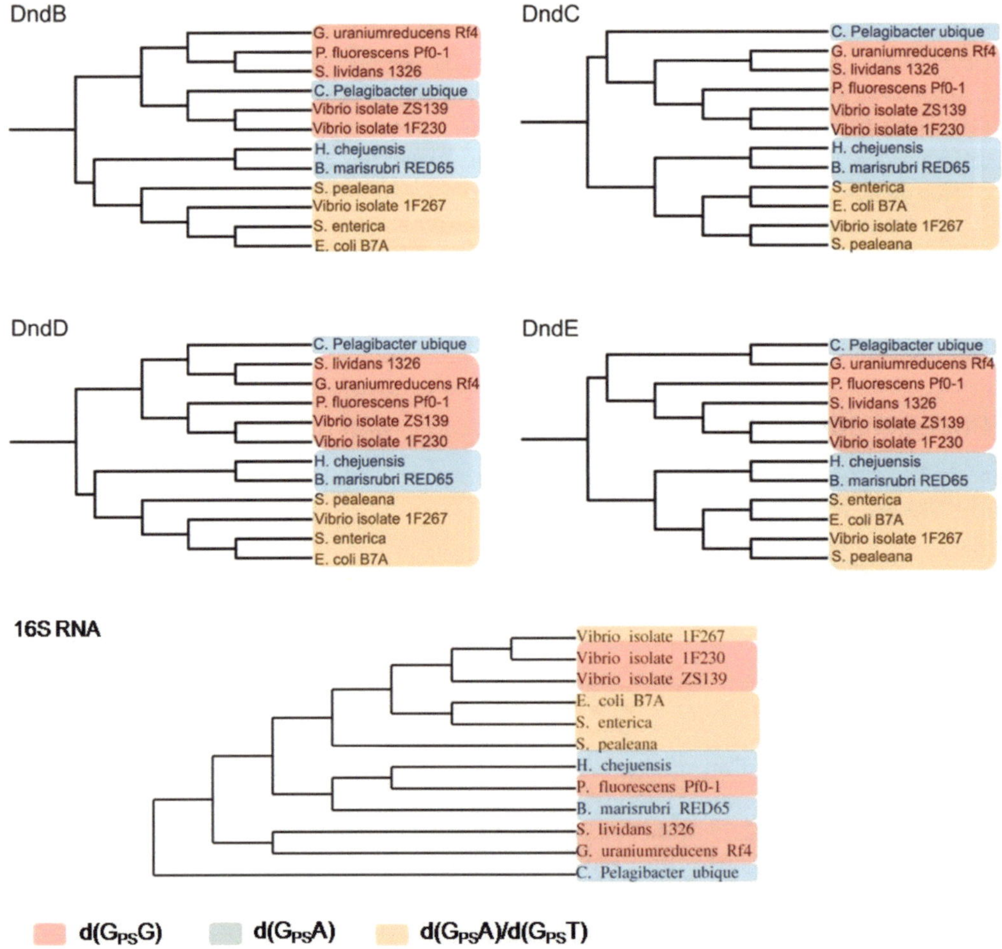

Fig. 6. Correlation between DNA phosphorothioate sequence contexts and Dnd proteins. DNA phopshorothioate modification follows the Dnd protein phylogenies but not species phylogenies (16S RNA tree), supporting horizontal rather than vertical gene transfer for *dnd* genes [2].

Besides *S. lividans*, 11 additional *dnd*$^+$ bacteria were analyzed by He *et al.* Remarkably, all *dnd* clusters lie on mobile genetic elements based on the characteristic features of G+C content, dinucleotide bias, direct repeats, and possession of intergrase and/or transposase (Figure 7). Ten of them lie within chromosomal genomic islands and one on a large plasmid. This indicates the dissemination of *dnd* genes in evolution and explains the ubiquitous occurrence of *dnd* clusters in taxonomically unrelated bacteria. It is still unclear how the *dnd* clusters evolved and disseminated across different bacterial species. He *et al.* suggested that the *dnd* cluster might be organized into a functional locus on a conjugative plasmid or other mobile element in very ancient times followed by extensive dissemination and diversification over the eons [17].

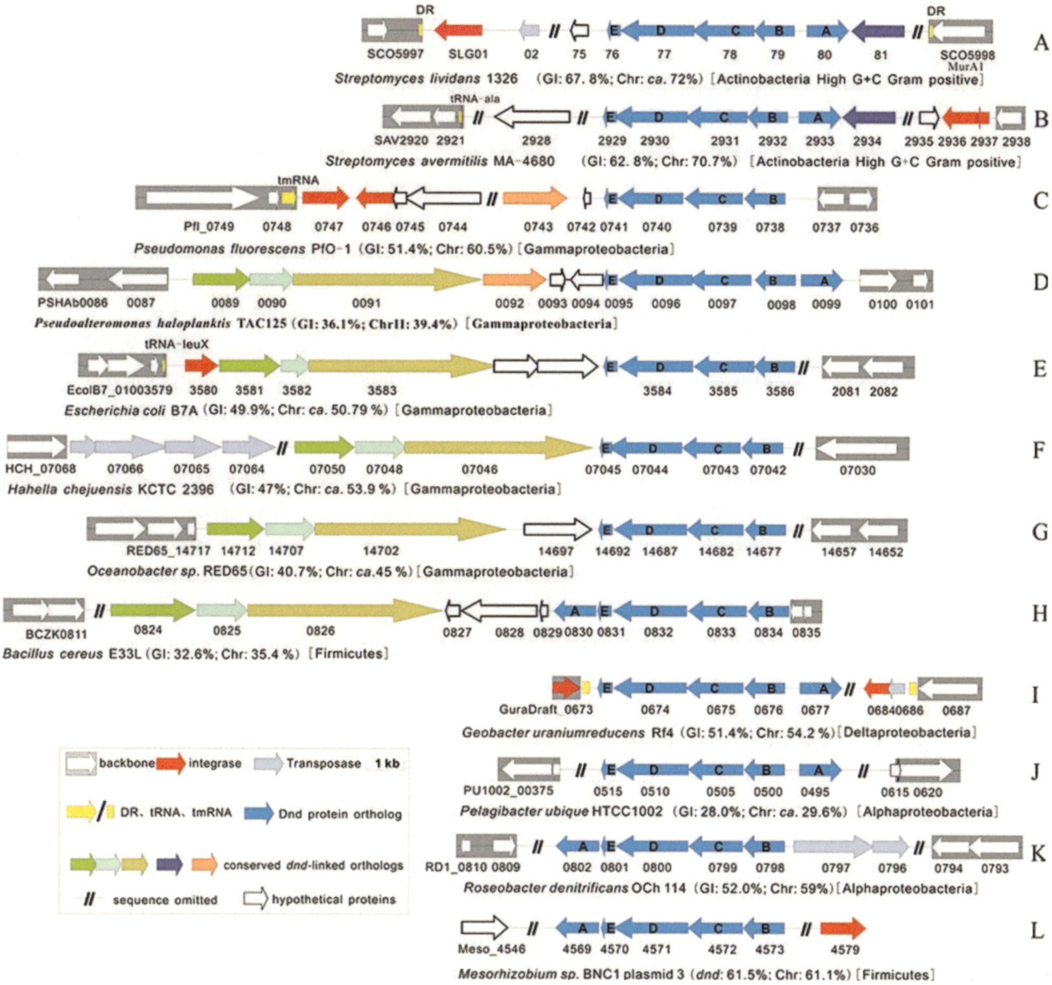

Fig. 7. Twelve *dnd* gene clusters on mobile elements. Blue arrows represent the *dnd* gene homologues. The characteristic elements of genomic islands, including integrase, transposase, direct repeats, insertion hotspots of tRNA, tmRNA sites are shown in red, purple and yellow colors [17]. Figure adapted from [17].

Ou *et al.* organized available data from experimental and bioinformatics analysis of the DNA phosphorothioation to assemble a *dndDB* database [26]. It contains detailed phosphorothioation-related information including the Dnd phenotype, *dnd* gene clusters, genomic islands harboring *dnd* genes, and Dnd proteins and conserved domains. The *dndDB* database provides a useful tool to effectively combine and interlink the genetics, biochemistry and functional aspects of *dnd* systems and related genomic islands.

9. Discussion

Chemically synthesized phosphorothioate internucleotide bonds had been in use for decades prior to the discovery of the physiological phosphorothioate modification in bacteria. Enzymes like snake venom phosphodiesterase, nuclease S1 and nuclease P1 recognize R_P and S_P phosphorothioate isomers differently, hydrolyzing one isomer more efficiently than the other. Therefore, phosphorothioate isomers have been utilized widely to elucidate the stereochemical action of different enzymes [27]. Other nucleases such as DNase I, DNase II, staphylococcal nuclease and spleen phosphodiesterase are unable to hydrolyse the internucleotidic linkage of either phosphorothioate diastereomer [28]. The significantly increased resistance of phosphorothioate linkage to nuclease hydrolysis inspired the extensive application of phosphorothioate oligonucleotide analogues in antisense therapy to treat a broad range of diseases, including viral infections, cancer and inflammatory diseases. It has been more than a decade since the approval of the first antisense drug Vitravene in 1998 by the FDA. The synthetic 21-mer oligonucleotide with phosphorothioate linkage is used in the treatment of cytomegalovirus retinitis (CMV) in immunocompromised patients, including those with AIDS [29].

Phosphorothioates can be introduced into oligonucleotides and DNA by both chemical synthesis and enzymatic polymerization. Currently, phosphorothioate-modified oligonucleotides are available via the oxathiaphospholane method, in which nucleoside 3′-*O*-(2-thio-1,3,2-oxathiaphospholane) derivatives are used as monomers. This method generates a racemic mixture of R_P and S_P stereoisomers at a close 1:1 ratio. The access to stereospecific phosphorothioate bearing oligonucleotides is still severely limited despite the considerable efforts that have been made [30]. Interestingly, the S_P diastereomer of dNTPαS can be accepted as a substrate by *E. coli* DNA polymerase I, and may be employed in polymerization reactions to produce phosphorothioate linkages of the R_P configuration [31]. This is consistent with the physiological configuration of phosphorothioation. However, the phosphorothioate modification modified by the *dnd* genes is post-replicative, requiring conserved core sequences and flanking sequences.

The desulfurization of phosphorothioate to a phosphate bond is an easy process. However, the reverse phosphorothioation is thought to be energetically uphill. It agrees well with the observed role of DndD which acts as an ATPase. Friz Eckstein proposed that the phosphorothioate modification might first require the activation of target phosphodiester bonds by alkylation, acylation, adenylation or phosphorylation followed by the successive substitution by a nucleophilic sulfur [32]. It is still unclear how the five Dnd proteins cooperate together to use L-cysteine and $SO4^{2-}$ as sulfur sources and transfer the sulfur to the DNA backbone sequence selectively and R_P specifically. Although the biochemical activity of several Dnd proteins has been assayed, additional insights are still needed to elucidate the role of each Dnd protein in the DNA phosphorothioation pathway and the interaction between Dnd proteins and target DNA regions. The *dnd* gene cluster is widespread in diverse and distantly related bacteria, however, a complete set of *dnd* homologs has not yet been found in eukaryotes.

Most of the commonly found structural changes in DNA are due to methylation of particular bases. In some viral DNAs, certain bases may be hydroxymethylated or glucosylated [33-35]. DNA phosphorothioation apparently is an unprecedented physiological modification, which renders DNA susceptible to Tris derivative leading to the characteristic Dnd phenotype.

It is such a surprise to find out that nature can synthesize a phosphorothioate-containing DNA backbone using the *dndABCDE* genes. Particularly, it is interesting that the modification occurs in a sequence-selective and stereo-specific manner. The discovery of physiological DNA phosphorothioation has revolutionized our view of the composition and structure of DNA, opening a new window that will stimulate research into novel aspects of DNA.

10. References

[1] Wang, L., et al., *Phosphorothioation of DNA in bacteria by dnd genes.* Nat Chem Biol, 2007. 3(11): p. 709-10.

[2] Wang, L., et al., *DNA phosphorothioation is widespread and quantized in bacterial genomes.* Proc Natl Acad Sci U S A. 108(7): p. 2963-8.

[3] Xu, T., et al., *A novel host-specific restriction system associated with DNA backbone S-modification in Salmonella.* Nucleic Acids Res. 38(20): p. 7133-41.

[4] Liu, G., et al., *Cleavage of phosphorothioated DNA and methylated DNA by the type IV restriction endonuclease ScoMcrA.* PLoS Genet. 6(12): p. e1001253.

[5] Zhou, X., et al., *Site-specific degradation of Streptomyces lividans DNA during electrophoresis in buffers contaminated with ferrous iron.* Nucleic Acids Res, 1988. 16(10): p. 4341-52.

[6] Evans, M., et al., *Characterization of a Streptomyces-lividans-type site-specific DNA modification system in the avermectin-producer Streptomyces avermitilis permits investigation of two novel giant linear plasmids, pSA1 and pSA2.* Microbiology, 1994. 140 (Pt 6): p. 1367-71.

[7] Ray, T., A. Mills, and P. Dyson, *Tris-dependent oxidative DNA strand scission during electrophoresis.* Electrophoresis, 1995. 16(6): p. 888-94.

[8] Dyson, P. and M. Evans, *Novel post-replicative DNA modification in Streptomyces: analysis of the preferred modification site of plasmid pIJ101.* Nucleic Acids Res, 1998. 26(5): p. 1248-53.

[9] Liang, J., et al., *DNA modification by sulfur: analysis of the sequence recognition specificity surrounding the modification sites.* Nucleic Acids Res, 2007. 35(9): p. 2944-54.

[10] Zhou, X., et al., *A novel DNA modification by sulphur.* Mol Microbiol, 2005. 57(5): p. 1428-38.

[11] Zhou, X., et al., *Streptomyces coelicolor A3(2) lacks a genomic island present in the chromosome of Streptomyces lividans 66.* Appl Environ Microbiol, 2004. 70(12): p. 7110-8.

[12] Xu, T., et al., *DNA phosphorothioation in Streptomyces lividans: mutational analysis of the dnd locus.* BMC Microbiol, 2009. 9: p. 41.

[13] You, D., et al., *A novel DNA modification by sulfur: DndA is a NifS-like cysteine desulfurase capable of assembling DndC as an iron-sulfur cluster protein in Streptomyces lividans.* Biochemistry, 2007. 46(20): p. 6126-33.

[14] Yao, F., et al., *Functional analysis of spfD gene involved in DNA phosphorothioation in Pseudomonas fluorescens Pf0-1.* FEBS Lett, 2009. 583(4): p. 729-33.

[15] Nakamura, Y., et al., *Complete genome structure of the thermophilic cyanobacterium Thermosynechococcus elongatus BP-1.* DNA Res, 2002. 9(4): p. 123-30.

[16] Kambampati, R. and C.T. Lauhon, *IscS is a sulfurtransferase for the in vitro biosynthesis of 4-thiouridine in Escherichia coli tRNA.* Biochemistry, 1999. 38(50): p. 16561-8.

[17] He, X., et al., *Analysis of a genomic island housing genes for DNA S-modification system in Streptomyces lividans 66 and its counterparts in other distantly related bacteria.* Mol Microbiol, 2007. 65(4): p. 1034-48.

[18] Zhang, Y., et al., *Pulsed-field gel electrophoresis study of Mycobacterium abscessus isolates previously affected by DNA degradation.* J Clin Microbiol, 2004. 42(12): p. 5582-7.

[19] Morris, R.M., et al., *SAR11 clade dominates ocean surface bacterioplankton communities.* Nature, 2002. 420(6917): p. 806-10.

[20] Chen, S., L. Wang, and Z. Deng, *Twenty years hunting for sulfur in DNA.* Protein Cell. 1(1): p. 14-21.

[21] Boyer, H.W., *DNA restriction and modification mechanisms in bacteria.* Annu Rev Microbiol, 1971. 25: p. 153-76.

[22] Wilson, G.G. and N.E. Murray, *Restriction and modification systems.* Annu Rev Genet, 1991. 25: p. 585-627.

[23] Juhas, M., et al., *Genomic islands: tools of bacterial horizontal gene transfer and evolution.* FEMS Microbiol Rev, 2009. 33(2): p. 376-93.

[24] Qiu, X., A.U. Gurkar, and S. Lory, *Interstrain transfer of the large pathogenicity island (PAPI-1) of Pseudomonas aeruginosa.* Proc Natl Acad Sci U S A, 2006. 103(52): p. 19830-5.

[25] Gaillard, M., et al., *The clc element of Pseudomonas sp. strain B13, a genomic island with various catabolic properties.* J Bacteriol, 2006. 188(5): p. 1999-2013.

[26] Ou, H.Y., et al., *dndDB: a database focused on phosphorothioation of the DNA backbone.* PLoS One, 2009. 4(4): p. e5132.

[27] Sayers, J.R., et al., *Strand specific cleavage of phosphorothioate-containing DNA by reaction with restriction endonucleases in the presence of ethidium bromide.* Nucleic Acids Res, 1988. 16(3): p. 803-14.

[28] Eckstein, F., *Phosphorothioate oligodeoxynucleotides: what is their origin and what is unique about them?* Antisense Nucleic Acid Drug Dev, 2000. 10(2): p. 117-21.

[29] Marwick, C., *First "antisense" drug will treat CMV retinitis.* JAMA, 1998. 280(10): p. 871.

[30] Oka, N., et al., *Solid-phase synthesis of stereoregular oligodeoxyribonucleoside phosphorothioates using bicyclic oxazaphospholidine derivatives as monomer units.* J Am Chem Soc, 2008. 130(47): p. 16031-7.

[31] Eckstein, F., *Nucleoside phosphorothioates.* Annu Rev Biochem, 1985. 54: p. 367-402.

[32] Eckstein, F., *Phosphorothioation of DNA in bacteria.* Nat Chem Biol, 2007. 3(11): p. 689-90.

[33] Hattman, S., *Unusual modification of bacteriophage Mu DNA.* J Virol, 1979. 32(2): p. 468-75.

[34] Hattman, S., *Specificity of the bacteriophage Mu mom+ -controlled DNA modification.* J Virol, 1980. 34(1): p. 277-9.

[35] Swinton, D., et al., *Purification and characterization of the unusual deoxynucleoside, alpha-N-(9-beta-D-2'-deoxyribofuranosylpurin-6-yl)glycinamide, specified by the phage Mu modification function.* Proc Natl Acad Sci U S A, 1983. 80(24): p. 7400-4.

4

Mitosis and DNA Replication and Life Origination Hydrate Hypotheses: Common Physical and Chemical Grounds

Ostrovskii Victor E.[1] and Kadyshevich Elena A.[2]
[1]*Karpov Institute of Physical Chemistry, Moscow,*
[2]*Obukhov Institute of Atmospheric Physics RAS, Moscow,*
Russia

1. Introduction

1.1 Formulation of the problem under consideration

We proceed from the assumptions that the Earth's living matter had originated on our planet from inorganic and simplest organic substances as an inevitable product of the atomistic world and that the same natural phenomenon underlies the processes of origination and reproduction of living matter. We believe that living matter was originating multiply and, maybe, originates now and that the diversity of the available forms of living matter is caused mainly by some variations in parameters of the native medium. In all probability, stable undisturbed conditions favor origination of the simplest living matter and this process proceeds so slowly that its direction is thermodynamically favorable. "Nature makes no jumps" (Nature non facit saltus (Lat.)): we had this Latin aphorism at our hearts when thinking over the problems of this paper.

The occurrence and reproduction of nucleic acids (deoxyribonucleic acid (DNA) and ribonucleic acid (RNA)) is the principal feature of living matter. Their molecules represent alternating phosphate–sugar chains, in which a hydroxyl of each sugar group is substituted with a so-called nitrogen base (N-base). As sugars, deoxy-D-riboses (DDR) and D-riboses (DR) enter the molecules of DNA and RNA, respectively. As N-bases, pyrimidines (cytosine (Cy), thymine (Th), and uracil (U)) and purines (guanine (G) and adenine (Ad) and, more rarely, xantine (X), hypoxantine (Hx)) and some quite rare N-bases are known. DNA molecules contain no U, and RNA molecules contain no Th. In the living organisms, DNA molecules are, at least most of the time, in the state of dimers, termed double helixes. The spatial arrangement of different components in the molecules of nucleic acids is strictly defined. For each organism, the occurrence of DNA molecules of a definite composition is the characteristic feature. It is commonly accepted that the heritage of living organisms is determined by the sequence of the N-bases in the DNA molecules.

The interest of the scientific community to the problem of the mechanism of living matter origination from mineral substances was triggered by the first-ever naturalistic hypothesis announced by A. Oparin (1924). It was twenty years before clarification of the facts that nucleic acids rather than proteins cause the diversity of living organisms and regulate their development. Oparin's hypothesis became the starting point for numerous works dedicated to this intriguing problem. With time, this problem was divided into two sub-problems: where did living matter originate, at the Earth or anywhere in the Universe beyond our planet, and how, i.e., by what mechanism, did it originate? We leave the first sub-problem out of our consideration and discuss the living matter origination mechanism, which can be applied, in our opinion, to any Universe region, where the appropriate conditions exist. Some authors think fit to regard imaginary processes of extended reproduction of some substances containing no nucleic acids or containing some of their surrogates that include silicon or other chemical elements, instead of carbon, as life. We risk of sounding tiresome and cold-blooded, but we believe that no other form of life but that similar to the Earth's one is possible and the other above-mentioned concepts have no scientific ground.

What is the physicochemical mechanism of cell replication? This is one of the central problems of our consideration. But is such a statement of the problem promising? May it be that none general physicochemical mechanism for the phenomenon of multi-step self-reproduction of a cell exists and each step is controlled by some different specific articles termed ferments, thousands of which are synthesized at right moments and carried to some definite points by some miraculous mode, following the plan once written independently of the physical and chemical laws? Who is the author of this plan? Is it the knowable Nature or a mysterious and unknowable Force that stays out of the natural laws and over them?

If this is Nature, all its manifestations are regulated by a rather limited number of physicochemical laws, which, taking a joint action on a cell located in a medium of any definite composition, temperature, and other ambient conditions, lead this cell to its inevitable replication, which may be precluded only by a critical variation in the conditions and (or) chemical composition of the medium. What is the key natural phenomenon that underlies the life-cycle repetition for any element of living matter termed cell? The answer for this question is just the aim to which we aspire. Nature is simple and, therefore, among the laws that determine running of any natural process, a leading one is usually specifiable. It is our opinion that the simplicity intrinsic to a natural phenomenon may be latent for the time being but is the reality noted by I. Newton (Newton, 1687), who wrote that "…Nature does nothing in vain, and more is in vain, when less will serve; for Nature is pleased with simplicity, and affects not the pomp of superfluous causes", i.e., it is simple and doesn't luxuriate in excessive sources. We are of the opinion that the most concise hypothetical way assumed to be the natural one gives the hypothesis the best chance to be correct. Indeed, most physicists believe that the hypothesis more laconic in its assumed steps and included substances is preferable against more complicated hypotheses, similarly to chess players who believe that the less is the number of pieces included into a chess problem, the more perfect it is. However, some researchers think otherwise. For example, Galimov argues that "…despite the remarkable inventiveness of nature in creating intricate biological mechanisms, their analysis indicates that almost each given result could be achieved by a simpler means" (Galimov, 2001, p. 218). He "forces" Nature, according to his hypothesis (Galimov, 2009), to create first adenosine triphosphate through a very multiple synthesis and to use it then for creation of living articles through no less multiple chain of syntheses.

If the today Nature has the "know how" allowing for creation living articles time and again, it should formerly perform the procedure of creation of the first living articles from mineral substances and this original procedure should be similar to that being repeated in our days. For a long time, this procedure could vary adapting itself to the environments but its principle law-obedience should be apparently conserved in time. Thus, the solutions of these two puzzles of Nature are interconnected.

Therefore, a revelation of the key phenomenon and leading law that determine events of living matter origination would approach us closely to a solution of the problem of cellular replication and, vice versa, a solution of the problem of cellular replication could supply us almost certainly with a magic wand capable of helping in clarification of the problem of living matter origination. We try to reveal the key physicochemical phenomenon and the leading natural law that determine both these problems and, on this basis, to describe the hypothetical mechanisms of living matter origination (the Life Origination Hydrate Hypothesis (the LOH-hypothesis)) and of cellular replication (the Mitosis and Replication Hydrate Hypothesis (the MRH-hypothesis)).

We develop the OK-hypothesis of the Universe development for the period from the Supernova explosion to the cellular living matter origination (OK is the abbreviation of the family names of the authors). This hypothesis includes the Solar System formation hypothesis (PFO–CFO hypothesis) (Ostrovskii & Kadyshevich, 2008, 2009a, 2009b, 2011; Kadyshevich & Ostrovskii, 2010a, 2010b; Kadyshevich, 2009a, 2009b), the hypothesis of formation of natural gas and some other localizations of minerals (Ostrovskii & Kadyshevich, 2007, 2008; Ostrovskii, 2010), and the LOH-hypothesis (Ostrovskii & Kadyshevich, 2000, 2002, 2006, 2007, 2009c, 2010; Kadyshevich & Ostrovskii, 2009, 2010c, 2010d; Kadyshevich, 2007) and the MRH-hypothesis (Kadyshevich & Ostrovskii, 2007; Kadyshevich, 2006).

The OK-hypothesis as a whole and each of its components taken separately are based on the notion that all natural phenomena proceed as a result of regular and inevitable chemical transformations regulated by universal physical and chemical laws. When reconstructing Nature's way, we are governed by the following main principles: (1) The Newton principle of simplicity. (2) The principle of repetition of supposed events and of the presence of individual features in the reproduced events. The matter is that, in Nature, there are many similar but somewhat differing events and there are no unique events without close analogues. (3) The principle of the unity of the event point. Separation of an event into several sub-events proceeding in different points with the subsequent interaction between the sub-events decreases the probability of the resulted event, because it multiply decreases the degree of repetition of the event as a whole.

1.2 Introduction into the life origination hydrate hypothesis

The processes that gave rise to life could not obey biological laws because they proceeded in the absence of biota. Hence, the origin of life is first and foremost a problem of chemistry and physics and a number of related scientific disciplines concerned with mechanisms underlying the development of the atomistic world.

Vitaly Ginzburg, who was awarded with the 2003 Nobel Prize, described the problem of the "reduction of the animate to the inanimate" in his Nobel lecture (Ginzburg, 2004) as one of the three great physical problems facing the 21st century. He formulated this thought in the following words (Ginzburg, 1999): "At present, we believe that we know what all alive consists of, meaning electrons, atoms, and molecules. We are aware of the structure of atoms and molecules and of the laws governing atoms, molecules, and radiation. Therefore, the hypothesis of reduction, i.e., the possibility of explaining the life on the basis of physics, of the already known physics, is natural. The main problems are those of the origin of life and of the appearance of consciousness (mentality). The problem is not solved, and I am inclined to think that it will be unreservedly solved only after 'life in a test-tube' is created."

We propose an original solution to the problem of the origin of living-matter simplest elements (LMSEs), i.e., N-bases and riboses, and of nucleic acids that ensure the protein synthesis and transmission of major traits of living organisms from one generation to another. Immanuel Kant contended that "To get knowledge from nature, the Mind should address to it, on the one hand, with his own principles, which are necessary for concordant phenomena to carry the force of law, and, on the other hand, with experiments intended in conformity with these principles." (Kant, 1997, pp. 85, 86). With this in mind, we described an experiment that could be used to verify our hypothesis if it is reproduced by several laboratories in a coordinated manner with the experimental conditions varied within a certain range (Ostrovskii & Kadyshevich, 2006, 2007). If the hypothesis proves valid, this experiment may yield precursors of nucleic acids and, possibly, DNA-like molecules. It can be expected that the LOH-hypothesis will contribute to realization of the cautious prediction by Ginzburg, who noted that he "would not be surprised if `life in a test tube' would be created in the 21st century" (Ginzburg, 1999).

We will first clarify our understanding of the borderline between the animate and inanimate. There is no consensus with regard to this issue. Thus, Oparin believed that life development started with the appearance of nucleotide sequences (nucleic acids) when the process of chemical evolution as the struggle among protobionts was coming to an end and competition in the growth rate turned into the struggle for existence (Oparin, 1924, 1957). Spirin maintains that "the origin of life in its present cellular form is reduced to the development of a mechanism of heritable protein synthesis" (Spirin, 2001), but leaves the problem of a cellular life beyond this definition. In the late 19th century, Friedrich Engels defined life as "the form of existence of protein bodies".

The problem of the border between the animate and inanimate is far from vain even if its discussion may seem to make no concrete sense. Drawing the line between the animate and inanimate determines the interpretation of viruses (DNA molecules containing genetic information and enclosed in a protein membrane), and viroids as subjects of biological (including biophysical) or organic and physicochemical studies. This problem has been discussed since 1935, when Stanley pioneered in isolation and crystallization of the tobacco mosaic virus. L. Pauling summarized the situation as follows: "in fact, there is no reason to consider this question as a scientific one; indeed, it reduces to the definition of the notion. If a living organism is defined as a material structure capable of self-reproduction, then plant viruses should be reckoned among living organisms. If it is assumed that living organisms must be capable of metabolism, then plant viruses must be regarded as mere molecules having a molecular weight of about 106 and a structure allowing them to catalyze, in a certain medium, a chemical reaction leading to the synthesis of molecules identical with them" (Pauling, 1970).

We emphasize that Pauling's opinion is not faultless in the light of modern knowledge. It has been many times demonstrated in the past 10 to 15 years (see, e.g., Orgel, 1992, 2000; Cech & Bass, 1986; Li & Nicolaou, 1994) that not only nucleic acids but even simpler organic substances are capable of self-replicating with consumption of certain chemical elements from the surrounding and excretion of nonutilized molecular residues. Should we call such a process "metabolism"? No reasoning can answer this question; the answer can be deduced only from the practice of using the term. Today, viruses and even viroids are regarded as biological substances and are studied by biologists, although a vast field of activity remains open to physicists and chemists. Each of these species contains DNA of a specific composition. In our opinion, it is therefore justified to regard the appearance of nucleic acids in the course of evolution as the onset of the simplest precellular life. Such a demarcation between the animate and inanimate is especially logical because, as noted by Kauffman, complex organic systems such as DNA and RNA inevitably become self-replicating and their self-replication proceeds through an autocatalytic mechanism (Kauffman, 1993). If a living system were devoid of nucleic acids, with its protein content preserved, the vital activity would surely cease; if a living system were devoid of its protein, with the nucleic acids preserved, the vital activity of the system supplied with nutrients might normalize with time.

Apparently, once nucleic acids had originated and propagated and a medium appropriate for their existence and replication had appeared, the appearance of cellular life was merely a matter of time. It follows from the foregoing that in our terminology, DNA and RNA are the simplest forms of precellular living matter, while N-bases and riboses are its simplest elements or constituents. We consider it appropriate to expound and substantiate our understanding of the border between the animate and inanimate, bearing in mind Kant's definition of physics as the theory field that should perceive natural objects by mind and that should determine them a priori and "purely, at least partially, and then should do it also on the basis of knowledge sources other than the mind" (Kant, 1997, p. 84).

Below, we briefly consider an important and rather intriguing question on dating the historic period when the first simplest living organisms appeared at the Earth. This question was recently developed as comprehensively as the today knowledge of the Archaean history of the Earth allows (Fedonkin, 2006, 2009). According to some authors (Hedges & Kumar, 2003; Mojzsis et al., 1996), the early divergence among prokaryotes was 3970 Myr ago (molecular time) or 3800 Myr ago (fossil time) and the origin of eukaryotes was 2730 Myr ago (molecular time) or 2150 Myr ago (fossil time). Note that the dates of divergence among prokaryotes were recently brought into question. The matter is that this conclusion was made on the basis of indirect data on the isotopic composition of the carbon inclusions within the apatite crystals mined from the Greenland Archaean beds. Meanwhile, according to others (Fedo & Whitehouse, 2002; van Zuilen et al, 2002), the apatite crystals and carbon inclusions could be formed much later as a result of metamorphism influenced by the hot fluids. We see that the molecular time and the fossil time differ rather significantly and that the periods of the starts of the Earth prokaryotization and eukaryotization are known rather approximately. These conclusions relate not only to the prokaryotes and eukaryotes ages. Fossil time measurements led to the conclusion that the earliest localities of invertebrate animals lived 600–550 Myr ago and that most of the species of invertebrate animals occurred in Cambrian period, i.e., their age is less than 510 Myr. However, the measurements of the molecular time give a period of 1500–1200 Myr ago for the development of the first Metazoa colonies and lead to the conclusion that the main branches of the invertebrates lived many hundreds of millions of years before Cambrian (Fedonkin, 2009). These data show that the today knowledge on the positions of different events on the time-scale is rather rough. Note that, multicellular organisms apparently appeared independently in the Earth history no less than 24 times (Buss, 1987).

Giving A. Oparin his due as the world's first researcher to consider living matter objects as the ones not differing fundamentally from the lifeless matter, we should note that his hypothesis could not be correct because it rested upon a pseudo-scientific statement. He thought mistakenly that the living matter entropy is so small that no decrease in the enthalpy could make the free energy change negative in chemical transformations of mineral substances to living matter. Therefore, Oparin believed that external energy in the form of electric discharges, heat of underground thermal water sources, etc. is necessary for such transformations. In addition, he, for some reason, thought that living matter could originate at ground–atmosphere or water–atmosphere phase boundaries. Meanwhile, the DNA and RNA molecules are very long, the chemical elements for their formation should be chosen very selectively, the atom groups should be located in strictly determined positions and should be limited in size, and some other special requirements should be performed in the process of their formation. The complexity of these conditions suggests the idea that such molecules could originate only under condition of the absence of heat, electrical, and weather perturbations, which are most likely capable of destroying any order rather than to create and maintain it. Therefore, the conditions at phase boundaries are hardly suited for origination of nucleic acids, which are necessary for subsequent formation of living matter. The Miller–Urey experiments showed that mineral substances could produce some amino-acids under the conditions that can be considered as those approached to the conditions of the Earth's primordial atmosphere, but nothing was synthesized that would be suitable for the subsequent RNA and DNA formation. Productions of DNA and RNA molecules from simple mineral substances by Oparin's mechanism represent extremely low-probability events, which cannot be realized in practice. In addition, this hypothesis gave no realistic assumption on a possible cause of the phenomenon of monochirality of biologically active substances.

Meanwhile, Russian physicist and biologist L. Blyumenfeld calculated the living matter entropy on the basis of the simple generalized approach of statistical physics and came to the unambiguous conclusion that "…according to physical criteria, any biological system is ordered no more than a rock piece of the same weight" (Blyumenfeld, 1981, 1996, 2002). Somewhat later, the standard values of the enthalpy of formation ($\Delta_f H^0$) and of the entropy (S^0) were obtained experimentally for different biologically active substances (Alberty, 2003; Ould-Moulaye et al., 2001; Lide, 1996; Boerio-Goates, 2005). We calculated the standard ($\Delta_f G^0$) values for a number of reactions leading to formation of nitrogen bases and riboses from minerals (Ostrovskii & Kadyshevich, 2006, 2007). It was stated that no external energy is necessary to synthesize biologically active substances from minerals, because the free-energy changes in such reactions are negative and rather great in magnitude. Unfortunately, the mistaken opinion by Oparin on the necessity of an external energy for origination of living matter from minerals is distributed among the researchers who try to understand the natural way from minerals to living matter, and several hypotheses that include this opinion in an explicit or implicit form are available.

The life origination hypotheses developed by Oparin and his followers are also criticized from another standpoint (Shapiro, 2000). Shapiro believes that the production of an information-bearing homopolymer within a complex mixture by chance cannot be excluded, but if such an event was required to start life, then its origin would have been an extremely improbable accident, and prospects for life elsewhere would be diminished. According to his opinion, "…a more likely alternative for the origin of life is one in which a collection of small organic molecules multiply their numbers through catalyzed reaction cycles, driven by a flow of available free energy" (Shapiro, 2006). More or less similar views on the life origination problem are available in the literature (e.g., Deamer, 1997; Segré et al. 1998; Parmon, 1999).

When considering the processes of metabolism of prokaryotes and eukaryotes, we try to reveal the central common natural physicochemical phenomenon underlying division of prokaryotic and somatic eukaryotic cells. Following Oparin, we consider living organisms as systems not differing fundamentally from the lifeless matter; i.e., we take that the intracellular processes are controlled by the universal physical and chemical laws. We proceed from the assumption that eukaryotic mitosis (Alberts et al., 2002 (Ch.4); Lodish et al., 2000 (Ch. 13) and prokaryotic binary fission (Alberts et al., 2002 (Ch.4); Lodish et al., 2000 (Ch. 12) are connected with the same definite fundamental natural physicochemical phenomenon that has them "in tow". In other words, the same physicochemical phenomenon is the prime cause of the eukaryotic mitosis and prokaryotic binary fission. Otherwise, we should evidently take that the first prokaryotes and the first eukaryotes had originated in nature independently and their subsequent metabolisms and evolutions were controlled by different physical and chemical regularities. In this case, these two branches of living matter should be, most likely, incompatible in their vital functions. Meanwhile, living organisms belonging to numerous species characterized by the anatomies and physiologies that are intermediate between those inherent in typical prokaryotes and eukaryotes are common in nature. This reasoning gives an indirect confirmation for our assumption on the similarity of the prime physicochemical causes underlying the mitosis and binary fission. We see additional confirmation for this assumption in the following fundamental common features of the anatomies and metabolisms of prokaryotes and eukaryotes. First, prokaryotes and eukaryotes transmit their principal hereditary characters from generation to generation through DNA molecules, which are similar in their chemical composition and molecular structure. Second, the eukaryotic mitosis and prokaryotic binary fission are principally similar in their results. Namely, either of them results in separation of genome into two identical halves and in subsequent cytokinesis leading to division of the cytoplasm and cell membrane into two identical new cells. Third, both the eukaryotic mitosis and prokaryotic binary fission are preceded by the DNA replication processes similar in their principal results. The MRH-hypothesis developed by us contains the supposition that formation of new nuclear envelopes and of cell membranes between two newly-formed cells in the processes of mitosis and cytokinesis is provided by precipitation of complex organo-mineral substances from oversaturated solutions. However, the central phenomenon providing the existence of living matter is not mitosis as such, but transmission of duplicated genomic information from parental genomes to daughter ones, i.e., the DNA replication. We suppose that DNA replication is initiated by the neutralization of the amide-amide interactions in DNA double helixes by water dipoles. Thus, two familiar and commonly-known natural phenomena (precipitation from oversaturated solutions and neutralization of the DNA–DNA dipole interactions by water dipoles) summarized with the phenomenon of continuous diffusion of water and organics into living cells from the outside represent the basis for the phenomenological content of living-matter reproduction.

However, each of these three phenomena proceeds monotonously in time and, therefore, the last statement as such is only a declaration that does not clarify metabolic processes. This paper represents an attempt to reveal the mechanisms of transformation of these monotonous processes into the cyclic ones providing development of living matter, including mitosis and DNA replication. We try to show that the so-called genetic code is nothing but manifestation of the universal physical and chemical laws guiding the chemical transformations in aqueous media containing organo-mineral substances of definite chemical compositions. We by no means take into account all factors influencing the processes under consideration but try to reveal the core phenomena controlling the directions of these processes. Finishing the introduction to this paper, we would like to say that the occurrence of individual organelles inside living cells is not necessarily caused by the usefulness of all these niceties for the metabolic processes. The occurrence of some of them might be caused by the natural processes of precipitation of one or another organic crystal structure from the saturated solution, and their disappearance in the course of mitosis or replication might be associated with swelling or dissolving caused by the concentration variations within the cell. The complexity of the structures of intracellular organelles and the repetition of the structures from cycle to cycle by no means contradict this opinion. Indeed, now that a lot of supramolecular crystals are synthesized artificially, we know well how daedal and fantastical the forms of precipitated crystal organics can be. Note that some organelles, such as chloroplasts and mitochondria (Henze & Martin, 2003) in eukaryotic plant and animal cells, have their own DNA and, evidently, use the intracellular medium just as the corresponding eukaryotic plant and animal cells use their environment.

2. The gas-hydrate matrix as the medium for living- matter origination and reproduction

2.1 Gas hydrates as a class of chemical substances

Gas-hydrates (Byk & Fomina, 1970; Atwood et al., 1996; Carroll, 2003; Chaplin, 2010) are honeycomb, solid or semi-liquid, mineral substances with cubic (structure I, a = 1.20 nm), face-centered cubic (structure II, a = 1.73 nm), or hexagonal (structure H, a = 1.23 nm and c = 1.02 nm) lattices composed of large and small cavities, where the waters (hosts) are the vertices of the cavities and other atoms, molecules, or atomic groups (guests) are housed within the cavities. As guests, particles of one type or two different types can be housed within the large cavities and, in addition, particles of a third type can be housed within the small cavities. Gas-hydrates that contain guest particles of two or more different chemical natures are termed mixed gas-hydrates. The structure type depends on the size of the guest particles or on the sizes of the guest particles if particles of two or three types are housed within the cavities. Gas hydrate structures can exist only under the condition that some guest particles are housed within no less than 80% of the cavities of any definite size; otherwise, the loose structure collapses and transforms to the usual dense ice. For example, in the hydrate structure II, the ideal water-to-guest ratio is equal to 17 and the critical one is equal to 20÷21. In gas-hydrates, the guest–H_2O interactions are provided by the Van-der-Waals (W-d-W) forces.

Figure 1 is designed in scale; it presents the gas-hydrate cavities of the hydrate structures I, II, and H. Structures I, II, and H contain 5^{12} and $5^{12}6^2$, 5^{12} and 6^4, and 5^{12}, $4^35^66^3$, and $5^{12}6^8$ cavities, respectively (over the structures, the lower-case figures mean the numbers of the edges of a facet and the superior figures mean the numbers of such facets that terminate the corresponding cavity). In Fig. 1, each vertex responds to the O atom of a H_2O molecule and each edge responds to the sum of the O–H valence bond of any H_2O molecule and the H····O hydrogen bond of this H_2O molecule with any adjacent H_2O molecule. Each of structures I and II has cavities of two types, and structure H has cavities of three types. Figure 1 gives also the sizes of particles capable of being housed within cavities of different types. Gas-hydrates are widely distributed in nature. For example, natural methane deposits exist frequently in the form of gas hydrates.

For crystal structures I, II, and H, the unit cell formulas, $(S)_2{\cdot}(L)_6{\cdot}46H_2O$, $(S)_{16}(L+)_8{\cdot}136H_2O$, and $(S)_5(L{+}{+}){\cdot}34H_2O$, respectively, are proposed (S is the small guest, L is the large guest, L+ is the larger guest, and L++ is the largest guest). Hydrate structures remain stable when the guest contents are below their stoichiometric values by 20–25%. Each unit crystal cell of the structure I, II, or H contains 2 small 5^{12} (20 waters) and 6 large $5^{12}6^2$ (24 waters) cavities, 16 small 5^{12} and 8 large $5^{12}6^4$ (28 waters) cavities, or 3 small 5^{12}, 2 small $4^35^66^3$ (20 waters) and

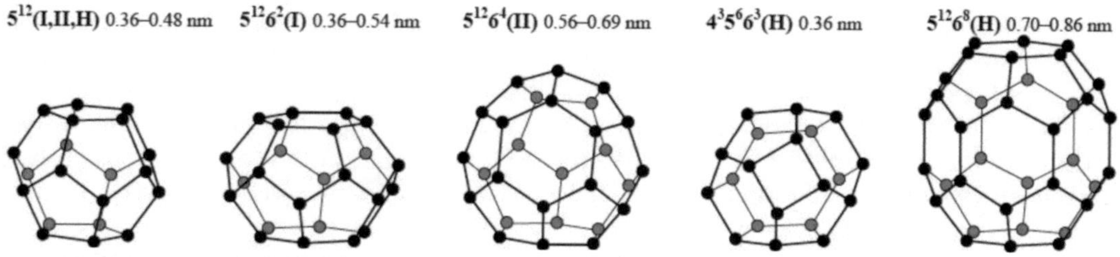

Fig. 1. Intra-structural cavities of hydrate structures I, II and H: the vertexes are the O-atoms of H_2O molecules, and the length of each edge corresponds to the sum of the lengths of the O–H valence bond in any H_2O molecule and H····O hydrogen bond between this and an adjacent H_2O molecule; above each cavity, its free diameter, the number of its facets (the superior figures) restricted with the definite number of the edges (the lower-case figures), and the indexes of the hydrate structures into which this cavity is included are given.

1 large $5^{12}6^{8}$ (36 waters) cavities, respectively. According to Chaplin (2010), the 5^{12}, $5^{12}6^{2}$, $5^{12}6^{4}$, $4^{3}5^{6}6^{3}$, and $5^{12}6^{8}$ cavities are capable of housing the molecules having diameters of 0.36–0.44 (such as Ar, O_2, N_2, and CH_4), 0.36–0.54 (such as CO_2 and C_2H_6), 0.56–0.62 (such as C_3H_8 and $(CH_3)_3CH$), 0.36 (such as CH_4), and 0.70–0.86 (such as $(CH_3)_3CC_2H_5$) nm, respectively. It was shown that water solutions of cyclic organic liquids consisting of rather large molecules, such as furan $(CH)_4O$ and tetrahydrofuran $(CH_2)_4O$, form solid hydrate structure II at temperatures below 298 K (Stackelberg & Meuthen, 1958). Sometimes, atoms of large-sized guest molecules partake in the formation of the "walls" of the cavities (Hagan, 1962), for example, in the so-called semi-clathrate hydrates, such as hydrates of n-propylamine and alkyl-amines (McMullan et al., 1967; Jordan & Mac, 1967). Many clathrate compounds of structure II with 17 "host" waters per one "guest" molecule are well known, e.g., $C_4H_4O{\cdot}17H_2O$ (Stackelberg & Meuthen, 1958), $(CH_2)_4O{\cdot}17H_2O$ (Pinder, 1965), $CH_3Cl{\cdot}17H_2O$ (Stackelberg & Muller, 1954), $C_3H_6{\cdot}17H_2O$ (Clarke et al., 1964), and so-called mixed hydrates, such as $C_3H_8{\cdot}2H_2S{\cdot}17H_2O$ (Platteeuw & Van-der-Waals, 1959), $(CH_2)_4O{\cdot}2H_2S{\cdot}17H_2O$ (Pinder, 1964), $C_3H_8{\cdot}2CH_4{\cdot}17H_2O$ (Van-der-Waals & Platteeuw, 1959), etc. According to Byk & Fomina (1970), each unit crystal cell of structure II has the size 1.74 nm and consists of 136 waters, which form 16 small and 8 large cavities with the free diameters 0.48 and 0.69 nm, respectively; the small and large cavities represent somewhat-depressed penta-dodecahedron and almost spherical hexa-decahedron, respectively. Just these structural parameters were used by us for the calculations presented below. Note that the free energy inherent in different hydrate structures is almost the same, and, therefore, they can metamorphose depending on the conditions and the nature of the guest particles.

At present, there are many under-seabed methane-hydrate deposits (Ginsburg & Soloviev, 1998). In 2004, the methane mass in the proven marine methane-hydrate deposits was estimated as (1÷5) mln. km^3 (Milkov, 2004), and this estimate grows continuously. Underground methane-hydrate deposits are also known.

Hydrate structures have a unique peculiarity. This peculiarity is caused by the fact that the structuring is provided by the weak V-d-W forces. Therefore, the molar free energies of the structured and unstructured states are rather close. As a result, variations in the relative concentrations of the components of both the host (water) and guest (substrate) can change the aggregate (structural) state of the systems. For example, when water slowly enters forcibly into an amorphous dried water–substrate system capable of structuring, a gas-hydrate structure arises and develops with a decrease in the free energy up to hydrate formation over the entire system; however, entering of excessive water leads to the disruption of the hydrate structure, which proceeds also with a decrease in the free energy. We will show below that this peculiarity of the gas-hydrate structures is of principal importance for the living matter origination and development; it is possible that this peculiarity is the cause of a number of derangements in the regular functioning of living cells and multi-cellular aggregates.

The capability for hydrate formation is a fundamental property of water; it can reveal itself in solid and highly-concentrated semi-liquid systems at sufficiently low temperatures and sufficiently high concentrations (or pressures) of particles of such sizes that correspond to the free sizes of the gas-hydrate cavities; the chemical nature of the guest particles is not of principal importance for the question on the possibility of hydrate formation in any substrate–water system.

2.2 Structuring of waters in the DNAs (and RNAs) vicinities in aqueous media

2.2.1 PAA–H_2O system as the model for studies of the mechanism of DNA–DNA interaction in aqueous media

Because of great importance of clarification of the mechanism of the purine–pyrimidine bond breakage in the process of DNA replication, information on water effects on the hydrogen DNA-DNA bonds in double helixes is of particular interest. Meanwhile, clarification of this process on the basis of water sorption or desorption in the DNA–H_2O system is difficult because of the occurrence of masking hydrophilic phosphate and ribose groups in the content of DNA molecules. Therefore, it is the practice to use polyacrylamide (PAA) as the model substance, because it is the polymer that contains functional groups similar to the amido-groups (AGs) of DNA. To make certain that the functional groups of PAA and DNA are similar in their chemical properties, we studied the available data on the valence angles and lengths of the valence bonds in the AGs of these two substances and made sure of their identity (Ostrovskii & Kadyshevich, 2000). We also studied water-vapor sorption and desorption in the PAA–H_2O system by adsorption and microcalorimetric methods (Ostrovskii & Tsurkova, 1997, 1998a, 1998b; Ostrovskii et al., 2000, 2001); most of the experiments were performed in undisturbed highly-concentrated semi-liquid aqueous media at about 290 K. Each substrate–water system intended for desorption measurements was aged before the experiments up to the equilibrium for no less than a week with no agitation. For comparison, H_2O sorption and desorption were also studied in the alanine–water and glycine–water systems (Kadyshevich & Ostrovskii, 2007). The techniques and procedures of these experiments are detailed in the works cited above in this paragraph; the original FOSKA microcalorimeter is described in Ostrovskii (2002). Some results and principal schemes of the portable sorption and desorption vacuum glass apparatuses are presented in Fig. 2. As far as we know, neither the differential heats of H_2O sorption nor the differential rates of H_2O sorption by PAA were studied until these experiments. The measurements of the integral heats of PAA dissolution in water yield negative and very small magnitudes (Silberberg et al., 1957; Day & Robb, 1981). In our experiments, the following specific features of H_2O sorption by polymers with functional AGs were revealed. When H_2O vapor contacts with PAA in air of almost 100% humidity at about 290 K, water sorption proceeds very slowly and terminates or, at least, moderates critically at a stoichiometry of $AG{\cdot}(17{\div}18)H_2O$; in desorption experiments, heightened molar differential heats of H_2O sorption are obtained at this composition of the PAA-H_2O system (Ostrovskii & Tsurkova, 1997, 1998a, 1998b).

In PAA, just AGs are the centers of H_2O sorption. It is obvious that some AGs of the dry polymer are inter-PAA or intra-PAA bound by pairs, forming quadrupoles (see Fig. 4d); the rest of the AGs are as dipoles. A small gain in the integral Gibbs energy during vapor sorption against the energy of vapor condensation on the surface of liquid water (the gain is small, as, under airless conditions, the polymer can be quickly dried out) is conditioned by the following causes. The dipole moment (in Debye, D) of AG is M_{AG} = 3.8 D (Thompson & LaPlanche, 1963), while that of a water molecule is M_W = 1.87 D (Pauling, 1970), so $M_{AG} > M_W$. Thus, the energy of a unit AG–AG interaction is somewhat higher than the energy of AG–H_2O interaction (in Fig. 2e, the differential heats of H_2O sorption are below the heat of water condensation). However, in the systems watered only slightly, localization of a water molecule in the vicinity of an AG group leads to a decrease in the water entropy as compared to that in its non-localized state and to a decrease in the Gibbs free energy change in this process to negative values. Therefore, the waters localize near the AG groups up to organization of the water continuum, i.e., the water phase. The AGs of PAA are rather large, bound to the carbon chain, and slow. Therefore, the coordination numbers of AGs is limited by steric hindrance. Furthermore, in a dry system, some AGs are not bound to any other AG. Thus, the dipole moments of AGs cannot be completely screened. As a consequence, dry PAA has some excessive energy as compared with the equilibrium energy that it would probably have after infinitely slow drying of the PAA–H_2O system.

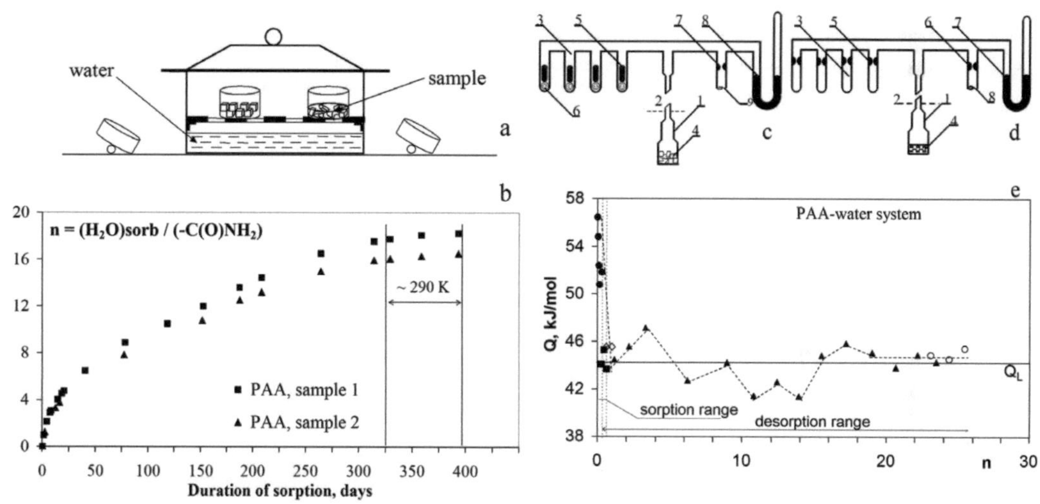

Fig. 2. (a) Water-vapor sorption by polyacrylamide (PAA) from air of 100% humidity at about 290 K; (b) degree of PAA wetting vs. duration of sorption; (c) apparatus for sorption experiments in the deaired PAA–water system: (1) calorimetric ampoule, (2) top of the calorimeter, (3) test tube, (4) sample for wetting, (5) "breaker", (6) sealed water-containing glass sphere, (7) neck, (8) mercury manometer, and (9) tube to vacuum setup; (d) apparatus for desorption experiments: (5) neck (for other notation, see (c)); (e) calorimetric molar heats of H_2O sorption: sorption by sample 8 (●) at 292 K and desorption from samples 7 (■), 9 (▲), 10 (◊), and 11 (○) at 292, 288, 297, and 291 K, respectively (samples 7, 9, 10, and 11 are aged before the experiments for 14, 9, 6, and 16 days, respectively); Q_L is the heat of H_2O vaporization from the pure water surface at 290 K.

The molar heat of water desorption (Fig. 2e) at high degrees of dilution is n-independent (n is the waters-to-AGs ratio in the PAA–H_2O system) at $n > 17$ and is equal to the tabulated value of the heat of H_2O vaporization (Q_L, horizontal line) from the pure H_2O surface. The peculiarities are observable at $0 < n < 17$. These peculiarities reflect the complicated transformations that proceed in the hydrate phase and are not caused by experimental inaccuracies. The last statement is confirmed by the low data spread in 7 experiments performed at high n values and by their close fit with the tabulated value of the heat of H_2O vaporization; it is well known that hydrates can have different stoichiometry depending on the H_2O content and that their different forms can somewhat differ one from another by the enthalpy and entropy.

At the initial step of wetting of dry PAA, waters diffuse into the PAA mass and interact with unpaired AGs. Therefore, the initial differential heats of water-vapor sorption are heightened. In our experiments, the heightened heats were observed up to $n \approx 0.4$; this value should depend on the degree of drying and on the rate of dehydration of the polymer.

Apparently, linearization of the polymer molecules, breaking of the irregular intramolecular and intermolecular AG–AG interactions, intramolecular structuring of each PAA molecule, and intermolecular structuring of the molecules 'filled' with water proceed as a result of the further water-vapor sorption. Note that straightening of the polymer globules in concentrated solutions of polymers with reorientation of the molecules and formation of aggregates or bundles, which contain polymer molecules packed parallel or almost parallel to each other, has been previously described (Kargin, 1962; Flory, 1962); such aggregates are considered as the germs of crystal phases. Figure 3 allows understanding a possible way to formation of the intermediate clathrate-like hydrate structure. This figure corresponds to $n = 2$.

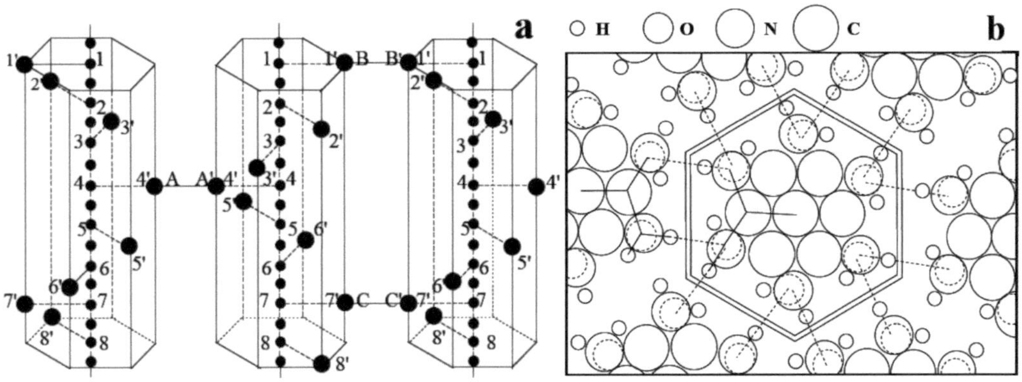

Fig. 3. Presumed intermediate clathrate-like structure for PAA·$2H_2O$.
(a) Longitudinal section: vertical rows of numerals denote the tertiary C-atoms of the main chains of the PAA molecules; primed numerals denote the centers of the AGs; AA', BB', and CC' segments denote the AG–AG bonds.
(b) Cross-section: double line restricts the area of the cross-section for a PAA molecule; dashed lines denote hydrogen O····H–N bonds binding the central PAA molecule with the neighboring ones; solid lines denote an example of H-binding of two neighboring AGs of the adjacent PAA molecules.

At the next step of water-vapor sorption, H_2O sorption occurs around each AG; therewith, the AG–AG bonds weaken and the AG-H_2O bonds harden gradually. In this period, the difference between the differential molar heat of H_2O vapor sorption in the PAA–H_2O system and the molar heat of water vapor condensation at the pure-water surface is determined by the difference between the molar heat consumption, which decreases with the degree of watering (because the AG–AG bonds become weaker with the degree of watering), and the molar heat liberation, which varies with the degree of watering following an unknown law. In Fig. 2e, it is seen that the differential heat of H_2O vapor sorption varies in a complicated way near the heat of water condensation and becomes equal to the heat of condensation at $n > (17 \div 18)$. This n value corresponds to the formation of hydrate structure II.

Figure 2b shows that water-vapor sorption from the air of almost 100% humidity terminates or, at least, moderates critically at the same n value, $n \approx 18$. It is seen that this result was reproduced with two PAA samples. The procedure of this experiment is simple; it is illustrated by Fig. 2a. Similar experiments showed that the approximately constant rates of H_2O-vapor sorption by glycine and alanine measured under the same conditions decreased by a factor of several units after $n \approx 20$ (Kadyshevich & Ostrovskii, 2007).

The results presented in this section, apparently, give grounds for the following conclusions. At the temperature about 290 K, at which the above described measurements were performed, PAA tends to hydrate formation in highly-concentrated semi-liquid aqueous systems. Specific H_2O sorption proceeds up to a water content of 17÷18 H_2O molecules per one AG. Only after achievement of such a composition of the system, water sorbs with the molar heat effect equal to the heat of H_2O condensation at the surface of pure water.

An analogous but less pronounced phenomenon is observable at water-vapor sorption by amino-acids. Most likely, the phenomenon of formation of hydrate structures around functional groups of monomers and around such molecules as amino-acids and other biologically important molecules in highly concentrated semi-liquid aqueous systems is more pronounced at lower temperatures. Unfortunately, such systems are difficult-to-study because of low rate of usual chemical processes at lower temperatures. However, the smallness of the rate doesn't stay in the way of a number of natural processes; moreover, the smallness of the rates creates the conditions when the processes could proceed selectively from one product to another and could strictly follow the sequence of gradual decreasing in the free energy of the reacting system from step to step.

2.2.2 The H_2O content in sperm as a criterion of structuring in DNA–H_2O systems

According to Josse et al. (1961), at 92% humidity, the DNA sample contained 147 parts of H_2O per 100 parts of DNA (the same data are given by others (Feughelman et al., 1955; Wilkins, 1961)). This content corresponds to 101 H_2O molecules per DNA fragment of composition $C_{39}N_{15}O_{24}P_4H_{49}$, which weigh 0.20516×10^{-20} g and contain two pairs of deoxyribose-phosphate groups and two pairs of H-bound bases (Th–Ad and Cy–G). However, there is no evidence that the H_2O-to-DNA ratio (Josse et al., 1961) corresponds to the equilibrium value; in addition, it is evident that the environmental humidity *in vivo* is close to 100%, and, thus, the H_2O content in DNA must be significantly higher than that in Wilkins (1961). Nevertheless, even the H_2O content of DNA samples reported by Wilkins (1961) contradicts the assumption that the equilibrium DNA structure *in vivo* is described by the Watson–Crick model (W–C model). Indeed, as shown below, the size of structural voids in the W-C model is too small to accommodate the above-mentioned water amount. According to the W–C model, the volume of the above mentioned DNA fragment is equal to $0.68 \cdot (1.29)^2 = 3.555$ nm^3. The value 1.29 nm is the radius of the cylinder occupied by a double helix within the sample and is equal to the sum of the half-distance between the P atoms (1.0 nm), P–O distance (0.154 nm), and the V-d-W radius of the O-atom (0.136 nm). The 0.68 nm is twice the distance between the N-bases. A void of volume of 3.555 nm^3 can accommodate only 118.8 H_2O molecules at a density of 1.0 g/cm^3. Actually, most of this void is occupied by the 131 atoms of the $C_{39}N_{15}O_{24}P_4H_{49}$ fragment of DNA. Therefore, the maximum H_2O content in the DNA fragment under consideration is much lower than 101 molecules. This means that, in order to accommodate the number of molecules that corresponds to the density measured by Josse et al. (1961), DNA must be packed more loosely than the W–C model predicts.

The point is that, the data on the parameters of the inter-molecular Cy–G and Th–Ad H-binding are based on the XRD studies of samples of crystal DNA (Arnott et al., 1965). It is common practice to apply such data for characterization of the DNA *in vivo,* although the validity of their extension to the equilibrium DNA state in the aqueous solutions is under question. This fact is important because the DNA molecule as a whole and its individual functional groups undoubtedly have a high affinity to water. According to Wilkins (1961), the procedure applied to the preparation of the samples studied in Arnott et al. (1965) by XRD provided 95–100% humidity. However, there is no direct evidence that the equilibrium was established before these measurements and was not violated during their performance. For example, in Josse et al. (1961), there is no evidence of the absence of H_2O desorption from sperm samples during their preparation and XRD measurements.

Meanwhile, our experiments (Ostrovskii & Tsurkova, 1997, 1998a, 1998b; Ostrovskii et al., 2000, 2001) with the PAA–H_2O system led us to the following conclusions. The approach of the system to the equilibrium is very slow: within 30 days, a sample of dry polymer sorbs only one-third of the equilibrium H_2O amount; the establishment of the complete equilibrium takes about a year. On the other hand, H_2O desorbed intensely from the equilibrium system when the atmospheric humidity decreased or when the system was heated by 1–2 K. Meanwhile, water influences significantly the structural parameters; according to Wilkins et al. (1953) and Wilkins (1961), the helix axis length per pair of N-bases increases with wetting from 0.255 nm in the A-form to 0.34 nm in the B-form. As was noted (Josse et al., 1961), the H_2O amounts in the DNA and nucleoprotein samples are not in agreement with the structure proposed. At a relative humidity of 92%, the densities of nucleic acid and nucleoprotein lie between 1.34 and 1.39 g/cm^3. Taking those molecules as distributed in water of a density of 1.0 g/cm^3, the authors obtained theoretical densities of 1.26 and 1.33 g/cm^3 (and H_2O contents of 147 and 85 weight parts per 100 weight parts of nucleic acid) for the samples of nucleic acid and nucleoprotein, respectively. The authors (Josse et al., 1961) explained this discrepancy by assuming that nucleic acid filaments were not well-crystallized and, therefore, the amorphous areas were characterized by a lower degree of hydration in comparison with crystalline areas. However, they did not substantiate this assumption. In our opinion, the equilibrium H_2O content is determined by the total content of hydrophilic groups, whereas the degree of crystallinity of the initial sample could influence only the rate of approach to the equilibrium in a humid medium.

After the work by Zimmerman & Pheiffer (1979), an opinion existed that the number of base pairs per turn of the DNA helix is the same in solids and in solutions. However, this work does not contain data sufficient for such a conclusion. First, the polarized-light technique applied in the work is insufficient to exclude the occurrence of bunches of very small diameters ranging within several tens of nanometers and is inapplicable to concentrated solutions. Second, the contact of the DNA fiber with water is too short-term to postulate that the equilibrium wetting of the DNA molecules is achieved and no data confirming the DNA–H_2O equilibrium (i.e., correlation with the DNA-to-H_2O ratio in sperm) are presented. The experiment does not reveal the amount of water actually bound with the DNA molecules. Meanwhile, at the first step of wetting, waters quickly elevate into the phase of DNA as a result of the capillary effect and an H_2O portion not bound with the DNA molecules might exist around them. Subsequent hydration proceeds slowly, since the process is limited by the rate of water diffusion in the thin capillary. Hydration of the phosphate groups of DNA proceeds apparently rather fast. This is caused by the fact that each positively polarized P-atom is located in the center of a tetrahedron formed by negatively polarized O-atoms and movable water dipoles neutralize O-atoms with a significant gain in energy. This process disperses the fiber DNA helixes from each other over the capillary cross-section. However, the equilibrium hydration of the DNA helixes should also include hydration of the N-bases by liquid water. This process is extremely slow and the equilibrium is being established for several months (Ostrovskii et al., 2000, 2001). Slowness of hydration of the $-NH_2\cdots O=$ bonds is caused by the steric hindrances and smallness of the energy gain for this process (Ostrovskii et al., 2000, 2001). Therefore, we think that the equilibrium hydration could not be achieved in the experiments of Zimmerman & Pheiffer (1979). This consideration shows that the conclusion of these authors on the equality of the number of the base pairs per one helix turn for solid and dissolved DNA has no ground.

It is commonly supposed that the B-DNA double helix characterizes the DNA state in living matter. However, its structural parameters obtained in different works differ noticeably. For example, values of 10.6 ± 0.1 (Rhodes & Klug, 1980), 10.4 ± 0.1 (Wang, 1979), 10.1 (Drew et al., 1980), and 9.95 (Zimmerman & Pheiffer, 1979) were obtained for the number of the purine and pyrimidine bases corresponding to the full turn of the double helix. Such a scatter in these values is too wide for works on specification of the structural parameters, and the nature of this scatter requires a special discussion.

The numerous experimental and calculated data considered above show that the DNA structure in the natural semi-liquid highly-concentrated aqueous systems depends on the H_2O concentration, that the water content in the crystal DNA samples used for specification of the DNA structure is much less than the water content in sperm, and that, therefore, the actual DNA structure differs from the well-known W-C model.

A new understanding of the H_2O effect in biological processes was proposed on the basis of the assumption on the principal role of water structuring and de-structuring around individual groups of biologically important substances in highly-concentrated semi-liquid H_2O-substrate systems (Ostrovskii & Kadyshevich, 2000, 2002). We paid attention to the surprising agreement between the sizes of the individual functional groups of the DNA (and RNA) molecules and the free sizes of the gas-hydrate structural cavities.

Figures 4b and 4e illustrate the size agreement between the large and small cavities of structure II and the N-bases and phosphate groups of DNA molecules, respectively. Each of these figures is given in scale. The sizes of ribose groups allow their housing within either small or large cavities. Final conclusion on the best agreement between the ribose size and the size of one of the kinds of these cavities should be made on the basis of the three-dimensional PC modeling.

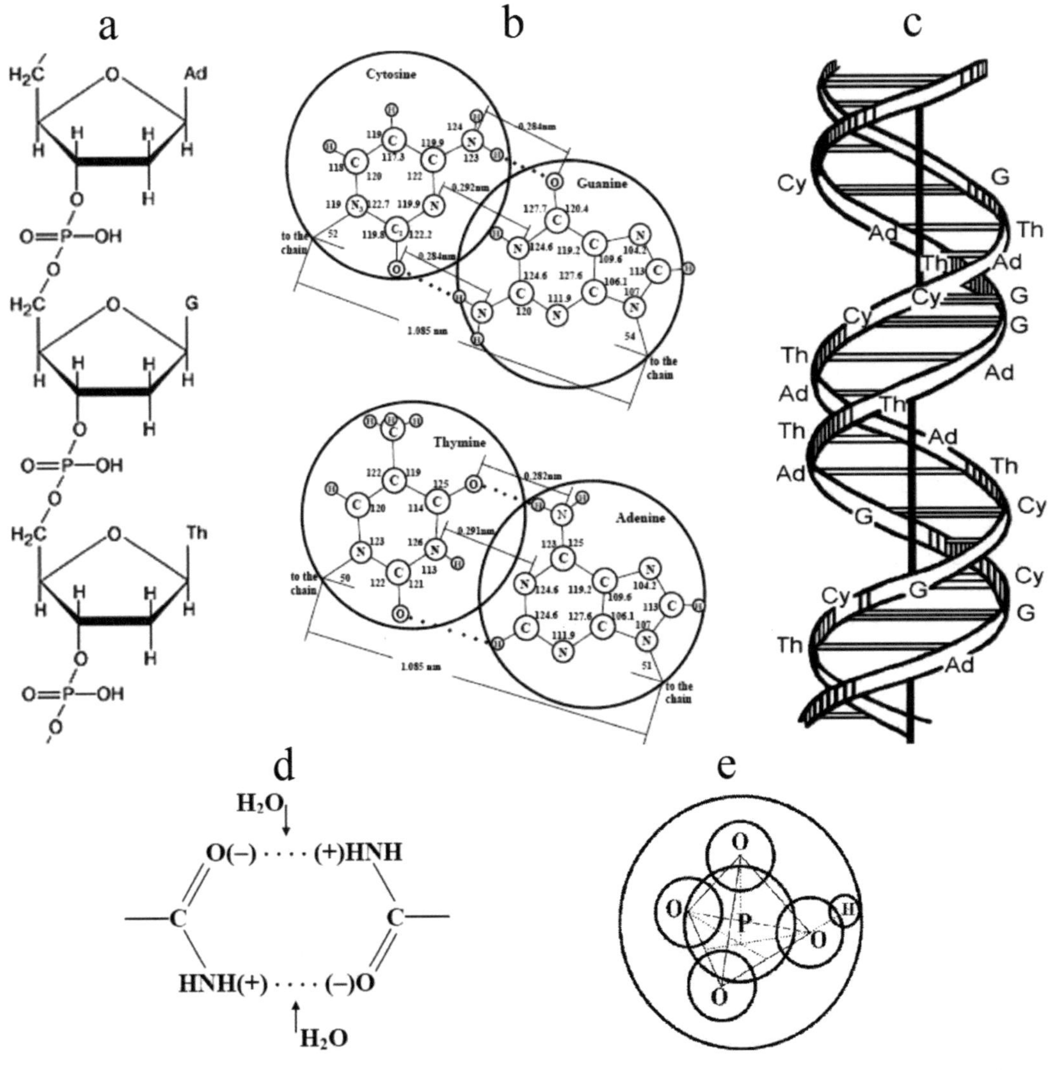

Fig. 4. (a) Fragment of a single DNA molecule; (b) scaled schematic representation of pairing between N-bases of two DNA molecules in the double helix structure; the valence angles are given in degrees, circles of diameter 0.69 nm correspond to the free diameter of the large cavity in the hydrate structure II; (c) schematic representation of a double-helix fragment formed by two DNA molecules; (d) scaleless scheme of AG–AG pairing of two adjacent PAA molecules; (e) scaled schematic representation of a phosphate group inside a small cavity of hydrate structure II (a circle of diameter 0.48 nm corresponds to the free diameter of the small cavity).

In Ostrovskii & Kadyshevich (2000, 2002), the following concept for the semi-liquid highly-concentrated structure of DNA-H_2O systems was developed. Each helix segment containing two pairs of N-bases can be housed in a volume of 5.268 nm^3 including 8 large and 16 small cavities of hydrate structure II formed by 136 water molecules. At the DNA-water equilibrium *in vivo*, hydrate structure II, whose large cavities are filled with fragments of

DNA, is formed. This structure corresponds to a complete neutralization of the affinity of DNA molecules with respect to each other. Therefore, when water penetrates into the equilibrium system from the outside, the double helix gradually unwinds and the DNA molecules begin to push off each other.

We calculate the DNA structure and the DNA-H_2O system density to have a possibility for their comparison with the available data. To compute the structural characteristics of the equilibrium state, we consider the transformation of the B-form of DNA (Wilkins, 1961), which we regard as nonequilibrium. The full diameter of the double helix of DNA (2.58 nm) is obtained by adding the distance between the axes of P atoms of two complementary DNA molecules (2.00 nm, (Wilkins, 1961)), the doubled O=P bond length (0.308 nm), and the doubled V-d-W oxygen radius (0.272 nm). Then, with a knowledge of the helix step (3.4 nm, (Wilkins, 1961)), we compute the helix length (the planar evolvent of the helix) per nitrogen base (0.879 nm). The following computations are performed by the method of successive iterations under the assumption that wetting of the B-form up to equilibrium does not change the helix diameter, but only increases the helix step. Varying the helix step, we compute the volume of the double helix, the number of pairs of nitrogen bases, and the number of large cavities in hydrate structure II per helix convolution. Then, we perform the iteration procedure up to a helix step corresponding to the 1/4 ratio between the number of large cavities and the number of pairs of N-bases. This computation is the critical point in our analysis. The resultant number of pairs of nitrogen bases per helix convolution is equal to 11.25. This value corresponds to a helix step of 5.67 nm and to 5.627 unit cubic cells of hydrate structure II per helix convolution. Our computation of the density of the equilibrium DNA–H_2O system gives a value of 1.161 g/cm^3. This result is significantly lower than a density of 1.34–1.39 g/cm^3 measured by Feughelman et al. (1955) for DNA wetted under nonequilibrium conditions. The application of the above-described notions of the DNA structure to the samples (Wilkins, 1961) characterized by 10 pairs of nitrogen bases per helix convolution, a helix step of 3.4 nm, and an above-specified diameter of 2.58 nm, gives a density value of 1.351 g/cm^3. Unlike the density reported by Wilkins (1961) (1.28 g/cm^3), which is based on the model proposed by Crick & Watson (1954), the value 1.351 g/cm^3, which we obtained based on our model, correlates well with the density of 1.34–1.39 g/cm^3 of the samples used by others (Watson & Crick, 1953; Crick & Watson, 1954; Feughelman et al, 1955) to formulate ideas about DNA structure. The density is calculated as the sum of the water and DNA contributions. Apparently, this calculation shows that the notion on the DNA–H_2O highly-concentrated media as on structured semi-liquid systems is justified, at least, no less than any other idea aimed at understanding such complicated and simple natural phenomenon as life. It is important that the notion on an equilibrium H_2O content in DNA–H_2O systems is a conventional one. The case is that it can be achieved only in the isolated DNA-H_2O systems under 100% humidity. Actually, when nutrients diffuse into a system, no equilibrium can be reached because the DNA molecules are at different steps of mitosis and the major portion of them are not completely watered.

Thus, at this step of our review, at least four statements weigh heavily the importance and, possibly, fundamental significance of the phenomenon of hydrate formation in the totality of the natural processes, which has the collective name "life".

1. No living matter exists in waterless media, and some other elements are necessary for its origination and existence; therewith, waters always tend to form hydrate structures within a narrow range of natural conditions when waters and other molecules are

already movable sufficiently to diffuse taking the thermodynamically-preferable positions and when other molecules, which are more chemically active, are already capable to react chemically with each other but have still so small reactive ability that they pass step-by-step all thermodynamically-possible steps of their chemical interaction until the heat of these reactions, diffusion of excessive water from outside, or any external phenomena or processes destroys the hydrate structures.

2. The sizes of individual functional groups of DNA (and RNA) coincide almost entirely with the free sizes of the cavities of hydrate structure II (until the special three-dimensional PC analysis is finished, we do not exclude that the hydrate structure H is also appropriate).
3. The results of sorption–desorption and calorimetric experiments weigh heavily the hydrate structure formation in the PAA–H_2O system at about 290 K.
4. The assumptions on the existence of the hydrate structure in the sperm–water system and on an unwinding (and "stretching" along the surface of the cylinder of constant diameter) of the DNA double helixes with wetting lead to realistic values of the DNA–H_2O-system density.

We will see somewhat later that, in fact, a number of other statements also count in favor of the significance of the hydrate-formation phenomenon for the processes that are under consideration in this review.

3. Life origination hydrate hypothesis (LOH-hypothesis)

3.1 Principal content of the LOH-hypothesis

According to the LOH-hypothesis, the LMSEs and proto-cells originated and, possibly, originate in our days from CH_4 (or other CH_4-hydrocarbons), niter, and phosphate under the Earth's surface or seabed within honeycomb structures of hydrocarbon hydrates. It is well known that CH_4 (and also aliphatic, alicyclic, and aliaromatic compounds) is capable of interacting with nitrate ions under pressure, yielding different organic substances (M. Konovalov's reaction, 1888 (Konovalov, 1893)). The underground deposits of CH_4 and other hydrocarbons could result from the reaction between H_2 and CO_2; CO_2 could be produced from carbonates as a result of their thermal decomposition induced by the gravitational compression of the young-Earth crust (Ostrovskii, 2010). Hydrogen could be desorbed from the solid aggregates of which the young Earth was composed; these aggregates had adsorbed H_2 from nebula before they were captured by the Earth's gravitational force in the period of the Earth origination as a planet body (Ostrovskii & Kadyshevich, 2007, 2008). Thus, the living-matter sources are H_2, carbonates, nitrates, and phosphates, which resulted from transformation of the nebula. The nebula that was the progenitrix for the Solar System arose after the supernova explosion (Kadyshevich & Ostrovskii, 2010b).

The LOH-hypothesis allows for answering the following questions (Kadyshevich & Ostrovskii, 2009, 2010c, 2010d; Ostrovskii & Kadyshevich, 2010, 2011). (1) In what phase did the LMSEs form? (2) From what substances did the LMSEs form? (3) By what mechanism did the N-bases, riboses, and nucleosides form? (4) Is Nature capable of synthesizing LMSEs from minerals with no external energy? (5) How had methane hydrate originated? (6) How did CH_4 and NO_3^- meet? (7) Why no substance but NO_3^- reacted with CH_4-hydrate? (8) How did DNA- and RNA-like molecules form from nucleosides? (9) Is there a relation between DNA and RNA formation, on the one hand, and the atmosphere composition, on the other hand? (10) Why do only five chemical elements usually enter the DNA and RNA composition? (11) Why are N-bases entering DNA and RNA similar in their composition and structure? (12) Why are N-bases and riboses limited in size? (13) Why are N-bases not identical? (14) Why do only five N-bases usually enter the DNA and RNA composition and why do other N-bases, such as X (xanthine), sometimes enter the DNA and RNA compositions? (15) Could DR, DDR, Th, and U exist simultaneously in a reaction mixture containing CH_4 and niter? (16) How had it happened that the sequences of N-bases in DNA and RNA molecules are not random? (17) Why did Nature choose DR and DDR, but not their L-enantiomers or mixtures of enantiomers for DNA and RNA syntheses? (18) How did proto-cells originate?

3.2 Several answers to the questions on living matter origination

Each of the above-listed questions is answered with comments in Ostrovskii & Kadyshevich (2007) and Kadyshevich & Ostrovskii (2009). Short answers on some of the questions are given in the first paragraph of Section 3.1. Several questions will be considered below.

First, let us dwell on question (4). The reaction of formation of the full set of N-bases and DR necessary for origination of an RNA molecule can be written in the form

$$a_1KNO_3 + a_2C_nH_m = a_3U + a_4Ad + a_5Cy + a_6G + 4DR + a_1KOH + a_7H_2O + a_8N_2, \quad (1)$$

where C_nH_m is the formula of a source aliphatic hydrocarbon and $a_1 \div a_8$ are the stoichiometric coefficients (therewith, the stoichiometric coefficients for KNO_3 and KOH are the same). (We showed by a thermodynamic consideration that, in the equilibrium system, the occurrence of U and DR means the occurrence of Th and DDR in the system (Kadyshevich & Ostrovskii, 2009)). Equation (1) shows how many molecules of each of the source substances are consumed and how many molecules of each of the products are produced counting on 4 DR molecules in the average over the chain. This equation corresponds to the situation when oxygen of niter reacts completely; i.e., O_2 is not produced. The calculations performed for the sets characterized by different r values ($r = (a_3 + a_4) / (a_5 + a_6)$) allow the following conclusions. The changes in the Gibbs free energy for the reactions of niter with CH_4, C_2H_6, C_3H_8, C_2H_4, and C_3H_6 are negative and rather great in magnitude and vary only slightly with the r value. For example, the Δ_iG^0 values for the reaction between niter and methane at $r = 0.0625$, 1.00, and 16.0 are equal to (kJ/mol) −8227, −8281, and −8336, respectively, and the Δ_iG^0 values for the reaction between niter and ethane at $r = 0.0625$, 1.00, and 16.0 are equal to −6050, −6104, and −6159, respectively. These results mean that the LMSEs could originate from methane hydrocarbons and niter at the expense of the internal energy of the source substances and that thermodynamics allows wide variations in relative yields of N-bases. Different sets of N-bases could originate in different historical periods in any one region or in any one historical period in different regions of the globe.

Our estimations are performed for the standard conditions. However, the Δ_iG^0 values for the reactions under consideration are so high in magnitude that there are no doubts that these reactions are feasible within the phases of hydrocarbon hydrates under real conditions.

CH_4 was captured by the Earth in the period of planet formation or was produced in intra-terrestrial reservoirs filled with the heated ($H_2 + CO_2$) mixtures by the following reaction (Ostrovskii & Kadyshevich, 2007; Kadyshevich & Ostrovskii, 2009):

$$4\,H_2(g) + CO_2(g) = CH_4(g) + 2\,H_2O\,(lq) \quad (2)$$

The change in the standard Gibbs energy for this reaction is rather high in magnitude and is equal to −130.6 kJ/mol; i.e., the reaction should proceed up to almost complete consumption of one of the source gases under rather wide variations in the reaction parameters. With time, the exothermal process of Earth's crust compacting was decaying and the Earth's crust was cooling. This phenomenon favored formation of CH_4-hydrate (and hydrates of other hydrocarbons) within underground reservoirs. Near some of the CH_4-hydrate deposits, niter deposits are located, for example, along the west coast of Central and South America. Apparently, the niter deposits were still more abundant in the Arhean period, because niter is H_2O-soluble. In the regions characterized by neighboring locations of CH_4-hydrate and niters, NO_3^--ions diffused into the CH_4-hydrate structures and reacted with methane.

CH_4 is a rather inert substance, and, under conditions of CH_4-hydrate stability, very few minerals are capable of interacting chemically with it. The CH_4-hydrate structure as if "swallows" selectively the NO_3^--ions and converts them to N-bases and riboses. Diffusion of NO_3^--ions into the structure is stimulated by the decrease in the Gibbs free energy in the process of chemical interaction of NO_3^- with CH_4. A similar situation arises when phosphate ions enter in contact with the hydrate structure filled with nucleosides. The foreign atoms rarely entering the DNA and RNA compositions in addition to C, N, P, O, and H come from the walls of the reservoirs filled with CH_4-hydrate, from admixtures to source CH_4 and H_2O, etc.

The sizes of each of the LMSEs were limited by the sizes of the cavities. The close agreement between the sizes of individual groups of DNAs and RNAs, on the one hand, and the free sizes of the cavities, on the other hand, testifies for this assumption (Fig. 4b, e). The large cavities are as if "moulds" for N-bases, and the small cavities are as if "moulds" for phosphate groups. As was mentioned above, riboses can be housed in small or large cavities. (The large cavities of structure H are somewhat "more roomy" than those of structure II, and we cannot exclude that structure H is the matrix for LMSE formation). Just the sizes of the structural cavities limit growing of the functional groups. They are similar because their formation proceeds from the same substances, in the cavities of the same size, slowly, step-by-step, decreasing the Gibbs energy over the entire CH_4-hydrate localization up to full filling of the cavities. The entire localization reaches its final state by the same time. N-bases are similar but not identical, and the cause of their nonidentity is as follows. Let one of the cavities be completely filled with a purine base in such a way that the atomic V-d-W radii of this N-base overstep the boundary of this cavity. In this case, the neighboring cavity should contain an N-base of a smaller size, because the distance between any two atoms of adjacent molecules should exceed the sum of their V-d-W radii.

Apparently, just the thermodynamics is instrumental in selection of N-bases to be further incorporated in the composition of nucleic acids. This opinion can be illustrated by the reaction between G and H_2O with formation of xanthine (X) and NH_3. For this reaction, $\Delta(G^0)$ = +7.32 kJ/mol. This value shows that, in a system, where reactions proceed in the vicinity of 273 K and so slowly that the equilibrium relations between reacting components keep constant in time, G should usually prevail over X but, under some conditions, the relative amounts of the last may be noticeable. We think that this is the cause of the usual significant prevailing of G over X in the DNA molecules (Kadyshevich & Ostrovskii, 2009).

As for the DNA and RNA monochirality, we assume that it is a natural inevitable consequence of the CH_4-hydrate matrix geometry. Apparently, only D-riboses are capable to "touch" both, an N-base and a phosphate group; this structural feature leads to the

consumption of the D-forms and to the shift of the equilibrium to formation of just D-molecules. This assumption should be verified by three-dimensional computer simulation.
The LMSEs formed within the structural cavities reacted with each other with formation of nucleosides. After diffusion of phosphates into the structure, the DNA- and RNA-like molecules formed. Then, as water, niter, and phosphates diffused into the system, the structure liquidized and transformed into a structured soup in which the simplest living organisms began the long history of their development and expansion over the world.
By analogy with the cellular cytoplasm, we term this soup super-cytoplasm. In the super-cytoplasm, all the substances necessary for the existence and development of the primary DNA- and RNA-like substances could be synthesized on the basis of CH_4 and of phosphates and niters that diffused from the environment. We have already cited articles in which nucleic acids were shown to self-replicate (Orgel, 1992, 2000; Cech & Bass, 1986; Li & Nicolaou, 1994). Under appropriate conditions, this led to an increase in the concentrations of nucleic acids and organophosphorous substances within the super-cytoplasm. Increasing in the concentrations to a certain critical level led to precipitation of phosphor-containing membranes around DNAs and to origination of proto-cells. Thus, in addition to the super-cytoplasm, intracellular cytoplasm appeared. After that, nucleic acids began to develop and replicate inside the cells and the cells began to divide similarly to the cells of the present prokaryotes. This assumed mechanism is described in more detail elsewhere (Ostrovskii & Kadyshevich, 2007).
Figure 5 gives the principal scheme for living-matter origination by the LOH-hypothesis.

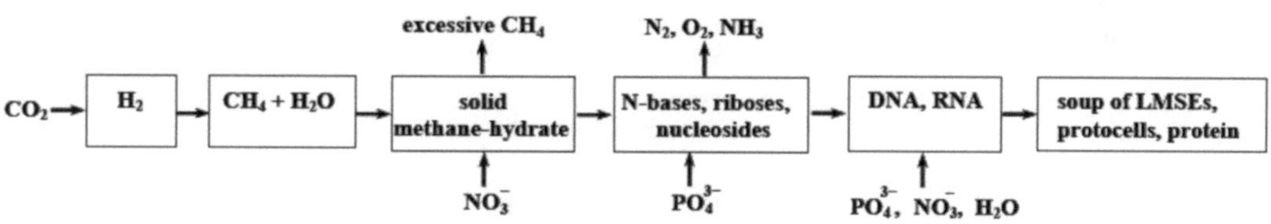

Fig 5. General hypothetical scheme of living-matter origination.

According to the LOH-hypothesis, living matter originated repeatedly. In any one localization, a multitude of different DNA- and RNA-like molecules and proto-cells could originate in the same time period, and, in different localizations, multitudes of progenitors of different species could originate in different time periods. The lengths and degrees of perfection of the DNA-like chains that originated within a hydrate structure were directly dependent on the period of their growth within an underground "incubator". Therefore, the first ancient prokaryotes appeared earlier than the eukaryotes with longer and more complicated DNA chains. New populations of both prokaryotes and eukaryotes appeared repeatedly in the Earth's history. Thus, the conclusion of Buss (1987) on the repeated originations of new species obtains a natural explanation. The LOH-hypothesis is capable of explaining the occurrence of numerous prokaryotic and eukaryotic species without Darwin's theory of evolution resulted from interspecific variations and natural selection as the leading causes of the species diversity of the prokaryotic and eukaryotic living matter. It cannot be excluded that living matter originates in our time.
In Ostrovskii & Kadyshevich (2007) and Kadyshevich & Ostrovskii (2009), it was shown that a number of natural phenomena (e.g., Schippers et al., 2005; MacDonald et al., 1996;

Davidson et al., 1986 ; Tresher et al.,1992; Oborin & Khmurchik, 2008) count in favor of this hypothesis. Menor-Salván et al. (2009) found that the repeated freezing–unfreezing cycles stimulate formation of some N-bases in urea solutions under the methane atmosphere. Apparently, this effect can be explained by hydrate-structure formation under freezing.

4. DNA replication, mitosis, and binary fission hypothesis (MRH-hypothesis)

4.1 The water state in living systems and the common physicochemical concept of DNA replication

An analysis performed by us (Ostrovskii & Kadyshevich, 2000, 2002) on the basis of available works and the data presented above led us to the following views on the water state in living systems. The processes of water structuring and de-structuring in living cells play a decisive role in the interactions of living cells with their environment. In definite periods of the cell cycle, water structuring within cells binds water diffusing into them and thus prevents excessive swelling and rupture of the cell. Namely, the intensity of water structuring is maximal when cells are "mature" and large and the danger for their rupturing is critical, while it is low when the cells are "young" and small and water diffusion from outside is not dangerous for their existence. The rate of cell swelling depends on the cell size, thickness and hydrostatic resistance of the semi-permeable membrane (plasma membrane with or without cell wall), composition of the cell interior, transport of environmental substances and metabolites, and degree of hydrate formation (of water structuring). The values of the osmotic pressure and of the Donnan effect are the external attendant integral manifestations of the exchange by waters, mineral and organic substances, and ions between living cells and their environment; the significance of artificial regulations of metabolism through variations of these effects is of common knowledge. The intracellular H_2O content varies depending on the phase of the cell cycle, and, at every instant, different cells are in different phases of the cell cycle. For ribose, phosphate groups, unpaired N-bases, and paired N-bases belonging to DNA, the *in-vivo* integral molar strength of water binding, excessive in comparison with the energy of H_2O condensation at the liquid pure-water surface, is different and depends on the degree of wetting of the corresponding functional groups of DNA. The H_2O content in a living cell at each phase of the cell cycle is strictly defined. Diffusion of excessive water into a cell leads to neutralization of the DNA–DNA interactions and moving apart of the paired DNA molecules. In water-deficient media, the DNA–DNA binding in double helixes is realized predominantly through AGs of N-bases. Decreasing in the environmental water concentration below some critical value leads to depression of the intracellular activity and to gradual degradation of the cells.

One of the phenomena that have stimulated the hypotheses considered in this section is the following one. As was mentioned above, the sizes of each of the N-bases entering the DNA and RNA molecules are equal to the free sizes of the large cavities of hydrate structure II (Fig. 4b, e). Thus, the sizes of the gas-hydrate structure II agree well with the sizes of all functional groups of DNA and RNA molecules. It is seldom that such agreements in Nature are causeless. Looks like Nature has a tea-set with "baking cups" ranged for each of the DNA and RNA functional groups.

The common physicochemical concept of replication is as follows. When waters and necessary nutrients enter continuously the system, each DNA double helix swells up to a critical (conventionally: equilibrium) state when the hydrate envelopes around the N-bases are formed completely. Under such conditions, DNA–DNA interactions are neutralized, the DNA double helix reaches its critical length, and the DNA mono-strands begin to move aside from each other, starting from their ends. The nutrients diffuse into the fresh vacancies and build a new complementary DNA molecule on each of the "orphaned" DNA mono-strands. Therewith, the newly formed N-bases displace waters because, at small degree of watering, the AG–AG bond is stronger than the AG–H_2O bond. After formation of two new DNA mono-strands, each paired with the corresponding maternal mono-strand, i.e., upon formation of two daughter double helixes, new waters diffuse to the AG–AG bonds. These waters weaken and destroy the AG–AG bonds, because excessively-watered hydrate structures are unstable. The newly-formed DNA double helixes move aside from each other. After that, the process repeats itself, but it includes now two daughter double helixes instead of the maternal one.

4.2 The processes of DNA replication and of formation of new cells in more detail

The present generally-accepted notion on the DNA-replication and mitosis mechanisms is formulated, to a great extent, on the basis of the light micrographs corresponding to different phases of the cell cycle (see, e.g., Oparin, 1927; Alberts, 2002). The NMR method gives no possibility to determine the sizes of different minor details, the special benefits of the confocal laser scanning microscopes against the non-laser optical microscopes are not principal for size measurements, and methods requiring treatment of samples by vacuum, hard radiation, or freezing give no possibility for controlling the temporal variations in sizes of cell components in living matter. As for the light micrographs, they, on frequent occasions, cannot be explained unambiguously. The point is that the maximum degree of magnification of light microscopes is limited by light diffraction, and the resolution of the best classic optical microscopes is no more than 200 nm. This means that an object of 200 nm in diameter is seen under microscopes as a point, which can be detailed by no photographic or PC means. Meanwhile, the C–C bond is about 0.15 nm; i.e., the carbon chain consisting of 1300 atoms or a graphite plane consisting of about $1.7 \cdot 10^6$ atoms is seen as a point, and the attempts to use PC software for revealing the interior structures of such points are questionable. Moreover, the light microscopes give almost no information on the intracellular transformations proceeding in the interphase covering about 90% of the cell-cycle period. Thus, the micrographs give limited information for estimating the comparative variations in the form and density of chromosomes in the course of the observable portion of cell cycles; however, they give no grounds for description of chromosome details smaller than 1300 atoms in length or $1.7 \cdot 10^6$ atoms in plane. Meanwhile, the examples of excessive insubstantial detailing of the chromosome-transformation phases are available in literature and can lead to erroneous views on the degree of clarification of the real mechanisms of intracellular processes if these views are presented as results of analyses of micrographs rather than as authors' suppositions.

Below, we propose a hypothetical physicochemical explanation for some processes proceeding in the course of mitosis and DNA replication. Our MRH-hypothesis relates to the maternal function of cells rather than to their function as a chemical factory producing organic materials. In this connection, we do not consider the outside–cell transport of organic substances and minerals and the chemical content of the intracellular reactions. We believe that a number of phenomena observable during mitosis and interphase can be explained on the basis of well-known physicochemical regularities inherent in the processes of continuous water diffusion into cells, formation and destruction of hydrate structures around N-bases belonging to the DNA molecules, and variations in the water concentration and precipitation and dissolution of organic substances in the cytoplasm.

In order for any chemical process to proceed in a fluid medium and to produce a desired product, the following conditions should be fulfilled: (1) the thermodynamics should allow proceeding of this process; (2) the concentrations of the reactants should be rather high; (3) the steric hindrances should not be insuperable; (4) the temperature should be rather high in order for the molecular mobility to be provided; (5) the rate of formation of the desired product should be higher than the rate of its subsequent transformations if the last are possible; and (6) no one of the source reactants should be consumed in any side reaction before its action in the desired reaction.

As was mentioned above, DNA replication is the central phenomenon inherent in living matter. Generally speaking, cells can duplicate or not duplicate, but duplication of chromosomes is necessary for the existence of living matter and transmission of the hereditary features. Apparently, DNA replication could proceed under some conditions without mitosis. (Similar ideas were expressed earlier (Orgel, 2000; Zielinski & Orgel, 1987)). Therefore, we will consider the cycles of replication and of cell division separately. Let the replication cycle proceed from the moment of separation of sister chromatids in a mother cell and formation there of two daughter chromosomes of the first generation to the moment of separation of sister chromatids in a daughter cell and formation there of two daughter chromosomes of the second generation, and let the cell-division cycle proceed from the moment of division of the mother cell to the moment of division of the daughter cell. Thus, in our consideration, the replication cycle does not coincide with the cell-division cycle.

Water is necessary for the processes of mitosis (in the case of prokaryotes, of binary fission) and DNA replication. It diffuses (in parallel with organic and inorganic substances) into living cells continuously from the outside through the cell membrane, and, as noted above, the rate of water diffusion is time-dependent. The water structuring within cells stimulates continuous water flow into cells.

Bearing in mind six conditions formulated above in this section and the involved data presented in the previous sections, we give the hypothetical explanation for the binary fission and DNA replication processes inherent in prokaryotes and in eukaryotes and consider their common features and peculiarities.

First we apply the MRH hypothesis to prokaryotes. Prokaryotes are the simplest cellular organisms, and analyses of their cell cycle can reveal the fundamental necessary and sufficient features of metabolism purified as much as possible of side processes and phenomena that are not necessary for metabolic processes. Meanwhile, the necessary and sufficient factors of metabolism of eukaryotes may be obscured by the occurrence of some intracellular organelles, the absence of which does not exclude the principal possibility of metabolism. It is known that each of the prokaryotic cells usually has one DNA double helix termed chromosome and consisting of two circular DNA mono-strands bound together through purine–pyrimidine H-bonds. The prokaryotic cell cycle includes replication of this chromosome and binary fission of the cell.

Consider the hypothetical mechanisms of the prokaryotic replication cycle. Before separation of sister chromatids into two daughter chromosomes, H_2O-dipole layers are formed along each of two coupled circular DNA double helixes. These double helixes repulse each other by an electrostatic force, the nature of which will be explained below, and two daughter chromosomes (of the first generation) move apart to the opposite sides of the cell and take up positions in immediate proximity to the plasma membrane. Just this moment is taken by us as the onset of the replication cycle. For the intra-cellular processes to go in the strict sequence, in accordance with the stepwise decrease in the free energy over the entire volume of the intra-cellular cytoplasm, waters should penetrate slowly into each double helix, envelope the N-bases, and house them into cavities similar to those existing in gas-hydrate structure II. Just such a process is in progress after formation of the daughter chromosomes. It starts about synchronously at several different locations of the chromosome, because different locations have no preferences for water structuring (this statement will be confirmed below). The first step of this process is thermodynamically caused and is analogous to the process of H_2O sorption by PAA (Fig. 2e) under conditions when the n value is somewhat higher than unity but is significantly lower than 17; the energy gain for this process is equal to the difference between the binding energy of two neighboring N-bases belonging to different DNA mono-strands and the algebraic sum of the binding energies of waters with two N-bases and the energy of electrostatic repulsion of two newly-formed water envelopes housing the N-bases. A similar process at 100% humidity goes spontaneously (Fig. 2b); i.e., it is characterized by a negative change in the Gibbs free energy. These experimental results give grounds to assert that the process of hydration of the AG–AG bonds is associated with a very small decrease in the Gibbs free energy and proceeds slowly and that formation of a water continuum and moving of AGs from each other should be thermodynamically caused when the water surrounding of neighboring N-bases is sufficiently extended. Figure 2e shows that the difference between the molar heat effects of H_2O sorption and H_2O condensation at the liquid pure-water surface is rather small in magnitude and can be positive or negative depending on the degree of wetting of the substrate, i.e., that H_2O sorption proceeds as a result of the entropy peculiarities. Each of the daughter chromosomes sorbs water intensively and the H_2O inflow to the cell from the outside becomes inadequate for covering their water demands. Therefore, the chromosomes sorb H_2O stored in the intracellular cytoplasm. Within the cell, two opposite H_2O flows directed from the central region of the cell to the daughter chromosomes arise. Because the H_2O density exceeds the densities of organic liquids, the H_2O outflows from the central region of the cell lead to a decrease in the fullness of this cell region and to a decrease in the density of the intracellular medium in it. In addition, H_2O depletion of the central cell region results in its supersaturation by phospholipids and other polymers. These phenomena initiate formation of a cleavage furrow and precipitation of excessive lipids in the equatorial plane of the cell and result finally in cell division in two daughter cells, each containing one daughter chromosome of the first generation. Thus, the binary fission realizes. Below, we consider one of the daughter cells.

The young daughter cell is small and water-deficient. However, the "water requirement" of the daughter chromosome is already satisfied partially and, therefore, the rate of water structuring around N-bases of this chromosome is decreased. As a result, the water inflow through the plasma membrane leads to swelling of the cell. Meanwhile, the water inflow enriches the peripheral cytoplasmic layer by water, thus increasing its density, and weakens the chromosome-to-membrane cohesion. As a result, the chromosome moves into the cell central region, which is enriched (as compared to the peripheral region) with organic substances and, therefore, has a decreased density. The so-called nucleoid forms. By this, the process of water structuring around N-bases of the chromosome DNA double-strand is yet not completed; however, in some chromosome locations, the DNA–DNA interactions are already neutralized by waters and the rate of water uptaking by the chromosome is minimized. Such a situation initiates a new step of the DNA replication.

In this period, the process of construction of DNA-replicas on the basis of each mono-strand of the daughter chromosome starts. This process is stimulated by the appearance of chromosome regions where several neighboring DNA–DNA H-bonds are neutralized, i.e., by the appearance of minor primitive water-filled capillaries, and by the organic and mineral substances taken up by the cell together with the water inflow. Apparently, the process of DNA replication starts almost simultaneously at different DNA locations where the DNA–DNA H-bonds are neutralized, because the circular-chromosome locations do not differ but in the degree of hydration of the N-bases responsible for the H-binding of two DNA mono-strands. The data (Sclafani & Holzen, 2007; Kornberg & Baker, 2005; Alberts et al., 2002) showing that eukaryotic chromosomes begin to replicate in different chromosome locations simultaneously count in favor of the analogous phenomenon of multiplicity of start locations of DNA watering and subsequent replication in prokaryotes. To understand the mechanism of the replication process, the well-known peculiarities of water behavior in contact with microcapillaries or microslots (the so-called capillary condensation) and the above-given information about smallness of the difference between the energies of AG–AG, AG–H_2O, and H_2O–H_2O interactions should be taken into consideration. It is well known that capillary condensation in solid–vapor systems starts at a relative humidity below 100% depending on the capillary diameter (more exactly, on the water-meniscus curvature). For the capillaries of a definite diameter, the start of capillary condensation is determined by the water concentration or, to be precise, by the water activity. In microcapillaries, when the capillary diameter and molecular interatomic distances are of the same order of magnitude, water capillary condensation can proceed in solutions with water activity significantly lower than unity. The process similar to the capillary condensation should proceed in living cells after the step of formation of H_2O envelopes around N-bases, because this step leads to some separation of the DNA mono-strands from each other and to some unwinding of the DNA double helixes. The process of capillary condensation of H_2O promotes formation of small water continuums in the volume between N-bases of the neighboring DNA mono-strands. Formation of these H_2O continuums leads to reorientation of water dipoles forming envelopes around N-bases, to partial neutralization of their dipole moment by the H_2O continuums, and, as a result, to weakening of the binding between the water envelopes and N-bases. Under such conditions, the H-interactions between the N-bases belonging to the DNA mono-strands and the nucleotides dissolved in the cytoplasm becomes more favorable thermodynamically than the H-binding between these N-bases and their water envelopes. Therefore, the nucleotides "moor" to these DNA mono-strands and form H-bonds with them, initiating formation of two sister chromatids of the second generation (as was said above, we do not consider the chemical content and, therefore, do not consider the details of this chemical process). So long as the N-bases are not enveloped by H_2O molecules, water sorption around them occurs on the basis of thermodynamics. Therefore, the H_2O continuum moves along the DNA mono-strand, enveloping gradually the pairs of N-bases; dissolved nucleotides move together with water, destroy water envelopes, and replace them. This process continues up to the confluence of the H_2O continuums moving towards each other from the different starting locations of DNA replication. During the process of replication, the water dipoles, entering between the DNA mono-strands of the daughter chromosome of the first generation, orient along each of them in such a way that the poles of the same polarity are directed to each of the newly-formed DNA double strands. Therefore, the outer facings of the H_2O-dipole layers surrounding each sister chromatids of the second generation have the same polarity. Thus, these chromosomes are affected by a repulsive electrostatic force, which unfolds them in a "double page" and pushes them apart as soon as the centromere-like region that has arisen between the sister chromatids of the second generation is replicated. The originated daughter chromosomes of the second generation move apart to the opposite walls of the cell. The replication cycle is finished.

The process of DNA replication proceeds for a rather long period, during which the segments consisting of two DNA double helixes and of one DNA double helix coexist along any one chromosome. In such a situation, there are no principal hindrances for simultaneous hydration of the segments of both types. Thus, replication of some segments of a newly-forming chromosome can start before complete replication of its parental chromosome. Evidently, the parental chromosome is somewhere multilayer and is increased in its cross-section; just this phenomenon makes the chromosomes sufficiently thick to be visible under optical microscopes.

The distinctions between eukaryotes and prokaryotes are essential and manifold; but, as was mentioned above, we think that the fundamental physicochemical regulations controlling the DNA replication and cell division for prokaryotes and eukaryotes are the same.

Thus, we described the hypothetical physicochemical mechanism of DNA replication and cell division for prokaryotes without notions on either enzymes or genetic code (therewith, we emphasize that we do not consider the chemical content of these processes). Note in this connection that an opinion that non-enzymatic replication is conceivable in a wide range of synthetic chemical systems was expressed in a number of works (e.g., Orgel, 1992, 2000).

Now we consider the principal peculiarities of the physicochemical mechanisms for the replication and cell-division cycles inherent in eukaryotic cells. Unlike the prokaryotic cells, the eukaryotic ones contain a chromosome family and each of the chromosomes has a linear (not circular) structure. Figure 6 presents the scheme of the eukaryotic cycle of chromosome replication for one pair of daughter chromosomes of the first generation, AC and BD (Fig. 6c); the capital letters A, B, C, D, F, G, and H under each of the DNA mono-strands individualize them and allow observation of their history. In this figure, we consider the chromosome region in the vicinity of the centromere. Figures 6c and 6f correspond to the start of replication cycle 1 in a mother cell, which is symbolized by one rectangle, and to the finish of this cycle in two daughter cells, which are symbolized by two rectangles, respectively. Figs. 6a and 6b respond to the prehistory of these daughter chromosomes in the previous replication cycle 0. Figs. 6a and 6d and Figs. 6b and 6e correspond to the DNA states after cytokinesis and after prophase, respectively. The physicochemical mechanism of replication for any eukaryotic chromosome consists in the processes of enveloping of the N-bases joining together the mono-strands in the DNA double helix, some unwinding of the DNA double helix, entering of waters and dissolved nucleotides into the capillaries thus formed, formation of a water continuum, "mooring" of the nucleotides to the corresponding sites at each of two DNA mono-strands, extrusion of water by the nucleotides, movement of the water continuum and dissolved nucleotides along the DNA double strand, and gradual duplication of each DNA mono-strand. The start of these processes is thermodynamically caused by a rather high H_2O activity (i.e., by a rather high H_2O concentration) in the cytoplasm; it occurs simultaneously at different chromosome locations (Sclafani & Holzen, 2007; Kornberg & Baker, 2005; Alberts et al., 2002) including two ends of the chromosome and induces no additional strain on the DNA double helix. For example, in Alberts et al.

(2002), the following confirmation of this phenomenon for human chromosomes is given: "An average-sized human chromosome contains a single linear DNA molecule of about 150 million nucleotide pairs. To replicate such a DNA molecule from end to end with a single replication fork moving at a rate of 50 nucleotides per second would require $0.02 \cdot 150 \cdot 10^6 = 3.0 \cdot 10^6$ seconds (about 800 hours). As expected, therefore, the autoradiographic experiments

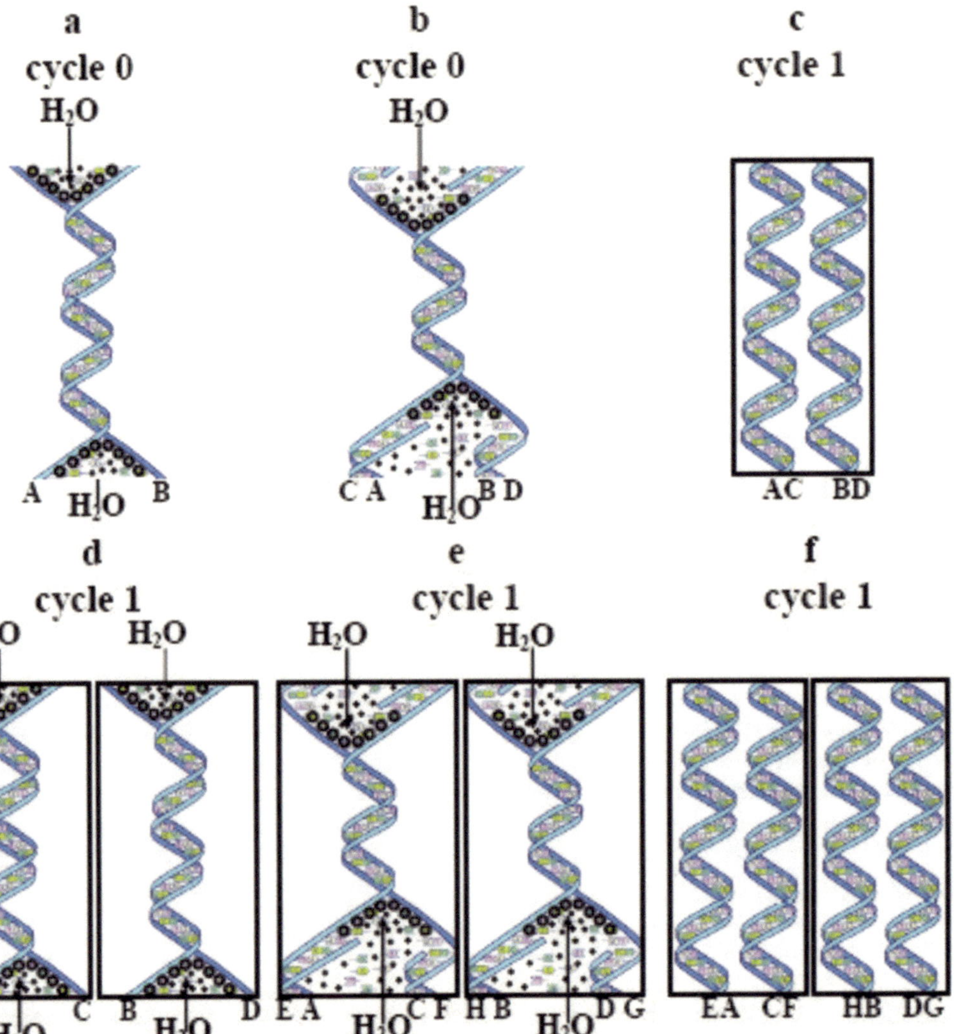

Fig. 6. Scheme of the DNA replication cycle in eukaryotic cells (in the centromere vicinity) (the letters A, B, C, D, E, F, G, and H under each of the DNA mono-strands individualize the DNA mono-strands): c–f: the replication cycle 1; c: start of replication cycle 1, late anaphase of cell cycle 1, just after chromosome dissociation along the centromere; d: replication cycle 1, just after cytokinesis of cell cycle 1; e: replication cycle 1, late prophase of cell cycle 2; f: finish of replication cycle 1, late anaphase of cell cycle 2; a: replication cycle 0, just after cytokinesis of cell cycle 0; b: replication cycle 0, late prophase of cell cycle 1; • is the water molecule, G, T, C, and A are different nucleotides; ○ is the H_2O envelope of an N-base.

... reveal that many forks are moving simultaneously on each eukaryotic chromosome." According to our views, the hydration and start of unwinding of chromosomes should proceed spontaneously and are in no want of extraneous support. Therefore, such enzymes as helicase and topoisomerase seem to be "jobless".

We consider some eukaryotic peculiarities on the basis of Fig. 7 showing schematically (not in proper scale) the chromosome sections II and III adjoining to one of the ends of the centromere I. Let A and B be the mono-strands of the chromosome under consideration. Water and nucleotides enter at the end of this chromosome between the DNA mono-strands (at the bottom of Fig. 7) and steadily move along them (in the upward direction in Fig. 7), unwinding the DNA double helix and duplicating each of the DNA mono-strands (in Fig. 7, the duplication of each of the mono-strands approaches to the boundary between the regions I and II). In the course of this process, nothing prevents duplication of the AC and BD double strands just formed; therefore, we believe that formation of new branches HB, DG, FC, and AE should begin. Later, two DNA double helixes begin to form on the basis of each of these double strands. A similar pattern occurs at the other end of the chromosome under consideration. Thus, we are of opinion that each of the DNA double helixes *in vivo* has a "branchy" structure with a rather long bare (not branchy) "stem", the central region of which is the centromere, and with branchings located at either end of this stem. We are of opinion that just such a branchy structure of the DNA double helixes and water structuring around each of their elements increase the cross-sections of chromosomes *in vivo* and make them visible under light microscopes. Two opposite fronts of DNA double-helix duplication move steadily to the centromere and shorten the chromosome section that binds the sister chromatids.

This process proceeds for so long that the central section of the centromere has time to be covered with an organic protein-like layer hampering the final separation of the sister chromatids. However, the protein-like layer eventually dissolves; the moment of dissolution terminates the replication cycle.

It was mentioned that, according to the available data, DNA replication begins at its different locations simultaneously. Therefore, it may seem strange that the centromere region is located in the vicinity of the central section of the chromosome. The MRH-hypothesis allows the following explanation of this phenomenon. The available light micrographs of living cells in early anaphase of mitosis (e.g., Davidson, 2004; Karkow, 2009) show that the central regions of chromosomes before their movement to the cell poles are located closely to each other, contrary to the end segments of these chromosomes, which are similar to two fans open widely on either side of the so-called mitotic spindle. Therefore, water and nucleotide diffusion to these central segments is hampered and their replication starts later than replication of the peripheral segments. Thus, it becomes clear why replication of the central segments terminates later than replication of the end segments.

Consider now the eukaryotic cell-division cycle, including mitosis. We consider the cell-division cycle as the time period between the moment right after cytokinesis in a cell cycle 0 (Fig. 6a) and the moment of cytokinesis in the following cell cycle 1 (Fig. 6d). The eukaryotic cell-division cycle differs fundamentally from the prokaryotic binary fission by the occurrence of a chromosome family instead of one chromosome, of a specific cell-cycle phase called interphase, and of a specific chromosome-family state termed chromatin and also by the formation of an envelope housing all newly-formed chromosomes within each newly-formed cell (the so-called nuclear envelope). Below, we describe the mechanism of the cell-division cycle, basing on the MRH-hypothesis.

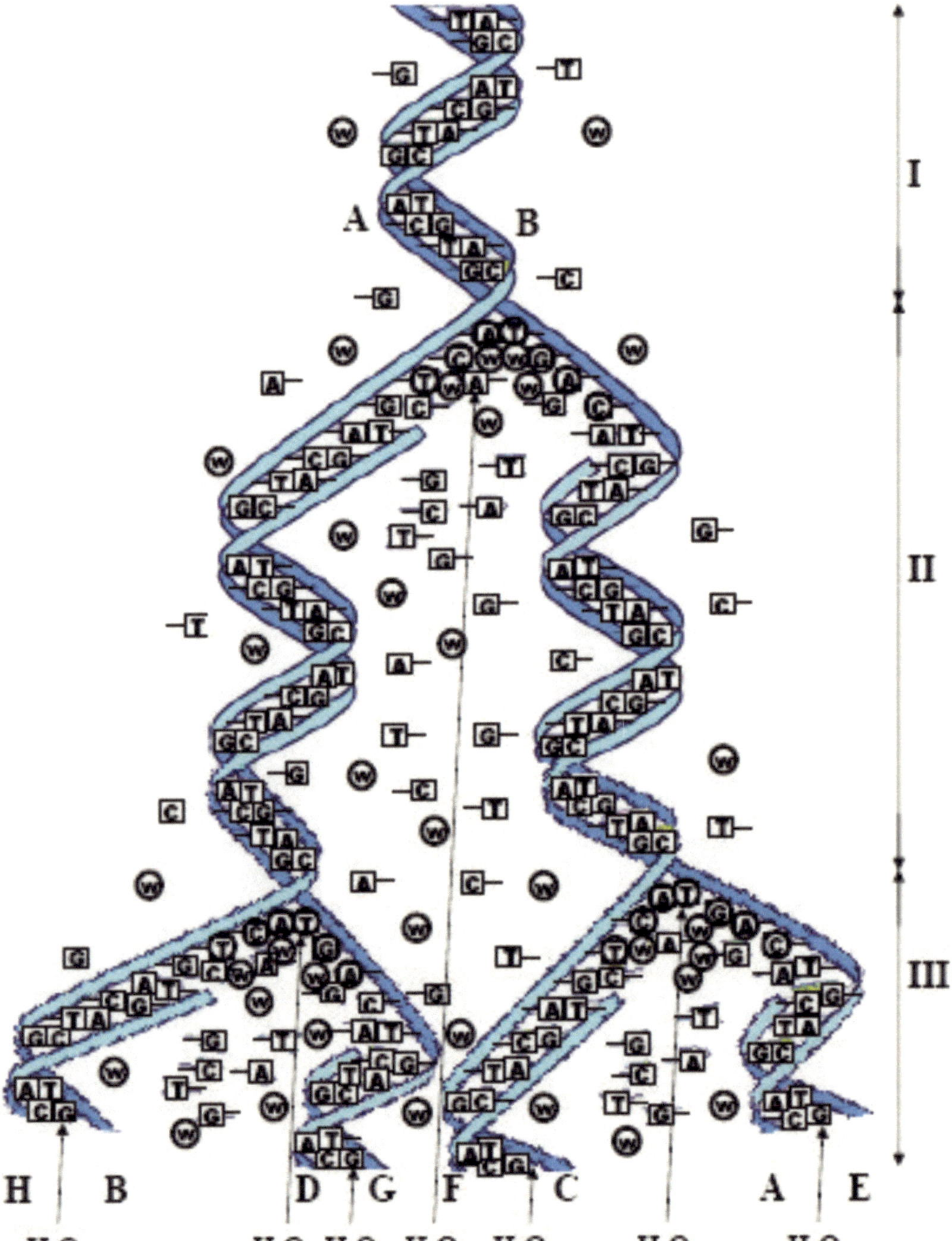

Fig. 7. Scheme of the "branchy" chromosome sections adjoining to one of the ends of the centromere: ⓦ are water molecules; for other denotations, see Fig. 6; II and III are the chromosome sections adjoining to one of the ends of centromere I.

By the beginning of the prophase, the cytoplasm is enriched with organic substances and the chromosomes are concentrated within the nuclear envelope, their end segments being duplicated. During the prophase, the chromosomes sorb H_2O and organic substances and become thicker as a result of formation of the hydrate-like structure inside double helixes, progressive duplication of their end segments, and branching. Active sorption of H_2O by the chromosomes intensifies H_2O diffusion into the cell from the outside, the H_2O concentration in the cell increases, the cell and its nucleus grow, and the nuclear envelope begins to dissolve as a result of dilution of the cytoplasm by water.

The disappearance of the nuclear envelope and formation of the so-called mitotic plate can be explained as follows. During prometaphase and metaphase, the chromosomes continue to duplicate, the H_2O concentration in the cell continues to increase, the nuclear envelope dissolves, the nucleus organics spill into the cell, the cytoplasm density in the equatorial plane of the cell decreases, and the chromosomes convene themselves in the zone of decreased density, forming the mitotic plate.

During anaphase, water continues to diffuse into the cell, the cytoplasm viscosity minimizes, chromosome replication along the centromere terminates, and each pair of sister chromatids dissociates into two daughter chromosomes moving apart to the opposite walls of the cell. Thus, two families of the newly-formed chromosomes arise. As was said above, the chromosomes are separated as a result of action of the electrostatic force induced by the H_2O-dipole layers surrounding each daughter chromosome. A number of authors (e.g., Alberts et al., 2002) hold the opinion that the daughter chromosomes move apart to the cell poles by the motors on microtubules; when a microtubule connects with the kinetochore, the motor activates, "crawls" up toward the centrosome, and the kinetochore provides separation of the sister chromatids. However, we think that this description is no more than one of the possible explanations of the observable phenomenon, because it is not clear how the microtubules learned to perform this complicated job. Besides, we refer to work (Reider et al., 2001), which claims that cells of different eukaryotic species can undergo mitosis (and interphase) without centrosomes (after their irradiation by laser); i.e., mitosis of eukaryotic cells can proceed normally without help of centrosomes. This work means that the cause-effect relation between the "motor" and movement of daughter chromosomes apart does not exist or it is opposite to the prevalent one. The prokaryotic binary fission proceeding with no developed organelles forces to be in earnest about this possibility. Apparently, the MRH-hypothesis allows simple and natural explanations for the process of separation of sister chromatids and for moving of the daughter chromosomes to the opposite cell poles.

During telophase and cytokinesis, chromosomes of each of two families are localized in opposite sides of the cell, are not connected to each other, and each chromosome sorbs water and nucleotides with minimal steric hindrances. As a result, two nuclei arise and the cell divides in two. Thus the cell cycle is complete.

In the course of telophase and cytokinesis of eukaryotic cells, a rather complicated hydrodynamic situation arises. Each family of chromosomes sucks in water from the center of the cell and from the region of the other family; in addition, H_2O diffuses into the cell from the outside, the flows being different near the chromosome families and in the central region of the cell, because each chromosome family functions as a pump and, the closer the pump, the stronger the H_2O diffusion flow; besides, the H_2O concentrations and cytoplasm compositions differ among cells. Above, when considering the mechanism of the prokaryotic binary fission, we qualitatively explained the formation of the cleavage furrow and the subsequent cell division. However, it is known that three different situations are possible in living cells: (1) the above-described situation typical for prokaryotes; (2) the situation most abundant for eukaryotes, when cytokinesis and mitosis occur in conjunction, i.e., formation of two new nuclear envelopes and of the intracellular membrane separating two new nuclei proceeds almost simultaneously; and (3) the situation observable for a number of eukaryotes, when cytokinesis and mitosis occur separately and single cells with multiple nuclei exist for a rather long time.

Apparently, each of these situations can be clarified on the basis of consideration of a rather complicated hydrodynamic problem responding to cells filled with a semi-liquid substance, the density of which varies along the cell diameter. We think that formation of the nuclear envelopes and intracellular membranes should be explained by the same phenomena of sedimentation of organo-mineral substances from oversaturated aqueous solutions under conditions when chromosomes sorb H_2O more rapidly than it diffuses into the cell from the outside. Analytical consideration of this problem is beyond this work; however, we think that all mentioned phenomena could be explained on the basis of such a physicochemical model. Evidently, the absence of nuclear envelopes in prokaryotic cells is caused by a rather high H_2O concentration in the cytoplasm during mitosis and by the occurrence of only one parental chromosome in each cell. Namely, the rate of H_2O sorption by each of the daughter prokaryotic chromosomes before binary fission is insufficient for formation of a region of oversaturated solution of organo-mineral substances around each of them. Meanwhile, the occurrence of nuclear envelopes in the cells of most species of eukaryotes is caused by a lower H_2O concentration in the cytoplasm of dividing cells and by the occurrence of a family of chromosomes in each of them. Namely, the H_2O flows directed to each of the chromosome families in a dividing eukaryotic cell are so intensive that they promote formation of regions of oversaturated solutions and precipitation of nuclear envelopes around each of the newly-formed chromosome families and subsequent formation of a similar region and precipitation of a membrane between the newly-formed nuclear envelopes. Thus, the phenomena observable in prokaryotic and eukaryotic cells can be understood on the basis of hydrodynamic considerations of the processes proceeding in aqueous solutions of organo-mineral substances whose concentrations vary near saturation conditions.

In this connection, we return to the idea that some organelles occurring in eukaryotic cells can be nothing but different organo-mineral crystals disappearing as a result of their swell and full dissolution or precipitating due to variations in the H_2O concentration in the cytoplasm. The occurrence of only primitive organelles in the cells of some prokaryotic species (Kerfeld et al., 2005) or the absence of organelles in the cells of other prokaryotic species can be, apparently, explained by the poorness of the organic composition of the prokaryotic cytoplasm and by a high H_2O concentration in it. As for such organelles as mitochondria and chloroplasts, which "live" inside eukaryotic cells and have their own DNA, their metabolism is evidently controlled by the regularities resembling those inherent in prokaryotic cells.

5. Conclusion

This chapter represents an attempt to understand the physicochemical grounds of DNA replication. Moreover, it is the first attempt to understand the processes of living matter origination and subsequent development and reproduction on the basis of one common natural phenomenon. This phenomenon is hydrate formation and destruction. Its physicochemical content is known in detail. The unique feature of this phenomenon, occurring within limited ranges of natural conditions, consists in the following. It is capable of supporting the process of chemical formation of germs of some substances with the definite sizes and very similar but identical chemical compositions and of supporting subsequent copying of these germs on the basis of diffusion of some source substances and water from outside into the system. The unique features of the hydrate phase as such consist in the facts that it is honeycomb, it is composed of the H_2O-matrix and intra-matrix guest substances, and its formation and destruction is thermodynamically supported and depends on the H_2O content in the system. Therefore, if H_2O and source substances enter the system and the guest products (chemically formed within the structural cavities) come off, the hydrate structure is capable of repeated formation and destruction with desorption of the same product.

The LOH-hypothesis differs principally from all living matter origination hypotheses previously published. These differences are not only factual but also represent an original world outlook and original philosophy. We consider the life origination process as a system of thermodynamically caused regular and inevitable chemical transformations, which are regulated by universal physical and chemical laws. We assume that living matter originated repeatedly in different localizations, and that each of them could give rise to a multitude of different living organisms. Different organisms consist of the cells that are similar in their constitution because they are built by Nature on the basis of the same mineral materials and the same physical and chemical laws.

Not proteins and not amino-acids, but the DNA and RNA molecules are the first carriers of life. Living matter originated and can originate now everywhere, where necessary minerals and necessary ambient conditions exist for long periods of time.

Our hypothesis includes an important notion on a "thermodynamic front", the temporal movement of which determines the gradual slow filling of the gas-hydrate cavities, step-by-step formation of almost the same N-bases and the same riboses within the cavities, and subsequent gradual and slow (on human life duration scale) growth and thermodynamic regularization of the DNA- and RNA-like molecules.

We also kept in mind the notion on the occurrence of a "thermodynamic front" when formulating the MRH-hypothesis. In our opinion, the same natural phenomenon of formation–destruction of hydrate structures underlies the living-matter origination and replication. However, the base lines of these two fronts pass on different levels of complexity of the source substances; if origination of the primary DNAs proceeded on the basis of simple minerals of an inorganic nature inside the matrix that contained initially only methane, replication of the DNAs in our days proceeds, in each case, on the basis of a definite primary DNA and on the basis of nutrients, which represent more complicated constructive parts. At that, just the effects of the "thermodynamic front" and of the hydrate matrix geometry create the conditions when, in the immediate vicinity of the maternal DNA mono-strand, only the mono-strand identical in its chemical composition and structure to the one that was paired with the maternal DNA mono-strand before the replication start can be formed. (The occurrence of the last effect should be verified by computer simulation.) With time and as a result of the natural selection, many of the DNAs adapted themselves to more complicated nutrients and higher temperatures as compared with those available to their archaean ancestry and their inter-replication periods became much shorter. Therewith, they learned to use only the necessary components of the nutrients for their replication, to preserve the surpluses in the form of proteins, and to throw out unusable remains. It goes without saying, the process of DNA replication is thermodynamically caused, similarly to the process of origination of the primary DNAs.

Before finishing this chapter, we consider necessary to formulate our principal opinion on the place of the so-called enzymes (and co-enzymes) in the cellular metabolism. *In corpore* consideration of the theme of enzymes is a special aim. However, we mentioned above some enzymes that, in the framework of our considerations, seem to be jobless and, therefore, we can not leave this theme without attention. Essentially, the today widely-distributed views on the intra-cellular processes connive at the occurrence of several lines of chemical interactions within each living cell. Those are, at least, interactions between DNA, enzymes, and co-enzymes; therewith, the objects of these interactions are divided in space, their chemical interactions are synchronized in time, and they diffuse to each other at a strictly determined moments, react, and go off. Up to now, no physical phenomenon that could determine these processes was proposed. Thus, all they were considered as random ones. However, the probability of the regular situations of such a kind is extremely low. In addition, many hundreds, and even thousands, of enzymes are housed within each cell and each of them is obliged to rub against DNA and to jump off giving place to another one; and all these events should proceed in a rather viscous medium characterized by a low rate of diffusion. It is quite possible that the formation–destruction of hydrate structures is just the phenomenon that is capable of providing the replication process and that the so-called enzymes or, at least, most of them are really nothing more than the initial surpluses and remains before their consolidation. Being out of living matter, some of them may be capable of catalyzing definite chemical processes under definite conditions.

The LOH-hypothesis allows for the living-world variety explanation from naturalistic positions. Each methane–niter–phosphate "incubator" yielded a great number of DNA- and RNA-like molecules close in their principal compositions but different in the sequences of the different N-bases. A great number of such "incubators" could exist during different periods at different sites of the Earth. Their occurrence on other planets cannot be excluded.

6. References

Alberts, B.; Johnson, A.; Lewis, J.; Raff, M.; Roberts, K. & Walter, P. (2002). *Molecular Biology of the Cell* (4th ed), Garland Science, Oxford, UK.

Alberty, R.A. (2003). Thermodynamics of Biochemical Reactions, Wiley, Hoboken, NJ, USA.

Arnott, S.; Wilkins, M.H.F.; Hamilton, L.D. & Langridge R. (1965). Fourier Synthesis Studies of Lithium DNA: Part III: Hoogsteen Models. *J.Mol.Biol.*, Vol. 11, No. 2, pp. 391–402.

Atwood, J.L. et al. (eds) (1996). *Comprehensive Supramolecular Chemistry.* Pergamon Press, N.Y., USA.

Blyumenfeld, L.A. (1996). Information, Thermodynamics, and the Structural Principles of Biological Systems. *Soros's Educat. J.*, No.7, pp. 88–92.

Blyumenfeld, L.A. (1981). *Problems of Biological Physics*, Springer-Verlag, Berlin.

Blyumenfeld, L.A. (2002). *Solvable and Unsolvable Problems of BiologicalPhysics*, Ch. 6. Editorial URSS, Moscow.

Boerio-Goates, J. (2005). Private communication.

Buss, L.W. (1987). *The Evolution of Individuality*, Princeton Univ. Press., Princeton, USA.

Byk, S.Sh. & Fomina, V.I. (1970). Gas Hydrates. In: *Progress in Science and Technology. Ser. Chemistry. Physical Chemistry, 1968*, VINITI, Moscow, Russia.

Carroll, J.J. (2003). *Natural Gas Hydrates: A Guide for Engineers* Amsterdam, Gulf Professional Publ., Amsterdam, Netherlands.

Chaplin, M. (2010). *Water Structure and Science.* http://www.lsbu.ac.uk/water/clathrat2.html; last updated 5 July 2010.

Clarke, E.C., Ford, R.W. & Glew, D.N., Propylene Gas Hydrate Stability. *Can. J. Chem.*, 1964, vol. 42, pp. 2027–2029.

Cech, T.R. & Bass, B.L. (1986). Biological Catalysis by RNA. *Annu. Rev. Biochem.*, Vol. 55, pp. 599–629.

Crick, F.H.C. & Watson, J.D. (1954). The Complementary Structure of Deoxyribonucleic Acid. *Proc. Roy. Soc. Lond. A*, Vol. 223, pp. 80-96.

Davidson D.W., Garg S.K., Gough S.R., Handa Y.P., Lawson W.F. et al. (1986). Laboratory Analysis of a Naturally Occurring Gas Hydrate from Sediment of the Gulf of Mexico, *Geochim. Cosmochim. Acta.*, V. 50. № 4. pp. 619–623.

Davidson, M.W. (2004). http://micro.magnet.fsu.edu/gallery/mitosis/earlyanaphase.html

Day, J.C. & Robb, I.D. (1981). Thermodynamic Parameters of Polyacrylamides in Water. *Polymer*, Vol. 22., No. 11, pp. 1530–1533.

Deamer, D.W. (1997). The First Living Systems: a Bioenergetic Perspective. *Microbiol. Mol. Biol. Rev.*, Vol. 61, No. 2, pp. 239-261.

Drew, H.; Takano, T.; Tanaka, S.; Itakura, K. & Dickerson, R. (1980). High-Salt d(CpGpCpG), a Left-Handed Z' DNA Double Helix. *Nature*, Vol. 286, No. 5773, pp. 567–573.

Fedo, C.M. & Whitehouse, M.J. (2002). Metasomatic Origin of Quartz-Pyroxene Rock, Akilia, Greenland, and Implications for Earth's Earliest Life. *Science*, Vol.296, pp.1448–1452.

Fedonkin, M.A. (2009). Eukaryotization of the Early Biosphere: a Biogeochemical Aspect. *Geochem. Intern.*, Vol. 47, No. 13, pp. 1265–1333.

Fedonkin, M.A. (2006). Two Chronicles of Living Matter. In: *Problems of geology and mineralogy*, (A.M. Pystin, ed.), Geoprint, Syktyvkar, pp. 331–350.

Feughelman, M.; Langridge, R.; Seeds, W.E.; Stokes, A.R.; Wilson, H.R.; Hooper, C.W.; Wilkins, M.H.F.; Barclay, R.K. & Hamilton, L.D. (1955). Molecular Structure of Deoxyribose Nucleic Acid & Nucleoprotein. *Nature*, Vol.175, No. 4463, pp. 834–838.

Flory, P.J. (1962). On the Morphology of the Crystalline State in Polymers. *J. Am. Chem. Soc.*, Vol. 84, No.15, pp. 2857–2867.

Galimov, E.M. (2001). *Phenomenon of Life*, Editorial URSS, Moscow, Russia.

Galimov, E.M. (2009). Concept of Sustained Ordering and ATP-related Mechanism of Life's Origin. *Int. J. Mol. Sci.*, Vol. 10., No. 5, pp. 2019-2030.

Ginsburg, G.D. & Soloviev, V.A. (1998). *Submarine Gas Hydrates*, Okeanologia, St. Petersburg, Russia, 220 p.

Ginzburg, V.L. (1999). What Problems of Physics and Astrophysics Seem Now to Be Especially Important and Interesting (Thirty Years Later, Already on the Verge of XXI Century)? *Physics-Uspekhi (Adv. Physical Sciences),* Vol. 42, No. 4, pp. 353–373.

Ginzburg, V.L. (2004). On Superconductivity and Superfluidity (What I Have and Have not Managed to Do), as Well as on the 'Physical Minimum' at the Beginning of the XXI Century. *Physics-Uspekhi (Adv. Physical Sciences),* Vol. 47, No. 11, pp. 1155–1170.

Gostev, B.V. & Ostrovskii, V.E. (1993). Calorimetric and Sorption Study of Water Sorption by Perfluorinated Membrane Materials. *Russ. J. Phys. Chem.*, Vol. 67, pp. 1255–1262.

Gostev, B.V. & Ostrovskii, V. (1994). Water Sorption by Perfluorinated Membrane Materials Treated by Ferric Chloride Water Solution. *Russ. J. Phys. Chem.* Vol. 68, pp. 668–675.

Hagan, M.M. (1962). *Clathrate Inclusion Compounds.* Reinhold Publ. Corp., New York, USA.

Hedges, S.B. & Kumar, S. (2003). Genomic Clocks and Evolutionary Timescales. *Trends in Genetics*, Vol. 19, No. 4, pp. 200–206.

Henze, K. & Martin, W. (2003). Evolutionary Biology: Essence of Mitochondria. Nature, *Vol. 426, pp. 127–128.*

Jordan, T.H. & Mac, T.C. (1967). Polyhedral Clathrate Hydrates. XII. The Structure of $(CH_3CH_2)_2NH{\cdot}8\frac{2}{3}H_2O$. *J. Chem. Phys.*, Vol. 47, No. 4, pp. 1222-1228.

Josse, J.; Kaiser, A.D. & Kornberg, A. (1961). Enzymatic Synthesis of Deoxyribonucleic Acid: VIII. Frequencies of Nearest Neighbor Base Sequences in Deoxyribonucleic Acid. *J. Biol. Chem.*, Vol. 236, pp. 864-875.

Kadyshevich, E.A. (2006). Mitosis: Does It Proceed According to an Enclosed Code or to Deterministic Physicochemical Regulations? In: *Abstracts of the XIVth ISBC Conference*, p. 49, Univ. Gdansk, Gdynia, Poland.

Kadyshevich, E.A (2007). Generalized Hydrate Hypothesis of Origin of Nucleic Acids and Hydrocarbons in Nature: Whether It Opens a New Page in Laboratory Syntheses of Biomaterials, In: *Adv. in Petrochem. Polymers, Proc.*, BB 1-4, Bangkok, Thailand.

Kadyshevich E.A. (2009a). The PFO-CFO Hypothesis of Planet Formation. *Meteorit.& Planet. Sci.*, Vol. 44, pp. A105.

Kadyshevich E.A. (2009b). The Planet Formation Hypothesis: Why Are the Solar System Planets Different in their Chemical Compositions? *EPSC Abstr.*, Vol. 4, EPSC2009-1.

Kadyshevich, E.A & Ostrovskii, V.E. (2007). Hypothetical Physicochemical Mechanisms of Some Intracellular Processes: The Hydrate Hypothesis of Mitosis and DNA Replication. *Thermochim. Acta*, Vol. 458, No. 1–2. pp. 148–161.

Kadyshevich, E.A & Ostrovskii, V.E. (2009). Hydrate Hypothesis of Living Matter Origination (LOH-Hypothesis): Thermodynamic Grounds of Formation of Living Matter Simplest Elements from Hydrocarbons and Niter. *J. Therm. Anal. Calor.*, Vol. 95, No. 2, pp. 571–578.

Kadyshevich, E.A & Ostrovskii, V.E. (2010a). Oxygen Isotopic Anomalies in the Rocks of Celestial Objects: Are They the Key to the Planet Formation Mechanism? *EPSC Abstracts*, Vol. 5, EPSC2010-3.

Kadyshevich, E.A & Ostrovskii, V.E. (2010b). Development of the PFO-CFO Hypothesis of Solar System Formation: Why Do the Celestial Objects Have Different Isotopic Ratios for Some Chemical Elements? *Proc. Int. Aston. Union,* Vol. 6, No. S274 (Advances in Plasma Astrophysics), pp. 95–101, Cambridge Univ. Press, UK.

Kadyshevich, E.A & Ostrovskii, V.E. (2010c). Hydrate Hypothesis of Living Matter Origination: Logical and Thermodynamic Grounds. In: *Degassing of the Earth: geotectonics, geodynamics, geofluids, oils, gases, hydrocarbons, and life.* pp. 195–198, GEOS, Moscow, Russia.

Kadyshevich, E.A & Ostrovskii, V.E. (2010d). Life Origination Hydrate Hypothesis (LOH-Hypothesis): What Questions Can Be Hypothetically Answered at Present? *EPSC Abstracts*, Vol. 5, EPSC2010-5.

Kant, I. (1997). *Critique of Practical Reason*, Cambridge Univ. Press, Cambridge (Transl. into English from *"Kritik der praktischen Vernunft"*, P. Reclam 1878, Leipzig, Germany.

Kargin, V.A. (1962). *Modern Problems of Polymer Science*. Moscow State Univ., Moscow, Russia.

Karkow, B. (2009). HAPS Histology Image Database.

Kauffman, S. (1993). *The Origin of Order Self Organization and Selection in Evolution*, Oxford Univ. Press., Oxford, UK.

Kerfeld, C.A.; Sawaya, M.R.; Tanaka, S.; Nguyen, C.V.; Phillips, M.; Beeby, M. & Yeates, T.O. (2005). Protein Structures Forming the Shell of Primitive Bacterial Organelles. *Science*, Vol. 309, pp. 936–938.

Konovalov, M.I. (1893). *Nitrating Action of Dilute Nitrous Acid at Hydrocarbons of Saturated Character*, Moscow, Russia.

Kornberg, A. & Baker, T.A. (2005). *DNA Replication*. 2nd. ed. Paperback Ed., p. 472, ISBN 978-1-891389-44-3, 932 p.

Lodish, H.; Berk, A.; Zipursky, L.; Matsudaira, P.; Baltimore, D. & Darnell, J. (2000). *Molecular Cell Biology* (4th ed.) W.H. Freeman, New-York, USA.

Li, T. & Nicolaou, K.C. (1994). Chemical Self-Replication of Palindromic Duplex DNA. *Nature*, Vol. 369, pp. 218–221.

Lide D.R. (ed.) (1996). *Handbook of Chemistry and Physics* (76th ed.), CRC Press, London, UK.

MacDonald I.R., Guinasso N.L., Brooks J.M., et al. (1994). Seafloor Gas-Hydrates: Video Documenting Oceanographic Influences on Their Formation and Dissociation. In: *Near Surface Expression of Hydrocarbon Migration. AAPG Hedberg Res. Conf. Abstracts*, Vancouver, B.C., Canada.

McMullan, R. K.; Jordan, T. H. & Jeffrey, G. A. (1967). Polyhedral Clathrate Hydrates. XII. The Crystallographic Data on Hydrates of Ethylamine, Dimethylamine, Trimethylamine, *n*-Propylamine (Two Forms), *Iso*-Propylamine, Diethylamine (Two Forms), and *Tert*-Butylamine. *J. Chem. Phys.*, Vol. 47, No. 4, pp. 1218–1223.

Menor-Salván, C.; Ruiz-Bermejo, M.; Osuna-Esteban, S. & Veintemillas-Verdaguer S. (2009). Efficient Synthesis of Pyrimidines and Triazines from Urea and Methane in Ice Matrix. *Orig. Life Evol. Biosph.*, Vol. 39, No. SI, pp. 250–251.

Milkov, A.V. (2004). Global Estimates of Hydrate-Bound Gas in Marine Sediments: How Much Is Really out There? *Earth-Sci Rev.*, Vol. 66, No. 3-4, pp. 183–197.

Mojzsis, S.J.; Arrhenius, G.; McKeegan, K.D.; Harrison, T.M.; Nutman, A.P. & Friend, C.R.L. (1996). Evidence for Life on Earth before 3,800 Million Years Ago. *Nature*, Vol. 384, pp. 55–59.

Newton, I. (1687). *Philosophiñ Naturalis Principia Mathematica*, Jussu Soc. Regiñ ac Typis Josephi Streater, Londini; [Translated into English: *Mathematical Principles of Natural Philosophy*, Univ. of California Press, Berkeley, Calif., 1999].

Oborin, A.A. & Khmurchik, V.T. (2008). Chemosynthesis at Deep Fluids as an Additional Source of Organic Matter in the Lithosphere. In: *Degassing of the Earth; geodynamics, geofluids, oil, gas, and their parageneses*, pp. 366–367. GEOS, Moscow, Russia.

Oparin, A.I. (1924). *The Origin of Life.* Moscow Worker publisher, Moscow, Russia, 71 p.
Oparin, A.I. (1957). *The Origin of Life on Earth* (3rd ed.). Acad. Press Inc., N.Y., USA 459 p.
Orgel, L.E. (2000). Self-Organizing Biochemical Cycles. *Proc. Nat. Acad. Sci.,* Vol. 97, No. 28, pp. 12503–12507.
Orgel, L.E. (1992). Molecular Replication. *Nature,* Vol. 358, pp. 203–209.
Ostrovskii, V.E. (2002). Differential Microcalorimeter for Isothermal Measurements of Heat Effects in Two-Phase Systems and Examples of Its Application. *Rev. Sci. Instr.,* Vol. 73, pp. 1304–1312.
Ostrovskii, V.E. (2010). Hypothesis of the Natural Gas Abiotic Origin in the Context of Living Matter Origination. In: *Gas Chemistry at the Present Stage of Development* (eds. A.I. Vladimirov, A.L. Lapidus), Gubkin RSU NG, pp. 35–69, Moscow, Russia.
Ostrovskii V.E.; Tsurkova B.V.; Kadyshevich E.A. & Gostev B.V. (2000). Differential Heat Effects, Kinetics, and Mechanisms for the Drying and Water Vapor Wetting of the Acrylamide–Water System. *Russ.J. Phys. Chem.,* Vol. 74, No. 2, pp. 191–201.
Ostrovskii, V.E.; Tsurkova, B.V.; Kadyshevich E.A. & Gostev B.V. (2001). Comparison Study of the Acrylamide–Water and Polyacrylamide–Water Systems: Differential Heat Effects, Kinetics, and Mechanisms of Drying and Vapor-Phase Wetting. *J. Phys. Chem. B,* Vol. 105, No. 50, pp. 12680–12687.
Ostrovskii, V.E. & Gostev, B.V. (1996). Heat Effects and Rates and Molecular Mechanisms of Water Sorption by Perfluorinated Polymer Materials Bearing Functional Groups. *J. Therm. Anal.,* Vol. 46. pp. 397-416.
Ostrovskii, V.E. & Kadyshevich, E.A. (2000). Use of Data on the Polyacrylamide–Water System in Analyzing the Equilibrium DNA–Water Structure. *Russ. J. Phys. Chem.,* Vol. 74, No. 7, pp. 1114–1124.
Ostrovskii, V.E. & Kadyshevich, E.A. (2002). Hydrate Model of the Equilibrium DNA–H_2O System. *Intern. J. Nanosci.,* Vol. 1, No. 2. pp. 101–121.
Ostrovskii, V.E. & Kadyshevich, E.A. (2006). Thermodynamics of Formation of Nitrogen Bases and D-ribose from Mineral Substances in Light of the Problem of Origination of Simplest Elements of Living Matter. *Thermochim. Acta,* Vol. 441, No. 1, pp. 69–78.
Ostrovskii, V.E. & Kadyshevich, E.A. (2007). Generalized Hypothesis of the Origin of the Living-Matter Simplest Elements, Transformation of the Archean Atmosphere, and the Formation of Methane-Hydrate Deposits. *Physics-Uspekhi (Advances in Physical Sciences),* Vol. 50, No. 2, pp. 175–196.
Ostrovskii, V.E. & Kadyshevich, E.A. (2008). Hypotheses of Hydrocarbon-Hydrate Formation and Living Matter Origination at the Earth. In: *Degassing of the Earth; geodynamics, geofluids, oil, gas, their parageneses,* pp. 374–377, GEOS, Moscow, Russia.
Ostrovskii, V.E. & Kadyshevich, E.A. (2009a). Hypothesis of Formation of Planets from Nebula: Why Are the Planets Different in Their Chemical Compositions? *Orig. Life. Evol. Biosp.,* Vol. 39, No. SI, pp. 217–219.
Ostrovskii, V.E. & Kadyshevich, E.A. (2009b). Solar System Formation Hypothesis: Why the Chemical Compositions of the Planets Are so Different? *Geochim. Cosmochim. Acta,* Vol. 73, pp. A 979.
Ostrovskii, V.E. & Kadyshevich, E.A. (2009c). Life Origination Hydrate Hypothesis (LOH-Hypothesis). *Orig. Life. Evol. Biosp.,* Vol. 39, No.SI, pp. 219–220.

Ostrovskii, V.E. & Kadyshevich, E.A. (2010). Life origination hydrate hypothesis (LOH-hypothesis): the content and chemical and thermodynamic grounds. In: *Chemical Evolution & Origin of Life, Intern. Workshop Proc.*, pp. 1-2, Jain Print., Roorkee, India.

Ostrovskii, V.E. & Kadyshevich, E.A. (2011). Physicochemical model of formation of the Solar System planets: the causes of differences in the chemical composition of planets. In: *"Physchemistry-2010", Selected works* (ed. A.S. Smolyanskii), LLC "Rosinatal", pp. 46–61, Obninsk, Russia.

Ostrovskii, V.E. & Tsurkova, B.V. (1997). Differential Heat Effects and Mechanisms of Interaction of Polyacrylamide with Water, *Russ. J. Phys. Chem.*, Vol. 71, pp. 967–973.

Ostrovskii. V.E., & Tsurkova, B.V. (1998a). The System Polyacrylamide-Water. Differential Heat Effects, Rates and Molecular Mechanisms of Wetting and Drying. *J. Therm. Anal.*, Vol. 51. pp. 369–381.

Ostrovskii, V.E. & Tsurkova, B.V. (1998b). The Polyacrylamide–Water System: Application of Differential Calorimetry to Study the Mechanisms of Dissolution. *Thermochim. Acta*, Vol. 316. pp. 111–122.

Ould-Moulaye, C.B.; Dussap C.G. & Gros J.B. (2001). A Consistent Set of Formation Properties of Nucleic Acid Compounds. Purines and pPyrimidines in the Solid State and in Aqueous Solution. *Thermochim. Acta*, Vol. 375. No. 1-2. pp. 93–107.

Parmon, V.N. (1999). Abiogenic Catalysts in Nature. *Col. Surf. A, Physicochem. Eng. Aspects*, Vol. 151, pp. 351–365.

Pauling, L. (1970). *General Chemistry* (3rd ed.), W.H. Free man, San Francisco, USA.

Platteeuw, J.C. & Van-der-Waals, J.H. (1959). Thermodynamic Properties of Gas Hydrates II: Phase Equilibria in the System H_2S-C_3H_8-H_2O at −3°C, *Rec. Trav. Chim.*, Vol. 78, No. 2, pp. 126–133.

Pinder, K.L. (1964). Time Dependent Rheology of the Tetrahydrofuran-Hydrogen Sulphide Gas Hydrate Slurry. *Can. J. Chem. Eng.*, Vol. 42, No. 3, pp. 132–138.

Pinder, K.L. (1965). A Kinetic Study of the Formation of the Tetrahydrofuran Gas Hydrate. *Can. J. Chem. Eng.*, Vol. 43, No. 5, pp. 271–274.

Reider, C.L.; Faruki, S. & Khodjakov, A. (2001). The Centrosome in Vertebrates: More than a Microtubule-Organizing Center. *Trends in Cell Biology*, Vol. 11, No. 10, pp. 413-419.

Rhodes, D. & Klug, A. (1980). Helical Periodicity of DNA Determined by Enzyme Digestion. *Nature*, Vol. 286, No. 5773, pp. 573-578.

Schippers, A.; Neretin, L.N.; Kallmeyer, J. et al. (2005). Prokaryotic Cells of the Deep Sub-seafloor Biosphere Identified as Living Bacteria. *Nature*, Vol. 433. pp. 861–864.

Sclafani, R.A. & Holzen, T.M. (2007). Cell Cycle Regulation of DNA Replication. *Annu. Rev. Genet.*, Vol. 41, pp. 237-280.

Segré, D.; Pilpel, Y. & Lancet, D. (1998). Mutual Catalysis in Sets of Prebiotic Organic Molecules: Evolution through Computer Simulated Chemical Kinetics. *Physica A (Amsterdam)*, Vol. 249, pp. 558–564.

Shapiro, R. (2000). A Replicator Was not Involved in the Origin of Life. *IUBMB Life*, Vol. 49, pp. 173–176.

Shapiro, R. (2006). Small Molecule Interactions Were Central to the Origin of Life. *The Quart. Review of Biology*, Vol. 81, pp. 105–125.

Silberberg, A; Eliassaf, J. & Katchalsky, A. (1957). Temperature-Dependence of Light Scattering and Intrinsic Viscosity of Hydrogen Bonding Polymers. *J. Polym. Sci.*, Vol. 23, No. 103, pp. 259–284.

Spirin, A.S. (2001). Protein Biosynthesis, the RNA World, and the Origin of Life. *Herald of the Russian Academy of Sciences,* Vol. 71, No. 2, pp. 146-153.

Stackelberg, M. & Muller, H. (1954). Solid Gas-Hydrate II. Structure and Stereochemistry. *Z. Electrochem.,* Vol. 58, No. 1, pp. 25–39.

Stackelberg, M. & Meuthen, B. (1958). Solid Gas-Hydrate VII. Water-Soluble Ether. *Z. Electrochem.*, Vol. 62, pp. 130–131.

Thompson, H.B. & LaPlanche, L.A. (1963). Electric Moments of N,N-disubstituted Amides. *J. Phys. Chem.*, Vol. 67, No. 10, pp. 2230—2231.

Tresher. J.; Durckworth, R. & Williams, A. (1992). The Identification of Three New Seepage Sites in the Gulf of Mexico, *Shallow Gas Group News Letters*, № 6.

Van-der-Waals, J.H. & Platteeuw, J.C. (1959) Clathrate Solutions. *Adv. Chem. Phys.*, Vol. 2, pp. 1–57.

van Zuilen, M.A.; Lepland, A. & Arrhenius, G. (2002). Reassessing the Evidence for the Earliest Traces of Life. *Nature*, Vol. 418, pp. 627–630.

Wang, J.C. (1979). Helical Repeat of DNA in Solution. *Proc. Natl. Acad. Sci. USA*, Vol. 76, No. 1, pp. 200-203.

Watson, J.D. & Crick, F.H.C. (1953). Molecular Structure of Nucleic Acids: A Structure for Deoxyribose Nucleic Acid. *Nature*, Vol. 171, No. 4356, pp. 737–738.

Wilkins, M.H.F.; Stokes, A.R. & Wilson, H.B. (1953). Molecular Structure of Nucleic Acids: Molecular Structure of Deoxypentose Nucleic Acids. *Nature*, Vol. 171, No. 4356, pp. 738–740.

Wilkins, M.H.F. (1961). The Molecular Structure of DNA. *J. Chim. Phys.*, Vol. 58, pp. 891–898.

Zielinski, W.S. & Orgel, L.E. (1987). Autocatalytic Synthesis of a Tetranucleotide Analogue. *Nature*, Vol. 327, No. 6120, pp. 346-347.

Zimmerman, S.B. & Pheiffer, B.H. (1979). Helical Parameters of DNA Do not Change when DNA Fibers Are Wetted: X-ray Diffraction Study. *Proc. Natl. Acad. Sci. USA.*, Vol. 76, No. 6, pp. 2703–2707.

Part 2

Mutations

5

Strand-specific Composition Bias in Bacterial Genomes

Feng-Biao Guo and Lu-Wen Ning
School of Life Science and Technology
University of Electronic Science and Technology of China
China

1. Introduction

In 1950, Chargaff experimentally found that nucleotides of G and C (or T and A) have the same abundance values when analyzing two DNA strands together (Chargaff, 1950). Three years later, Watson and Crick (1953) published the DNA double helix model and the base-pairing rule in the model explained such equivalent frequencies. This is called the first rule of Chargaff or parity rule 1. Surprisingly, Lin and Chargaff (1967) observed approximately equivalent frequencies of complementary nucleotides within each single DNA strand. This is called the second rule of Chargaff or parity rule 2. The rule 2 is theoretically explained as follows. When mutation and selection are symmetric with respect to the two strands of DNA, parity rule 1 holds the following six pairs of substitution rate to be equal, $r_{GC}=r_{CG}$, $r_{TA}=r_{AT}$, $r_{GA}=r_{CT}$, $r_{AG}=r_{TC}$, $r_{CA}=r_{GT}$, $r_{AC}=r_{TG}$, where, r_{GC} means the substitution rate of G to C in a specific strand and so on (Lobry, 1995). Having the six pairs of equal substitution rates, it is formally derived that complementary nucleotides within each strand have the same occurrence frequencies. Indeed, parity rule 2 only exists when there are not any strand biases of mutation or selection. Therefore, parity rule 2 is a natural derivation of parity rule 1 at the equilibrium state between two strands. And any deviation from parity rule 2 implies substitutional strand biases: the result of different mutations (and or repair) rates, different selective pressures, or both, between the two strands of DNA (Lobry and Sueoka, 2002). In the past two decades, these deviations from intra-strand equimolarities have been extensively studied in eukaryotes (Niu et al., 2003) and their organelles (Krishnan et al. 2004), viruses (Mrazek and Karlin, 1998), particularly in bacteria and archaea (Necsulea and Lobry, 2007). In bacteria, the observed deviations switch sign at the origin and terminus of replication. This chapter reviews the subject of strand-specific composition bias in bacterial genomes, varying strength of it in different species, the underlying mechanisms and the analyzing methods.

2. Strand-specific composition bias in bacterial genomes

2.1 Strand-specific substitution and composition biases

DNA replication is a semi-conservative process (Rocha, 2004). The two strands of the parental duplex are separated, and each serves as a template for the synthesis of a new partner strand. The parental duplex is replaced with two daughter duplexes, each of which consists of one parental strand and one newly synthesized strand. Because of the duplex structure of the parental strands, one daughter strand would be synthesized in a 5' -> 3' direction and the other would have to be copied in a 3' -> 5' direction. However, DNA polymerases can only catalyze synthesis in the 5'-3' direction. Thus, the 5'->3' strand (known as the Leading strand), is continuously synthesized. For the 5'->3' strand (known as the lagging strand), the solution is addressed by adopting discontinuous synthesis. That is to say, lagging strand replication proceeds through the synthesis of relatively short polynucleotide segments (Okazaki fragments) that are then joined together to form a continuous strand (Rocha, 2004).

As mentioned above, the deviations from parity rule 2 observed in bacteria switch sign at the origin and terminus of replication. That is to say, the substitution bias occurs between the two replicating strands, namely leading and laggings strands. There are two major ways for studying asymmetric substitutions: observation of rate bias of substitutions between homologous sequences and direct detection of composition deviations from parity rule 2 (Frank and Lobry, 1999).

Wu and Maeda (1987) used the first method to test for asymmetric substitution in certain regions of chromosomal sequences from six primates. They obtained homologous sequences of the beta-globin complex for the six primates and then calculated the substitution matrix. After comparing the substitution rates of complementary nucleotides, they obtained the first observation of strand asymmetry. The sequence comparisons even allowed them to make predictions about the positions of replication origins. But in later studies, the examination of longer sequences (Bulmer, 1991) did not show the existence of strand asymmetry. Francino et al. (1996) used the same method to investigate asymmetric substitution in the bacterium *Escherichia coli*. They found no differences in substitution rates between leading and lagging strands. However, an excess of C -> T changes was observed on the coding strand when compared to the non-coding strand. Based on this result, they suggested that strand bias of substitution mainly resulted from transcription coupled mutation or repair. The two works were the early reports on asymmetry substitution between leading and lagging strands or between coding and non-coding strands. Rocha et al. (2006) evaluated substitution biases between leading and lagging strands in seven bacteria. Significant biases existed in all seven genomes. Among them, in *E. coli* the C -> T substitution is much higher in the leading strand than in the lagging strand. This result contradicts previous ones partly (Francino et al., 1996) and the contradiction may be caused by the very small size of gene samples used by Francino and colleagues. Recently, different substitution (C to T, A to G, and G to T) rates between coding strands and non-coding strands were also observed for 1630 human genes (Mugal et al., 2009).

The substitution bias could be reflected by the different occurrence frequencies of the four nucleotides between the two strands. The second method builds on the analysis of the DNA sequences for deviations from A=T and G=C. Such deviations in SV 40 were found to have a polarity switch at the origin of replication and thus were taken as evidence for asymmetric mutation in the replication process (Filipski, 1990). The strand nucleotide composition bias was then found in genomes of echinoderm and vertebrate mitochondria (Asakawa et al., 1991). Strand composition biases were observed in the genome of *Haemophilus influenzae* and in parts of the *E. coli* and *Bacillus subtilis* genomes by using the method of GC skew and AT skew (Lobry, 1996). In these genomes the leading strands are relatively enriched in G over C and T over A. However, the case is reversed for the lagging strands. McLean et al. (1998) examined GC skew and AT skew at the third codon position along genomic regions in completely sequenced prokaryotes at that time. Among nine bacteria, eight have GC and AT skews that change sign at the origin of replication. The leading strand in DNA replication is G richer (over C) and T richer (over A) at codon position 3 in six eubacteria, but C and T richier in two *Mycoplasma* species. Tiller and Collins (2000) investigated the relative contributions of replication orientation, gene direction, and signal sequences to base composition asymmetries in 13 bacterial genomes by using qualitative graphical presentations and quantitative statistical analyses. The effect of replication orientation, i.e., the gene is locacted on the leading or lagging strand, was found to contribute a significant proportion of the GC and AT skews. This effect is independent of, and can have opposite signs to the effects of transcriptional or translational processes, such as selection for codon usage, expression levels. With the rapid growth in the number of sequenced genomes, more and more bacteria are described with strand composition bias. Here, *Chlamydia muridarum* (Guo and Yu, 2007) is taken as an example to illustrate strand-specific composition bias at the three codon positions of genes and results are shown in Table 1. As can be seen, the G versus C bias is statistically significantly (Paried t-test, $p<0.01$) different between the two repicating strands, whereas the T verus A bias is not (Paried t-test, $p>0.05$).

	Leading strand					
	a	c	g	t	g-c	t-a
1st codon position	0.26	0.18	0.33	0.23	0.16	-0.03
2nd codon position	0.30	0.21	0.17	0.32	-0.04	0.02
3rd codon position	0.28	0.12	0.21	0.38	0.09	0. 10
Overall	0.28	0.17	0.24	0.31	0.07	0.03
	Lagging strand					
1st codon position	0.28	0.22	0.27	0.23	0.05	0.05
2nd codon position	0.30	0.24	0.14	0.32	-0.10	0.10
3rd codon position	0.31	0.20	0.14	0.36	-0.06	0.06
Overall	0.30	0.22	0.18	0.30	-0.04	0.04

Table 1. Strand specific composition bias in the *C. muridarum* genome.

2.2 Methods used to elucidate the bias and to predict replication origins

For un-annotated bacterial genomes, information on the localization of the replication origin is not available. Therefore, it is unknown whether a gene is located on the leading or lagging strands and quantitative results as in Table 1 could not be obtained. In this circumstance, the strand composition biases, i.e. deviations from parity rule 2, are usually studied by graphical methods. GC-skew (and or AT-skew), cumulative GC-skew and Z curve are three such methods.

GC skews were first used to study mitochondrial strand asymmetry and then widely used to bacterial genomes (Lobry, 1996). The GC skew calculation is performed by the following equation:

$$\text{GC-skew}=(G-C)/(G+C) \quad (1)$$

where G and C denote the occurrences of the corresponding bases in a given sequence with given length. The skew values along a long sequence were studied often by using a sliding window. The window length is fixed and two adjacent windows may overlap partly in some cases. Take the chromosomal position as horizontal axis and the vertical axis denotes the skew value, a line chart could be drawn. In that way, a GC skew plot for *E. coli* K12 is obtained and shown in Figure 1. As can be seen from the figure, there is composition asymmetry along the chromosome. The skew switches signs at two sites and hence divides the genome into three parts. In fact, the two switching points correspond to experimentally determined replication termini and origins. So, the three regions are leading strand, lagging strand and leading strands, respectively. As can be seen, the leading strand has positive GC skew values and the region that is a lagging strand has negative GC skew values in the *E. coli* genome.

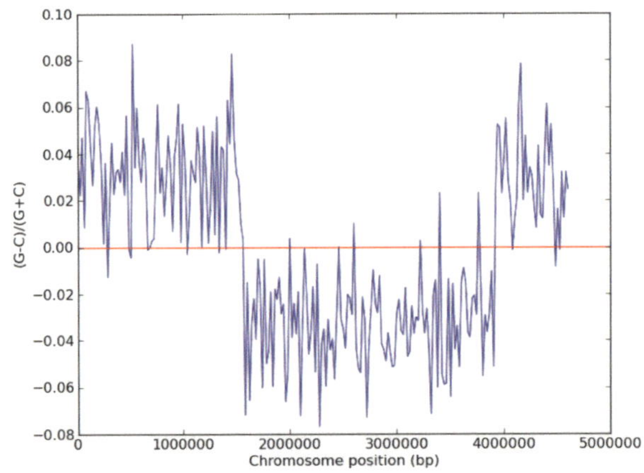

Fig. 1. GC skew for the *E. coli* K12 genome.

Although the window-based GC skew method is extensively used, the proper window size is hard to adjust. Such plots may not always be very illustrative due to many visible fluctuations for a small window size, while larger windows may hide precise coordinates of polarity switches. Therefore, an optimal window size does not exist in many cases. To address this point, a more convenient skew diagram was later proposed by Grigoriev (1998). He suggested to calculate directly the sum of (G–C)/(G+C) in adjacent windows from an arbitrary start to a given point in a sequence. Although this method is based on a sliding window, the diagram of cumulative GC skew tends to be smoother because it adopts the form of a sum. To avoid the dependence on the window size w and chromosome length c, Grigoriev (1998) suggested that the cumulative skew values are multiplied by w/c. A cumulative skew diagram for *E. coli* K12 is shown in Figure 2. As can be seen, there indeed are much less fluctuations than in Figure 1. It also shows that the switching points become peaks. The maximum skew value corresponds to the replication terminus and the minimum corresponds to the replication origin.

TA skew or cumulative TA skew could be calculated and plotted by replacing the symbol G by T and C by A in the equation (1). Similarly, keto-amino or purine-pyrimidine skew may be obtained by making appropriate replacements.

Both GC skew and cumulative GC skew are based on sliding windows. The Z curve is one method that thoroughly gets rid of sliding window. We briefly describe the Z curve method

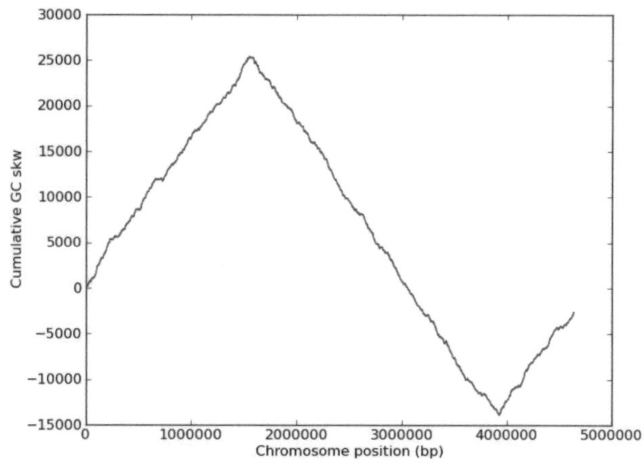

Fig. 2. Cumulative GC skew diagram for the *E. coli* K12 genome.

as follows. The Z curve is a three dimensional space curve constituting the unique representation of a given DNA sequence in the sense that for the curve or for the sequence each can be uniquely reconstructed from the other (Zhang and Zhang, 2003). Consider a DNA sequence read from the 5′-end to the 3′-end with N bases, inspecting the sequence one base at one time, and beginning with the first base. The number of inspecting steps could be denoted by n, i.e., n =1, 2,. . . , N. In the *n*th step, let us count the cumulative numbers of the bases A, C, G, and T, occurring in the subsequence from the first to the *n*th base and denote them by A_n, C_n, G_n, and T_n, respectively. The Z curve consists of a series of nodes P_n, where n =1, 2,. . . , N, whose coordinates are denoted by x_n, y_n, and z_n. It was shown that (Zhang and Zhang, 2003)

$$\begin{aligned} Xn &= (An + Gn) - (Cn + Tn) \equiv Rn - Yn \\ yn &= (An + Cn) - (Gn + Tn) \equiv Mn - Kn \\ zn &= (An + Tn) - (Cn + Gn) \equiv Wn - Sn \\ n &= 0, 1, 2, ..., N,\ \ xn, yn, zn \in [-N,N], \end{aligned} \tag{2}$$

where $A_0 = C_0 = G_0 = T_0 = 0$ and hence $x_0 = y_0 = z_0 = 0$. The symbols R, Y, M, K, W, and S represent the puRines, pYrimidines, aMino, Keto, Weak hydrogen bonds and Strong hydrogen bonds, respectively, according to the Recommendation 1984 by the NC-IUB (Cornish-Bowden, 1984). The connection of the nodes P_0 (P_0 = 0), P_1, P_2, ..., until P_N one by one sequentially by straight lines is called the Z curve for the DNA sequences inspected. The Z curve defined above is a 3-D space curve, having three independent components, i.e., x_n, y_n and z_n (Zhang and Zhang, 2003).

When being used for predicting replication origin or studying strand composition bias, only the x and y components of the 3-D Z curve are involved (Guo and Yu, 2007). According to equation (1), the x component curve denotes the plus of cumulative excess of G over C and A over T. Whereas, the y component curve represents the opposite number of the plus of cumulative excess of G over C and T over A. In short, the x component denotes the cumulative excess of purine over pyrimidine and the y component means the opposite number of cumulative excess of keto over amino. As an example, the x and y component curves for the *E. coli* K12 chromosome are shown in Figure 3. As can be seen, there are two peaks in both of the two curves and they correspond to the replication terminus and the replication origin, respectively.

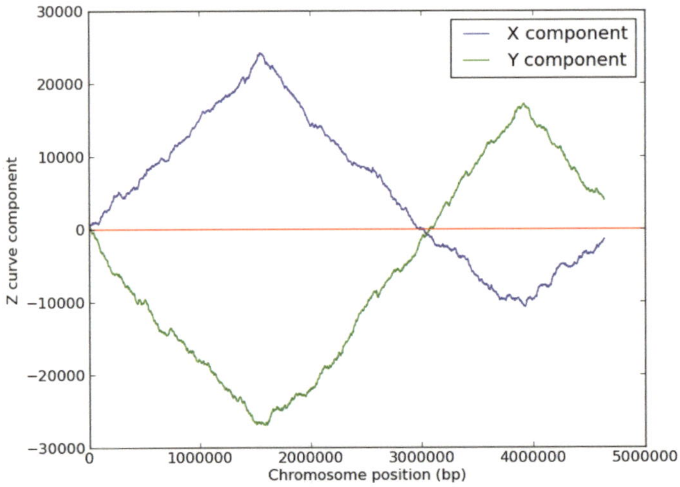

Fig. 3. X and Y component curves of the Z curve method for *E. coli* K12 genome.

According to analyses on bacterial genomes with experimentally replication origin, skew or Z curve plots for almost all of them inflect the sign or polarity at the sites of replication origins. This is the result of different nucleotide composition biases between the two replicating strands. Based on that fact, replication origins may be putatively predicted by using such methods in newly sequenced bacterial genomes. Indeed, during the annotation process for most of sequenced prokaryotes, replication origins were identified by using one, two or all three of these methods. Therefore, theoretically predicting replication origins is one of the practical applications from the universal phenomenon of strand composition bias in bacterial genomes.

2.3 Consistent direction and varying strengths of strand composition bias

Almost all of the literatures reporting significant strand composition bias revealed an excess of G over C in the leading strands in bacterial genomes. However, C over G excess in the leading strand is very rarely observed. Necsulea and Lobry (2007) performed a thorough analysis of base skew in 360 sequenced bacterial genomes. In this work, they investigated the direction or sign of bias between complementary nucleotides. Table 2 summarizes their results. Among 360 bacteria, only 33 chromosomes show no significant effect of replication. The absence of direct replication effects on base composition bias seems to be more frequent in certain bacterial families, such as *Cyanobacteria,* where 7 out of 17 chromosomes show no effect of replication on nucleotide skews, and Mollicutes (10 out of 16 chromosomes). Another noteworthy point is that only two out of 360 genomes have excess of C over G in the leading strands. Therefore, the direction (or sign) of G versus C bias is the same in nearly 100% of bacterial species. Comparatively, the bias of T versus A is not so consistent. As can be seen, about 14% (35/253) of chromosomes differ from the collective with statistically significant (randomisation test, $p < 0.05$) excess of T over A in the leading strands. Therefore, the directions of G versus C and T versus A biases are generally consistent in most bacterial genomes.

	A>T	A=T	A<T
G>C	33	73	205
G=C	1	33	13
G<C	1	1	0

Table 2. Numbers of bacteria with various composition biases in the leading strand (adapted from Necsulea and Lobry, 2007)

However, the strength of specific composition biases varies from genome to genome in bacteria. Rocha (2004) once used one quantitative method to evaluate the strength of strand composition bias in 58 completely sequenced prokaryotes. The accuracy of the discrimination of the leading strand genes and proteins based on their nucleotide compositions is employed as the index measuring strand bias. If there are no composition biases between the two strands, the expected accuracy is about 50%. According to their results, *Streptomyces coelicolor* has the least bias and the classification accuracy is less than 60%. The accuracies of most genomes vary in the ranges between 60% and 90%. Most interestingly, three obligate intracellular parasites have the accuracy higher than 90%. That means they have very strong composition biases between the two replicating strands. Among them, *Borrelia burgdorferi*, has the highest accuracy of 95% when differentiating genes on the two strands based solely on the amino acid content and 97% using nucleotide composition.

Prior to Rocha, the different nucleotide compositions between genes on the two replicating strands of *B. burgdorferi* had been observed using graphical methods (Mcinerney, 1998). If the strand composition bias is strong enough, the individual nucleotide biases could propagate into higher-order biases in a correlated way, thereby changing the relative frequencies of codons and even amino acids of genes and encoded proteins in each of the replicating strands. Therefore, codon usage analysis could reflect the nucleotide composition in bacterial genomes with strong strand bias. In Mcinerney (1998), a correspondence analysis (COA) was made first for codon usages of all genes in *B. burgdorferi*. Then a scattering plot was drawn by using the two most important axes of COA. In the plot, points denoting about 567 genes were divided into two clusters. These two clusters appeared to be quite distinct, with very little overlap. And this meant that they had different nucleotide compositions or codon usages. On inspection, it was shown that these two groups defined the genes that were located on the leading or on the lagging strands. This was the first observation of separate codon usage associated with replication in bacterial genomes. In the past decade, another 10 bacterial genomes were also found to have extremely strong composition bias (Wei and Guo, 2010). In other words, genes on the two replicating strands were found to have separate base/codon usages in genomes of 11 bacteria including *B. burgdorferi*.

Among the 11 bacteria with extremely strong strand composition bias, the observations for three are from our group: *Chlamydia muridarum* (Guo and Yu, 2007), *Lawsonia intracellularis* (Guo and Yuan, 2009) and *Ehrlichia canis* (Wei and Guo, 2010). Here we take *Lawsonia intracellularis* as an example and briefly describe our work in the following. As an obligate intracellular bacterium, *Lawsonia intracellularis* could cause ileum inflammation in most animals, especially in pigs. The genome of *L. intracellularis* PHE/MN1-00 was determined in

2006. The complete genome sequence of *L. intracellularis* was downloaded from GeneBank. According to the annotation, the chromosome contains 1180 protein-coding genes. Most analyses were carried out using codonW. This software was used to determine the major source of variation of codon usage among the genes on the chromosome. Only those codons for which there is a synonymous alternative were used in the analysis. Hence, the three termination codons and the codons that encode Methionine and Tryptophan were excluded. Consequently, each gene is described by a vector of 59 variables (codons). COA plots all the genes analyzed in their 59-dimensional space and attempts to identify a series of new orthogonal axes accounting for the greatest variation among genes. The first principal axis is chosen to maximize the standard deviation of the derived variable and the second principal axis is the direction that maximizes the standard deviation among directions un-correlated with the first, and so forth.

Here, Figures 4 shows the positions of the genes along the first and second major axes produced by COA on codon counts. The closeness of any two genes on the plot reflects the similarities of their codon usages. As can be seen, the first axis individually could separate the genes into two clusters with little overlap. The following two facts indicate that the two groups correspond to genes on the leading and lagging strands of replication, respectively. (i) The first axis is found to strongly correlate with GC and AT skews. At the left end of the first axis, genes are characterized by richness in nucleotides G and T, whereas the case is opposite at the right end. (ii) The coordinates of individual genes along the first axis of COA are plotted against the chromosomal locations of the corresponding genes in Figure 5. Genes on the direct strand and those on the reverse complement strand are denoted by red and blue squares, respectively. It is found that genes on the left side of sequenced direct strand and genes on the right side of the reverse complement strand have lower coordinate values of the first axis, whereas, for the other genes, the opposite occurs. In fact, genes on the left side of direct strand and those on the right side of the reverse complement strand just correspond to genes on the leading strand, whereas the other ones correspond to the lagging strand. Therefore, it is reasonable to say that two clusters in Figure 4 correspond to genes on the leading strands and lagging strands, respectively. After marking genes located on the leading, lagging strands by different symbols in Figure 4, the speculation is confirmed.

A Chi-square test was then performed for comparing RSCU values of genes located on the two replicating strands and results are listed in Table 3. RSCU (Relative Synonymous Codon Usage) is defined in Equation 3. where x_{ij} is the occurence number of the *j*th codon for the *i*th amino acid, and n_i denotes the degree of codon degeneracy for the *i*th amino acid.

$$\mathrm{RSCU}\,ij = \frac{x_{ij}}{\frac{1}{n_i}\sum_{j=1}^{n_i} x_{ij}} \tag{3}$$

In the table 3, the symbl ++ indicates that the leading strand genes used the codon more frequently than the lagging strand genes, and the symbol -- indicates the lagging strand genes used the codon more frequently than the leading strand genes, whereas xx indicates that there is no significant difference in usage of the codon on either strand. In total, 49 among 59 codons are found to be significantly different between genes on the leading strand from those on the lagging strand. Among the 23 codons used more frequently in the leading strand, 19 are G-ending or T-ending and the exceptions are TTA, ACA, AGA and GCA.

Among the 26 codons used more frequently in the lagging strand, 16 are C-ending, 8 are A-ending and codons CTT and ACT constitute the outliers. Results of the chi-square test confirm that there is a bias towards G, T in the leading strand, and towards C, A in the lagging strand. Therefore, it could be concluded that in *L. intracellularis*, the leading and lagging strands of replication display an asymmetry in the compositions and this bias is the most important source of codon usage variation.

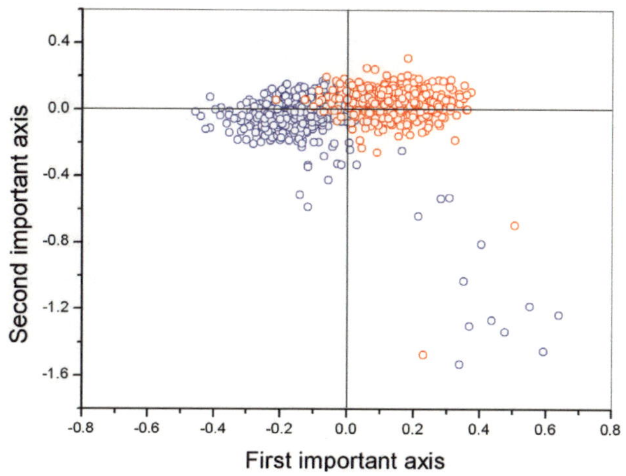

Fig. 4. Plot of the two most important axes after COA on codon counts for the 1180 genes on the *L. intracellularis* chromosome.

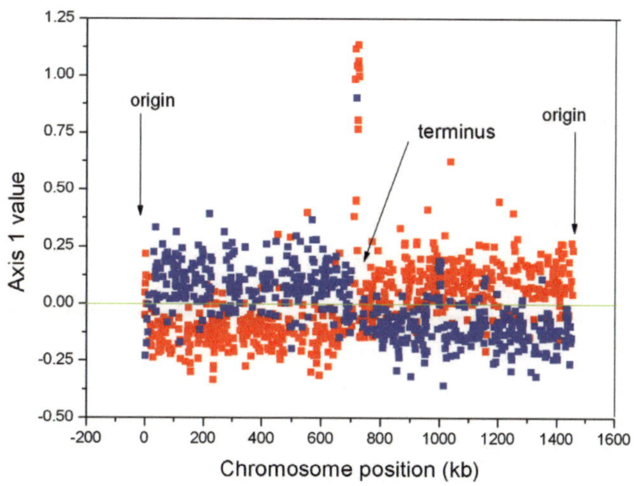

Fig. 5. Plot of axis 1 values of chromosomal genes against the corresponding chromosomal locations in the *L. intracellularis* genome.

AA	Codon	RSCU Leading	Significant	RSCU Lagging	AA	Codon	RSCU Leading	Significant	RSCU Lagging
Phe	UUU	1.81	++	1.64	Ser	UCU	2.21	XX	2.25
	UUC	0.19	--	0.36		UCC	0.23	--	0.39
Leu	UUA	2.53	++	1.86		UCA	1.47	--	1.60
	UUG	0.60	++	0.20		UCG	0.14	++	0.08
Tyr	UAU	1.74	++	1.60	Cys	UGU	1.77	++	1.59
	UAC	0.26	--	0.40		UGC	0.23	--	0.41
ter	UAA	0.00	XX	0.00	ter	UGA	0.00	XX	0.00
ter	UAG	0.00	XX	0.00	Trp	UGG	1.00	XX	1.00
Leu	CUU	1.98	--	2.44	Pro	CCU	2.08	XX	2.06
	CUC	0.17	--	0.46		CCC	0.18	--	0.30
	CUA	0.56	--	0.89		CCA	1.64	XX	1.59
	CUG	0.15	XX	0.14		CCG	0.10	XX	0.05
His	CAU	1.75	++	1.61	Arg	CGU	2.24	XX	2.18
	CAC	0.25	--	0.39		CGC	0.26	--	0.51
Gln	CAA	1.41	--	1.74		CGA	0.74	--	1.02
	CAG	0.59	++	0.26		CGG	0.25	XX	0.20
Ile	AUU	1.72	++	1.59	Thr	ACU	1.33	--	1.39
	AUC	0.26	--	0.41		ACC	0.24	--	0.36
	AUA	1.02	XX	1.01		ACA	2.24	++	2.14
Met	AUG	1.00	XX	1.00		ACG	0.19	++	0.12
Asn	AAU	1.66	++	1.49	Ser	AGU	1.58	++	1.24
	AAC	0.34	--	0.51		AGC	0.36	--	0.45
Lys	AAA	1.47	--	1.76	Arg	AGA	1.88	++	1.75
	AAG	0.53	++	0.24		AGG	0.63	++	0.34
Val	GUU	1.93	++	1.82	Ala	GCU	1.85	XX	1.84
	GUC	0.29	--	0.47		GCC	0.25	--	0.36
	GUA	1.40	--	1.51		GCA	1.78	++	1.73
	GUG	0.37	++	0.20		GCG	0.12	XX	0.08
Asp	GAU	1.73	++	1.60	Gly	GGU	1.67	++	1.41
	GAC	0.27	--	0.40		GGC	0.32	--	0.41
Glu	GAA	1.43	--	1.73		GGA	1.46	--	1.76
	GAG	0.57	++	0.27		GGG	0.55	++	0.42

Table 3. Chi-square results of RSCU of genes on the leading and lagging strands.

2.4 The underlying mechanism for the composition bias in bacterial genomes

As mentioned above, almost all the bacterial genomes have significant strand-specific composition biases. It is necessary and important to investigate the underlying mechanisms of such biases. Two published papers reviewed numerous explanations for the base composition bias in bacterial genomes (Frank and Lobry, 1999; Rocha, 2004). These hypotheses could be divided into two major categories (Necsulea and Lobry, 2007). The first hypothesis supposes that the replication mechanism is a direct cause of base composition asymmetry. The different mutation frequencies between the two replicating strands result in the nucleotide composition bias (Powdel et al., 2009). The second hypothesis states (Powdel et al., 2009) that the deviations from PR2 are associated with the strand asymmetry of the transcription mechanism, in combination with the gene distribution bias encountered in bacterial chromosomes (most protein-coding genes were located on the leading strands). This theory also falls back on mutation bias for detail interpretation. During transcription, template strand and non-template strand have different mutation probabilities and subsequent repair. As for the main cause of these asymmetries, numerous authors have provided many solid evidence in favour of the mutationist view by demonstrating that the base skews are mainly expressed at the third codon positions of genes as well as in non-coding regions where selective pressure is minimal (Lobry, 1996). For either mutationist views, cytosine deamination of single-stranded DNA performs a vital role in the generation of strand composition bias. The deaminiation of cytosine leads to the formation of uracil. Because of the Watson-Crick base paring, cytosine is effectively protected against deamination in normal circumstances in vivo. However, the rate of cytosine deamination increases 140 times in the single-stranded DNA (Beletskii and Bhagwat, 1996). If the resulting uracil is not replaced with cytosine, C -> T mutations occur. During the process of replication, the leading strand is exposed more time in the single-stranded state than the lagging strand. Therefore, C to T mutations occur more frequently in the leading strand than in the lagging strand and then the excesses of G(C) relative to C(G) and T(A) relative to A(T) are produced in the leading(lagging) strand. During transcription, the coding strand is more exposed in the single-stranded state. Therefore, it has more G over C.

Extensive evidence has been proposed to support the replication mechanism as a direct cause of base composition asymmetries (Necsulea and Lobry, 2007). As mentioned above, the analyses of the codon usage patterns, through correspondence analysis or other statistical methods, showed that in some bacterial species genes located on the replicating strands can be distinguished by their synonymous codon choice (McInerney, 1998; Wei and Guo, 2010). Using the ANOVA method on GC and AT skews, with gene direction and replication orientation as the explanatory variables, Tillier and Collins showed that the nucleotide composition of a bacterial gene is significantly influenced by its position on the leading or the lagging strand for replication (Tillier and Collins, 2000). Lobry and Sueoka (2002) performed one thorough analysis on 43 prokaryotic chromosomes and confirmed that deviations from parity rule 2 differ significantly between leading and lagging strands. This is one of the convincing evidences. Worning et al. (2006) suggested that the sign of AT-skew is determined by the polymerase alpha subunit that replicates the leading strand. In bacteria such as *Firmicutes,* where both genes are present the AT-skew is positive on the leading strand, whereas it is negative in genomes that contain only *dnaE*. Qu et al. (2010) confirmed this conclusion based on a larger dataset.

The second hypothesis also has its supporting evidence. Francino et al. (1996) concluded that the substitution patterns were similar on the leading and lagging strands, but significantly different between the coding and non-coding strands, based on the observation of several genes in E. coli K12. Therefore, they suggested that a process linked to transcription rather than the mode of replication caused the nucleotide asymmetry. Note that a partly contradictory result was obtained by Rocha et al. (2006), at the whole genomic scale in the same species. According to them, the C to T substitution is much higher in leading strands than in lagging strands in *E. coli.* Nikolaou and Almirantis (2005) contributed an interesting work to the area, in favour of the latter type of mechanism. In order to produce a perfect gene orientation bias, they used the method of artificially rearranging the bacterial chromosome. In the case of *Nostoc* sp. the rearrangement generated a strong trend in base composition asymmetry. Thus, Nikolaou and Almirantis (2005) suggested that the gene orientation bias would be the main factor responsible for the existence of the nucleotide skews in this bacterium, and replication only had an indirect role on base asymmetry.

Based on the artificial genome rearrangement proposed by Nikolaou and Almirantis, Necsulea and Lobry (2007) developed one novel method to distinguish the replication and transcription effects on base composition asymmetry. Their results suggested that the effect of replication on the GC-skew is generally very strong. For numerous species, the AT-skew is caused by coding sequence-related mechanisms. Therefore, the cause of base composition bias in bacterial genomes would be the superposed effect of replication and transcription. The superposed effect of the two processes may be the sum or the difference. In other words, transcription-associated asymmetries can either increase or decrease replication-associated strand asymmetries, depending on the transcription direction and the position of the gene relative to the origin of replication (Necsulea and Lobry, 2007; Mugal et al., 2009). See also the chapter by Seligmann in this book.

2.5 Why there exists extremely strong strand composition bias in obligate intracellular parasites?

As mentioned above, 11 bacteria have been found to have extremely strong strand composition bias (Wei and Guo, 2010). The bias is strong enough to divide base and codon usages according to whether genes are located on the leading or lagging strands. Their names are *Borrelia burgdorferi, Treponema pallidum, Chlamydia trachomatis, Buchnera aphidicola, Blochmannia floridanus, Bartonella henselae, Bartonella quintana, Tropheryma whipplei, Chlamydia muridarum, Lawsonia intracellularis* and *Ehrlichia canis*, respectively. Among them, the replication associated codon usage seperation for the last three bacteria are reported by our group (Guo and Yu, 2007; Guo and Yuan, 2009; Wei and Guo, 2010). Investigating the common characters of 11 bacteria may be interesting and important.

As reported in many cases, the living environment and living styles may exert influence on the genomic G+C content and on codon usgaes of genes. Based on this consideration, we compare the living habitation of the 11 bacteria. Among them, 9 belong to oligate intracellular parasites and this means they live permanently in the cell of their host. Due to this safe habitation in the living cell, they would suffer less damage on DNA from ultraviolet radiation or other physical, chemical factors than freely living bacteria. After long-term evolution, some or most genes coding for DNA repair enzymes may be lost from these species. Due to the loss of such genes or enzymes, mutations generated during the replication process are not effectively corrected. The replicaiton associated mutation in obligate intracellular parasites would accumulate much more than in freely living bacteria. Such mutations might be a major cause for the strand composition bias in bacterial genomes. So, more mutations, more bias. The above deduction is our speculation. Its correctness should be validated by a large scale test in the future.

Secondly, chromosomes of the 11 bacteria are all shorter than 2000 kb. According to statistics on fully sequenced genomes, bacterial chromosomes vary from 160 kb to more than 10000 kb. However, all 11 species have small genome sizes although some of these bacteria are not endosymbionts. Hence, we supposed that small genome size is a necessary condition to generate strong enough strand-specific mutational bias. Perhaps in small bacterial genomes that have suffered reductive evolution, the repair mechanism of replication may be inefficient. Alternatively, in bacteria with larger chromosome, the mutation pressure is hard to prevail over translational selection.

Thirdly, all of the 11 bacteria have medium or low genomic G+C content. Among them, *B. aphidicola* has the lowest G+C content (26%), whereas *T. pallidum* has the highest G+C content (52%). Perhaps, the environment of high G+C contents is adverse to the generation of strong strand mutation biases. Future experimental works are required to clarify the relationship between the asymmetric mechanism of replication and genomic GC content or genome size.

Fourthly, the strong mutation bias may be associated with the absence of certain genes involved in chromosome replication. As suggested by Klasson and Andersson (2006), the strong strand-specific mutational bias in endosymbiont genomes coincides with the absence of genes associated with replication restart. After a comparative analysis on 20 gamma-proteobacterial genomes, it was found that endosymbiont bacteria lacking *recA* and other genes coding for the replication restart pathway, such as *priA*, displayed the strongest strand bias. Following that study, here we investigate the absence of *mutH, priA, topA, dnaT, fis* and *recA*, which are all associated with replication initiation and the re-initiation pathway. Consequently, genes *mutH, dnaT* and *fis* are found to be absent in all 11 bacterial genomes with extreme strand asymmetry bias. Comparatively, all of the three genes exist in *E. coli* and other -proteobacteria, which have medium mutation biases. Klasson and Andersson (2006) suggested that cytosine deaminations accumulate during single-strand exposure at stalled replication forks and the extent of strand composition bias may depend on the time spent in repairing such lesions. Inefficient re-start mechanisms result in the replication fork to be arrested for longer time and hereby lead to higher DNA strand asymmetry. As a common character of the 11 genomes, we believe that genes associated with the replication restart pathway are very likely to be absent in the other genomes, found in the future, with strong strand mutational bias.

Finally, Figure 6 shows the y component curves of the Z curve defined in equation (2) for five representatives of the 11 bacteria with extremely strong strand composition bias. For comparison, the y component curve of the *E. coli* K12 chromosome is also shown. In *E. coli*, there also exists strand specific composition bias, however it is not strong enough to generate separate codon usages. As can be seen, all of the y component curves for the five bacteria are much smoother than for *E. coli*. The latter's y component curve has many prickles (or local fluctuations) along the chromosome. As shown in Grigoriev (1998), local fluctuations in the chromosome diagrams often correspond to sequence inversions or direct

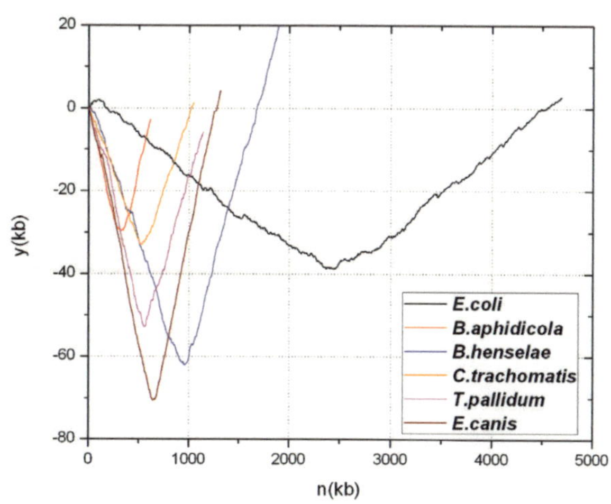

Fig. 6. Y component curves for 5 bacteria with extremely strong strand composition bias and that for the free-living bacterium *E.coli* K12.

translocations to another half of a chromosome, or integration of foreign DNA into the chromosome. Note that protection against mutations by secondary strcuture formation also explains such strand asymmetries (Krishnan et al., 2004). In other words, chromosome rearrangements often are exhibited as little prickles in the y component curves. Therefore, we could make the conclusion that the 11 bacterial chromosomes are highly stable and have very few rearrangements. According to Rocha (2004), lower rearrangement frequency are just the most likely reasons for the appearance of seperate codon usages in some obligate intracellular parasites. Our results confirmed this speculation.

3. Strand composition bias in eukaryotes, organelles, archaea and plasmids

Compared with bacterial genomes, studies on strand composition bias in eukaryotic genomes are limited. Most analyses of eukaryotic genomes did not show strand compositional asymmetry at chromosome scale (Grigoriev, 1998; Gierlik et al., 2000). It is probably a result of a relative excess of autonomously replicating sequences (ARS) and of random choice of these sequences in each replication cycle (Gierlik et al., 2000). However, the examination of three contigs from human genomes gave some evidence of strand compositional asymmetries. In addition, local asymmetries have been found in the last ARS from both ends of chromosomes of *Saccharomyces cerevisiae* (Grigoriev, 1998; Gierlik et al., 2000). In these regions, replicons may be longer. To circumvent the predicament of the lack of known replication origin, Niu et al. (2003) resorted to neighboring gene pairs that are located on different strands of nuclear DNA. Such gene pairs are most probably coded on two replicating strands. It was found that the relative frequencies of T versus A and of G versus C are significantly skewed in most studied eukaryotes when examining the introns and the fourfold degenerate sites of codons in the genes of each pair. After using quadrant diagrams to distinguish the effects of replication and transcription, the study demonstrated that there are different causes in studied genomes although the composition bias existed in most of them. For example, both transcription-associated mutation bias and replication-associated mutation bias may play an important role in causing strand asymmetry in *S. cerevisiae*. In *Schizosaccharomyces pombe*, transcription asymmetry is more likely to be the major cause of the DNA strand bias. In *A. thaliana*, transcription-associated asymmetric A to T or A to C to T substitution may be the genuine cause of the bias (Niu et al., 2003).
As for human genomes, Francino and Ochman (2000) failed to detect the asymmetry of some replicons by the phylogenetic comparisons. Analysis of the whole set of human genes revealed that most of them presented TA and GC skews (Touchon et al., 2003). The two kinds of biases are correlated to each other and they are specific to gene sequences, exhibiting sharp transitions between transcribed and non-transcribed regions. At the same time, Green et al. (2003) also described a qualitatively different transcription-associated strand asymmetry in humans. In their study, human orthologous sequences were generated by aligning with eight other mammals. The authors saw pronounced asymmetric transition substitutions in the transcribed regions of human chromosome 7. The transitions of A to G were 58% more frequent than T to C and G to A transitions were 18% more frequent than C to T. With 'maximal segment' analysis, they showed that the strand asymmetry was associated specifically with transcribed regions. Two years later, Touchon et al. (2005) analyzed intergenic and transcribed regions flanking experimentally identified human replication origins and the corresponding mouse and dog homologous regions. They demonstrated that there existed compositional strand asymmetries associated with replication. By using wavelet

transformations of skew profiles, the authors revealed the existence of 1000 putative replication origins associated with randomly distributed termination sites in human genome (Touchon et al., 2005). Around these putative origins, the skew profile displayed a characteristic jagged pattern which was also observed in mouse and dog genomes. By analyzing the nucleotide composition of intergenic sequences larger than 50 kb by cumulative skew diagrams, Hou et al. (2006) found replication-associated strand asymmetry in vertebrates including humans. Therefore, they proposed that transcription-associated strand asymmetries masked the replication-associated ones in the human genome. Huvet et al. (2007) found with multi-scale analysis that the base skew profile presented characteristic patterns consisting of successions of N-shaped structures in more than one-quarter of the human genome. These N domains are bordered by putative replication origins. Wang et al. (2008) illustrated that transcription-associated strand compositional asymmetries and replication-associated ones coexist in most vertebrate (including human) large genes although in most cases the former conceals the latter. The three most frequent types of asymmetric substitution, C to T, A to G, and G to T, were examined in the human genome (Mugal et al., 2009). All three rates were found to be on average higher on the coding strands than on the transcribed. Such finding points to the simultaneous action of rate increasing effects on the coding strands, such as increased adenine and cytosine deamination, and transcription-coupled repair as a rate-reducing effect on the transcribed strands. Furthermore, the author showed that the rate asymmetries of genes are to some extent also produced by the process of replication, depending on the distance to the next ORI and the relative direction of transcription and replication (Mugal et al., 2009). With the help of the very recently published work by Chen et al. (2011), we conclude that strand composition asymmetry (bias) is the superposed effect of replication and transcription asymmetries in the human genome. Among them, transcription associated mutation and or repair bias exert effects on transcribed regions. However, replication induced mutation and repair biases act on the whole chromosome. This is quite similar to bacterial genomes.

As for eukaryotic organelles, there are quite a few reports of strand bias. For example, Seligmann and colleagues observed strand asymmetric gradients in various mitochondria and investigated in the past five years how properties of replication origins affect the gradients (Seligmann, 2010; Seligmann and Krishnan, 2006; Seligmann et al., 2006a, 2006b).

Regarding archaea, a few have shown significant strand composition skews, which are associated with replication. Among them, some are determined or predicted to contain a single replication origin, while others have multiple origins of replication, similar to eukaryotes. According to Necsulea and Lobry (2007), 18 out of 29 archaeal chromosomes showed significant effects of replication on nucleotide skews

Usually, it is believed that bacterial plasmids replicate using a different mechanism than that of the chromosome of their host cell. In 2000, cumulative skew diagrams showed that plasmid and chromosome of *B. burgdorferi* adopted a similar bi-directional replication (Picardeau et al., 2000). Recently, our group performed skew analysis on the largest plasmid of *L. Intracellularis*. As shown in Figure 7, the cumuliatve GC-skew diagram shows two peaks, at two points, around 27 kb and 115 kb in the replicon. And this suggests that the plasmid replicates bi-directionally from an internal origin as the chromosome does. Leading strands and lagging strands are hence determined based on the putative origin and terminus. Result of COA shows that genes on the two replicating strands have distinct codon usages. Note that similar results were observed in genes on the chromosome. Based on these two facts, we suppose that common asymmetric replication would be involved in the chromosome and the largest plasmid of *L. intracellularis*. Not only both replicate bi-directionally from an internal origin, but also they have biased mutation/repair rates between the two replicating strands. Recently, Arakawa et al. (2009) performed thorough analyses on skew profiles of hundreds of plasmids. Their results suggested the existence of rolling-circle replication in plasmids. Correlation of skew strength between plasmids and their corresponding host chromosomes, which was observed by the authors on 302 host chromosomes and 606 plasmids, suggested that within the same strain, these replicons had reproduced using the same replication machinery.

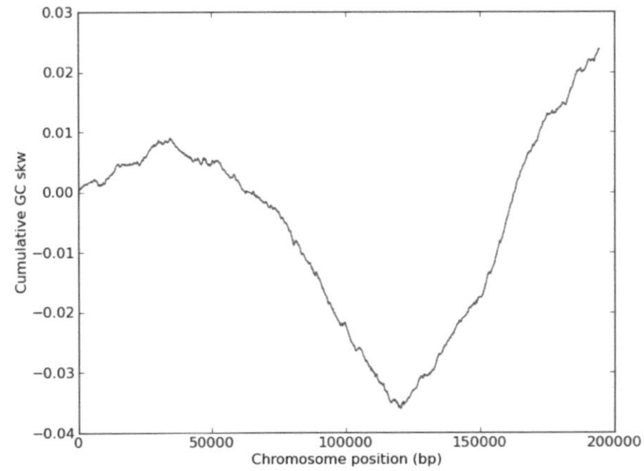

Fig. 7. Cumulative GC skew for the largest plasmid of *L. Intracellularis*.

4. Conclusion and future research

Strand composition bias has been found in various genomes for 20 years. The cause of base composition bias in bacterial genomes is supposed to be the superposed effect of replication and transcription asymmetries in mutation biases. In some species, the former mechanism is mainly responsible for the bias, while in some others the latter constitutes the major force driving the bias. In others, the two mechanisms have equally important effects. Transcription-associated asymmetries can either increase or decrease replication-associated strand asymmetries, depending on the transcription direction and the position of the gene relative to the origin of replication. Theoretically predicting replication origins is one of the practical applications of the universal phenomenon of strand composition bias in bacterial genomes. Future work should focus on the following aspects: (1) Investigation of the common characters and mechanisms of the biases between prokaryotic and eukaryotic genomes; (2) The cause for the varying strength of composition bias in different bacterial genomes; (3) More works should be performed on strand composition bias in eukaryotes other than *Homo* sapiens and in archaeal genomes.

5. Acknowledgment

The present study was supported by the National Natural Science Foundation of China (grant 60801058 and 31071109), and the Fundamental Research Fund for the Central Universities of China (grant ZYGX2009J082).

6. References

Arakawa K., Suzuki H. & Tomita M. (2009). Quantitative analysis of replication-related mutation and selection pressures in bacterial chromosomes and plasmids using generalised GC skew index. BMC Genomics, Vol. 10, (December 2009), 10: 640, ISSN 1471-2164

Asakawa S., Kumazawa Y., Araki T., Himeno H., Miura K. & Watanabe K. (1991). Strand-specific nucleotide composition bias in echinoderm and vertebrate mitochondrial genomes. Journal of Molecular Evolution, Vol. 32, No. 6, (June 1991), pp. 511-520, ISSN 0022-2844

Beletskii A. & Bhagwat A.S. (1996). Transcription-induced mutations: increase in C to T mutations in the nontranscribed strand during transcription in Escherichia coli. Proceedings of the National Academy of Sciences of the United States of America, Vol. 93, No. 24, (November 1996), pp. 13919-13924, ISSN 0027-8424

Bulmer M. (1991). Strand symmetry of mutation rates in the beta-globin region. Journal of Molecular Evolution, Vol. 33, No. 4, (October 1991), pp. 305-310, ISSN 0022-2844

Chargaff E. (1950). Chemical specificity of nucleic acids and mechanism of their enzymatic degradation. Experientia, Vol. 6, No. 6, (June 1950), pp. 201-209, ISSN 0014-4754

Chen C.L., Duquenne L., Audit B., Guilbaud G., Rappailles A., Baker A., Huvet M., d'Aubenton-Carafa Y., Hyrien O., Arneodo A., & Thermes C. (2011). Replication-associated mutational asymmetry in the human genome. Molecular Biology Evolution, [Epub ahead of print], (March 2011), ISSN 0737-4038

Cornish-Bowden A. (1985). Nomenclature for incompletely specified bases in nucleic acid sequences: Recommendation 1984. Nucleic Acids Research, Vol. 13, Issue 9, (May 1985), pp. 3021-3030, ISSN 0305-1048

Filipski J. (1990). Evolution of DNA sequence, contributions of mutational bias and selection to the origin of chromosomal compartments. Advances in Mutagenesis Research 2, Publisher Springer, (February 1991), pp. 1–54, ISBN-10 3540524281

Frank A.C. & Lobry J.R. (1999). Asymmetric substitution patterns: a review of possible underlying mutational or selective mechanisms. Gene, Vol. 238, Issue 1, (September 1999), pp. 65-77, ISSN 0378-1119

Francino M.P., Chao L., Riley M.A., & Ochman H. (1996). Asymmetries generated by transcription-coupled repair in enterobacterial genes. Science, Vol. 272, No. 5258, (April 1996), pp. 107-109, ISSN 0036-8075

Francino M.P. & Ochman H. (2000). Strand symmetry around the beta globin origin of replication in primates. Molecular Biology Evolution, Vol. 17, Issue 3, (March 2000), pp. 416–422, ISSN 0737-4038

Gierlik A., Kowalczuk M., Mackiewicz P., Dudek M.R., & Cebrat S. (2000). Is there replication-associated mutational pressure in the Saccharomyces cerevisiae genome? Journal of Theoretical Biology, Vol. 202, Issue 4, (February 2000), pp. 305–314, ISSN 0022-5193

Green P., Ewing B., Miller W., Thomas P.J., NISC Comparative Sequencing Program & Green E.D. (2003). Transcription-associated mutational asymmetry in mammalian evolution. Nature Genetics, Vol. 33, No. 4, (April 2003), pp. 514-517, ISSN 1061-4036

Grigoriev A. (1998). Analyzing genomes with cumulative skew diagrams. Nucleic Acids Research, Vol. 26, Issue 10, (April 1998), pp. 2286-2290, ISSN 0305-1048s

Guo F.B. & Yu X.J. (2007). Separate base usages of genes located on the leading and lagging strands in Chlamydia muridarum revealed by the Z curve method. BMC Genomics, Vol. 8, (October 2007), 8: 366, ISSN 1471-2164

Guo F.B. & Yuan J.B. (2009). Codon usages of genes on chromosome, and surprisingly, genes in plasmid are primarily affected by strand-specific mutational biases in Lawsonia intracellularis. DNA Research, Vol. 16, Issue 2, (January 2009), pp. 91-104, ISSN 1340-2838.

Hou W.R., Wang H.F. & Niu D.K. (2006). Replication-associated strand asymmetries in vertebrate genomes and implications for replicon size, DNA replication origin, and termination. Biochemical Biophysical Research Communications, Vol. 344, Issue 4, (June 2006), pp. 1258-1262, ISSN 0006-291X

Huvet M., Nicolay S., Touchon M., Audit B., d'Aubenton-Carafa Y., Arneodo A. & Thermes C. (2007). Human gene organization driven by the coordination of replication and transcription. Genome Research, Vol. 17, Issue 9, (September 2007), pp. 1278-1285, ISSN 1465-6906

Klasson L. & Andersson S.G. (2006). Strong asymmetric mutation bias in endosymbiont genomes coincide with loss of genes for replication restart pathways. Molecular Biology Evolution, Vol. 23, Issue 5, (February 2006), pp. 1031-1039, ISSN 0737-4038

Krishnan, N.M, Seligmann, H., Raina, S.Z., Pollock, D.D. (2004) Detecting gradients of asymmetry in site-specific substitutions in mitochondrial genomes. DNA Cell Biol. 23, 707–714.

Lin H.J. & Chargaff E. (1967). On the denaturation of deoxyribonucleic acid: II. Effects of concentration. Biochimica Biophysica Acta, Vol. 145, Issue 2, (September 1967), pp. 398-409, ISSN 0006-3002

Lobry, J.R. (1995). Properties of a general model of DNA evolution under no-strand-bias conditions. Journal of Molecular Evolution, Vol. 40, No. 3, (December 1994), pp. 326–30, ISSN 0022-2844

Lobry J.R. (1996). Asymmetric substitution patterns in the two DNA strands of bacteria. Molecular Biology Evolution, Vol. 13, No. 5, (May 1996), pp. 660–665, ISSN 0737-4038

Lobry J.R. & Sueoka N. (2002). Asymmetric directional mutation pressures in bacteria. Genome Biology, Vol. 3, Issue 10, (September 2002), research0058.1-research0058.14, ISSN 1465-6906

Mcinerney J.O. (1998). Replicational and transcriptional selection on codon usage in Borrelia burgdoreferi. Proceedings of the National Academy of Sciences of the United States of America, Vol 95, No. 18, (June 1998), pp. 10698-10703, ISSN 0027-8424

McLean J.M., Wolfe K.H. & Devine K.M. (1998). Base composition skews, replication orientation and gene orientation in 12 prokaryote genomes. Journal of Molecular Evolution, Vol 47, No. 6, (June 1998), pp. 691–696, ISSN 0022-2844

Mrazek, J., Karlin, S. (1998) Strand compositional asymmetry in bacterial and large viral genomes. Proc. Nat. Acad. Sci. USA 95, 3720-3725.

Mugal C.F., von Grünberg H.H. & Peifer M. (2009). Transcription-induced mutational strand bias and its effect on substitution rates in human genes. Molecular Biology Evolution, Vol .26, Issue 1, (October 2008), pp. 131-142, ISSN 0737-4038

Necsulea A. & Lobry J.R. (2007). A new method for assessing the effect of replication on DNA base composition asymmetry. Molecular Biology Evolution, Vol. 24, Issue 10, (July 2007), pp. 2169-79, ISSN 0737-4038

Nikolaou C. & Almirantis Y. (2005). A study on the correlation of nucleotide skews and the positioning of the origin of replication: different modes of replication in bacterial species. Nucleic Acids Research, Vol. 33, Issue 21, (November 2005), pp. 6816-6822, ISSN 0305-1048

Niu D.K., Lin K. & Zhang D.Y. (2003). Strand compositional asymmetries of nuclear DNA in eukaryotes. Journal of Molecular Evolutian, Vol. 57, No. 3 (April 2003), pp. 325-334, ISSN 0022-2836

Qu H., Wu H., Zhang T., Zhang Z., Hu S., & Yu J. (2010), Nucleotide compositional asymmetry between the leading and lagging strands of eubacterial genomes. Research in Microbiology, Vol. 161, Issue 10, (December 2010), pp. 838-846, ISSN 0923-2508

Picardeau M., Lobry J.R. & Hinnebusch B.J. (2000), Analyzing DNA strand compositional asymmetry to identify candidate replication origins of Borrelia burgdorferi linear and circular plasmids. Genome Research, Vol 10, (July 2000), pp. 1594-604, ISSN 1088-9051

Powdel B.R., Satapathy S.S., Kumar A., Jha P.K., Buragohain A.K., Borah M. & Ray S.K. (2009). A study in entire chromosomes of violations of the intra-strand parity of complementary nucleotides (Chargaff's second parity rule). DNA Research, Vol. 16, (October 2009), pp. 325-343, ISSN 1340-2838

Rocha E.P.C. (2004). The replication-related organization of bacterial genomes. Microbiology, Vol. 150, (2004), pp. 1609-1627, ISSN 1350-0872

Seligmann, H. (2010) The ambush hypothesis at the whole-organism level: Off frame, 'hidden' stops in vertebrate mitochondrial genes increase developmental stability. Comp. Biol. Chem. 34, 80-85.

Seligmann, H., Krishnan, N.M. (2006) Mitochondrial replication origin stability and propensity of adjacent tRNA genes to form putative replication origins increase developmental stability in lizards. J. Exp. Zool. 306B, 433-439.

Seligmann, H., Krishnan, N.M., Rao, B.J. (2006a) Mitochondrial tRNA sequences as unusual replication origins: Pathogenic implications for Homo sapiens. J. Theor. Biol. 243, 375-385.

Seligmann, H., Krishnan, N.M., Rao, B.J. (2006b) Possible multiple origins of replication in Primate mitochondria: alternative role of tRNA sequences. J. Theor. Biol. 241, 321-332.

Tillier E.R. & Collins R.A. (2000). The contributions of replication orientation, gene direction, and signal sequences to base-composition asymmetries in bacterial genomes. Journal of Molecular Evolution, Vol 50, No. 3, (March 2000), pp. 249–257, ISSN 0022-2836

Touchon M., Nicolay S., Arneodo A., d'Aubenton-Carafa Y. & Thermes C. (2003). Transcription-coupled TA and GC strand asymmetries in the human genome. FEBS Letters, Vol. 555, Issue 3, (December 2003), pp. 579-582, ISSN 0014-5793

Touchon M., Nicolay S., Audit B., Brodie of Brodie E.B, d'Aubenton-Carafa Y. Arneodo A., & Thermes C. (2005). Replication-associated strand asymmetries in mammalian genomes: toward detection of replication origins. Proceedings of the National

Academy of Sciences of the United States of America, Vol 102, No. 28, (July 2005), pp. 9836-9841, ISSN 0027-8424

Wang H.F., Hou W.R. & Niu D.K. (2008). Strand compositional asymmetries in vertebrate large gens. Molecular Biology Reports, Vol 35, (April 2007), pp. 163-169, ISSN 1573-4978

Watson J.D. & Crick F.H.C. (1953). Molecular structure of nucleic acids: a structure for deoxyribose nucleic acid. Nature, Vol 171, Issue 4356, (April 1953), pp. 737-738, ISSN 0028-0836

Wei W. & Guo F.B. (2010). Strong strand composition bias in the genome of Ehrlichia canis revealed by multiple methods. The Open Microbiology Journal, Vol 4, (October 2010), pp. 98-102, ISSN 1874-2858

Worning P., Jensen L.J., Hallin P.F., Staerfeldt H.H. & Ussery D.W. (2006). Origin of replication in circular prokaryotic chromosomes. Environmental Microbiology, Vol. 8, Issue 2, (February 2006), pp. 353–361, ISSN 1462-2912

Wu C.I. & Maeda N. (1987). Inequality in mutation-rates of the two strands of DNA. Nature, Vol 327, Issue 6118, (May 1987), pp. 169-170, ISSN 0028-0836

Zhang R. & Zhang C.T. (2003). Multiple replication origins of the archaeon Halobacterium species NRC-1. Biochemical and Biophysical Research Communications, Vol 302, Issue 4, (March 2003), pp. 728-734, ISSN 0006-291X

6

Mutation Patterns Due to Converging Mitochondrial Replication and Transcription Increase Lifespan, and Cause Growth Rate-Longevity Tradeoffs

Hervé Seligmann
[1]*Herpetological Collection National Natural History Collections (NNHC), The Hebrew University of Jerusalem,*
[2]*Center for Ecological and Evolutionary Synthesis, University of Oslo,*
[3]*Department of Life Sciences, Ben Gurion University,*
[1,3]*Israel*
[2]*Norway*

1. Introduction

DNA replication and RNA transcription share many properties (Little et al., 1993; Hassan & Cook, 1994; Marczynski and Shapiro 1995; Mohanty et al., 1996; Prado & Aguilera 2005), notably in mitochondria (Nass 1995; Lee & Clayton, 1997). The joint occurrence of transcription and replication on DNA apparently necessitates coordination (Gilbert, 2001; MacAlpine at al., 2004), among others because collisions occur between the replication and transcription complexes on the same DNA strand (Mirkin & Mirkin, 2005). This coordination may be part of the regulation of gene expression (Patnaik, 1997) and the rates of both processes (Morton, 1999). This predicts the structural organization of genes on chromosomes around replication origins in relation to functional pressures (Schwaiger & Schubeler, 2006): highly expressed genes are located close to replication origins, those expressed in few tissues are more distant (Huvet et al., 2007). Such functional pressures seem strong enough to cause convergences in genome organization between very distant organisms such as yeast (*Saccharomyces cerevisiae*) and *Caulobacter*, despite that the proteins involved in their replication and transcription are basically unrelated (Brazhnik & Tyson, 2006). For that reason, transcription-associated genes are frequently located close to replication origins (Couturier and Rocha, 2006). The conserved arrangements of mitochondrial tRNA genes in vertebrates also seems to optimize between early replication of tRNAs whose anticodons have high probability to mutate in the single strand state (Seligmann et al., 2006a) and early transcription of tRNAs with frequently used cognate amino acids (Satoh et al., 2010). Note that this principle of optimizing between two competing processes exists also at the level of translation, between initiation and elongation (Xia et al., 2007), and might apply to many other molecular processes.

1.1 Replication and transcription in mitochondria

Both mitochondrial rRNA genes, the only transcription genes coded by vertebrate mitochondrial genomes, are located next to the mitochondrial control region. Indeed, the mitochondrial D-loop, according to the frequently observed collinearity between replication and transcription in prokaryotes (Nikolaou & Almirantis, 2005), includes the regions that initiate replication of the heavy strand (OH) and transcription (Shadel & Clayton, 1997; Fernandez-Silva et al., 2003), fitting the model that all transcription enhancers also enhance replication and vice versa (Boulikas, 1995). The major regulatory sequences in the D-Loop contain the only mitochondrial promoters, for both light- and heavy-strand transcription, in addition to the origin of heavy strand replication (Chang and Clayton, 1984). Biochemical evidence indicates that the primers generated by the light-strand promoter are used for replication priming (Chang & Clayton, 1985; Chang et al., 1985). This close association between the two processes in mitochondria expresses itself by the fact that some Alzheimer-associated mutations in the mitochondrial control region suppress both mitochondrial replication and transcription (Coskun et al., 2004). Hence, mitochondria, because of their involvement in ageing (Martin & Grotewiel 2006; Yu & Chung 2006), are a good system in which to study the putative relationship existing between the connection (and level of connection) of replication and transcription with ageing processes.

1.2 Mitochondria and ageing

Several properties of mitochondrial genomes have already been shown to associate with lifespan, presumably because of cumulative DNA damage due to free radicals produced by the normal function of mitochondria in the cell's energetic metabolism (Wiesner et al., 2006). It seems that evolution of vertebrate longevities (and in general, the associated evolution of their life history strategies) causes accelerated rates of amino acid replacements in mitochondrion-encoded protein coding genes (Rottenberg, 2006, 2007). Mutagenesis independent of free oxidative radicals also affects mitochondrion-associated ageing: in mitochondrial genomes, the number of direct repeats, a factor causing deletions, correlates negatively with mammalian lifespan (Samuels, 2004; Samuels et al., 2004; Khaidakov et al., 2006). Using a similar comparative approach, Samuels (2005) showed that lifespan increases proportionally to the stability of hybridization between complementary mitochondrial DNA strands, estimated by free energies. This property is proportional to the probability of opening up and expansion of single-stranded mtDNA bubbles. Negative selection on repeats (Samuels, 2005; Khaidakov et al., 2006) explains the exceptional status of most vertebrate mitochondrial genomes as breaking Chargaff's second parity rule (complementary nucleotides are met with almost equal frequencies in single stranded DNA), fitting the hypothesis that inversions and inverted transposition could be a major contributing if not dominant factor in the almost universal validity of this rule (Albrecht-Buehler, 2006).

These single stranded bubbles are more likely to occur where direct repeats exist, causing deletions (Khaidakov et al., 2006), but this probably also increases mutation rates in the single stranded sequences forming the bubble when the bubble is not enzymatically excised. This is because hydrolytic deaminations of cytosine to thymine and adenine to guanine, both transitions, occur proportionally to time spent single stranded (D_{ssh}) by the genome (as shown for example during replication in primate mitochondrial genomes, Krishnan et al., 2004a, b).

1.3 Developmental stabilities

Developmental stabilities, typically estimated by the level of symmetry of bilateral traits (Seligmann, 2000) usually increase with correlates of fitness (Moller, 1997, 1999). Hence it is sensible that rationales similar to those for longevity and ageing apply to developmental stabilities. In mitochondria, the chemical stability of rRNA increases developmental stability (Seligmann, 2006a), and the structural stability of the regular light strand origin of replication (OL) also increases developmental stability. So does usage of tRNAs adjacent to the regular OL as additional OLs (Seligmann and Krishnan 2006). Densities of off frame stops in mitochondrial genomes also increase developmental stability, probably because off frame stops stop early translation after unprogrammed ribosomal frameshifts, which produce dysfunctional proteins (Seligmann, 2010a). It hence makes sense to expect that connections between mitochondrial transcription and replication could affect developmental stability as well as lifespan.

1.4 Mutation gradients across genomes

Deamination gradients exist along mitochondrial genomes proportionally to D_{ssh} during replication (D_{ssh}r). In several independent taxa, inversion of the mitochondrial control region inverts the directions of these gradients (Hassanin et al., 2005).

D_{ssh} during transcription (D_{ssh}t) also creates deamination gradients along genomes or sections of genomes. The relative dominance of replication- versus transcription-associated gradients varies among genome regions and organisms (Francino et al., 1996; Baran et al., 2003), especially in bacteria (Mackiewicz et al., 1999). It seems that in nuclear vertebrate genomes, transcription-associated gradients mask the replication-associated ones (Hou et al., 2006), and more complex analyses are required to detect them (Touchon et al., 2005). These nuclear vertebrate transcription-associated gradients even reveal genes that are otherwise undetected because of their long introns and low sequence conservation (Glusman et al., 2006). Replication-associated deamination gradients are usually present in bacteria (Mrazek & Karlin, 1998). Transcription-associated ones have also been detected in bacteria (Francino & Ochman, 2001). In an adenovirus, gradients in nucleotide composition asymmetries between strands exist where replication and transcription share directions, but are basically nonexistent where they have opposite directions (Grigoriev, 1999).

In the latter case, this lack of a clear gradient does not signify that no mutations occur during replication and transcription, but rather that maximal and minimal mutation rates of each process coexist in the same region, increasing the range of the genome that is affected by high mutation regimes from at least one of the two processes. This might be adaptive in viruses, by maximizing evolvability (see for example Aldana et al., 2007; Feder, 2007; Jones et al., 2007). But, it is no surprise that both processes are frequently collinear in other organisms, as this limits maximal mutation rates to a specific region that might have relatively high mutational robustness, decreasing mutational constraints on the rest of the genome (Ciliberti et al., 2007; Elena et al., 2007; Wagner & Wright, 2007). It also makes sense that replication and transcription gradients, reflecting the relative frequencies of each process, are approximately balanced in prokaryotes. Hence the tendency for dominance of transcription-related gradients in nuclear genomes of eukaryotes would result from their generally lower cell replication rates. According to this, their mitochondria should resemble bacteria.

1.5 Convergence of replication and transcription in mitochondria

The level of collinearity, also termed here convergence, between replication and transcription is expected to slow ageing and ageing-related processes. Vertebrate

mitochondrial genomes seem good candidates for testing this hypothesis, because a) data are available for many species, b) they affect ageing and c) mitochondrial replication and transcription are at least partially collinear.
Indeed, in vertebrate mitochondria, the distance from the D-loop determines $D_{ssh}t$, while $D_{ssh}r$ results from calculating relative distances from the OH, also in the D-loop, and the light strand replication origin (OL, see Seligmann et al., 2006b for details on D_{ssh} calculations, and Seligmann, 2008). Usually, one considers that mitochondrial genomes have a single OL located in the WANCY region, a cluster of 5 tRNA genes (Desjardins & Morais, 1990; Clayton, 2000), resulting in $D_{ssh}rW$. Both processes are only partially collinear when solely the WANCY region functions as OL, but the probabilistic combination of multiple tRNA clusters distributed across the genome that putatively act as OLs (Seligmann et al., 2006b; Seligmann, 2008; Seligmann, 2010b) can result in an overall replication gradient ($D_{ssh}rX$) collinear with the transcription gradient ($D_{ssh}t$). In Figure 1, $D_{ssh}rX$ (as it is expected after integrating with equal weights all putative tRNA clusters as OLs into $D_{ssh}r$ calculations) is highly correlated with the distance from the Dloop. As compared to $D_{ssh}rW$, this $D_{ssh}rX$ has only one region with high mutation risks (this region codes for ND6 and CytB), while for $D_{ssh}rW$, there is an additional region (coding for ND1 and ND2), ranging

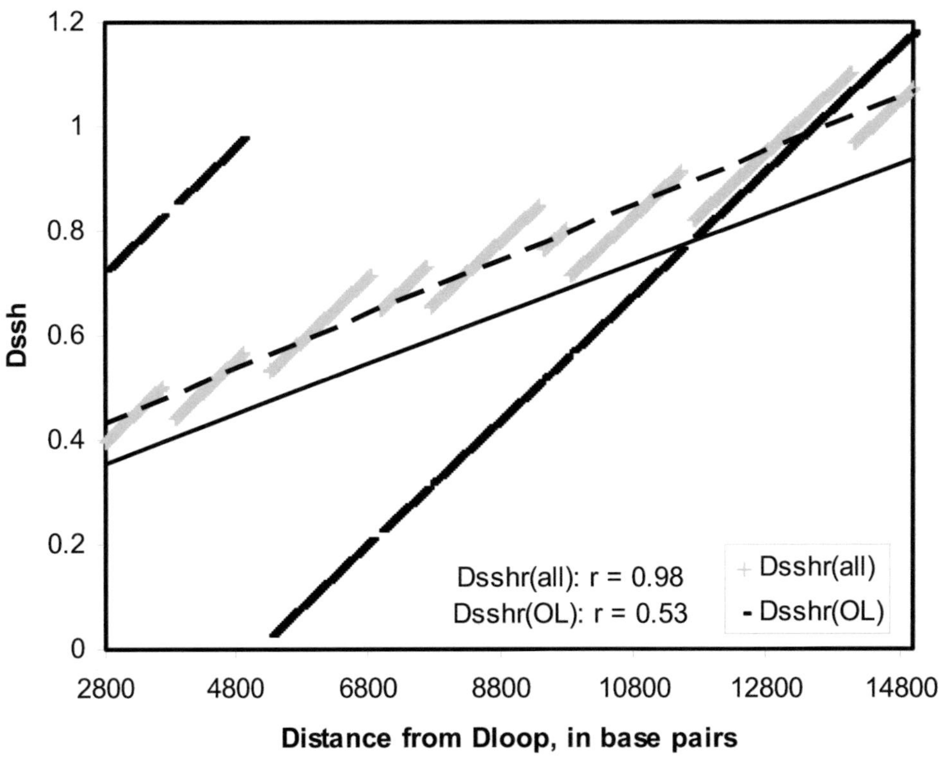

Fig. 1. Duration of time spent single stranded during replication ($D_{ssh}r$) as a function of distance in number of base pairs from the heavy strand promoter in the mitochondrial D-loop. Black- $D_{ssh}r$ assuming a single light strand origin of replication, OL, in the WANCY region, termed $D_{ssh}rW$ in the text; grey- $D_{ssh}rX$, assuming that all DNA regions coding for tRNAs function at equal weights as additional OLs.

over 4 of all 13 mitochondrially encoded protein coding genes and both rRNAs. Hence, one could expect that evolution of multiple OLs in mitochondrial genomes, especially in taxa with long lifespan, would tend towards increasing collinearity of $D_{ssh}rX$ with $D_{ssh}t$, reducing the extent of DNA regions with high mutation risks. Multiple OLs would regulate $D_{ssh}r$->$D_{ssh}t$ convergence. These interactions between mitochondrial replication and transcription would be an additional process interacting with mitochondrial transcription (Bonawitz et al., 2006).

1.6 Alternative replication mechanisms

This is in line with studies suggesting that multiple OLs exist in vertebrate mitochondria (Brown et al., 2005; Brown & Clayton 2006; Clayton & Brown 2006). The hypothesis that mitochondrial light strands are replicated at multiple locations by Okazaki fragments (Holt et al., 2000) as the lagged strand in nuclear genomes is also compatible with the statistical patterns observed by Seligmann et al., (2006b). In fact, the deamination gradients detected by comparative analyses are considered as strong evidence in favor of the unidirectional replication mechanisms (Gibson, 2005). My interpretation is that the unidirectional replication is relatively rare, but it leaves at evolutionary scales a clear imprint on genomes because it causes biases in mutation patterns, and that at least one other replication process, putatively similar to the one in nuclei, exists. That process is more frequent and effective, affecting less the genome at evolutionary scale. Indeed, some evidence on mitochondrial transcription factors suggests that two replication modes coexist, and that the modes of mitochondrial replication are regulated by mitochondrial metabolism (Pohjoismaki et al., 2006). Results and conclusions will be also interpreted according to this hypothesis, considering that only one replication mechanism, the unidirectional one, creates replication deamination gradients.

1.7 Lifespan and convergence of replication and transcription

Heavy strand sequences of mitochondrial tRNA genes tend to form OL-like structures and seem to assist the "recognized" vertebrate mitochondrial OL in the WANCY region (Seligmann & Krishnan, 2006). $D_{ssh}rX$ resembles $D_{ssh}t$ more than does $D_{ssh}rW$ (see Figure 1, and Seligmann et al., 2006b). Pathogenic mutations, as compared to non-pathogenic polymorphisms in human mitochondrial tRNAs, disturb the fine balance of $D_{ssh}rX$ by altering which tRNAs function and which do not function as alternative OLs (Seligmann et al., 2006b). These observations strengthen the hypothesis that collinearity between these processes increases longevity by slowing ageing.

A further observation in line with this hypothesis is that nucleotide contents of heavy strand DNA sequences coding for the first and second positions of tRNA anticodons in vertebrate mitochondrial genomes correlate with $D_{ssh}t$ calculated according to the highly conserved tRNA arrangement along the vertebrate mitochondrial genome. When mitochondrial replication and transcription are collinear, as observed in *Homo sapiens* after integrating all putative OLs in $D_{ssh}rX$ calculations, overall deamination risks at sites coding for the first two anticodon positions are minimized (Seligmann et al., 2006b), not only during transcription, but also during replication because replication is collinear with transcription in this case. It hence makes sense that ageing-related processes, such as developmental stability and lifespan, are affected by convergence between replication and transcription. I test this hypothesis and discuss alternative hypotheses that could account for the patterns described below.

2. Materials and methods

In order to test this ageing-related collinearity hypothesis, I calculated rt, the correlation coefficient between C or T contents at third codon positions for all 13 protein coding genes (methodology as in Seligmann et al., 2006b) and $D_{ssh}t$; and rW, the correlation coefficient between C or T contents as above, and $D_{ssh}rW$. I used the light strand sequences, coding Cs by "1" and Ts by zero, so that the gradient reflects the slower deamination reaction of A to G that occurs during replication on the heavy strand as a function of D_{ssh}. I did also similar calculations for the other gradient, coding light strand As by "1" and Gs by zero, reflecting the heavy strand gradient due to the faster deamination of C to T. Results were generally qualitatively similar for this gradient, but are not presented here.

I used for D_{ssh} calculations the numbering system of Genbank for nucleotide sites, also used by Tanaka and Ozawa (1994) and Seligmann et al., (2006b). $D_{ssh}t$ is the relative distance of the base pair from the starting point of the transcription, meaning the number assigned to that base pair following that numbering system divided by the total length of the genome:

$$D_{ssh}t = b/N,$$

where b is the distance in bases of the nucleotide position from the genome numbering starting point and N is the total mitochondrial genome length.

I calculated $D_{ssh}rW$ of ND1 and ND2 genes using the equation:

$$D_{ssh}rW = ((N-W)*2+b-(N-b))/N,$$

where W is the position at mid-location of the sequence forming the classical light strand replication origin. In species lacking the classical origin, I used for W the mid-location of the sequence located between the two tRNAs that normally flank the regular light strand replication origin, tRNA-Asn and tRNA-Cys. For other genes, I calculated $D_{ssh}rW$ according to the equation:

$$D_{ssh}rW = (b-W)*2/N.$$

Note that visual examinations of gradients in single species, such as those shown in Figure 2, are based on gene-wise averages of the binary C and T contents of that gene at third codon position. Analyses based on such averages would probably yield qualitatively similar results. I opt for the method using site specific nucleotide contents, without averaging over genes in order to maximize the amount of information used from the raw sequence data. It is possible that reducing data by averaging following the natural units of protein coding sequences might reveal additional phenomena or aspects of the main phenomenon examined, a point that should be kept in mind. The gene-wise averaging method has clear advantages for graphical presentation and is therefore used here in various Figures.

$D_{ssh}r$ calculations for tRNA clusters different from the WANCY region containing the classical light strand replication origin are done following Seligmann et al., (2006b). These calculations were not used besides for Figure 1, for other analyses presented here, only $D_{ssh}rW$ and $D_{ssh}rt$ were used. $D_{ssh}r$ calculations for the various tRNA clusters as light strand replication origins, as they were used to estimate $D_{ssh}rX$ in Figure 1, are calculated following the principles described by Seligmann (2008).

This was done for a number of mammalian and reptilian taxa, notably for 26 complete Primate mitochondria, and two outgroups, *Cynocephalus variegatus* and *Tupaia belangeri*. The

correlation coefficients, rt and rW are used here as estimates of gradient strengths. In Primates, I tested for correlations of rt and rW each, with the maximal lifespan of these taxa (lifespan data from http://genomics.senescence.info/species/ (de Magalhaes & Costa, 2009), besides for *Chlorocebus sabaeus* (Sade and Hildrech 1965), *Procolobus badius* (http://www.missouri.edu/~anthmark/courses/mah/factfiles/redcolubus.htm) and *Pongo abelii* (Wich et al., 2004)). In other groups, I only tested for the correlation of rt-rW with lifespan. The use of maximal lifespan for animals in captivity is a reasonable proxy for longevity, as well as maximal lifespan in the wild, as was shown at least in geckos (Werner et al., 1993). Before using correlation coefficients as variables in analyses, they were z transformed in order to linearize their scales (Amzallag, 2001) considering sample sizes (Seligmann et al., 2007). Analyses were done for various groups for which the relevant genomic and life history data were available for a sufficient number of species. For lizards, correlations with lifespan were tested, as well as correlations with estimates of developmental stabilities, when such were available (Seligmann et al., 2003). Two independent sets of lizard species were used: Amphisbaenidae, (*Bipes biporus, Bipes canaliculatus, Bipes tridactylus, Diplometopon zarudnyi, Rhineura floridana*), using the number of intercalated annuli on the ventral side of these animals (Seligmann & Krishnan, 2006) as a measure of developmental instability (the association with maximal longevity was not tested in this group because of lack of longevity data), and species for which both complete genome sequences and estimates of maximal lifespan* or fluctuating asymmetry$ in subdigital lamellae under the fourth toe were available (Agamidae, *Calotes versicolor**$; Anguidae, *Abronia graminea*$; Cordylidae, *Cordylus warreni**; Eublepharidae, *Coleonyx variegatus**$; Gekkonidae, *Gekko gecko**$, *Gekko vitattus*$; Helodermatidae, *Heloderma suspectum**$; Iguanidae, *Iguana iguana**$; Lacertidae, *Lacerta viridis**$, *Takydromus tachydromoides*$; Scincidae, *Eumeces egregius*$; Sceloporidae, *Sceloporus occidentalis*$; Xantusiidae, *Lepidophyma flavimaculatum**$). D_{ssh} calculations for species possessing duplicate Dloops are not straightforward and deserve special treatment. Such species (i.e. *Varanus niloticus, Sphenodon punctatus*) were excluded from analyses.
I also tested for correlations of rt-rW, termed collinearity between gradients or $D_{ssh}r$->$D_{ssh}t$ convergence, with the length of the gestation period. Information on gestation periods is also from http://genomics.senescence.info/species/.

3. Results and discussion

3.1 Replication versus transcription gradients in various species

Examining graphs plotting the mean C/T ratio at third codon position for each gene as a function of $D_{ssh}t$ and as a function of $D_{ssh}rW$, one finds that for a majority of species, $D_{ssh}rW$ is the better predictor of nucleotide contents at third codon positions and there is no evidence for a gradient resembling the one that would be expected due to transcription, whether due to replication convergent with transcription or transcription itself (for example the greater white-toed shrew *Crocidura russula* in Figure 2a). In some species, usually relatively long lived, such as in the western gorilla and the Yangtze river dolphin *Lipotes vexillifer* (Figures 2b, c), the situation is less clear, with both $D_{ssh}t$ and $D_{ssh}rW$ explaining a significant amount of variation in nucleotide contents, although $D_{ssh}rW$ is the better predictor and hence can be considered as the major cause of the gradient (meaning, the WANCY region would be the most commonly used OL). In some rarer cases, such as in the yellow-spotted night lizard *Lepidophyma flavimaculatum* (Figure 2d), the correlation

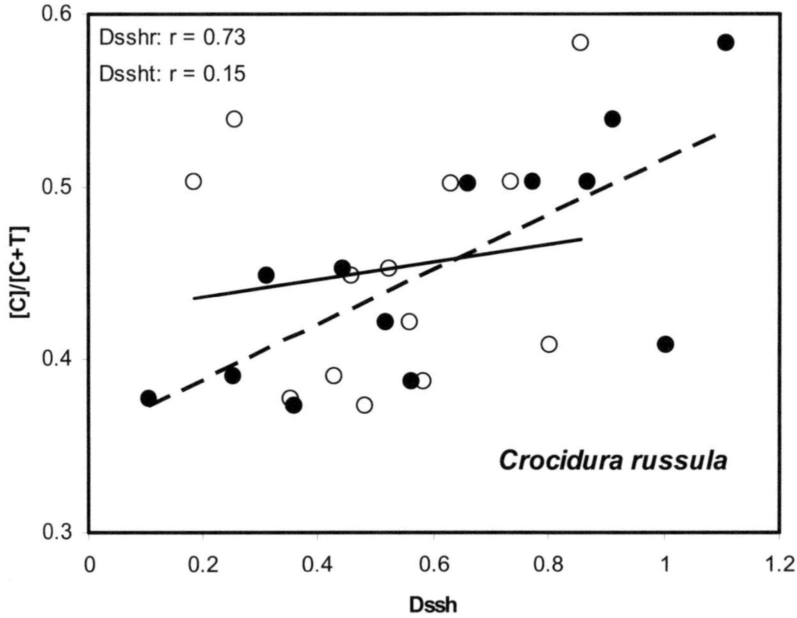
Dsshr: r = 0.73
Dssht: r = 0.15
Crocidura russula
[C]/[C+T]
Dssh
0.6
0.5
0.4
0.3
0
0.2
0.4
0.6
0.8
1
1.2

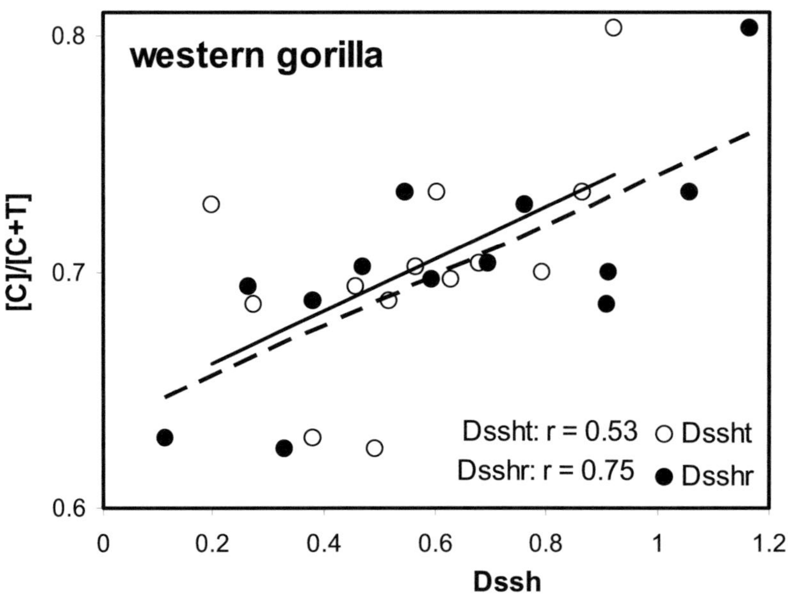
western gorilla
Dssht: r = 0.53
Dsshr: r = 0.75
Dssht
Dsshr
[C]/[C+T]
Dssh
0.8
0.7
0.6
0
0.2
0.4
0.6
0.8
1
1.2

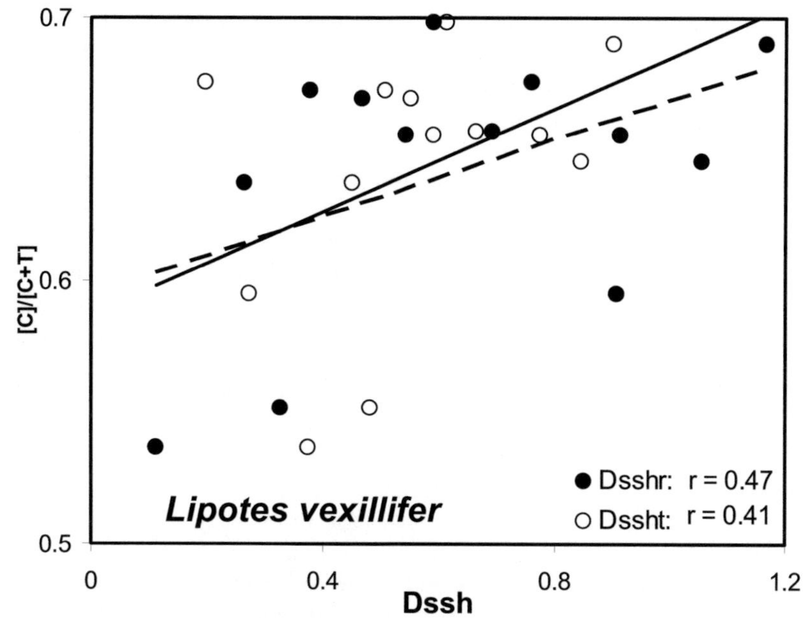

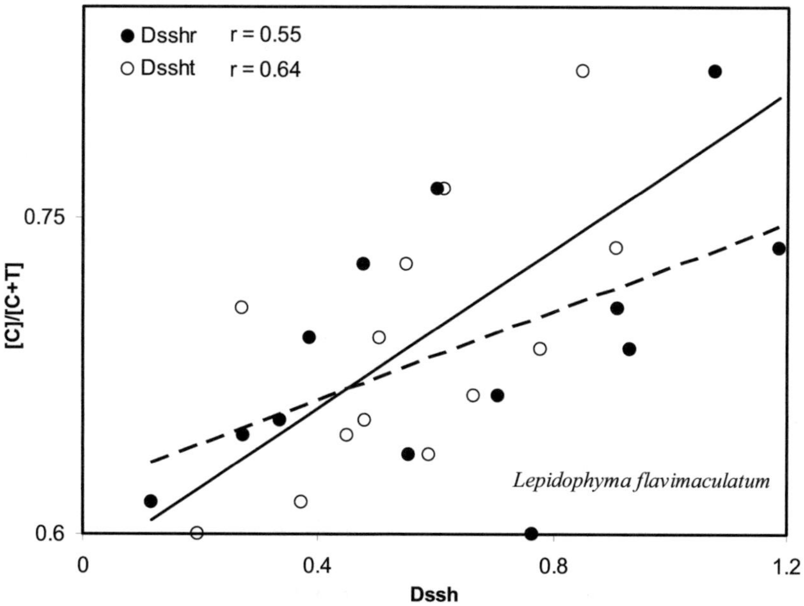

Fig. 2. Proportion of cytosine at third codon positions as a function of time spent single stranded during transcription ($D_{ssh}t$) and replication ($D_{ssh}r$) in 13 mitochondrial protein coding sequences: a) in the insectivore *Crocidura russula*, a typical example where the replication gradient is by far stronger than the transcription-like gradient; b) in the western gorilla, where the transcription-like gradient is apparent, but weaker than the replication gradient; c) in the cetacean *Lipotes vexillifer*, where both gradients are similar; and d) in the lizard *Lepidophyma flavimaculatum*, where the transcription-like gradient is stronger than the replication one.

of nucleotide contents with $D_{ssh}t$ is better than with $D_{ssh}rW$, indicating that in that species, processes causing deamination gradients due to the time spent single stranded tend to start usually within the Dloop. This could either indicate that in that species the frequency of transcriptions is overwhelmingly larger than of replications, or that replication does relatively rarely start in the region of the regular OL. The latter option is in line with the fact that there is no recognized OL sequence in that lizard species at the regular OL location, between tRNA-Asn and tRNA-Cys, and that in this species, unlike in other lizards lacking a recognized OL sequence between these tRNAs, the adjacent 5′ arm of tRNA-Asn and 3′ arm of tRNA-Cys, including the short intergenic sequence, do not form OL-like structures as those found in *Trogonophis* (Seligmann & Krishnan, 2006) and other lizards (Macey et al., 1997). Hence it is likely that patterns are due to replication resembling (converging with) transcription, rather than due to transcription itself. This point is further discussed below.
These observations suggest that variation exists among species in the extent that $D_{ssh}r$ converges with $D_{ssh}t$, and that this variation might associate with life history: in the examples presented, regular replication gradients starting at the recognized OL sequence are observed in short lived species with high metabolic rates (shrew), while the convergence between replication and transcription increases for more long lived species with lower metabolisms (gorilla, dolphin, lizard), paralleling the dichotomy noted above for gradients between prokaryotes (where patterns remind more those found in mitochondria of short lived mammals) and eukaryotes (resembling more those found in mitochondria of long lived animals with slower metabolisms). This justifies testing whether the extent of $D_{ssh}r$->$D_{ssh}t$ convergence correlates with lifespan and other ageing-related processes.

3.2 Gradient convergence and lifespan in Primates

In Primates, the strength of the replication gradient that considers only the recognized OL (rW) does not correlate with maximal lifespan ($r = 0.11$, $P = 0.29$, one tailed test, not shown); the strength of the transcription gradient (rt) increases with maximal lifespan ($r = 0.318$, $P = 0.049$, one tailed test, not shown). This improvement in the correlation with lifespan fits the prediction that the actual replication gradient, calculated having considered all putative OLs and not only the one in the WANCY region, is to some extent collinear with the transcription gradient, and hence the strength of the transcription gradient, rt, is a better estimate of the strength of the replication gradient than rW. In this case, and as expected by the working hypothesis, the extent by which rt is stronger than rW would measure the extent by which $D_{ssh}rX$ resembles $D_{ssh}t$.
I quantified this extent by calculating the residuals of rt for each Primate species from the regression between rt (dependent) and rW (independent) ($rt = 0.822*rW+0.04$, $r = 0.83$, $P < 0.001$). These residuals are unlikely, from a statistical point of view, to correlate with lifespan because rt correlates with lifespan: they represent only a small fraction of the variation inherent to rt because rW explains 69% of the variation in rt. Nevertheless, results show that they correlate better than rt with maximal lifespan ($r = 0.405$, $P = 0.016$, 1 tailed test; see Figure 3), indicating that the extent of $D_{ssh}r$->$D_{ssh}t$ convergence affects lifespan. Analyses reveal similar patterns in other groups, such as Carnivora (Figure 4, analyses excluding Pinnipedia). In these cases, no residual analyses were done, and rW was simply subtracted from rt. The correlation is positive as expected for a pool of groups excluding Mustelidae and other closely related groups. Patterns in Mustelidae closely resemble those for other Carnivora, besides for an outlier, the Eastern spotted skunk (*Spilogale putorius*), whose maximal lifespan is lower than expected considering its relatively high $D_{ssh}r$->$D_{ssh}t$ convergence.

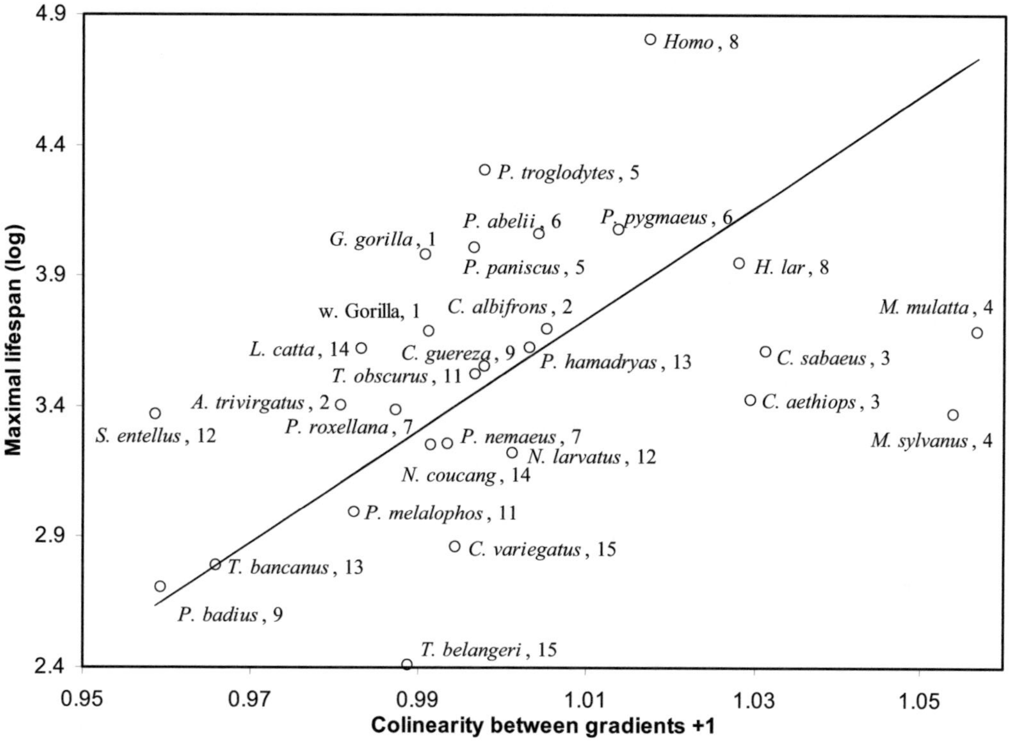

Fig. 3. Maximal primate lifespan as a function of a measure of convergence between replication and transcription in primate mitochondrial genomes. The x axis is the residual of rt, the strength of the transcriptional deamination gradient, with rW, the strength of the replicative deamination gradient calculated considering only the classically recognized OL in the WANCY region. Gradient strengths are estimated by Pearson correlation coefficients (see also text for further explanations). Species names are followed by numbers that indicate pairing in phylogenetic contrast analyses, then by NCBI (genbank) entries for species that were not used by Seligmann et al. 2006a: *Aotus trivirgatus*[2]; *Cebus albifrons*[2]; *Chlorocebus aethiops*[3]; *Chlorocebus sabaeus*[3], NC_008066; *Colobus guereza*[9]; *Cynocephalus variegatus*[15], NC_004031; *Gorilla gorilla*[1]; *western Gorilla*[1]; *Homo sapiens*[8]; *Hylobates lar*[8]; *Lemur catta*[14]; *Macaca mulatta*[4]; *Macaca sylvanus*[4]; *Nasalis larvatus*[12], NC_008216; *Nycticebus coucang*[14]; *Pan paniscus*[5]; *Pan troglodytes*[5]; *Papio hamadryas*[13]; *Pongo abelii*[6]; *Pongo pygmaeus*[6]; *Presbytis melalophos*[11], NC_008217; *Procolobus badius*[9]; *Pygathrix nemaeus*[7], NC_008220; *Pygathrix roxellana*[7], NC_008218; *Semnopithecus entellus*[12], NC_008215; *Tarsius bancanus*[13]; *Trachypithecus obscurus*[11]; *Tupaia belangeri*[15], NC_002521.

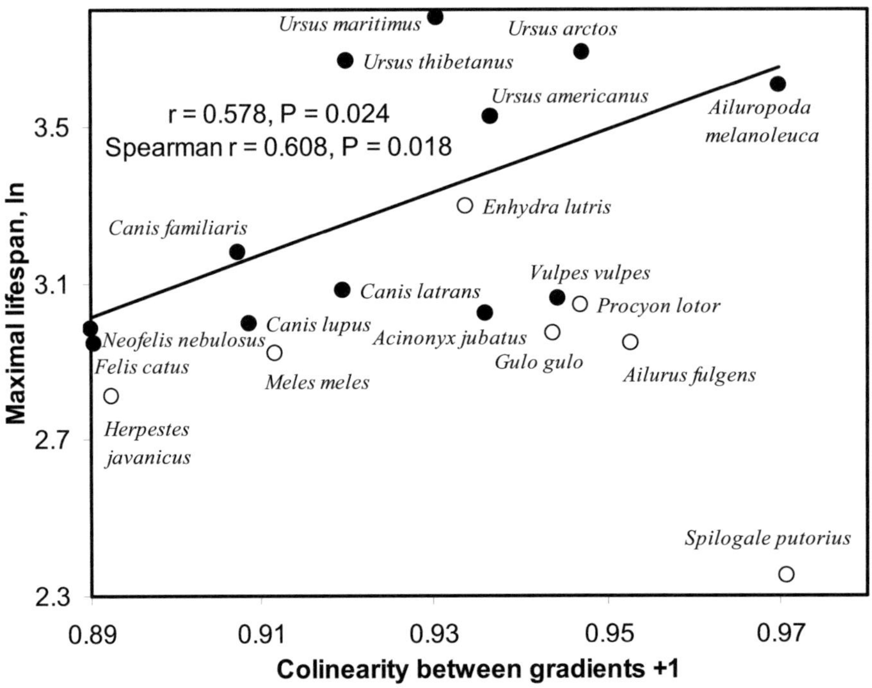

Fig. 4. Maximal lifespan as a function of a measure of convergence between replication and transcription in mitochondrial genomes of two groups of Carnivora, excluding Pinnipedia. The x axis is the subtraction of rW, which estimates the strength of the regular replication gradient, from rt, which estimates the strength of the transcription-like gradient. Species names are followed by NCBI (genbank) entries. Full symbols are for Carnivora excluding Mustelidae and consorts: *Acinonyx jubatus*, NC_005212; *Ailuropoda melanoleuca*, NC_009492; *Canis familiaris*, NC_002008; *Canis latrans*, NC_008450; *Canis lupus*, NC_008066; *Felis catus*, NC_008450; *Neofelis nebulosus*, NC_008450; *Ursus arctos*, NC_003427; *Ursus americanus*, NC_003426; *Ursus maritimus*, NC_003428; *Ursus thibetanus*, NC_009431; *Vulpes vulpes*, NC_008434. Open symbols are for Mustelidae and consorts: *Ailurus fulgens*, NC_009691; *Enhydra lutris*, NC_009692; *Gulo gulo*, AM711901; *Herpestes javanicus*, NC_004031; *Meles meles*,NC_009677; *Procyon lotor*, NC_009126; *Spilogale putorius*, AM711988. Correlation analyses exclude Mustelidae.

3.3 Convergence of replication towards transcription

Analyses between the various life history traits and gradient strengths presented and discussed in the rest of this study did not detect any significant correlation with rW, while those with rt were systematically stronger and sometimes statistically significant. This is despite the strong mathematically trivial correlation existing between rt and rW, which is also apparent from Figure 1. But the strongest correlations were systematically with rt-rW, confirming that the factor that is most relevant to life history is the extent of convergence of replication towards transcription, rather than the extent of the transcription-like replication gradient. This is the main point of the hypothesis presented here.

3.4 Too extreme convergence between replication and transcription decreases lifespan

Closer examinations of Figures 3 and 4 reveal that for species with relatively high (or even extreme) convergence between gradients (rt>rW: *Cercopithecus aethiops*, *C. sabaeus*, *Macaca mulatta* and *M. sylvanus* in Primates; Figure 3; similar patterns exist in Mustelidae, Figure 4), lifespan is sometimes much below the general trend expected according to other species with lower convergence levels.

This suggests that at high $D_{ssh}r$->$D_{ssh}t$ convergence levels, another factor decreases lifespan. It is plausible that collinearity between the processes increases the frequency of collisions between replication and transcription forks. This decreases the respective rates of these processes, increasing the overall time spent single stranded, causing more mutations. This increase might be greater than the relative decrease in mutation rate due to collinearity between the processes, especially at high collinearity levels. Figure 5 plots lifespan in

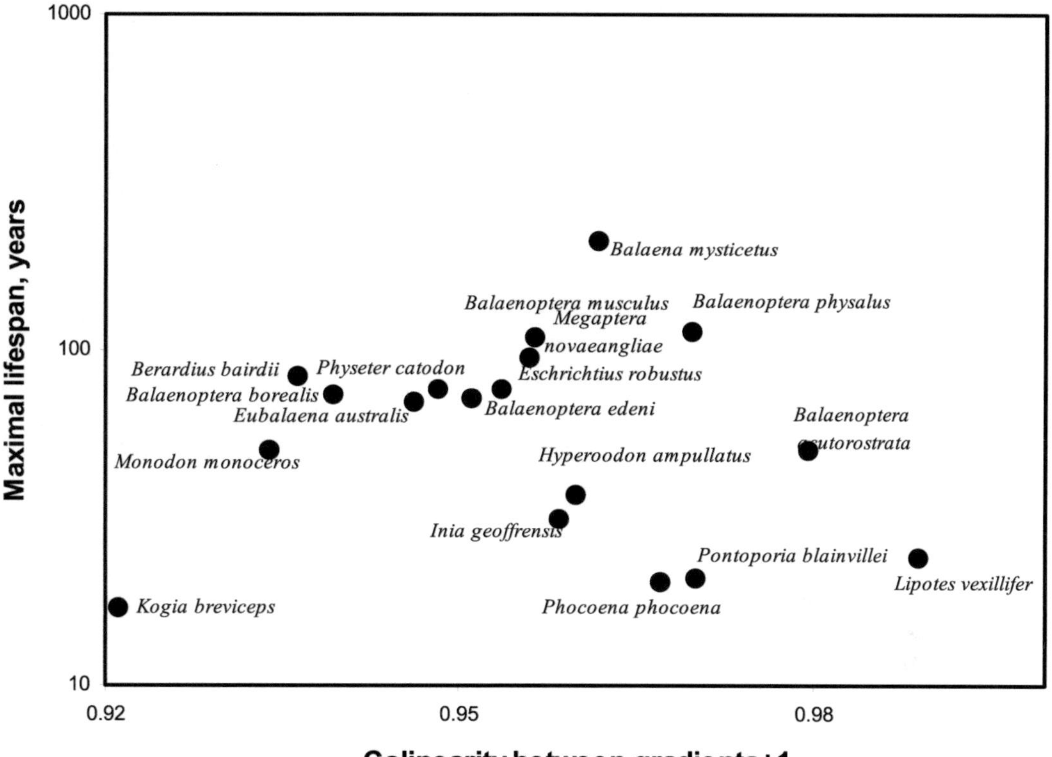

Fig. 5. Maximal lifespan as a function of a measure of convergence between replication and transcription in mitochondrial genomes in Cetacea. Axes are as in Figure 3. Species names are followed by NCBI (genbank) entries: *Balaena mysticetus*, NC_005268; *Balaenoptera acutorostrata*, NC_005271; *Balaenoptera borealis*, NC_006929; *Balaenoptera edeni*, NC_007938; *Balaenoptera musculus*, NC_001601; *Balaenoptera physalus*, NC_001321 ; *Balaenoptera bairdii*, NC_005274; *Eschrichtius robustus*, NC_005279; *Eubalaena australis*, NC_006930; *Hyperoodon ampullatus*, NC_005273; *Inia geoffrensis*, NC_005276; *Kogia breviceps*, NC_005272; *Lipotes vexillifer*, NC_007629; *Megaptera novaeangliae*, NC_006927; *Monodon monoceros*, NC_005279; *Phocoena phocoena*, NC_005280; *Physeter catodon*, NC_002503; *Pontoporia blainvillei*, NC_005277.

Cetacea as a function of $D_{ssh}r$->$D_{ssh}t$ convergence. At low convergence levels, lifespan increases with convergence until a threshold region in $D_{ssh}r$->$D_{ssh}t$ convergence. Beyond that threshold, lifespan decreases with $D_{ssh}r$->$D_{ssh}t$ convergence. It is hence not a surprise to find a negative correlation between $D_{ssh}r$->$D_{ssh}t$ convergence and maximal lifespans in lizards (Figure 6). Hence the few outliers found in Figures 3 and 4a would reflect the same phenomenon as the one observed for a larger part of species in Cetacea (those for which a negative correlation of lifespan with convergence for high convergence levels exists) or for lizards (Figure 6).

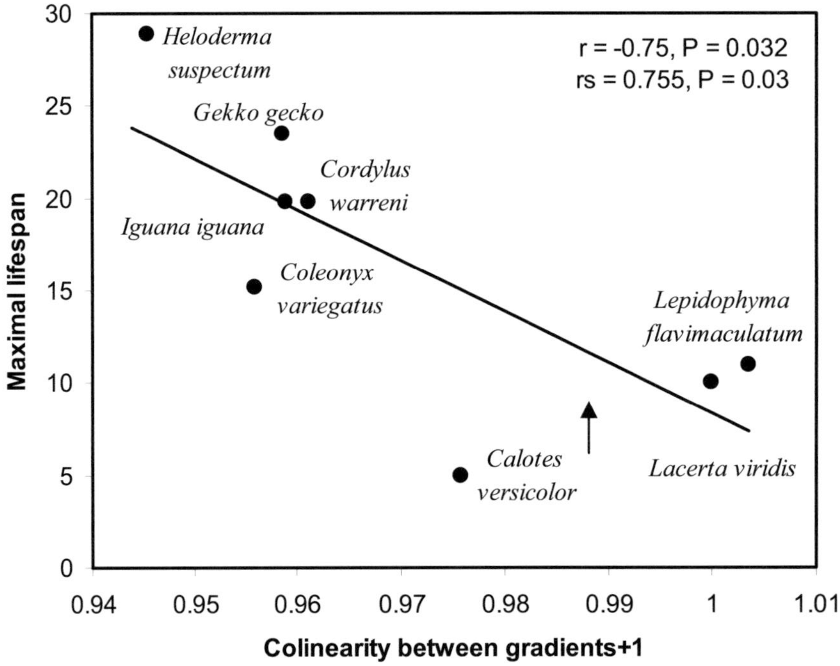

Fig. 6. Maximal lifespan as a function of a measure of convergence between replication and transcription in lizard mitochondrial genomes possessing only one Dloop region. Axes are as in Figure 4. Species names are followed by NCBI (genbank) entries: *Calotes versicolor* (NC_009683), *Coleonyx variegatus* (NC_008774), *Cordylus warreni* (NC_005962), *Gekko gecko* (NC_007627), *Heloderma suspectum* (NC_008776), *Iguana iguana* (NC_002793), *Lacerta viridis* (NC_008328) and *Lepidophyma flavimaculatum* (NC_008775).

3.5 Developmental stability and convergence between transcription and replication

Analyses testing for correlations between $D_{ssh}r$->$D_{ssh}t$ convergence and developmental stabilities yield qualitatively similar results to those found for associations with maximal lifespan: in some groups, convergence decreases stability (in a pool of lizards from several families, r = -0.52, Figure 7), and in others, convergence decreases instability (Amphisbaenia, r = - 0.76, Figure 8).

3.6 Rates of development and convergence between replication and transcription

As noted above, convergence between replication and transcription increases the frequency of collisions between these processes, hence decreasing their respective rates. Ultimately, decreased replication and transcription rates should impede on an organism's development, decreasing its differentiation and growth rates. I used the length of the gestation period as an estimate inversely proportional to differentiation rate and tested for the expected positive correlation between gestation period and $D_{ssh}r$->$D_{ssh}t$ convergence levels (see the example for Insectivora in Figure 9). Because maximal lifespan, together with brain size, correlates positively with the length of the gestation period (Sacher & Staffeld, 1974; Jones & MacLarnon, 2004), this result does not independently confirm the $D_{ssh}r$->$D_{ssh}t$ convergence hypothesis, despite that the mechanisms assumed to cause the correlations with lifespan and those with gestation length differ: lifespan is presumed to increase because convergence increases mutational robustness (only extreme convergence decreases mutational robustness and lifespan); at the same time, convergence decreases the rates of replication and transcription,, and presumably also developmental rates.

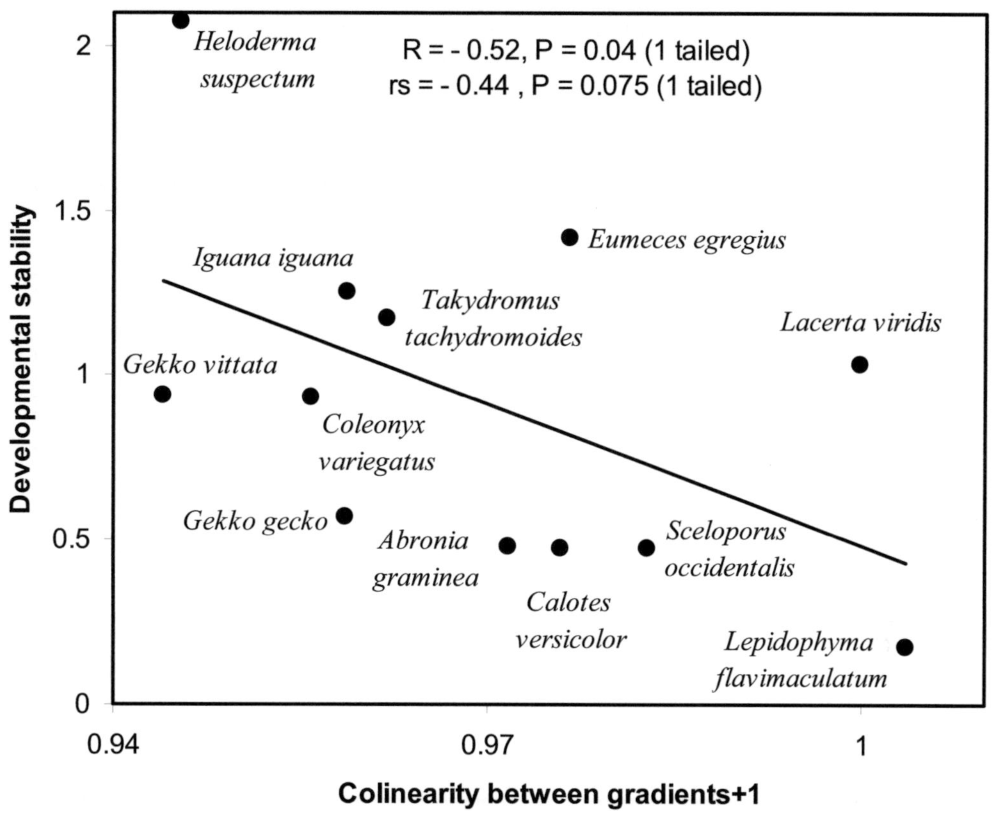

Fig. 7. Developmental stability in subdigital lamellae counts as a function of a measure of convergence between replication and transcription in lizard mitochondrial genomes possessing only one Dloop region. X axis is as in Figure 4. Species names are followed by NCBI (genbank) entries: *Abronia graminea* (NC_005958), *Calotes versicolor* (NC_009683), *Coleonyx variegatus* (NC_008774), *Eumeces egregius* (NC_000888), *Gekko gecko* (NC_007627), *Gekko vittatus* (NC_008772), *Heloderma suspectum* (NC_008776), *Iguana iguana* (NC_002793), *Lacerta viridis* (NC_008328), *Lepidophyma flavimaculatum* (NC_008775), *Sceloporus occidentalis* (NC_005960), *Takydromus tachydromoides* (NC_008773).

However, the rationale that $D_{ssh}r$->$D_{ssh}t$ convergence affects both lifespan and gestation yields a prediction that is not trivial, despite the strong positive correlation that exists between lifespan and the length of the gestation period: in groups of species with high fertility and rates of development (short gestation), considered as r-strategists, one expects that $D_{ssh}r$->$D_{ssh}t$ convergence adaptively coevolved with the length of gestation, while in groups of species with low fertility and rates of development (long gestation and lifespan), considered as K-strategists, it makes sense to expect adaptive coevolution between $D_{ssh}r$->$D_{ssh}t$ convergence and lifespan. Hence, despite that lifespan and the length of gestation are highly correlated, a testable, independent, nontrivial prediction exists, which is that correlations between $D_{ssh}r$->$D_{ssh}t$ convergence and lifespan should be weaker in r strategists than those between $D_{ssh}r$->$D_{ssh}t$ convergence and the length of gestation, while in K strategists, the opposite is expected. This is estimated by subtracting the z transformed correlation coefficient between $D_{ssh}r$->$D_{ssh}t$ convergence and the length of gestation from the z transformed correlation coefficient between $D_{ssh}r$->$D_{ssh}t$ convergence and lifespan in that group (z transformation was adjusted for differences in sample sizes between different

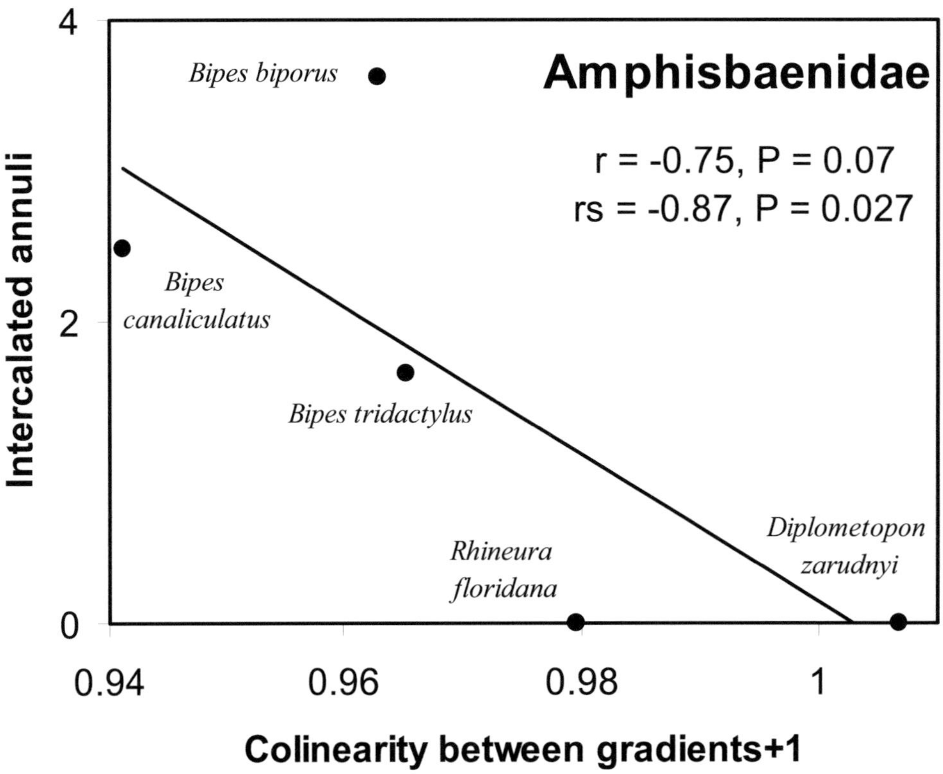

Fig. 8. Number of intercalated annuli on the ventral side of Amphisbaenidae, a measure of developmental instability in serpentiform reptile species (see Seligmann and Krishnan 2006), as a function of colinearity between replication and transcription. X axis is as in Figure 4. Species names are followed by NCBI (genbank) entries: *Bipes biporus* (NC_006287); *Bipes canaliculatus* (NC_006288); *Bipes tridactylus* (NC_006286), *Diplometopon zarudnyi* (NC_006283) and *Rhineura floridana* (NC_006282).

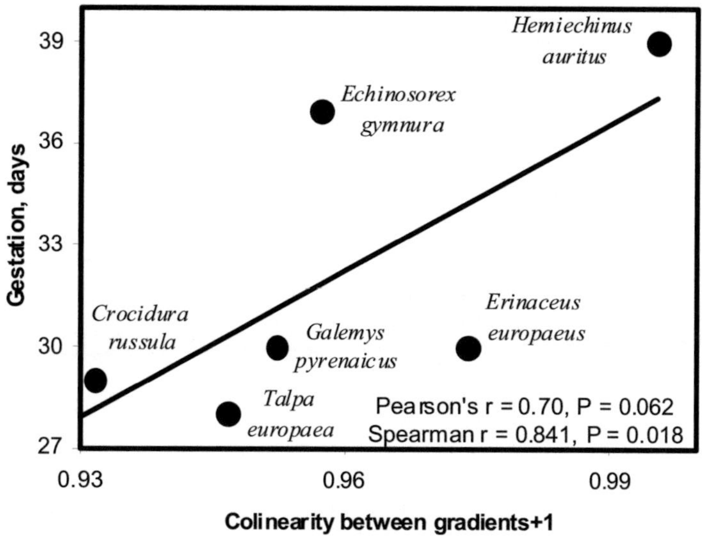

Fig. 9. Gestation period as a function of a measure of convergence between replication and transcription in mitochondrial genomes of Insectivora. X-Axis is as in Figure 3. Species names are followed by NCBI (genbank) entries: *Crocidura russula*, NC_006893; *Echinosorex gymnura*, NC_002808; *Erinaceus europaeus*, NC_002080; *Galemys pyrenaicus*, NC_008156; *Hemiechinus auritus*, NC_005033; *Talpa europaea*, NC_002391.

taxonomic groups, see method in Seligmann et al., 2007). Figure 10 tests this prediction by plotting this subtraction as a function of the mean maximal lifespan for that taxonomic group, used here as an estimate of the extent that the group is a relatively r- or K-strategist (short and long maximal lifespans, respectively). Results in Figure 10 fit the expectation that correlations with lifespan, relative to those with the length of the gestation period, increase along the r-K gradient. The increase in the subtraction is approximately gradual along the r-K gradient (which is estimated by the mean maximal lifespan in that group). According to this result, patterns from more than 100 mitochondrial genomes follow the complex predictions from a simple hypothesis.

4. General discussion

4.1 Replication versus transcription gradients in various species

Results show that species vary widely in extents of convergence between replication and transcription gradients. In many species, the replication gradient starting at the recognized OL is the only or the major gradient detected, as found for *Crocidura* (Figure 2a). In these species, no gradient resembling the transcription gradient, whether due to transcription or replication, was detected. This observation, considering that transcription occurs in all species, suggests that most mutations on mitochondrial DNA occur during replication. The lack of detection of gradients that resemble what could be interpreted as a transcription-related gradient suggests that in those fewer species where significant correlations occur between nucleotide contents and $D_{ssh}t$, these reflect mutations occurring during replication,

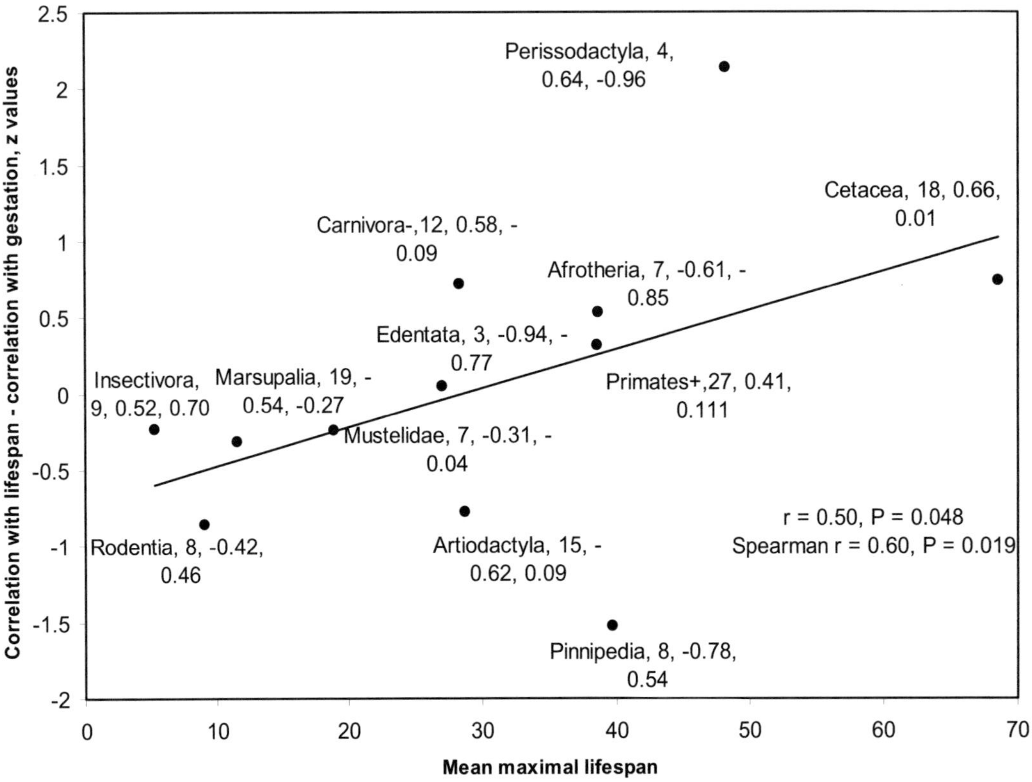

Fig. 10. Difference between strength of association of convergence between replication and transcription gradients with maximal lifespan and with length of gestation period as a function of the mean maximal lifespan in that mammalian taxonomic group. For each taxonomic group, the Pearson correlation coefficient of gradient convergence with length of gestation in that group was subtracted from its correlation coefficient with maximal lifespan. Group names are indicated near datapoints, followed by the number of species used for the lifespan analyses, and the correlation coefficients with lifespan and length of gestation, respectively. Values used for the y axis, but not for those indicated inside the figure, are z transformed correlation coefficients, taking into account sample sizes (see text). Carnivora- indicates that analyses were done excluding Mustelidae and Pinnipedia, and Primates+ indicates that analyses of this group included *Cynocephalus* and *Tupaia*.

with replication origins distributed such that the overall replicational gradient (integrating over different replication origins) resembles the one caused by transcription. It is possible that because transcription is much more frequent than replication, the reactions that create the gradients are saturated, and hence no gradient is detected at the time scales the phenomenon is observed here. Hence while the comparative methodology used seems adequate to detect replication gradients, other methods should be used in order to detect transcription gradients. This means that at this evolutionary time scale, replication is the main phenomenon, and transcription is probably a secondary phenomenon, whose detection necessitates more sophisticated methods, as explained for some cases from the literature in the Introduction.

The correlation between convergence of replication gradient with transcription gradient with lifespan was r = 0.80 in Chiroptera (5 species), but this group is not included in Figure 10 because only for 2 Chiroptera both genomic and gestation period data were available. Results presented for lizards (Figure 9) are not included because there is no gestation *per se* in these groups.

4.2 Transcription or replication?

For the sake of simplicity, I consider that the major cause for the observed gradients in nucleotide contents with $D_{ssh}t$ is replication, meaning that in these cases replication converged with transcription, but that transcription itself is not responsible for the observed gradients. Although this is at this point a rough simplification, there are several reasons beyond those given above justifying this assumption. It makes sense that the polymerization rates by the gamma polymerase, the enzyme replicating mitochondrial DNA, and by the mitochondrial RNA polymerase (Bonawitz et al., 2006) differ, because these are very different enzymes and the functional requirements differ for each process: the frequency of transcription is much greater than that of replication, and its rate is also probably much greater. However, the impact of errors during RNA polymerization is lower than that during DNA replication and hence RNA and DNA polymerase fidelities are also probably very different. Deamination gradients result from time spent single stranded during these processes, but because one can assume that transcription is much faster than replication, it is likely that the properties of the mutation gradient resulting from transcription differ from those of the replication gradient. Hence effects of one D_{ssh} unit on nucleotide contents should differ between gradients caused by transcription or replication. Examining the various graphs in Figure 2, one can see that this is not the case: the slopes found for gradients with $D_{ssh}rW$ and $D_{ssh}t$ are very similar when gradients are detected with each $D_{ssh}rW$ and $D_{ssh}t$ (see for example the western gorilla, Figure 2b). This justifies the simplifying assumption that replication is the major cause of the observed gradients, and this approach should be considered as a satisfying approximation at this point.
This does not mean that this assumption should not be tested later, especially that exploring this issue might yield valuable information on the relative regulations of transcription, replication, and/or various types of replication, which are at the heart of the mitochondrial replication controversy and ageing-related pathologies. Note that even at that level of distinguishing between deamination gradients caused by transcription and those caused by replication in a situation where both are confounded because replication is collinear with transcription, bioinformatics analyses can be helpful. Two deamination gradients exist on the heavy strand, one caused by the chemical reaction C->T, and one by A->G (both hydrolytic deaminations). The former is the faster reaction, and therefore the latter saturates less quickly, also from an evolutionary point of view (see Krishnan et al., 2004a, b). Therefore each of these two mutation types reacts differently to D_{ssh}. Hence the ratio between the slopes of each of these gradients should differ if the gradients are due to transcription (C->T should be less saturated and more similar to the A->G gradient because transcription is faster than replication) than when deamination gradients are due to replication. Hence such analyses could determine which process, transcription or replication, created the detected gradient(s), even when both processes are collinear and apparently confounded.

4.3 Gradient convergence and lifespan in Primates

Results in Figure 3 suggest that convergence between replication and transcription slows ageing-related processes in Primates. Note that Figure 3 shows that relative to other Primates, longevity in *Homo sapiens* is greater than expected according to convergence between replication and transcription. This would be congruent with the hypothesis that human longevities increased recently, due to factors other than convergence of $D_{ssh}r$->$D_{ssh}t$, but suggests that future evolution increasing this convergence could still increase longevity.

The correlation in Figure 3 also remains significant after applying the method of phylogenetic contrasts (Felsenstein, 1985) to the data, suggesting that the results are statistically valid independently of phyletic constraints ($r = 0.50$, $P = 0.03$, one tailed test). It makes sense that results of regular correlations, with and without accounting for phylogenetic contrasts are qualitatively similar because evolution of tRNAs functioning as OLs tends to be saltatory (Seligmann et al., 2006b).

Gestation time, despite its association with maximal lifespan in Primates ($r = 0.67$, $P < 0.01$), only slightly increases with the level of $D_{ssh}r$->$D_{ssh}t$ convergence ($r = 0.11$, $P < 0.1$). This suggests that collinearity between replication and transcription might cause interferences, slowing down both processes and ultimately developmental rates. Even a weak effect on developmental rates (inversely proportional to gestation length) could be a potent selective pressure in natural populations, counterbalancing pressures against cumulating excess mutations that favor collinearity between the processes.

This effect on growth rates is probably relatively weak in Primates and in general K-strategists, which maximize lifespan rather than developmental rates (Brookfield, 1986). The opposite is expected in groups that are, relatively to Primates, more r-strategy-oriented, a strong prediction corroborated in Figure 10 and discussed below.

4.4 Correlations between molecular and whole organism levels

One should note that several correlations between life history parameters and molecular indices characterizing metabolic strategies of cells have already been described, specifically for Primates: the length of the gestation period with cost minimization of nuclear amino acid usages (Seligmann, 2003), cost minimization of mitochondrial ribosomal frameshifts (Seligmann & Pollock, 2004), slopes of (regular) mitochondrial replication gradients (Raina et al., 2005); and now maximal lifespan with convergence between mitochondrial replication and transcription. Seligmann & Krishnan (2006) discuss how whole organism properties probably result from many different, coadapted cellular processes, so that the wealth of significant correlations detected between molecular properties and whole organism features should be of no surprise. In addition, it is notable that nuclear genome size is not related to life-history traits in Primates (Morand & Ricklefs, 2005), so that effects of mitochondrial properties are more likely to be detected in this group.

4.5 Too extreme convergence between replication and transcription

The examination of Figures 3 and 4 shows that the trend between maximal lifespan and $D_{ssh}r$->$D_{ssh}t$ convergence has outliers, and that these outliers are usually placed in the same relative area of the graph: these are species with relatively high convergence but lower than expected lifespan. It is possible that this situation results from asymmetry in inaccuracies in maximal lifespan estimations, as sampling error can only cause lower values than the real maximal lifespan. However it makes little sense that the well studied *Macaca* species, for example, have a lifespan that is much greater than in Figure 3, although these species are clearly outliers in respect to the general trend in Figure 3. This situation was also observed in other taxonomic groups (results not presented graphically here but used in Figure 10), and it is remarkable that there were never cases of outliers with low convergence but high lifespan. Hence the hypothesis of statistical artifact is unlikely here, and this situation is most probably biologically meaningful. It indicates that low convergence between replication and transcription does not enable to reach a long lifespan, but that high convergence is not necessarily a sufficient condition to enable a long lifespan, and that other factors affect this. The results for Cetacea (Figure 5) indeed show that high convergence might in fact limit lifespan. Presumably, this is because at high convergence levels, the decrease in mutations due to collinearity between replication and transcription might be smaller than the increase due to longer D_{ssh} because of increasing delays due to collisions between replication and transcription. This could explain the relatively sharp boundary between the region where convergence increases lifespan, and the one where a negative correlation is observed in Cetacea, and would account for outliers in figures presenting results for other taxa.

4.6 Rates of development and convergence between replication and transcription

The hypothesis that collisions decrease rates of replication and transcription when both processes are collinear predicts that rates of development decrease with $D_{ssh}r$->$D_{ssh}t$ convergence. The cause for this would differ from the correlation between $D_{ssh}r$->$D_{ssh}t$ convergence and lifespan. For lifespan, convergence decreases cumulation of mutations and in general, increases mutational robustness; for developmental rates, they are the direct result of decreased replication and transcription rates because of increased collision frequencies between replication and transcription forks. It is notable that this rationale yields a molecular mechanism for the well known negative association between metabolic rates and longevities, as described in Insects (Antler flies, Bonduriansky & Brassil, 2005; Drosophila, Marden et al., 2003; Novoseltsev et al., 2005; Mockett & Sohal, 2006), nematodes (Jenkins et al., 2004; Chen et al., 2007; Lee et al., 2006; Hughes et al., 2007) and mice (Cargill et al., 2003; and others, Bonsall, 2006). Some ecological data explaining the tradeoffs exist (Bonduriansky & Brassil, 2005), and results suggest the tradeoff is due to dietary metabolism (Partridge et al., 2005a,b; Speakman, 2005a,b; Kaeberlein et al. 2006; Ruggiero & Ferrucci, 2006; Szewczyk et al., 2006; Wolkow & Iser, 2006). Other evidence shows that this rule might not be universal (Van Voorhies et al., 2004; Khazaeli et al., 2005; Johnston et al., 2006), stressing the need for unifying hypotheses. Several molecular or biochemical mechanisms have been proposed (Balaban et al., 2005; Bartke ,2005; Knauf et al., 2006; Powers et al., 2006) but no general molecular model exists, stressing the importance to link the $D_{ssh}r$->$D_{ssh}t$ convergence hypothesis with the lifespan-growth rate tradeoff. Making a meaningful test for this prediction that $D_{ssh}r$->$D_{ssh}t$ convergence decreases developmental rates (hence increases the length of gestation) is not straightforward because of the strong positive association that exists between maximal lifespan and gestation length. However, using evolutionary ecology theory on r and K strategists, the simple molecular mechanism makes complex predictions on the relative strengths of association of $D_{ssh}r$->$D_{ssh}t$ convergence with lifespan and gestation length, respectively. The fact that these predictions are overall verified by the analysis of a large number of species and groups of species in Figure 10 is strong support for the $D_{ssh}r$->$D_{ssh}t$ convergence hypothesis and its coevolution with major life history traits.

4.7 Causal interpretations of correlations between lifespan and convergence between replication and transcription

The hypothesis that collisions decrease rates of replication and transcription when both processes are collinear enables to predict the occurrence of species that seem outliers in graphical analyses. However, the longevity-growth rate tradeoff hypothesis suggests the possibility that the causal interpretation of the association of $D_{ssh}r$->$D_{ssh}t$ convergence with maximal lifespan is opposite to the direction assumed. This is because offspring fitness decreases with parental age (Kern, 2001; Priest et al., 2002; Moore & Harris, 2003; Moore & Sharma, 2005), putatively due to ontogenetic cumulation of mutations, especially in mothers (McIntyre & Gooding, 1998; Hercus & Hoffmann, 2000), which are inherited by offspring. This issue is particularly relevant to mitochondria. Indeed, species with long lifespan probably have relatively high transcription/replication ratios. Hence what appears to be convergence of replication gradients towards transcription gradients could be the result of increased lifespan, rather than its cause. This interpretation assumes that the gradients observed are transcription-, rather than replication ones, which remains possible despite the arguments against this in previous sections. Notwithstanding these arguments, this interpretation is not compatible with other predictions presented here about developmental rates, the relatively frequent outlying species characterized by high convergence and lower than expected lifespan, and the threshold phenomenon observed in Figure 5. In addition, this individual-based observation is a stabilizing feedback mechanism where increased longevity causes inheritance of mutations that decrease offspring longevity. This would rather predict negative correlations, or no correlation at time scales larger than that of single generations, such as in the inter-species comparisons described in the Results.

The specific situation in *Homo*, where recent evolution caused a rapid increase in lifespan that is not paralleled by a proportionately high $D_{ssh}r$->$D_{ssh}t$ convergence, could be interpreted both ways: lifespan, which is known to have increased recently by man-made environmental changes and not cell metabolism (Larkin, 2000), does not fit what would be expected according to cell metabolism (as measured by $D_{ssh}r$->$D_{ssh}t$ convergence), suggesting that in other species where no such fast changes occurred, $D_{ssh}r$->$D_{ssh}t$ convergence explains lifespan. Alternatively, one could speculate that in *Homo*, the recent man-made increase in lifespan did not yet alter the relative strengths of transcription versus replication gradients, following the hypothesis that a long lifespan increases more the number of transcriptions than of replication. According to that scenario, the relatively recently increased transcription/replication ratio did not yet result in stronger transcription gradients in *Homo*, explaining the position of that species in Figure 3. Besides that the latter interpretation is based on a more complex rationale than the former, it also seems less likely because if the causal mechanism underlying the $D_{ssh}r$->$D_{ssh}t$ convergence-lifespan association is that increased lifespan causes more transcription-related deaminations, this is due to mutations cumulating ontogenetically (see the effects of parental age on offspring quality referred to above). However, following this rationale, gradients should almost immediately react to the increase in lifespan, which is not the case in *Homo*.

4.8 Developmental stability and convergence between transcription and replication

It is interesting to note that the principles observed for the association between $D_{ssh}r$->$D_{ssh}t$ convergence and lifespan are also valid for that between $D_{ssh}r$->$D_{ssh}t$ convergence and developmental stability. This observation fits the general trend that developmental instability associates with low fitness and pathologies. It would be interesting to explore whether this hypothesis of convergence of replication with transcription fits with the "double-agent" unifying hypothesis of ageing and diseases based on the tradeoff between oxidative stress inducing genetic reaction mechanisms against stress and its effect on ageing and age-related disease (Lane, 2003). The molecular processes presented provide mechanistic explanations for these similarities.

5. Conclusions

I present the original hypothesis that heavy strand sequences of tRNA-coding genes functioning as additional light strand replication origins tend to increase the similarity of mutational patterns resulting from replication with those due to transcription, putatively decreasing cumulation of mutations during the two processes. Variation exists among mitochondrial genomes in the extent that replication mutation gradients resemble transcription gradients; in most species (mainly short lived with high metabolism), replication gradients do not resemble transcription gradients. The similarity of replication mutation gradients to transcription ones correlates positively with maximal lifespan in Primates and other taxa. Systematically, outliers to these trends have replication mutation gradients relatively resembling transcription gradients but are for short lived species, the opposite (long lived outliers with replication gradients not resembling transcription gradients) does not occur. In some taxa such as Cetacea, this phenomenon is enhanced with two clearcut ranges in similarity between replication and transcription, one with relatively low similarities, where maximal lifespan increases with the similarity of replication gradients to transcription gradients, and another region where similarities are highest and maximal lifespan decreases with similarity. These patterns suggest that low convergence does not enable high maximal lifespans, but too high convergence limits lifespan, probably because too many collisions between replication and transcription forks decrease both replication and transcription rates, increasing durations spent single stranded, and mutation frequencies. The length of gestation periods increases also with convergence, notably, in r strategists; in K strategists, the convergence levels coevolve more with maximal lifespan, fitting the rationale that the molecular machinery is adapted for high metabolism and fertility in r strategists, and high survival in K strategists. Results are interpreted assuming that the observed phenomena are due to replication that sometimes resembles transcription, but are not due to transcription. Evidence supporting this is presented: in species possessing two gradients, one according to the classical replication origin, and one resembling transcription, both mutation gradients have very similar slopes, which is more compatible with a single enzymatic machinery (the mitochondrial gamma DNA polymerase) causing both gradients, rather than each due to a different polymerase. A method based on differences in the respective rates of replication and transcription for distinguishing between replication and transcription gradients is suggested, where the ratios between slopes of mutation gradients of purines versus pyrimidines should vary when mutation gradients are due to replication resembling transcription rather than transcription itself. The hypothesis that results are due to a causal relationship opposite to the one proposed (high longevity causes high transcription/replication ratios and hence transcription gradients dominate replication ones) is examined and discussed. This interpretation is unlikely, not only because gradients seem to be due to a single enzymatic process, but also because this hypothesis is less compatible with patterns in the data: among others it does not predict the patterns observed for outliers and the differences between r- and K-strategists.

6. Acknowledgments

I am very thankful to Neeraja M. Krishnan for manifold help in the preparation and improvement of this manuscript. Morphological data could not have been gathered without considerable curatorial help at the various herpetological collections I visited: American Museum of Natural History, New York; California Academy of Sciences, San Francisco; Field Museum, Chicago; Hebrew University of Jerusalem; Museum of Natural History, London; Museum of Vertebrate Zoology, Berkeley; Peggy Notebaert Nature Museum, Chicago Academy of Sciences; Tel Aviv University.

7. References

Albrecht-Buehler, G. (2006) Asymptotically increasing compliance of genomes with Chargaff's second parity rules through inversions and inverted transpositions. *Proc. Nat. Acad. Sci.* USA, 103, 17828-17833.

Aldana, M., Balleza, E., Kauffman, S., Resendiz, O. (2007) Robustness and evolvability in genetic regulatory networks. *J. Theor. Biol.* 245, 433-448.

Amzallag, G.N. (2001) Data analysis in plant physiology: are we missing the reality? *Plant Cell. Env.* 24, 881-890.

Balaban, R.S., Nemoto, S., Finkel, T. (2005) Mitochondria, oxidants, and aging. *Cell* 120, 483-495.

Baran, R.H., Ko, H., Jernigan, R.N. (2003) Methods for comparing sources of strand compositional asymmetry in microbial chromosomes. *DNA Res.* 10, 85-95.

Bartke, A. (2005) Minireview: Role of the growth hormone/insulin-like growth factor system in mammalian aging. *Endocrinology* 146, 3718-3723.

Bonawitz, N.D., Clayton, D.A., Shadel, G.S. (2006) Initiation and beyond: multiple functions of the human mitochondrial transcription machinery. *Mol. Cell.* 24, 813-825.

Bonduriansky, R., Brassil, C.E. (2005) Reproductive ageing and sexual selection on male body size in a wild population of antler flies (*Protopiophila litigata*). *J. Evol. Biol.* 18, 1332-1340.

Bonsall, M.B. (2006) Longevity and ageing: appraising the evolutionary consequences of growing old. *Phil. Trans. Royal Soc. B-Biol. Scie.* 361, 119-135.

Boulikas, T. (1995) A model of transcription replication enhancers. *Oncol. Rep.* 2, 171-181.

Brazhnik, P., Tyson, J.J. (2006) Cell cycle control in bacteria and yeast - A case of convergent evolution? *Cell Cycle* 5, 522-529.

Brookfield, J.F.Y. (1986) The evolution of r-strategies and K-strategies. *Biol. J. Linn. Soc.* 27, 165-178.

Brown, T.A., Clayton, D.A. (2006) Genesis and wanderings - Origins and migrations in asymmetrically replicating mitochondrial DNA. *Cell Cycles* 5, 917-921.

Brown, T.A., Cecconi, C., Tkachuk, A.N., Bustamante, C., Clayton, D.A. (2005) Replication of mitochondrial DNA occurs by strand displacement with alternative light-strand origins, not via a strand-coupled mechanism. *Genes & Dev.* 19, 2466-2476.

Cargill, S.L., Carey, J.R., Muller, H.G., Anderson, G. (2003) Age of ovary determines remaining life expectancy in old ovariectomized mice. *Aging Cell* 2, 185-190.

Chang,D.D., Clayton,D.A. (1984) Precise identification of individual promoters for transcription of each strand of human mitochondrial DNA. *Cell* 36, 635-643.

Chang, D.D., Clayton, D.A. (1985) Priming of human mitochondrial DNA replication occurs at the light-strand promoter. *Proc. Natl. Acad. Sci. USA* 82, 351-355.

Chang, D.D., Hauswirth, W.W., Clayton, D.A. (1985) Replication priming and transcription initiate from precisely the same site in mouse mitochondrial DNA. *EMBO J.* 4: 1559-1567.

Chen, J.J., Senturk, D., Wang, J.L., Muller, H.G., Carey, J.R., Caswell, H., Caswell-Chen, E.P. (2007) A demographic analysis of the fitness cost of extended longevity in *Caenorhabditis elegans*. *J. Geront. A-Biol. Scie. & Med. Scie.* 62, 126-135.

Ciliberti, S., Martin, O.C., Wagner, A. (2007) Robustness can evolve gradually in complex regulatory gene networks with varying topology. *PLOS Comp. Biol.* 3, 164-173.

Clayton, D.A. (2000) Transcription and replication of mitochondrial DNA. Hum. Reprod. 15, 11-17.

Clayton, D.A., Brown, T.A. (2006) Replication of mammalian mitochondrial DNA occurs by strand displacement with alternative light-strand origins. *FASEB J* 20, A453-A453.

Coskun, P.E., Beal, M.F., Wallace, D.C. (2004) Alzheimer's brains harbor somatic mtDNA control-region mutations that suppress mitochondrial transcription and replication. *Proc. Nat. Ac. Sci. USA* 101, 10726-10731.

Couturier, E., Rocha, E.P.C. (2006) Replication-associated gene dosage effects shape the genomes of fast-growing bacteria but only for transcription and translation genes. *Mol. Microbiol.* 59, 1506-1518.

de Magalhaes, J. P., and Costa, J. (2009) A database of vertebrate longevity records and their relation to other life-history traits. *J. Evol. Biol.* 22, 1770-1774.

Desjardins, P., Morais, R. (1990) Sequence and gene organization of the chicken mitochondrial genome - a novel gene order in higher vertebrates. *J. Mol. Biol.* 212, 599-634.

Elena, S.F., Wilke, C.O., Ofria, C., Lenski, R.E. (2007) Effects of population size and mutation rate on the evolution of mutational robustness. *Evolution* 61, 666-674.

Feder, M.E. (2007) Evolvability of physiological and biochemical traits: evolutionary mechanisms including and beyond single-nucleotide mutation. *J. Exp. Biol.* 210, 1653-1660,

Felsenstein, J. (1985) Phylogenies and the comparative method. *Am. Nat.* 125, 1-15.

Fernandez-Silva, P., Enriquez, J.A., Montoya, J. (2003) Replication and transcription of mammalian mitochondrial DNA. *Exp. Physiol.* 88, 41-56.

Francino, M.P., Chao, L., Riley, M.A., Ochman, H. (1996) Asymmetries generated by transcription-coupled repair in enterobacterial genes. *Science* 272, 107-109.

Francino, M.P., Ochman, H. (2001) Deamination as the basis of strand-asymmetric evolution in transcribed *Escherichia coli* sequences. *Mol. Biol. Evol.* 18, 1147-1150.

Gibson, A.P. (2005) *Comparative analysis of vertebrate mitochondrial genomes*. PhD thesis, University of Manchester, UK.

Gilbert, D.M. (2001) Making sense of eukaryotic DNA replication origins. *Science* 294, 96-100.

Glusman, G., Qin, S.Z., El-Gewely, R., Siegel, A.F., Roach, J.C., Hood, L., Smit, A.F.A. (2006) A third approach to gene prediction suggests thousands of additional human transcribed regions. *PLOS Comp. Biol.* 2, 160-173.

Grigoriev, A. (1999) Strand-specific compositional asymmetries in double-stranded DNA viruses. *Virus Res.* 60, 1-19.

Hassan, A.B., Cook, P.R. (1994) Does transcription by RNA-polymerase play a direct role in the initiation of replication? *J. Cell. Sci.* 107, 1381-1387.

Hassanin, A., Leger, N., Deutsch, J. (2005) Evidence for multiple reversals of asymmetric mutational constraints during the evolution of the mitochondrial genome of Metazoa, and consequences for phylogenetic inferences. *Syst. Biol.* 54, 277-298.

Hercus, M.J., Hoffmann, A.A. (2000) Maternal and grandmaternal age influence offspring fitness in Drosophila. *Proc. Royal Soc. London B-Biol. Scie.* 267, 2105.

Holt, I.J., Lorimer, H.E., Jacobs, H.T. (2000) Coupled leading- and lagging-strand synthesis of mammalian mitochondrial DNA. *Cell* 105, 515-524.

Hou, W.R., Wang, H.F., Niu, D.K. (2006) Replication-associated strand asymmetries in vertebrate genomes and implications for replicon size, DNA replication origin, and termination. *Biochem. Biophys. Res. Comm.* 344, 1258-1262.

Hughes, S.E., Evason, K., Xiong, C.J., Kornfeld, K, (2007) Genetic and pharmacological factors that influence reproductive aging in nematodes. *PLOS Genetic* 3, 254-265.

Huvet, M., Nicolay, S., Touchon, M., Audit, B., d'Aubenton-Carafa, Y., Arneodo, A., Thermes, C., (2007) Human gene organization driven by the coordination of replication and transcription. *Genom. Res.* 17, 1278-1285.

Jenkins, N.L., McColl, G., Lithgow, G.J. (2004) Fitness cost of extended lifespan in *Caenorhabditis elegans. Proc. Royal Soc. London B-Biol. Scie.* 271, 2523-2526.

Jones, A.G., Arnold, S.J., Burger, R. (2007) The mutation matrix and the evolution of evolvability. *Evolution* 61, 727-745.

Jones, K.E., MacLarnon, A.M. (2004) Affording larger brains: Testing hypotheses of mammalian brain evolution on bats. *Amer. Nat.* 164, E20-E31.

Johnston, S.L., Grune, T., Bell, L.M., Murray, S.J., Souter, D.M., Erwin, S.S., Yearsley, J.M., Gordon, I.J., Illius, A.W., Kyriazakis, I., Speakman, J.R. (2006) Having it all: historical energy intakes do not generate the anticipated trade-offs in fecundity. *Proc. Royal. Soc. B-Biol. Scie.* 273, 1369-1374.

Kaeberlein, T.L., Smith, E.D., Tsuchiya, M., Welton, K.L., Thomas, J.H., Fields, S., Kennedy, B.K., Kaeberlein, M. (2006) Lifespan extension in *Caenorhabditis elegans* by complete removal of food *Aging Cell* 5, 487-494.

Kern, S., Ackermann, M., Stearns, S.C., Kawecki, T.J. (2001) Decline in offspring viability as a manifestation of aging in *Drosophila melanogaster*. *Evolution* 55, 1822-1831.

Khaidakov, M., Siegel, E.R., Reis, R.J.S. (2006) Direct repeats in mitochondrial DNA and mammalian lifespan. *Mech. Ageing Dev.* 127, 808-812.

Khazaeli, A.A., Van Voorhies, W., Curtsinger, J.W. (2005) Longevity and metabolism in *Drosophila melanogaster*: Genetic correlations between life span and age-specific metabolic rate in populations artificially selected for long life. *Genetics* 169, 231-242.

Knauf, F., Mohebbi, N., Teichert, C., Herold, D., Rogina, B., Helfand, S., Gollasch, M., Luft, F.C., Aronson, P.S. (2006) The life-extending gene Indy encodes an exchanger for Krebs-cycle intermediates. *Biochem. J.* 397, 25-29.

Krishnan, N.M, Seligmann, H., Raina, S.Z., Pollock, D.D. (2004a) Detecting gradients of asymmetry in site-specific substitutions in mitochondrial genomes. *DNA Cell Biol.* 23, 707–714.

Krishnan N.M, Seligmann, H., Raina, S.Z., Pollock, D.D. (2004b) Phylogenetic analyses detect site-specific perturbations in asymmetric mutation gradients. *Curr. Computa. Mol. Biol.* 2004, 266–267.

Larkin, M. (2000) Is the human lifespan limitless? *Lancet* 356, 1249-1249.

Lane, N. (2003) A unifying view of ageing and disease: the double-agent theory. *J. Theor. Biol.* 225, 531-540.

Lee, D.Y., Clayton, D.A. (1997) RNase mitochondrial RNA processing correctly cleaves a novel R loop at the mitochondrial DNA leading-strand origin of replication. *Genes Dev.* 11,582-592.

Lee, G.D., Wilson, M.A., Zhu, M., Wolkow, C.A., de Cabo, R., Ingram, D.K., Zou, S.G. (2006) Dietary deprivation extends lifespan in *Caenorhabditis elegans. Aging Cell* 5, 515-524.

Little, R.D., Platt, T.H.K., Schildkraut, C.L. (1993) Initiation and termination of DNA replications in human ribosomal-RNA genes. *Mol. Cell Biol.* 13, 6600-6613.

MacAlpine, D.M., Rodriguez, H.K., Bell, S.P. (2004) Coordination of replication and transcription along a Drosophila chromosome. *Genes Dev.* 18, 3094-3105.

Macey, J.R., Larson, A., Ananjeva, N.B., Fang, Z., Papenfuss, T.J. (1997) Two novel gene orders and the role of light-strand replication in rearrangement of the vertebrate mitochondrial genome. *Mol. Biol. Evol.* 14, 91-104.

Mackiewicz, P., Gierlik, A., Kowalczuk, M., Dudek, M.R., Cebrat, S. (1999) How does replication-associated mutational pressure influence amino acid composition of proteins? *Genome Res.* 9, 409-416.

Marczynski, G.T., Shapiro, L. (1995) The control of asymmetric gene-expression during *Caulobacter* cell-differentiation. *Arch. Microbiol.* 163, 313-321.

Martin, I., Grotewiel, M.S. (2006) Oxidative damage and age-related functional declines. *Mech. Ageing Dev.* 127, 411-423.

Marden, J.H., Rogina, B., Montooth, K.L., Helfand, S.L. (2003) Conditional tradeoffs between aging and organismal performance of Indy long-lived mutant flies. *Proc. Nat. Acad. Scie. USA* 100, 3369-3373.

McIntyre, G.S., Gooding, R.H. (1998) Effect of maternal age on offspring quality in tsetse (Diptera : Glossinidae). *J. Med. Entom.* 35, 210-215.

Mirkin, E.V., Mirkin, S.M. (2005) Mechanisms of transcription-replication collisions in bacteria. *Mol. Cell Biol.* 25, 888-895.

Mockett, R.J., Sohal, R.S. (2006) Temperature-dependent trade-offs between longevity and fertility in the Drosophila mutant, Methuselah. *Exp. Geront.* 41, 566-573.

Mohanty, B.K., Sahoo, T., Bastia, D. (1996) The relationship between sequence-specific termination of DNA replication and transcription. *Embo J.* 15, 2530-2539.

Moller, A.P. (1997) Developmental stability and fitness: A review. *Am. Nat.* 149:916-932.

Moller, A.P. (1999) Developmental stability is related to fitness. *Am. Nat.* 153:556-560.

Moore, P.J., Harris, W.E. (2003) Is a decline in offspring quality a necessary consequence of maternal age? *Proc. Royal Soc. London B-Biol. Scie.* 270: S192-S194.

Moore, P.J., Sharma, S. (2005) A delay in age at first mating results in the loss of future reproductive potential via apoptosis. *Evol. & Dev.* 7, 216-222.

Morand, S., Ricklefs, R.E. (2005) Genome size is not related to life-history traits in Primates. *Genome* 48: 273-278.

Morton, B.R. (1999) Strand asymmetry and codon usage bias in the chloroplast genome of *Euglena gracilis. Proc. Nat. Acad. Sci.* USA 96, 5123-5128.

Mrazek, J., Karlin, S. (1998) Strand compositional asymmetry in bacterial and large viral genomes. *Proc. Nat. Acad. Sci. USA* 95, 3720-3725.

Nass, N.M.L. (1995) Precise sequence assignment of replication origin in the control region of chick mitochondrial-DNA relative to 5'-D-loop-ends and 3'-D-loop-ends, secondary structure, DNA-synthesis, and protein-binding. *Curr. Genet.* 28, 401-409.

Nikolaou, C., Almirantis, Y. (2005) A study on the correlation of nucleotide skews and the positioning of the origin of replication: different modes of replication in bacterial species. *Nuc. Acids Res.* 33, 6816-6822.

Novoseltsev, V.N., Arking, R., Carey, J.R., Novoseltseva, J.A., Yashin, A.I. (2005) Individual fecundity and sensescence in Drosophila and Medfly. *J. Geront.* 60A, 953-962.

Partridge, L., Gems, D., Withers, D.J. (2005a) Sex and death: What is the connection? *Cell* 120, 461-472.

Partridge, L., Piper, M.D.W., Mair, W. (2005b) Dietary restriction in Drosophila. *Mechan. in Ageing & Dev.* 126, 938-950.

Patnaik, P.K. (1997) Studies with artificial extrachromosomal elements in trypanosomatids: Could specificity in the initiation of DNA replication be linked to that in transcription? *Parasitol. Today* 13, 468-471.

Pohjoismaki, J.L.O., Wanrooij, S., Hyvarinen, A.K., Goffart, S., Holt, I.J., Spelbrink, J.N., Jacobs, H.T. (2006) Alterations to the expression level of mitochondrial transcription factor A, TFAM, modify the mode of mitochondrial DNA replication in cultured human cells. *Nuc. Acids Res.* 34, 5815-5828.

Powers, R.W., Kaeberlein, M., Caldwell, S.D., Kennedy, B.K., Fields, S. (2006) Extension of chronological life span in yeast by decreased TOR pathway signaling. *Genes & Dev.* 20, 174-184.

Prado, F., Aguilera, A. (2005) Impairment of replication fork progression mediates RNA polII transcription-associated recombination. *Embo J.* 24, 1267-1276.

Priest, N.K., Mackowiak, B., Promislow, D.E.L. (2002) The role of parental age effects on the evolution of aging. *Evolution* 56, 927-935.

Rottenberg, H. (2006) Longevity and the evolution of the mitochondrial DNA-coded proteins in mammals. *Mech. Ageing Dev.* 127, 748-760.

Rottenberg, H. (2007) Coevolution of exceptional longevity, exceptionally high metabolic rates, and mitochondrial DNA-coded proteins in mammals. *Exp. Geront.* 42, 364-373.

Ruggiero, C., Ferrucci, L. (2006) The endeavor of high maintenance homeostasis: Resting metabolic rate and the legacy of longevity. *J. Geront. A-Biol. Scie. & Med. Scie.* 61, 466-471.

Sacher, G.A., Staffeld, E.F. (1974) Relation of gestation time to brain weight for placental mammals - implications for theory of vertebrate growth. *Amer. Nat.* 108, 593-615.

Sade, D.S., Hildrech, R.W. (1965) Notes on Green Monkey (*Cercopithecus aethiops sabaeus*) on St. Kitts, West Indies. *Caribbean J. Sci.* 5, 65-81.

Samuels, D.C. (2004) Mitochondrial DNA repeats constrain the life span of mammals. *TRIGS* 20, 226-229.

Samuels, D.C. (2005) Life span is related to the free energy of mitochondrial DNA. *Mech. Ageing Dev.* 126, 1123-1129.

Samuels, D.C., Schon, E.A., Chinnery, P.F. (2004) Two direct repeats cause most human mtDNA deletions. *TRIGS* 20, 393-398.

Satoh , T.P., Sato, Y., Masuyama, N., Miya, M., Nishida, M. (2010) Transfer RNA gene arrangement and codon usage in vertebrate mitochondrial genomes: a new insight into gene order conservation. *BMC Genomics* 11, 479.

Schwaiger, M., Schubeler, D. (2006) A question of timing: emerging links between transcription and replication. *Curr. Opin. Gen. & Dev.* 16, 177-183.

Szewczyk, N.J., Udranszky, I.A., Kozak, E., Sunga, J., Kim, S.K., Jacobson, L.A., Conley, C.A. (2006) Delayed development and lifespan extension as features of metabolic lifestyle alteration in *C.elegans* under dietary restriction. *J. Exp. Biol.* 209, 4129-4139.

Seligmann, H. (2003) Cost minimization of amino acid usage. *J. Mol. Evol.* 56, 151-151.

Seligmann, H. (2006) Error propagation across levels of organization: from chemical stability of ribosomal RNA to developmental stability. *J. Theor. Biol.* 242, 69-80.

Seligmann, H. (2010a) The ambush hypothesis at the whole-organism level: Off frame, 'hidden' stops in vertebrate mitochondrial genes increase developmental stability. *Comp. Biol. Chem.* 34, 80-85.

Seligmann, H. (2010b) Mitochondrial tRNAs as light strand replication origins: similarity between anticodon loops and the loop of the light strand replication origin predicts initiation of DNA replication. *Biosystems* 99, 85-93.

Seligmann, H., Krishnan, N.M. (2006) Mitochondrial replication origin stability and propensity of adjacent tRNA genes to form putative replication origins increase developmental stability in lizards. *J. Exp. Zool.* 306B, 433-439.

Seligmann, H., Krishnan, N.M., Rao, B.J. (2006a) Mitochondrial tRNA sequences as unusual replication origins: Pathogenic implications for *Homo sapiens*. *J. Theor. Biol.* 243, 375-385.

Seligmann, H., Krishnan, N.M., Rao, B.J. (2006b) Possible multiple origins of replication in Primate mitochondria: alternative role of tRNA sequences. *J. Theor. Biol.* 241, 321-332.

Seligmann, H., Pollock, D.D. (2004) The ambush hypothesis: hidden stop codons prevent off-frame gene reading. *DNA & Cell Biol.* 23, 701-705.

Shadel, G.S., Clayton, D.A. (1997) Mitochondrial DNA maintenance in vertebrates. *Ann. Rev. Biochem.* 66, 409-435.

Speakman, J.R. (2005a) Body size, energy metabolism and lifespan. *J. Exp. Biol.* 208, 1717-1730.

Speakman, J.R. (2005b) Correlations between physiology and lifespan - two widely ignored problems with comparative studies. *Aging Cell* 4, 167-175.

Tanaka, M., Ozawa, T. (1994) Strand asymmetry in human mitochondrial mutations. *Genomics* 22, 327–335.

Touchon, M., Nicolay, S., Audit, B., Bordie of Brodie, E.B., d'Aubenton-Carafa, Y., Arneodo, A., Thermes, C. (2005) Replication-associated strand asymmetries in mammalian genomes: Toward detection of replication origins. *Proc. Nat. Acad. Sci. USA* 102, 9836-9841.

Van Voorhies, W.A., Khazaeli, A.A., Curtsinger, J.W. (2004) Testing the "rate of living" model: further evidence that longevity and metabolic rate are not inversely correlated in *Drosophila melanogaster*. *J. Appl. Physiol.* 97, 1915-1922.

Wagner, A., Wright, J. (2007) Alternative routes and mutational robustness in complex regulatory networks. *Biosystems* 88, 163-172.

Werner, Y.L., Frankenberg, E., Volokita, M., Harari, R. (1993) Longevity of geckos (Reptilia, Lacertilia, Gekkonoidea) in captivity - an analytical review incorporating new data. *Isr. J. Zool* 39, 105-124.

Wich, S.A., Utami-Atmoko, S.S., Mitra Setia, T.M., Rijksen, H.D., Schuermann, C., van Hooff, J.A.R.A.M., van Schaik, C.P. (2004) Life history of wild Sumatran orangutans (*Pongo abelii*). *J. Hum. Evol.* 47, 385-398.

Wiesner, R.J.,, Zsurka, G., Kunz W. (2006) Mitochondrial DNA damage and the aging process-facts and imaginations. *Free Radical Res.* 40, 1284-1294.

Wolkow, C.A., Iser, W.B. (2006) Uncoupling protein homologs may provide a link between mitochondria, metabolism and lifespan. *Ageing Res. Rev.* 5, 196-208.

Xia, X., Huang, H., Carullo, M., Betrán, M., Moriyama, E.N. (2007) Conflict between translation initiation and elongationj in vertebrate genomes. *PLoS* 2, e227.

Yu, B.P., Chung, H.Y. (2006) Adaptive mechanisms to oxidative stress during aging. *Mech. Ageing Dev.* 127. 436-443.

7

Mitochondrial DNA Replication in Health and Disease

Nadezda Apostolova[1,2] and Juan V. Esplugues[1,2,3]
[1]*Departamento de Farmacología, Facultad de Medicina, Universidad de Valencia,*
[2]*Centro de Investigación Biomédica en Red-Enfermedades Hepáticas y Digestivas (CIBERehd), Valencia,*
[3]*Fundación para la Investigación Dr. Peset, Valencia,*
Spain

1. Introduction

Mitochondria are dynamic, semi-autonomous organelles that play a diverse role in cellular physiopathology, being involved in bioenergetics, ROS generation/signaling and redox balance, β-oxidation of free fatty acids, Ca^{2+} homeostasis, thermogenesis, and essential anabolic pathways (fatty acids, cholesterol, urea, haem and bile acids). They contain their own, mitochondrial DNA (mtDNA) which is one of the main points in favor of the hypothesis of the endosymbiotic origin of these organelles (Lang et al., 1999). The human mitochondrial genome, a 16.5 kb circular DNA consisting of a heavy and a light chain, contains 37 genes, 13 of which encode proteins involved in the mitochondrial electron transport chain (ETC), 22 of which encode transfer RNA and the remaining 2 genes encode ribosomal RNA. A mammalian somatic cell contains between 1000 and 10000 copies of mtDNA arranged in covalently closed circular molecules. There are considerable physiological variations in the mtDNA content in any given human tissue, however the mechanism of these modulations and their clinical relevance are still not clear. Like bacterial chromosomal DNA, mtDNA is organized in DNA-protein structures called nucleoids. Several proteins seem to be involved in the maintenance of these structures. The most widely studied is Transcription Factor A (TFAM) which has a clear structural role and is necessary for nucleoid stabilization.

2. Replication of mtDNA

The replication of mtDNA is wholly dependent on the nucleus. The minimal mtDNA replication apparatus consists of DNA polymerase γ (Pol γ) and two replication factors: mitochondrial single-stranded DNA binding protein (SSB) and the Twinkle helicase. Pol γ is the only known DNA polymerase present in mammalian mitochondria (there are 16 DNA polymerases in the eukaryotic cell) and carries out both DNA replication and DNA repairing function (Bebenek & Kunkel, 2004; Sweasy et al., 2006). The presence of a specific mitochondrial DNA polymerase was suggested in the late 1960s with the discovery of a polymerase in mitochondrial fractions that exhibited distinct characteristics from known mammalian DNA polymerases (Kalf et al., 1968). Several years later, a novel human polymerase was identified in HeLa cells that could utilize DNA/RNA primer templates

(Fridlender et al., 1972) which was eventually identified as mitochondrial DNA polymerase (Bolden et al., 1977). The holoenzyme of Pol γ consists of a catalytic subunit encoded by *POLG* (located at the chromosomal locus 15q25) and a dimeric form of an accessory subunit p55 encoded by *POLG2* (located at the chromosomal locus 17q24.1), which all together form the Pol γ holoenzyme (Yakubovskaya et al., 2006). Pol γ is a 140kDa enzyme that possesses DNA polymerase but also additional intrinsic activities such as 3´-5´ proofreading exonuclease activity and 5´ deoxyribonucleic phosphate lyase activity, which are responsible for base excision repair (Graziewicz et al., 2006) (Fig.1). Initial pre-steady state kinetic analyses of Pol γ demonstrated that the catalytic subunit of this enzyme alone was somewhat inefficient, with relatively weak binding to DNA (39nM) and a slow maximum rate of polymerization ($3.5s^{-1}$). Processivity of the enzyme was estimated to be about 50-100 nucleotides (Graves et al., 1998; Longley et al., 1998). Thus, it became clear that the catalytic subunit was insufficient for successful DNA replication. An accessory subunit was purified and described as a 55kDa protein required for tight DNA binding and processing DNA synthesis (Lim et al., 1999). Kinetic analysis showed that the accessory and the catalytic subunit bind with a K_d of 35nM and that this association enhances enzyme processivity from several hundreds to thousands of nucleotides. This enhancement was not linked to a significant decrease in the dissociation rate of the holoenzyme from the primer/template (Johnson et al., 2000). However, the accessory subunit provides a 3.5-fold increase in DNA binding affinity and a 6-fold decrease in K_d for dATP incorporation. The accessory subunit has also been suggested to play a role in primer recognition (Fan et al., 1999) and its ability to bind nucleic acids, particularly dsDNA, has also been demonstrated, which is very uncommon for processing factors. This feature points to a function of the accessory unit not directly related with mtDNA synthesis; namely it has been suggested to have a role in maintenance of the mitochondrial genome, specifically by organization of mtDNA in nucleoids (Di Re et al., 2009). Pol γ has high base substitution fidelity due to high nucleotide selectivity and 3´-5´ exonucleolytic proofreading. It is particularly efficient in base incorporation in short repetitive sequences in which a missinsertion has been estimated to occur only once in every 500000 nucleotides (Longley et al., 2001). However, for copying homopolymeric sequences longer than 4 nucleotides, Pol γ has lower frameshift fidelity, which can lead to replication errors and frameshift mutations in mtDNA. Importantly, Pol γ contains an intrinsic 3´-5´ exonuclease activity that contributes to its replication fidelity.

The exonuclease activity is also efficient in repairing buried mismatches. Several additional factors have also been reported to contribute to mtDNA replication and/or repair, such as mitochondrial DNA-directed RNA polymerase (POLRMT), RNA-DNA hybrid-specific RNase, Topoisomerase I and IIIα, 5´-3´ Flap endonuclease, 5´-3´ exonuclease, uracil DNA glycosylase and 8-oxo-dG glycosylase, among others (Table 1)(Copeland, 2010).

Pol γ has three main roles related to disease.

- Synthesis and repair, the origin of most spontaneous mtDNA mutations are believed to be due to errors produced by Pol γ. Comparison of the mutation spectrum from *in vivo* sources with DNA copied *in vitro* by purified human Pol γ has revealed that over 85% of the *in vivo* mutations can be recapitulated *in vitro* (Zheng et al., 2006).
- Inherited mutations in *POLG*- more than 150 disease-associated mutations have been described in this gene (Copeland, 2010).
- Mitochondrial toxicity induced by NRTI drugs- Pol γ is the only DNA polymerase that is sensitive to the nucleoside analogues used for HIV treatment (Lim et al., 2003; Lewis et al., 2006).

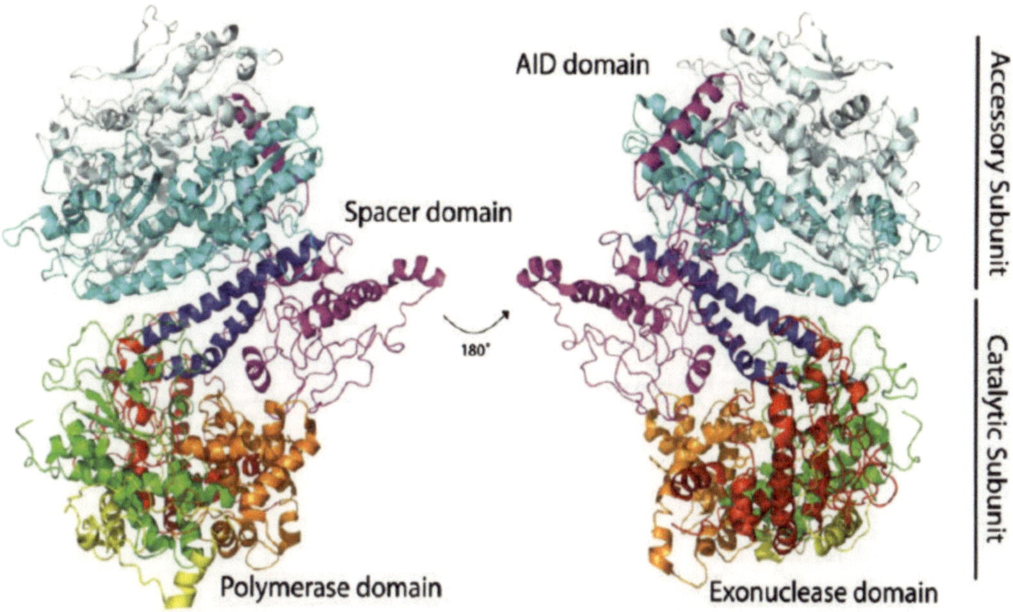

Fig. 1. Crystal structure of the Pol γ holoenzyme. Canonical right hand organization of the polymerase domain: fingers (orange), palm (green) and thumb (blue). Additional domains: mitochondrial localization sequence (yellow), exonuclease (red) and spacer (purple). Dimeric accessory subunit: proximal (cyan) and distal (light cyan) monomers (From Bailey & Anderson, 2010).

2.1 Mechanism of mtDNA replication and repair

Although mtDNA replication was identified as far back as 1972, it was only in the last decade that researchers began to understand its complex mechanism. Basically, two models have been proposed for replication of the mitochondrial genome: the strand-displacement theory and the strand-coupled theory. The strand-displacement theory suggests that replication is performed in one direction in a continuous manner without requiring the processing of Okazaki fragments on the displaced strand (Clayton, 1982). Copying of the mitochondrial genome begins at the origin of replication of the heavy strand DNA in the non-coding D-loop region of the mitochondrial genome, displacing the light chain until progressing two thirds of the way around the circular DNA. Synthesis of the light chain then begins after the formation of a stem-loop structure of the displaced heavy chain which forms the replication origin of the light strand DNA (Shadel et al., 1997). The strand-coupled model suggests that the synthesis occurs bidirectionally from multiple sites of initiation in a zone near the origin of the heavy chain replication (Holt et al., 2000; Bowmaker et al., 2003). Of note, there is a high prevalence of ribonucleotides in the lagging strand during mtDNA replication, which has more recently led to an alternative view of the strand-displacement theory termed RITOLS (RNA incorporated throughout the lagging strand) replication (Yasukawa et al., 2006; Holt, 2009). In this process, large patches of RNA protect the displaced strand during one-directional DNA synthesis. Short RNA templates are used as primers to complete replication of the lagging strand. This phenomenon may explain the lag between synthesis of the heavy and light chains of mtDNA.

Function	Gene	Protein	Size (kDa)	Chromosome locus
Core replication	POLG	DNA polymerase γ	140	15q25
	POLG2	DNA polymerase γ accessory subunit	55	17q23-24
	SSB	Single stranded DNA binding protein	15	7q34
	PEO1 (Twinkle)	Helicase	77	10q24
Replication and repair	DNA ligase III	Ligase	96	17q11.2-12
	RNase H1	RNA-DNA hybrid specific RNase	32	19p13.2
	Topo I	Topoisomerase I	67	8q24.3
	Topo IIIα	Topoisomerase IIIα	112	17p12-11.2
	Fen-1	5´-3´Flap endonuclease	43	11q12
	DNA2	5´-3´DNA/RNA endonuclease/exonuclease	130	10q21.3-q22.1
	ExoG	5´-3´exonuclease	41	3p21.3
DNA repair	UDG	Uracil DNA glycosylase	27.5	12q23-q24.1
	OGG1	8-oxo-dG glycosylase	38	3p26.2
	NTH1	Thymine glycol glycosylase	34	16p13.3
	MUTYH	glycosylase	60	1p34.3-p32.1
	NEIL1	Fapy glycosylase	44	15q4.2
	APE1	Ap endonuclease	35	14q11.2-q12
	APE2	Ap endonuclease	57	Xp11.22

Table 1. Gene products required for mtDNA replication and repair. Ap (apurinic, apyrimidinic); Fapy (2,6-diamino-4-hydroxy-formamido-pyrimidine) (Modified from Copeland, 2010).

mtDNA repair is limited to base excision repair (BER), for which the mitochondrion is equipped with several glycosylases that recognize base damage. Mitochondrial excision base repair can be performed via two pathways: single-nucleotide-BER (SN-BER) and long-patch BER (LP-BER) (Copeland & Longley, 2008). In both repair pathways, a damaged base is recognized and cleaved by a specific glycosylase, leaving an abasic site that is further cleaved on the 5´ end by AP nuclease to generate a nick with a 5´ deoxyribose phosphate (dRP) flap. During SN-BER, Pol γ fills the gap and cleaves the 5´dRP moiety prior to ligation. LP-BER seems to need the activity of additional proteins such as 5´-3´Flap endonuclease (FEN-1) (Liu et al., 2008) and 5´-3´DNA/RNA endonuclease/exonuclease (DNA2) (Zheng et al., 2008).

Current efforts are focused not only on elucidating the process of replication but particularly on identifying the factors involved in mtDNA repair and maintenance. This special interest is due to the observation that mtDNA depletion and/or mutation underlies a constantly growing list of human pathologies (Wanrooij & Falkenberg, 2010).

3. Inherited mitochondrial diseases which involve impaired DNA replication

Mitochondrial depletion syndrome (MDS) is a heterogeneous group of inherited disorders, characterized by a decreased amount of mtDNA in a specific tissue. The most severely affected organs include the brain, muscle and liver. This syndrome includes a wide spectrum of clinical disorders ranging from well-known diseases such as progressive external ophthalmoplegia (PEO) to rare tricarboxylic acid (TCA) cycle abnormalities. Typically, MDS are devastating and usually lethal diseases of infancy or early childhood and show autosomal recessive inheritance (Suomalainen & Isohanni, 2010). Since 1999, a dozen genes linked to MDS and related disorders have been described including mutations in the essential genes of mtDNA replication machinery: *POLG*, *POLG2* and *TWINKLE*. *POLG* is the most common of the genes that cause MDS and is believed to be the cause of 25% of described mitochondriopathies. Nearly 150 pathogenic mutations have been found in *POLG* (Copeland, 2010) which result in highly heterogenous disorders, such as PEO, Parkinson´s disease, Alpers syndrome, sensory ataxic neuropathy, mitochondrial neurogastrointestinal encephalomyopathy, dysarthria, Charcot-Marie-Tooth syndrome and ophthalmoparesis. In addition, mutations in several nuclear genes encoding enzymes involved in the mitochondrial nucleotide metabolism can cause depletions of mtDNA, resulting in mitochondrial syndromes. These include mitochondrial thymidine kinase (TK2), a pyrimidine nucleoside kinase essential to post-mitotic cells for phosphorylation of pyrimidine nucleosides, deoxyguanosine kinase (DGUOK), an enzyme necessary for mitochondrial purine nucleoside salvage pathways, adenine nucleotide translocator (ANT1), and mitochondrial deoxynucleotide carrier (DNC) (Suomalainen & Isohanni, 2010). Indeed, the fact that many genes involved in nucleotide salvage pathways and nucleotide transport are responsible for mitochondrial diseases suggests that imbalanced nucleotide pools are detrimental to mtDNA replication. The inherited mitochondrial diseases involving mtDNA replication are characterized by a long range of overlapping and progressing clinical symptoms, most commonly lactic acidosis, muscle weakness and myopathy which can lead to ataxia, polyneuropathy with epilepsy, cognitive delay and sensory impairment (ophthalmoplegia, deafness) as well as liver and gastrointestinal alterations (dysmotility) (Copleand, 2008; Copeland, 2010). According to the manifestations of the disease, MDS can be divided into three categories: myopathic, encephalomyopathic and hepatocerebral. To illustrate these effects, two inherited *POLG*-originated diseases are described. PEO, a mitochondrial disorder characterized by mtDNA depletions and/or accumulation of mutated mtDNA, has a late onset (between 18 and 40 years of age) and results in progressive weakening of the external eye muscles, leading to blepharoptosis and ophthalmoparesis (Copeland, 2008). PEO patients also manifest skeletal muscle weakness and wasting accompanied by exercise intolerance. This disease is also associated with specific neurologic syndromes such as familial forms of spastic paraplegia, spinocerebellar disorders, and sensorimotor peripheral neuropathy. The variants of this disorder involve both autosomal dominant (adPEO) and recessive (arPEO) forms, as both the nuclear and the mitochondrial genome are implicated in this pathogenesis. Importantly, several mutations in *POLG*, the first of which was described in 2001, are involved in the development of PEO. Alpers syndrome is another disease caused by mutations in *POLG* (Copeland, 2008). This is a rare but very severe and usually lethal autosomal recessive MDS disease that appears within the first few years of life. Patients exhibit progressive spastic quadri-paresis, progressive cerebral degeneration leading to mental deterioration, cortical blindness, deafness and liver failure.

4. mtDNA replication and NRTI

The most widely studied class of drugs that inhibit mtDNA replication, thus generating drug-related toxicities, are the nucleoside analog reverse transcriptase inhibitors (NRTI) (Fig.2). This was the first family of drugs approved by FDA for treatment of HIV infection (zidovudine, 1987). The combined antiretroviral approach currently employed in HIV therapeutics was introduced in 1996 and is known as Highly Active Antiretroviral Therapy (HAART) or Combination Antiretroviral Therapy (cART). It involves the use of one or two NRTI and one Non-Nucleoside Analogue Reverse Inhibitor (NNRTI) or one protease inhibitor (Zolopa, 2010). In this way, NRTI constitute the cornerstone of current HIV therapy. They are administered as prodrugs that must be transported into the cell and phopshorylated to the metabolically active triphosphate in order to exert their therapeutic effect. These drugs are pharmacological analogues of native nucleosides that can be

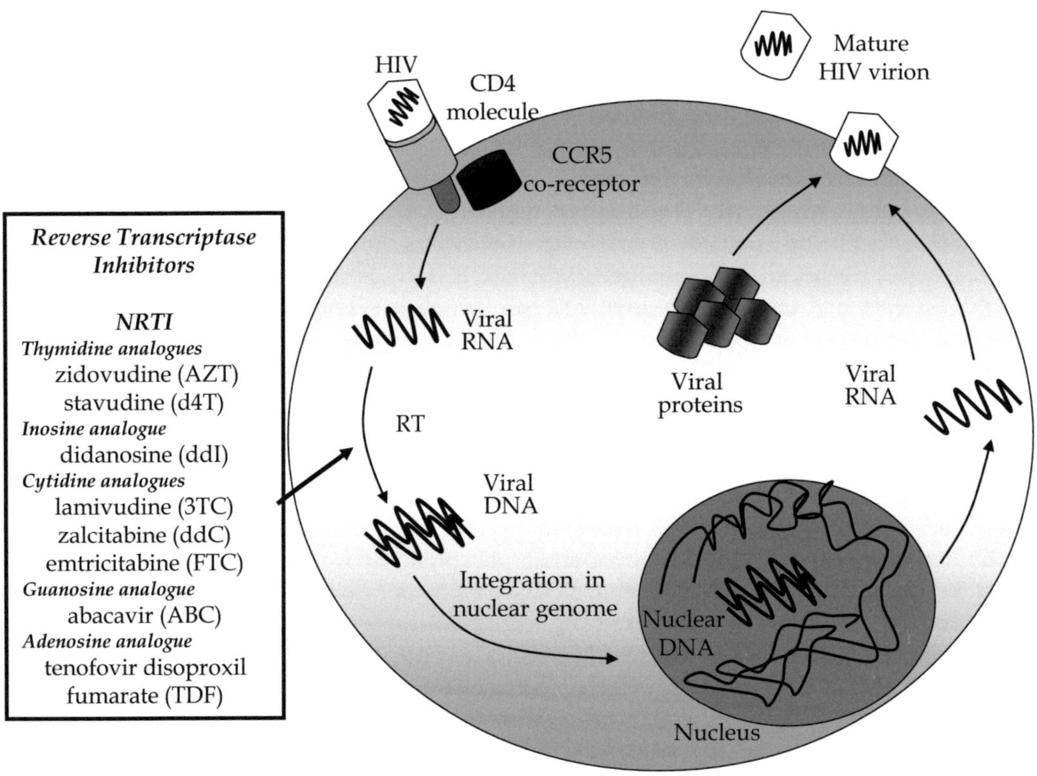

Fig. 2. The interference of NRTI drugs with the life cycle of HIV.
Reverse Transcriptase Inhibitors are a group of antiretroviral drugs which inhibit the viral reverse transcriptase, a crucial enzyme of the HIV life cycle. This enzyme reverse-transcribes the viral RNA genome into DNA, which is then integrated into the host genome and replicated along with it. This drug group comprises nucleoside analogues (NRTI) and non-nucleoside analogues (NNRTI). NRTI are administered as prodrugs and act as competitive inhibitors whereas NNRTI which do not require intracellular activation exert a non-competitive inhibitory action by acting at an allosteric, non-substrate binding site and thereby inducing a conformational change which impairs the enzyme's catalytic activity.

incorporated into proviral DNA during DNA replication by reverse transcriptase. Because they lack the 3´-OH group, their incorporation results in the termination of viral DNA replication. However, the triphosphate forms of the analogues have also been shown to be substrates for Pol γ and can also provoke termination of the DNA chain during mtDNA replication, an effect which can alter mitochondrial function. It has been postulated that NRTI inhibits Pol γ through several mechanisms or a combination of them: 1) termination of the mtDNA chain due to incorporation of NRTI in the growing strand without the 3´-OH group; 2) direct competitive inhibition of Pol γ without incorporation in the nascent DNA chain, as they compete with natural nucleotides for such incorporation; 3) alteration of Pol γ synthesis fidelity -induction of errors during mtDNA replication by inhibition of the exonucleolytic proof-reading function of Pol γ; 4) decrease in mtDNA reparatory exonuclease activity as NRTI resists exonucleolytic removal. Additional effects on mtDNA synthesis have also been suggested. Regardless of the mechanism by which mtDNA replication is compromised, it ultimately interferes with the synthesis of essential proteins of the mitochondrial ETC (Chiao et al., 2009).

The "Pol γ hypothesis" holds that NRTI treatment disrupts the OxPhos process thereby generating an energy defect and triggering subsequent alterations in the mitochondrial function such as increase in ROS production, reduced ATP synthesis, electron leakage, changes in the mitochondrial membrane potential and ROS generation, alterations which lead to further cellular damage (Fig.3),(Kohler & Lewis, 2007). Clinical experience with NRTI-including therapy has revealed the appearance of several side effects ranging from hyperlactatemia and lactic acidosis to lipodystrophy, myopathy, peripheral neuropathy, bone marrow suppression, insulin resistance and diabetes, as well as hepatosteatosis and pancreatitis, some of which develop into life-threatening condition (Kakuda, 2000). The first report of NRTI-induced mitochondrial effects, described in 1990, was myopathy in patients treated with zidovudine, who exhibited ragged red muscle fibers and reduced mtDNA content (Dalakas et al., 1990). Cardiomyopathy and bone marrow suppression were also described.

Kinetic *in vitro* studies have reported that dideoxynucleotides can be substrates for Pol γ nearly as efficiently as natural deoxynucleotides and thus the proposed hierarchy of mitochondrial toxicity for the approved NRTI is: zalcitabine >didanosine >stavudine >> lamivudine >tenofovir >zidovudine >abacavir (Lim & Copeland, 2001). Once incorporated into DNA, terminal NRTI can be removed by the intrinsic exonuclease activity of Pol γ, however this action is quite inefficient particularly in the case of dideoxynucleotides. For, example, zidovudine is unlikely to be incorporated into DNA by Pol γ, but once incorporated its removal is very inefficient which may explain the strong zidovudine-induced mtDNA depletion observed *in vitro* (Lim et al., 2003).

In contrast, removal of 3´- terminal lamivudine residues is 50% as efficient as natural 3´-termini. This, together with the lower degree of lamivudine incorporation in the mtDNA chain, predicts reduced toxicity for this analogue, a finding which is supported by *in vivo* observations. Pol γ discrimination against specific NRTI drugs, as illustrated in the examples, is considered the basis of the mitochondrial toxicity induced by these compounds and is a major rationale in the design of new antiretroviral nucleoside analogs.

Three aminoacid residues in human Pol γ (Tyr951, Tyr955 and Glu895) are thought to account for the selection of dNTPs and, therefore, NRTI (Lim et al., 2003). For example, a

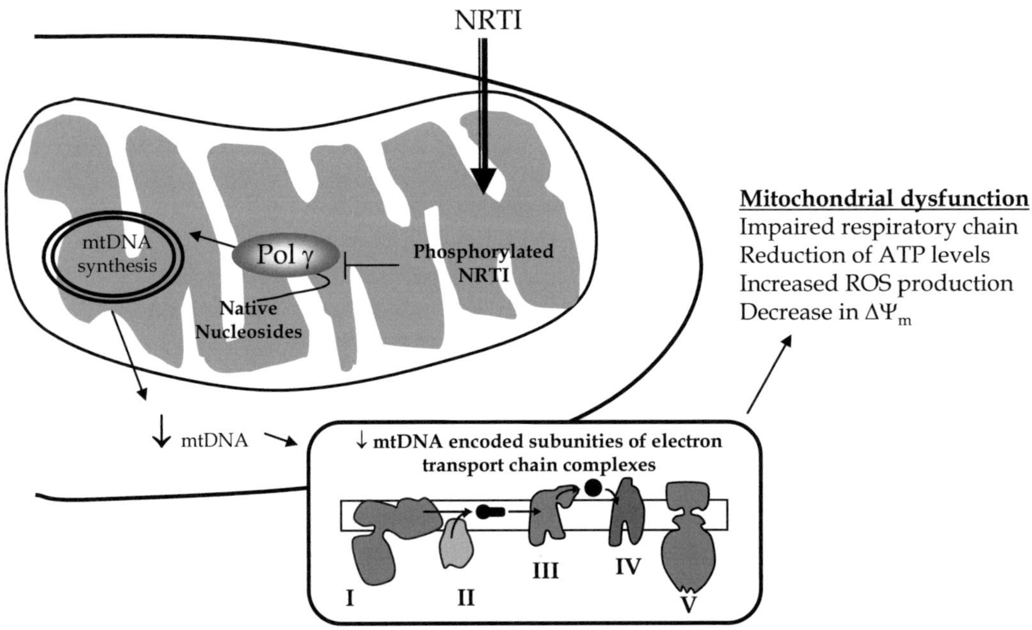

Fig. 3. The effect of NRTI drugs on Pol γ and its consequences for mitochondrial function. NRTI drugs are prodrugs which are phosphorylated intracellularly and the generated triphosphate form inhibits Pol γ in a competitive fashion. This undermines mtDNA synthesis with a consequent depletion of the mtDNA-encoded subunits of the mitochondrial electron transport chain. Such an effect leads to impairment of the mitochondrial function manifested as compromised oxidative phosphorylation, a reduction in mitochondrial membrane potential and induction of oxidative stress.

single tyrosine in motif B of human Pol γ, Tyr951, has been shown to cause dideoxynucleoside and stavudine sensitivity. Substitution of this Tyr residue with phenylalanine reduces the inhibition by dideoxynucleotides or stavudine by several thousand-fold with only minor effects on the overall function of Pol γ (Lim et al., 2003). It was hypothesized that the phenolic hydroxyl group of the tyrosine residue could substitute the missing 3´-OH of the bound ddNTP, thus allowing its efficient incorporation. Tyr955 and Glu895 seem to interact with the rigid sugar rings of stavudine and abacavir. Interestingly, discrimination against zidovudine does not seem to be related to any of these aminoacid residues at the active site of Pol γ. Moreover HIV-1 reverse transcriptase mutants derived from zidovudine-resitant viruses harbor changes in aminoacid residues outside the active site and the drug resistance conferred by these mutations could be due to subtle structural changes in Pol γ (Lim et al., 2003).
Additional effects of NRTI on mtDNA synthesis have also been suggested. Therefore, given that conversion of the monophosphate to the triphosphate form of NRTI inside the mitochondria is rather inefficient, it is possible that the monophosphorylated forms can accumulate within the mitochondrial matrix reaching extremely high (mM) levels which could have unspecific inhibitory effects on mtDNA synthesis, such as decreased mtDNA replication fidelity induced by the inhibition of the exonuclease function of Pol-γ, and inhibition of mtDNA replication, mediated by the reduction of thymidine phosphorylation,

a necessary substrate for DNA synthesis (Walker et al., 2003). *In vivo* millimolar accumulation has been shown for the phosphorylated form of zidovudine (Frick et al., 1988). Moreover, interactions with host proteins during the process of activation of NRTI inside the cell, allow additional mechanisms for mitochondrial toxicity of these drugs.

4.1 Pol-γ independent mitochondrial action of NRTI

HAART has dramatically reduced AIDS-related morbidity and mortality and has converted HIV-infection into chronic rather than a mortal disease (in the pre-HAART era a HIV-infected individual was expected to survive only 7 years). However, the adverse reactions associated with the long-term use of this therapy (rash and hypersensibility reactions, hepatotoxicity, metabolic disturbances including lipodystrophy, hyperlactatemia, and CNS toxic effects) have become a major concern. As a result, research efforts are now focused on understanding the cellular mechanisms underlying these effects. Most of NRTI-induced side effects have been attributed to their mitotoxic potential which has mainly been believed to originate from the inhibitory action of these drugs on Pol γ. However, other mitochondrial mechanisms and targets responsible for NRTI-induced mitotoxicity have also been suggested. There is evidence of NRTI-induced mitochondrial dysfunction unrelated to mtDNA depletion. Zidovudine has been shown to inhibit thymidine phopshorylation, ADP/ATP translocase and adenylate kinase, to provoke a decrease in cytochrome *c* oxidase (Complex IV) expression, and to enhance oxidative stress (Maagaard & Kvale, 2009). *In vivo* studies have demonstrated that treatment with this drug leads to a disrupted cardiac mitochondrial ultrastructure and a diminished expression of mitochondrial cytochrome b mRNA, as well as induction of oxidative stress in heart mtDNA (Sardao et al., 2008). In addition, in cultured rat hepatocytes, stavudine, but not zidovudine or zalcitabine, impairs fatty acid oxidation in the absence of mtDNA depletion (Igoudjil et al., 2008). Moreover, mitochondrial import of nucleoside drugs may also be related to their toxicity in this organelle. Some of the nucleoside channels have been shown to transport stavudine, zalcitabine, zidovudine and didanosine (Yamamoto et al., 2007; Baldwin et al., 2005) and nucleoside drugs are also the subject of several other transporters, including organic cation and anion transporters and multi-drug-resistant proteins with potential implication in toxicity (Leung & Tse, 2007). Recently, mitochondrial bioenergetics has been directly linked to NRTI-induced mitotoxicity, independently of mtDNA replication. *In vitro* exposure to zidovudine has revealed a direct interaction with cellular bioenergetics by impairing mitochondrial respiration through inhibition of Complex I of the ETC (Lund & Wallace, 2008).

Hepatotoxicity has emerged as one of the most common adverse events associated with HAART and constitutes a major problem in the management of HIV-patients. In certain clinical trials, up to 10% of patients receiving cART exhibited a severely increased liver enzymes level which is a major cause of therapy discontinuation (Jain, 2007). The implication of mitochondria in these events and particularly the drug-induced mitochondrial effects that occur independently of Pol γ is still not clear. We employed a human hepatoma cell line, Hep3B (ATCC HB-8064) to assess the potential direct and Pol γ–independent involvement of mitochondria in hepatic side effects. Preliminary studies were performed in which cells were treated with NRTI (Sequoia Research Products) at therapeutic concentrations during a short period of time in order to avoid any effects due to a decrease in mtDNA content. Subsequently, several parameters of mitochondrial function including mitochondrial respiration, generation of ATP and mitochondrial ROS production were determined. Electrochemical measurement of oxygen (O_2) consumption was performed using a Clark-type O_2 electrode (Rank Brothers, Bottisham, UK). Cells (3-5x10^6) were placed in a gas-tight chamber containing 1mL respiration buffer (Hank's balanced salt solution, HBSS) and agitated at 37°C. Measurements were recorded using the Duo.18 data acquisition device (WPI, Stevenage, UK), immediately after addition of the drugs. The adenosine triphosphate (ATP) concentration (nmol/mg protein) was determined using Bioluminescence Assay Kit HSII (Roche, Mannheim, Germany) and a Fluoroskan microplate reader (Thermo Labsystems, Thermo Scientific, Rockford, IL). For these measurements, cells were incubated for 1h with the NRTI under study. Protein concentrations were determined with the BCA protein assay kit. ROS production was analyzed in cells seeded in a black 96-well plate. The fluorescent probe DCFH-DA (2´,7´-dichlorodihydrofluorescein diacetate, 2.5 μM) was added for 30 minutes, cells were washed with HBSS before addition of the NRTI drug and fluorescence was detected at 5-minute intervals over a 1h period using a Fluoroskan. Rotenone (100 μM) or exogenous hydrogen peroxide (H_2O_2, 100 μM) were used as a positive control. We observed that abacavir but not lamivudine significantly reduced mitochondrial respiration and ATP production (Fig.4). However no significant changes were detected regarding ROS production with either of the drugs (results not shown) (Blas-Garcia, 2010). Other preliminary studies conducted in our laboratory have revealed that clinically relevant concentrations of another NRTI, didanosine, also lead to alterations in the mitochondrial function of Hep3B cells, detected as decreased O_2 consumption and ATP generation, but in the absence of an increase in ROS production (unpublished data).

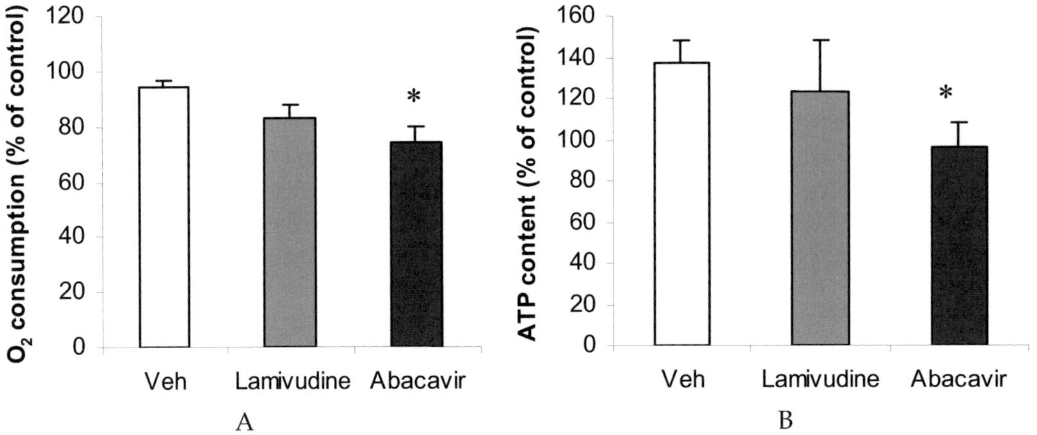

Fig. 4. Acute and Pol γ-independent effect of NRTI drugs (lamivudine and abacavir) on mitochondrial function in Hep3B cells. A) Rate of mitochondrial O_2 consumption determined in a Clark-type O_2 electrode. 10μM of lamivudine or abacavir were added to the chamber immediately after addition of the cell suspension. B) Intracellular ATP concentration studied with a bioluminescence assay in cells treated with 10μM of lamivudine or abacavir for 1h. Data are mean±SEM of 5-6 experiments and are shown as % of the control value (i.e. the value obtained in untreated cells, considered to be 100%). Statistical analysis was performed using the Student´s t-test, *$p<0.05$, vs Vehicle (Veh)-treatment.

These preliminary data lead to several important observations: i) some NRTI, at their clinically employed concentrations, have the potential to directly inhibit the mitochondrial oxidative phosphorylation process, and this occurs in a drug-specific manner; ii) further studies need to be carried out with the aim of analyzing whether these effects are transient or accumulate over time, particularly regarding ROS accumulation which does not seem to be acutely affected. However prolonged and/or more severe impairment of mitochondrial respiration can lead to a progressive increase in ROS generation and the subsequent appearance of oxidative stress; iii) the pathophysiological relevance of the mitochondrial effects elicited by NRTI is unclear and awaits the findings of more detailed studies.

4.2 Factors influencing NRTI-induced mitotoxicity

Several general factors directly influence NRTI-induced mitochondrial toxicities, both related and un-related to mtDNA depletion: i) the subcellular abundance of NRTI, as there is a concentration threshold beyond which these compounds compete with natural moieties; ii) the ability of cellular nucleoside kinases to create nucleoside triphosphate, which is responsible for mtDNA toxicity, and the interaction of nucleoside analogues with the resident proteins during the process of their activation; iii) the existence of a functional threshold as most cells contain a substantial number of mitochondria and therefore, manifestations of cellular injury appear only when a substantial number of malfunctional mitochondria is reached; and iv) the "mtDNA threshold effect" in relation with tissue specificity of OxPhos dependence. The majority of cells have a surplus of mtDNA copies and can withstand significant mtDNA depletion before mitochondrial dysfunction occurs (60-80% of basal levels). In the case of mutations, the threshold varies from 60% for large scale mtDNA deletions to 90% in tRNA point mutations. Nevertheless, the relationship between mtDNA content and NRTI-induced adverse events is unclear. Until recently, quantification of mtDNA in peripheral blood mononuclear cells (PBMC) was employed as a marker of mitochondrial toxicity in HIV patients. However, the accuracy of this measurement regarding toxicity is controversial since several studies have failed to report a decrease in the mtDNA content of PBMC or fat tissue in patients experiencing adverse events such as lipoatrophy (Maagaard & Kvale, 2009). Finally, v) recent advances in pharmacogenomics suggest a link between specific genetic polymorphisms and NRTI toxicity; for instance, R964C (Yamanaka et al., 2007) and E1143G polymorphisms (Chiappini et al., 2009) have been associated with an increased stavudine-induced mitotoxicity whereas mitochondrial haplogroup T has been related to increased peripheral neuropathy in treatment with stavudine and didanosine (Hulgan et al., 2005).

5. Conclusion

Mitochondria contain their own DNA which encodes 13 proteins which are involved in the mitochondrial ETC. The replication of mtDNA is performed by Pol γ, the only mitochondrial DNA polymerase, which consists of a catalytic subunit and a dimeric form of an accessory subunit p55, and operates in conjunction with two replication factors, SSB and Twinkle. A decreased amount of mtDNA, often due to mutations in *POLG*, is a hallmark of mitochondrial depletion syndrome, a heterogeneous group of several severe and usually deadly inherited disorders. Mitochondrial DNA depletion and, consequently, mitochondrial dysfunction are also considered to be the basis of the side effects induced by a class of drugs known as nucleoside analogue reverse transcriptase inhibitors. These drugs are the cornerstone of the current therapeutic approach employed for treatment of HIV infection. It is believed that the adverse events related to NRTI-containing treatments are mainly due to the mitochondrial toxicity that arises as a result of the inhibitory effect of these drugs on Pol γ. However, Pol γ-independent mitochondrial targets and mechanisms of NRTI-induced toxicity have also been suggested. Using a human hepatic cell line, our group has recently provided *in vitro* evidence of a direct inhibitory effect on mitochondrial respiration and ATP production induced by an acute exposure to certain NRTI such as abacavir and didanosine. No such changes were observed with lamivudine, thus indicating a drug- rather than a class-specific effect. A detailed analysis of these effects is paramount to a better understanding of NRTI-related adverse events. This is of particular clinical relevance given the existence of NRTI that do not exhibit a strong Pol γ -inhibitory action.

6. Acknowledgement

The authors thank Brian Normanly for his English language editing. The study was supported by grants PI081325 and PI070091 from "Fondo de Investigacion Sanitaria", and ACOMP2010/207 y PROMETEO/2010/060 from Generalitat Valenciana, Spain.

7. References

Bailey, C.M. & Anderson, K.S. (2010). A mechanistic view of human mitochondrial DNA polymerase gamma: providing insight into drug toxicity and mitochondrial disease. *Biochimica et Biophysica Acta*, Vol.1804, No.5, (May, 2010), pp.1213-1222, ISSN: 0006-3002

Baldwin, S.A.; Yao, S.Y.; Hyde, R.J.; Ng, A.M.; Foppolo, S.; Barnes, K.; Ritzel, M.W.; Cass, C.E. & Young, J.D. (2005). Functional characterization of novel human and mouse equilibrative nucleoside transporters (hENT3 and mENT3) located in intracellular membranes. *The Journal of Biological Chemistry*, Vol.280, No.16, (April 22, 2005), pp. 15880-15887, ISSN: 0021-9258

Bebenek, K. & Kunkel, T.A. (2004). Functions of DNA polymerases. *Advances in Protein Chemistry*, Vol.69, (December, 2004), pp. 137-165, ISSN: 0065-3233

Blas-García, A.; Apostolova, N.; Ballesteros, D.; Monleón, D.; Morales, J.M.; Rocha, M.; Victor, V.M. & Esplugues, J.V. (2010). Inhibition of mitochondrial function by efavirenz increases lipid content in hepatic cells. *Hepatology*. Vol.52, No.1, (July, 2010), pp. 115-125, ISSN: 0270-9139

Bolden, A.; Noy, G.P. & Weissbach, A. (1977). DNA polymerase of mitochondria is a gamma-polymerase. Journal of Biological Chemistry, Vol.252, No.10, pp. 3351-3356.

Bowmaker, M.; Yang, M.Y.; Yasukawa, T.; Reyes, A.; Jacobs, H.T.; Huberman, J.A. & Holt, I.J. (2003). Mammalian mitochondrial DNA replicates bidirectionally from an initiation zone. *The Journal of Biological Chemistry*, Vol.278, No.51, (December 19, 2003), pp. 50961-50969, ISSN: 0021-9258

Chiao, S.K.; Romero, D.L. & Johnson D.E. (2009). Current HIV therapeutics: mechanistic and chemical determinants of toxicity. *Current opinion in drug discovery & development*, Vol. 12, No.1, (January, 2009), pp. 53-60, ISSN: 1367-6733

Chiappini, F.; Teicher, E.; Saffroy, R.; Debuire, B.; Vittecoq, D. & Lemoine, A. (2009). Relationship between polymerase gamma (POLG) polymorphisms and antiretroviral therapy-induced lipodystrophy in HIV-1 infected patients: a case-control study. *Current HIV Research,* Vol.7, No.2, (March, 2009), pp. 244-253, ISSN: 1570-162X

Clayton, D.A. (1982). Replication of animal mitochondrial DNA. *Cell.* Vol.28, No.4, (April, 1982), pp. 693-705, ISSN: 0092-8674

Copeland, W.C. (2008). Inherited mitochondrial diseases of DNA replication. *Annual review of medicine,* Vol.59, pp. 131-146, ISSN: 0066-4219

Copeland, W.C. & Longley, M.J. (2008). DNA2 resolves expanding flap in mitochondrial base excision repair. Molecular Cell Vol.32, No.4, (November 21, 2008), pp 457-458, ISSN: 1097-2765

Copeland, W.C. (2010). The mitochondrial DNA polymerase in health and disease. *Subcellular Biochemistry,* Vol.50, pp. 211-222, ISSN: 0306-0225

Dalakas, M.C.; Illa, I.; Pezeshkpour, G.H.; Laukaitis, J.P.; Cohen, B. & Griffin, J.L. (1990). Mitochondrial myopathy caused by long-term zidovudine therapy. *The New England Journal of Medicine,* Vol.322, No.16, (April 19, 1990), pp. 1098-1105, ISSN 0028-4793

Di Re, M.; Sembongi, H.; He, J.; Reyes, A.; Yasukawa, T.; Martinsson, P.; Bailey, L.J.; Goffart, S.; Boyd-Kirkup, J.D.; Wong, T.S.; Fersht, A.R.; Spelbrink, J.N. & Holt, I.J. (2009). The accessory subunit of mitochondrial DNA polymerase gamma determines the DNA content of mitochondrial nucleoids in human cultured cells. *Nucleic Acids Research,* Vol.37, No.17, (September, 2009), pp. 5701-5713, ISSN: 0305-1048

Fan, L.; Sanschagrin, P.C.; Kaguni, L.S. & Kuhn, L.A. (1999). The accessory subunit of mtDNA polymerase shares structural homology with aminoacyl-tRNA synthetases: implications for a dual role as a primer recognition factor and processivity clamp. *Proceedings of National Academy of Sciences of the United States of America,* Vol.96, No17, (August 17, 1999), pp. 9527-9532, ISSN-0027-8424

Frick, L.W.; Nelson, D.J.; St Clair, M.H.; Furman, P.A. & Krenitsky, T.A. (1988). Effects of 3'-azido-3'-deoxythymidine on the deoxynucleotide triphosphate pools of cultured human cells. *Biochemical and Biophysical Research Communications,* Vol.154, No.1, (July 15, 1988), pp. 124-129, ISSN: 0006-291X

Fridlender, B.; Fry, M.; Bolden, A. & Weissbach, A. (1972). A new synthetic RNA-dependent DNA polymerase from human tissue culture cells (HeLa-fibroblast-synthetic oligonucleotides-template-purified enzymes). *Proceedings of National Academy of Sciences of the United States of America,* Vol.69, No.2, (February, 1972), pp. 452-455, ISSN-0027-8424

Graves, S.W.; Johnson, A.A. & Johnson, K.A. (1998). Expression, purification, and initial kinetic characterization of the large subunit of the human mitochondrial DNA polymerase. *Biochemistry,* Vol.37, No.17, (April 28, 1998), pp. 6050-6058, ISSN: 0006-2960

Graziewicz, M.A.; Longley, M.J. & Copeland, W.C. (2006). DNA polymerase gamma in mitochondrial DNA replication and repair. *Chemical Reviews,* Vol.106, No.2, (February, 2006), pp. 383-405, ISSN: 0009-2665

Holt, I.J.; Lorimer, H.E. & Jacobs, H.T. (2000). Coupled leading- and lagging-strand synthesis of mammalian mitochondrial DNA. *Cell,* Vol.100, No.5, (February, 2006), pp. 515-524, ISSN: 0092-8674

Holt, I.J. (2009). Mitochondrial DNA replication and repair: all a flap. *Trends in Biochemical Sciences,* Vol.34, No.7, (July, 2009), pp. 358-365, ISSN: 0968-0004

Hulgan, T.; Haas, D.W.; Haines, J.L.; Ritchie, M.D.; Robbins, G.K.; Shafer, R.W.; Clifford, D.B.; Kallianpur, A.R.; Summar, M. & Canter, J.A. (2005). Mitochondrial haplogroups and peripheral neuropathy during antiretroviral therapy: an adult AIDS clinical trials group study. *AIDS.* Vol.19, No.13, (September 2, 2005), pp. 1341-1349, ISSN: 0269-9370

Igoudjil, A.; Massart, J.; Begriche, K.; Descatoire, V.; Robin, M.A. & Fromenty, B. (2008). High concentrations of stavudine impair fatty acid oxidation without depleting mitochondrial DNA in cultured rat hepatocytes. *Toxicology In Vitro,* Vol.22, No.4, (Juny, 2008), pp. 887-898, ISSN: 0887-2333

Jain, M.K. (2007). Drug-induced liver injury associated with HIV medications. *Clinics in Liver Disease,* Vol.11, No.3, (August, 2007) pp. 615-39, vii-viii, ISSN: 1089-3261

Johnson, A.A.; Tsai, Y.; Graves, S.W. & Johnson, K.A. (2000). Human mitochondrial DNA polymerase holoenzyme: reconstitution and characterization. *Biochemistry.* Vol.39, No.7, (February 22, 2000), pp. 1702-1708. ISSN: 0006-2960

Kakuda, T.N. (2000). Pharmacology of nucleoside and nucleotide reverse transcriptase inhibitor-induced mitochondrial toxicity. *Clinical Therapeutics,* Vol.22, No.6, (Juny, 2000), pp. 685-708, ISSN: 0149-2918

Kalf, G.F. & Ch'ih, J.J. (1968). Purification and properties of deoxyribonucleic acid polymerase from rat liver mitochondria. *The Journal of Biological Chemistry,* Vol.243, No.18, (September 25, 1968), pp. 4904-4916, ISSN: 0021-9258

Kohler, J.J. & Lewis, W. (2007). A brief overview of mechanisms of mitochondrial toxicity from NRTIs. *Environmental and Molecular Mutagenesis,* Vol.48, No.(3-4), (April-May, 2007), pp. 166-172, ISSN: 0893-6692

Lang, B.F.; Gray, M.W. & Burger, G. (1999). Mitochondrial genome evolution and the origin of eukaryotes. *Annual Review of Genetics,* Vol.33, (December, 1999), pp. 351-97, ISSN: 0066-4197

Leung, G.P. & Tse, C.M. (2007). The role of mitochondrial and plasma membrane nucleoside transporters in drug toxicity. *Expert Opinion on Drug Metabolism & Toxicology,* Vol.3, No.5, (October, 2007), pp. 705-718, ISSN: 1742-5255

Lewis, W.; Kohler, J.J.; Hosseini, S.H.; Haase, C.P.; Copeland, W.C.; Bienstock, R.J.; Ludaway, T.; McNaught, J.; Russ, R.; Stuart, T. & Santoianni, R. (2006). Antiretroviral nucleosides, deoxynucleotide carrier and mitochondrial DNA: evidence supporting the DNA pol gamma hypothesis. *AIDS,* Vol.20, No.5, (March 21, 2006), pp. 675-684, ISSN: 0269-9370

Lim, S.E.; Longley, M.J. & Copeland, W.C. (1999). The mitochondrial p55 accessory subunit of human DNA polymerase gamma enhances DNA binding, promotes processive DNA synthesis, and confers N-ethylmaleimide resistance. *The Journal of Biological Chemistry,* Vol. 274, No.53, (December 31, 1999), pp. 38197-38203, ISSN: 0021-9258

Lim, S.E. & Copeland, W.C. (2001). Differential incorporation and removal of antiviral deoxynucleotides by human DNA polymerase gamma. *The Journal of Biological Chemistry,* Vol.276, No.26, (Juny 29, 2001), pp. 23616-23623, ISSN: 0021-9258

Lim, S.E.; Ponamarev, M.V.; Longley, M.J. & Copeland, W.C. (2003). Structural determinants in human DNA polymerase gamma account for mitochondrial toxicity from nucleoside analogs. *Journal of Molecular Biology,* Vol.329, No.1, (May 23, 2003), pp. 45-57, ISSN: 0022-2836

Liu, P.; Qian, L.; Sung, J.S.; de Souza-Pinto, N.C.; Zheng, L.; Bogenhagen, D.F.; Bohr, V.A.; Wilson, D.M. 3rd.; Shen, B. & Demple, B. (2008). Removal of oxidative DNA damage via FEN1-dependent long-patch base excision repair in human cell mitochondria. *Molecular and Cellular Biology,* Vol.28, No.16, (August, 2008), pp. 4975-4987, ISSN: 0270-7306

Longley, M.J.; Ropp, P.A.; Lim, S.E. & Copeland, W.C. (1998). Characterization of the native and recombinant catalytic subunit of human DNA polymerase gamma: identification of residues critical for exonuclease activity and dideoxynucleotide sensitivity. *Biochemistry.* Vol.37, No.29, (July 21, 1998), pp. 10529-10539, ISSN: 0006-2960

Longley, M.J.; Nguyen, D.; Kunkel, T.A. & Copeland, W.C. (2001). The fidelity of human DNA polymerase gamma with and without exonucleolytic proofreading and the p55 accessory subunit. *The Journal of Biological Chemistry,* Vol.276 No.42, (October 19, 2001), pp. 38555-38562, ISSN: 0021-9258

Lund, K.C. & Wallace, K.B. (2008). Adenosine 3',5'-cyclic monophosphate (cAMP)-dependent phosphoregulation of mitochondrial complex I is inhibited by nucleoside reverse transcriptase inhibitors. *Toxicology and Applied Pharmacology,* Vol.226, No.1, (January 1, 2008), pp. 94-106, ISSN: 0041-008X

Maagaard, A. & Kvale, D. (2009). Long term adverse effects related to nucleoside reverse transcriptase inhibitors: clinical impact of mitochondrial toxicity. *Scandinavian Journal of Infectious Diseases,* Vol.41, No.11-12, pp. 808-817, ISSN: 0036-5548

Sardão, V.A.; Pereira, S.L. & Oliveira, P.J. (2008). Drug-induced mitochondrial dysfunction in cardiac and skeletal muscle injury. *Expert Opinion on Drug Safety,* Vol.7, No.2, (March, 2008), pp. 129-146, ISSN: 1474-0338.

Shadel, G.S. & Clayton, D.A. (1997). Mitochondrial DNA maintenance in vertebrates. *Annual Review of Biochemistry,* Vol.66, (July, 1997) pp. 409-435, ISSN: 0066-4154

Suomalainen, A. & Isohanni, P. (2010). Mitochondrial DNA depletion syndromes-Many genes, common mechanisms. *Neuromuscular Disorders* Vol.20, (July, 2010), pp. 429-437, ISSN: 0960-8966

Sweasy, J.B.; Lauper, J.M. & Eckert, K.A. (2006). DNA polymerases and human diseases. *Radiation Research.* Vol.166, No.5, (November, 2006), pp. 693-714, ISSN: 0033-7587

Walker, U.A.; Venhoff, N.; Koch, E.C.; Olschewski, M.; Schneider, J. & Setzer, B. (2003). Uridine abrogates mitochondrial toxicity related to nucleoside analogue reverse transcriptase inhibitors in HepG2 cells. *Antiviral Therapy,* Vol.8, No.5, (October, 2003), pp. 463-470, ISSN: 1359-6535

Wanrooij, S. & Falkenberg, M. (2010). The human mitochondrial replication fork in health and disease. *Biochimica et Biophysica Acta,* Vol.1797, No.8, (August, 2010), pp. 1378-88, ISSN: 0006-3002

Yakubovskaya, E.; Chen, Z.; Carrodeguas, J.A.; Kisker, C. & Bogenhagen, D.F. (2006). Functional human mitochondrial DNA polymerase gamma forms a heterotrimer. *The Journal of Biological Chemistry.* Vol. 281, No.1, (January 6, 2006), pp. 374-82, ISSN: 0021-9258

Yamamoto, T.; Kuniki, K.; Takekuma, Y.; Hirano, T.; Iseki, K. & Sugawara, M. (2007). Ribavirin uptake by cultured human choriocarcinoma (BeWo) cells and Xenopus laevis oocytes expressing recombinant plasma membrane human nucleoside transporters. *The European Journal of Pharmacology,* Vol. 557, No.1, (February 14, 2007), pp 1-8, ISSN: 0014-2999.

Yamanaka, H.; Gatanaga, H.; Kosalaraksa, P.; Matsuoka-Aizawa, S.; Takahashi, T.; Kimura, S. & Oka, S. (2007). Novel mutation of human DNA polymerase gamma associated with mitochondrial toxicity induced by anti-HIV treatment. *The Journal of Infectious Disease,* Vol.195, No.10, (May 15, 2007), pp. 1419-1425, ISSN: 0022-1899

Yasukawa, T.; Reyes, A.; Cluett, T.J.; Yang, M.Y.; Bowmaker, M.; Jacobs, H.T. & Holt, I.J. (2006). Replication of vertebrate mitochondrial DNA entails transient ribonucleotide incorporation throughout the lagging strand. *The EMBO Journal.* Vol.25, No.22, (November 15, 2006), pp. 5358-5371, ISSN: 0261-4189

Zheng, W.; Khrapko, K.; Coller, H.A.; Thilly, W.G. & Copeland, W.C. (2006). Origins of human mitochondrial point mutations as DNA polymerase gamma-mediated errors. *Mutation Research,* Vol.599, No.(1-2), (July 25, 2006), pp. 11-20, ISSN: 0027-5107

Zheng, L.; Zhou, M.; Guo, Z.; Lu, H.; Qian, L.; Dai, H.; Qiu, J.; Yakubovskaya, E.; Bogenhagen, D.F.; Demple, B. & Shen, B. (2008). Human DNA2 is a mitochondrial nuclease/helicase for efficient processing of DNA replication and repair intermediates. *Molecular Cell,* Vol. 32, No.3, (November 7, 2008), pp. 325-36, ISSN: 1097-2765.

Zolopa, A.R. (2010). The evolution of HIV treatment guidelines: current state-of-the-art of ART. *Antiviral Research,* Vol.85, No.1, (January, 2010), pp. 241-244, ISSN: 0166-3542

8

Damage and Replication Stress Responses

Haiying Wang[1], Ping Shen[2] and Wei-Guo Zhu[1]
[1]*Key laboratory of Carcinogenesis and Translational Research (Ministry of Education), Department of Biochemistry and Molecular Biology, Peking University Health Science Center,*
[2]*Department of Applied linguistics, Peking University Health Science Center, China*

1. Introduction

The character of DNA replication is high fidelity. Precise and complete DNA replication is critical for the maintenance of genetic stability. Failures in these processes are major sources of genomic instability and will lead to cancer or other diseases. A wide variety of factors, such as DNA replication errors, spontaneous chemical reactions, reactive metabolic products, exogenous environmental agents or some anticancer therapeutics e.g. 5′-aza-2′-deoxycytidine (5-Aza-CdR), can cause DNA damage (Wang et al, 2008; Zhu et al, 2004; Chai et al, 2008; Hoeijmakers, 2009). It is estimated that DNA damage occurs at a rate of 1,000 to 1,000,000 molecular lesions per cell per day (Lodish, 2004). In order to deal with problems under which the genome is vulnerable to injury or replication stress, eukaryotic cells elaborate a genomic maintenance apparatus, which is termed the DNA damage response (DDR) and replication stress response, including various checkpoint, signal-transduction and effectors system, which monitor problems and trigger a comprehensive cellular response pathway to prevent genome integrity. The extent of DNA damage depends on the type of environment to which it is exposed (Hoeijmakers, 2001). So, organisms must be capable of recognizing and dealing with each type of damage. It is not surprising that there are various different types of DNA damage response and repair systems.

ATM and ATR are at the top of the DNA damage pathways. Although a cross-talk exists between the ATM and ATR pathways, ATM primarily seems to be involved in the detection of DNA double-strand breaks via Mre11/Rad50/Nbs1 complex (MRN), ATR is critical for cellular responses to a variety of DNA damage and stalled replication forks (Hefferin & Tomkinson, 2005). When these protein kinases activated, they eventually phosphorylate and modulate the downstream effectors (e.g., Chk1 and Chk2) and multiple additional substrates that initiate the cellular responses.

Dynamic changes in protein post-translational modifications play a significant role in most cellular signalling pathways. More and more proteins were found in a variety of post-translational modifications in response to DNA damage and genotoxic stress, such as phosphorylation, acetylation, sumolyation, methylation and ubiquitylation. Recent studies indicate that a crosstalk between multiple protein modifications exists, which collaboratively regulates signal transduction of DNA damage and genetic stresses.

Actually, the DNA damage and replication stress response consists of multiple interconnected pathways, which impact the cell cycle, DNA replication, DNA repair, transcriptional regulation, chromatin remodelling, metabolic and other cellular biological processes (Rouse & Jackson, 2002; Zhou & Elledge, 2000). In this chapter, we focus on recent findings of DNA damage response signalling pathways.

2. The DNA damage response pathways

The ability of cells to respond to DNA damage and replication stress response is critical for cellular survival. The evidence indicates that DNA damage and replication stress response are a cascade signal transductional process, which consists of multiple interconnected pathways through which sense damage or replication stress, transduce the damage signals, and trigger cellular responses, including cell cycle arrest, DNA repair or apoptosis (Shiloh, 2003; Bakkenist & Kastan, 2004; McGowan & Russell, 2004). In mammalian cells, PI3K family members, ATM and ATM-Rad3-related (ATR) are central to the entire DNA damage response (Elledge, 1996). All types of DNA lesions induce responses to these two main signalling pathways. Next, we will summarize the model of cells dealing with DNA damage and replication stress through these two pathways.

2.1 ATM dependent cellular response to DNA double strand breaks pathway

The DNA double strand breaks (DSBs) are the most dangerous damage type for the organisms because they are prone to cause genomic rearrangements, cancer predisposition, and cell death if not repaired correctly (Wyman & Kanaar, 2006). Many endogenous and exogenous factors may induce DSBs, such as IR, UV, reactive oxygen species (ROS) or topoisomerases inhibitors (Tanaka, 2006; Tanaka, 2007). Cellular responses to DSBs, include complex signal-transduction, cell-cycle-checkpoint and repair pathways, play a pivotal role in maintenance of the genome integrity. It is accepted that ATM is a central component of the DSB signalling cascade (Khanna & Jackson, 2001; Shiloh, 2001; Abraham, 2001).

2.1.1 ATM

ATM is the gene product mutated in ataxia telangiectasia discovered in 1995 and characterized by progressive cerebellar ataxia, immune deficiencies, radiation sensitivity, and an increased risk of cancer (Lavin & Shiloh, 1997; Savitsky et al, 1995). ATM is a serine-threonine kinase which belongs to the phosphatidylinositol-3-kinase (PI3K) like protein kinases (PIKK) family. In normal condition, ATM exists in an inactive form of dimer or multimer. Following DSBs, ATM was dissociated into an active monomer through autophosphorylation (Bakkenist & Kastan, 2003). Upon activation, ATM is recruited to DNA breaks where it initiates phosphorylation of several substrates such as p53, Mdm2, BRCA1, Chk2 and Nbs1 to initiate cell cycle arrest, DNA repair, and apoptosis (Lukas et al., 2003; Shiloh Y, 2006).

2.1.2 Mechanism for the activation of ATM

Many progresses have been made on understanding how DSBs activates ATM. Several investigations suggest that the Mre11-Rad50-Nbs1 (MRN) complex is involved in ATM activation and recruitment to the sites of DSBs (Uziel et al, 2003; Cerosaletti & Concannon, 2004), because attenuated activation and no recruitment of ATM to DSBs upon damage were found in Mre11- and Nbs1- deficient cell lines. Earlier studies have shown that MRN lies

downstream of the ATM mediated DNA damage signalling pathway because ATM can phosphorylate the components of the MRN complex in response to IR (Lim & Ki, 2000; Wu & Ranganathan, 2000; Zhao & Weng, 2000). However, further analyses demonstrate that the MRN complex is more like an upper actor of ATM pathway (Uziel et al, 2003；Difilippantonio et al, 2005; Carson et al, 2003). Because the MRN complex was reported to play a role in early detection of DSBs which initiates the localization of ATM to DSBs (Lee & Paull, 2004, 2005). It is now established that ATM at DSBs is a spatio-temporal dynamics mechanism. At first, change in chromatin structure caused by DNA DSB partially activates ATM (Berkovich et al, 2007). Activated ATM rapidly phosphorylates H2AX on its C-terminus, and γ-H2AX subsequently recruits MDC1 (mediator of DNA damage checkpoint protein 1) to bind to it and acts as a scaffold, in turn, recruits MRN at the flanking chromatin of DSBs (Burma et al, 2001; Stucki & Jackson, 2006; Lou et al, 2006; Stucki et al, 2005), which promotes accumulation of ATM to sites of DSBs, where it is fully activated (Lavin, 2008). In addition, MDC1 also mediates the interaction between ATM and γ-H2AX, which contributes to the extended phosphorylation of H2AX and the maintenance of the DSB response (Huen & Chen J, 2008).
Autophosphorylation has been proposed as the other mechanism for ATM activation. Three phosphatases, PP2A, PP5 and WIP1, have been reported to be involved in the control of ATM activation. Autophosphorylation on Ser367, Ser1893, Ser1981 and a new site S2996 are present on activated ATM through dissociation of the inactive dimeric ATM to an active monomeric form (Bakkenist & Kastan, 2003; Kozlov et al, 2010). Recent reports indicate that there is a Nbs1-independent ATM activation pathway which regulates ATM activity through its effect on ATM autophosphorylation (Kanu & Behrens, 2007; Sun et al., 2005, Gupta et al., 2005; Richard et al, 2008). Interestingly, notwithstanding the difference on the importance of ATM autophosphorylation in humans and in mice, this is certainly the case in human cells that autophosphorylation of ATM at serine 1981 is required for the interaction of ATM with MDC1, which stabilizes ATM at DSBs and thereby promotes a full-scale response to DNA damage (Sairei et al, 2009). Once activated, ATM directly or indirectly phosphorylates approximately 30 substrates, such as Chk2, p53, BRCA1, RPAp34, H2AX, SMC1, HDMX, FANCD2, Rad17, Artemis or Nbs1, which are involved in cell cycle checkpoint control, apoptotic responses and DNA repair.

2.2 "two-man rule" of ATR in response to DNA damage

Like ATM, ATR (ATM- and Rad3-related) is a nuclear Ser/Thr kinase which belongs to the PIKK family (Bentley et al, 1996). ATR forms a stable heterodimer with its interacting partner ATRIP which can be activated by DNA damage (Cliby et al, 1998; Wright et al, 1998). Compared with the ATM, ATR can respond to a broader spectrum of genotoxic stimuli including DNA replication inhibitors (such as hydroxyurea), UV radiation, ionizing radiation, and agents that induce DNA interstrand cross-links and generate single-stranded DNA (Wright et al, 1998; Yang et al, 2003; Costanzo & Gautier, 2003; Wang et al, 2008). Once the break occurs, ATR is recruited by ATR-IP to the sites of DNA damage and interacts with RPA to initiate the response (Zou & Elledge, 2003b; Cortez et al, 2001; Wang et al, 2008).

2.2.1 Mechanisms of ATR activation

ATR is involved in many different types of DNA damage responses. The common feature is that ATR is activated by single strand DNA (ssDNA), which is a common intermediate structure that can be formed at sites of DNA damage and replication stress, or induced by

most cancer chemotherapies (Costanzo & Gautier, 2003; Zou & Elledge, 2003b). A study shows that both ssDNA and a 5′ junction are sufficient to activate ATR signalling (MacDougall et al, 2007). ATR activation requires assembly of a protein complex on ssDNA, which begins with ATR-ATRIP complex loading on the RPA-coated ssDNA (Stokes et al, 2002; MacDougall et al, 2007; Byun et al, 2005). Earlier works have shown that RPA binds to ssDNA and then recruits ATR-ATRIP by interacting with ATRIP (Cortez et al, 2001; Ball et al, 2007). However, the recruitment to ssDNA is not sufficient for ATR activation (Ball et al., 2005; Namiki & Zou, 2006; Yoshioka et al., 2006), it requires additional ATR regulator, Rad9-Rad1-Hus1 (9-1-1) complex, a heterotrimeric ring-shaped structure like PCNA (Parrilla-Castellar et al., 2004). The 9-1-1 complex recognizes a DNA end that is adjacent to a stretch of RPA-coated ssDNA through working with RFC-RAD17 (Ellison & Stillman, 2003; Zou et al., 2003a; Bermudez et al., 2003). Current models for ATR activation suggest that the 9-1-1 mediated recruitment of TopBP1 to the ATR-ATRIP complex, and the ATR-activating domain of TopBP1 activates the kinase activity of ATR (Harper & Elledge, 2007; Cimprich & Cortez, 2008; Shiotani & Zou, 2009; Yan & Michael, 2009). In addition to be an activator of ATR, TopBP1 is also a substrate of ATR. The phosphorylation of TopBP1 on residue S1131 by ATM enhanced the interaction of it with ATR-ATRIP, which suggests that TopBP1 promotes a feed-forward signalling loop to amplify ATR-mediated signals (Yoo et al., 2007). Thus, sustained co-localization of the ATR-ATRIP and 9-1-1-TopBP1 complexes at the DNA damage site may increase their local concentration so that ATR activation is stimulated continually by TopBP1. However, recruitment of the ATR-ATRIP and 9-1-1-TopBP1 complexes to sites of DNA damage or stalled replication forks is independent events (Bonilla et al, 2008; Kondo et al, 2001; Melo et al, 2001; Zou et al, 2002; You et al, 2002; Lee et al, 2003). Therefore, there is the two-man rule in TopBP1-dependent regulation of ATR activity, by which ATRIP and 9-1-1 together control the TopBP1 to initiate ATR signalling.
As described above, activation of ATM involves its autophosphorylation, which helps it convert an inactive dimmer form into an active monomers form. Some phosphorylation sites on ATR and ATRIP have been found (Cimprich & Cortez, 2008), unlike ATM, as yet, none of these identified modifications has been reported to contribute to ATR activation and the oligomerization status of ATR-ATRIP.

2.3 Interplay between ATM and ATR pathway

It was previously thought that ATM and ATR had overlapping but distinct roles in response to DNA damage. However, a current study demonstrate a high degree of cross-talk and connectivity. For instance, ATM and ATR collaborate in the IR-induced G2/M checkpoint, but incomplete DNA replication in mammalian cells can prevent M phase entry independent of ATR (Brown & Baltimore, 2003). Recently, Trenz et al indicate that both ATM and ATR promote Mre11-dependent restart of collapsed replication forks and prevent accumulation of DNA DSBs (Trenz et al, 2006). Another study showed that ATR is activated rapidly by IR, and both ATM and Mre11 enhance ATR signalling (Myers & Cortez, 2006). The new data demonstrate that ATR is required for the response to either replication stress or IR without any role for ATM (Paul et al. 2004).

3. DNA damage response pathways and cell cycle checkpoints

The maintenance of genome stability is critical to the survival and propagation of all cellular organisms. The cell cycle is required for cell growth and cell division into two daughter cells. Cell cycle checkpoints are regulatory pathways that control the cell cycle events in the right order. DNA is vulnerable to diverse types of injury throughout the cell cycle. In response to DNA damage, checkpoint surveillance mechanisms initiate a cascade of events which coordinate cell cycle arrest and facilitate DNA repair pathways. These checkpoints include the G1/S, intra-S and G2/M of the cell cycle and are controlled by the ATM/Chk2 and ATR/Chk1 pathways. We will discuss the progresses of different signalling pathways involved in different checkpoints.

3.1 G1 Checkpoint

G1 checkpoint is the first checkpoint making the key decision of whether the cell should divide or arrest, which prevents the damaged DNA from being replication (Bartek & Lukas, 2001). The major player in the G1 checkpoint is the p53 protein. In normal cells, p53 is maintained at low levels due to interaction with MDM2, which targets p53 for degradation in the cytoplasm (Alarcon-Vargas & Ronai, 2002). In response to distinct or partially overlapping types of DNA damage, p53 is activated by ATM or ATR through phosphorylating different Ser/Thr residues directly and indirectly (Matsuoka et al., 2000; Maya et al., 2001; Shieh et al., 2000). The phosphorylation of Ser15 appears important in enhancing p53 transcriptional transactivation activity (Dumaz & Meek, 1999; Wang et al, 2008). The result of p53 activation is the up-regulation of various target genes (such as MDM2, GADD45a, and $p21^{Waf1/Cip1}$), some of which are involved in the DNA damage response. $p21^{Waf1/Cip1}$ elicits G1 arrest through suppressing Cyclin E/Cdk2 kinase activity (Bartek & Lukas, 2001). In other p53 target genes, such as Gadd45 and BIG2, also lead to G1 arrest. p53 lead to G1 checkpoint arrest in multiple pathways, now, p53 is reported to contribute to maintain G1 checkpoint control via activating microRNAs directly.

3.2 S-phase Checkpoint

The S-phase checkpoint monitors cell cycle process and lowers the rate of DNA replication after DNA damage. ATM plays a primary role in contributing to S-phase checkpoints although it overlapping with the ATR dependent pathway in maintenance of the S-phase checkpoint. In response to ionizing radiation, ATM phosphorylates Nbs1 and Chk2 and triggers two parallel cascades of the DNA damage responses to activate the S-phase checkpoint. One is the ATM-Chk2-Cdc25A pathway; the other is the ATM dependent NBS1/BRCA1/SMC1 pathway, though the mechanism of this pathway is not well understood (Falck et al., 2002). On the other hand, the ATR-Chk1 pathway is also involved in the S-phase checkpoint arrest auxiliary in response to IR. Furthermore, the ATR-Chk1 pathway plays a dominant role in directing S-phase checkpoint arrest in response to UV damage and replication errors (Abraham, 2001).

3.3 G2 Checkpoint

The G2 cell cycle checkpoint is an important control point which functions to prevent damaged DNA from being segregated into daughter cells. This checkpoint activation depends on the maintenance of Cdc2 phosphorylation on T14 and Y15 (Rhind et al., 1997). ATM and ATR both indirectly modulate the phosphorylation status of these sites in response to DNA damage. Different from other checkpoints, ATR mainly controls the response to UV damage and replication blocks. The response to IR is also mediated primarily by ATR while ATM plays a supporting role (Graves et al, 2000). Upon DNA

damage, ATR and ATM phosphorylate their downstream kinases Chk1 and Chk2, respectively, and then phosphorylate the phosphatase Cdc25C on Ser216 (Peng et al., 1997). The phosphorylated Cdc25C binds with 14-3-3 protein and is sequestered in the cytoplasm, which prevents Cdc25C from dephosphorylating Cdc2 in the nucleus and the cells remain arrested in the G2 phase (Lopez-Girona et al., 1999; Peng et al., 1997).
p53 also plays a role in the G2/M checkpoint (Passalaris et al., 1999). Activated p53 in response to DNA damage results in G2/M checkpoint arrest through induction of GADD45 (Zhan et al., 1994). In addition, p53-dependent transcriptional repression of cdc2 and cyclin B may also contribute to the G2/M checkpoint (Passalaris et al., 1999).

4. DNA damage response and protein post-modifications

Post-translational modifications play a vital role in harmonizing cellular response to DNA damage. More and more proteins were found occurring in a variety of post-translational modifications including phosphorylation, acetylation, methylation and ubiquitylation in response to DNA damage or genotoxic stress. Recent research suggests that a crosstalk exists between multiple protein modifications. Here, we will summarize recent findings of protein post-translational modifications in coordinating the DNA damage response signalling cascade.

4.1 Protein phosphorylation modification in response to DNA damage

Signal transduction is predominantly mediated by a cascade of protein phosphorylation and dephosphorylation reactions, which is of prime importance for the organisms to sense the external and internal stimuli and generate the appropriate responses. Protein phosphorylation plays the same role in cellular DNA damage response. As indicated above, in responding to DSB signalling, ATM undergoes autophosphorylation, which seems to be instrumental in the monomerization and activation of ATM. It seems that DNA lesions activate various protein kinases, such as ATM and ATR, which transduce the damage signalling by directly phosphorylating or mediating the phosphorylation and activation of numerous substrates involved in the DNA repair machinery, the cell cycle checkpoints and apoptosis (Abraham, 2001; Osborn et al., 2002). So far, more than 700 proteins have been identified to be phosphorylated in response to DNA damage (Matsuoka et al., 2007). A signalling cascade is initiated starting with the phosphorylation of H2AX (γ-H2AX). γ-H2AX is a chromatin-based signal that regulates the assembly of DNA damage response proteins at the break sites and induction of DNA repairs (Lavin, 2008; Cook et al., 2009). So, the H2AX phosphorylation level is not only important as a marker of the DNA damage response, but also involve in DNA repair processes (van Attikum & Gasser, 2009).
The effector p53 stands at the cross-roads of cellular responses to various stresses (Appella & Anderson, 2001; Bode & Dong, 2004). DNA damage leads to specific phosphorylation modifications of p53 protein. Up to date, at least 20 phosphorylation sites have been detected in the p53 molecule in human cells following DNA damage (Bode & Dong, 2004). Some of which were phosphorylated by ATM in response to irradiation and chemotherapeutic drugs (Banin et al, 1998; Canman et al, 1998), whereas some are phosphorylated by ATR when cells are treated with UV or anti-cancer drugs (Appella & Anderson, 2001; Wang, 2008). Phosphorylation of p53 usually modulates its stability and sequence-specific DNA binding activity (Bode & Dong, 2004). Two major phospho-binding modules, the BRCA1 C-terminal repeat (BRCT) and the forkhead-associated (FHA) domain,

which are present in many proteins are involved in the cellular response to DNA damage, and facilitated protein-protein interactions in the recruitment and activation of damage signalling (Yu et al, 2003; Hofmann & Bucher, 1995; Li et al, 2002).

4.2 Protein acetylation in response to DNA damage

Phosphorylation is not the only post-translational modification in cellular response to DNA damage. For instance, following DSB, ATM is activated in the vicinity of the break and is recruited to the break site by the MRN complex where it is fully activated, facilitated by not only autophosphorylation but also acetylation of ATM (Bakkenist & Kastan, 2003; Sun et al, 2007). The study showed that after DNA damage, CK2 phosphorylates and releases HP1β from chromatin which recruits a ATM-Tip60 complex to MRN at the break site. This promotes interaction between Tip60 acetyltransferase and the unbound histone H3 K9me3 leading to acetylation and activation of ATM (Sun et al, 2009). A single site at Lys3016 is acetylated by Tip60 acetyltransferase. This mutation inhibits the monomerization and up-regulation of ATM activation by DNA damage, further prevents ATM-dependent phosphorylation of p53 and checkpoint kinase-2 (Chk2) (Sun et al, 2005, 2007).

As the recruitment of the Tip60 acetyltransferase, the deacetylase enzymes HDAC1, HDAC2, HDAC4, SIRT1, and SIRT6 also have been observed at DSB sites in mammalian cells (Kao et al. 2003; Oberdoerffer et al. 2008; Kaidi et al. 2010; Miller et al. 2010). For instance, the MRN complex serves as a sensor for the detection of DSBs and is involves in the S phase checkpoint (Paull & Lee, 2005; van den Bosch et al, 2003). The acetylation level of NBS1 was recently reported to be tightly regulated by deacetylase SIRT1 (Yuan et al., 2007). Moreover, SIRT6-dependent deacetylation of the CtIP in response to DSBs stimulates the RPA and RAD51 foci, thus promoting ATR signalling and DSB repair (Kaidi et al. 2010). Furthermore, histone acetylation can regulate the dynamics of DDR factors in the vicinity of DNA breaks.

p53 acetylation also plays important roles in response to various types of DNA damage (Gu & Roeder, 1997; Lill et al, 1997; Nag et al, 2007). Transcription factors with histone acetyltransferase activity, p300/CBP, p300/CBP-associated factor (PCAF), and Tip60 are reported to be mainly responsible for the p53 acetylation (Liu et al., 1999; Sykes et al.,2006; Tang et al., 2006, 2008). p53 acetylation can increase its sequence-specific DNA binding capacity (Gu & Roeder, 1997; Zhao et al, 2006; Luo et al, 2004) or enhance its stabilization by inhibiting ubiquitination of p53 mediated by MDM2 (Li et al, 2002; Ito et al, 2002). Recently our studies indicate that histone deacetylase inhibitors and other chemical agents also induce p53 acetylation through the DNA damage response pathway (Zhao et al, 2006; Wang et al, 2008). Novel discoveries further confirm that p53 acetylation is an indispensable event for mediating the p53 response (Kruse & Gu, 2009). However, the regulatory mechanisms involving in this posttranslational modification are still largely unknown.

4.3 Protein ubiquitylation in response to DNA damage

Ubiquitylation is the process by which the 76-amino-acid polypeptide ubiquitin is attached to the target protein singly (monoubiquitylation) or in the form of polyubiquitin chains (polyubiquitylation) via the covalent bond. This is an enzyme cascade reaction which is involved by ubiquitin E1, E2 and E3 ligase proteins (Pickart, 2001). A growing number evidences have shown that ubiquitylation and deubiquitylation are important regulatory mechanisms in response to DNA damage and genotoxic stresses. Assembly of DNA damage response proteins at the break site is catalyzed by the E3 ubiquitin ligases.

Consistent with these actions, several ubiquitin ligases have been shown to accumulate at sites of DNA breaks in mammalian cells, including BRCA1, RNF8, RNF168, RAD18, HERC2, and PRC1 (Polycomb-repressive complex 1) (Scully et al. 1997; Kolas et al. 2007; Doil et al. 2009; Huang et al. 2009; Stewart et al. 2009; Bekker-Jensen & Mailand, 2010; Chou et al., 2010; Lavin, 2008). For example, phosphorylation of MDC1 at ATM consensus sites promotes interaction with RNF8, the E3 ubiquitin ligase, which in turn ubiquitylates H2A, leading to the accumulation of 53BPI, BRCA1, and other proteins at the site of damage (Kolas et al, 2007; Mailand et al, 2007). Ubiquitylated H2A serves as an interacting partner for RNF168 that further propagates the ubiquitylation of H2A and other unknown targets at the double-strand break site (Doil et al, 2009; Stewart, 2009). In addition, FANCD2 (Fanconi anemia complementation group D2) is monoubiquitinated during the S phase (Taniguchi et al. 2002) and in response to various DNA damaging agents, which is required for its localization to DNA damage foci (Garcia-Higuera et al. 2001). It is demonstrated that ATR is required for efficient FANCD2 monoubiquitination and foci assembly in response to various genotoxic stresses, including IR and MMC. Another example is p53, which is kept at low level in unstressed cells through Mdm2-mediated polyubiquitination, which leads to nuclear export of p53 and subsequent proteasomal degradation. DNA damage attenuates polyubiquitination of p53, thereby stabilizes and activates p53 as a transcription factor, up-regulating expression of numerous proteins involved in cell cycle control, apoptosis and senescence (Toledo & Wahl, 2006; Bode & Dong, 2004).

Besides ubiquitylation, deubiquitylation has also been documented as an opposite way to regulate protein stability in response to genotoxic stress. A number of de-ubiquitylating enzymes (DUBs) were identified at double-strand breaks including USP3, USP28 and BRCC36. BRCC36 antagonizes RNF8-dependent ubiquitylation to maintain steady state levels required for appropriate signalling (Sobhian et al, 2007; Chen et al, 2006; Shao et al, 2009). USP3 is a chromatin-associated DUB that also antagonizes RNF8-mediated ubiquitylation (Nicassio et al, 2007). USP28 is a major regulator of DNA damage-induced apoptosis. It was shown that USP28 stabilizes CHK2, 53BP1 and a number of other DNA damage responsive proteins upon irradiation (Wu-Baer et al, 2003).

4.4 Crosstalk between post-translational modifications in response to DNA damage

Recent researches suggest that a crosstalk exists among multiple protein modifications, which collaboratively to regulate signal transduction of DNA damage and genetic stresses. p53, is subjected to multiple posttranslational modifications in response to genotoxic stress, which results in the accumulation of p53 and triggers its transcriptional activities. The damage-induced phosphorylation of p53 seems to be a signal for subsequent acetylation, because phosphorylation enhances its association with the CBP/p300 and PCAF to induce p53 acetylation in response to DNA damage, which results in p53 acetylation and further stabilized (Wang, 2008). Recent reports revealed that the Set8/Pr-Set7 methyltransferase suppresses p53 function in response to DNA damage (Shi et al. 2007), and lysine methylation of p53 by Set7/9 methyltransferase is important for its subsequent acetylation, which results in stabilization of the p53 protein (Ivanov et al., 2007). We also demonstrate that Set7/9 interacts with Sirt1 and induces a decrease in binding of Sirt1 to p53, and this relatively enhances p53 transactivity(Liu et al, 2011).

Apart from the above mentioned, H2AX, a variant form of H2A, is known to be acetylated by Tip60 acetyltransferase following DNA damage. Acetylated H2AX is required for its subsequent ubiquitylation via the ubiquitin-conjugating enzyme UBC13 (Ikura et al., 2007).

They suggested that acetylation-dependent ubiquitination by the Tip60-UBC13 complex leads to the release of H2AX from damaged chromatin, which enhanced histone dynamics and in turn stimulates a DNA damage response.

5. Conclusion

In summary, instability of genome is a constant problem of organisms. The coordination of DNA damage response (DDR) processes is required to maintain cellular viability and prevent diseases. The ATM and ATR protein kinases are master regulators of the DNA damage response. To further understand the molecular mechanisms through which the DDR operates, elucidate the genetic interactions between different DDR pathways and between DDR pathways and other cellular pathways, will be helpful for therapeutic strategies to treat many human disease.

6. Acknowledgment

This article was supported by National Natural Science Foundation of China 90919030 and 31070691 to Wei-Guo Zhu and 31071117 to Haiying Wang, and Beijing Natural Science Foundation 7112081(Study on the mechenism of HDAC inhibitor depsipeptide in cancer treatment) to Haiying Wang.

7. Abbreviations

The abbreviations used are: ATM, ataxia-telangiectasia mutated; ATR, ATM and Rad3-related; Chk, Checkpoint kinase; IR, ionizing radiation; PIKK, phosphoinositide-3 kinase-related kinases; ATR-IP, ATR-interacting protein; ROS, reactive oxygen species; DSB, double strand break ; 5-Aza-CdR,5′-aza-2′-deoxycytidine; DDR, DNA damage response; MRN, Mre11/Rad50/Nbs1; ssDNA, single strand DNA; 9-1-1, Rad9-Rad1-Hus1; FHA, forkhead-associated; BRCT, BRCA1 C-terminal; PRC1, Polycomb-repressive complex 1; DUBs, de-ubiquitylating enzymes.

8. References

Abraham RT (2001) Cell cycle checkpoint signaling through the ATM and ATR kinases. *Genes Dev* 15(17):2177-2196.

Alarcon-Vargas D & Ronai Z (2002) p53-Mdm2--the affair that never ends. *Carcinogenesis* 23(4):541-547.

Appella E & Anderson CW (2001) Post-translational modifications and activation of p53 bygenotoxic stresses. *Eur J Biochem* 268(10):2764-2772.

Bakkenist CJ & Kastan MB (2003) DNA damage activates ATM through intermolecular autophosphorylation and dimer dissociation. *Nature* 421(6922):499-506.

Bakkenist CJ & Kastan MB (2004) Initiating cellular stress responses. *Cell* 118(1):9-17.

Ball HL, Ehrhardt MR, Mordes DA, Glick GG, Chazin WJ & Cortez D. (2007) Function of aconserved checkpoint recruitment domain in ATRIP proteins. *Mol Cell Biol* 27(9):3367-3377.

Ball HL, Myers JS, & Cortez D (2005) ATRIP binding to replication protein A-single-stranded DNA promotes ATR-ATRIP localization but is dispensable for Chk1 phosphorylation. *Mol Biol Cell* 16(5):2372-2381.

Banin S, Moyal, L, Shieh, S, Taya, Y, Anderson, C W, Chessa, L, Smorodinsky, N I, Prives, C, Reiss, Y, Shiloh, Y, & Ziv, Y (1998) Enhanced phosphorylation of p53 by ATM in response to DNA damage. *Science* 281(5383):1674-1677.

Bartek J & Lukas J (2001) Mammalian G1- and S-phase checkpoints in response to DNA damage. *Curr Opin Cell Biol* 13(6):738-747.

Bekker-Jensen S & Mailand N (2010) Assembly and function of DNA double-strand break repair foci in mammalian cells. *DNA Repair* 9(12):1219-1228.

Bentley NJ, Holtzman DA, Flaggs G, Keegan KS, DeMaggio A, Ford JC, Hoekstra M& Carr AM. (1996) The Schizosaccharomyces pombe rad3 checkpoint gene. *Embo J* 15(23):6641-6651.

Berkovich E, Monnat RJ, Jr., & Kastan MB (2007) Roles of ATM and NBS1 in chromatin structure modulation and DNA double-strand break repair. *Nat Cell Biol* 9(6):683-690.

Bermudez VP, Lindsey-Boltz LA, Cesare AJ, Maniwa Y, Griffith JD, Hurwitz J & Sancar A.(2003) Loading of the human 9-1-1 checkpoint complex onto DNA by the checkpoint clamp loader hRad17-replication factor C complex in vitro. *Proc Natl Acad Sci U S A* 100(4):1633-1638.

Bode AM DZ (2004) Post-translational modification of p53 in tumorigenesis. *Nat Rev Cancer.* 4(10):793-805.

Bonilla CY, Melo JA, & Toczyski DP (2008) Colocalization of sensors is sufficient to activate the DNA damage checkpoint in the absence of damage. *Mol Cell* 30(3):267-276.

Brown EJ & Baltimore D (2003) Essential and dispensable roles of ATR in cell cycle arrest and genome maintenance. Genes Dev 17(5):615-628.

Burma S, Chen BP, Murphy M, Kurimasa A, & Chen DJ (2001) ATM phosphorylates histone H2AX in response to DNA double-strand breaks. *J Biol Chem* 276(45):42462-42467.

Byun TS, Pacek M, Yee MC, Walter JC, & Cimprich KA (2005) Functional uncoupling of MCM helicase and DNA polymerase activities activates the ATR-dependent checkpoint. *Genes Dev* 19(9):1040-1052.

Canman CE, Lim, DS, Cimprich, KA, Taya, Y, Tamai, K, Sakaguchi, K, Appella, E, Kastan, M B & Siliciano, JD. (1998) Activation of the ATM kinase by ionizing radiation and phosphorylation of p53. *Science* 281(5383):1677-1679.

Carson CT, Schwartz RA, Stracker TH, Lilley CE, Lee DV & Weitzman MD. (2003) The Mre11 complex is required for ATM activation and the G2/M checkpoint. *Embo J* 22(24):6610-6620.

Cerosaletti K & Concannon P (2004) Independent roles for nibrin and Mre11-Rad50 in the activation and function of Atm. *J Biol Chem* 279(37):38813-38819.

Chai G, Li L, Zhou W, Wu L, Zhao Y, Wang D, Lu S, Yu Y, Wang H, McNutt MA, Hu YG, Chen Y, Yang Y, Wu X, Otterson GA & Zhu WG. (2008) HDAC inhibitors act with 5-aza-2'-deoxycytidine to inhibit cell proliferation by suppressing removal of incorporated abases in lung cancer cells. *PLoS One* 3(6):e2445.

Chen X, Arciero CA, Wang C, Broccoli D, & Godwin AK (2006) BRCC36 is essential for ionizing radiation-induced BRCA1 phosphorylation and nuclear foci formation.*Cancer Res* 66(10):5039-5046.

Chou DM, Adamson B, Dephoure NE, Tan X, Nottke AC, Hurov KE, Gygi SP, Colaiacovo MP & Elledge SJ. (2010) A chromatin localization screen reveals poly (ADP ribose)-regulated recruitment of the repressive polycomb and NuRD complexes to sites of DNA damage. *Proc Natl Acad Sci U S A* 107(43):18475-18480.

Cimprich KA & Cortez D (2008) ATR: an essential regulator of genome integrity. *Nat Rev Mol Cell Biol* 9(8):616-627.

Cliby WA, Roberts CJ, Cimprich KA, Stringer CM, Lamb JR, Schreiber SL & Friend SH. (1998) Overexpression of a kinase-inactive ATR protein causes sensitivity to DNA-damaging agents and defects in cell cycle checkpoints. *Embo J* 17(1):159-169.

Cook PJ, Ju BG, Telese F, Wang X, Glass CK & Rosenfeld MG.. (2009) Tyrosine dephosphorylation of H2AX modulates apoptosis and survival decisions. *Nature* 458(7238):591-596.

Cortez D, Guntuku S, Qin J, & Elledge SJ (2001) ATR and ATRIP: partners in checkpoint signaling. *Science* 294(5547):1713-1716.

Costanzo V & Gautier J (2003) Single-strand DNA gaps trigger an ATR- and Cdc7-dependent checkpoint. *Cell Cycle* 2(1):17.

Difilippantonio S, Celeste A, Fernandez-Capetillo O, Chen HT, Reina San Martin B, Van Laethem F, Yang YP, Petukhova GV, Eckhaus M, Feigenbaum L, Manova K, Kruhlak M, Camerini-Otero RD, Sharan S, Nussenzweig M & Nussenzweig A. (2005) Role of Nbs1 in the activation of the Atm kinase revealed in humanized mouse models. *Nat Cell Biol* 7(7):675-685.

Doil C, Mailand N, Bekker-Jensen S, Menard P, Larsen DH, Pepperkok R, Ellenberg J, Panier S, Durocher D, Bartek J, Lukas J & Lukas C. (2009) RNF168 binds and amplifies ubiquitin conjugates on damaged chromosomes to allow accumulation of repair proteins. *Cell* 136(3):435-446.

Dumaz N & Meek DW (1999) Serine15 phosphorylation stimulates p53 transactivation but does not directly influence interaction with HDM2. *Embo J* 18(24):7002-7010.

Elledge SJ (1996) Cell cycle checkpoints: preventing an identity crisis. *Science* 274(5293):1664-1672.

Ellison V & Stillman B (2003) Biochemical characterization of DNA damage checkpoint complexes: clamp loader and clamp complexes with specificity for 5' recessed DNA. *PLoS Biol* 1(2):E33.

Falck J, Petrini JH, Williams BR, Lukas J, & Bartek J (2002) The DNA damage-dependent intra-S phase checkpoint is regulated by parallel pathways. *Nat Genet* 30(3):290-294.

Garcia-Higuera I, Taniguchi T, Ganesan S, Meyn MS, Timmers C, Hejna J, Grompe M & D'Andrea AD. (2001) Interaction of the Fanconi anemia proteins and BRCA1 in a common pathway. *Mol Cell* 7(2):249-262.

Graves PR, Yu L, Schwarz JK, Gales J, Sausville EA, O'Connor PM & Piwnica-Worms H. (2000) The Chk1 protein kinase and the Cdc25C regulatory pathways are targets of the anticancer agent UCN-01. *J Biol Chem* 275(8):5600-5605.

Gu W &Roeder RG (1997) Activation of p53 sequence-specific DNA binding by acetylation of the p53 C-terminal domain. *Cell* 90(4):595-606.

Gupta A, Sharma GG, Young CS, Agarwal M, Smith ER, Paull TT, Lucchesi JC, Khanna KK,
Ludwig T& Pandita TK. (2005) Involvement of human MOF in ATM function. *Mol Cell Biol* 25(12):5292-5305.

Harper JW & Elledge SJ (2007) The DNA damage response: ten years after. *Mol Cell* 28(5):739-745.

Hefferin ML & Tomkinson AE (2005) Mechanism of DNA double-strand break repair by non-homologous end joining. *DNA Repair (Amst)* 4(6):639-648.

Hoeijmakers JH (2009) DNA damage, aging, and cancer. *N Engl J Med* 361(15):1475-1485.Hoeijmakers JH (2001) Genome maintenance mechanisms for preventing cancer. *Nature* 411(6835):366-374.

Hofmann K & Bucher P (1995) The FHA domain: a putative nuclear signalling domain found in protein kinases and transcription factors. *Trends Biochem Sci* 20(9):347-349.

Huang J, Huen MS, Kim H, Leung CC, Glover JN, Yu X & Chen J. (2009) RAD18 transmits DNA damage signalling to elicit homologous recombination repair. *Nat Cell Biol* 11(5):592-603.

Huen MS & Chen J (2008) The DNA damage response pathways: at the crossroad of protein modifications. *Cell Res* 18(1):8-16.

Ikura T, Tashiro S, Kakino A, Shima H, Jacob N, Amunugama R, Yoder K, Izumi S, Kuraoka I, Tanaka K, Kimura H, Ikura M, Nishikubo S, Ito T, Muto A, Miyagawa K, Takeda S, Fishel R, Igarashi K & Kamiya K. (2007) DNA damage-dependent acetylation and ubiquitination of H2AX enhances chromatin dynamics. *Mol Cell Biol* 27(20):7028-7040.

Ito A KY, Lai CH, Kovacs JJ, Higashimoto Y, Appella E, Yao TP (2002) MDM2-HDAC1-mediated deacetylation of p53 is required for its degradation. *EMBO J.* 21(22):6236-6245.

Ivanov GS, Ivanova T, Kurash J, Ivanov A, Chuikov S, Gizatullin F, Herrera-Medina EM, Rauscher F 3rd, Reinberg D & Barlev NA. (2007) Methylation-acetylation interplay activates p53 in response to DNA damage. *Mol Cell Biol* 27(19):6756-6769.

Kaidi A, Weinert BT, Choudhary C, & Jackson SP (2010) Human SIRT6 promotes DNA end resection through CtIP deacetylation. *Science* 329(5997):1348-1353.

Kanu N & Behrens A (2007) ATMIN defines an NBS1-independent pathway of ATM signalling. *Embo J* 26(12):2933-2941.

Kao GD, McKenna WG, Guenther MG, Muschel RJ, Lazar MA & Yen TJ. (2003) Histone deacetylase 4 interacts with 53BP1 to mediate the DNA damage response. *J Cell Biol* 160(7):1017-1027.

Khanna KK & Jackson SP (2001) DNA double-strand breaks: signaling, repair and the cancer connection. *Nat Genet* 27(3):247-254.

Kolas NK, Chapman JR, Nakada S, Ylanko J, Chahwan R, Sweeney FD, Panier S, Mendez M, Wildenhain J, Thomson TM, Pelletier L, Jackson SP & Durocher D. (2007) Orchestration of the DNA-damage response by the RNF8 ubiquitin ligase. *Science* 318(5856):1637-1640.

Kondo T, Wakayama T, Naiki T, Matsumoto K, & Sugimoto K (2001) Recruitment of Mec1 and Ddc1 checkpoint proteins to double-strand breaks through distinct mechanisms. *Science* 294(5543):867-870.

Kozlov SV, Graham ME, Jakob B, Tobias F, Kijas AW, Tanuji M, Chen P, Robinson PJ, Taucher-Scholz G, Suzuki K, So S, Chen D & Lavin MF. (2011) Autophosphorylation and ATM activation: additional sites add to the complexity. *J Biol Chem* 286(11):9107-9119.

Kruse JP & Gu W (2009) Modes of p53 regulation. *Cell* 137(4):609-622.

Kumagai A, Lee J, Yoo HY, & Dunphy WG (2006) TopBP1 activates the ATR-ATRIP complex. *Cell* 124(5):943-955.

Lavin MF & Shiloh Y (1997) The genetic defect in ataxia-telangiectasia. *Annu Rev Immunol* 15:177-202.

Lavin MF (2008) Ataxia-telangiectasia: from a rare disorder to a paradigm for cell signalling and cancer. *Nat Rev Mol Cell Biol* 9(10):759-769.

Lee J, Kumagai A, & Dunphy WG (2003) Claspin, a Chk1-regulatory protein, monitors DNA replication on chromatin independently of RPA, ATR, and Rad17. *Mol Cell* 11(2):329-340.

Lee JH & Paull TT (2004) Direct activation of the ATM protein kinase by the Mre11/Rad50/Nbs1 complex. *Science* 304(5667):93-96.

Lee JH & Paull TT (2005) ATM activation by DNA double-strand breaks through the Mre11-Rad50-Nbs1 complex. *Science* 308(5721):551-554.

Li J, Williams BL, Haire LF, Goldberg M, Wilker E, Durocher D, Yaffe MB, Jackson SP & Smerdon SJ. (2002) Structural and functional versatility of the FHA domain in DNA-damage signaling by the tumor suppressor kinase Chk2. *Mol Cell* 9(5):1045-1054.

Li M LJ, Brooks CL, Gu W (2002) Acetylation of p53 inhibits its ubiquitination by Mdm2. *J Biol Chem.* 277(52):50607-50611.

Lill NL GS, Ginsberg D, DeCaprio J, Livingston DM. (1997) Binding and modulation of p53 by p300/CBP coactivators. *Nature.* 387(6635):823-827.

Lim DS & Kim ST. (2000) ATM phosphorylates p95/nbs1 in an S-phase checkpoint pathway. *Nature* 404(6778):613-617.

Liu L SD, Trievel RC, Zhang HB, Marmorstein R, Halazonetis TD, Berger SL (1999) p53 sites acetylated in vitro by PCAF and p300 are acetylated in vivo in response to DNA damage. *Mol Cell Biol.* 19(2):1202-1209.

Liu X, Wang D, Zhao Y, Tu B, Zheng Z, Wang L, Wang H, Gu W, Roeder RG & Zhu WG. (2011) Methyltransferase Set7/9 regulates p53 activity by interacting with Sirtuin 1 (SIRT1). Proc Natl Acad Sci U S A 108(5):1925-1930.

Lodish H, Berk A, Matsudaira P, Kaiser CA, Krieger M, Scott MP, Zipursky SL & Darnell J.(2004). Molecular Biology of the Cell, p963. WH Freeman: New York, NY. 5th ed.

Lopez-Girona A, Furnari B, Mondesert O, & Russell P (1999) Nuclear localization of Cdc25 is regulated by DNA damage and a 14-3-3 protein. *Nature* 397(6715):172-175.

Lou Z, Minter-Dykhouse K, Franco S, Gostissa M, Rivera MA, Celeste A, Manis JP, van Deursen J, Nussenzweig A, Paull TT, Alt FW & Chen J. (2006) MDC1 maintains genomic stability by participating in the amplification of ATM-dependent DNA damage signals. *Mol Cell* 21(2):187-200.

Lukas C, Falck J, Bartkova J, Bartek J, & Lukas J (2003) Distinct spatiotemporal dynamics of mammalian checkpoint regulators induced by DNA damage. *Nat Cell Biol* 5(3):255-260.

Luo J, Li, M., Tang, Y., Laszkowska, M., Roeder, R. G. & Gu, W. (2004) Acetylation of p53 augments its site-specific DNA binding both in vitro and in vivo. *Proc Natl Acad Sci U S A* 101(8):2259-2264.

MacDougall CA, Byun TS, Van C, Yee MC, & Cimprich KA (2007) The structural determinants of checkpoint activation. *Genes Dev* 21(8):898-903.

Mailand N, Bekker-Jensen S, Faustrup H, Melander F, Bartek J, Lukas C & Lukas J. (2007) RNF8 ubiquitylates histones at DNA double-strand breaks and promotes assembly of repair proteins. *Cell* 131(5):887-900.

Matsuoka S, Rotman G, Ogawa A, Shiloh Y, Tamai K & Elledge SJ. (2000) Ataxia telangiectasia-mutated phosphorylates Chk2 in vivo and in vitro. *Proc Natl Acad Sci U S A* 97(19):10389-10394.

Matsuoka S, Ballif BA, Smogorzewska A, McDonald ER 3rd, Hurov KE, Luo J, Bakalarski CE, Zhao Z, Solimini N, Lerenthal Y, Shiloh Y, Gygi SP & Elledge SJ. (2007) ATM and ATR substrate analysis reveals extensive protein networks responsive to DNA damage. *Science* 316(5828):1160-1166.

Maya R, Balass M, Kim ST, Shkedy D, Leal JF, Shifman O, Moas M, Buschmann T, Ronai Z, Shiloh Y, Kastan MB, Katzir E & Oren M. (2001) ATM-dependent phosphorylation of Mdm2 on serine 395: role in p53 activation by DNA damage. *Genes Dev* 15(9):1067-1077.

McGowan CH & Russell P (2004) The DNA damage response: sensing and signaling. *Curr Opin Cell Biol* 16(6):629-633.

Melo JA, Cohen J, & Toczyski DP (2001) Two checkpoint complexes are independently recruited to sites of DNA damage in vivo. *Genes Dev* 15(21):2809-2821.

Miller KM, Tjeertes JV, Coates J, Legube G, Polo SE, Britton S & Jackson SP. (2010) Human HDAC1 and HDAC2 function in the DNA-damage response to promote DNA nonhomologous end-joining. *Nat Struct Mol Biol* 17(9):1144-1151.

Myers JS & Cortez D (2006) Rapid activation of ATR by ionizing radiation requires ATM and Mre11. *J Biol Chem* 281(14):9346-9350.

Nag A, Germaniuk-Kurowska A, Dimri M, Sassack M, Gurumurthy CB, Gao Q, Dimri G, Band H, & Band V (2007) An essential role of human ADA3 in p53 acetylation. *J Biol Chem*. 282,8812–8820.

Nakanishi K, *et al.* (2002) Interaction of FANCD2 and NBS1 in the DNA damage response. *Nat Cell Biol* 4(12):913-920.

Namiki Y & Zou L (2006) ATRIP associates with replication protein A-coated ssDNA through multiple interactions. *Proc Natl Acad Sci U S A* 103(3):580-585.

Nicassio F, Taniguchi T, Ranganathan V, New HV, Moreau LA, Stotsky M, Mathew CG, Kastan MB, Weaver DT & D'Andrea AD. (2007) Human USP3 is a chromatin modifier required for S phase progression and genome stability. *Curr Biol* 17(22):1972-1977.

Oberdoerffer P, Michan S, McVay M, Mostoslavsky R, Vann J, Park SK, Hartlerode A, Stegmuller J, Hafner A, Loerch P, Wright SM, Mills KD, Bonni A, Yankner BA, Scully R, Prolla TA, Alt FW & Sinclair DA. (2008) SIRT1 redistribution on chromatin promotes genomic stability but alters gene expression during aging. *Cell* 135(5):907-918.

Osborn AJ, Elledge SJ, & Zou L (2002) Checking on the fork: the DNA-replication stress-response pathway. *Trends Cell Biol* 12(11):509-516.

Pandita TK, Lieberman HB, Lim DS, Dhar S, Zheng W, Taya Yand Kastan MB. (2000) Ionizing radiation activates the ATM kinase throughout the cell cycle. *Oncogene* 19(11):1386-1391

Parrilla-Castellar ER, Arlander SJ, & Karnitz L (2004) Dial 9-1-1 for DNA damage: the Rad9-Hus1-Rad1 (9-1-1) clamp complex. *DNA Repair (Amst)* 3(8-9):1009-1014.

Passalaris TM, Benanti JA, Gewin L, Kiyono T, & Galloway DA (1999) The G(2) checkpoint is maintained by redundant pathways. *Mol Cell Biol* 19(9):5872-5881.

Paul R, Andreassen, Alan D. D'Andrea & Toshiyasu Taniguchi.. (2004) Cell cycle-dependent dynamic localization of a bacterial response regulator with a novel di-guanylate cyclase output domain. *Genes Dev* 18(6):715-727.

Paull TT & Lee JH (2005) The Mre11/Rad50/Nbs1 complex and its role as a DNA double-strand break sensor for ATM. *Cell Cycle* 4(6):737-740.

Peng CY, Graves PR, Thoma RS, Wu Z, Shaw AS & Piwnica-Worms H. (1997) Mitotic and G2 checkpoint control: regulation of 14-3-3 protein binding by phosphorylation of Cdc25C on serine-216. *Science* 277(5331):1501-1505.

Pickart CM (2001) Mechanisms underlying ubiquitination. *Annu Rev Biochem* 70:503-533.

Rhind N, Furnari B, & Russell P (1997) Cdc2 tyrosine phosphorylation is required for the DNA damage checkpoint in fission yeast. *Genes Dev* 11(4):504-511.

Richard DJ, Bolderson E, Cubeddu L, Wadsworth RI, Savage K, Sharma GG, Nicolette ML, Tsvetanov S, McIlwraith MJ, Pandita RK, Takeda S, Hay RT, Gautier J, West SC, Paull TT, Pandita TK, White MF & Khanna KK. (2008) Single-stranded DNA-binding protein hSSB1 is critical for genomic stability. *Nature* 453(7195):677-681.

So S, Davis AJ, & Chen DJ (2009) Autophosphorylation at serine 1981 stabilizes ATM at DNA damage sites. *J Cell Biol* 187(7):977-990.

Savitsky K, Bar-Shira A, Gilad S, Rotman G, Ziv Y, Vanagaite L, Tagle DA, Smith S, Uziel T, Sfez S, Ashkenazi M, Pecker I, Frydman M, Harnik R, Patanjali SR, Simmons A, Clines GA, Sartiel A, Gatti RA, Chessa L, Sanal O, Lavin MF, Jaspers NG, Taylor AM, Arlett CF, Miki T, Weissman SM, Lovett M, Collins FS & Shiloh Y. (1995) A single ataxia telangiectasia gene with a product similar to PI-3 kinase. *Science* 268(5218):1749-1753.

Scully R, Chen J, Ochs RL, Keegan K, Hoekstra M, Feunteun J & Livingston DM. (1997) Dynamic changes of BRCA1 subnuclear location and phosphorylation state are initiated by DNA damage. *Cell* 90(3):425-435.

Shao G, Lilli DR, Patterson-Fortin J, Coleman KA, Morrissey DE & Greenberg RA. (2009) TheRap80-BRCC36 de-ubiquitinating enzyme complex antagonizes RNF8-Ubc13-dependent ubiquitination events at DNA double strand breaks. *Proc Natl Acad Sci U S A* 106(9):3166-3171.

Shi X, Kachirskaia I, Yamaguchi H, West LE, Wen H, Wang EW, Dutta S, Appella E & Gozani O.(2007) Modulation of p53 function by SET8-mediated methylation at lysine 382. *Mol Cell* 27(4):636-646.

Shieh SY, Ahn J, Tamai K, Taya Y, & Prives C (2000) The human homologs of checkpoint kinases Chk1 and Cds1 (Chk2) phosphorylate p53 at multiple DNA damage-inducible sites. *Genes Dev* 14(3):289-300.

Shiloh Y (2001) ATM and ATR: networking cellular responses to DNA damage. *Curr Opin Genet Dev* 11(1):71-77.

Shiloh Y (2003) ATM and related protein kinases: safeguarding genome integrity. *Nat Rev Cancer* 3(3):155-168.

Shiloh Y (2006) The ATM-mediated DNA-damage response: taking shape. *Trends Biochem Sci* 31(7):402-410.

Shiotani B & Zou L (2009) ATR signaling at a glance. *J Cell Sci* 122(Pt 3):301-304.

Sobhian B, Shao G, Lilli DR, Culhane AC, Moreau LA, Xia B, Livingston DM & Greenberg RA. (2007) RAP80 targets BRCA1 to specific ubiquitin structures at DNA damage sites. *Science* 316(5828):1198-1202.

Stewart GS (2009) Solving the RIDDLE of 53BP1 recruitment to sites of damage. *Cell Cycle* 8(10):1532-1538.Stokes MP, Van Hatten R, Lindsay HD, & Michael WM (2002) DNA replication is required for the checkpoint response to damaged DNA in Xenopus egg extracts. *J Cell Biol* 158(5):863-872.

Stucki M, Clapperton JA, Mohammad D, Yaffe MB, Smerdon SJ & Jackson SP. (2005) MDC1 directly binds phosphorylated histone H2AX to regulate cellular responses to DNA double-strand breaks. *Cell* 123(7):1213-1226.

Stucki M & Jackson SP (2006) gammaH2AX and MDC1: anchoring the DNA-damage-responsemachinery to broken chromosomes. *DNA Repair (Amst)* 5(5):534-543.

Sun Y, Jiang X, Chen S, Fernandes N, & Price BD (2005) A role for the Tip60 histoneacetyltransferase in the acetylation and activation of ATM. *Proc Natl Acad Sci U S A* 102(37):13182-13187.

Sun Y, Xu Y, Roy K, & Price BD (2007) DNA damage-induced acetylation of lysine 3016 of ATM activates ATM kinase activity. *Mol Cell Biol* 27(24):8502-8509.

Sun Y, Jiang X, Xu Y, Ayrapetov MK, Moreau LA, Whetstine JR & Price BD. (2009) Histone H3 methylation links DNA damage detection to activation of the tumour suppressor Tip60. *Nat Cell Biol* 11(11):1376-1382.

Sykes SM, Mellert HS, Holbert MA, Li K, Marmorstein R, Lane WS & McMahon SB. (2006) Acetylation of the p53 DNA-binding domain regulates apoptosis induction. *Mol Cell* 24(6):841-851.

Tanaka T, Halicka HD, Huang X, Traganos F, & Darzynkiewicz Z (2006) Constitutive histone H2AX phosphorylation and ATM activation, the reporters of DNA damage by endogenous oxidants. *Cell Cycle* 5(17):1940-1945.

Tanaka T, Huang X, Halicka HD, Zhao H, Traganos F, Albino AP, Dai W & Darzynkiewicz Z. (2007) Cytometry of ATM activation and histone H2AX phosphorylation to estimate extent of DNA damage induced by exogenous agents. *Cytometry A* 71(9):648-661.

Tang Y, Luo J, Zhang W, & Gu W (2006) Tip60-dependent acetylation of p53 modulates the decision between cell-cycle arrest and apoptosis. *Mol Cell* 24(6):827-839.

Tang Y, Zhao W, Chen Y, Zhao Y, & Gu W (2008) Acetylation is indispensable for p53 activation. *Cell* 133(4):612-626.

Taniguchi T, Garcia-Higuera I, Andreassen PR, Gregory RC, Grompe M & D'Andrea AD. (2002) S-phase-specific interaction of the Fanconi anemia protein, FANCD2, with BRCA1 and RAD51. *Blood* 100(7):2414-2420.

Tibbetts RS, Brumbaugh KM, Williams JM, Sarkaria JN, Cliby WA, Shieh SY, Taya Y, Prives C & Abraham RT. (1999) A role for ATR in the DNA damage-induced phosphorylation of p53. *Genes Dev* 13(2):152-157.

Toledo F & Wahl GM (2006) Regulating the p53 pathway: in vitro hypotheses, in vivo veritas. *Nat Rev Cancer* 6(12):909-923.

Trenz K, Smith E, Smith S, & Costanzo V (2006) ATM and ATR promote Mre11 dependent restart of collapsed replication forks and prevent accumulation of DNA breaks. *Embo J* 25(8):1764-1774.

Uziel T, Lerenthal Y, Moyal L, Andegeko Y, Mittelman L & Shiloh Y. (2003) Requirement of the MRN complex for ATM activation by DNA damage. *Embo J* 22(20):5612-5621.
van Attikum H & Gasser SM (2009) Crosstalk between histone modifications during the DNA damage response. *Trends Cell Biol* 19(5):207-217.
van den Bosch M, Bree RT, & Lowndes NF (2003) The MRN complex: coordinating and mediating the response to broken chromosomes. *EMBO Rep* 4(9):844-849.
Wang H, Zhao Y, Li L, McNutt MA, Wu L, Lu S, Yu Y, Zhou W, Feng J, Chai G, Yang Y & Zhu WG.(2008) An ATM- and Rad3-related (ATR) signaling pathway and a phosphorylation-acetylation cascade are involved in activation of $P53/P21^{Waf1/Cip1}$ in response to 5-aza-2'-deoxycytidine treatment. *J Biol Chem* 283(5):2564-2574.
Wright JA, Keegan KS, Herendeen DR, Bentley NJ, Carr AM, Hoekstra MF & Concannon P. (1998) Protein kinase mutants of human ATR increase sensitivity to UV and ionizing radiation and abrogate cell cycle checkpoint control. *Proc Natl Acad Sci U S A* 95(13):7445-7450.
Wu X & Ranganathan V. (2000) ATM phosphorylation of Nijmegen breakage syndrome protein is required in a DNA damage response. *Nature* 405(6785):477-482.
Wu-Baer F, Lagrazon K, Yuan W, & Baer R (2003) The BRCA1/BARD1 heterodimer assembles polyubiquitin chains through an unconventional linkage involving lysine residue K6 of ubiquitin. *J Biol Chem* 278(37):34743-34746.
Wyman C & Kanaar R (2006) DNA double-strand break repair: all's well that ends well. *Annu Rev Genet* 40:363-383.
Yan S & Michael WM (2009) TopBP1 and DNA polymerase alpha-mediated recruitment of the 9-1-1 complex to stalled replication forks: implications for a replication restart-based mechanism for ATR checkpoint activation. *Cell Cycle* 8(18):2877-2884.
Yang J, Yu Y, Hamrick HE, & Duerksen-Hughes PJ (2003) ATM, ATR and DNA-PK: initiators of the cellular genotoxic stress responses. *Carcinogenesis* 24(10):1571-1580.
Yoo HY, Kumagai A, Shevchenko A, & Dunphy WG (2007) Ataxia-telangiectasia mutated (ATM)-dependent activation of ATR occurs through phosphorylation of TopBP1 by ATM. *J Biol Chem* 282(24):17501-17506.
Yoshioka K, Yoshioka Y, & Hsieh P (2006) ATR kinase activation mediated by MutSalpha and MutLalpha in response to cytotoxic O6-methylguanine adducts. *Mol Cell* 22(4):501-510.
You Z, Kong L, & Newport J (2002) The role of single-stranded DNA and polymerase alpha in establishing the ATR, Hus1 DNA replication checkpoint. *J Biol Chem* 277(30):27088-27093.
Yu X, Chini CC, He M, Mer G, & Chen J (2003) The BRCT domain is a phospho-protein binding domain. *Science* 302(5645):639-642.
Yuan Z, Zhang X, Sengupta N, Lane WS, & Seto E (2007) SIRT1 regulates the function of the Nijmegen breakage syndrome protein. *Mol Cell* 27(1):149-162.
Zhan Q, Bae I, Kastan MB, & Fornace AJ, Jr. (1994) The p53-dependent gamma-ray response of GADD45. *Cancer Res* 54(10):2755-2760.
Zhao S & Weng YC. (2000) Functional link between ataxia-telangiectasia and Nijmegen breakage syndrome gene products. *Nature* 405(6785):473-477.
Zhao Y, Lu S, Wu L, Chai G, Wang H, Chen Y, Sun J, Yu Y, Zhou W, Zheng Q, Wu M, Otterson GA & Zhu WG. (2006) Acetylation of p53 at lysine 373/382 by the histone

deacetylase inhibitor depsipeptide induces expression of p21(Waf1/Cip1). *Mol Cell Biol* 26(7):2782-2790.

Zhou BB & Elledge SJ (2000) The DNA damage response: putting checkpoints in perspective. *Nature* 408(6811):433-439.

Zhu WG, HT, Ke Y, Wang P, Lu S, Duan W, Dai Z, Tong T, Villalona-Calero MA, Plass C & Otterson GA (2004) 5-aza-2'-deoxycytidine activates the p53/p21Waf1/Cip1 pathway to inhibit cell proliferation. *J Biol Chem.* 279(15):15161-15166.

Zou L, Cortez D, & Elledge SJ (2002) Regulation of ATR substrate selection byRad17-dependent loading of Rad9 complexes onto chromatin. *Genes Dev* 16(2):198-208.

Zou L, Liu D, & Elledge SJ (2003a) Replication protein A-mediated recruitment and activation of Rad17 complexes. *Proc Natl Acad Sci U S A* 100(24):13827-13832.

Zou L & Elledge SJ (2003b) Sensing DNA damage through ATRIP recognition of RPA-ssDNA complexes. *Science* 300(5625):1542-1548.

Part 3

Replication Origins, Forks, Chromatine Organization

9

Relationship between Fork Progression and Initiation of Chromosome Replication in *E. coli*

Elena C. Guzmán[1] et al.*
[1]*Departamento de Bioquímica, Biología Molecular y Genética, Facultad de Ciencias, Universidad de Extremadura, 06071-Badajoz Spain*

1. Introduction

Ribonucleoside diphosphate reductase (RNR) of *Escherichia coli* is the prototype of the class I reductases common to most prokaryotes and eukaryotes from viruses to man. It is the only specific enzyme required, under aerobic growth, for the enzymatic formation of deoxyribonucleotides, the precursors for DNA synthesis. DNA replication requires a balanced supply of the four dNTPs, which explains the complex allosteric control of the enzyme (reviewed in Nordlund & Reichard, 2006). The active enzyme is a 1:1 complex of two subunits called proteins R1 and R2, each consisting of two polypeptide chains, coded by the genes *nrdA* and *nrdB*, respectively (Hanke & Fuchs, 1983). Although about 3000 nucleotides have to be consumed per second when a bacterium replicates its chromosome with two replication forks, only a very small pool of dNTP is accumulated in the cells. This pool would permit replication for no longer than half a minute (Werner, 1971; Pato, 1979). Channeling of the biosynthesis and compartmentation of the precursors has been proposed as explanations of how this shortage may be circumvented (Mathews, 1993; Kim et al., 2005) To satisfy the changing demand for the four deoxynucleotides, RNR must be closely associated with the replication machinery. In the aforementioned studies, Mathews et al., found evidence for the association of this enzyme with others related to the precursor biosynthesis, and coined the term dNTP-synthesizing complex (Mathews, 1993).
The best-known defective RNR mutant in *E. coli* contains a thermolabile R1 subunit, coded by the *nrdA101* allele. This allele carries a missense mutation, causing a change in amino acid 89 (L89P) (Odsbu et al., 2009). This leucine-to-proline substitution is close to the ATP cone domain that is located in the N-terminal region of the R1 protein and is, according to the holoenzyme model, located close to the R1-R2 interaction surface (Uhlin & Eklund, 1994), although no structural analysis of the mutant protein has been performed.

---

* Israel Salguero[2], Carmen Mata Martín[1], Elena López Acedo[1], Estrella Guarino[2],
Mª Antonia Sánchez-Romero[3], Vic Norris[4] and Alfonso Jiménez-Sánchez
[2]*Department of Zoology, University of Oxford, South Parks Road, Oxford OX1 3PS, United Kingdom.*
[3]*School of Biosciences. University of Birmingham. Edgbaston. Birmingham B15 2TTUK.*
[4]*Laboratoire d'Assemblages moléculaires: modélisation et imagerie SIMS, EA 3829, Faculté des Sciences de l'Université de Rouen, 76821 Mont Saint Aignan Cedex, France.*

The RNR101 protein is inactivated at 42ºC *in vitro* after 2 min (Fuchs et al., 1972), although a thermoresistant period of 50 min has been observed *in vivo* sustaining a relative increase in the amount of DNA up to 45-50% in the *nrdA101* mutant strain (Guzmán et al., 2002). Furthermore, it has been shown by flow cytometry that the *nrdA101* mutant is able to replicate the entire chromosome in the presence of rifampicin at 42ºC (Guzmán et al., 2002; Fig. 1). The pool of free dNTPs is not responsible for this DNA synthesis, as inhibition of RNR activity by hydroxyurea caused an immediate cessation of dNTP incorporation either in the presence or in absence of rifampicin (Fig. 1). Marker frequency analysis and flow cytometry show that this chain elongation of DNA replication in the *nrdA101* mutant does not end at the terminus of replication but stops stochastically throughout the chromosome (Guzmán et al., 2002).

These results are consistent with RNR having a thermoresistance period due to protection by some subcellular structure. This enzyme has been proposed to be part of a complex for the biosynthesis of dNTP (Mathews, 1993) therefore the association with this complex might explain such protection. We have proposed that, as a component of the replication hyperstructure, the RNR101 protein would be protected from thermal inactivation and that this would suffice to allow chromosome replication for 50 min in restrictive conditions (Guzmán et al., 2002; 2003, Molina & Skarstad, 2004; Guarino et al., 2007a; 2007b; Riola et al., 2007).

Supporting this model, RNR has been colocalized with the replisome-associated proteins DnaB helicase and DNA polymerase τ subunit, and with the fork-associated protein SeqA (Fig. 2) (Sánchez-Romero et al., 2010).

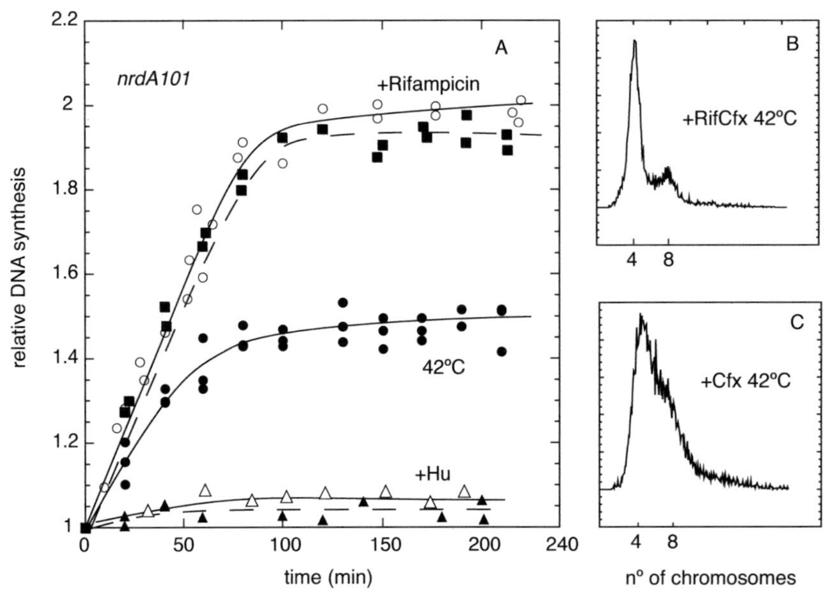

Fig. 1. (A) Runout DNA synthesis of the *nrdA101* strain in the presence of rifampicin (open circles) or in the presence of rifampicin and hydroxyurea at 30ºC (open triangles), or after a shift from 30ºC to 42ºC in the absence (closed circles) or in the presence of rifampicin (closed squares) or in the presence of rifampicin and hydroxyurea (closed triangles). Flow cytometry profile after 4h in cephalexin at 42ºC with (B) or without (C) rifampicin. Data were adapted from Guzmán et al. 2002.

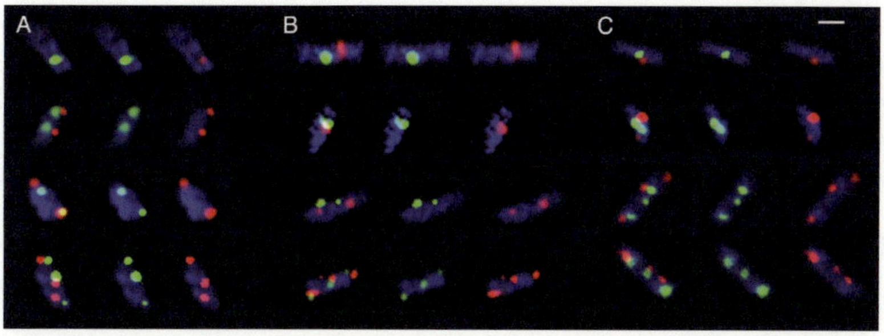

Fig. 2. Fluorescence microscopy of tagged-NrdB and SeqA or DnaB or DnaX. Fluorescence microscopy images of (A) CMT935 (nrdB::3×FLAG dnaB::HA) immunolabeled with Cy3-anti-FLAG (red) and FITC-anti-HA (green), (B) CMT936 (nrdB::3×FLAG dnaX::HA) immunolabeled with the same antibodies, (C) CMT931 (nrdB::3×FLAG) immunolabeled with Cy3-conjugated anti-FLAG (red) and FITC-anti-SeqA (green) antibodies (C). Cells were also stained with Hoechst 33258 for nucleoid visualization. Each group of cells shows nucleoid (blue) and, from left to right: both green and red, only green, and only red fluorescence. The bar represents 1 µm. Data were adapted from Sánchez-Romero et al., 2010.

Furthermore, a hyperstructure containing RNR101 impairs replication fork progression even at the permissive temperature (Guarino et al., 2007a). Arrest of replication forks is known to cause double-strand breaks, DSBs (Bierne & Michel, 1994; Kuzminov, 1995). We have shown that the number of DSBs in the *nrdA101 recB* strain is greater than that in the strain *nrdA+ recB*, consistent with an increase in the number of the stalled forks due to the presence of the deficient replication fork reversal (RFR) even at the permissive temperature. These DSBs are generated by RuvABC, a specific resolvase for Holliday junctions. According to the RFR model (Michel et al., 2004), these results indicate the occurrence of replication fork reversal as the mechanism for restarting stalled replication forks. These results indicate that the lengthening of the C period in the *nrdA101* mutant strain growing at 30ºC results not only from the reduced activity of RNR101 but also from the impaired progression of replication forks. The Tus protein is known to arrest replication forks through specific interaction with *ter* sequences by antagonizing the activity of the replicative helicase (reviewed by Bussiere & Bastia, 1999). Hence, the progression of the replication forks might be improved by the absence of this protein. In support of this idea we have found a decrease in the number of stalled replication forks in a *nrdA101 recB Dtus* triple mutant strain (Table 1).

Relevant phenotype	% linear DNA [a]	
nrdA+	4.58	±2.51
nrdA+ recB	15.18	±2.83
nrdA+ recB ruvABC	6.74	±2.60
nrdA101	5.72	±1.41
nrdA101 recB	24.79	±7.05
nrdA101 recB Dtus	12.64	±4.70
nrdA101 recB ruvABC	5.94	±2.19

Table 1. Growing the *nrdA101 recB* mutant strain at 30ºC increases RuvABC-dependent DSBs. [a] The *% linear DNA* is expressed by its mean ± standard deviation. Data were adapted from Guarino et al., 2007a.

It is intriguing that rifampicin or cloramphenicol addition, as well as the presence of a *dnaAts* allele, allowed the completion of chromosome replication in the *nrdA101* mutant at the high temperature (Guzmán et al., 2002, Salguero et al., 2011). Inhibition of RNA and of protein synthesis, and inactivation of the DnaA protein all inhibit initiation of chromosome replication; therefore, completion of chromosome replication in the *nrdA101* strain at 42ºC could be ascribed to the inhibition of new DNA initiations (Salguero et al., 2011). We suggest that the replication of the entire chromosome that occurs at the non-permissive temperature when new initiations are inhibited is due to a more efficient elongation as a consequence of the decreasing number of forks per chromosome.

In studying replication in the *nrdA101* mutant, we used several conditions to reduce the overlap of replication rounds (*n*, Sueoka & Yoshikawa, 1965) and, consequently, the number of replication forks per chromosome (2^{n+1}–2). We found an inverse correlation between this overlap and the amount of DNA that can be synthesized by the *nrdA101* strain at the restrictive temperature.

Consequently, we propose that a reduction in the number of forks replicating the chromosome results in an improvement in the quality of replication that allows the deficient replication hyperstructure of the *nrdA101* strain to be more processive at the high temperature. This proposal points toward the co-regulation of the elongation rate and the initiation frequency as a general control mechanism in prokaryotic and eukaryotic replication.

2. Reduction in the overlap of replication rounds improves fork progression at the restrictive temperature in a *nrdA101* strain

We have previously shown that, due to an elongation of the replication period lasting more than twice the cell cycle at 30ºC (C = 186 min, τ = 79 min), the *nrdA101* strain undergoes multifork replication resulting in two thirds of cells containing one or two chromosomes with 6 forks per chromosome, and one third of cells with a chromosome containing 14 forks (Guzmán et al., 2002). After a temperature shift from 30ºC to 42ºC, these cells replicate their DNA for 50 min, giving a runout synthesis of 52 per cent (Table 2). To test whether a reduction in the number of replication forks at 30ºC could improve the ability of forks to replicate the chromosome at 42ºC in the *nrdA101* strain, we reduced that number by different methods.

2.1 Experimental approach

In contrast with eukaryotic organisms, the time required to replicate a single chromosome (C) in *E. coli* can be longer than the generation time (τ), and in these conditions an overlap of replication rounds is obtained. The degree of overlap can be quantified by n, defined as the C to τ ratio (Sueoka & Yoshikawa, 1965; Cooper & Helmstetter, 1968). n was determined by using the ΔG value, which is defined as the relative runout DNA synthesized after inhibiting new initiation events, while ongoing forks are allowed to finish (Pritchard & Zaritsky, 1970). This experimental condition can be achieved by the addition of rifampicin (150μg/ml), which inhibits RNA polymerase whose activity is known to be required for the initiation step. From the experimental ΔG value, n can be calculated from the algorithm $\Delta G=[2^n n \ln 2/(2^n-1)]-1$ (Sueoka & Yoshikawa, 1965). Thus, the relative amount of the DNA synthesized after inhibition of initiation of replication only depends on the number of replication cycles per chromosome before the inhibition. The ΔG values under any growth

condition were obtained according to Pritchard and Zaritsky (Pritchard & Zaritsky, 1970; Zaritsky & Pritchard, 1971), and *n* was obtained by the use of a computer software developed in our lab (Jiménez-Sánchez & Guzmán, 1988). As the ΔG algorithm requires the completion of chromosome replications under any treatment, additional flow cytometry analysis is necessary to verify this completion. Flow cytometry analysis was performed in the presence of rifampicin (150 μg/ml) and cephalexin (50μg/ml) to inhibit cell division. Thus at the end of the treatment with the drugs, cells should contain $2^{(\text{integer } n)}$ or $2^{(\text{integer } n+1)}$ fully replicated chromosomes if they display synchronous initiation (Skarstad et al., 1985).
As explained above, the overlap of the replication rounds depends on two parameters, the generation time, τ, and the *C* period. In this study we used conditions that affect both parameters. The generation time was altered by growing the cells in glycerol or arabinose media. The *C* period was reduced by several methods such as by the presence of the *dnaA174* allele, by increasing the number of copies of *datA* sites in a plasmid, or by deletion of the DARS2 reactivating sequence. To determine the effect of several replication overlaps on DNA synthesis in the *nrdA101* strain at 42°C, we compared the residual DNA synthesis at 42°C relative to the runout after rifampicin at 30°C (i.e. 42°C/ΔG at 30°C) with the *n* value (the C to τ ratio).

2.2 Increasing the generation time

We lowered *n* by increasing the generation time using different carbon sources, such as glucose, arabinose or glycerol. Cultures of the *nrdA101* strain were grown at 30°C, in MM9 media containing one of the carbon sources, in the presence of ^{3}H-thymidine to label the newly synthesized DNA. When cultures reached mid-exponential phase (0.1 OD_{550}), two samples were taken, one to be incubated at 42°C, the non-permissive temperature, and the second one to be treated with rifampicin (150μg/ml) at 30°C to inhibit new initiations of chromosome replication. DNA synthesis was measured for 4 h (as the acid-precipitable radioactive material) and the values relative to the radioactive material incorporated at the beginning of treatment were represented. The values obtained in several strains and growth media are given in Table 2. To verify the completion of replication rounds, flow cytometry analysis was performed in the presence of rifampicin (150μg/ml) and cephalexin (50μg/ml), which inhibits cell division (data not shown).
As expected from growing the bacteria in a carbon source different from glucose, a lengthening of the generation time and a lowering in the number of overlapped replication rounds, *n*, were observed (Table 2). After the shift to 42°C in these media, the amount of synthesized DNA was inversely correlated with the number of previous overlaps. These results suggest that a reduction in the overlap of the replication rounds increases the capability to synthesize DNA for a longer period of time after the shift to 42°C.

2.3 Reducing the C period

2.3.1 By the presence of *dnaA* defective alleles

The presence of *dnaA* defective alleles has been reported to reduce the time required for chromosomal elongation (C period) at permissive conditions and this effect might suppress the defects in replication of some DNA elongation mutants (Torheim et al., 2001; Skovgaard & Lobner-Olesen, 2005). We used the *dnaA174* allele, which codes for a non-thermosensitive DnaA protein with a high ATPase activity, which in turn maintains a low DnaA-ATP level associated with a decreased the C period (Gon et al., 2006). We found the *nrdA101 dnaA174* double mutant had an overlap of replication cycles at 30°C that decreased from 2.36 to 1.37

and a five fold increased capability to synthesize DNA at 42°C relative to the *nrdA101* single mutant (Fig. 3, Table 2).
When incubated for 4 h at 42°C in the presence of cephalexin, the DNA content per cell in *nrdA101 dnaA174* double mutant is higher than observed under completion of the ongoing chromosome replication rounds; although the flow cytometry profile showed a broad distribution with no discrete peaks corresponding to completed chromosomes, as observed in the *nrdA101* strain (Fig. 3).
We have verified that the number of overlapped replication forks per chromosome at 30°C could be also lowered by introducing *dnaA46, dnaA5* or *dnaA508* alleles in the *nrdA101* background (Table 2; Salguero et al., 2011). After incubation at 42°C, all *nrdA101 dnaAts* strains exhibited a relative DNA synthesis and a thermoresistant period similar to those obtained by rifampicin addition either at 30°C or 42°C. As DnaA protein is required for chromosomal initiation and as all these alleles code for a thermosensitive DnaA protein, the runout value at the restrictive condition is the highest value that can be expected.
These results suggest that a lowering in the number of replication forks running along the chromosome could improve the progression of replication in the *nrdA101* mutant at the restrictive condition. DnaA is also known to have a regulatory control in the transcription of several genes, including *dnaA, mioC, rpoH* and the *nrdAB* operon (reviewed in Messer & Weigel, 2003; Gon et al., 2006; Herrick & Sclavi, 2007; Olliver et. al., 2010); moreover, the *nrdA* gene is over-expressed in the presence of a defective DnaA protein (Gon et al., 2006, Lobner-Olesen et al., 2008). This over-expression is, however, unlikely to be responsible for the high residual DNA synthesis found in the *nrdA101* strain at 42°C since the chromosome is fully replicated at 42°C in all studied *nrdA101 dnaA* strains even in the absence of protein synthesis (and hence absence of overproduced NrdA) (Salguero et al., 2011).
In addition, over-expression of the *nrdAB* operon from a plasmid, leading to a doubling of enzyme activity as measured in cell-free extracts, causes only a doubling of the dATP, dCTP and dTTP pools without any increase in the dGTP pool (Wheeler et al., 2005). Consequently, an increase in the replication rate should not be expected as dGTP pool would be limiting. Moreover, it is far from certain that an overproduction of RNR outside the replication

Strains	τ	ΔG30°C	42°C	42°C/ΔG30°C	n	ori/ter	C
nrdA+	78	0.55	nt	nt	1.37	2.58	107
nrdA101	79	1.03	0.52	0.50	2.36	5.13	186
nrdA101 arabinose	105	0.59	0.83	1.40	1.46	2.75	153
nrdA101 glycerol	112	0.35	0.58	1.65	0.91	1.87	102
nrdA101 dnaA174	78	0.55	1.40	2.54	1.37	2.58	107
nrdA101 dnaA46	80	0.45	0.48	1.06	1.15	2.21	92
nrdA101 dnaC2	82	1.00	0.45	0.45	2.30	4.92	188
nrdA101/pMOR6	81	0.73	0.70	0.95	1.76	3.38	142
nrdA101 DARS2	85	0.55	0.95	1.80	1.26	2.39	107

Table 2. Cell cycle parameters from the *nrdA101* strain growing in MM9 with different carbon sources or containing a second mutant allele. All strain were grown in MM9 medium with glucose except otherwise indicated. ΔG30°C, relative increase of the amount of DNA after rifampicin addition at 30°C. 42°C, relative increase of the amount of DNA after a shift to 42°C. *n*, number of replication rounds per chromosome or overlapping degree. ori/ter= 2^n or number of origins per chromosome. *C* elongation time (min) from C= $n\tau$.

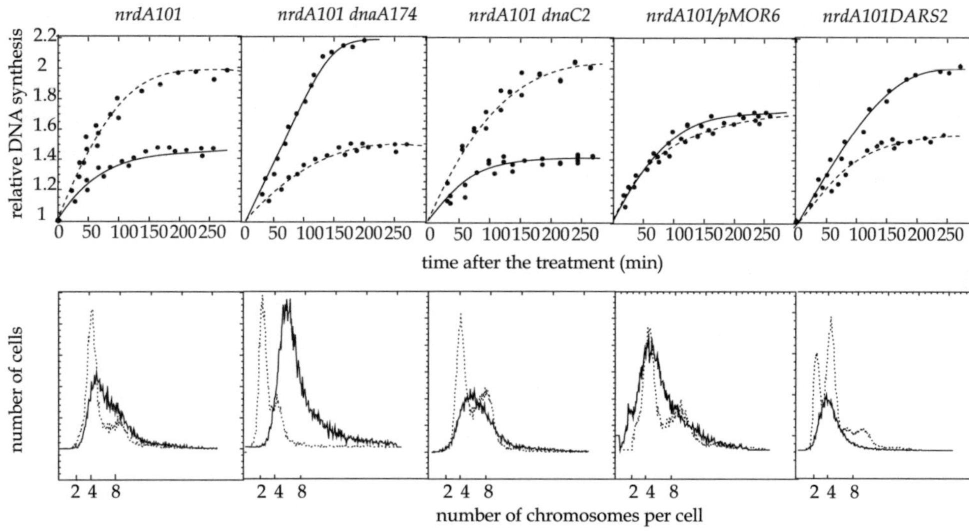

Fig. 3. DNA synthesis (upper panels) after rifampicin addition (dashed line) or incubation at 42°C (solid line), and flow cytometry profiles (lower panels) after 4 hours of incubation at 30°C in the presence of rifampicin and cephalexin (dashed line) or after 4 hours at 42°C in the presence of cephalexin (solid line) in strains *nrdA101, nrdA101 dnaA174, nrdA101 dnaC2, nrdA101/pMOR and nrdA101 DARS2*

hyperstructure would increase the supply of dNTP to the replication enzymes (Pato, 1979; Mathews, 1993).

It has been shown that the *nrdAB* operon is also over-expressed in a *dnaC2* mutant and that, when incubated at the high temperature, 18 per cent of the cells failed to complete chromosome replication (Lobner-Olesen et al., 2008). This observation has been explained by the implication of the DnaC protein in the restart of stalled replication forks during elongation (Maisnier-Patin et al., 2001). We measured DNA synthesis at 30°C with rifampicin and at 42°C in the *nrdA101 dnaC2* strain; this strain had about the same τ and C, hence n, at 30°C as the parental *nrdA101* strain (Table 2). As expected from these cell cycle parameters, the amount of DNA synthesized at 42°C was also similar (Fig. 3). Consequently, over-expression of the *nrdAB* operon cannot explain the extensive thermoresistant replication found in the *nrdA101* strain when new initiations are prevented.

2.3.2 By increasing the number of copies of the *datA* sequence

The *E. coli* genome contains 308 DnaA boxes (TTAT(C/A)CA(C/A)A) with variable affinity to DnaA (Schaper & Messer 1995). A strong DnaA-binding region, *datA* (from *DnaA titration*) containing five boxes, has been identified among them (Kitagawa et al., 1996). The *datA* site titrates unusually large amounts of DnaA protein *in vivo* (Kitagawa et al., 1996) and it has been suggested that the *datA*-bound DnaA molecules act as a reservoir of DnaA (Kitagawa et al., 1998). Recently, it has been found that high levels of *datA* completely shut down initiation of replication, whilst moderate levels of *datA* increase the replication rate relative to that of the wild type (Morigen et al., 2001; 2003). Using this feature we constructed an *nrdA101* strain harboring the pMOR6 plasmid, a derivative of the moderate copy number plasmid pACYC177 (Morigen et al., 2001). We found a shortened *C* period and a lower overlap of replication cycles (Table 2, Fig. 3). Consistent with this, the *nrdA101/pMOR6* strain synthesizes more DNA at the restrictive temperature than its *nrdA101* parental strain (Fig. 3). After 4 h of incubation at 42ºC we found similar amount of DNA synthesis, either in the presence or in the absence of rifampicin at restrictive conditions. This result differs from that obtained in the *nrdA101* mutant, whose DNA synthesis at 42ºC is half of the observed at 42 ºC when new initiations were inhibited (Table 2) (Salguero et al., 2011). As DNA initiation is not inhibited in the *nrdA101/pMOR6* strain after the shift to 42ºC, none fully replicated chromosomes were detected at 42ºC (Fig. 3).

2.3.3 By deleting the DARS sequence

The DnaA protein is a member of the AAA+ ATPase family and has an exceptionally high affinity for ATP/ADP (Sekimuzu et al., 1987; Kaguni, 2006). The level of cellular ATP-DnaA oscillates during the replication cycle, peaking around the time of initiation (Kurokawa et al., 1999).

Katayama's group has recently found two chromosomal intergenic regions termed DARS1 and DARS2 (*DnaA-r*eactivating *s*equence) that directly promote regeneration of ATP-DnaA from ADP-DnaA by nucleotide exchange resulting in the promotion of replication initiation *in vitro* and *in vivo*. Deletion of DARS results in decrease in the ATP-DnaA level, causing synthetic lethality with *dnaAts* and suppression of over-initiation in defective *seqA*, *datA* and *hda* mutants (Fujimitsu et al., 2009). These effects led us to infer that, in the absence of DARS sequences, the *nrdA101 DARS* mutant would decrease DnaA effective protein and consequently a reduction of the C period would be expected. We found the expected decrease in the C period and in the overlap of replication cycles at 30ªC, with a reduction in the number of chromosomes per cell (Table 2, Fig. 3). After 4 hours of incubation at 42ºC, the flow cytometry profile showed a broad distribution of the DNA content per cell, although the capability to synthesize DNA at the restrictive temperature increased three times relative to the single mutant *nrdA101* (Table 2, Fig. 3).

Our data show that decreasing the number of replication rounds (*ori/ter* ratio) correlates with an improved capacity to synthesize DNA in the *nrdA101* mutant at the restrictive temperature (Fig. 4). Given that the progression of the replisome is affected in this mutant (Guarino et al., 2007a), we propose there is an improvement in the progression of the replication forks at 42ºC as a consequence of lowering the number of the replication rounds along the chromosome (*ori/ter* ratio). According to the model where the RNR is a component of the replication hyperstructure (Guzmán et al., 2002), it is reasonable to think that the defective fork progression observed in this mutant can be alleviated by reducing the number of replication forks running along the chromosome. Consistent with this, the presence of *dnaA* defective alleles, *dnaA(Sx)*, suppresses the detrimental effect on DNA replication observed in mutants that have problems with the progression of forks due to the presence of defective subunits of DNA polymerase III coded by the *dnaX* gene (Gines-Candelaria et al., 1995; Blinkova et al., 2003; Skovgaard & Lobner-Olesen 2005).

Furthermore, a lower availability of wild type DnaA protein induced by the presence of extra copies of the *datA* sequence alleviates replication problems in both the *dnaX* (Skovgaard & Lobner-Olesen, 2005) and the *nrdA101* mutant (this work), whilst initiation defects caused by deletion of DnaA box R4 suppress replication elongation defects (Stepankiw et al., 2009).

These observations, together with our data, are consistent with the idea that the progression of replication forks is not merely responsive to elongation factors (dNTP pools or proteins engaged in elongation) but also to the number of forks running along the chromosome. We suggest that the best explanation for the reduction of the C period in the results discussed above is a reduction in the number of forks per chromosome or a decrease in the extent of overlapping of replication rounds. Thus, under conditions where *ori/ter* is high the cells could experience at least two changes. One could be a possible scarcity of hyperstructure components such that increasing the number of hyperstructures increases the probability that they are incomplete and relatively ineffective; hence, reciprocally, restricting the number of replication hyperstructures would increase the probability they contain all the components needed for fully effective replication. In this sense, the suppression of *dnaE* mutation by the deficiency of enzymes engaged in the glycolysis in *Bacilus subtilis*, has been explained by a differential composition of the replication hyperstructures that would affect the replication rate (Jannière et al., 2007). Another change could be in the structural constraints caused by the proximity of the replication forks belonging to overlapped replication rounds (Odsbu et al., 2009). In agreement with our explanation, Zaritsky A. et al. have proposed the existence of an 'eclipse' in terms of a minimal distance (*l*min) that the replication forks must move away from *oriC* before *oriCs* can 'fire' again (Zaritsky et al., 2007). Our explanation can readily accommodate the proposal of an obligatory, minimal distance between replication forks. The greater the number of the replication rounds per chromosome, the shorter the distance between the replication forks. Thus, the distance between the replication forks could explain the differential progression of the forks along the chromosome in the strains discussed here.

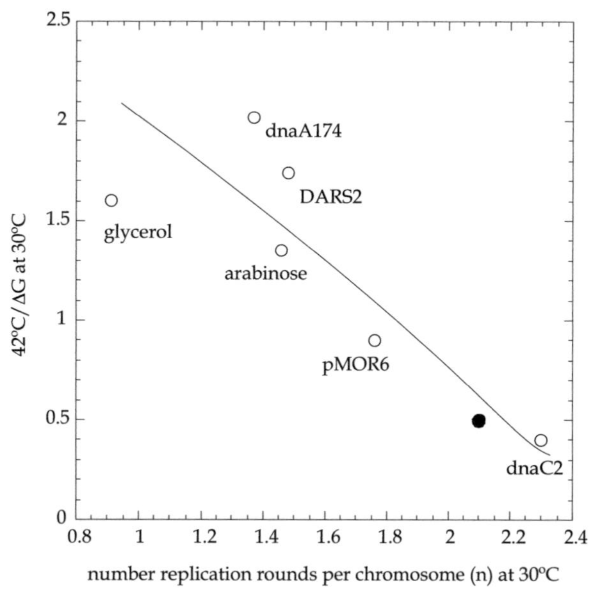

Fig. 4. Relationship between the residual DNA synthesis at 42°C relative to the runout after rifampicin at 30°C (i.e. 42°C/ΔG at 30°C and the *n* value (the C to τ ratio) in *nrdA101* strain growing in the indicated media or containing the depicted alleles growing in glucose MM9 medium. The black point shows the value of this relationship in the *nrdA101* strain growing in glucose MM9 medium.

3. Stalled multifork chromosomes as the cause of aberrant DNA segregation and cell death in the *nrdA101* mutant at the restrictive temperature

Growth of *nrdA101* strain at the restrictive temperature causes aberrant nucleoid segregation (Guzmán et al., 2003; Riola et al., 2007; Odsbu et al., 2009). This aberrant nucleoid segregation leads to breakdown of the coupling between replication and cell division (Dix & Helmstetter, 1973; Riola et al., 2007) causing filamentation and cell death. These problems could be related to the fact that DNA replication stops stochastically in the *nrdA101* strain at 42°C to generate stalled replication forks along the multiforked chromosome (Fig. 3). Similar problems have been observed under other conditions, including UV irradiation, thymine starvation, and mitomycin treatments, inversion of the Ter sequences (Jaffe et al., 1986; Hill et al., 1997), and in *dnaN59ts* and *dnaG2903ts* mutants, where the problems have also been attributed to stalled replication forks (Kawakami et al., 2001; Grompe et al., 1991).

Cell viability was studied in all the growth media and strains described above. Cells were grown at 30°C and when the cultures reached mid-logarithmic phase (about 0.1 OD_{550}), an aliquot of each culture was incubated at 42°C and the number of viable cells were estimated by serial dilution and plating on rich medium at 30°C. Viability is expressed relative to the onset of treatment. Growing *nrdA101* cells in different carbon sources resulted in different values of cell cycle parameters with a higher number of replication overlaps in glucose than in glycerol medium (Table 2) and a greater lethality after the incubation at 42°C (Fig. 5). Loss of viability of the *nrdA101* strain at the high temperature was completely suppressed by the presence of *dnaA174* allele, by extra copies of *datA,* or by deleting DARS2 sequence from the chromosome (Fig. 6). The ensemble of these results (Table 2, Fig. 5, Fig. 6) reveals a direct correlation between lethality at high temperature and replication overlapping. This correlation might be explained by either the higher number of sensitive targets (i. e. the replication forks) at 42°C, the greater vulnerability of sensitive targets due to more replication overlaps, or by an increase in the number of defective replication hyperstructures. These explanations are not mutually exclusive and we consider all as equally likely.

Nucleoid segregation analysis was performed in aliquots of the cultures incubated at 42°C in the presence of cephalexin (50 μg/ml) for 4 hours plus, during the last 20 min, chloramphenicol addition(200μg/ml) to condense nucleoids. Micrographs of DAPI stained cells show a high number of cells containing an abnormal number of nucleoids randomly distributed along the filaments (Fig. 5) (Riola et al., 2007). An increased number of cells containing normal and well-segregated nucleoids were found in cells grown in arabinose or in glycerol (Fig. 5). The anomalous number and distribution of nucleoids found in the *nrdA101* strain grown at 42°C were almost fully suppressed by the presence of *dnaA174* allele, by the presence of plasmid pMOR6, which increases the *datA* sequence copy number, or by the absence of DARS sequences (Fig. 6).

The above results reveal a good correlation between the overlap of replication rounds and aberrant nucleoid segregation and cell lethality. This correlation is consistent with the hypothesis that these problems are associated with a highly forked chromosome structure. The detrimental effects of such chromosomes are reduced or eliminated by any environmental or genetic modification that reduces replication overlap. We therefore suggest that the observed morphological alterations of *nrdA101* strain at 42°C could be ascribed to the activity of an inaccurate replication apparatus. The impaired replication hyperstructure made with a deficient RNR101 protein (Guarino et al., 2007a) stops more frequently than a wild type hyperstructure. In cells with a high degree of replication

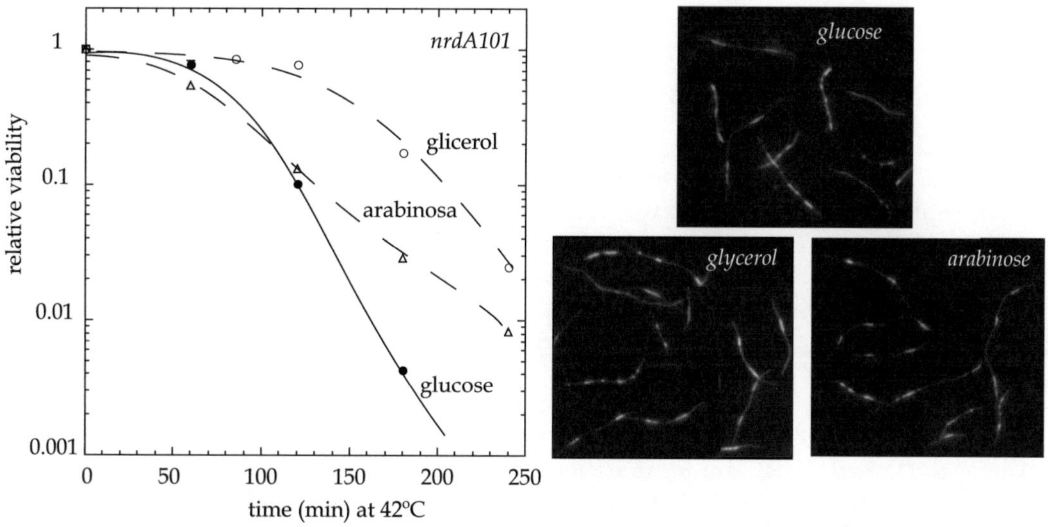

Fig. 5. Cell viability and nucleoid segregation of *nrdA101* growing with different carbon sources after the shift to 42°C.

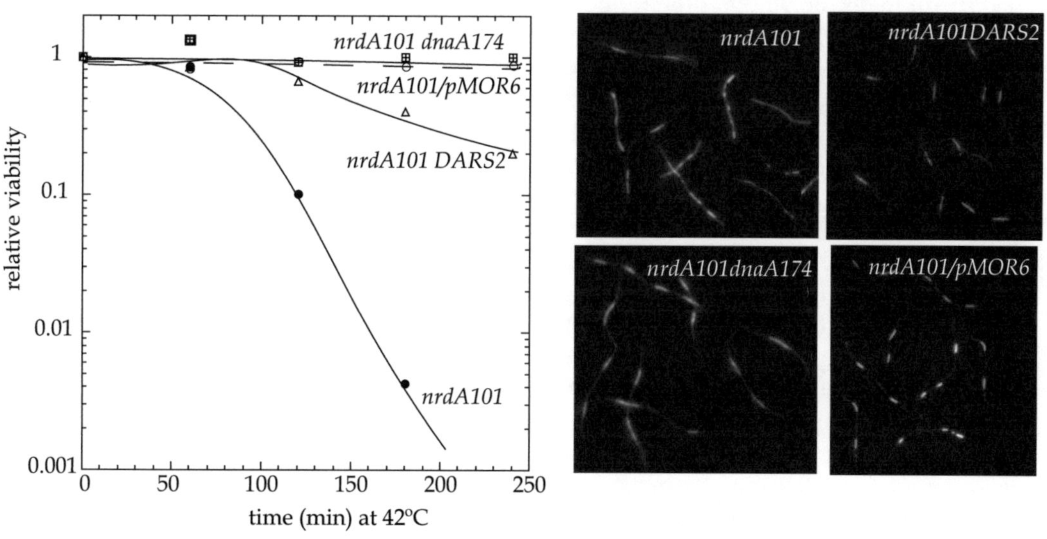

Fig. 6. Cell viability and nucleoid segregation of *nrdA101* derivatives after the shift to 42°C.

overlaps, stalled forks have less opportunity to be repaired and restarted and this interferes with subsequent forks. This results in chromosomal abnormalities, disrupted chromosome and nucleoid segregation, loss of cell division, and, finally, cell death.

DNA topology has been found to play an important role in the segregation of duplicated chromosomes (Dasgupta et al., 2000; Holmes & Cozarelli, 2000). Consequently, a disturbed DNA topology due to a highly forked chromosome structure, could contribute to the altered nucleoid segregation observed in the *nrdA101* mutant at 42°C. Fork collisions and topological changes would be reduced, or even prevented, in *nrdA101* strains at 42°C by inhibiting new initiations of replication (Salguero et al., 2011), or by diminishing the overlap of replication rounds.

4. The number of replication rounds in the chromosome limits the replication rate of individual forks

In the *nrdA101* strain growing at the permissive temperature we have found that the number of forks per chromosome was reduced and the elongation rate was increased by the presence of the *dnaA174* allele or of extra copies of *datA* and by the deletion of the DARS2 sequence (Table 2). Reduction of chromosome replication overlaps, with the associated lowering of the *ori/ter* ratio, together with an increased replication rate, have been also found in strains containing different defective *dnaA* alleles, such as *dnaA204* (Torheim et al., 2001), *dnaA46, dnaA174,* and *dnaA345* (Gon et al., 2006; Morigen et al., 2009), as well as in wild type cells containing extra copies of *datA* sequence which is believed to reduce the availability of DnaA protein (Morigen et al., 2003). Similar results have also been obtained in studies of *hns* (Atlung & Hansen, 2002) and *ihf* mutants (von Freiesleben et al., 2000). Additionally, we have also shown by growing the *nrdA101* mutant in poor media at 30ºC, that the improvement in the replication fork progression is accompanied by a decrease in replication overlap.The correlation between these effects has been well established but the mechanism remains elusive.

It is difficult to decide whether the reduction in the number of forks is the consequence of an increased replication rate (as *ori/ter*=2^n, n=C/τ), or whether the increase in the replication rate is the consequence of the reduction of the number of forks (*ori/ter* ratio). The first proposition implies that the activities of DnaA, HNS, and IHF affect the elongation rate directly or indirectly. This is plausible as DnaA protein has 308 binding sites in the bacterial genome (Schaper & Messer, 1995) and, furthermore, it is a transcriptional regulator controlling the expression of several replication genes (reviewed in Messer & Weigel, 2003). Therefore, deficiency of DnaA protein, as well as HNS and IHF, might well allow the replication forks to run faster. Moreover, a deficiency of DnaA protein increases *nrdAB* operon expression (Lobner-Olesen et al., 2008; Gon et al., 2006), which might also increase the velocity of the replication forks (Herrick & Sclavi, 2008). However, as explained above (2.3.1 this chapter), the over-expression of the *nrdAB* operon does not necessarily increase the actual supply of the dNTPs used in DNA replication. In addition, the growth of cells in poor carbon source media is not known to affect *nrdAB* gene expression, and a decrease in replication rate in wild type cells has been observed under poor media conditions (Michelsen et al., 2003). Furthermore, it has been reported that deletion of DnaA box R4 suppresses replication elongation defects in *gyrB* mutant strains as a consequence of the lowering of initiation frequency (Stepankiw et al., 2009) indicating that no transcriptional factor is required to increase the replication rate. Hence the first proposition, in which faster replication forks are responsible for there being fewer forks, is difficult to justify.

The second proposition is that the elongation rate increased as a consequence of the reduction of the number of forks or the replication overlap. This reduction in the number of the forks would be caused by the deficiency of any factor required for the initiation step since this would result in the delay of the initiation of replication.

In the above work, we have shown that a decrease in the growth rate of the *nrdA101* mutant, due to growth on poor carbon sources, improves the elongation rate of chromosome replication, which is the same as to say that *C* decreases when τ increases. From the

algorithm $C = n\tau$ one can conclude that any increase in the cell doubling time, should lead to a decrease in the n value, or the number of forks per chromosome. Nevertheless, we have shown that increasing τ also decreases the C value. Even though elongation rate in wild type strains is expected to be lower under decreased growth rate (Michelsen et al., 2003) we can infer that a reduction in the number of forks per chromosome in the *nrdA101* strain with a extremely slow replication rate could also be a cause of improvement of the replication rates.
An unified explanation for all the results presented here is difficult to find. Clearly though, the underlying mechanism should explain the precise correlation between initiation and elongation that tunes DNA replication to any environmental circumstance. Whatever the nature of this mechanism, reduction in the number of forks per chromosome or decreased overlapping of consecutive replication rounds might increase the elongation rate by providing *i*) a better overall chromosome structure, including discrete regional organization and supercoiling domains, *ii*) an increased availability of a limiting constituent required for replication and/or for segregation, and *iii*) an increased time for the repair and restart of a stalled fork so as to avoid collision with the next fork. This homeostatic regulation between the numbers and velocities of forks would also explain how the replication rate compensates for widely varying replication origins and activities in eukaryotes (Conti et al., 2007).

5. Balance between the number of origins and elongation rates as a general regulatory mechanism in the control of eukaryotic cell cycle

In eukaryotic cells, the DNA replication program is organized according to multiple tandem replicons that span each chromosome. Each replicon is replicated bidirectionally by a pair of replication forks that increase their rates up to three fold towards the end of S phase. Furthermore, the rate of the replication fork progression varies up to ten-fold or more depending on the distance between origins in different conditions or cell types (Housman & Huberman, 1975; reviewed in Herrick, 2010). Two replication regimes with distinct kinetics govern duplication of the genome: in the first half of the S phase, when the gene-rich euchromatin is predominantly replicated, the density of the activated replication origins steadily increases to about twice the initial value; during the second half of the S phase, when the gene-poor heterochromatin tends to be replicated, the density of active replication origins increases substantially by about ten fold (Herrick & Bensimon, 2008). It has been proposed that this mechanism would guarantee the rapid and complete duplication of the genome. Nevertheless, in mammalian cells the relationship between origin activation, the size of replicons (50-300kb) and the existence of multiple potential origins remains to be elucidated (Herrick, 2010).
The efficient duplication of the eukaryotic genome depends on the orderly activation of the origins, estimated to be ten thousand, and on the proper progression of their forks. The coordinated activation of origins is insufficient on its own to account for timely completion of genome duplication when interorigin distances vary significantly and fork velocities are constant. Therefore the coordination and compensation between origin spacing and fork progression may be one of the mechanisms for the complete duplication of the genome in the limited amount of time of the S phase. By using a single-molecule approach based on molecular combing, the interorigin distances and replication fork velocities over extensive regions of the genome have been measured in both primary keratinocytes and cancer cells (Conti et al., 2007). This study provides evidence for the direct correlation between the interorigin distances and the replication rates, insofar as the further the origins are from one

another, the faster the forks progress. These results are in agreement with the results of this and other studies of *E. coli*, which show a correlation between the frequency of initiation (*ori/ter* ratio) and the replication fork rates.

Figure 3 in Conti et al., 2007 shows a significant linear correlation between these two parameters in eukaryotic cells, consistent with a biological mechanism that coordinates replication fork progression with interorigin distance. The mechanism that allows replication forks to adjust their speed is unknown. Nevertheless the possibilities for the nature of this mechanism are similar to the ones proposed above for *E. coli*. A feedback mechanism might be based on the accumulation of torsional strain as incoming fork approach each other and the length of DNA to be replicated decreases. However, a mechanism based only on mechanical stress would strongly limit the possibility of modification and adaptation of the fork rates. The concentration of dNTP could also play a role in regulating fork velocity (Anglana et al., 2003). Supporting this notion, it has been shown that the kinase Chk1 plays an essential role in S phase progression through regulation of RNR2 expression (Naruyama et al., 2008), although ectopic expression of RNR2 failed to rescue the S phase arrest observed in Chk1-depleted cells, suggesting the presence of Chk1 target(s) for completion of S phase in addition to or other that RNR2. The observation of dynamically regulated adjacent forks also supports the idea that dNTP pool sizes alone are not implicated in the observed changes in fork velocity (Conti et al., 2007). Additionally, intracellular dNTP pool sizes are expected to increase (as replication rate increase), rather than decrease, during S phase (Malinsky et al., 2001). Therefore, although the size of the dNTP pool could be globally responsible for fork velocity, it would not be responsible for the local control and dynamic correlation between adjacent forks; this must involve other factors, for example, the processivity of DNA helicases and toposiomerases (Conti et al., 2007).

6. Concluding remarks

In this work we show that reducing the number of replication forks per chromosome in *E. coli* improves the amount of DNA that a thermosensitive *nrdA* mutant strain is able to synthesize at restrictive conditions. Activity of the RNR101 at 42ºC has been proposed to be maintained due to the protection of the thermolabile protein by the replication hyperstructure; therefore, the effect we have found may be related to the processivity of the replication hyperstructure. More specifically, in our hypothesis, the processivity of the replication hyperstructure is improved by the lowering of the number of the replication forks along the chromosome, i.e. by reducing the overlap. Such a relationship between processivity and the number of replication forks could be explained by 1) variations in the availability of some limiting hyperstructure component which might lead to assembly of an inefficient hyperstructure when a high number of forks compete for this component, or 2) the structural constraints caused by a chromosome undergoing several rounds of replication running at the same time. Results from other research groups, reviewed above, and comparison with DNA replication in eukaryotes provide further evidence that, in widely different systems, the initiation and the elongation of chromosome replication are not independent processes.

7. Acknowledgements

We are very grateful to Kirsten Skarstad and Tsutomu Katayama for bacterial strains and plasmids. We especially thank Encarna Ferrera for her technical help. This work was supported by grant BFU2007-63942 from the Ministerio de Ciencia e Innovación. IS, CM and MAS-R acknowledge the studentship from Junta de Extremadura.

8. References

Anglana, M., Apiou, F., Bensimon, A. & Debatisse, M. (2003). Dynamics of DNA replication in mammalian somatic cells: nucleotide pool modulates origin choice and interorigin spacing. *Cell* 114: 385-94.

Atlung, T. & Hansen, F.G. (2002). Effect of different concentrations of H-NS protein on chromosome replication and the cell cycle in *Escherichia coli. J Bacteriol* 184: 1843-1850.

Blinkova, A., Hermandson, M. & Walker J. R. (2003). Suppression of Temperature-Sensitive Chromosome Replication of an *Escherichia coli dnaX*(Ts) Mutant by Reduction of Initiation Efficiency. *J Bacteriol.* 185: 3583-3595.

Bierne, H. & Michel, B. (1994). When replication forks stop. *Mol Microbiol.* 13: 17-23.

Bussiere, D.E. & Bastia, D. (1999). Termination of DNA replication of bacterial and plasmid chromosomes. *Mol Microbiol.* 31: 1611-1618.

Conti, C., Sacca, B., Herrick, J., Lalou, C., Pommier, Y. & Bensimon, A. (2007). Replication fork velocities at adjacent replication origins are coordinately modified during DNA replication in human cells. Molecular Biology of the Cell. 18: 3059–3067.

Cooper, S. & Helmstetter, C.E. (1968). Chromosome replication and the division cycle of *Escherichia coli B/r. J Mol Biol* 31: 519-540.

Dasgupta, S., Maisnier-Patin, S. & Nordstrom, K. (2000). New genes with old modus operandi. The connection between supercoiling and partitioning of DNA in *Escherichia coli. EMBO Rep* 1: 323–327.

Dix, D. E. & Helmstetter, C. E. (1973). Coupling between chromosome completion and cell division in *Escherichia coli. J Bacteriol* 115: 786-95.

Fuchs, J. A., Karlstrom, H. O., Warner, H. R. & Reichard, P. (1972). Defective gene product in dnaF mutant of *Escherichia coli. Nat New Biol* 238: 69-71.

Fujimitsu K, Senriuchi T, Katayama, T. (2009). Specific genomic sequences of *E. coli* promote replicational initiation by directly reactivating ADP-DnaA. *Genes Dev.* 23: 1221-33.

Gines-Candelaria, E., Blinkova, A. & Walker, J. R. (1995). Mutations in *Escherichia coli dnaA* which suppress a *dnaX*(Ts) polymerization mutation and are dominant when located in the chromosomal allele and recessive on plasmids. *J Bacteriol* 177: 705-715.

Gon, S., Camara, J.E., Klungsoyr, H.K., Crooke, E., Skarstad K. & Beckwith, A.J. (2006). A novel regulatory mechanism couples deoxyribonucleotide synthesis and DNA replication in *Escherichia coli. EMBO J* 25: 1137–1147.

Grompe, M., Versalovic, J., Koeuth, T. & Lupski, J.R. (1991). Mutations in the Escherichia coli *dnaG* gene suggest coupling between DNA replication and chromosome partitioning. *J Bacteriol.* 173: 1268-1278.

Guarino, E., Jiménez-Sánchez, A. & Guzmán, E. C. (2007). Defective ribonucleoside diphosphate reductase impairs replication fork progression in *Escherichia coli. J Bacteriol* 189: 3496-501.

Guarino, E., Salguero, I., Jiménez-Sánchez, A. & Guzmán, E. C. (2007). Double-strand break generation under deoxyribonucleotide starvation in *Escherichia coli. J Bacteriol* 189: 5782-6.

Guzmán, E. C., Caballero, J. L. & Jiménez-Sánchez, A. (2002). Ribonucleoside diphosphate reductase is a component of the replication hyperstructure in *Escherichia coli. Mol Microbiol* 43: 487-95.

Guzmán, E. C., Guarino, E., Riola, J. & Jiménez-Sánchez, A. (2003). Ribonucleoside diphosphate reductase is a functional and structural component of the replication hyperstructure in *Escherichia coli. Rec Res Devel Mol Biol* 1: 29-43.

Hanke, P. D. & Fuchs, J. A. (1983). Regulation of ribonucleoside diphosphate reductase mRNA synthesis in *Escherichia coli. J Bacteriol* 154: 1040-1045.

Herrick, J. (2010) The dynamic replicon: adapting to a changing cellular environment. *Bioessays* 32:153-64.

Herrick, J. & Sclavi, B. (2007). Ribonucleotide reductase and the regulation of DNA replication: an old story and an ancient heritage. *Mol Microbiol* 63: 22-34.

Herrick, J. & Bensimon, A. (2008). Global regulation of genome duplication in eukaryotes: an overview from the epifluorescence microscope. *Chromosoma* 117: 243-260.

Hill, T.M, Sharma, B., Valjavec-Gratian, M. & Smith, J. (1997). sfi-independent filamentation in *Escherichia coli* is *lexA* dependent and requires DNA damage for induction. *J Bacteriol* 179 :1931-9.

Holmes, V.F. & Cozzarelli, N.R. (2000). Closing the ring: links between SMC proteins and chromosome partitioning, condensation, and supercoiling. Proc Natl Acad Sci USA 97: 1322–1324.

Housman, D., & Huberman, J.A. (1975). Changes in the rate of DNA replication fork movement during S phase in mammalian cells.*J Mol Biol* 94: 173–181.

Jaffe, A., D'Ari, R. & Norris, V. (1986). SOS-independent coupling between DNA replication and cell division in *E. coli. J. Bacteriol.*165, 66-71.

Jannière, L., Canceill, D, Suski, C., Kanga, S., Dalmais B, Lestini, R., Monnier, A.F., Chapuis, J., Bolotin, A., Titok, M., Le Chatelier, E. & Ehrlich, S.D. Genetic evidence for a link between glycolysis and DNA replication. (2007). *PLoS One* 2(5):e447.

Jiménez-Sánchez, A. & Guzmán, E.C. (1988). Direct procedure for the determination of the number of replication forks and the reinitiation fraction in bacteria. *Comput Appl Biosci* 4: 431-433.

Kawakami, H., Iwura, T., Tanaka, M. & Sekimizu, T. (2001). Arrest of cell division and nucleoid partition by genetic alterations in the sliding clamp of the replicase and in DnaA. *Mol. Genet. Genomics* 266: 167-79.

Kaguni, J. M. (2006). DnaA: Controlling the Initiation of Bacterial DNA Replication and More. *Annu. Rev. Microbiol* 60: 351–71.

Kim, J., Wheeler, L.J., Shen, R., & Mathews, C.K. (2005). Protein-DNA interactions in the T4 dNTP synthetase complex dependent on gene 32 single-stranded DNA-binding protein. *Mol Microbiol* 55: 1502-1514.

Kuzminov, A. (1995). Collapse and repair of replication forks in *Escherichia coli. Mol Microbiol* 16: 373-384.

Kitagawa, R., Mitsuki, H, Okazaki T. & Ogawa, T. (1996). A novel DnaA protein-binding site at 94.7 min on the *Escherichia coli* chromosome. *Mol Microbiol* 19:1137-47.

Kitagawa, R., Ozaki, T., Moriya, S. & Ogawa, T. (1998). Negative control of replication initiation by a novel chromosomal locus exhibiting exceptional affinity for *Escherichia coli* DnaA protein. *Genes Dev* 12 :3032-43.

Kurokawa, K., Nishida, S., Emoto, A., Sekimizu, K., & Katayama, T. (1999). Replication cycle-coordinated change of the adenine nucleotide-bound forms of DnaA protein in Escherichia coli. Embo J 18: 6642-6652.

Løbner-Olesen, A., Slominska-Wojewodzka, M., Hansen, F. G. & Marinus, M. G. (2008). DnaC Inactivation in Expression of Nucleotide Biosynthesis Genes. *PLoS ONE* 3(8): e2984.

Malínsky, J., Koberna, K., Staněk, D., Masata, M., Votruba, I. & Raska, I. (2001). The supply of exogenous deoxyribonucleotides accelerates the speed of the replication fork in early S-phase. *J Cell Sci.* 114 :747-50.

Maisnier-Patin, S., Nordstrom, K., y Dasgupta, S. (2001). Replication arrests during a single round of replication of the *Escherichia coli* chromosome in the absence of DnaC activity. *Mol Microbiol* 42: 1371-1382.

Mathews, C. K. (1993). Enzyme organization in DNA precursor biosynthesis. *Prog Nuc Ac Res* 44: 167-203.

Messer, W. & Weigel, C. (2003). DnaA as a transcription regulator. *Methods Enzymol.* 370: 338-49.

Michel, B., Grompone, G., Flores, M.J., & Bidnenko, V. (2004). Multiple pathways process stalled replication forks. *Proc Natl Acad Sci U S A* 101: 12783-12788.

Michelsen, O., Teixeira de Mattos, M.J, Jensen, P.R. & Hansen, F.G. (2003). Precise determinations of C and D periods by flow cytometry in *Escherichia coli* K-12 and B/r. *Microbiology* 149: 1001-10.

Molina, F. & Skarstad, K. (2004). Replication fork and SeqA focus distributions in *Escherichia coli* suggest a replication hyperstructure dependent on nucleotide metabolism. *Mol Microbiol* 52: 1597-612.

Morigen, Boye, E., Skarstad, K. & Løbner-Olesen A. (2001). Regulation of chromosomal replication by DnaA protein availability in *Escherichia coli*: effects of the *datA* region. *Biochem. et Bioph. Acta* 1521: 73-80.

Morigen, Løbner-Olesen, A. & Skarstad K. (2003). Titration of the *Escherichia coli* DnaA protein to excess *datA* sites causes destabilization of replication forks, delayed replication initiation and delayed cell division. *Mol Microbiol* 50: 349-62.

Morigen, Odsbu, I., Skarstad, K. (2009). Growth rate dependent numbers of SeqA structures organize the multiple replication forks in rapidly growing *Escherichia coli. Genes Cells* 14: 643–657.

Naruyama H, Shimada M, Niida H, Zineldeen DH, Hashimoto Y, Kohri K, Nakanishi M (2008). Essential role of Chk1 in S phase progression through regulation of RNR2 expression. *Biochem Biophys Res Commun.* 374: 79-83.

Nordlund, P. & Reichard, P. (2006). Ribonucleotide reductases. *Annu. Rev. Biochem* 75: 681–706.

Odsbu, I., Morigen & Skarstad, K. (2009). A reduction in ribonucleotide reductase activity slows down the chromosome replication fork but does not change its localization. *PLoS One* 4 (10), e7617.

Olliver, A., Saggioro, C., Herrick, J. & Sclavi, B. (2010). DnaA-ATP acts as a molecular switch to control levels of ribonucleotide reductase expression in *Escherichia coli. Mol Microbiol* 76: 1555-71.

Pato, M. L. (1979). Alterations of deoxyribonucleoside triphosphate pools in *Escherichia coli*: effects on deoxyribonucleic acid replication and evidence for compartmentation. *J Bacteriol* 140: 518-24.

Pritchard, R.H. & Zaritsky, A. (1970). Effect of Thymine Concentration on the replication velocity of DNA in a thymineless mutant of *Escherichia coli. Nature* 226: 126-130.

Riola, J., Guarino, E., Guzmán, E. C. & Jiménez-Sánchez, A. (2007). Differences in the degree of inhibition of NDP reductase by chemical inactivation and by the thermosensitive mutation *nrdA101* in *Escherichia coli* suggest an effect on chromosome segregation. *Cell Mol Biol Lett* 12: 70-81.

Salguero, I, López Acedo, E. & Guzmán, E. C. (2011). Overlap of replication rounds disturbs the progression of replicating forks in a ribonucleotide reductase mutant of *Escherichia coli*. Microbiology 157: 1955-1967.

Sánchez Romero, M.A., Molina, F. & Jiménez-Sánchez, A. (2010). Correlation between ribonucleoside-diphosphate reductase and three replication proteins in *Escherichia coli. BMC Molecular Biology* doi: 10.1186/1471-2199-11-11.

Sekimizu, K., Bramhill, D. & Kornberg A. (1987). ATP activates DnaA protein in initiating replication of plasmids bearing the origin of the *E. coli* chromosome. *Cell* 50: 259-65.

Schaper, S. & Messer, W. (1995). Interaction of the initiator protein DnaA of *Escherichia coli* with its DNA target. *J Biol Chem.* 270: 17622-6.

Skarstad, K., Steen, H. B. & Boye, E. (1985). *Escherichia coli* DNA distributions measured by flow cytometry and compared with theoretical computer simulations. *J Bacteriol* 163: 661-8.

Skovgaard, O. & Lobner-Olesen, A. (2005). Reduced initiation frequency from *oriC* restores viability of a temperature-sensitive *Escherichia coli* replisome mutant. *Microbiology* 151: 963-73.

Stepankiw, N., Kaidow, A., Boye, E. & Bates, D. (2009). The right half of the *Escherichia coli* replication origin is not essential for viability, but facilitates multi-forked replication. *Mol Microbiol.* 74: 467-479.

Sueoka, N. & Yoshikawa, H. (1965). The chromosome of *Bacillus subtilis*. I. Theory of marker frequency analysis. *Genetics* 52: 747-757.

Torheim, N.K, Boye , E., Løbner-Olesen, A., Stokke, T. & Skarstad, K. (2000). The *Escherichia coli* SeqA protein destabilizes mutant DnaA204 protein. *Mol Microbiol.* 37: 629-38.

Uhlin, U. & Eklund, H. (1994). Structure of ribonucleotide reductase protein R1. *Nature* 13: 533-539.

Von Freiesleben, U., Rasmussen, K.V., Atlung, T., & Hansen, F.G. (2000). Rifampicin-resistant initiation of chromosome replication from *oriC* in *ihf* mutants. *Mol Microbiol* 37: 1087-1093.

Werner, R. (1971). Nature of DNA precursors. *Nature New Biol* 233: 99-103.

Wheeler, L.J., Rajagopal, I. & Mathews, C. K. (2005). Stimulation of mutagenesis by proportional deoxyribonucleoside triphosphate accumulation in Escherichia coli. DNA repair 4, 1450-1456.

Zaritsky, A. & Pritchard, R.H. (1971). Replication time of the chromosome in thymineless mutants of *Escherichia coli*. *J Mol Biol* 60: 65–74.

Zaritsky, A., N. Vischer & Rabinovitch, A. (2007). Changes of initiation mass and cell dimensions by the 'eclipse'. *Mol Microbiol* 63: 15-21.

10

Replication Origin Selection and Pre-Replication Complex Assembly

Kusic-Tisma Jelena and Stefanovic Dragana
Institute of Molecular Genetics and Genetic Engineering, University of Belgrade, Serbia

1. Introduction

The most important replication proteins, their structural and functional assembly with each other and with DNA, and the whole mechanism that ensures complete and accurate duplication of DNA, are highly conserved during eukaryotic evolution. Prior to initiation of DNA replication, a multiprotein assembly called pre-replication complex (pre-RC) forms at replication origins. Formation of the pre-RC is initiated by the eukaryotic initiator Origin Recognition Complex (ORC). ORC recognizes origin DNA and recruits Cdc6, Cdt1, and MCM complex to origins (review Blow & Dutta, 2005). The selection of particular locations within the eukaryotic chromosome for initiation is poorly understood. The whole process of origin recognition includes complex interplay between factors affecting ORC assembly on replication origins and structural constrains of bound DNA. Given that replication origins of higher eukaryots do not have common consensus sequences, specificity of protein-DNA interactions does not play a central role in origin recognition. However, origin transfer studies show that origins have some genetic elements comprised in different modules which are essential for origin activity and are functionally interchangeable between origins (review Aladjem, 2007). The quite obscure step of origin selection is followed by origin remodeling which is promoted by pre-RC. Origin remodeling opens DNA for replication proteins and prepares the origin to be activated and to accommodate the double replisome. The complete sequence of events from origin recognition to activation involves multiple protein-protein and protein-DNA interactions. Identification of all abovementioned components and their interactions will ultimately lead to understanding of the complex mechanism which governs origin selection and ensures accurate initiation in eukaryotic cells.

2. Eukaryotic replication origins

Replication origins are DNA sites at which replication initiates during the S phase. Using different approaches, these sites were identified in simple eukaryotes and in metazoa. In yeast, specific origin sequences were identified by their ability to confer autonomous replication to small circular plasmids. The same assay employed in multicellular systems reviled that virtually any DNA fragment not smaller than 10kb had origin activity (Krysan, 1993). Real replication origins of metazoa were identified by alternative procedures, but they are not numerous and not yet well understood, due to extreme genome complexity and cell-to-cell heterogeneity in origin selection (Hamlin et al., 2008). Recent development of genome-scale methods for identifying hundreds or thousands of new origins may compensate for this lack of data and thus provide information regarding the recognition features of complex origins (Eaton et al., 2010; MacAlpin et al., 2010).

The best understood replication origins belong to budding yeast. They are composed of AT-rich sequences of about 150bp, termed ARS elements. ARS elements were discovered because of their capacity to confer high-frequency transformation of plasmids in *S. cerevisiae* (ARS assay). As shown by systematic mutation analysis, full replicator activity requires multiple DNA elements. These are origin recognition elements A and B, elements that exclude nucleosomes, and DUE or DNA unwinding elements (review Aladjem et al., 2006). DNA elements A and B1 bind the origin recognition complex (ORC). The A element contains an 11-bp essential ACS, (A/TTTTAYRTTT(A/T) that tolerates at maximum 2 mismatches, and adjacent nonconserved sequences. Point mutations in the ACS reduce or inactivate ARS function, origin activity and ORC binding in vitro (Bell, 2002). The B domain consists of several elements (B1-B4) positioned 3′ to the T-rich strand of the A element. Individual B elements are not essential for replicator function and their arrangement within the domain varies. However, these elements contribute significantly to origin efficiency (Huang and Kowalski, 1996). Asymmetric AT-rich sequences, with clusters of A's on one strand and T's on the other, are present in many ARS elements and enriched in nucleosome-free DNA (Yuan et al., 2005). Cooperatively, these and other sequences facilitate replicator chromatin opening, which is functionally important, as illustrated by the observation that forced positioning of the nucleosome over the A element inactivates origin function (Simpson, 1990).

Fission yeast *Schizosaccharomyces pombe*, a very distant relative of budding yeast, has considerable larger (500 – 1000 bp) and less understood replicators. Fission yeast replicators also consist of AT-rich sequences, initiate autonomous replication on plasmids, and bind a six-subunit ORC complex. However, fission yeast can initiate replication from any sufficiently extensive stretch of AT-rich DNA without any apparent sequence preference (Cotobal et al., 2010; Dai et al., 2005). Several *S. pombe* replicators contain two or three required regions consisting of asymmetric AT-rich sequences. In *ars*2004 there are three such regions that can be replaced by 40bp fragments of poly(dA/dT) (Okuno et al., 1997), which shows that the distribution of AT elements, rather than their specific sequences may contribute to origin function.

Different origin mapping procedures have revealed that replication origins of metazoa belong to two categories. Some of them contain unique high-frequency initiation sites, while the others have extensive zones with numerous initiation sites (Aladjem, 2007) and diffuse initiation pattern. Within such zones each site is activated only in a fraction of cell cycles which means that, once initiated at one site, replication forks just pass through the others. In beta-globin genes (HBB), the replication origin contains two adjacent initiation sites which are activated in different cell cycles (Wang et al., 2004). It therefore seems that combined data suggest that replication origins in metazoa generally contain few or more nonrandom initiation sites which could be activated in different cell cycles. Some of these sites are strong and initiate DNA replication at high frequency while the others are not and initiate DNA at low frequency. It, however, seems that initiation sites do not contain any common DNA motif, which is consistent with the apparent lack of sequence specificity of metazoa ORCs *in vitro*. In contrast to that, deletion and origin transfer studies demonstrate some role for DNA sequence composition in positioning origins. In the same manner, the analysis that compares the position of origins with the positions of evolutionary conserved regions (CRs) in mammalian genomes, suggests that replication origins contain sequence motifs under selective constraints (Cadoret, 2008).

Analysis of HBB *ori* provided the first evidence that origins in metazoa contain specific sequences: origin activity was abolished by deletion of the 8-kb origin, which forced the locus to replicate from an unidentified upstream origin (Kitsberg et al, 1993). Deletion experiments were followed by transfer of putative replicators to ectopic chromosomal regions and testing for replication initiation at the new locations. Following this procedure, specific origin sequences were shown to be both necessary and sufficient to direct initiation of replication when transferred to ectopic locations. Replicators that exhibit ectopic origin activity include those near the *Drosophila* chorion genes (Lu et al., 2001), DHFR ori-β (Altman and Fanning, 2001), the human HBB (Aladjem et al., 2002), lamin B2 (Paixao et al., 2004), c-myc (Liu et al., 2003) and possibly HRPT (Cohen et al., 2004), which exhibits origin activity when replacing its murine orthologue. Combined, origin transfer studies show that at least some replication origins have modular structure, with each module being essential for origin activity and functionally interchangeable between origins (Paixao et al., 2004). The following structural features of origin modules could be important for origin activation:

a. Sequences rich in A+T are abundant in eukaryotic origins and could have roles in facilitating DNA unwinding. Asymmetric AT stretches are present in the hamster DHFR origin and in the human LMNB2, HBB and DHFR origins. Such sequences are recognized by proteins, such as SpORC4 that has the relevant AT hooks (Kong & DePamphilis, 2002). Interestingly, even its human homologue displays a similar preference for asymmetric AT stretches (Stefanovic et al., 2003). The other AT rich elements that could be important for initiation of DNA replication are matrix attachment sites. Matrix attachment regions are required for maintenance of plasmid replication in human cells and could be part of metazoan replication origins. In addition, different AT elements could build unorthodox structures similar to one detected in the asymmetric AT-rich stretch of the LMNB2 origin (Kusic et al., 2005).
b. In some promoters CpG islands are correlated with open chromatin structure and it is believed that they could have similar roles in replication origins. Human nascent DNA is 10-fold enriched in CpG islands (Delgado et al., 1998), whereas removal of a CpG island significantly decreases the efficiency of ectopic LMNB2 origin (Paixao et al., 2004).
c. Unusual DNA structures could form from origin elements that are not AT rich. Palindromes were found in hamster DHFR and human HBB and LMNB2 origins. Different unorthodox structures were detected in the hamster DHFR origin (Bianchi et al., 1990) including one bent element important for DHFR ectopic activity, which indicated a correlation between origin topology and its function (Altamn & Fanning, 2004).

In summary, replication origins in metazoa are determined by a complex, poorly understood set of structural and topological features of DNA in which no single-sequence module has a key role.

3. Origin recognition complex

The Origin Recognition Complex (ORC) was first discovered and purified from budding yeast, based on its ability to specifically bind to replication origins (Bell & Stillman, 1992).

Shortly thereafter, the corresponding genes were cloned and orthologues of Orc1-Orc5 were identified in organisms such as *Drosophila melanogaster* (Gossen et al., 1995), *Arabidopsis thaliana* (Diaz-Trivino et al., 2005) and *Homo sapiens* (Dhar & Dutta, 2000), which strongly suggested that these genes could exist in all eukaryotes. ORC6 genes are relatively well conserved between metazoa and fission yeast, but there is insufficient identity to conclude that they are homologous to budding yeast Orc6 (Dhar & Dutta, 2000).

ORC-like proteins are not just confined to eukaryotes. Studies of archeal Orc1/cdc6 proteins, as well as DnaA have provided important structural information about ORC-DNA interactions. DnaA, like ORC, acts as an initiator of DNA replication, and whereas DnaA and the archeal Orc1/cdc6 proteins share little sequence identity, structural studies have shown that they do have a high degree of similarity in some of their functional domains (Mott & Berger, 2007). Moreover, a study of *Drosophila* ORC structure suggested that DnaA and ORC wrap DNA in a similar manner (Clarey et al., 2008).

ORC function is tightly controlled by ATP binding and hydrolysis. Three of the ORC subunits (Orc1, 4, and 5) are members of AAA+ family of ATPases. Recent studies suggest that ORC2 and ORC3 represent more distant relatives of the AAA+ proteins that lack the key conserved elements of the ATP-binding site (Speck et al., 2005). In *S. cerevisiae* and *Drosophila* the ATP-binding activity of Orc1 is essential and regulates DNA binding. Although not essential, mutations in the *S. cerevisiae* Orc5 ATP-binding motif cause defects in the apparent complex stability (Takahashi et al., 2004). In contrast, mutations of the Orc1, Orc4 or Orc5 ATP-binding motifs inhibit the ability of human ORC to activate replication in ORC-depleted *Xenopus* egg extracts (Giordano-Coltart et al., 2005). Direct DNA binding studies of human ORC show that addition of ATP stimulates ORC-DNA interaction (Vashee et al., 2003). DNA has a significant effect on the ATP binding and hydrolysis functions of ORC. In *S. cerevisiae*, double-stranded origin DNA stabilizes ATP binding and inhibits ATP hydrolysis, whereas single-stranded DNA of any sequence stimulates ATPase activity (Lee et al., 2000). Similar findings have been made for Drosophila ORC (Chesnokov et al., 2001).

Although formally a member of ORC, Orc6 does not share similar structural features or a common evolutionary origin with Orc1-5 (Duncker et al., 2009). Nevertheless, its association with the other five subunits is required to promote the initiation of DNA replication and it is considered an ORC protein.

It appears that all six ORC subunits remain associated with chromatin throughout the cell cycle in *S. cerevisae*, but not in metazoan cells. In human cells ORC was detected on replication origins in G1 and S phases, while missing in the M phase. Orc1 protein leaves the replication complex when DNA synthesis starts (DePamphilis, 2005). When the cells move into the S phase the pre-replicative complex is restructured into the smaller post-replicative form. The transition from the pre- to the post-replicative complex is accompanied by displacement of the ORC subunit (Abdurashidova et al., 2003). Immunofluorescent detection of Orc2-green fluorescent protein (GFP) in *Drosophila* neuroblasts and live-cell imaging in embryos show no ORC2 in chromosomes in the period from prophase to anaphase (Baldinger & Gossen, 2009). Fluorescent loss in photobleaching analysis in hamster cells suggests less static interaction of ORC subunits with chromatin and shows a highly dynamic interaction of both Orc1 and Orc4 with chromatin throughout the cell cycle (McNairn et al., 2005).

Assembly of the human recombinant ORC subunits was investigated *in vitro* (Giordano-Coltart et al., 2005; Siddiqui & Stillman, 2007) and it was demonstrated that human ORC follows an ordered pathway of assembly. First subunits 2 and 3 bind to each other and then recruit Orc5. The Orc2/3/5 complex recruits Orc4 then Orc1. Mutations in the ATP binding sites of Orc4 and Orc5 impair complex assembly, whereas Orc1 does not require ATP binding. It is possible than in living cells additional regulatory mechanisms operate at the level of the ORC complex assembly and disassembly and not only at the level of protein-DNA interaction or preRC activation.

4. Mechanisms of replication initiation site selection

Selection of DNA replication origins may be regulated by various factors and may be achieved at different levels. Replication initiates at many sites along linear chromosomes, which ensures complete genome duplication within a single S phase, but the number of activated origins does not match the number of prereplication complexes previously assembled on DNA (review Gilbert, 2010). From the large pool of all assembled pre-RCs only a subset is chosen for subsequent initiation while the rest remain dormant. Two-step mechanism or mechanisms that select preRCs for initiation or govern the pre-RC assembly remain unknown.

In budding yeast, ORC binds the corresponding ARS element in a sequence specific manner. One component of the recognition site is the 11-bp ACS. As shown by analysis of modified DNA substrates, DNA-bound ORC primarily interacts with the A-rich strand of the ACS. It is not yet clear which subunit of ORC determines DNA binding, but protein-DNA cross-linking studies show four out of six ORC subunits (Orc1, Orc2, Orc4 and Orc5) in close association with origin DNA (Lee & Bell, 1997).

In *S. pombe* replication origins are recognized by ORC via a species-specific AT-hook in the ORC4 subunit (Chuang & Kelly, 1999). SpORC binds to preferred DNA sites containing multiple runs of three A's or T's in vitro. In fission yeast structural elements are redundant and could compensate for deletion of one of the many ORC-binding sites.

ARS function appears to be governed primarily by AT content and length (Dai et al., 2005). Whether the replicator length is needed to include the required DNA elements or to provide spacing between them is not clear. DNA appears to wrap around ORC (Gaczynska et al., 2004), suggesting a possible spacing length requirement between ORC-binding sites. Intervening deletion mutations could affect replicator function by either shortening the spacing length between elements or by removing elements.

S. pombe Orc4 could bind to origin DNA even in the absence of other ORC subunits. The AT hook motif is known to bind to the minor groove of AT where it can recognize or induce structural changes. The N-terminal domain of *S. pombe* Orc4 may function to tether the ORC complex to origins of DNA replication and this interaction is independent of ATP. However, the tethered complex may also make ATP-dependent contacts with additional sites in the origin to nucleate formation of the initiation complex. As demonstrated by recent studies, SpORC binds DNA in at least two steps (Houchens et al., 2008). The first step, possibly mediated by electrostatic interactions between the AT-hook motifs of SpOrc4 subunit and AT tracts in replication origin, results in formation of a salt sensitive SpORC-DNA complex, which is then slowly converted to a salt-stable form.

In the metazoan model system ORC-DNA interactions were first explored in *Drosophila*. As demonstrated by imunofluorescent studies, the *Drosophila* DNA element ACE3 (Amplification Control Element 3) alone directed ORC to the region of chorion amplification

(Austin et al., 1999). Moreover, chromatin imunoprecipitation studies indicated that ACE3 can target *Drosophila* ORC not only to sites within the ACE3 element itself but also to sites within adjacent DNA sequences. In contrast to that, ORC purified from *Drosophila* embryos or reconstituted from recombinant proteins, bound origin DNA in an ATP-dependent manner but with little sequence specificity (Remus et al, 2004), insufficient to target the ORC to origins of replication.

Similar to *Drosophila* ORC, reconstituted, highly purified human ORC exhibits ATP stimulated DNA-binding and preference for either natural or synthetic AT rich sequences, (Vashee et al., 2003). However, it is generally assumed that origin specification in metazoa involves mechanisms other than simple recognition of DNA sequence by ORC. Thus DmORC exhibits 30-fold higher affinity for negatively supercoiled DNA as compared to relaxed or linear DNA (Remus et al., 2004). Binding of DmORC is accompanied by changes in DNA topology, suggesting that ORC-DNA complexes contain underwound DNA. Purified human ORC induces similar topological changes in origin DNA (Houchens et al., 2008), indicating conservation of this property of ORC during eukaryotic evolution.

Interestingly, human ORC and human Orc4 exhibit similar DNA binding properties, such as preference for negatively supercoiled DNA (Kusic or Tomic unpublished), preference for AT rich DNA and the ability to distinguish between different AT-rich DNA structures. HsOrc4 protein also exhibits preference for triple stranded DNA (Kusic et al., 2010) and the ability to stimulate formation of noncanonical oligonucleotide structures (Stefanovic et al., 2008). Such HsOrc4 properties could play part in origin selection through directing ORC to DNA sequences able to adopt unorthodox structures.

Pre-RC factors other than ORC may also contribute to origin recognition. In budding yeast, Cdc6 ATPase activity contributes to stabile and specific binding of the ORC-Cdc6 complex to the origin (Speck & Stillman, 2007), whereas in fission yeast Cdt1 and Cdc6 proteins facilitate SpORC-DNA interactions (Houchens et al., 2008).

In addition to origin structure and preRC components, chromatin structure could significantly affect replication origin selection. As revealed by ChIP-seq for ORC in budding yeast, many consensus sequences are not bound by ORC (Eaton et al., 2010). A genome-wide analysis of nucleosome architecture of replication origins in budding yeast, aligned by their ORC-binding sites, suggested a model in which the underlying DNA sequence at replication origins occludes nucleosomes. This creates a permissive environment for ORC binding, after which ORC positions nucleosomes in regular array on both sides (Berbenetz et al., 2010). In addition, only a subset of nucleosome free regions (NFR) with specific flanking sequence features - which allow the ORC to position nucleosomes with sufficient space for MCM protein loading - can promote binding of ORC. Accordingly, by genome-scale mapping of *D. melanogaster* ORC localization, ORC was found in previously mapped NFRs. The sites of rapid nucleosome turnover were found to align with ORC (MacAlpine et al., 2010). Consistent with *in vitro* binding data, specific sequence motifs were not identified, but an *in silico* learning approach revealed a complex code of short sequences that could simultaneously predict ORC binding and NFR.

Transcription factors may also play a role in localization of ORC. Thus, at the chorion loci of *Drosophila* folicule cells, transcription factors containing the Myb protein facilitate DNA replication at the ACE3 and ori-β replication origins (Beal et al., 2002). Specific RNA recruits ORC to the Epstein-Barr virus (EBV) replicator, *ori*P by linking *ori*P-bound nuclear antigen-1 (EBNA-1) and ORC (Norseen et al., 2008).

5. Assembly of Pre-RC complexes

Originally identified by *in vivo* DnaseI protection assay (Diffley et al., 1994), the multiprotein assembly formed at all potential origins of replication was termed the pre-RC. Pre-RC formation can only occur during late M and G1 phases of the cell cycle and only preexisting pre-RCs can be activated in the subsequent S phase. Pre-RC formation requires at least 4 different entities: the origin recognition complex (ORC), Cdc6, Cdt1, and the MCM complex. Since the pre-RC complex acts as eukaryotic replicative helicase, pre-RC formation is equivalent to helicase loading event (Chong et al., 2000).

In pre-RCs formed *in vivo* or *in vitro* multiple MCM complexes are assembled at each origin. Depending on the organism, the MCM:origin DNA ratio varies between 10:1 and 40:1 (Takahachi et al., 2005). Since each replication fork requires at least one MCM complex, the role of additional MCMs remains unclear. The MCM complex has no affinity for origin DNA and its association with the origin requires the action of ORC, Cdc6 and Cdt1. Once assembled, MCM does not require Cdc6 and Cdt1 proteins and they are released from chromatin (Hua & Newport, 1998). After loading, MCM DNA association is independent of other components (Bowers et al., 2004), possibly due to the ring shape structure of MCM which could be closed around origin DNA. Since loaded MCM complexes direct initiation in the apparent absence of other pre-RC components, ORC, Cdc6 and Cdt1 could be considered MCM loading factors. It is important to note that ten of the fourteen protein components of the pre-RC belong to the AAA+ family of ATPases (Mcm2-7, ORC1, Orc4, Orc5, and Cdc6). Consequently the pre-RC formation requires ATP and is inhibited by its of nonhydrolyzable analogs (Harvey & Newport, 2003).

A similarity of ORC subunits and Cdc6 to sliding clamp loaders and the ring shaped structure of MCM have led to the proposal of a model for MCM origin loading (Speck & Majka, 2009). Loading initiates by association of ORC with origin DNA in the ATP-bound state. ORC-ATP recruits Cdc6, stimulates its association with ATP and subsequent recruitment of Cdt1 and the MCM proteins. According to the model, this leads to the opening of the MCM ring thus exposing a previously hidden DNA-binding site. MCM binding to DNA triggers Cdc6 ATP hydrolysis which leads to two events: the release of Cdc6 and Cdt1, and closing of the MCM ring around the DNA.

6. Conclusion

As suggested by extensive conservation of replication factors, the basic mechanism of DNA replication is evolutionally conserved. However, regulation of origin firing in higher eukaryotes is much more complex than in lower eukaryotes. Consequently, in order to understand what specifies the metazoan origins one must look far beyond simple linear sequences and take into account combinatorial interaction of multiple components that make up the initiation machinery and insert it in the cell cycle regulatory network. The main entity that initiates preRC formation, protein complex ORC, does not have the ability to select origins in metazoa based solely on its own affinity for specific DNA sequences. In this function it could be aided by other pre-RC proteins, DNA topology, and even unorthodox DNA structures. Characteristics and state of chromatin structure in specific regions of the genome, nucleosome positioning, binding of transcription factors and degree of DNA supercoiling may restrict the area in which initiation could occur. Altogether these features could play a critical role in initiation of DNA replication by the mechanism that requires many precise small steps leading to a single goal.

7. Acknowledgments

This work was supported by grants from the Ministry of Science and Technological Development, Serbia (173008) and the International Centre for Genetic Engineering and Biotechnology, Italy (CRP/YUG08-01).

8. References

Abdurashidova G, Danailov MB, Ochem A, Triolo G, Djeliova V, Radulescu S, Vindigni A, Riva S, Falaschi A. (2003) Localization of proteins bound to a replication origin of human DNA along the cell cycle. *EMBO J.* 22(16):4294-4303.

Aladjem M.I., Falaschi A., Kowalski D. (2006) Eukaryotic DNA Replication Origins, In *DNA Replication and human desease* DePamphilis M., 31-61, Cold Spring Harbor Laboratory Press, ISBN 0-87969-766-0 , New York

Aladjem MI, Rodewald LW, Lin CM, Bowman S, Cimbora DM, Brody LL, Epner EM, Groudine M, Wahl GM. (2002) Replication initiation patterns in the beta-globin loci of totipotent and differentiated murine cells: evidence for multiple initiation regions. *Mol Cell Biol.* 22(2):442-452.

Aladjem MI. (2007) Replication in context: dynamic regulation of DNA replication patterns in metazoans. *Nat Rev Genet.* 8(8):588-600.

Altman AL & Fanning E. (2004) Defined sequence modules and an architectural element cooperate to promote initiation at an ectopic mammalian chromosomal replication origin. *Mol Cell Biol.* 24(10):4138-50.

Altman AL, Fanning E. (2001) The Chinese hamster dihydrofolate reductase replication origin beta is active at multiple ectopic chromosomal locations and requires specific DNA sequence elements for activity. *Mol Cell Biol.* 21(4):1098-1110

Austin RJ, Orr-Weaver TL, Bell SP. (1999) Drosophila ORC specifically binds to ACE3, an origin of DNA replication control element. *Genes Dev.* 13(20):2639-2649.

Author last name, Author initial. (Year of publication). Name of paper. *Name of Journal in Italics,* Vol. volume number, No. issue number, (month and year of the edition), pp. (first-last page numbers), ISSN

Baldinger T & Gossen M. (2009) Binding of Drosophila ORC proteins to anaphase chromosomes requires cessation of mitotic cyclin-dependent kinase activity. *Mol Cell Biol.* J 29(1):140-149.

Beall EL, Manak JR, Zhou S, Bell M, Lipsick JS, Botchan MR. (2002) Role for a Drosophila Myb-containing protein complex in site-specific DNA replication. *Nature.* 420(6917):833-837.

Bell SP & Stillman B. (1992) ATP-dependent recognition of eukaryotic origins of DNA replication by a multiprotein complex. Nature. 357(6374):128-134.

Bell SP. (2002) The origin recognition complex: from simple origins to complex functions. *Genes Dev.*16(6):659-672.

Berbenetz NM, Nislow C, Brown GW. (2010) Diversity of eukaryotic DNA replication origins revealed by genome-wide analysis of chromatin structure. *PLoS Genet.* 6(9). pii: e1001092.

Bianchi A, Wells RD, Heintz NH, Caddle MS. (1990) Sequences near the origin of replication of the DHFR locus of Chinese hamster ovary cells adopt left-handed Z-DNA and triplex structures. *J Biol Chem.* 265(35):21789-21796.

Blow JJ & Dutta A. (2005) Preventing re-replication of chromosomal DNA. *Nat Rev Mol Cell Biol.* 6(6):476-486.

Bowers JL, Randell JC, Chen S, Bell SP. (2004) ATP hydrolysis by ORC catalyzes reiterative Mcm2-7 assembly at a defined origin of replication. *Mol Cell.* 16(6):967-978.

Cadoret JC, Meisch F, Hassan-Zadeh V, Luyten I, Guillet C, Duret L, Quesneville H, Prioleau MN. (2008) Genome-wide studies highlight indirect links between human replication origins and gene regulation. *Proc Natl Acad Sci U S A.* 105(41):15837-15842

Chesnokov I, Remus D, Botchan M. (2001) Functional analysis of mutant and wild-type Drosophila origin recognition complex. *Proc Natl Acad Sci U S A.* 98(21):11997-2002.

Chong JP, Hayashi MK, Simon MN, Xu RM, Stillman B. (2000) A double-hexamer archaeal minichromosome maintenance protein is an ATP-dependent DNA helicase. *Proc Natl Acad Sci U S A.* 97(4):1530-5.

Chuang RY & Kelly TJ. (1999) The fission yeast homologue of Orc4p binds to replication origin DNA via multiple AT-hooks. *Proc Natl Acad Sci U S A.* 96(6):2656-2661.

Clarey MG, Botchan M, Nogales E.() Single particle EM studies of the Drosophila melanogaster origin recognition complex and evidence for DNA wrapping. *J Struct Biol.* 164(3):241-249.

Cohen SM, Hatada S, Brylawski BP, Smithies O, Kaufman DG, Cordeiro-Stone M. (2004) Complementation of replication origin function in mouse embryonic stem cells by human DNA sequences. *Genomics.* 84(3):475-484.

Cotobal C, Segurado M, Antequera F. (2010) Structural diversity and dynamics of genomic replication origins in Schizosaccharomyces pombe. *EMBO J.* 29(5):934-942.

Dai J, Chuang RY, Kelly TJ. (2005) DNA replication origins in the Schizosaccharomyces pombe genome. *Proc Natl Acad Sci U S A.* 102(2):337-342.

Delgado S, Gómez M, Bird A, Antequera F. (1998) Initiation of DNA replication at CpG islands in mammalian chromosomes. *EMBO J.*17(8):2426-2435.

DePamphilis ML.(2005) Cell cycle dependent regulation of the origin recognition complex. *Cell Cycle.* 4(1):70-79.

Dhar SK & Dutta A. (2000) Identification and characterization of the human ORC6 homolog. *J Biol Chem.* 275(45):34983-34988.

Diaz-Trivino S, del Mar Castellano M, de la Paz Sanchez M, Ramirez-Parra E, Desvoyes B, Gutierrez C. (2005) The genes encoding Arabidopsis ORC subunits are E2F targets and the two ORC1 genes are differently expressed in proliferating and endoreplicating cells. *Nucleic Acids Res.* 33(17):5404-5414.

Diffley JF, Cocker JH, Dowell SJ, Rowley A. (1994) Two steps in the assembly of complexes at yeast replication origins in vivo. *Cell.* 78(2):303-316.

Duncker BP, Chesnokov IN, McConkey BJ. (2009) The origin recognition complex protein family. *Genome Biol.* 10(3):214-214.8.

Eaton ML, Galani K, Kang S, Bell SP, MacAlpine DM. (2010) Conserved nucleosome positioning defines replication origins. *Genes Dev.* 24(8):748-753.

Gaczynska M, Osmulski PA, Jiang Y, Lee JK, Bermudez V, Hurwitz J. (2004) Atomic force microscopic analysis of the binding of the Schizosaccharomyces pombe origin recognition complex and the spOrc4 protein with origin DNA. *Proc Natl Acad Sci U S A.* 101(52):17952-17957.

Gilbert DM. (2010) Evaluating genome-scale approaches to eukaryotic DNA replication. *Nat Rev Genet.* 11(10):673-684.

Giordano-Coltart J, Ying CY, Gautier J, Hurwitz J. (2005) Studies of the properties of human origin recognition complex and its Walker A motif mutants. *Proc Natl Acad Sci U S A.* 102(1):69-74.

Gossen M, Pak DT, Hansen SK, Acharya JK, Botchan MR. (1995) A Drosophila homolog of the yeast origin recognition complex. *Science.* 270(5242):1674-1677..

Hamlin JL, Mesner LD, Lar O, Torres R, Chodaparambil SV, Wang L. (2008) A revisionist replicon model for higher eukaryotic genomes. *J Cell Biochem.* 105(2):321-329.

Harvey KJ & Newport J. (2003) Metazoan origin selection: origin recognition complex chromatin binding is regulated by CDC6 recruitment and ATP hydrolysis. *J Biol Chem.* 278(49):48524-48528.

Houchens CR, Lu W, Chuang RY, Frattini MG, Fuller A, Simancek P, Kelly TJ. (2008) Multiple mechanisms contribute to Schizosaccharomyces pombe origin recognition complex-DNA interactions. *J Biol Chem.* 283(44):30216-30224

Hua XH & Newport J. (1998) Identification of a preinitiation step in DNA replication that is independent of origin recognition complex and cdc6, but dependent on cdk2. *J Cell Biol.* 140(2):271-281.

Huang RY & Kowalski D. (1996) Multiple DNA elements in ARS305 determine replication origin activity in a yeast chromosome. *Nucleic Acids Res.* 24(5):816-823.

Kitsberg D, Selig S, Keshet I, Cedar H. (1993) Replication structure of the human beta-globin gene domain. *Nature.* 366(6455):588-590.

Kong D & DePamphilis ML. (2002) Site-specific ORC binding, pre-replication complex assembly and DNA synthesis at Schizosaccharomyces pombe replication origins. *EMBO J.* 21(20):5567-5576.

Krysan PJ, Smith JG, Calos MP. (1993) Autonomous replication in human cells of multimers of specific human and bacterial DNA sequences. *Mol Cell Biol.* 13(5):2688-2696.

Kusic J, Kojic S, Divac A, Stefanovic D. (2005) Noncanonical DNA elements in the lamin B2 origin of DNA replication. *J Biol Chem.* 280(11):9848-9854.

Kusic J, Tomic B, Divac A, Kojic S. (2010) Human initiation protein Orc4 prefers triple stranded DNA. *Mol Biol Rep.* 37(5):2317-2232.

Lee DG & Bell SP. (1997) Architecture of the yeast origin recognition complex bound toorigins of DNA replication. *Mol Cell Biol.* 17(12):7159-7168.

Lee DG, Makhov AM, Klemm RD, Griffith JD, Bell SP. (2000) Regulation of origin recognition complex conformation and ATPase activity: differential effects of single-stranded and double-stranded DNA binding. *EMBO J.* 19(17):4774-4782.

Liu G, Malott M, Leffak M. (2003) Multiple functional elements comprise a Mammalian chromosomal replicator. *Mol Cell Biol.* 23(5):1832-1842.

Lu L, Zhang H, Tower J. (2001) Functionally distinct, sequence-specific replicator and origin elements are required for Drosophila chorion gene amplification. *Genes Dev.* 15(2):134-146.

MacAlpine HK, Gordân R, Powell SK, Hartemink AJ, MacAlpine DM. (2010) Drosophila ORC localizes to open chromatin and marks sites of cohesin complex loading. *Genome Res.* 20(2):201-211.

McNairn AJ, Okuno Y, Misteli T, Gilbert DM. (2005) Chinese hamster ORC subunits dynamically associate with chromatin throughout the cell-cycle. *Exp Cell Res.* 308(2):345-356.

Mott ML & Berger JM. (2007) DNA replication initiation: mechanisms and regulation in bacteria. *Nat Rev Microbiol.* 5(5):343-354.

Norseen J, Thomae A, Sridharan V, Aiyar A, Schepers A, Lieberman PM. (2008) RNA-dependent recruitment of the origin recognition complex. *EMBO J.* 27(22):3024-3035.

Okuno Y, Okazaki T, Masukata H. (1997) Identification of a predominant replication origin in fission yeast. *Nucleic Acids Res.* 25(3):530-537.

Paixão S, Colaluca IN, Cubells M, Peverali FA, Destro A, Giadrossi S, Giacca M, Falaschi A, Riva S, Biamonti G. (2004) Modular structure of the human lamin B2 replicator. *Mol Cell Biol.* 24(7):2958-2967.

Remus D, Beall EL, Botchan MR. (2004) DNA topology, not DNA sequence, is a critical determinant for Drosophila ORC-DNA binding. *EMBO J.* 23(4):897-907.

Siddiqui K & Stillman B. (2007) ATP-dependent assembly of the human origin recognition complex. *J Biol Chem.* 282(44):32370-32383

Simpson RT. (1990) Nucleosome positioning can affect the function of a cis-acting DNA element in vivo. *Nature.* 343(6256):387-389.

Speck C & Majka J. (2009) The Action of AAA+ ATPases in Loading Replication Factors, In *Molecular Themes in DNA Replication*, Edited by Cox LS. 22-46, RSC, UK

Speck C & Stillman B. (2007) Cdc6 ATPase activity regulates ORC x Cdc6 stability and the selection of specific DNA sequences as origins of DNA replication. *J Biol Chem.* 282(16):11705-11714.

Speck C, Chen Z, Li H, Stillman B. (2005) ATPase-dependent cooperative binding of ORC and Cdc6 to origin DNA. *Nat Struct Mol Biol.* 12(11):965-971.

Stefanovic D, Kusic J, Divac A, Tomic B. (2008) Formation of noncanonical DNAstructures mediated by human ORC4, a protein component of the origin recognition complex. *Biochemistry.* 47(33):8760-8767.

Stefanovic D, Stanojcic S, Vindigni A, Ochem A, Falaschi A. (2003) In vitro protein-DNA interactions at the human lamin B2 replication origin. *J Biol Chem.* 278(44):42737-42743.

Takahashi N, Yamaguchi Y, Yamairi F, Makise M, Takenaka H, Tsuchiya T, Mizushima T. (2004) Analysis on origin recognition complex containing Orc5p with defective Walker A motif. *J Biol Chem.* 279(9):8469-8477.

Takahashi TS, Wigley DB, Walter JC. (2005) Pumps, paradoxes and ploughshares: mechanism of the MCM2-7 DNA helicase. *Trends Biochem Sci.* 30(8):437-444.

Vashee S, Cvetic C, Lu W, Simancek P, Kelly TJ, Walter JC. (2003) Sequence-independent DNA binding and replication initiation by the human origin recognition complex.

Genes Dev. 17(15):1894-1908Wang L, Lin CM, Brooks S, Cimbora D, Groudine M, Aladjem MI. (2004) The human beta-globin replication initiation region consists of two modular independent replicators. *Mol Cell Biol.* 24(8):3373-3386.

Yuan GC, Liu YJ, Dion MF, Slack MD, Wu LF, Altschuler SJ, Rando OJ. (2005) Genome-scale identification of nucleosome positions in S. cerevisiae. *Science*. 309(5734):626-630.

11

The Coordination between DNA Replication Initiation and Other Cell Cycle Events

Shijiao Huang and Chuanmao Zhang
The Education Ministry Key Laboratory of Cell Proliferation and Differentiation and the State Key Laboratory of Bio-membrane and Membrane Bio-engineering, College of Life Sciences, Peking University, Beijing China

1. Introduction

The cell cycle is the process of accurate self-reproduction and proliferation of a cell. It is the basis of the growth, development, heredity and evolution of organisms. Misregulation of the cell cycle may result in malignant cell proliferation, tumorigenesis or cell death. In this chapter, we mainly discuss the coordination regulations between DNA replication initiation and other cell cycle events that ensure genomic integrity. Recent breakthroughs have uncovered more and more DNA replication licensing machinery proteins (ORC, Cdc6, Cdt1, geminin, etc.) functioning in other cell cycle events, including centrosome replication, mitotic events, transcription and so on.

2. The connections between DNA replication and other cell cycle events

DNA replication occurs once and only once per cell cycle mainly regulated by DNA replication initiation factors in eukaryotic cells. The pre-replication complex (pre-RC) assembly or the DNA replication licensing is the first step in DNA replication initiation, characterized by the sequential recruitment of ORCs, Cdc6, Cdt1 and MCMs to the DNA replication origins to form the pre-RC at the end of mitosis (Bell and Dutta 2002). The replication licensing is suppressed during G2 phase and mitosis to prevent DNA re-replication within one cell cycle by down-regulating the Cdt1 activity in metazoans achieved mainly by degradation of Cdt1 or through its inhibitor geminin (Nishitani et al. 2006). Geminin inhibits Cdt1 by binding to Cdt1 and interfering with the interaction of Cdt1 and MCM proteins, thus preventing Cdt1 from recruiting MCM2-7 proteins to the replication origins (Wohlschlegel et al. 2000, Yanagi et al. 2002). The precise regulations of pre-RC protein levels and assembly are effective ways to prevent reassembly of *de novo* MCM2-7 onto the replicated origins to re-license and re-replicate the genomic DNA in the subsequent phases of the same cell cycle (Figure 1). In addition to DNA replication licensing, pre-RC proteins are also involved in the centrosome duplication in the S phase, chromosomes alignment and segregation in mitosis and cytokinesis and RNA transcription throughout the cell cycle.

2.1 Coordination of centrosome duplication and DNA replication

The centrosome in an animal cell is composed of two centrioles and the surrounding pericentriolar material (PCM). Centrosome duplication and separation also take place once and only once in one cell division cycle as does DNA replication, and accordingly the process of centrosome duplication and separation is recognized as the centrosome duplication cycle or centrosome cycle. Mis-regulation of centrosome duplication causes multiple centrosomes, multipolar spindle and chromosome misalignment. Centrosome duplication initiates simultaneously with the initiation of DNA replication. Both centrosome duplication and chromosome replication have to be coordinated to produce proper centrosome numbers for a normal cell cycle. Although the coordination between these two cycles has been noticed for a long time (Mazia 1987), the underlying mechanism is still largely unknown.

2.1.1 The centrosome cycle

Through electron microscopy (Kuriyama and Borisy 1981), the centrosome cycle has been recognized to comprise the following steps: the centriole disengagement, the centriole duplication and elongation, and the centrosome maturation and separation. From the mitotic exit to the early G1 phase, the centrioles change their orthogonal configuration and are in preparation of a pre-duplication state (Alvey 1985, Piel et al. 2000). The centriole duplication initiates with the nucleation of the daughter centrioles at the late G1 phase and elongates during the S and G2 phases, resulting in two new centrosomes paired in one PCM. The maturation and separation of the two centrosomes occurs during the G2/M transition along with the chromatin condensation. Considering the behaviour of the centrosome cycle, it might be possible that there is a licensing mechanism for regulating that centrosome duplication occurs once per cell cycle similar to the DNA replication licensing (Figure 1). Several proteins possibly function in the licensing process of centrosome duplication. Overexpression of Plk4, nucleophosmin (NPM/B23) and SAS-6 leads to centrosome amplification (Bettencourt-Dias et al. 2005, Habedanck et al. 2005, Leidel et al. 2005, Dammermann et al. 2004). The expression level of the Plk4 protein peaks at mitosis and is minimal in the G1 phase (Fode, Binkert and Dennis 1996). It is possible that the protein level of Plk4 is strictly down-regulated after centrosome duplication starts in order to avoid centrosome re-duplication in one cell cycle, similar to the down-regulations of the DNA replication licensing proteins Cdt1 and Cdc6 after DNA replication initiation in S and G2 phases. B23 (also named as Nucleophosmin (NPM)), a multifunctional nucleolar protein, is also probably involved in the licensing system of the centrosome duplication. B23 partially binds to unduplicated centrosomes in the G1 phase, dissociates from the centrosomes by cyclin E-CDK2 phosphorylation at the late G1 phase and triggers centriole duplication initiation (Okuda et al. 2000, Tokuyama et al. 2001). In S and G2 phases, B23 is prevented from re-association with centrosomes due to phosphorylation until mitosis (Okuda et al. 2000, Tokuyama et al. 2001, Zatsepina et al. 1999). Induction of the unphosphorylated B23 by microinjection of anti-B23 monoclonal antibody or expression of the non-phosphorylated form of B23 results in persistent centrosome binding of B23 and inhibits centrosome duplication initiation at the very early step of the centriole disengagement (Okuda et al. 2000, Tokuyama et al. 2001). SAS-6 is a coiled-coil protein which localizes to centrosomes and is recruited to centrioles at the onset of the centrosome cycle (Leidel et al. 2005). Centrosome duplication once per cell cycle requires the activity of SAS-6. Overexpression of SAS-6 results in excess foci-bearing centriolar markers, while RNAi knockdown of this protein interferes with the normal centrosome duplication (Leidel et al. 2005).

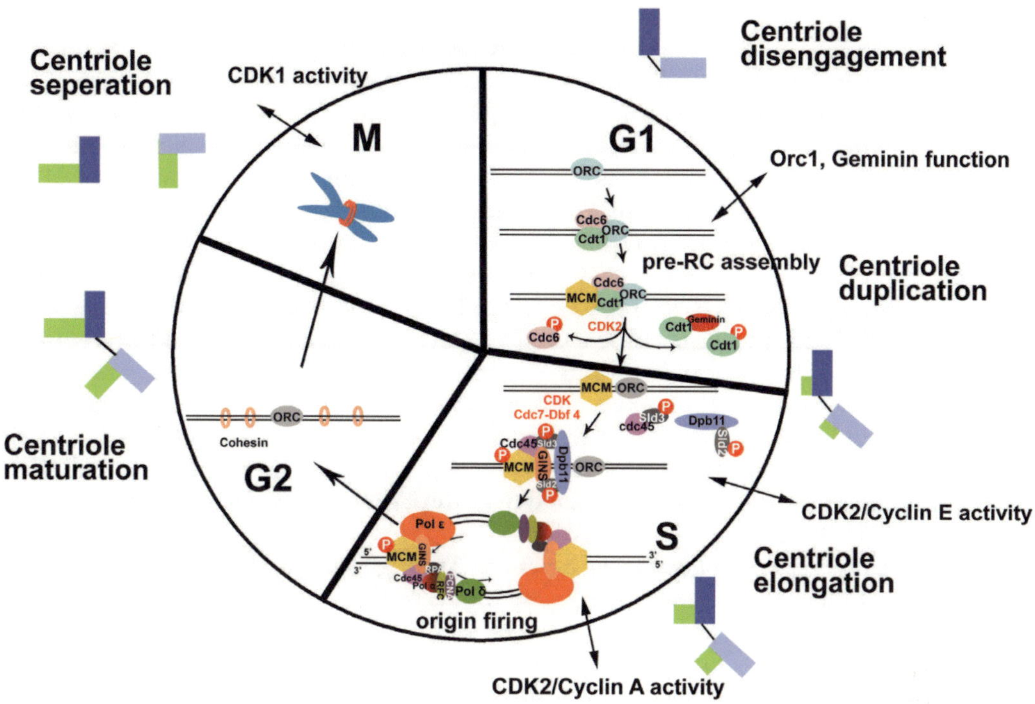

Fig. 1. The DNA replication cycle and the centrosome duplication cycle
The DNA replication cycle is shown inside the circle, while the centrosome replication cycle is shown outside the circle. The proteins with double-arrows denote their function in coordinating both cycles. **Inside the circle**. At the late M and G1 phases, ORC, Cdc6 and Cdt1 recruit MCM helicases to the replication origins to form pre-replication complex (pre-RC). Once the pre-RC is assembled, the origin is licensed to replicate. Upon entry into the S phase, Cdc45 and GINS are recruited to the replication origins dependent on Dpb11, sld2 and sld3 under the regulations of CDK2/cyclin E and Cdc7 kinases. The phosphorylated MCM2-7 helicase, together with Cdc45 and GINS, forms a CMG complex and functions to unwind the DNA replication origin site. Subsequently, Pol ε and Pol δ are recruited to the replication fork, and DNA replication initiates. The replicated DNA duplexes are held together by cohesin in the G2 phase and separate in mitosis; **Outside the circle**. During the G1/S transition in the same cell cycle, centrosome duplication initiates from centriole disengagement and takes place during the S phase. CDK2/cyclin E activity is required for centrosome duplication initiation. The replication licensing factors ORC1, geminin and maybe the others function by preventing the centrosome re-duplication after centrosome duplication initiation. Centriole elongation and maturation occur during the S and G2 phases. At the G2-M phase, the duplicated centrosomes are segregated to form the poles of the bipolar spindles to execute mitosis.

In addition to centrosome-localized proteins which may be involved in the licensing of the centrosome cycle, some other regulators including the DNA replication licensing system proteins may also participate in the licensing process of the centrosome cycle.

2.1.2 The roles of the DNA replication licensing system proteins in Centrosome duplication

Accumulated evidences show that several DNA licensing system proteins and regulators also play important roles in the centrosome duplication licensing system. ORC2, one of the origin recognizing complex proteins for DNA replication initiation is reported to localize to centrosomes throughout the cell cycle. ORC2 depletion leads to abnormal centrosome copy numbers, chromosomes misalignment and multipolar spindle in addition to DNA replication defects (Prasanth et al. 2004). In addition, transfected ORC1 is also found to localize to centrosomes. When co-expressed with the cyclin A in cells, the centrosomal localized proportion of the transfected ORC1 is elevated. ORC1 controls centrosome duplication through cyclin E to prevent reduplication of centriole and centrosomes. Depletion of ORC1 results in increased cyclin E level and cyclin E-dependent centriole reduplication. Accordingly, cyclin E can override the ORC1 inhibition of centrosome reduplication, rather than cyclin A or cyclin B. Simultaneous depletion of cyclin E and ORC1 inhibits the reduplication of centrioles caused by ORC1 depletion (Hemerly et al. 2009). Moreover, MCM5 also localizes to centrosomes depending on its interaction with CLS domain of cyclin E and prevents centrosome over-duplication in S phase-arrested cells by interacting with cyclin E (Ferguson and Maller 2008).

Geminin is a DNA replication licensing inhibitor. Through targeting Cdt1 and interfering with Cdt1-MCM interaction, geminin prevents the recruitment of MCM2-7 by Cdt1 to the chromatin. Geminin is targeted for destruction by APC in M phase (McGarry and Kirschner 1998) and accumulates in late G1 phase, S phase and G2 phase when APC is inactivated. Consequently, DNA replication licensing is prohibited in S phase and G2 phase largely by the geminin inhibiting mechanism in metazoans (Wohlschlegel et al. 2000). Depletion of geminin leads to substantial re-replication in primary cells and mouse embryos (Melixetian et al. 2004, Gonzalez et al. 2006).

Recent studies show that DNA replication licensing inhibitor geminin might also function in the centrosome duplication licensing system as an inhibitor. Geminin-depleted cells show over-duplication of centrosomes without the passage through mitosis, suggesting that geminin might function as a licensing inhibitor of centrosome duplication in a similar manner to its function in DNA replication licensing during S and G2 phase (Tachibana et al. 2005). We further found that geminin is also localized to centrosomes through the mediation of Arp1, one subunit of the dynein-dynactin complex. The centrosomal localization of geminin is dependent on the integrity of the dynein-dynactin complex and intact microtubules. The coiled-coil domain of geminin is responsible for its centrosome localization and interaction with Arp1 and is required for the inhibition of centrosome re-duplication (Lu et al. 2009). Although a number of reports (Hemerly et al. 2009, Ferguson and Maller 2008, Tachibana et al. 2005, Lu et al. 2009) indicate that the same partners in DNA licensing play roles in centrosome duplication, their functional cooperation in centrosome duplication and preventing re-duplication are not yet described.

2.1.3 The roles of the key regulators of the DNA replication licensing system in centrosome duplication

The key regulators that prevent DNA re-replication, such as the S phase kinase CDK2, also regulate centrosome duplication and reduplication. High CDK2 activity in S phase prevents the pre-RC reassembly through different ways in different organisms. In yeast, the rising

CDK2 activity at the onset of the S phase prevents DNA replication relicensing by targeting and inactivating all the initiation proteins of the licensing system in different ways. ORC2 and ORC6 are phosphorylated and inhibited by CDK2 (Nguyen, Co and Li 2001). Cdc6 in *S. cerevisiae* (or Cdc18 in *S. pombe*) is phosphorylated by CDK2 and subsequently degrades in S phase after licensing (Jallepalli et al. 1997, Elsasser et al. 1999). Cdt1 in *S. pombe* is subject to degradation following CDK2 phosphorylation with a similar fate to Cdc6. In *S. cerevisiae*, MCM2-7 exports out of the nucleus by CDK2 phosphorylation (Nguyen et al. 2000). Cdt1 is also excluded from the nucleus by association with MCM2-7 during S, G2 phases and early mitosis (Tanaka and Diffley 2002). All these CDK2 dependent controls prevent the access of these licensing factors to the chromatins and thus prevent relicensing during the cell cycle effectively. These controls by CDK2 are redundant, for all the controls have to be destroyed simultaneously in order to induce significant re-replication (Nguyen et al. 2000). In metazoans cells, CDK2/cyclin A interacts with and phosphorylates ORC1 (Mendez et al. 2002). Excess Cdc6 is translocated to the cytoplasm in the S phase due to CDK2 phosphorylation (Saha et al. 1998). Cdt1 is targeted for destruction via the SCF^{skp2} ubiquitin pathway by CDK2 phosphorylation (Takeda, Parvin and Dutta 2005). There is evidence suggesting that the phosphorylation of proteins by cyclin A-CDK1/CDK2 is responsible for blocking re-replication in Emi (early mitotic inhibitor) depletion induced re-replication (Machida and Dutta 2007).

Cyclin E and cyclin A, the activators of CDK2, have also been implicated in regulating centrosome duplication by targeting likely centrosome duplication licensing proteins and coupling the initiation of centrosome duplication and DNA replication initiation. Cyclin E localizes at the centrosome through its centrosome localization signal (CLS), and CDK2/cyclin E activity is required for centrosome duplication. Studies in S phase frog egg extract support multiple rounds of centrosome reproduction and found that inactivation of CDK2/cyclin E blocks centrosome reduplication (Hinchcliffe et al. 1999, Matsumoto and Maller 2004). Notably, B23 is identified to be a substrate of CDK2/cyclin E in centrosome duplication. CDK2/cyclin E phosphorylates threonine 199 of B23 and releases B23 from the unduplicated centrosomes to initiate centrosome duplication (Okuda et al. 2000, Tokuyama et al. 2001). Besides, cyclin E interacts directly with MCM5 through its CLS domain and recruits MCM5 to the centrosomes. Over-expressing MCM5 or the domain of MCM5 which is responsible for cyclin E interaction inhibits the centrosome re-duplication of S phase arrested cells (Ferguson and Maller 2008). All these data indicate that CDK2/cyclin E functions in centrosome duplication. The possible mechanism will be that, at the late G1 phase, CDK2/cyclin E phosphorylates and releases its substrates including B23 from the unduplicated centrosome to initiate centrosome duplication; during the progress of the centrosome duplication in the S phase, CDK2/cyclin E activity is not needed and suppressed by another series of proteins such as ORC1 and MCM5 as reported (Hemerly et al. 2009, Ferguson and Maller 2008). So far the reported inhibitor proteins for CDK2/cyclin E are mostly DNA replication licensing proteins. These inhibitor proteins, which are either promoted by CDK2/cyclin A to localize at the centrosome, such as ORC1, or directly phosphorylated and recruited to centrosome by CDK2/cyclin E such as MCM5, are enriched at the centrosomes to suppress CDK2/cyclin E activity and prevent centrosome reduplication (Figure 2). Accordingly, depletion of these proteins such as ORC1, ORC2 and geminin leads to centrosome reduplication and multiple centrosome copy numbers

(Hemerly et al. 2009, Prasanth et al. 2004, Tachibana et al. 2005). Notably, it has been demonstrated that centrosome reduplication by ORC1 depletion is in a cyclin E dependent way, and cyclin E could override the prevention of ORC1 on centrosome over-duplication (Hemerly et al. 2009). Depletion of ORC2 and geminin also resulted in centrosome reduplication (Prasanth et al. 2004, Tachibana et al. 2005). It is not clear if ORC2 and geminin cooperate with cyclin E to regulate centrosome duplication. In contrast to their licensing roles in DNA replication, ORC1, geminin, MCM5 and so on, take an inhibitory role for centrosome over-duplication. The fact that overexpression of these proteins could inhibit centrosome re-duplication in S phase arrested cells is probably by suppressing the constant high CDK2/cyclin E activity in S phase-arrested cells.

The possible mechanism of centrosome duplication initiation and prevention of centrosome reduplication involves two subsets of proteins and is likely to be separated into two steps. One subset of the licensing proteins including B23 associates with the unduplicated centrosome and licenses it to duplicate. Upon phosphorylation by CDK2/cyclin E, the licensing proteins are dissociated from the centrosome to allow it to initiate duplication. Persistent association of these proteins with the centrosome will inhibit the initiation of centrosome duplication. Another subset of licensing proteins for centrosome duplication plays an inhibitory role to prevent relicensing of the centrosome duplication, probably by suppressing the kinase activity of CDK2/cyclin E (Figure 2). It is likely that this subset of proteins, mostly the DNA replication licensing proteins including ORC1, ORC2, MCM5 and geminin, coordinates DNA replication and centrosome duplication in the same cell cycle. CDK2/cyclin A is also required for centrosome duplication. Depletion of CDK2 or cyclin A and cyclin E abolishes centriole separation (Lacey, Jackson and Stearns 1999). Cyclin A also directly interacts with MCM5 and ORC1. Persistent centrosome localization of MCM5 is dependent on cyclin A (Ferguson, Pascreau and Maller 2010). These results indicate that cyclin E and cyclin A sequentially function in centrosome duplication. CDK2/cyclin E initiates centrosome duplication by phosphorylating its substrates, such as B23. CDK2/cyclin A subsequently prevents centrosome re-duplication by phosphorylating MCM5, ORC1 and possibly additional DNA replication licensing proteins and targeting them to the centrosome to prevent it from reduplication through suppressing CDK2/Cycin E activity (Figure 2). Moreover, Rb and E2F are also involved in both DNA replication and centrosome duplication (Meraldi et al. 1999). These functions may be performed by regulating gene transcription of DNA replication licensing proteins.

In summary, the centrosome duplication cycle and the DNA replication cycle in a cell are coordinated tightly to occur once and only once per cell cycle. These two cycles take place in the same time window with initiation during the late G1 phase, proceeding in the S phase and inhibition of re-duplication in S and G2 phases. They use the same licensing proteins and are subject to the same regulators of CDK2/cyclin E and CDK2/cyclin A. The mechanism for DNA replication licensing is well understood, while the detailed mechanism for centrosome duplication licensing and initiation remains unclear. Despite the identification of several DNA replication licensing proteins and kinases involved in centrosome duplication, how these licensing proteins and kinases additionally regulate centrosome duplication licensing and duplication processes, especially how cyclin E and cyclin A in the S phase sequentially regulate the same apparatus of DNA replication licensing proteins to coordinate the DNA replication and the centrosome duplication, remains largely unknown.

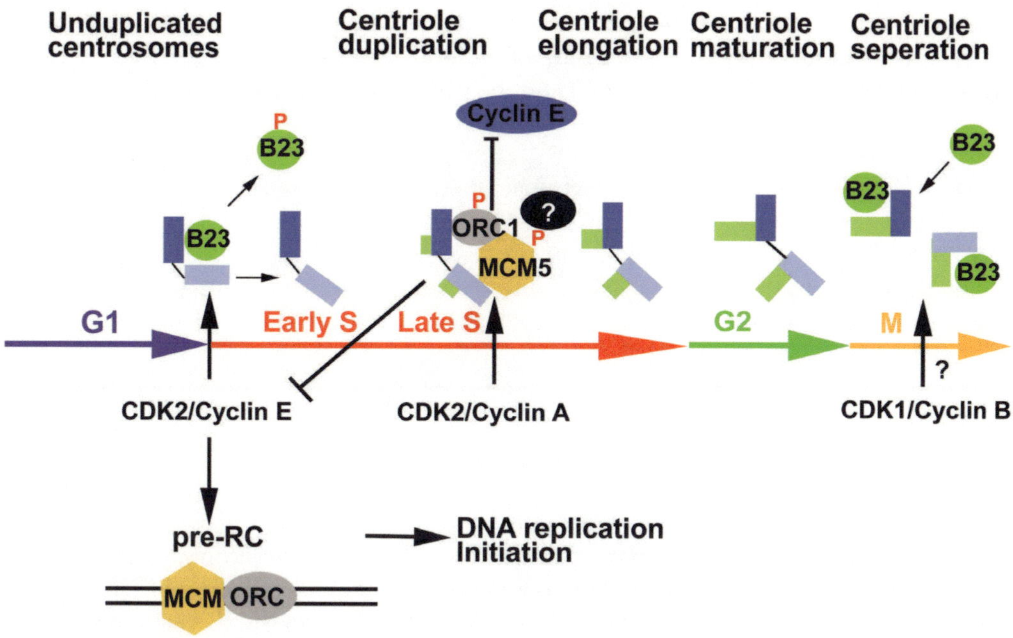

Fig. 2. An emerging model for centrosome duplication licensing
Centrosome duplication initiates during the late G1 phase. CDK2/cyclin E phosphorylates its substrates including B23 to release them from the unduplicated centrosome to initiate centrosome duplication. CDK2/cyclin E also promotes the transition of pre-RC to pre-IC and activates DNA replication initiation along with initiation of centrosome duplication. During the process of centrosome duplication in S phase, CDK2/cyclin A comes to prevent centrosome re-duplication by phosphorylating MCM5, ORC1 and other DNA replication licensing proteins and targeting them to the centrosome to suppress the local CDK2/Cycin E activity. Once the centrosomes separated after duplication in mitosis, B23 relocalizes to the centrosomes to prepare for a new round of duplication in the next cell cycle, possibly regulated by CDK1/cyclin B phosphorylation.

2.2 The coordination of mitotic events and DNA replication

To ensure genomic integrity, the cell enters mitosis only when it has finished its DNA replication. This coordination between DNA replication and mitosis is controlled partially by checkpoints, including the "intra-S phase checkpoint" when DNA damage occurs and the "S-M checkpoint" in a normal cell cycle which ensures DNA replication completes before mitotic entry. Accumulating evidences show that lack of DNA replication licensing proteins causes aberrant mitotic cells and implicate that the DNA replication licensing proteins directly coordinate both DNA replication and mitosis.

2.2.1 The mitosis events and their key regulators

Mitosis is the process by which a eukaryotic cell segregates its chromosomes in its nucleus into two genetically identical daughter sets to two nuclei. The mitosis is generally followed by cytokinesis to faithfully separate the two nuclei and the cytoplasm with its organelles and cell membranes into daughter cells. This process of the mitosis is achieved by elaborate regulatory mechanisms and apparatus assembly during the process. The central molecular engines coordinating mitosis are a series of mitotic kinases, including CDK1/cyclin B, Aurora kinase and Polo-like kinase (Plks) and their partner phosphotases (Figure 3).

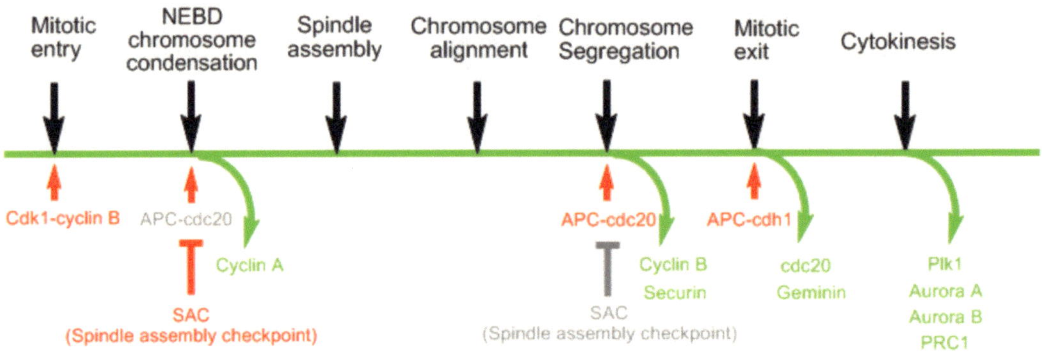

Fig. 3. The mitotic events and its key regulators
The orderly activation and destruction of different regulators and accordingly the orderly progression of the mitotic events are shown. Red arrows denote the activated CDK or APC; green arrows denote degraded proteins. At mitotic entry, CDK1-cyclin B is activated. During the nuclear envelope breakdown (NEBD), APC-cdc20 is partially activated to degrade cyclin A, yet is mostly inhibited by Spindle assembly checkpoint (SAC) (the red SAC stands for the activated SAC and the grey APC-cdc20 stands for the inhibited APC-cdc20). After the onset of the anaphase, most SAC proteins are inactivated, while the APC-cdc20 is activated to degrade its substrate proteins including cyclin B and securin (the red APC-cdc20 stands for the activated APC-cdc20 and the grey SAC for the inactivated SAC). Soon after securin degradation, separase activity is released to cleave cohesin and initiate segregation of the sister-chromatids. Cyclin B1 degradation inactivates CDK1 and APC-cdc20, and activates the second APC activator cdh1. APC-cdh1 then targets additional substrates including cdc20 and geminin for degradation during mitotic exit. During cytokinesis, Plk1, Aurora kinases and PRC1 are degraded by APC-cdh1.

CDK1 is activated by cyclin B. Cyclin B translocates into the nucleus after the G2 phase checkpoint prior to mitosis and triggers mitotic entry initiation (Toyoshima-Morimoto et al. 2001). Cyclin B is not destroyed until anaphase by the anaphase promoting complex or cyclosome (APC/C). During the interval from mitotic entry to anaphase, active CDK1/cyclin B promotes chromosome condensation, spindle assembly and chromosome segregation sequentially, and prevents the onset of cytokinesis until anaphase. Through cyclin B1 degradation by APC/C during the transition from metaphase to anaphase, CDK1 is inactivated, and accordingly, mitotic exit and cytokinesis of the cell take place to generate the two genetically identical daughter cells (Malumbres and Barbacid 2009).

Aurora kinases are a family of serine–threonine protein kinases, consisting of Aurora A, Aurora B and Aurora C in mammals. Aurora A localizes to centrosomes during the G2 phase and mitosis and distributes to the mitotic spindle in mitosis. In contrast, Aurora B localizes to centromeres and chromosome arms in early mitosis, concentrates further on centromeres in prometaphase, relocates to spindle midzone in anaphase and concentrates at the midbody of chromosomes at telophase and cytokinesis. Both Aurora A and Aurora B are targets of APC/C and are destructed during mitotic exit (Littlepage and Ruderman 2002,

Stewart and Fang 2005). Aurora A promotes centrosome maturation and separation, spindle assembly and mitotic entry, while Aurora B regulates chromosome condensation and segregation, metaphase to anaphase transition and cytokinesis. Despite the high similarity in protein sequences and structures between Aurora A and B, Aurora kinases exhibit different subcellular localization and correspondingly divergent functions in mitotic events. We found that a single amino acid residue change is adequate to convert Aurora A to Aurora B in partners binding and cellular function (Fu et al. 2009).

Polo-like kinases (Plks) also comprise a family of serine/threonine kinases. The family members include Plk1, Plk2, Plk3 and Plk4 in vertebrates, although they differ in structure and function. The Plk protein consists of a Polo-box domain (PBD) responsible for substrate recognition and a kinase domain for catalyzing its substrate. Plk1 is the best known member of the Plks (Sunkel and Glover 1988, Llamazares et al. 1991, Strebhardt and Ullrich 2006). It functions essentially in mitosis, regulating a variety of the mitosis events including bipolar spindle formation, chromosome segregation, centrosome maturation, CDK1 activation, APC regulation and cytokinesis execution. During mitotic exit, Plk1 is degraded by APC-cdh1 (Lindon and Pines 2004). Plk1 recognizes its substrates by consensus recognition sequences in the PBD domain and usually requires a phosphopriming by prime kinases such as CDKs and mitogen-activated protein kinase. From prophase to metaphase, Plk1 phosphorylates INCENP, BUB1 and Nedd1 after phosphopriming by CDK1 (Zhang et al. 2009). However, from anaphase to cytokinesis when CDK1 is inactive, Plk1 promotes its own recognition of the substrates such as central spindle proteins MKLP2 and PRC1 (Carmena et al. 1998).

2.2.2 The roles of the checkpoints in coordination of DNA replication with mitosis

Coordination between DNA replication and mitosis is executed by different checkpoints. When the DNA double strand break (DSB) occurs in S phase, unfired replication origins are specifically inhibited by "intra-S phase checkpoint" to acquire S phase delay. Two pathways are involved in the intra-S phase checkpoint. One is the ATM-MDC1-MRN (especially NBS1) dependent phosphorylation of SMC1 (structural maintenance of chromosomes-1) (Yazdi et al. 2002), although how the phosphorylated SMC1 interferes with DNA replication is unclear. Another one is ATM/ATR-mediated Cdc25A phosphatase proteolysis that inhibits CDK2-cyclin E/cyclin A kinase activity. The inhibited CDK2-cyclin E/cyclin A in turn prevents the loading of Cdc45, the key co-activator of DNA helicase MCM 2-7, to the unfired replication origins and thereby inhibits the DNA replication (Falck et al. 2002).

Another "DNA replication checkpoint" also functions during DNA damage in S phase by stalling the replication fork to delay the S phase. This checkpoint is mainly mediated by ATR/CHK1 activation. Although the mechanism for this checkpoint and the substrates of ATR/CHK1 are poorly understood, the ATR/CHK1-dependent CDK2-cyclin E/cyclin A inhibition through Cdc25A degradation at least partially contributes to the slow down of the overall replication rates. Many DNA replication proteins at the replication forks including RPC (replication factor C complex), RPA1/2, the MCM2-7 complex, MCM10 and several DNA polymerases are phosphorylated by ATR (Cortez, Glick and Elledge 2004, Liu, Kuo and Melendy 2006); however, the functions of these phosphorylation events are largely unclear.

Besides the checkpoints in response to DNA damage mentioned above, the "S-M checkpoint" is also an intrinsic mechanism required for normal cell cycle progression. The S-M checkpoint ensures that cells faithfully finish genome replication before entry into mitosis. The S-M checkpoint is mediated by ATR and prevents mitotic entry by inhibiting

CDK1/cyclin B kinase activity. In *Xenopus* egg extracts, ATR depletion may result in early mitotic entry without completing DNA replication (Hekmat-Nejad et al. 2000). CHK1-Knocking out in ES cells also causes premature mitotic entry with incomplete DNA replication (Niida et al. 2005). Although the precise pathway by which ATR functions in the unperturbed S phase is largely unknown, it is noticeable that the ATR/CHK1 pathway can limit excessive firing of replication origins (Shechter, Costanzo and Gautier 2004) and that the inhibition of CHK1 causes increased origin firing and Cdc45 loading (Syljuasen et al. 2005). It will be intriguing in the future to reveal how the checkpoint proteins which function in DNA damage checkpoint regulate normal DNA replication and prevent premature entry into mitosis.

2.2.3 The roles of DNA replication licensing proteins in coordination of DNA replication with mitosis

Many DNA replication licensing proteins play multiple roles in coordinating DNA replication and mitosis in addition to DNA replication licensing. As reported, depletion of the DNA licensing machinery proteins ORC1, ORC2, ORC6 and geminin results in aberrant mitosis. Depletion of ORC1 by siRNA leads to mitotic arrest and centrosome amplification. ORC1 depletion also results in reduced MCM3 loading onto chromatin and activates DNA damage responses (Hemerly et al. 2009). Depletion of ORC2 also leads to increased mitotic cells and over-amplified centrosomes, abnormal chromosomes condensation, defects of chromosomes allignment and multipolar spindles in mitosis (Prasanth et al. 2004). ORC6, also an origin recognition complex protein, localizes to the kinetochores during mitosis and to the midbody region of the chromosome during cytokinesis (Prasanth, Prasanth and Stillman 2002). ORC6 depletion leads to decreased DNA replication, multipolar spindles, misalignment chromosomes, cytokinesis failure and multinucleated cells (Prasanth et al. 2002, Bernal and Venkitaraman 2011), indicating that ORC6 might coordinate DNA replication, chromosomes segregation and cytokinesis.

Geminin and Cdc6 also play important roles in coordinating DNA replication and mitosis. Depletion of geminin results in multiple mitotic defects in addition to DNA replication defects. Geminin inactivation causes overduplicated centrosomes in one cell cycle (Melixetian et al. 2004). When using caffeine to override the G2-M checkpoint and induce mitosis, geminin-depleted cells showed bipolar spindles with multiple centrosomes and unattached chromosomes or multipolar spindles with multiple centrosomes (Tachibana et al. 2005). Cdc6 in yeast can prevent cells from progressing into mitosis before maturation by directly interacting with CDK1 and inhibiting its kinase activity (Weinreich et al. 2001). Cdc6 also coordinates DNA replication and mitosis in human cells. Overexpressed Cdc6 causes checkpoint kinase Chk1 to be phosphorylated and activated to prevent premature mitotic entry before DNA replication is completed (Clay-Farrace et al. 2003) (Figure 4). Cdc6 also plays important roles in mitosis. Depletion of Cdc6 causes abnormal spindles, misaligned chromosomes and multinucleated cells in addition to defects of DNA replication; however, no Chk1 activation was detected upon Cdc6 depletion (Lau et al. 2006). Depletion of Cdc6 in mouse oocytes also leads to spindle assembly defects (Anger, Stein and Schultz 2005). Cdc6 is phosphorylated by Plk1 at T37 in mitosis and colocalizes with Plk1 to the central spindle in anaphase. Phosphorylation of Cdc6 by Plk1 promotes its interaction with CDK1 and inhibition of CDK1 activity, releases the separase activity and chromosome segregation (Yim and Erikson 2010) (Figure 4).

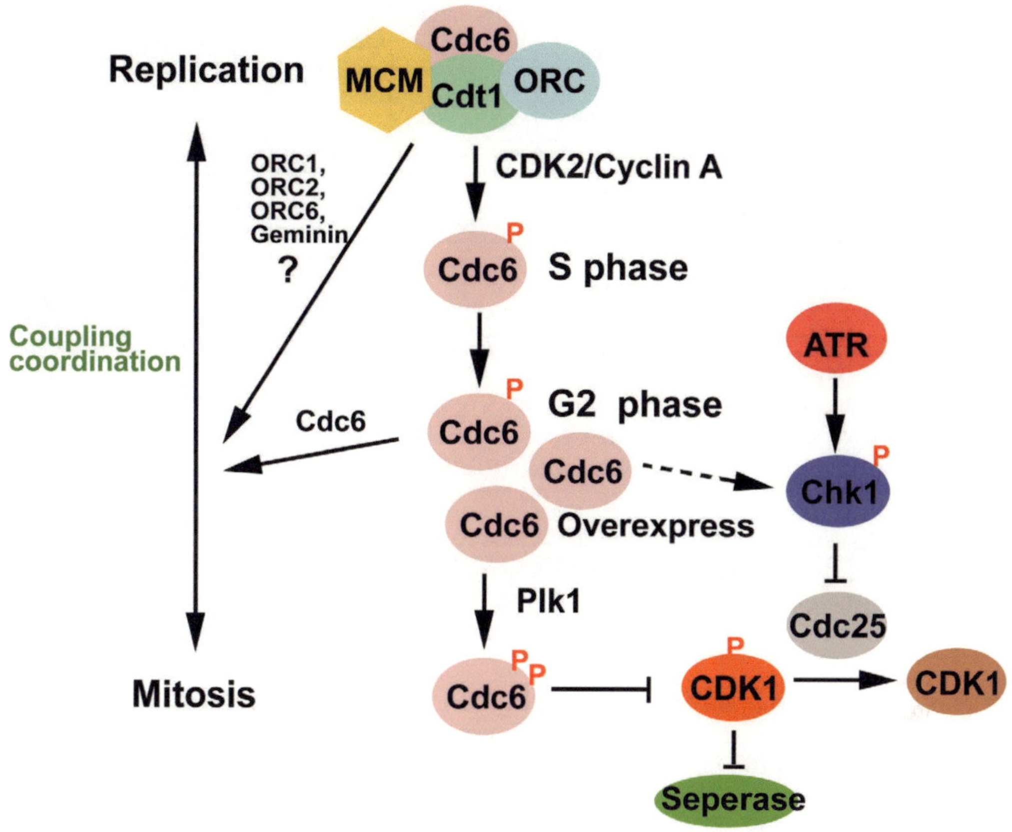

Fig. 4. The coordination of DNA replication and mitosis by DNA replication licensing proteins
DNA replication licensing protein Cdc6 is phosphorylated during the S phase by CDK2/cyclin A. Aberrant overexpression of Cdc6 in the G2 phase activates Chk1 and prevents mitotic entry. In mitosis, Plk1 phosphorylates Cdc6 and promotes the interaction between Cdc6 and CDK1. The phosphorylated Cdc6 promotes chromosome segregation by inhibiting CDK1 and the release of separase activity. Depletion of the other DNA replication licensing proteins can also lead to multiple mitotic defects.

In conclusion, in addition to the roles in DNA replication, most DNA licensing machinery proteins function in multiple mitotic events to coordinate DNA replication and mitosis. These functions are summarized in Table 1. As shown in Table 1, the defects of DNA replication and mitosis progression caused by depletion of DNA replication licensing proteins indicate that DNA replication and mitotic events are coordinated directly by the same machinery, although the mechanisms are largely unknown. Moreover, the Rb-E2F pathway which targets transcription of DNA replication licensing proteins was important for coupling DNA replication with mitosis. Rb depletion in the adult mouse liver led to aberrant accumulation of DNA replication licensing proteins, over-replication of DNA without mitotic condensation and decreased cyclin B1 level at G2/M checkpoint (Bourgo et al. 2011).

Depletion of DNA replication licensing proteins	Increase of mitotic cells	Centrosome amplifi-cation	Abnormal chromo-somes conden-sation	Misallign-ment chromo-somes	Multipolar spindles	Cytokinesis	Multi-nucleated cells
ORC1	+	+	*	*	*	*	*
ORC2	+	+	+	+	+	*	*
ORC6	*	*	*	+	+	+	+
Cdc6	*	*	*	+	+	+	+
geminin	*	+	*	+	+	*	*

Table 1. Mitotic defects caused by the depletion of DNA replication licensing proteins (+ denotes "Yes"; * denotes "Not reported")

It has been reported that depletion of many DNA replication licensing proteins can lead to multiple mitotic defects. The phenomena caused by depletion of the respectively DNA replication licensing proteins are summarized in Table 1.

2.3 The coordination of transcription and DNA replication

DNA replication and transcription are fundamental processes essential for normal cell cycle progression and cell proliferation. They are both carried out by assembled protein complexes machinery proceeding at DNA templates.

2.3.1 The pre-initiation complex assembly of RNA transcription and DNA replication

DNA replication can be divided into two stages: the pre-RC assembly with licensing at replication origins; and the pre-IC (pre-initiation complex) assembly with replication origin firing. ORC, Cdc6 and Cdt1 are assembled at origins to recruit MCM helicases to form pre-RC at origins. After replication initiation in S phase, MCM2-7 proteins are displaced from origins and proceed along with replication forks as the DNA helicase (Labib, Tercero and Diffley 2000). The pre-RC assembly and the licensing on origins mark these origins as candidates for DNA replication initiation. Activation of DNA replication initiation on origins, which is also named "origin firing", requires additional factors assembled to pre-RC to form pre-IC. CDK2 and DDK (Dbf4-dependent cdc7 kinase) promote MCM to form a CMG complex with GINS (a complex of Sld5-Psf1-Psf2-Psf3) and Cdc45 at origins. With the assembly of the CMG complex, the DNA helicase activity is performed, the DNA replication origin is melted and DNA unwinding is initiated (Figure 5).

Recruitment of Cdc45 to replication origins plays a key role for the subsequent initiation complex formation and DNA polymerase loading. DNA unwinds and RPA binds to the single strand DNA only in the presence of Cdc45. RPA binding is required for DNA polymerase α to load to the chromatin. The interaction between Cdc45 and DNA polymerase α is also important for the loading of DNA polymerase α (Mimura et al. 2000). The loading of leading strand processive polymerase ε also depends on Cdc45 (Mimura et al. 2000, Masumoto, Sugino and Araki 2000). In the lagging strand, after recruitment, DNA polymerase α begins to synthesize short nascent DNA segments following primer RNA synthesis. Then, replication factor C (RFC) recognizes nascent DNA 3′ end and functions as a clamp loader to load PCNA (proliferating cell nuclear antigen). Finally, the lagging strand processive polymerase δ is loaded to chromatin by PCNA. Subsequently, DNA replication proceeds from origins as replication forks with processive DNA polymerase (Figure 5).

Transcriptions of chromatin includes the transcription of rRNA genes by RNA polymerases (Pols) I, protein-encoding genes by Pol II and short untranslated genes of 5S rRNA, tRNA and so on by Pol III. Pol I transcription contributes up to about 70% of the nuclear transcription in the growing cells, Pol II transcription takes up to about 20% and Pol III transcription takes up to about 10%. Pols execute transcription of genes from the promoter regions of respective genes. Similar to DNA polymerases, RNA polymerases have no intrinsic ability to recognize specific DNA sequences of the promoters. A pre-initiation complex (PIC) which is made up of transcription factors is required to assemble at the promoter to recruit RNA polymerases. Complexes of TBP (TATA-box binding protein) and TBP-associated factors (TAF) assembled at the promoter regions are required for the initiation of transcription by all three Pols, despite the variation of respective TAFs. In pol II transcription, the TBP-TAF complex TFIID recognizes the TATA boxes and the promoter sequences. Interactions between TAFs and Pol II recruit Pol II and other factors to form the PIC and then Pol II transcription initiates (Verrijzer and Tjian 1996). Pol III is recruited to the promoters by its TBP-TAF complex TFIIIB and the PIC-containing Pol III is assembled to initiate the Pol III transcription (Geiduschek and Kassavetis 2001, Schramm and Hernandez 2002). Distinct from Pol II and Pol III transcription, Pol I transcription is confined to the nucleolus and is activated by PIC assembly. UBF (upstream binding factor), which binds to the UCE (upstream control element) and core promoter, appears to be the first step in PIC formation, followed by the recruitment of the TBP-TAF complex (Learned et al. 1986, Bell et al. 1988). SL1 (promoter-selectivity factor, mouse TIF-IB) is the TBP-TAF complex of Pol I. SL1 recruits Pol I to the promoter through the interaction of TIF-IA with Pol I (Miller et al. 2001). After PIC assembly, Pol I transcription initiates from the promoter of the rRNA genes. Therefore, DNA replication initiation and RNA transcription initiation share the mechanisms that recruit polymerases by an orderly assembled protein complex (Figure 5). Coordination between the two fundamental assembly events and the coupling between DNA replication and RNA transcription in cycling cells to coordinate cell growth are an intriguing issue; however, the mechanism remains to be elucidated.

2.3.2 The roles of DNA replication initiation proteins in RNA transcription

It has been noticed that MCM proteins are involved in RNA transcription, which implicates the coordination of RNA transcription and DNA replication (Figure 5). MCM proteins might be components of the Pol II transcriptional apparatus, as MCM2 and other MCMs can be co-purified with Pol II and other general transcription factors in the holoenzyme complex of *Xenopus* oocytes and HeLa cells. Moreover, microinjection of MCM2 antibody specifically inhibits Pol II transcription in *Xenopus* oocytes. The association of MCMs with the holoenzyme partly depends on its amino acids 168-230 and the C-terminal domain of Pol II (Yankulov et al. 1999). Mutations in amino acids 169-212 of MCM2 disrupt its binding to Pol II and to general transcription factors *in vivo* (Holland et al. 2002). MCM2 and MCM5 are also required for general transcription, and their depletion may lead to transcription defects. MCM2-7 proteins also co-localize with Pol II on constitutively transcribing genes. Notably, MCM5 is required for the elongation of Pol II. Moreover, MCM5 functions in Pol II transcription and requires integrity of the MCM complex and helicase activity of MCM5 (Snyder, Huang and Zhang 2009). MCM also functions in cytokine-induced gene transcription activation. Stat1 translocates into the nucleus in response to IFN-γ and recruits MCM3 and MCM5 to enhance the stat1-mediated transcription activation. The amino acids R732 and K734 of MCM5 are important residues required for the interaction with Stat1 and stat1-mediated transcription activation. The enhancement of Stat1-mediated transcription activation also requires ATPase activity and helicase activity of MCM5 (DaFonseca, Shu and Zhang 2001). Further study (Snyder, He and Zhang 2005) shows that MCM5 and other members of MCMs are recruited directly to the gene promoters targeted by Stat1 upon cytokine stimulation. MCMs move along with Pol II during transcription elongation. Furthermore, MCM5 is essential for Stat1-targeted gene transcription elongation. The domain responsible for MCM5 and stat1 interaction is also identified, and expression of this domain interferes with the interaction between MCM5 and Stat1 and represses Stat1 mediated transcription (Snyder et al. 2005). In conclusion, the DNA licensing machinery MCM proteins also play important roles in the activation of RNA transcription. It is possible that other DNA licensing machinery proteins are also involved in the transcription process and coordinate DNA replication and RNA transcription.

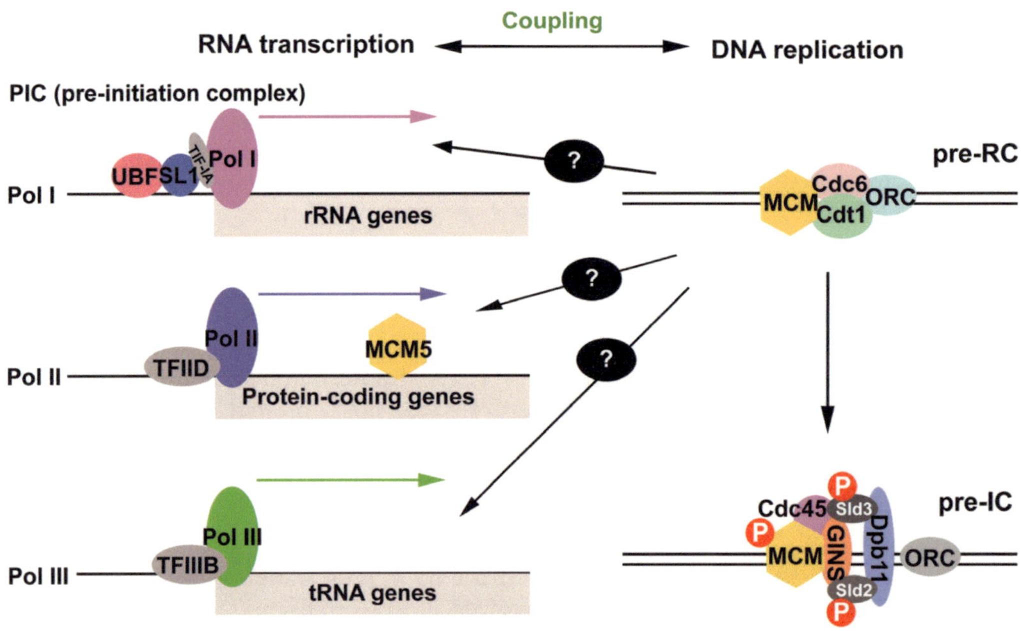

Fig. 5. Coordination of RNA transcription and DNA replication by DNA replication licensing proteins
ORCs, Cdc6 and Cdt1 are assembled at the DNA replication origins to recruit MCM helicases to form the pre-RC. The activation of DNA replication initiation at the origins, known as the "origin firing", requires additional factors to be recruited to the pre-RC to from the pre-IC. Polymerases are recruited by an orderly assembled protein complex in similar ways in both DNA replication and RNA transcription. The pre-initiation complex (PIC) assembly at the promoter is required for the recruitment of the RNA polymerases. The complex assembly of TBP and TBP-associated factors (TAF) at the promoter regions are required for the initiation of transcription by all three Pols, with variation of respective TAFs of SL1 in Pol I transcription, TFIID in Pol II transcription and TFIIIB in Pol III transcription. Pol I is recruited by UBF and SL1 through interaction with TIF-IA of the SL1 complex. DNA replication licensing protein MCM5 is required for Pol II transcription and elongation. It is possible that other DNA replication licensing machinery proteins are involved in RNA transcription and couple these two fundamental events of RNA transcription and DNA replication (indicated in by the question marks).

3. Conclusion

DNA replication, centrosome duplication and mitosis are the basic events in a cell cycle to ensure proper cell division and proliferation. RNA transcription is also a basic event which takes place throughout the whole cell cycle to provide continuous protein synthesis. In this chapter, we reviewed evidence for coordination between these basic events. Centrosome duplication and DNA replication use the same licensing proteins and are subject to the same regulators of CDK2/cyclin E and CDK2/cyclin A. Similarly, in correlation with mitosis, several DNA licensing machinery proteins have been demonstrated to function in multiple mitotic events and coordinate DNA replication and mitotic entry. Besides, DNA replication initiation proteins such as MCM proteins are involved in RNA transcription and might coordinate RNA transcription and DNA replication. In summary, accumulated evidence shows that the same set of regulators is implied in regulating these connected cell cycle events to ensure genomic integrity and sheds lights on the molecular mechanisms connecting these cell cycle events.

4. Acknowledgments

We thank all the other members of our laboratory for useful comments. This work was supported by funds provided to C.Z. from the National Natural Science Foundation of China (NSFC) (30900726, 31071188, 30721064, 31030044 and 90913021) and the State Key Basic Research and Development Plan (2006CB910101, 2007CB914502 and 2010CB833705). All correspondence should be addressed to Chuanmao Zhang (E-mail: zhangcm@pku.edu.cn).

5. References

Alvey, P. L. (1985). An investigation of the centriole cycle using 3T3 and CHO cells. J Cell Sci, Vol.78, pp. 147-62.

Anger, M., P. Stein & R. M. Schultz (2005). CDC6 requirement for spindle formation during maturation of mouse oocytes. Biol Reprod, Vol.72, pp. 188-94.

Bell, S. P. & A. Dutta (2002). DNA replication in eukaryotic cells. Annu Rev Biochem, Vol.71, pp. 333-74.

Bell, S. P., R. M. Learned, H. M. Jantzen & R. Tjian (1988). Functional cooperativity between transcription factors UBF1 and SL1 mediates human ribosomal RNA synthesis. Science, Vol.241, pp. 1192-7.

Bernal, J. A. & A. R. Venkitaraman (2011). A vertebrate N-end rule degron reveals that Orc6 is required in mitosis for daughter cell abscission. J Cell Biol, Vol.192, pp. 969-78.

Bettencourt-Dias, M., A. Rodrigues-Martins, L. Carpenter, M. Riparbelli, L. Lehmann, M. K. Gatt, N. Carmo, F. Balloux, G. Callaini & D. M. Glover (2005). SAK/PLK4 is required for centriole duplication and flagella development. Curr Biol, Vol.15, pp. 2199-207.

Bourgo, R. J., U. Ehmer, J. Sage & E. S. Knudsen (2011). RB deletion disrupts coordination between DNA replication licensing and mitotic entry in vivo. Mol Biol Cell, Vol.22, pp. 931-9.

Carmena, M., M. G. Riparbelli, G. Minestrini, A. M. Tavares, R. Adams, G. Callaini & D. M. Glover (1998). Drosophila polo kinase is required for cytokinesis. J Cell Biol, Vol.143, pp. 659-71.

Clay-Farrace, L., C. Pelizon, D. Santamaria, J. Pines & R. A. Laskey (2003). Human replication protein Cdc6 prevents mitosis through a checkpoint mechanism that implicates Chk1. EMBO J, Vol.22, pp. 704-12.

Cortez, D., G. Glick & S. J. Elledge (2004). Minichromosome maintenance proteins are direct targets of the ATM and ATR checkpoint kinases. Proc Natl Acad Sci U S A, Vol.101, pp. 10078-83.

DaFonseca, C. J., F. Shu & J. J. Zhang (2001). Identification of two residues in MCM5 critical for the assembly of MCM complexes and Stat1-mediated transcription activation in response to IFN-gamma. Proc Natl Acad Sci U S A, Vol.98, pp. 3034-9.

Dammermann, A., T. Muller-Reichert, L. Pelletier, B. Habermann, A. Desai & K. Oegema (2004). Centriole assembly requires both centriolar and pericentriolar material proteins. Dev Cell, Vol.7, pp. 815-29.

Elsasser, S., Y. Chi, P. Yang & J. L. Campbell (1999). Phosphorylation controls timing of Cdc6p destruction: A biochemical analysis. Mol Biol Cell, Vol.10, pp. 3263-77.

Falck, J., J. H. Petrini, B. R. Williams, J. Lukas & J. Bartek (2002). The DNA damage-dependent intra-S phase checkpoint is regulated by parallel pathways. Nat Genet, Vol.30, pp. 290-4.

Ferguson, R. L. & J. L. Maller (2008). Cyclin E-dependent localization of MCM5 regulates centrosome duplication. J Cell Sci, Vol.121, pp. 3224-32.

Ferguson, R. L., G. Pascreau & J. L. Maller (2010). The cyclin A centrosomal localization sequence recruits MCM5 and Orc1 to regulate centrosome reduplication. J Cell Sci, Vol.123, pp. 2743-9.

Fode, C., C. Binkert & J. W. Dennis (1996). Constitutive expression of murine Sak-a suppresses cell growth and induces multinucleation. Mol Cell Biol, Vol.16, pp. 4665-72.

Fu, J., M. Bian, J. Liu, Q. Jiang & C. Zhang (2009). A single amino acid change converts Aurora-A into Aurora-B-like kinase in terms of partner specificity and cellular function. Proc Natl Acad Sci U S A, Vol.106, pp. 6939-44.

Geiduschek, E. P. & G. A. Kassavetis (2001). The RNA polymerase III transcription apparatus. J Mol Biol, Vol.310, pp. 1-26.

Gonzalez, M. A., K. E. Tachibana, D. J. Adams, L. van der Weyden, M. Hemberger, N. Coleman, A. Bradley & R. A. Laskey (2006). Geminin is essential to prevent endoreduplication and to form pluripotent cells during mammalian development. Genes Dev, Vol.20, pp. 1880-4.

Habedanck, R., Y. D. Stierhof, C. J. Wilkinson & E. A. Nigg (2005). The Polo kinase Plk4 functions in centriole duplication. Nat Cell Biol, Vol.7, pp. 1140-6.

Hekmat-Nejad, M., Z. You, M. C. Yee, J. W. Newport & K. A. Cimprich (2000). Xenopus ATR is a replication-dependent chromatin-binding protein required for the DNA replication checkpoint. Curr Biol, Vol.10, pp. 1565-73.

Hemerly, A. S., S. G. Prasanth, K. Siddiqui & B. Stillman (2009). Orc1 controls centriole and centrosome copy number in human cells. Science, Vol.323, pp. 789-93.

Hinchcliffe, E. H., C. Li, E. A. Thompson, J. L. Maller & G. Sluder (1999). Requirement of Cdk2-cyclin E activity for repeated centrosome reproduction in Xenopus egg extracts. Science, Vol.283, pp. 851-4.

Holland, L., L. Gauthier, P. Bell-Rogers & K. Yankulov (2002). Distinct parts of minichromosome maintenance protein 2 associate with histone H3/H4 and RNA polymerase II holoenzyme. Eur J Biochem, Vol.269, pp. 5192-202.

Jallepalli, P. V., G. W. Brown, M. Muzi-Falconi, D. Tien & T. J. Kelly (1997). Regulation of the replication initiator protein p65cdc18 by CDK phosphorylation. Genes Dev, Vol.11, pp. 2767-79.

Kuriyama, R. & G. G. Borisy (1981). Centriole cycle in Chinese hamster ovary cells as determined by whole-mount electron microscopy. J Cell Biol, Vol.91, pp. 814-21.

Labib, K., J. A. Tercero & J. F. Diffley (2000). Uninterrupted MCM2-7 function required for DNA replication fork progression. Science, Vol.288, pp. 1643-7.

Lacey, K. R., P. K. Jackson & T. Stearns (1999). Cyclin-dependent kinase control of centrosome duplication. Proc Natl Acad Sci U S A, Vol.96, pp. 2817-22.

Lau, E., C. Zhu, R. T. Abraham & W. Jiang (2006). The functional role of Cdc6 in S-G2/M in mammalian cells. EMBO Rep, Vol.7, pp. 425-30.

Learned, R. M., T. K. Learned, M. M. Haltiner & R. T. Tjian (1986). Human rRNA transcription is modulated by the coordinate binding of two factors to an upstream control element. Cell, Vol.45, pp. 847-57.

Leidel, S., M. Delattre, L. Cerutti, K. Baumer & P. Gonczy (2005). SAS-6 defines a protein family required for centrosome duplication in C. elegans and in human cells. Nat Cell Biol, Vol.7, pp. 115-25.

Lindon, C. & J. Pines (2004). Ordered proteolysis in anaphase inactivates Plk1 to contribute to proper mitotic exit in human cells. J Cell Biol, Vol.164, pp. 233-41.

Littlepage, L. E. & J. V. Ruderman (2002). Identification of a new APC/C recognition domain, the A box, which is required for the Cdh1-dependent destruction of the kinase Aurora-A during mitotic exit. Genes Dev, Vol.16, pp. 2274-85.

Liu, J. S., S. R. Kuo & T. Melendy (2006). Phosphorylation of replication protein A by S-phase checkpoint kinases. DNA Repair (Amst), Vol.5, pp. 369-80.

Llamazares, S., A. Moreira, A. Tavares, C. Girdham, B. A. Spruce, C. Gonzalez, R. E. Karess, D. M. Glover & C. E. Sunkel (1991). polo encodes a protein kinase homolog required for mitosis in Drosophila. Genes Dev, Vol.5, pp. 2153-65.

Lu, F., R. Lan, H. Zhang, Q. Jiang & C. Zhang (2009). Geminin is partially localized to the centrosome and plays a role in proper centrosome duplication. Biol Cell, Vol.101, pp. 273-85.

Machida, Y. J. & A. Dutta (2007). The APC/C inhibitor, Emi1, is essential for prevention of rereplication. Genes Dev, Vol.21, pp. 184-94.

Malumbres, M. & M. Barbacid (2009). Cell cycle, CDKs and cancer: a changing paradigm. Nat Rev Cancer, Vol.9, pp. 153-66.

Masumoto, H., A. Sugino & H. Araki (2000). Dpb11 controls the association between DNA polymerases alpha and epsilon and the autonomously replicating sequence region of budding yeast. Mol Cell Biol, Vol.20, pp. 2809-17.

Matsumoto, Y. & J. L. Maller (2004). A centrosomal localization signal in cyclin E required for Cdk2-independent S phase entry. Science, Vol.306, pp. 885-8.

Mazia, D. (1987). The chromosome cycle and the centrosome cycle in the mitotic cycle. Int Rev Cytol, Vol.100, pp. 49-92.

McGarry, T. J. & M. W. Kirschner (1998). Geminin, an inhibitor of DNA replication, is degraded during mitosis. Cell, Vol.93, pp. 1043-53.

Melixetian, M., A. Ballabeni, L. Masiero, P. Gasparini, R. Zamponi, J. Bartek, J. Lukas & K. Helin (2004). Loss of Geminin induces rereplication in the presence of functional p53. J Cell Biol, Vol.165, pp. 473-82.

Mendez, J., X. H. Zou-Yang, S. Y. Kim, M. Hidaka, W. P. Tansey & B. Stillman (2002). Human origin recognition complex large subunit is degraded by ubiquitin-mediated proteolysis after initiation of DNA replication. Mol Cell, Vol.9, pp. 481-91.

Meraldi, P., J. Lukas, A. M. Fry, J. Bartek & E. A. Nigg (1999). Centrosome duplication in mammalian somatic cells requires E2F and Cdk2-cyclin A. Nat Cell Biol, Vol.1, pp. 88-93.

Miller, G., K. I. Panov, J. K. Friedrich, L. Trinkle-Mulcahy, A. I. Lamond & J. C. Zomerdijk (2001). hRRN3 is essential in the SL1-mediated recruitment of RNA Polymerase I to rRNA gene promoters. EMBO J, Vol.20, pp. 1373-82.

Mimura, S., T. Masuda, T. Matsui & H. Takisawa (2000). Central role for cdc45 in establishing an initiation complex of DNA replication in Xenopus egg extracts. Genes Cells, Vol.5, pp. 439-52.

Nguyen, V. Q., C. Co, K. Irie & J. J. Li (2000). Clb/Cdc28 kinases promote nuclear export of the replication initiator proteins Mcm2-7. Curr Biol, Vol.10, pp. 195-205.

Nguyen, V. Q., C. Co & J. J. Li (2001). Cyclin-dependent kinases prevent DNA re-replication through multiple mechanisms. Nature, Vol.411, pp. 1068-73.

Niida, H., S. Tsuge, Y. Katsuno, A. Konishi, N. Takeda & M. Nakanishi (2005). Depletion of Chk1 leads to premature activation of Cdc2-cyclin B and mitotic catastrophe. J Biol Chem, Vol.280, pp. 39246-52.

Nishitani, H., N. Sugimoto, V. Roukos, Y. Nakanishi, M. Saijo, C. Obuse, T. Tsurimoto, K. I. Nakayama, K. Nakayama, M. Fujita, Z. Lygerou & T. Nishimoto (2006). Two E3 ubiquitin ligases, SCF-Skp2 and DDB1-Cul4, target human Cdt1 for proteolysis. EMBO J, Vol.25, pp. 1126-36.

Okuda, M., H. F. Horn, P. Tarapore, Y. Tokuyama, A. G. Smulian, P. K. Chan, E. S. Knudsen, I. A. Hofmann, J. D. Snyder, K. E. Bove & K. Fukasawa (2000). Nucleophosmin/B23 is a target of CDK2/cyclin E in centrosome duplication. Cell, Vol.103, pp. 127-40.

Piel, M., P. Meyer, A. Khodjakov, C. L. Rieder & M. Bornens (2000). The respective contributions of the mother and daughter centrioles to centrosome activity and behavior in vertebrate cells. J Cell Biol, Vol.149, pp. 317-30.

Prasanth, S. G., K. V. Prasanth, K. Siddiqui, D. L. Spector & B. Stillman (2004). Human Orc2 localizes to centrosomes, centromeres and heterochromatin during chromosome inheritance. EMBO J, Vol.23, pp. 2651-63.

Prasanth, S. G., K. V. Prasanth & B. Stillman (2002). Orc6 involved in DNA replication, chromosome segregation, and cytokinesis. Science, Vol.297, pp. 1026-31.

Saha, P., J. Chen, K. C. Thome, S. J. Lawlis, Z. H. Hou, M. Hendricks, J. D. Parvin & A. Dutta (1998). Human CDC6/Cdc18 associates with Orc1 and cyclin-cdk and is selectively eliminated from the nucleus at the onset of S phase. Mol Cell Biol, Vol.18, pp. 2758-67.

Schramm, L. & N. Hernandez (2002). Recruitment of RNA polymerase III to its target promoters. Genes Dev, Vol.16, pp. 2593-620.

Shechter, D., V. Costanzo & J. Gautier (2004). ATR and ATM regulate the timing of DNA replication origin firing. Nat Cell Biol, Vol.6, pp. 648-55.

Snyder, M., W. He & J. J. Zhang (2005). The DNA replication factor MCM5 is essential for Stat1-mediated transcriptional activation. Proc Natl Acad Sci U S A, Vol.102, pp. 14539-44.

Snyder, M., X. Y. Huang & J. J. Zhang (2009). The minichromosome maintenance proteins 2-7 (MCM2-7) are necessary for RNA polymerase II (Pol II)-mediated transcription. J Biol Chem, Vol.284, pp. 13466-72.

Stewart, S. & G. Fang (2005). Destruction box-dependent degradation of aurora B is mediated by the anaphase-promoting complex/cyclosome and Cdh1. Cancer Res, Vol.65, pp. 8730-5.

Strebhardt, K. & A. Ullrich (2006). Targeting polo-like kinase 1 for cancer therapy. Nat Rev Cancer, Vol.6, pp. 321-30.

Sunkel, C. E. & D. M. Glover (1988). polo, a mitotic mutant of Drosophila displaying abnormal spindle poles. J Cell Sci, Vol.89 (Pt 1), pp. 25-38.

Syljuasen, R. G., C. S. Sorensen, L. T. Hansen, K. Fugger, C. Lundin, F. Johansson, T. Helleday, M. Sehested, J. Lukas & J. Bartek (2005). Inhibition of human Chk1 causes increased initiation of DNA replication, phosphorylation of ATR targets, and DNA breakage. Mol Cell Biol, Vol.25, pp. 3553-62.

Tachibana, K. E., M. A. Gonzalez, G. Guarguaglini, E. A. Nigg & R. A. Laskey (2005). Depletion of licensing inhibitor geminin causes centrosome overduplication and mitotic defects. EMBO Rep, Vol.6, pp. 1052-7.

Takeda, D. Y., J. D. Parvin & A. Dutta (2005). Degradation of Cdt1 during S phase is Skp2-independent and is required for efficient progression of mammalian cells through S phase. J Biol Chem, Vol.280, pp. 23416-23.

Tanaka, S. & J. F. Diffley (2002). Interdependent nuclear accumulation of budding yeast Cdt1 and Mcm2-7 during G1 phase. Nat Cell Biol, Vol.4, pp. 198-207.

Tokuyama, Y., H. F. Horn, K. Kawamura, P. Tarapore & K. Fukasawa (2001). Specific phosphorylation of nucleophosmin on Thr(199) by cyclin-dependent kinase 2-cyclin E and its role in centrosome duplication. J Biol Chem, Vol.276, pp. 21529-37.

Toyoshima-Morimoto, F., E. Taniguchi, N. Shinya, A. Iwamatsu & E. Nishida (2001). Polo-like kinase 1 phosphorylates cyclin B1 and targets it to the nucleus during prophase. Nature, Vol.410, pp. 215-20.

Verrijzer, C. P. & R. Tjian (1996). TAFs mediate transcriptional activation and promoter selectivity. Trends Biochem Sci, Vol.21, pp. 338-42.

Weinreich, M., C. Liang, H. H. Chen & B. Stillman (2001). Binding of cyclin-dependent kinases to ORC and Cdc6p regulates the chromosome replication cycle. Proc Natl Acad Sci U S A, Vol.98, pp. 11211-7.

Wohlschlegel, J. A., B. T. Dwyer, S. K. Dhar, C. Cvetic, J. C. Walter & A. Dutta (2000). Inhibition of eukaryotic DNA replication by geminin binding to Cdt1. Science, Vol.290, pp. 2309-12.

Yanagi, K., T. Mizuno, Z. You & F. Hanaoka (2002). Mouse geminin inhibits not only Cdt1-MCM6 interactions but also a novel intrinsic Cdt1 DNA binding activity. J Biol Chem, Vol.277, pp. 40871-80.

Yankulov, K., I. Todorov, P. Romanowski, D. Licatalosi, K. Cilli, S. McCracken, R. Laskey & D. L. Bentley (1999). MCM proteins are associated with RNA polymerase II holoenzyme. Mol Cell Biol, Vol.19, pp. 6154-63.

Yazdi, P. T., Y. Wang, S. Zhao, N. Patel, E. Y. Lee & J. Qin (2002). SMC1 is a downstream effector in the ATM/NBS1 branch of the human S-phase checkpoint. Genes Dev, Vol.16, pp. 571-82.

Yim, H. & R. L. Erikson (2010). Cell division cycle 6, a mitotic substrate of polo-like kinase 1, regulates chromosomal segregation mediated by cyclin-dependent kinase 1 and separase. Proc Natl Acad Sci U S A, Vol.107, pp. 19742-7.

Zatsepina, O. V., A. Rousselet, P. K. Chan, M. O. Olson, E. G. Jordan & M. Bornens (1999). The nucleolar phosphoprotein B23 redistributes in part to the spindle poles during mitosis. J Cell Sci, Vol.112 (Pt 4), pp. 455-66.

Zhang, X., Q. Chen, J. Feng, J. Hou, F. Yang, J. Liu, Q. Jiang & C. Zhang (2009). Sequential phosphorylation of Nedd1 by Cdk1 and Plk1 is required for targeting of the gammaTuRC to the centrosome. J Cell Sci, Vol.122, pp. 2240-51.

12

The Organisation of Replisomes

Anna Ligasová and Karel Koberna
Institute of Experimental Medicine, Academy of Sciences of the Czech Republic
Czech Republic

1. Introduction

The eukaryotic chromosomal DNA is divided into hundreds to thousands of independent replication segments called replicons. Each replicon is replicated from one replication origin. In the S phase of the cell cycle, individual replicons are gradually activated and subsequently replicated (Edenberg & Huberman, 1975; Hand, 1978). The size of particular replicons varies and is usually within the range of 30–450 kbp. On the other hand, much smaller (shorter than 10 kbp) or much longer (longer than 1 Mbp) replicons have also been observed (Berezney et al., 2000; Edenberg & Huberman, 1975; Hand, 1978; Hyrien & Mechali, 1993; Jackson & Pombo, 1998; Yurov & Liapunova, 1977). It is supposed that several adjacent replicons are synchronously activated in the S phase (Edenberg & Huberman, 1975; Hand, 1978), whereas the number of replicons in one such group is lower than ten (Jackson & Pombo, 1998; Ma et al., 1998). The evidence of such replicon organisation comes mainly from studies mapping the newly-synthesised DNA on stretched DNA fibres (Edenberg & Huberman, 1975; Hand, 1978; Jackson & Pombo, 1998).

The replication of replicons proceeds bi-directionally by means of two replication forks and is terminated when the replication forks of two adjacent replicons meet (Blow & Dutta, 2005; Heintz, 1996). The so-called "licensing" of replication origins is performed before the actual initiation of DNA synthesis. First, many different proteins such as the ORC complex, Cdc6 protein, Cdt1 protein, MCM 2-7 protein complex bind in that exact order at the sites of replication origins (Bell & Dutta, 2002; Blow & Dutta, 2005; DePamphilis, 2003; Diffley, 2004; Chesnokov, 2007; Lei & Tye, 2001; Sasaki & Gilbert, 2007; Stillman, 2005; Takahashi et al., 2005). Later, due to the regulation mechanisms, some of the proteins are removed and other new proteins are bound to DNA instead of them. Examples include the Cdc45 protein, MCM10 protein or GINS protein complex (Bauerschmidt et al., 2007; Diffley & Labib, 2002). Cyclin-dependent kinases and Dbf4-dependent kinase are important for the changes in the protein-DNA interactions (Bauerschmidt et al., 2007; Diffley & Labib, 2002). All of these processes result in the formation of two replication complexes, also referred to as replisomes, at the site of the active replication origin that ensure the synthesis of DNA in mutually opposite directions (Baker & Bell, 1998; Johnson & O'Donnell, 2005; Waga & Stillman, 1998). The main components of replisomes are a helicase complex enabling the unwinding of the parental DNA strands, DNA polymerases responsible for the duplication of DNA, and a complex of polymerase and primase (Langston et al., 2009). It is supposed that the MCM2-7 protein complex, which is necessary for the "licensing" of replication origins, plays also the role of a helicase in the common complex with Cdc45 protein and GINS complex (Aparicio et al., 2006).

On the cellular level, the individual active replicons or groups of simultaneously replicated replicons were localised to the discrete domains (Dimitrova & Gilbert, 1999; Fox et al., 1991; Hozak et al., 1993; Leonhardt et al., 2000; Ma et al., 1998; Nakamura et al., 1986; Nakayasu & Berezney, 1989; O'Keefe et al., 1992). At the light microscopy level (LM), these domains are referred to as replication foci. In the case of electron microscopy (EM) localisation, these domains are commonly called replication factories. Presently, the term replication factory is used also for the description of the complex of replication proteins and is frequently substituted by the term replisome. Alternatively, replication factory can designate a complex where besides replication proteins other proteins such as proteins for DNA recombination and DNA repair are present (Migocki et al., 2004). It is evident that the number, size and localisation of the replication foci are changed during the S phase whereas several different replication patterns have been described by various groups. Some of them distinguish between three basic replication patterns (Jackson, 1995; Manders et al., 1992; Nakayasu & Berezney, 1989), others describe five replication patterns (Dimitrova & Gilbert, 1999; O'Keefe et al., 1992; van Dierendonck et al., 1989). Basically, at the onset of the S phase, small replication foci scattered throughout the nucleoplasm except the nucleoli are observed. In the middle part of the S phase, the foci are less numerous; on the other hand, they are larger and localised mainly in the perinucleolar and perinuclear parts of the cell nucleus. At the end of the S phase, heterochromatin is replicated. In this part of the S phase, replication typically proceeds via large and not very numerous foci. The number and size of replication foci was measured by means of several techniques of light microscopy (Ma et al., 1998; Nakayasu & Berezney, 1989; Tomilin et al., 1995). The use of various techniques contributed to the high variability in the obtained numbers and sizes of replication foci in the early replicated cells (0.1–0.5 µm; 120–1500; Jackson, 1995; Ma et al., 1998; Mills et al., 1989; Nakamura et al., 1986; Nakayasu & Berezney, 1989; Tomilin et al., 1995).

Replisome complexes are of course assembled not only in eukaryotic cells but also in prokaryotic cells. In both of the groups of organisms, there are two basic views of the organisation of sister replisomes during replication. According to the first one, the sister replisomes move independently in opposite directions along the DNA (Bates & Kleckner, 2005; Berkmen & Grossman, 2006; Hiraga et al., 2000; Kongsuwan et al., 2002; Reyes-Lamothe et al., 2008; Yardimci et al., 2010). On the contrary, the second view supposes that the sister replisomes are tightly associated during replication (Dingman, 1974; Falaschi, 2000; Jensen et al., 2001; Kitamura et al., 2006; Lau et al., 2003; Lemon & Grossman, 2000; Ligasová et al., 2009; Migocki et al., 2004; Pardoll et al., 1980; Wessel et al., 1992).

In the chapter, a procedure enabling the distinction between the above-mentioned models of replisome organisation in human HeLa cells is described. This procedure can be used universally for other eukaryotic systems. The method is based on the pulse-chase labelling of the short segments of DNA and their localisation by means of the pre-embedding approach followed by electron tomography. Presently, the pre-embedding approach is the only method that allows the localisation of labelled DNA in the sections and provides 3D information at sufficient resolution by means of the EM tomography. The EM tomography approach is based on the stepwise tilting of the section in the electron beam followed by the mathematical analysis of the obtained data. This method provides high resolution of structures (5-10 nm) in three dimensions as the plastic sections are cut enough (200-1,000 nm) to contain the sufficient amount of information. In the case of serial sections, the resolution of the third dimension (the depth of the section) cannot be more than twice the thickness of the section (McEwen & Marko, 2001). The thickness of the common EM sections is about 70 nm, although it is possible to prepare sections with approximately 10-nm thickness (McEwen & Marko, 2001). However, the resolution is still 20 nm as opposed to 5-10 nm for EM tomography. Moreover, an obligatory problem is the ordering of the serial section by processing the data.

The whole experiment is illustrated in Figure 1. From the scheme, it is apparent that the most significant difference between both models is a change in the number of the labelled domains after the different lengths of incubation: in the case of independent replisomes, the number of the labelled domains in mitosis is at most doubled; in the tightly associated replisomes, this number is almost quadrupled (Figure 1).

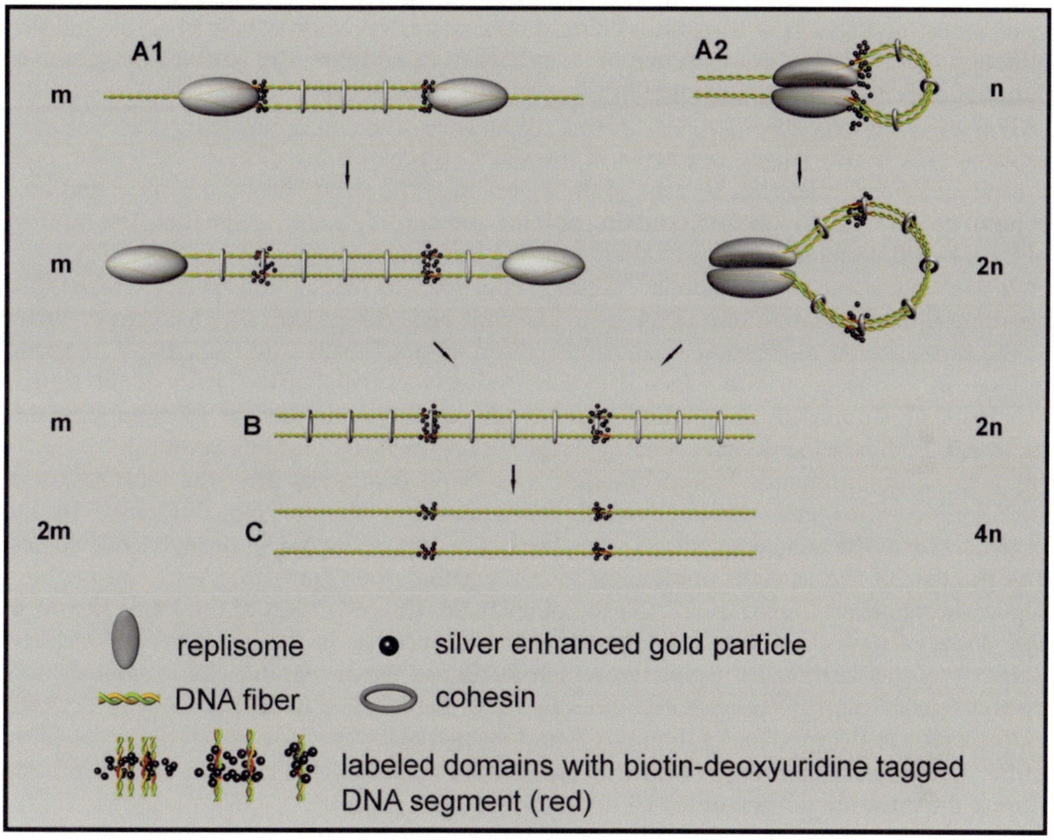

Fig. 1. The explanatory scheme depicting two models of the arrangement of "sister" replisomes in HeLa cells and the effect of different organisations of the biotin-16-2′-deoxy-uridine-tagged segments on the number of labelled domains during various pulse-chase experiments.

The scheme shows the expected results of the consecutive mapping (indicated by arrows) of the segments tagged during a short pulse of biotin-16-2′-deoxy-uridine-5′-triphosphate (biotin-dUTP) in the early S phase followed by the chase period of a different length from the time immediately after the pulse (the upper part of the scheme) to the complete mitotic segregation of the sister chromatids (the lower part of the scheme). Note that some clusters of silver-enhanced gold particles belonging to the mutually close segments can "fuse". Therefore, the domain labelled by silver-enhanced gold particles, used as markers in the present study, can contain between one and four segments, depending on the model and the

length of the chase. This "fusion" is a result of the "large" size of the antibody complex with the silver-enhanced gold particle as against the distance between the segments. The expected number of domains for the individual stages of replicon organisation is shown as a multiple of the initial number of domains. The initial number is designated by **m** for the model of replisome singles and by **n** for the model of replisome couples. Note that the number of labelled domains is doubled in the model of replisome singles (A1) and quadrupled in the model of replisome couples (A2) in mitosis. In fact, the increase in the model of replisome couples is lower as the labelled segments of replicons early after initiation cannot contribute to this increase (see below). Several simplifications have been used in the model such as chromatin being shown as a DNA double helix in all the models, although the DNA in chromatin is more condensed. In addition, the partial segregation of chromatids is not taken into account in the model before mitosis.
(A1) A model of replisome singles. "Sister" replisomes move in opposite directions during replication. The two tagged segments of the sister chromatids are close to each other both during and after replication because of the cohesion of the sister chromatids mediated by a cohesin complex. Each labelled domain contains one pair of "sister" segments. The number of the labelled domains remains unaltered during this process.
(A2) A model of replisome couples. "Sister" replisomes form a closely associated complex, resulting in the formation of a DNA loop. The four tagged segments are in close proximity at the time of their replication and are visualised as one labelled domain. Later, the loop inflates, as a consequence of which the distance between both "sister" pairs of the tagged segments of chromatids is gradually prolonged and the number of labelled domains increases. Each labelled domain contains only one pair of segments at this point.
(B) Two sister chromatids bound together by cohesin complexes after the termination of replicon synthesis and dissociation of replisomes are shown. No difference in the organisation of the tagged segments is visible in the case of the model of replisome singles. The number of the labelled domains is also the same when compared with the ongoing replicon replication shown in A1. On the other hand, the relaxation of the loops shown in the model of replisome couples (A2) resulted in an increase in the distances between the pairs of tagged chromatin segments, which facilitates the recognition of previously less distant "sister" pairs. Consequently, the number of the labelled domains is nearly doubled with respect to the number of domains found immediately after the biotin-dUTP labelling pulse. The increase is lower as labelled segments of replicons which began DNA synthesis during the pulse are not separated by non-labelled DNA strand.
(C) In mitosis, sister chromatid cohesion is broken and the pairs of the tagged segments separate. Mitotic segregation results in the twofold increase of labelled domains with respect to (B). Each individual domain contains only one biotin-16-2'-deoxy-uridine-tagged (biotin-dU) chromatin segment. (From Ligasová, et al., 2009).

2. EM tomography analysis of the organisation of replisomes in human HeLa cells

2.1 Material and methods

2.1.1 Cell culture and synchronisation

Human HeLa cells were incubated in cell culture flasks or on coverslips in Dulbecco's modified Eagle's medium with L-glutamine supplemented with 10% fetal calf serum 1% gentamicin and 0.85 g/l $NaHCO_3$ at 37 °C in a humidified atmosphere containing 5% CO_2.

In the most of experiments, the cells were synchronised at the G1/S border by means of the double block with 2'-deoxytymidine (dT; Koberna et al., 2005). After the release from the block, the cells were labelled with biotin-dUTP (Koberna et al., 1999; Ligasová et al., 2009). In short, the cells were rinsed with the hypotonic buffer (30 mM KCl, 10 mM Hepes, pH 7.4) and subsequently incubated in the hypotonic buffer supplemented with 0.2 mM biotin-dUTP for 10 minutes. Next, the cells were incubated in culture medium for 10 minutes unless otherwise stated.

For the analysis of mitotic chromosomes, the cells were first synchronised by means of a double block with dT. Then, the cells were incubated for 100 minutes in fresh medium. After the 100-minute incubation, biotin-dUTP was introduced into the cells by means of hypotonic delivery. The cells were subsequently incubated for 9 hours in fresh medium and then the medium was changed for a medium supplemented with nocodazol (0.04 µg/ml, 5 hours; Zieve et al., 1980).

2.1.2 Antibodies

The rabbit anti-biotin primary antibody (Enzo Biochem Inc.) and secondary antibody conjugated with 1nm gold particles (Aurion) were used for the detection of incorporated biotin-dU.

2.1.3 Electron tomography and the evaluation of the tomograms

The ultrastructural localisation of the biotin-tagged DNA was performed using the synchronised cells by means of the pre-embedding approach (Koberna et al., 2005). Briefly, the cells were fixed by 2% formaldehyde and subsequently permeabilised by 0.2% Triton X-100. After the incubation with primary and secondary antibodies and silver intensification of the ultra-small gold following Dancher (Danscher, 1981), the samples were dehydrated and embedded in Epon resin. After the polymerisation, ultra-thin sections (of 70 and 200 nm) were cut on a Leica UltraCut S microtome with a diamond knife and then contrasted in 3% uranyl acetate. The 70-nm-thick sections were cut as a ribbon of three and more adjacent sections. The sections were analysed by means of a Morgagni 268 transmission electron microscope equipped with a Megaview II camera (a resolution: 1280 × 1024 pixels, a magnification: 14,000×). The mutual position of the neighbouring sections was adjusted by means of the Adobe Photoshop software. The electron tomography analysis of the 200-nm sections was performed by means of a Tecnai G2 Sphera electron tomography microscope equipped with a Gatan Ultrascan camera 894 US1000 (resolution: 2048 × 2048 pixels, magnification: 5000×) at 200 kV. The picture series were scanned within the range of angles −64° to +64° with the increment of 2°. The scanned picture series were reconstructed in IMOD software (Kremer et al., 1996). The final 3D models were created in Amira software (Figure 2).

To minimise the possible inaccuracies at the edges of the tomograms, every side of the original tomogram was reduced by 10–20 nm. The 300–500 labelled domains in the 3D model were measured in the case of the evaluation of the size of labelled domains. In this evaluation, we have excluded those domains found at the borders of the tomogram. The length of the labelled domains was measured as the longest distance between the outer margins of silver-enhanced gold particles. In the case of the analysis of the number of labelled domains, we did not evaluate the domains crossing the left, bottom and front sides of the model. In both analyses, we have analysed 100 sections from more than fifty different cells.

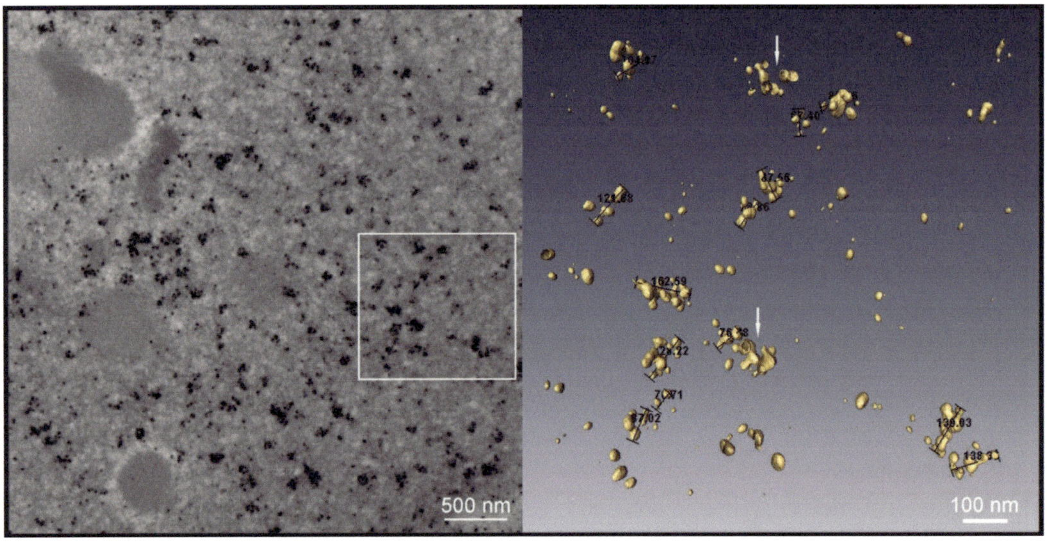

Fig. 2. A 3D reconstruction of the labelled domains.
The original image of a 200-nm-thick section of the cell nucleus from the 2-h experiment is shown on the left (scale bar: 500 nm), whereas a 3D reconstruction of the labelled domains reconstructed from the insert is shown on the right (scale bar: 100 nm). Only clusters of silver-enhanced gold particles in the outlined area of the electron microscopy image were reconstructed using Amira software. The length measurement is demonstrated. The arrows indicate the labelled domains traversing the section faces. (From Ligasová, et al., 2009).

The whole volume of the cell nuclei in the S-phase cells and the volume of mitotic cells was calculated by means of Cavalieri's method (Gundersen et al., 1988). An analysis was performed on fifteen cells from three different experiments.
In order to evaluate the distance between the pairs of labelled domains, we analysed only such pairs that had similar size (the difference in their length was smaller than 20%), similar labelling intensity (the difference in the labelling intensity was below 25%), similar shape and whose mutual distance was less than 400 nm. The number of domains in pairs was calculated as a percentage of the domains in pairs to the overall number of labelled domains.

2.2 Results

2.2.1 Around 5400 domains in one cell nucleus are labelled in the 10-minute experiment

Data from our experiments showed that around twenty-one labelled domains are in 1 μm^3 of the cell nucleus in the early S phase after the 10-minute labelling pulse. Every such domain represents several tagged segments of DNA (Koberna et al., 2005; Figure 1). As the total volume of the cell nucleus in the early S phase was 260 ± 44 μm^3, the number of labelled domains in one cell nucleus was 5460 ± 923. In fact, the number of the labelled domains of concurrently active replicons is lower, because some of the labelled domains contain also the tagged segments of the replicons which began synthesis during the labelling pulse. To determine the number of domains labelled during the pulse, we supposed that this number is inversely proportional to the length of the replication of one average replicon and directly proportional to the length of labelling (for a more detailed description of the calculation see Ligasová et al., 2009). On the basis of the performed calculations, it is clear that the average number of the labelled domains after the above-mentioned correction was 4890 ± 827 and the number of the domains labelled during the pulse was 570.

An analysis of the size of the labelled domains after the ten-minute labelling pulse showed that the average size of these domains was 113 ± 40 nm. This value was corrected with respect to the size of the antibody complex used for the detection of biotin-dU-tagged DNA segments and also with respect to the different degree of the intensification of the ultra-small gold particles (for the more detailed explanation see Ligasová et al., 2009). The maximum diameter of the tagged segments of DNA in domains after this correction was ≥ 74 ± 45 nm. This data surprisingly corresponds to the thickness of one or two pairs of 30 nm-chromatin fibres associated for example with the help of cohesin molecules and sister replisomes (cf. Fig. 1A1 and A2).

2.2.2 The number of the labelled domains is doubled after the two-hour labelling pulse and quadruples after the sister chromatid separation in mitosis.

To assess which of the two models of the mutual organisation of replisomes is correct, it was crucial to determine the number of domains after the various lengths of the incubation of cells in medium after a biotin pulse (see Fig. 1). In this case, the cells were incubated in the culture medium alternatively for 30 minutes, 1 hour, 2 hours or until mitosis (approximately fourteen hours, Figure 3). The number of domains after the 30-minute incubation was similar to that found in the ten-minute experiment. This finding is in absolute agreement with our conclusion that the pool of biotin-dUTP introduced into the cells during the hypotonic shift is depleted in less than 10 minutes (for a more detailed description see Ligasová et al., 2009).

In the case of the one-hour and two-hour experiments, we observed a gradual increase of the number of labelled domains (around 7040 ± 1191 and 11,000 ± 1875 domains were labelled in one cell nucleus in one-hour and two-hour experiments, respectively). Moreover, during the analysis of the tomograms, we found the presence of pairs of labelled domains with a similar shape and intensity of labelling. These pairs of domains were observed mainly in the two-hour experiment. In the analysis of the distances between the paired domains, we evaluated only pairs with a similar size, similar intensity of labelling, shape and with a mutual distance of less than 400 nm. The average measured distance was approximately 227 ± 96 nm (Fig. 3). When we take into account that the replication of an average replicon is around one hour (for example Jackson & Pombo, 1998; Manders et al., 1992; Nakamura et al., 1986) and the speed of replication fork in the S phase is 0.6 kbp/minute (Malinsky et al., 2001), then the average size of the replicon in the early S phase does not exceed 72 kbp. The length of a 2.6 kbp-long fragment of stretched DNA is around 1 μm (Jackson & Pombo, 1998). As the compactation of a 30-nm chromatin fibre is around 40 (Wagner et al., 2005), the length of a 72-kbp-long replicon in the form of a 30-nm fibre is around 700 nm. The determined distance between domains in pairs would then correspond to one-third of such a replicon. It is a very realistic estimation that indicates the possibility that the maximum condensation of a replicon during its replication is not higher than the condensation of a 30-nm chromatin fibre, at least at the replicon level.

These results strongly support the model of associated replisome pairs (Model A2 in the Fig. 1). If we take into account that the sister replisomes operate as independent units, the

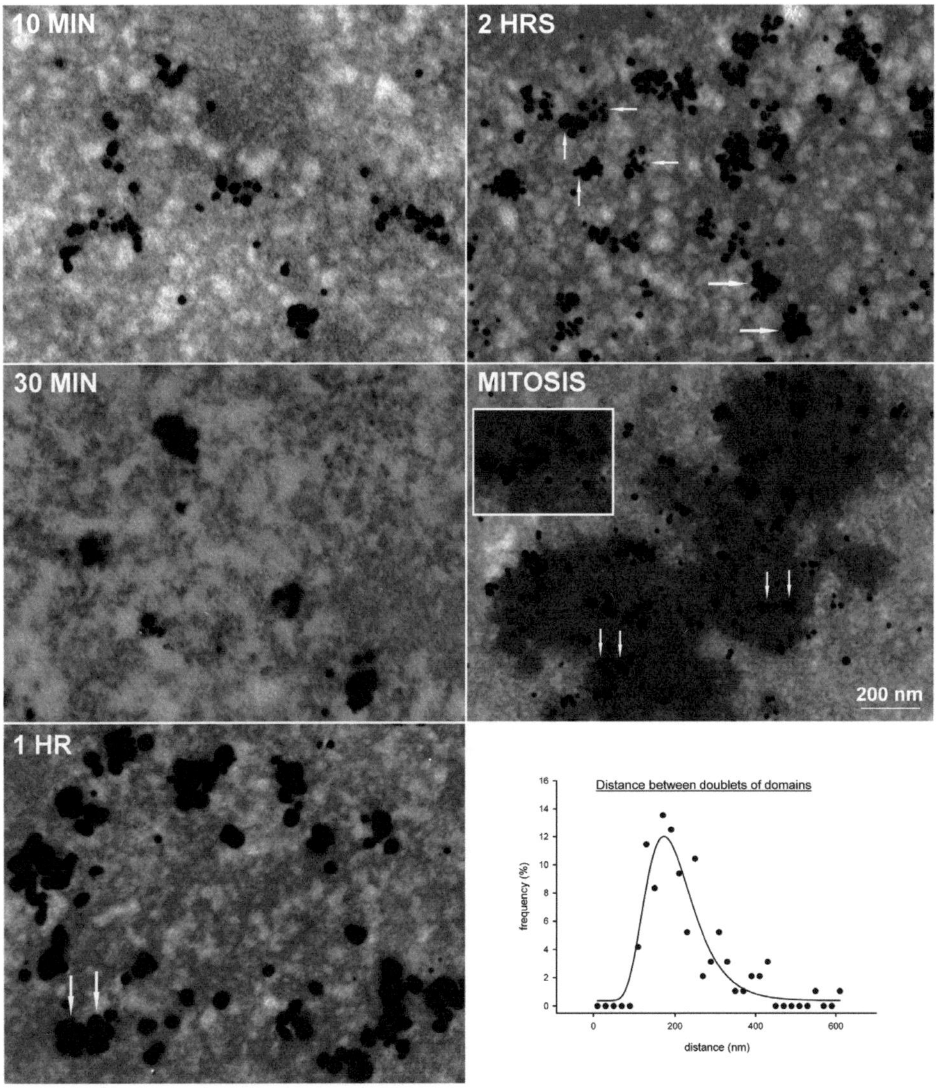

Fig. 3. EM images of thin sections of HeLa cell nuclei with labelled domains and a graph of the distances between the doublets of labelled domains.
Images of the 70-nm-thick sections of the nuclei from the 10-min, 30-min, 1-h, 2-h and mitotic experiments are shown. The clusters of the silver-enhanced gold particles correspond to the labelled domains. The number of the labelled domains increases substantially between the 1-h and mitotic experiments. The arrows in the images from the 1- and 2-h and mitotic experiments indicate doublets of the labelled domains. The insert in the image of the mitotic-cell nucleus shows an example of a cluster of several labelled domains from a different cell. Seventy-nanometre sections were chosen instead of 200-nm sections as they have higher contrast and accommodate a much lower number of labelled domains. In this respect, they are much more suitable for the demonstration of individual doublets although they cannot reflect their overall organisation. Scale bar: 200 nm. The graph shows the frequency of the distances between the doublets of "sister" domains from the 2-h experiment. (From Ligasová, et al., 2009).

double increase of the number of labelled domains would correspond to the complete separation of sister chromatids. However, regarding the fact that the analysed cells were in the S phase, it is unlikely. This conclusion is also in complete agreement with the results obtained from the analysis of the mitotic cells. To achieve the complete segregation of sister chromatids, we analysed the number of labelled domains in metaphase cells (Rieder & Cole, 1999). We found that a 1-μm^3 mitotic cell contains eleven labelled domains. The volume of mitotic cells was around 1919 ± 310 μm^3, thus the total number of labelled domains in mitotic cells was around 21,109 ± 3420. Our theoretic calculation of the number of labelled domains after sister-chromatid segregation was 20,700 (4 × 4890 + 2 × 570) for the model of replisome pairs, which is in agreement with the measured value.

Besides the number of labelled domains, we also analysed the size of these domains for each experiment. The values after the correction of the effect of the various sizes of the gold-enhanced particles (Ligasová et al., 2009) in the individual experiments were: 92 ± 45 nm for the 10-minute experiment, 85 ± 46 nm for the 30-minute experiment, 83 ± 58 nm for the 1-hour experiment, 90 ± 48 nm for the 2-hour experiment and 48 ± 26 nm for mitotic cells. The similar size of the domains in the 10-minute to 2-hour experiments is in absolute agreement with the possibility that the maximum size of the labelled domains corresponds to the thickness one or two pairs of tightly associated 30-nm chromatin fibres. This hypothesis is also in agreement with our previous results showing that the size of the domains is independent of the time of the incorporation of biotin-dUTP in the 3- and 10-minute experiments (Koberna et al., 2005). According to the model of replisome couples (Fig. 1A2), two pairs of 30 nm fibres can be found in most labelled domains in the 10-min experiment. Later, as the segment pairs are moved away from the replisomes and the loop is finally relaxed, each labelled domain contains only one pair of the segments. In mitotic cells, only one labelled segment is accommodated in the labelled domain. The reduction in the number of segments in the individual domains between the 2-h and mitotic experiments is reflected in the steep decrease in the size of the domains labelled. Such a decrease was not observed between the 10-min and 2-h experiments, likely due to the similar thickness of the bundle of 4 or 2 parallel segments.

2.2.3 Model of replisome pairs

All of the above-mentioned data showed that in HeLa cells the sister replisomes are tightly associated during replication. Another important finding concerning the organisation of the DNA loops that are formed during replication was the same number of labelled domains in 10- and 30-minute experiments. On the basis of this result, we suppose that the arms of DNA loops are tightly associated during and even for a certain time after the replication of the replicon. According to these data, we have proposed the model of newly replicated DNA (Fig. 4).

3. Conclusions

Our results are in complete agreement with the model showing that sister replisomes are organised as tightly associated pairs. Similar findings have been published also for other organisms, both prokaryotic (Jensen et al., 2001; Lau et al., 2003; Lemon & Grossman, 2000; Migocki et al., 2004) and eukaryotic (Kitamura et al., 2006). On the other hand, there are several studies showing a high degree of independence of sister replisomes (Reyes-Lamothe et al., 2008; Yardimci et al., 2010). Moreover, some studies showing that the sister replisomes

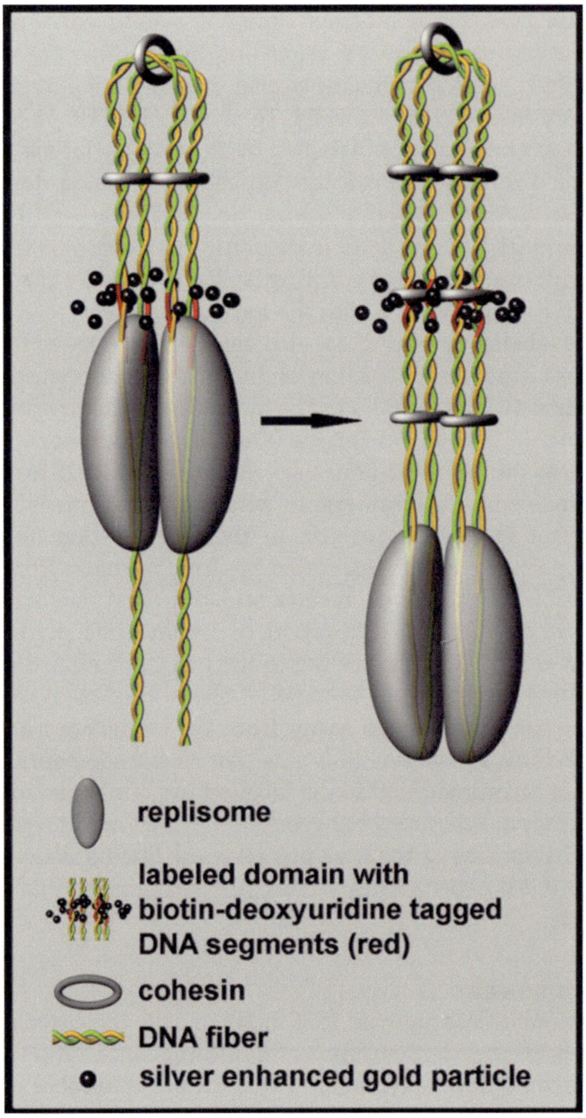

Fig. 4. The model of zipping loops.
The zipping of a DNA loop is shown. During replication, replisome couples produce a loop with the associated (zipped) arms probably in the form of four tightly associated 30-nm fibres. According to this model, "sister" pairs of biotin-dU-tagged segments of chromatids do not separate before the termination of the DNA synthesis of the replicon and the relaxation of the zipped arms. Immediately after labelling, the four tagged segments are present in one labelled domain (the left part of the image). Such an organisation of the tagged segments persists during the synthesis of the whole replicon (the right part of the image). Although the mutual changes of the replisome position between the left and right part of the figure can result in the impression of a movement of the replisome along DNA, this model does not reflect whether DNA or the replisome complex is moving during the replication. (From Ligasová, et al., 2009).

are tightly associated suppose the movement of DNA instead of DNA polymerase (Dingman, 1974; Lemon & Grossman, 1998, 2000; Pardoll et al., 1980). According to the above-mentioned studies, DNA is pulled through the static replisome and the newly-synthesised daughter DNA strains are released from the replication complex. The model of the coupled replisomes is also supported by the results of a time-lapse microscopic study focused on the microscopic analysis of the expressed GFP-PCNA in cell nuclei. This study (Leonhardt et al., 2000) showed that the replication foci form and again disintegrate during DNA replication, but no direct movement was observed.

Three basic studies dealing with the mutual position of sister replisomes were performed in eukaryotic cells. In the first one (Kitamura et al., 2006), the method that enables the tracking of specific chromosomal loci in an individual live cell was used to determine the organisation of replisomes in *Saccharomyces cerevisiae* yeast. The general disadvantage of such methods is the necessity of manipulation with the original genetic information of various proteins using GFP tags. Therefore, a high number of controls are required. Moreover, the number of cells inspected is usually relatively low and the resolution of light microscopy need not be sufficient, because chromatin is highly compacted in the cell nuclei.

In the study described here, we have used the labelling of short DNA segments and analysed them during replication and mitosis. These tagged segments were analysed by means of electron tomography. Electron-microscopic studies generally provide high resolution. In addition, with respect to the possibility of using stereological approaches for evaluation, the obtained data are not burdened by high error owing to the high number of analysed cells. On the other hand, it is necessary to work with fixed and permeabilised cells, which results in volume changes and a corresponding error, whose value depends on the many factors. Apparently, the ratio values are less burdened by this error than the absolute values. From this point of view, the number of domains was selected as the crucial parameter for the testing of both models in the described approach. Independently of the methods used and their limitations, both studies brought data supporting the model of mutually associated replisomes.

In contrast to the above-mentioned studies, Yardimci et al. (Yardimci et al., 2010) tracked replication in an *in vitro* system. In this case, they used biotinylated DNA of λ phage, which was attached by one or both ends to the streptavidin-coated microfluid flow cell. The cell-free system based on the *Xenopus* egg extract was used to replicate these DNA molecules. From the results obtained, it was obvious that the studied DNA was replicated by two independent replication complexes. Despite the advantages of the mentioned arrangement consisting mainly in the high control of the described system, the main problem is the interpretation of the obtained data in terms of their application to the processes proceeding in the complex structure of the cell nucleus. In this respect, it seems that the nuclear structures are necessary for the replication of replicons by means of the pairs of tightly associated replisomes. These nuclear structures are, however, absent in the cell extracts (Yardimci et al., 2010).

In order to answer the question of the mutual organization of sister replisomes definitively, the development of a new approach enabling the acquisition of 3D data sets from well preserved cells at high resolution seems to be the next necessary step. In this regard, the recently developed procedure of labelling DNA via the incorporation of 5-ethynyl-2'-deoxyuridine represents a very promising base (Salic & Mitchison, 2008).

Independently of the question of the mutual organisation of replisomes, our results have shown that the method used has enabled distinction between individual replicons. The observed number of labelled domains in the 10-minute experiment was around 5000. This number is several times higher than the number of the replication foci/factories published in the previous studies (120–1500; Jackson, 1995; Jackson & Pombo, 1998; Ma et al., 1998; Mills et al., 1989; Nakamura et al., 1986; Nakayasu & Berezney, 1989; Tomilin et al., 1995). It is supposed that at any time of the S phase approximately 10–15% of all the replicons are active (Jackson, 1995; Jackson & Pombo, 1998) and that the total number of replicons is around 40,000 (Singer et al., 1996). This is in absolute agreement with our results of the analysis of the number of labelled domains.

Our data also allowed us to speculate about the organisation of the replicon during its replication as well as to propose the model of the organisation of the replicon during replication. We suppose that the arms of DNA loop created during the duplication of replicon are tightly associated. The mechanism and the reason for this association remain unclear, and it is also not obvious whether the association of newly-replicated DNA is characteristic also for other organisms. Although our data have made it possible to test the model of the mutual organisation of replisomes in human cells, this method has not made it possible to decide whether the sister replisomes are moving during replication or not. In this respect, several studies have supposed that replisomes are attached e.g. to the nucleoskeleton in eukaryotic cells (Cook, 1999; Falaschi, 2000) or to cell structures such as the plasmatic membrane or cell wall in the gram-positive bacteria *Bacillus subtilis* (Lemon & Grossman, 2000) and that there are molecular motors mediating the movement of DNA. However, the direct evidence for such connection of replisomes does not exist.

4. Acknowledgement

This project was supported by the following grants: CZ: GAČR: 204/09/0973, CZ: GA ASCR: KAN 200520801 and by AV0Z 50390512 and AV0Z 50390703. Parts of the research results were published in the Journal of Structural Biology, Volume: 165, Authors: Ligasová, A., Raška, I., Koberna, K., Title: Organization of human replicon: singles or zipping couples?, pp. 204-213, Copyright Elsevier (2009).

5. References

Aparicio, T., Ibarra, A. & Mendez, J. (2006). Cdc45-MCM-GINS, a new power player for DNA replication. *Cell Div*, Vol. 1, (August), ISSN: 1747-1028.

Baker, T. A. & Bell, S. P. (1998). Polymerases and the replisome: machines within machines. *Cell*, Vol. 92, No. 3, (February), pp. 295-305, ISSN: 0092-8674.

Bates, D. & Kleckner, N. (2005). Chromosome and replisome dynamics in E. coli: loss of sister cohesion triggers global chromosome movement and mediates chromosome segregation. *Cell*, Vol. 121, No. 6, (June), pp. 899-911, ISSN: 0092-8674.

Bauerschmidt, C., Pollok, S., Kremmer, E., Nasheuer, H. P. & Grosse, F. (2007). Interactions of human Cdc45 with the Mcm2-7 complex, the GINS complex, and DNA polymerases delta and epsilon during S phase. *Genes Cells*, Vol. 12, No. 6, (June), pp. 745-758, ISSN: 1356-9597.

Bell, S. P. & Dutta, A. (2002). DNA replication in eukaryotic cells. *Annu Rev Biochem*, Vol. 71, (July), pp. 333-374, ISSN: 0066-4154.

Berezney, R., Dubey, D. D. & Huberman, J. A. (2000). Heterogeneity of eukaryotic replicons, replicon clusters, and replication foci. *Chromosoma*, Vol. 108, No. 8, (March), pp. 471-484, ISSN: 0009-5915.

Berkmen, M. B. & Grossman, A. D. (2006). Spatial and temporal organization of the Bacillus subtilis replication cycle. *Mol Microbiol*, Vol. 62, No. 1, (October), pp. 57-71, ISSN: 0950-382X.

Blow, J. J. & Dutta, A. (2005). Preventing re-replication of chromosomal DNA. *Nat Rev Mol Cell Biol*, Vol. 6, No. 6, (June), pp. 476-486, ISSN: 1471-0072.

Cook, P. R. (1999). The organization of replication and transcription. *Science*, Vol. 284, No. 5421, (June), pp. 1790-1795, ISSN: 0036-8075.

Danscher, G. (1981). Localization of gold in biological tissue. A photochemical method for light and electronmicroscopy. *Histochemistry*, Vol. 71, No. 1, (March), pp. 81-88, ISSN: 0301-5564.

DePamphilis, M. L. (2003). The 'ORC cycle': a novel pathway for regulating eukaryotic DNA replication. *Gene*, Vol. 310, (May), pp. 1-15, ISSN: 0378-1119.

Diffley, J. F. & Labib, K. (2002). The chromosome replication cycle. *J Cell Sci*, Vol. 115, No. Pt 5, (March), pp. 869-872, ISSN: 0021-9533.

Diffley, J. F. (2004). Regulation of early events in chromosome replication. *Curr Biol*, Vol. 14, No. 18, (September), pp. R778-786, ISSN: 0960-9822.

Dimitrova, D. S. & Gilbert, D. M. (1999). The spatial position and replication timing of chromosomal domains are both established in early G1 phase. *Mol Cell*, Vol. 4, No. 6, (December), pp. 983-993, ISSN: 1097-2765.

Dingman, C. W. (1974). Bidirectional chromosome replication: some topological considerations. *J Theor Biol*, Vol. 43, No. 1, (January), pp. 187-195, ISSN: 0022-5193.

Edenberg, H. J. & Huberman, J. A. (1975). Eukaryotic chromosome replication. *Annu Rev Genet*, Vol. 9, (December), pp. 245-284, ISSN: 0066-4197.

Falaschi, A. (2000). Eukaryotic DNA replication: a model for a fixed double replisome. *Trends Genet*, Vol. 16, No. 2, (February), pp. 88-92, ISSN: 0168-9525.

Fox, M. H., Arndt-Jovin, D. J., Jovin, T. M., Baumann, P. H. & Robert-Nicoud, M. (1991). Spatial and temporal distribution of DNA replication sites localized by immunofluorescence and confocal microscopy in mouse fibroblasts. *J Cell Sci*, Vol. 99 No. Pt 2, (June), pp. 247-253, ISSN: 0021-9533.

Gundersen, H. J., Bendtsen, T. F., Korbo, L., Marcussen, N., Moller, A., Nielsen, K., Nyengaard, J. R., Pakkenberg, B., Sorensen, F. B., Vesterby, A. & et al. (1988). Some new, simple and efficient stereological methods and their use in pathological research and diagnosis. *APMIS*, Vol. 96, No. 5, (May), pp. 379-394, ISSN: 0903-4641.

Hand, R. (1978). Eucaryotic DNA: organization of the genome for replication. *Cell*, Vol. 15, No. 2, (October), pp. 317-325, ISSN: 0092-8674.

Heintz, N. H. (1996). DNA Replication in Mammals. In: *DNA Replication in Eukaryotic Cells*, M. L. DePamphilis, (Ed.), pp. 983-1004, Cold Spring Harbor Laboratory Press, ISBN: 0-87969-459-9, New York, USA.

Hiraga, S., Ichinose, C., Onogi, T., Niki, H. & Yamazoe, M. (2000). Bidirectional migration of SeqA-bound hemimethylated DNA clusters and pairing of oriC copies in Escherichia coli. *Genes Cells*, Vol. 5, No. 5, (May), pp. 327-341, ISSN: 1356-9597.

Hozak, P., Hassan, A. B., Jackson, D. A. & Cook, P. R. (1993). Visualization of replication factories attached to nucleoskeleton. *Cell*, Vol. 73, No. 2, (April), pp. 361-373, ISSN: 0092-8674.

Hyrien, O. & Mechali, M. (1993). Chromosomal replication initiates and terminates at random sequences but at regular intervals in the ribosomal DNA of Xenopus early embryos. *EMBO J*, Vol. 12, No. 12, (December), pp. 4511-4520, ISSN: 0261-4189.

Chesnokov, I. N. (2007). Multiple functions of the origin recognition complex. *Int Rev Cytol*, Vol. 256, pp. 69-109, ISSN: 0074-7696.

Jackson, D. A. (1995). S-phase progression in synchronized human cells. *Exp Cell Res*, Vol. 220, No. 1, (September), pp. 62-70, ISSN: 0014-4827.

Jackson, D. A. & Pombo, A. (1998). Replicon clusters are stable units of chromosome structure: evidence that nuclear organization contributes to the efficient activation and propagation of S phase in human cells. *J Cell Biol*, Vol. 140, No. 6, (March), pp. 1285-1295, ISSN: 0021-9525.

Jensen, R. B., Wang, S. C. & Shapiro, L. (2001). A moving DNA replication factory in Caulobacter crescentus. *EMBO J*, Vol. 20, No. 17, (September), pp. 4952-4963, ISSN: 0261-4189.

Johnson, A. & O'Donnell, M. (2005). Cellular DNA replicases: components and dynamics at the replication fork. *Annu Rev Biochem*, Vol. 74, (July), pp. 283-315, ISSN: 0066-4154.

Kitamura, E., Blow, J. J. & Tanaka, T. U. (2006). Live-cell imaging reveals replication of individual replicons in eukaryotic replication factories. *Cell*, Vol. 125, No. 7, (June), pp. 1297-1308, ISSN: 0092-8674.

Koberna, K., Stanek, D., Malinsky, J., Eltsov, M., Pliss, A., Ctrnacta, V., Cermanova, S. & Raska, I. (1999). Nuclear organization studied with the help of a hypotonic shift: its use permits hydrophilic molecules to enter into living cells. *Chromosoma*, Vol. 108, No. 5, (September), pp. 325-335, ISSN: 0009-5915.

Koberna, K., Ligasova, A., Malinsky, J., Pliss, A., Siegel, A. J., Cvackova, Z., Fidlerova, H., Masata, M., Fialova, M., Raska, I. & Berezney, R. (2005). Electron microscopy of DNA replication in 3-D: evidence for similar-sized replication foci throughout S-phase. *J Cell Biochem*, Vol. 94, No. 1, (January), pp. 126-138, ISSN: 0730-2312.

Kongsuwan, K., Dalrymple, B. P., Wijffels, G. & Jennings, P. A. (2002). Cellular localisation of the clamp protein during DNA replication. *FEMS Microbiol Lett*, Vol. 216, No. 2, (November), pp. 255-262, ISSN: 0378-1097.

Kremer, J. R., Mastronarde, D. N. & McIntosh, J. R. (1996). Computer visualization of three-dimensional image data using IMOD. *J Struct Biol*, Vol. 116, No. 1, (January), pp. 71-76, ISSN: 1047-8477.

Langston, L. D., Indiani, C. & O'Donnell, M. (2009). Whither the replisome: emerging perspectives on the dynamic nature of the DNA replication machinery. *Cell Cycle*, Vol. 8, No. 17, (September), pp. 2686-2691, ISSN: 1551-4005.

Lau, I. F., Filipe, S. R., Soballe, B., Okstad, O. A., Barre, F. X. & Sherratt, D. J. (2003). Spatial and temporal organization of replicating Escherichia coli chromosomes. *Mol Microbiol*, Vol. 49, No. 3, (August), pp. 731-743, ISSN: 0950-382X.

Lei, M. & Tye, B. K. (2001). Initiating DNA synthesis: from recruiting to activating the MCM complex. *J Cell Sci*, Vol. 114, No. Pt 8, (April), pp. 1447-1454, ISSN: 0021-9533.

Lemon, K. P. & Grossman, A. D. (1998). Localization of bacterial DNA polymerase: evidence for a factory model of replication. *Science*, Vol. 282, No. 5393, (November), pp. 1516-1519, ISSN: 0036-8075.

Lemon, K. P. & Grossman, A. D. (2000). Movement of replicating DNA through a stationary replisome. *Mol Cell*, Vol. 6, No. 6, (December), pp. 1321-1330, ISSN: 1097-2765.

Leonhardt, H., Rahn, H. P., Weinzierl, P., Sporbert, A., Cremer, T., Zink, D. & Cardoso, M. C. (2000). Dynamics of DNA replication factories in living cells. *J Cell Biol*, Vol. 149, No. 2, (April), pp. 271-280, ISSN: 0021-9525.

Ligasová, A., Raška, I. & Koberna, K. (2009). Organization of human replicon: singles or zipping couples? *J Struct Biol*, Vol. 165, No. 3, (March), pp. 204-213, ISSN: 1095-8657.

Ma, H., Samarabandu, J., Devdhar, R. S., Acharya, R., Cheng, P. C., Meng, C. & Berezney, R. (1998). Spatial and temporal dynamics of DNA replication sites in mammalian cells. *J Cell Biol*, Vol. 143, No. 6, (December), pp. 1415-1425, ISSN: 0021-9525.

Malinsky, J., Koberna, K., Stanek, D., Masata, M., Votruba, I. & Raska, I. (2001). The supply of exogenous deoxyribonucleotides accelerates the speed of the replication fork in early S-phase. *J Cell Sci*, Vol. 114, No. Pt 4, (February), pp. 747-750, ISSN: 0021-9533.

Manders, E. M., Stap, J., Brakenhoff, G. J., van Driel, R. & Aten, J. A. (1992). Dynamics of three-dimensional replication patterns during the S-phase, analysed by double labelling of DNA and confocal microscopy. *J Cell Sci*, Vol. 103, No. Pt 3, (November), pp. 857-862, ISSN: 0021-9533.

McEwen, B. F. & Marko, M. (2001). The emergence of electron tomography as an important tool for investigating cellular ultrastructure. *J Histochem Cytochem*, Vol. 49, No. 5, (May), pp. 553-564, ISSN: 0022-1554.

Migocki, M. D., Lewis, P. J., Wake, R. G. & Harry, E. J. (2004). The midcell replication factory in Bacillus subtilis is highly mobile: implications for coordinating chromosome replication with other cell cycle events. *Mol Microbiol*, Vol. 54, No. 2, (October), pp. 452-463, ISSN: 0950-382X.

Mills, A. D., Blow, J. J., White, J. G., Amos, W. B., Wilcock, D. & Laskey, R. A. (1989). Replication occurs at discrete foci spaced throughout nuclei replicating in vitro. *J Cell Sci*, Vol. 94, No. Pt 3, (November), pp. 471-477, ISSN: 0021-9533.

Nakamura, H., Morita, T. & Sato, C. (1986). Structural organizations of replicon domains during DNA synthetic phase in the mammalian nucleus. *Exp Cell Res*, Vol. 165, No. 2, (August), pp. 291-297, ISSN: 0014-4827.

Nakayasu, H. & Berezney, R. (1989). Mapping replicational sites in the eucaryotic cell nucleus. *J Cell Biol*, Vol. 108, No. 1, (January), pp. 1-11, ISSN: 0021-9525.

O'Keefe, R. T., Henderson, S. C. & Spector, D. L. (1992). Dynamic organization of DNA replication in mammalian cell nuclei: spatially and temporally defined replication of chromosome-specific alpha-satellite DNA sequences. *J Cell Biol*, Vol. 116, No. 5, (March), pp. 1095-1110, ISSN: 0021-9525.

Pardoll, D. M., Vogelstein, B. & Coffey, D. S. (1980). A fixed site of DNA replication in eucaryotic cells. *Cell*, Vol. 19, No. 2, (February), pp. 527-536, ISSN: 0092-8674.

Reyes-Lamothe, R., Possoz, C., Danilova, O. & Sherratt, D. J. (2008). Independent positioning and action of Escherichia coli replisomes in live cells. *Cell*, Vol. 133, No. 1, (April), pp. 90-102, ISSN: 1097-4172.

Rieder, C. L. & Cole, R. (1999). Chromatid cohesion during mitosis: lessons from meiosis. *J Cell Sci*, Vol. 112, No. Pt 16, (August), pp. 2607-2613, ISSN: 0021-9533.

Salic, A. & Mitchison, T. J. (2008). A chemical method for fast and sensitive detection of DNA synthesis in vivo. *Proc Natl Acad Sci U S A*, Vol. 105, No. 7, (February), pp. 2415-2420, ISSN: 1091-6490

Sasaki, T. & Gilbert, D. M. (2007). The many faces of the origin recognition complex. *Curr Opin Cell Biol*, Vol. 19, No. 3, (June), pp. 337-343, ISSN: 0955-0674.

Singer, J. D., Manning, B. M. & Formosa, T. (1996). Coordinating DNA replication to produce one copy of the genome requires genes that act in ubiquitin metabolism. *Mol Cell Biol*, Vol. 16, No. 4, (April), pp. 1356-1366, ISSN: 0270-7306.

Stillman, B. (2005). Origin recognition and the chromosome cycle. *FEBS Lett*, Vol. 579, No. 4, (February), pp. 877-884, ISSN: 0014-5793.

Takahashi, T. S., Wigley, D. B. & Walter, J. C. (2005). Pumps, paradoxes and ploughshares: mechanism of the MCM2-7 DNA helicase. *Trends Biochem Sci*, Vol. 30, No. 8, (August), pp. 437-444, ISSN: 0968-0004.

Tomilin, N., Solovjeva, L., Krutilina, R., Chamberland, C., Hancock, R. & Vig, B. (1995). Visualization of elementary DNA replication units in human nuclei corresponding in size to DNA loop domains. *Chromosome Res*, Vol. 3, No. 1, (January), pp. 32-40, ISSN: 0967-3849.

van Dierendonck, J. H., Keyzer, R., van de Velde, C. J. & Cornelisse, C. J. (1989). Subdivision of S-phase by analysis of nuclear 5-bromodeoxyuridine staining patterns. *Cytometry*, Vol. 10, No. 2, (March), pp. 143-150, ISSN: 0196-4763.

Waga, S. & Stillman, B. (1998). The DNA replication fork in eukaryotic cells. *Annu Rev Biochem*, Vol. 67, (July), pp. 721-751, ISSN: 0066-4154.

Wagner, G., Bancaud, A., Quivy, J. P., Clapier, C., Almouzni, G. & Viovy, J. L. (2005). Compaction kinetics on single DNAs: purified nucleosome reconstitution systems versus crude extract. *Biophys J*, Vol. 89, No. 5, (November), pp. 3647-3659, ISSN: 0006-3495.

Wessel, R., Schweizer, J. & Stahl, H. (1992). Simian virus 40 T-antigen DNA helicase is a hexamer which forms a binary complex during bidirectional unwinding from the viral origin of DNA replication. *J Virol*, Vol. 66, No. 2, (February), pp. 804-815, ISSN: 0022-538X.

Yardimci, H., Loveland, A. B., Habuchi, S., van Oijen, A. M. & Walter, J. C. (2010). Uncoupling of sister replisomes during eukaryotic DNA replication. *Mol Cell*, Vol. 40, No. 5, (December), pp. 834-840, ISSN: 1097-4164.

Yurov, Y. B. & Liapunova, N. A. (1977). The units of DNA replication in the mammalian chromosomes: evidence for a large size of replication units. *Chromosoma*, Vol. 60, No. 3, (April), pp. 253-267, ISSN: 0009-5915.

Zieve, G. W., Turnbull, D., Mullins, J. M. & McIntosh, J. R. (1980). Production of large numbers of mitotic mammalian cells by use of the reversible microtubule inhibitor nocodazole. Nocodazole accumulated mitotic cells. *Exp Cell Res*, Vol. 126, No. 2, (April), pp. 397-405, ISSN: 0014-4827.

13

Eukaryotic Replication Barriers: How, Why and Where Forks Stall

Jacob Z. Dalgaard[1], Emma L. Godfrey[1] and Ramsay J. MacFarlane[2]
[1]*Warwick Medical School, Clinical Science Research Institute, Gibbet Hill Campus, University of Warwick, Coventry,*
[2]*North West Cancer Research Fund Institute, College of Natural Sciences, Bangor University, Memorial Building, Deiniol Road, Bangor, Gwynedd, United Kingdom*

1. Introduction

Maintaining genetic fidelity is paramount for all living organisms. The process of replicating DNA is especially dangerous for cells. Not only must the genetic sequence be replicated precisely by the replicative polymerases, but stalled replication forks and single-stranded DNA present at the forks increase risks of chromosome breakage leading to rearrangements. Also, once the cell commits itself to the replication process it has to be fully completed before chromosomes can be disentangled and condensed prior to their proper segregation in the subsequent mitosis. Many processes have evolved that ensure the precision and stability of the replication process; helicases remove bound proteins in front of the fork, topoisomerases ensure that topological entanglements generated during replication are resolved; checkpoint activation in response to stalled replication forks controls an array of molecular responses, repair polymerases and proteins to be recruited to stalled replication forks to allow replication restart; moreover, origin firing is controlled such that firing of origins is delayed in response to the replication checkpoint and dormant origins can be activated if replication is not completed. It is at first hand therefore surprising that at specific loci in the genome, molecular mechanisms exist where deliberate pausing or termination of the replication fork occur. This wonder is further confounded by the fact that several studies have shown that these replication barriers cause genetic instability (see MacFarlane, Al-Zeer and Dalgaard, Chapter 16). What the evolutionary benefits of these replication barriers might be remains a major question. More and more evidence is accumulating that indicates many replication barriers have opposing effects on genome stability; on one hand they promote genetic stability though a controlled stalling of the replication fork at specific sites or situations, however, in doing so they potentially cause fork collapse and genetic instability. In many cases these barriers "coordinate" transcription and replication, preventing collisions between the two types of enzymatic complexes, suggesting that such collisions are more detrimental to the stability of the genome than the instability induced by stalling at a replication barrier (references are given in the main text). Thus, one might argue that most replication barriers evolved to promote genetic stability while allowing "controlled" genetic instability, although other functions of replication barriers are also evident. Here, we review what different types of natural replication impediments are known, how they prevent replication fork progression, and what potential biological function they have.

2. Epstein-Barr virus protein EBNA-1

Epstein-Barr virus or human herpes virus 4 DNA is replicated once per cell-cycle in latently infected cells. Here the DNA binding EBNA-1 protein plays several important roles for viral replication. First, EBNA-1 binds to inverted repeats at the *cis*-acting *OriP* sequence, where it acts to recruit cellular ORC proteins and as a consequence, other replication factors required for replication. Binding to the *OriP* sequence occurs at a region with dyad symmetry containing four low-affinity binding sites for EBNA-1 (Ambinder, et al. 1990). However, EBNA-1 also interacts with another region within *OriP* called *FR* (family of repeats), which contains twenty 30-bp high-affinity sites for the EBNA-1 dimer (Rawlins, et al. 1985). When replication is initiated at *OriP* it proceeds in a bi-directional manner but the replication fork moving toward *FR* is stalled by the bound EBNA-1, thus converting the bi-directional replication process into an uni-directional replication one. Reducing the number of *FR* repeats from 20 to 15, 6, 2 or 0 showed that 6, 15 or 20 copies promoted barrier activity (Dhar & Schildkraut, 1991). The *FR* region with bound EBNA-1 acts both as a barrier for the cellular MCM replicative helicase during viral replication as well as the SV40 large T-antigen for SV40 plasmids. The latter barrier activity has been observed both *in vitro* and *in vivo* (Dhar & Schildkraut, 1991, Ermakova, et al. 1996, Aiyar, et al. 2009). EBNA-1 also prevents strand unwinding by both the SV40 large T-antigen 3′ to 5′ helicase and the *E. coli* dnaB 5′ to 3′ helicase (Ermakova, et al. 1996). Interestingly, FR/EBNA-1 complexes containing 20 or 40 repeats also act as a barrier to RNA polymerase II transcription, and since a viral transcript (although catalysed by RNA polymerase III; Howe & Shu, 1989; Howe & Shu, 1993) is oriented toward *FR*, the *FR*/EBNA-1 barrier could have a role in preventing collisions between transcription and replication forks (Aiyar, et al. 2009). In addition to its role in replication, the *FR*/EBNA-1 element is also required for maintenance and partitioning of viral DNA. The element tethers the viral episome to a cellular chromosome, thereby allowing appropriate segregation into the daughter cells (Marechal, et al. 1999; Sears, et al. 2003; Sears, et al. 2004). Interestingly, the FR/EBNA-1 element also has a negative effect on plasmid maintenance; puromycin resistance encoding plasmids containing 20 or more copies of the element are not efficiently maintained in cell culture (Aiyar, et al. 2009). Thus, the *FR*/EBNA-1 replication barrier element might have both negative and positive effects on viral copy number.

3. rDNA replication barriers

Most organisms share the same basic arrangement of the rDNA, consisting of one or more arrays of a genetic unit, where each unit contains a RNA polymerase I transcribed pre-curser rRNA encoding the 25-28S large rRNA, the 16-18S small rRNA as well as the 5.8 S rRNAs. The latter is separated from the origin of replication by a non-transcribed spacer (NTS). This NTS contains one or more replication barriers that pause or stall replication forks, thus preventing them from entering the polymerase I transcribed unit. Such barriers have been described in many different organisms, including fission yeast (*Schizosaccharomyces pombe*), budding yeast (*Saccharomyces cerevisiae*), ciliated protozoa (*Tetrahymena thermophila*), Pea

(*Pisum sativum*), frog (*Xenopus laevis*), mouse (*Mus musculus*) and human (see below for references). Generally these barriers are thought to prevent collisions (and therefore genetic instability) between the polymerase I transcription bubbles and the replication forks moving in opposite directions, but data suggests that they have both a positive and a negative effect on genome stability (see below).

3.1 Pea rDNA barriers

2D-gel analysis of the rDNA of *P. sativum* detected several replication barriers in the NTS, located just downstream the RNA polymerase I transcript. The *P. sativum* replication barrier region maps to a 27 base pair direct repeat region with the consensus sequence TCCGCC(T/A)CTTGT-ATTCGTTGCGTTG(A/C)A that is either present in 9 or 3 copies in two different classes of arrays (Hernandez, et al. 1988; Hernandez, et al. 1993; Lopez-Estrano, et al. 1999). This repeated sequence motif shows some similarity with the sequence that mediates barrier activity in *S. cerevisia* (Hernandez, et al. 1993), and mobility shifts indicate that an unknown transacting factor(s) can bind to the repeats (Lopez-Estrano, et al. 1999).

3.2 Ciliate rDNA barriers

In *T. thermophila* the rDNA barriers are developmentally regulated. In the germ line micronucleus the 10.3 kb rDNA is present in a single copy, while in the differentiated macro nucleus the rDNA has been excised from the genome, arranged into an inverted repeat (the two polymerase I transcripts arranged in opposite directions), telomeres are added and the repeat is amplified 10000 fold (Reviewed in Tower, 2004). This amplification occurs within one cell cycle. Interestingly, here the 5′ NTS contains three replication barriers that pause the replication fork in a polar manner (MacAlpine, et al. 1997). These barriers are located between the site of replication initiation (that occurs at two sites flanking the centre of the inverted repeat) and the polymerase I transcript. Thus, here the barriers are upstream of the RNA polymerase I transcript. The consensus sequence of the three *cis*-acting sequences is 5′ A(A/T)TTTCANNNNNNNNNNNNNNNNNNNA(A/G)TTTCATTCANNNNNNNNNNTTT TTTTT 3′. These replication pause sites are active both during vegetative growth and when amplification occurs. In addition to the three pause sites, an additional replication barrier is present which only acts during amplification and not during vegetative growth. This barrier is present in the middle of the palindrome and acts to stall the fork until a converging replication fork initiated at the other side of the palindrome arrives to promote termination (Zhang, et al. 1997). Interestingly, this central barrier element is required for both proper excision of the rDNA before amplification in the macronucleus, as well as for maintaining genetic stability at the unamplified rDNA gene in the micronucleus (Yakisich & Kapler, 2006). In the absence of the barrier element breakage occurs at the loci leading to loss of the chromosome arm, which again has a dominant effect on the stability of the homologues chromosome present in the diploid nucleus.

3.3 Frog rDNA barriers

Similarly, developmentally regulated replication barriers have been described in *X. laevis*. Firstly, a barrier is present at the RNA polymerase I termination region. This barrier can be detected in cell culture and tissues where the rDNA is highly transcribed, but not in early embryos and in egg extracts where transcription is low or absent (Hyrien & Mechali, 1993; Wiesendanger, et al. 1994; Hyrien, et al. 1995). Secondly, 15 weaker pause sites distributed over the rDNA unit appear during the midgastrula stage, for then to disappear again at the neurula stage (Maric, et al. 1999). The appearance of these pause sites was proposed to reflect chromatin remodelling associated with the developmental regulation of polymerase I transcription.

3.4 Budding yeast rDNA barriers

The replication barrier in the rDNA of *S. cerevisiae* was the first to be described (Brewer & Fangman, 1987; Linskens & Huberman, 1988). Like the other barriers it is located in one of two NTS regions downstream of both the coding regions of the polymerase I transcribed 35S rRNA and the RNA polymerase III transcribed 5S rRNA. However, unlike the other eukaryotic systems, the barrier activity is not mediated by the Reb1 factor involved in Polymerase I transcription termination (*S. cerevisiae* Reb1 is related to Mammalian TTF1 and *S. pombe* Reb1; see below) (Reeder, et al. 1999). Instead the barrier activity is mediated by an unrelated *S. cerevisiae* factor Fob1 that binds to the DNA at a region closer to the origin (Kobayashi & Horiuchi, 1996) and about 90% of replication forks are stalled at this barrier (Brewer et al. 1992). Barrier activity is independent of transcription (Brewer, et al. 1992) and Fob1 interacts with three sites, RFB1-3, where the latter two are the minor barrier sites (Brewer, et al. 1992; Gruber, et al. 2000; Ward, et al. 2000; Kobayashi, 2003). The *cis*-acting sequences show phylogenetic conservation between *Saccharomyces* species (Ganley, et al. 2005). Fob1 possesses a Zn^{2+}-finger domain and a domain with similarity to integrases (Dlakic, 2002); mutations in the former affect DNA binding activity, barrier activity and HOT1 (HOT1 is a recombination hot spot in the rDNA) activity, whilst a mutation of the putative catalytic residue D291A of the integrase domain has no effect (Kobayashi, 2003). Using Atomic Force Microscopy (AFM) it was shown that Fob1 interacts with the barrier sequence in a fashion where the DNA is wound around the protein (Kobayashi, 2003). Moreover, the same data suggest that Fob1 acts as a dimer interacting with two sequences at the same time. The position of the stalled replication fork has been precisely mapped (Gruber, et al. 2000); the 3′ end of the leading-strand and the 5′ end of the lagging-strand map three nucleotides apart, 41 and 38 nucleotides in front of the sequences required for pausing at RFB1, respectively. However, weaker signals due to fork stalling were also observed in a region between RFB1 and RFB2 (Figure 1).

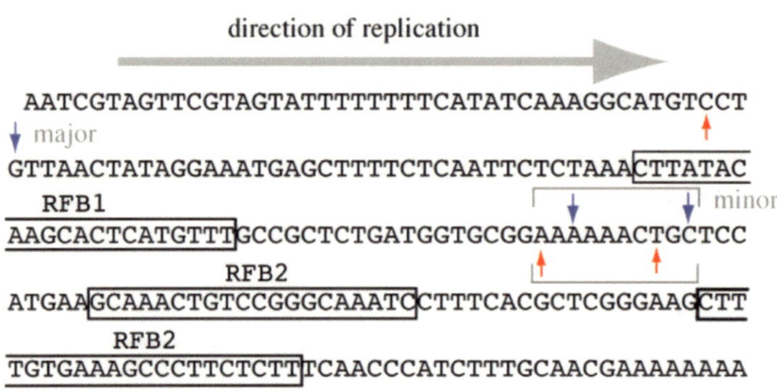

Fig. 1. Positions of the sites of replication stalling for the *S. cerevisiae* rDNA barrier. Positions of stalling of the leading-strand polymerase (red arrows) and 5′-ends of the last lagging-strand Okazaki fragment (blue arrows) are shown relative to the binding sites of Fob1.

AFM analysis also shows that the RNA primer at the lagging-strand has been removed in the stalled replication complex. (Kobayashi, 2003). Stalling of the replication fork at the Fob1 barrier depends on Tof1 (*S. pombe* Swi1/Human TIMELESS) and Csm3 (*S. pombe* Swi3/ Human TIPIN), but not Mrc1 (*S. pombe* Mrc1/ Human Claspin) (Mohanty, et al. 2006). When the replication fork is stalled at the Fob1 barrier located at an ectopic site (Calzada, et al. 2005) the replisome (Mrc1, Tof1, MCM-Cdc45, GINS and DNA polymerases α and ε) is maintained intact, thus allowing the replication fork to restart. The stability of the stalled replication fork was also shown not to depend on replication checkpoint kinases Mec1 and Rad53 or the Sml1 factor (See Section 6.0), nor does the replication restart depend on the Rad52 recombinase. Stalling leads to the recruitment of the Rrm3 helicase, which was suggested to mediate restart. These data and suggestions were later verified by a study that showed that replication stalling was dependent on Tof1 and Csm3, but partly restored in *Δtof1 Δrrm3* and *Δcsm3 Δrrm3* mutants (Mohanty, et al. 2006). It was proposed that Tof1 and Csm3 mediate stalling by counteracting Rrm3, but since Rrm3 is required for efficient replication past many non-histone DNA binding proteins (See Section 10.0), the effect could be unspecific (Mohanty, et al. 2006). Similarly, the requirement for two other helicases, Sgs1 and Srs2, was tested in the absence of Tof1 but neither affected barrier activity. Another study looked at Sgs1, Top3, Dnl4 and Rad52 with again no major effects on barrier activity, although in all the mutants there was an increase in the amount of single-stranded DNA at the fork measured using electron microscopy (Fritsch, et al. 2010). However, increased barrier activity was observed in a Dna2 mutant, a helicase implicated in Okazaki fragment maturation, suggesting that events at the lagging strand affect the stalled fork (Weitao, et al. 2003a; Weitao, et al. 2003b). The biological function of the Fob1 barrier has been an area of intense research and resulted in some key findings. Firstly, Fob1 barrier activity promotes recombination between repeats in the rDNA array and has a role in repeat expansion through induction of recombination and unequal sister-chromatid exchange (Kobayashi & Horiuchi, 1996; Kobayashi, et al. 1998; Mayan-Santos, et al. 2008; Ganley, et al. 2009). Double stranded breaks have been detected at the barrier and related to replication fork pausing, potentially due to fork collapse (Weitao, et al. 2003a; Weitao, et al. 2003b; Fritsch, et al. 2010). Secondly, barrier activity acts to prevent collisions between the DNA replication fork and the polymerase I transcription forks, leading to fluctuations in copy numbers and formation of extra chromosomal rDNA circles (ERCs) (Takeuchi, et al. 2003). Thirdly, Fob1 barrier activity has also been implicated in ageing as its fork barrier activity leads to formation of ERCs that accumulate in the mother cell, as well as in an increased loss of heterozygosity of markers distal to the rDNA array on chromosome XII (Defossez, et al. 1999; Lindstrom, et al. 2011). However, recent data suggest that age related replication stress underlies the ageing process, and not the formation of ERCs (Lindstrom, et al. 2011). Forthly, Fob1 also has a role in silencing of the rDNA through the recruitment of the regulator of nucleolar silencing and telophase exit (RENT) complex that includes Net1, Sir2, CDC14, Tof2, Lrs4 and Csm1 as well as Cohesin (Huang & Moazed, 2003), but this role is independent of the replication barrier activity of the protein (Bairwa, et al. 2010). The RENT complex inhibits polymerase II transcription and represses recombination (Kobayashi, et al. 2004; Kobayashi & Ganley, 2005). Lastly, Fob1 also regulates the activity of Topoisomerase I, as Fob1 dependent but replication independent topoisomerase I catalysed nicks have been mapped within the replication barrier region (Burkhalter & Sogo, 2004; Di Felice, et al. 2005).

3.5 Mammalian rDNA barriers

Replication barriers have also been identified in human and mouse rDNA arrays (Little, et al. 1993b; Langst, et al. 1998; Lopez-estrano, et al. 1998b). The barrier signals were detected by 2D-gel analysis of replication intermediates and map to the binding sites of the TTF-I transcription factor within the NTS region located downstream of the 38S rRNA polymerase I transcribed regions. The TTF-1 transcription factor belongs to the same family of proteins as *S. pombe* Rtf1 and Reb1 and *S. cerevisiae* Reb1 (see Figure 2). TTF-I mediates termination of polymerase I transcription, but also has additional roles in polymerase II termination as well as both polymerase I transcription activation and silencing (Langst, et al. 1998; Wang & Warner, 1998). TTF-I binds to ten 18 base-pair long or eleven 11 base-pair long *Sal-boxes* in mouse and human cells, respectively, which are located within the NTS region of the rDNA. TTF-I binding mediates polar polymerase I transcription termination (Grummt, et al. 1985a; Grummt, et al. 1985b; Lang, et al. 1994; Reeder & Lang, 1994). However, TTF-I *Sal*-box binding also promotes replication barrier activity. 2D-gel analysis of replication intermediates isolated from the human cell cultures suggests that the rDNA replication barriers are bi-polar, stalling forks moving in both directions (Little, et al. 1993a). A similar analysis of the mouse barriers showed that in this system the TTF-I dependent barriers are polar, mediating replication stalling at each of the four clusters of *Sal-boxes* of replication forks moving in the opposite direction to that of the flanking RNA polymerase I transcription (Lopez-estrano, et al. 1998a). Finally, an *in vitro* study suggests that only *Sal-box 2* acts as a strong replication barrier (Gerber, et al. 1997). Using the SV40 *in vitro*

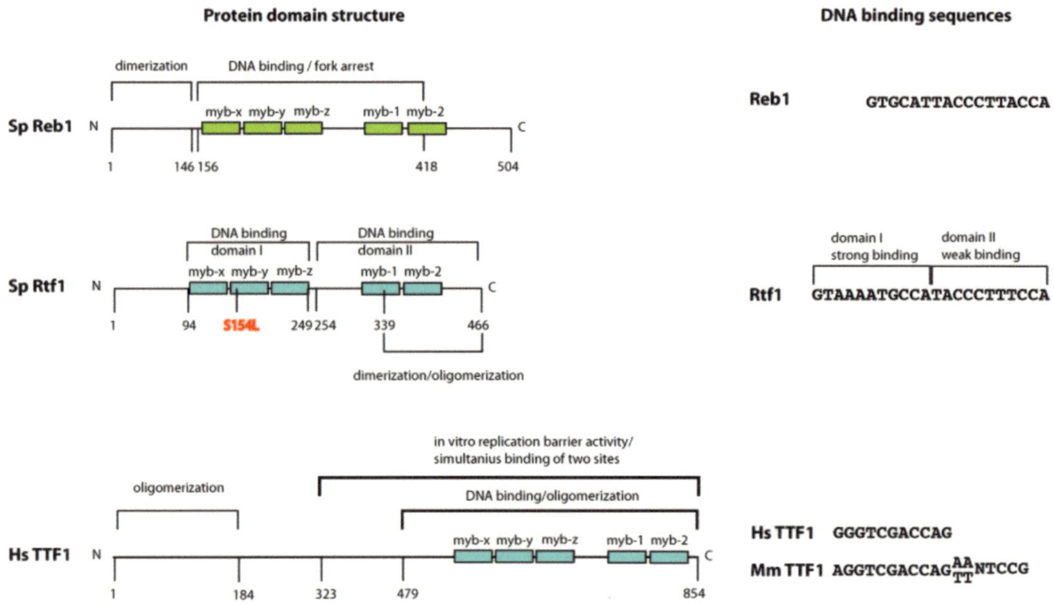

Fig. 2. Protein domains and DNA interaction sequences of the related TTF-I, Reb1 and Rtf1 factors. Left, the positions of the structural myb DNA-binding motifs identified by a hidden Markov model analysis are shown (Eydmann, et al. 2008); Domains with defined functions are indicated by square horizontal brackets. The position of the Rtf1-S154L mutation that changes the polarity of the *RTS1* element is indicated in red. Right, DNA recognition sequences of Reb1 and Rtf1 and Human/Mouse TTF-I.

replication system, this study also defined the *Sal-box 2 cis*-acting sequence requirements for site-specific replication termination, and verified the TTF-I dependence for barrier activity. When bound to *Sal-box 2,* TTF-I counteracts the strand displacement activity of the SV40 large-T antigen 3'-5' helicase (Putter & Grummt, 2002b). Three *cis*-acting elements are required for full activity of *Sal-box 2*. Firstly, the *in vitro* barrier activity depends on the *Sal-box 2* sequences that mediate TTF-I binding (Grummt, et al. 1985a; Putter & Grummt, 2002b). Secondly, this binding site is flanked by a GC-rich box that consists of 20 cytosine residues followed by a GC-rich stretch at the origin-proximal side. Introduction of point mutations within this region, shortening the stretch of cytosines (dC stretch), or inverting this region relatively to the *Sal-box,* abolished replication barrier activity and contra-helicase activities (Gerber, et al. 1997; Putter & Grummt, 2002a). The 20 base pair long dC stretch potentially forms a secondary structure, a poly dG-dG-dC triple helix that can act as a barrier for the progressing helicase or polymerase (Putter & Grummt, 2002a). Thirdly, flanking the GC rich sequence is a stretch of 26 thymidines that acts as an enhancer of the barrier activity; deletion of the thymidines causes a ~30% reduction in activity (Putter & Grummt, 2002a). The position of the *in vitro* leading-strand replication termination site has been mapped to 28 nucleotides from the *Sal-box* just in front of the long stretch of dC residues (Gerber, et al. 1997).

Several studies of the 883 amino acid long TTF-I factor have been performed. Two regions within the protein have been implicated in polymerization of the protein (Sander, et al. 1996a; Gerber, et al. 1997), (Figure 2). A 323 N-terminal truncated version of TTF-I is fully active for both *in vitro* transcription and replication termination, while a 445 amino acids N-terminal truncation leads to loss of both activities. Neither of these truncations affect the DNA binding of the protein, however, the region between residue 323 and 445 is required for polymeric TTF-1 to interact simultaneously with two DNA sites (Sander & Grummt, 1997; Evers & Grummt, 1995; Sander, et al. 1996b; Gerber, et al. 1997). Similar to the other replication barriers described below, the data suggest that passive binding of TTF-1 is not sufficient to cause replication barrier activity, but that in addition specific interactions with replication fork proteins must occur. Furthermore, dimerization or polymerization of TTF-I might be important for replication termination as observed recently for *S. pombe* Reb1 (see 3.6). Interestingly, TTF-I binds both in the promoter region and, as described above, in the transcription termination region of the polymerase I transcribed element, and a 3C analysis shows that these two regions interact by a mechanism that depends on TTF-I (Nemeth, et al. 2008). This interaction has been proposed to be important for regulation of transcription initiation; TTF-1 recruits the chromatin remodelling complex NoRC to the promoter region through a direct interaction in the N-terminal part of TTF-I to silence rDNA transcription (Nemeth, et al. 2004). The N-terminal domain of TTF-I has a negative effect on DNA binding through an interaction with the DNA binding domain. This inhibition is relieved through the interaction in *trans* with NoRC (Nemeth, et al. 2004). The described interaction between TTF-I molecules bound at the promoter and termination regions, also opens up the possibility that there might be coordination between transcription initiation at the promoter and replication barrier activity at the transcription termination region.

The proteins Ku70 and Ku86 have also been implicated in replication barrier activity at the mammalian rDNA (Wallisch, et al. 2002). Using affinity purification with a bait that consisted of the GC-rich region that flanks the *Sal box 2*, a protein fraction was isolated which stimulated *in vitro* replication termination. The stimulating activity could be depleted from the HeLa cell extracts using an oligonucleotide sequence containing the GC rich region bound to DYNA beads, and subsequently the depleted extracts could be complemented by addition of recombinant Ku70/Ku86. Thus, Ku70/Ku86 binding promotes replication termination at the *Sal-box 2*, potentially involving the formation of secondary structures when the DNA is unwound by the helicase or replicated by the polymerase.

3.6 Fission yeast rDNA barriers

The rDNA barrier region of *S. pombe* is more complex than the other systems described, in that four different barrier elements have been defined; *RBF1-4*. These barrier elements are clustered downstream of the coding region of the 25S rRNA gene in the NTS. Again the elements act as polar barriers for replication forks initiated at the origin and moving toward the RNA polymerase I transcribed unit, thus preventing collisions between the two types of enzymatic complexes. Two different *trans*-acting factors have been identified that serve as barriers at these sites, Reb1 and Sap1.

Sap1 is responsible for the barrier activity at the *RFB1* site, which in one study was delineated to a 21 bp region (Krings & Bastia, 2005) and in another to a 30 bp region (Mejia-Ramirez, et al. 2005). Sap1 is an essential DNA binding protein involved in chromatin formation, checkpoint activation and maintenance of genome stability (Arcangioli & Klar, 1991; Ghazvini, et al. 1995; de Lahondes, et al. 2003; Noguchi & Noguchi, 2007). Loss of Sap1 causes chromosomal segregation defects, while overexpression causes toxic DNA replication dependent chromosome fragmentation and abnormal mitosis. Due to the fact that Sap1 is essential, the evidence for Sap1 binding at the *RFB1* site is indirect. Firstly, Sap1 was purified from crude extracts as a factor that binds the *cis*-acting sequences at *RFB1* (Mejia-Ramirez, et al. 2005). Secondly, *RFB1* point mutations that affect Sap1 binding *in vitro* also affect barrier activity *in vivo* (Krings & Bastia, 2005). Lastly, supershifts can be achieved with antibodies against tagged-Sap1 in EMSA experiments (Krings & Bastia, 2005). Binding of the dimeric Sap1 protein to the *RFB1* site causes a slight bending of the DNA *in vitro* (Krings & Bastia, 2005). Replication fork stalling at *RFB1* is dependent of the *trans*-acting factors Swi1 and Swi3 (Mejia-Ramirez, et al. 2005). Sap1 also binds the *SAS1* sequence required for mating-type switching (Arcangioli & Klar, 1991), but does not cause barrier activity at this locus (Kaykov, et al. 2004; Krings & Bastia, 2005; see Section 8.1). A comparison of the interactions between Sap1 and these two *cis*-acting sequences showed that the Sap1 dimer bound differently to the two sites; the interaction of the Sap1 protein with *RFB1* covered successive major grooves, had translational symmetry and occurred with higher affinity; while the interaction with SAS1 was a minor groove interaction, occurred with a relatively lower affinity and had rotational symmetry (Krings & Bastia, 2006).

Reb1 was identified as mediating barrier activity at the two *cis*-acting sites *RFB2* and *RFB3* (Sanchez-Gorostiaga, et al. 2004). Reb1 also mediates Polymerase I termination at the same sequences (Melekhovets, et al. 1997). Reb1 belongs to the same family of factors as Human/Mouse TTF1, *S. cerevisiae* Reb1 and *S. pombe* Rtf1, which are characterized by the presence of a repeated myb domain (Eydmann, et al. 2008) Figure 2). Reb1 acts as a dimer that dimerizes through a 146 amino acid long N-terminal domain (Biswas & Bastia, 2008). This dimerization allows the dimeric protein to interact with two recognition sites at the same time (Singh, et al. 2010). When the two sites are in *cis* the intervening DNA is looped out, however, the dimeric protein can also interact with two sites in *trans*. In the latter case, "chromosome kissing" was observed between a Reb1 dependent barrier on chromosome 2, Ter344314, and two sites on chromosome 1, Ter4257637 (Cyp8) and Ter4680236 (Srw1/Ste9)

(Singh, et al. 2010). Furthermore, using weakened binding sites at the Ter344314 and Ter4680236 sites it was shown that this "chromosome kissing" was important for barrier activity. Only the middle 156-418 AA Section of Reb1 is absolutely required for barrier activity. Barrier activity at *RFB2* and *RFB3* depends on both Swi1 and Swi3, however, a Swi1 mutation (*swi1-rtf*) that abolishes barrier activity at the *RTS1* element does not affect barrier activity at the *RFB1-4* (see Section 8.0; Krings & Bastia, 2004). Interestingly, when the 156-418 AA Reb1 segment was expressed in *S. cerevisia*, it was unable to act as a barrier even though it was binding to the RFB3 sequence (Biswas and Bastia, 2008). Finally, Reb1 has also been shown to be important for gene regulation; Reb1 binding at the promoter of *Ste9* is required for transcriptional activation and G1 arrest (Rodriguez-Sanchez, et al. 2011). Reb1 also acts as a replication barrier at this site.

The RFB4 barrier is the weakest of the four barriers, and has been proposed to be generated by collisions between the polymerase I transcription machinery and the DNA replication machinery (Krings & Bastia, 2004). The intensity of the RFB4 barrier signal increases in the absence of Swi1, Swi3 or Reb1, potentially because more replication forks are colliding with the transcription machinery. Also, RFB4 does not act as a replication barrier when the region is moved onto a plasmid.

4. Centromeric and telomeric replication barriers

Replication pause sites have been described at both the *S. cerevisiae* telomeres and centromeres. At the Y' elements of the telomeres the replication fork pauses at internal $C_{1\text{-}3}A/TG_{1\text{-}3}$ telomeric sequences as well as at the terminal $C_{1\text{-}3}A/TG_{1\text{-}3}$ repeats. The internal $C_{1\text{-}3}A/TG_{1\text{-}3}$ sequences promote stalling independent of the orientation relative to of the progressing replication fork, and the replication pausing is intensified in absence of the Rrm3 helicase (Ivessa, et al. 2002; Makovets, et al. 2004, Makovets, 2009). In the *rrm3* mutant strain, pausing can also be observed at an inactive *ARS* element in the subtelomeric region. Insertion of *Tetrahymena* telomeric repeats in the subtelomeric region of *S. cerevisiae* did not lead to pausing suggesting that it is the binding of a *trans*-acting factor that leads to the barrier activity and not the repeat sequences themselves (Makovets, et al. 2004). However, mutation of the sub-telomeric binding sites of Tbf1 and Reb1, deletion of the *Rif1, Rif2, Sir2* or *Sir3* genes, or introduction of a C-terminal truncated version of Rap1, do not affect the replication pause (Makovets, et al. 2004; Makovets, 2009). Tbf1 and Reb1 act at chromatin barriers in the subtelomeric region, while Sir2 mediates silencing at the telomeres and Rap1 binds directly the telomeric repeats when they are double stranded. The C-terminal truncated version of Rap1 is unable to interact with the Rif proteins and deficient in the recruitment of Sir proteins to the telomeres, although DNA binding to the telomeric repeats is unaffected. Thus, it is argued that it is most likely Rap1 binding per se, potentially through the interaction with other unknown protein(s), which mediate the pause activity. Since the strength of the replication pause is dependent on the length of the telomeres, a potential role of the pause is to regulate the time in which the telomeres can be elongated; short telomeres do not cause pausing and are therefore replicated faster, thus giving telomerase longer time for elongation.

Several replication pause sites have also been observed at the sub-telomeric regions of *S. pombe*, however, it is not known what proteins mediate pausing at these sites (Miller, et al. 2006). In addition, a protein that binds the telomeric repeats, named Taz1, has been attributed an interesting role; in the absence of Taz1 replication defects are observed at the telomeric repeats, leading to loss of telomeric sequences and chromosome entanglement. In addition, in the absence of Taz1, replication pausing is observed at the junction between the telomeric repeats and the sub-telomeric region, as well as at repeats located internally within the chromosome. In the latter case, the requirement is independent of the orientation of the repetitive sequence (Miller, et al. 2006). One possibility is that Taz1 has a role in recruiting replicative helicases that act to aid fork progression through the repeats. With respect to this, it is interesting to note that the human homologues of Taz1, TRF1 and TRF2, have also been shown to affect telomeric replication, although in a different manner (Ohki & Ishikawa, 2004). Using the SV40 *in vitro* replication system, it was shown that addition of recombinant TRF1 and TRF2 lead to stalling of the replication fork at the telomeric region of the linear SV40 DNA. Similarly, overexpression of TRF1 in HeLa cells, leads to an increase of replication foci that overlap with telomeric signals, suggesting an increase of replication forks stalled at telomeres.

Replication pausing is also observed at the *S. cerevisiae* centromeres *CEN1*, *CEN3* and *CEN4*, and presumably replication pausing occurs at all centromeres (Greenfeder & Newlon, 1992). Interestingly, pausing at the centromeric DNA is bipolar and thus occurs independently of the direction by which the replication fork enters the centromeric DNA. A mutational analysis of the *cis*-acting sequences showed that the barrier activity is dependent on the ability of the centromeric DNA to form a nuclease resistant core protein structure, suggesting that it is the interaction with centromeric proteins that causes the pause to replication fork progression (Greenfeder & Newlon, 1992). It is not known whether replication pausing is important for centromere function. Interestingly, recent papers describing the genome-wide localization of phosphorylated histone H2A show accumulation at the centromeric regions of both *S. cerevisiae* and *S. pombe,* thus, potentially replication stalling occurs at centromeres in both yeasts (see Section 11.0).

5. Replication barriers at tRNA genes, retrotransposons and LTRs

Early work identified replication pause sites at *Ty1-LTRs* and tRNA genes in *S. cerevisiae* (Greenfeder & Newlon, 1992, Deshpande & Newlon, 1996). These tRNA gene replication barrier activities were shown to be polar only stalling replication forks moving in one direction, that opposite to the direction of Polymerase III transcription. *Cis*- and *trans*-acting mutations that reduce or abolish the efficiency of transcription initiation correspondingly reduced or abolished replication barrier activity. Indeed, a temperature sensitive mutation in the large subunit of RNA polIII, that affects transcription initiation but not the formation of the initiation complex consisting of TFIIIC and TFIIIB at the tRNA gene also abolished barrier activity. Therefore, the replication barrier activity most likely results from a direct interaction between the transcription machinery and the progressing replication fork complex, although a build up of supercoiling between the approaching transcription and replication forks was also proposed as a potential mechanism for fork pausing (Deshpande & Newlon, 1996). Importantly, a later study showed that barrier activity is abolished in a *Δtof1* mutant (*S. pombe* Swi1/Human TIMELESS), but is restored in the *Δtof1 Δrrm3* double mutant (Mohanty, et al. 2006). In the same study, increased stalling was observed at the tRNA gene in the absence of the Rrm3 helicase.

S. pombe tRNA^{GLU} and *sup3-e* tRNA genes have also been shown to pause replication forks. However, in this system the tRNAs act as bi-polar barriers stalling replication forks moving in both orientations. Furthermore, the tRNA gene barrier activity is independent of Swi1 function (McFarlane & Whitehall, 2009; Pryce, et al. 2009). Similarly, polar replication pausing has been observed at *S. pombe* retrotransposons *Tf2 LTRs* (Zaratiegui, et al. 2011). Interestingly, replication pausing at these elements is abolished by the *sap1-c* mutation. The *sap1-c* allele was isolated as a spontaneous mutation that restored growth and improves viability to a double mutant strain of the two CENP-B homologues Abp1 and Cbh1. The *Δabp1 Δcbh1* double mutant has poor viability due to increased levels of unreplicated regions and/or recombination structures, and the *sap1-c* allele was isolated as a spontaneous mutation that restored growth and viability. The *sap1-c* mutation reduces the Sap1 proteins ability to bind DNA. Thus, Abp1 and Cbh1 have roles preventing genetic instability and replication defects induced by Sap1 barrier activity. *Δabp1* and *Δcbh1* single mutants slightly increase the intensity of the Sap1 dependent barrier signal, and in the *Δabp1 Δcbh1* double mutant recombination intermediates can also be observed by 2D-gel analysis of replication intermediates (Zaratiegui, et al. 2011). Abp1 also localizes to tRNA genes suggesting that it might have a role in maintaining genome stability at these replication barriers as well. Abp1 interacts with Mcm10 that has been shown to have primase activity (Locovei, et al. 2006), thus Abp1 might promote replication restart after pausing through a priming event.

6. Replication slow zones

Replication slow zones have been described in *S. cerevisiae* and are characterized by increased amounts of replication intermediates as measured by 2D-gel analysis (Cha & Kleckner, 2002). These zones are regularly spaced throughout the genome between active origins, except at the centromere. The replication slow zones were identified as regions of genetic instability in the *mec1* mutant background. Mec1 is the homologue of Human ATR and *S. pombe* Rad3, and has multiple roles in DNA replication, replication checkpoint activation, DNA damage repair and recombination. Interestingly, the genetic instability is suppressed by a *Δsml1* mutation, suggesting that the instability is due to low levels of dNTPs. Sml1 is an inhibitor of ribonucleotide reductase, and the lack of Sml1 leads to an increase in dNTP levels. Similarly, the *Δrrm3* mutation partly suppresses the genetic instability observed at replication slow zones, which is correlated with a decrease in the Sml1 protein level (Hashash, et al. 2011). Thus, the data suggest that low levels of dNTPs cause replication forks to slow down even in an unperturbed S-phase, and that Mec1 is important for maintaining the stability of these slow moving forks, potentially via the function of Mec1 in regulating the nucleotide pools through inhibition of Sml1 and in intra-S and G2-M checkpoint activation. Whether replication slow zones are important for genome stability in higher organism has yet to be established.

7. Replication barriers mediated by DNA structures or repetitive sequences

Inverted repeats and micro repeats, through formation of triplexes and G-quartets have all been shown to inhibit DNA polymerase progression *in vitro* (for a review see Mirkin & Mirkin, 2007). Similarly, there is growing *in vivo* evidence that structures and repetitive sequences in the DNA are difficult templates, which promote replication fork stalling and as a consequence genetic instability. Since formation of structures distinct to the double helix are not energetically favoured, especially in front of the replication fork where there is supercoiling, it is most likely that the structures are formed in the lagging-strand template (Mirkin & Mirkin, 2007). Sequences that have been shown to mediate fork stalling include inverted repeats as well as (CAG)n/(CTG)n, (CGG)n/(CCG)n, and (GAA)n/(TTC)n repeat sequences. In the case of the inverted repeats, a very elegant recent study showed that while two Alu sequences oriented as direct repeats did not affect replication fork progression, the same sequences oriented as inverted repeats caused fork stalling in *E. coli*, *S. cerevisiae* and a mammalian cell line (Voineagu, et al. 2008). In *E. coli* and the mammalian cell lines the ability of the inverted repeats to mediate stalling was dependent on the homology between the inverted sequences, and it gradually decreased with decreasing homology, thus supporting the idea that structures formed at the sequences were responsible for the pause. Furthermore, by varying the distance between the inverted sequences the authors were able to show they were most likely due to formation of hairpins in the lagging-strand template and not by cruciforms formed in front of the replication fork. The foundation of this conclusion was the fact that similar barrier activity was observed even in the presence of a 12 bp spacer, which would either reduce or abolish the ability of the repeated sequence to form a cruciform structure. Interestingly, *S. cerevisiae* Tof1 and Mrc1 (homologues of *S. pombe* Swi1 and Mrc1 and Human Timeless and Claspin) are required for efficient passage through the repeats and mutation of these factors leads to an increase in the intensity of the replication pause signal, an effect which is opposite to that observed at protein-mediated barriers. The repetitive sequences d(CGG)n, d(CCG)n d(CTG) and d(CAG) are also thought to form hairpin structures with both Watson-Crick and nonWatson-Crick base pairs, and d(CGG) sequences can form quartets (Chen, et al. 1995, Gacy, et al. 1995, Zheng, et al. 1996, Mariappan, et al. 1998). Both (CAG)n/(CTG)n and (CGG)n/(CCG)n repeats have been shown to stall replication forks in *S. cerevisiae* and mammalian cells, while (GAA)n/(TTC)n have been shown to stall forks in *S. cerevisiae* (Pelletier, et al. 2003; Krasilnikova & Mirkin; 2004a, Krasilnikova & Mirkin, 2004b; Kim, et al. 2008). The barrier activity was length dependent, although there were differences between systems; 10 (CGG)/(CCG) repeats were sufficient to stall replication forks in *S. cerevisiae* but 40 were required in mammalian cells (Voineagu, et al. 2009). Similarly, 60 (GAA)/(TTC) repeats do not cause any barrier activity, while increased barrier activity can be observed with increasing number of repeats (120, 230 and 340 units). There are also variations in whether the orientation of the repetitive sequences are important for barrier activity; in *S. cerevisiae* (GAA)n/(TTC)n barrier activity is orientation-dependent, whilst (CGG)n/(CCG)n repeats pause the replication fork in both orientations (Pelletier, et al. 2003; Kim, et al. 2008): In mammalian cells (CGG)n/(CCG)n repeats act as a barrier in both orientations (Voineagu, et al. 2009). Again, both *S. cerevisiae* factors Tof1 and Mrc1 were required for efficient replication through the repeat sequences as observed for an inverted repeat. Interestingly, a mutant Mrc1 protein ($Mrc1^{AQ}$) that can not be phosphorylated by the checkpoint kinases did not affect the barrier activity, thus the authors concluded that it is not the checkpoint function of Mrc1, but this factor's role in stabilizing stalled replication forks that is required (Voineagu, et al. 2009). Instability of stalled replication forks at repeat sequences is thought to underlie a range of Human diseases including fragile X-syndrome, Fraxe, Huntinton's disease and myotonic dystrophy (reviewed in Pearson, et al. 2005).

8. Cellular differentiation involving replication barriers: Mating-type switching in fission yeast

In the fission yeast *S. pombe,* a program of mating-type switching is mediated by a replication-coupled recombination event. Three different replication barriers are involved in setting up this cellular program of differentiation, where the expressed mating-type specific cassette at the *mat1* locus is replaced with a gene cassette expressing the information of the opposite mating-type. The information is copied from one of the two transcriptionally silenced centromere-distally located donor loci, *mat2P* and *mat3M*, into to the expressed *mat1* locus. In order for this program of cellular differentiation to occur, the *mat1* locus has to be replicated in a centromere-distal direction. The unidirectional replication of the *mat1* locus is maintained by the *RTS1* element, which is located at the centromere-proximal side of *mat1* and which acts as a polar replication terminator. Replication forks that move in the centromere-distal direction are terminated at the *RTS1* element, while forks moving in the centromere-proximal direction are allowed to pass through unhindered (Dalgaard & Klar, 2001). At the sequence level the *RTS1* element consists of two *cis*-acting regions that cooperate for function (Codlin & Dalgaard, 2003); a 446 base pair region named region B that contains four repeated ~55 bp long motifs as well as a 64 bp enhancer region called region A of similar length. Each of the repeated motifs of region B contributes to the overall barrier activity. A linker substitution analysis of region-B-motif-4 established that only a 20 bp region within the 55 bp long repeat is required for activity. This 20 base pair region shows similarity to the *S. pombe* Reb1 recognition site (Figure 2). Region A on the other hand is characterized by an uneven distribution of purines and pyrimidines on the two strands. In the absence of region A, the presence of each of the repeated motifs of region B has an additive effect on overall barrier activity. In the presence of region A, the region B motifs cooperate for function leading to a four-fold increase in overall barrier activity. Individually, region A does not possess any barrier activity. A recent study showed that the factor Sap1 binds to the enhancer region A (Zaratiegui, et al. 2011), however, it is not known whether Sap1 binding contributes to enhancer activity. Several factors have been identified that are required for efficient replication termination at the *RTS1* element. Rtf1 is a member of the family of factors that include *S. cerevisiae* Reb1, *S. pombe* Reb1 and human/mouse TTF-I (Eydmann, et al. 2008, see Sections 3.4 & 3.5; Figure 2). Deletion of the *rtf1* gene abolishes *RTS1* barrier activity. This protein family is characterized by the presence of two myb-domains that respectively contain three and two myb DNA interacting motifs. Each of the two Rtf1-myb domains have been expressed and purified separately and have been shown to have DNA binding activity; Rtf1-domain I binds *RTS1* DNA *in vitro*, interacting both with the repeated motifs of region B and the enhancer region A (Eydmann, et al. 2008). The Kd for the interaction with region A is 3467 nM, while the interaction with the repeated motif is somewhat stronger with a Kd for the interaction at 549 nM. A ten base pair substitution that abolishes barrier activity of the region B motif 4 *in vivo* strongly reduces binding of the Rtf1-domain I *in vitro*. Rtf1-domain II on the other hand only interacts weakly with the region B motif 4. A 10 bp substitution of the region flanking the binding site of domain I, that abolishes barrier activity of motif 4 *in vivo*, also abolishes binding of the Rtf1-domain II *in vitro*. Amino acid substitutions have been identified in both Rtf1-domain I and II that abolish barrier function, establishing genetically that they are of functional importance (Eydmann, et al. 2008). In addition, a point mutation has been identified in Rtf1-domain I (S154L) that changes the polarity of the *RTS1* barrier, such that instead of terminating replication forks moving in the centromere-distal direction, it acts as a pause site for replication forks moving in the centromere-proximal direction. The Rtf1-domain I-S154L mutation slightly enhances the domain affinity for region A and motif 4, such that the Kd is now 343 nM for region A and 265 nM for the motif 4. This observation suggests that the Rtf1-S154L protein is binding the *RTS1* element, but that it is unable to stall the replication fork, thus a protein-protein interaction(s) between Rtf1 and the progressing replication fork may be important for barrier activity. In addition, a dominant Rtf1-mutation has been identified that abolishes termination of replication. This non-sense mutation truncates the Rtf1 protein such that 120 amino acids of the C-terminus are missing. Two-hybrid analysis of this 120 AA C-terminal Rtf1 tail shows that it can interact with itself. This discovery suggests that Rtf1 self-interactions are required for barrier activity and that the tail-less Rtf1 allele interferes with the action of the wild-type protein at *RTS1* (Eydmann, et al. 2008).

In addition to DNA binding proteins other factors have been shown to be required for *RTS1* function (Inagawa, et al. 2009). Rtf2 is required for efficient termination of DNA replication at the *RTS1* element. An epistasis analysis of the enhancer region A deletion and the *Δrft2* mutation suggest that Rtf2 acts through the region A deletion. In the absence of Rtf2 replication forks pause in an Rtf1-dependent manner, but are restarted again. This replication restart is dependent on the Srs2 helicase, but not the Rqh1 helicase. Potentially, Srs2 acts by removing Rtf1 from the DNA in front of the replication fork, in a manner similar to its role in preventing recombination by removing Rhp51/Rad51 from single-stranded DNA (Krejci, et al. 2003; Veaute, et al. 2003). Rtf2 is the defining member of a family of proteins that are conserved from *S. pombe* to humans, which are characterized by the presence of a novel type of C2HC2 ring finger motif that potentially only binds one Zn^{2+} atom. A similar Ring finger motif, named the SP motif, with only one Zn^{2+}-atom binding site, is found in many E3 SUMO ligases including *S. cerevisiae* Siz1, Siz2; *S. pombe* Pli1, Nse2; human PIAS1, PIASxβ, PIAS3, PIASy, Mms21 (Watts, et al. 2007; Yunus & Lima, 2009) and an epistasis analysis suggests that Rtf2 and SUMO (*pmt3*) might act together in the same pathway (Inagawa, et al. 2009). However, Rtf2 also seems to have a role that is independent of SUMO, as slow moving replication forks are present at the *RTS1* element in the Rtf2 single mutant that are absent in the SUMO single mutant. In addition, Rtf2 interacts with proliferating cell nuclear antigen (PCNA) and might be travelling with the replication fork. Sumorylation and ubiquitination of PCNA at residues K127 and K164 has in *S. cerevisiae* been shown to affect molecular events at stalled forks (Stelter & Ulrich, 2003). Of these residues only K164 is conserved in *S. pombe* PCNA (gene *pcn1*). Interestingly, when lysine K164 is mutated to an alanine, it has no effect on barrier activity measured by genetic assays, which utilize efficiency of sporulation as the readout (Figure 3B). Thus most likely, Rtf2 targets either other residues of PCNA or other replication proteins for SUMOylation. Finally, both Swi1 and Swi3 are required for barrier activity at the *RTS1* element (Dalgaard & Klar, 2000). Swi1 and Swi3 travel with the replication fork as part of the Replication Progression Complex (RPC) and genetic evidence suggests that Swi1 might interact directly with Rtf1 to mediate replication barrier activity; a point mutation in Swi1, *swi1-rtf3* G2785A, has been identified that abolishes termination of *RTS1* but does not affect other replication barriers such as the rDNA barrier and the *mat1* pause site *MPS1* (Dalgaard & Klar, 2000; Krings & Bastia, 2004). Recent work has demonstrated that *in vitro* the hetromeric complex of Swi1 and Swi3 can interact with double-stranded DNA (Tanaka, et al. 2010). In addition, a super-shift can be achieved through an interaction with purified Mrc1, a replication checkpoint protein that is also traveling with the RPC. Furthermore, data suggested that the *swi1-rtf3* G2785A mutation affects the super-shift caused by Mrc1 binding, thus providing a possible mechanism for the loss of barrier activity at *RTS1* (Tanaka, et al. 2010). However,

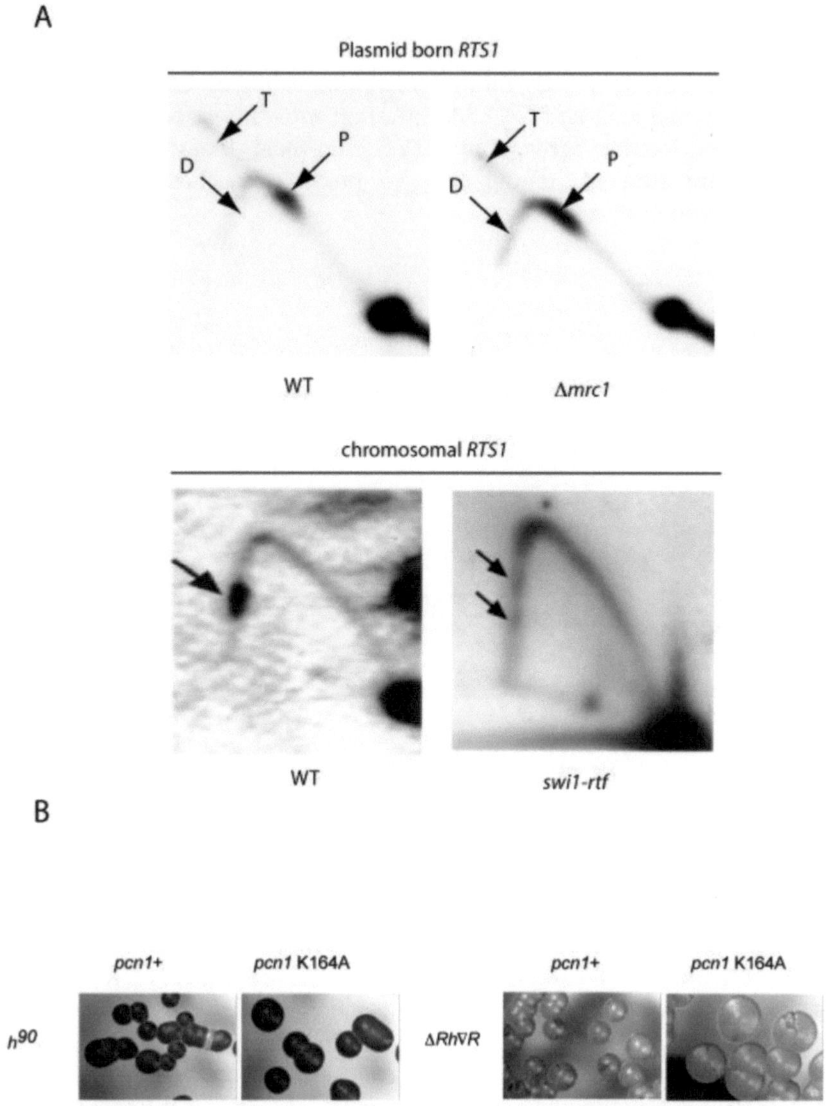

Fig. 3. A. Comparison of the effect on barrier activity of the *Δmrc1* mutation and the *swi1-rtf* mutation. The upper two panels show replication intermediates that have been digested with *Sac*I and *Pst*I and separated on a 2D-gel as described earlier. T is a termination signal, D the descending arc and P the pause signal. The analysed *RTS1* element is present on a plasmid (pBZ142) (Method is described in Codlin & Dalgaard, 2003). Below, as comparison, the effect of the *swi1-rtf* mutation on the *RTS1* element at it wild-type genomic position is shown (reproduced from (Dalgaard & Klar, 2000). B. Sporulation assays used for identifying effects on replication pausing at the *MPS1* element (left two panels) and replication termination at the *RTS1* element (right two panels). In the first case a reduction of replication pausing will lead to reduced sporulation, while in the second case reduced termination will lead to increased sporulation (For a description of the assay see Codlin & Dalgaard, 2003) .

our analysis of a Δ*mrc1* strain shows that this mutation does not affect the overall *RTS1* barrier activity, although the region of stalling does seem to be slightly expanded and the intensity of the descending arc is slightly more intense suggesting an increase of replication restart (Figure 3A). Thus, the *swi1-rtf3* G2785A mutation must affect other protein-protein interactions required for barrier activity at *RTS1,* the most likely candidate for the interacting partner being Rtf1. A model for the possible mechanism of replication termination at *RTS1* is given in Figure 4.

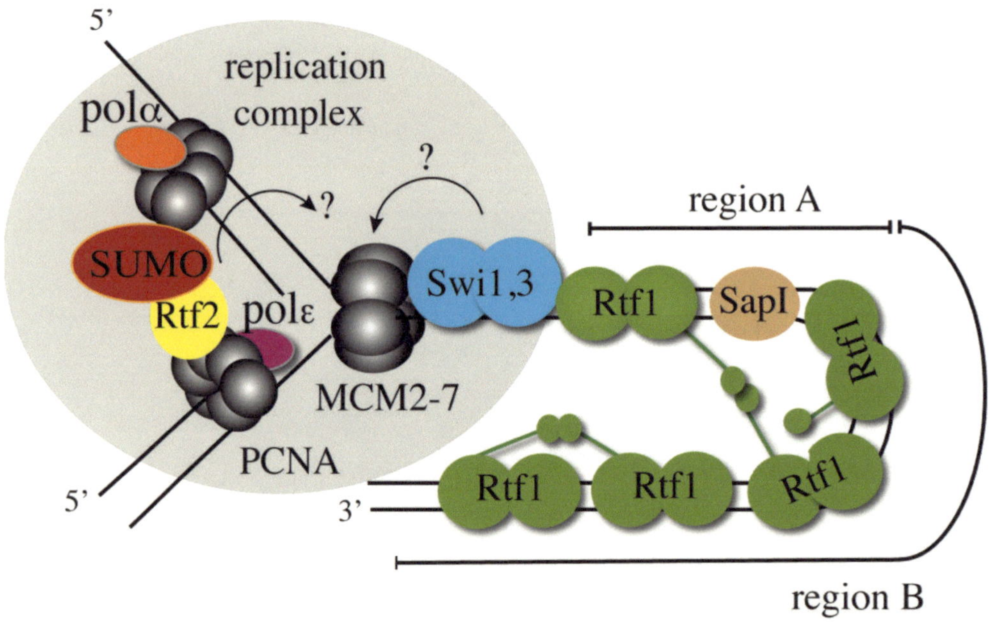

Fig. 4. Model for the molecular mechanism of replication termination at the *RTS1* element. Rtf1 molecules interact with the repeated motifs present in the *RTS1* element as well as the enhancer region A. Potentially, C-terminal interactions of Rtf1 are important for stabilizing the interactions and can provide additional constraints when the DNA template is unwound by the approaching helicase. The function of the interaction of Sap1 with the enhancer region (region A) is unknown. When the replication complex approaches the *RTS1* element, protein-protein interactions stall the progression. These protein-protein interactions are most likely between Rtf1-domain I and Swi1. The interactions potentially lead to inhibition of DNA unwinding by the MCM2-7 replicative helicase. The stalled replication fork is stabilized by the action of Rtf2, potentially by SUMOylation of other replication factors (Inagawa, et al. 2009) .

8.1 Molecular differentiation of sister chromatids through replication pausing

Another replication barrier required for *S. pombe* mating-type switching is the *MPS1* site required for imprinting at the *mat1* locus (Dalgaard & Klar, 1999; Dalgaard & Klar, 2000; Vengrova & Dalgaard, 2004). *mat1* imprinting is required for mating-type switching. At *MPS1* the replication forks are paused but then all re-started again. All *cis-* and *trans-*acting mutations that abolish replication pausing at *MPS1* also abolish imprinting, suggesting a mechanistic role between imprinting and replication pausing. Also, inversion of the *mat1* locus relative to the *RTS1* element so that it is replicated in the opposite orientation, abolishes both pausing and imprinting (Dalgaard & Klar, 1999). The *cis*-acting sequences that are required for pausing at the *MPS1* are named the *abc* region (Sayrac, et al. 2011). Replication pausing can be observed both in P and M cells and interestingly the required sequences are located within the two Plus (P) and Minus (M) DNA cassettes that are swapped during the switching process (Dalgaard & Klar, 2000; Vengrova & Dalgaard, 2004). Thus, different *cis*-acting sequences mediate barrier activity in the two cell-types. Generally there is no sequence similarity between the P and M cassettes, however, within the *abc* region there is some sequence similarity (Sayrac, et al. 2011). The part of the *abc* region that is required for pausing is about 60 bp long and is located approximately 30 nucleotides from where the imprint is introduced. Both the *P-* and *M-abc* regions act as pause sites for the replication fork when they are located on a plasmid. Furthermore, competition experiments suggest that a *trans*-acting factor is binding to the *abc* region to mediate pausing; introduction of two multi-copy plasmids each containing 10 copies of the *M-* or *P-abc* regions cause a 30-40% reduction in sporulation (the sporulation efficiency is dependent on the efficiency of mating-type switching and mating). Importantly, the data does suggest that the factor(s) binding to the *abc* region is present in the cells in a significant number of molecules. Interestingly, the *abc* region does not mediate replication pausing at the transcriptionally silenced donor *loci,* even though *mat2P* is replicated in the correct orientation for pausing. This observation is important as it establishes a mechanism by which replication barriers can be regulated in other systems through the regulation of heterochromatin formation.

As mentioned above, replication pausing at *MPS1* is required for introduction of an imprint that marks switchable cells of *S. pombe.* This imprint has been shown to consist of two ribonucleotides incorporated into the DNA (Vengrova & Dalgaard, 2004; Vengrova & Dalgaard, 2005; Vengrova & Dalgaard, 2006). Several *cis*-acting regions have been identified that are required for the introduction of the imprint. First, there is a small *cis*-acting sequence located distal to *mat1* that is named *SAS1* (Arcangioli & Klar, 1991). *SAS1* mediates binding of the *trans*-acting factor Sap1 that is required for barrier activity at the rDNA and *LTRs* (see Sections 3.6 & 5.0). However, the deletion of a 264 bp region (*Msmt0*) that includes *SAS1* does not affect replication pausing at *MPS1,* suggesting that Sap1 has another role during imprinting (Dalgaard & Klar, 2000). A study of the interaction between Sap1 and its binding sites *SAS1* and in the rDNA suggests that the protein might be interacting differently with the DNA at the two sites and that this might cause the difference in whether the protein mediates barrier activity (see Section 3.6). Another *cis*-acting sequence that is required for the introduction of the imprint is a 204 bp spacer region that is located centromere-proximal to the *abc* region and the site of imprinting (Sayrac, et al. 2011). Deletion of this region leads to abolishment of imprinting but only a small decrease in the intensity of the *MPS1* signal. Replacing the region with a randomized sequence only has a small effect on both imprinting and pausing. Similarly, gradually reducing the length of the spacer region gradually reduces imprinting. High-resolution Southern blot analysis of replication intermediates from the strain carrying the spacer deletion mapped the position both of the 3′ end of the leading-strand and the 5′ end of the lagging-strand to the imprinting site, suggesting that the imprint consists of ribonucleotides that originate from the priming of an Okazaki fragment. Furthermore, the high-resolution Southern blot analysis also detected a centromere-proximal lagging-strand priming site about 350 nucleotides from the site of the imprint in the wild-type strain, which also previously has been detected by RIP mapping (Vengrova & Dalgaard, 2004; Sayrac, et al. 2011). This priming site is absent in the spacer deletion strain (instead a diffuse set of priming sites are observed closer to the imprint), but restored when the spacer is replaced by a random sequence (Sayrac, et al. 2011). The analysis also showed that while the sequences within the *abc* region are required, there is no sequence requirement for the region where the imprint is introduced. The data suggest that the imprint is formed in response to a site-specific priming event induced by replication pausing, and that the position of subsequent priming sites for subsequent replication fork restart is important for the formation of the imprint. Potentially, topological restraints could prevent access of factors if the priming site chosen after the release of the fork is too close to the imprinting site. This is the first example of a *cis*-acting region affecting the position of priming sites and suggests that chromatin could affect primer localization during lagging-strand replication. Importantly, the data provide a mechanism by which replication barriers can act to differentiate sister-chromatids for cellular differentiation.

The *mat1* imprint/ribonucleotides are maintained in the DNA for one cell-cycle, potentially through the binding of a *trans*-acting factor to flanking *cis*-acting sequences and act themselves as a replication barrier in the S-phase of the next cell-cycle (the 3'-end of the leading-strand was mapped to the nucleotide preceeding the ribonucleotides), thus leading to induction of the replication-coupled recombination event that drives mating-type switching (Vengrova & Dalgaard, 2004). Ribonucleotides have been shown to frequently be incorporated during DNA replication (Nick McElhinny, et al. 2010a; Nick McElhinny, et al. 2010b) and to stall DNA polymerases when present in the replication template *in vitro* (Vengrova & Dalgaard, 2004). Interestingly, only a single ribonucleotide present in a DNA template has been show to act as a barrier for DNA polymerase ε (Nick McElhinny, et al. 2010). However, RNA can template DNA repair *in vivo* and both *S. cerevisiae* polymerases α and δ can use templates containing four ribonucleotides in a row, although with decreased efficiency (Storici, et al. 2007).

9. Interference between RNA polymerase II transcription and the DNA replication machinery

In *S. cerevisiae,* RNA polymerase II transcription has been shown to interfere with DNA replication fork progression. Transcription associated recombination (TAR) increased when the orientation of polymerase II transcribed genes was head-on to the progressing replication fork (Prado & Aguilera, 2005). Using cell-cycle specific promoters they also showed that this increase was dependent on the S-phase. The study also detected a replication barrier by 2D-gel analysis of replication intermediates within the recombination substrate that was dependent on polymerase II transcription. The intensity of the replication barrier signal was increased in an Rrm3 mutant. Importantly, more recent data suggest that it is the formation of RNA-DNA hybrids (R-loops) that are the cause of TAR and not the collision of the two types of forks (Aguilera & Gomez-Gonzalez, 2008; Gonzalez-Aguilera, et al. 2008). Also, several mutations affecting the maturation of mRNPs increase TAR. While these experiments were done using a *CEN*-plasmid, a genome wide study identified 96 sites where there were high levels of DNA polymerase binding (Azvolinsky, et al. 2009). A significant number of these were genes highly transcribed by RNA Polymerase II. However, there was no correlation between the direction of replication and transcription at these sites. The sites also correlated with high occupancy of the Rrm3 helicase, but the absence of Rrm3 did not lead to an increase in the DNA polymerase occupancy. Similarly, 2D-gel analysis of replication intermediates detected replication fork barriers at some of these sites, but the absence of Rrm3 did not lead to an increase in pausing at these barriers. R-loops have also been proposed to act as barriers for replication fork progression in human cells (Tuduri, et al. 2009; Tuduri, et al. 2010). Topoisomerase 1 (Top1) together with ASF/SF2, a splicing factor of the SR family, act to suppress the formation of DNA-RNA hybrids during transcription, thus preventing these R-loops from interfering with the progression of replication forks. In Top1 deficient cells γH2AX, a phosphorylated specialized histone (see Section 11.), accumulates at genes that are highly expressed during S-phase such as histone genes. The Top1 deficiency might affect fork progression in two ways; through Top1's role in releasing super-coiling between two types of converging forks, and through Top1's role in regulation of mRNP assembly, presumably by binding and phosphorylating splicing factors of the SR family (Rossi, et al. 1996; Soret, et al. 2003; Malanga, et al. 2008). It has long been known that in bacterial genomes highly-expressed genes are oriented such that transcription does not interfere with replication and it has been proposed that this might also be true for a large fraction of the human genome (Huvet, et al. 2007).

10. The Rrm3 helicase mediated replication progression at non-nucleosomal protein-DNA barriers

The *S. cerevisiae* Rrm3 5′ to 3′ helicase has been shown to have an important function at replication barriers. Rrm3, which is a member of a family conserved from yeast to humans (Zhou, et al. 2002), was originally identified because its absence caused an increase in recombination and formation of extra chromosomal circles at the rDNA array (Keil & McWilliams, 1993; Ivessa, et al. 2000). Rrm3 travels with the replication fork, interacts *in vivo* with Pol2 (the catalytic subunit of DNA polymerase ε) and has a role in replication at all the yeast chromosomes (Azvolinsky, et al. 2006). Importantly, in the absence of Rrm3 replication pausing/stalling is observed (or increased) at an estimated 1400 sites in the genome, including centromeres, tRNA genes, inactive replication origins, and the silent mating-type loci, as well as telomeric and rDNA sites (Ivessa, et al. 2003). Potentially, Rrm3 is required for proper replication through all stable, non-nucleosomal protein-DNA complexes. Replication through the rDNA is generally impaired in a *Δrrm3* mutant leading to replication stalling at several sites including the polymerase III transcribed 5S rRNA gene, at inactive origins and at the beginning and end of the RNA polymerase I transcription unit (Ivessa, et al. 2000). In addition, the intensity of the Fob1-dependent replication barrier significantly increased and more replication termination was observed at the barrier. Rrm3 also affects replication at the telomeres and internal tracts of $C_{1\text{-}3}A/TG_{1\text{-}3}$ telomeric DNA; in the absence of Rrm3 replication slowing at the repeats were increased and in addition replication stalling was observed at multiple sites within the sub-telomeric regions including in active origins (Ivessa, et al. 2002). At the silent mating-type regions and at the tRNA genes the Rrm3-dependent stalling was shown to be dependent on the presence of the associated protein complexes (Ivessa, et al. 2003). Also, loss of the ATPase function of Rrm3 has the same effect as deletion alleles, establishing that the catalytic activity of the helicase is needed for this function. Due to the increased genetic instability of Rrm3 mutants, their viability is dependent on *mrc1, mre11, rad50, sgs1, srs2, top3, xrs2* and *dia2*, genes involved in activation of the inter-S phase checkpoint and replication fork restart (Torres, et al. 2004; Morohashi, et al. 2009). Interestingly, Dia2 is an F-box protein (E3 ubiquitin ligase) that also travels with the replication fork and might have a role at stalled DNA replication forks at protein-DNA barriers, perhaps by interaction with key substrates (Mimura, et al. 2009; Morohashi, et al. 2009). However, a recent study looking at the Fob1-dependent barrier using 2D-gel analysis of replication intermediates did not detect any effect on intensity of the barrier signal in a Δ*dia2* mutant (Bairwa, et al. 2011).

11. γ-H2A.X formation at stalled replication forks

Stalling of replication forks generally leads to the activation of the protein kinases of the PI(3) kinase-like kinase (PIKK) family, *S. pombe* Rad3, *S. cerevisiae* Mec1 and Mammalian ATR. One function of the activation of these kinases is to stabilize replication forks to prevent their collapse (Desany, et al. 1998; Lopes, et al. 2001). The PIKK mediated phosphorylation of a specialized histone called H2A.X (mammalian) or H2A (yeast) might help stabilize the stalled fork (Cobb, et al. 2005; Papamichos-Chronakis & Peterson, 2008) but also recruits DNA damage repair proteins (Mammalian Mdc1 and *S. pombe* Crb2 and Brc1; Du, et al. 2006; Williams, et al. 2010). Two studies have utilized this molecular beacon for identifying sites of replication stalling genome wide (Szilard, et al. 2010; Rozenzhak et al. 2010). In *S. cerevisiae,* γ-H2A (the phosphorylated form of H2A) enriched loci are concentrated at the rDNA locus, telomeres, DNA replication origins, *LTRs*, tRNA genes and centromeres, all of which are known replication barriers, but also at actively repressed protein-coding genes (Szilard, et al. 2010). In the latter case, the analysis showed that actively repressed genes, which are notably enriched for the transcription factors Sum1 and Ume6 that are known to recruit the two Hst1 and Rpd3 histone deacetylases (HDACs) (Kadosh & Struhl, 1997; Xie, et al. 1999; Robert, et al. 2004). This observation suggests that hetero-chromatin may pose an obstacle to progression of DNA replication forks. Importantly, loss of Hst1 or Rpd3 histone deacetylase activity abolished the γ-H2A enrichment at genes specifically regulated by Hst1 or Rpd3. Generally, γ-H2A enrichment was depended on both Mec1 and Tel1 (the latter is activated by double-stranded breaks), suggesting that both replication fork stalling as well as collapse occurred at the identified loci. Also, increased γ-H2A enrichment was observed in a *Δrrm3* mutant background, suggesting a decreased ability of replication forks to pass through the barriers, thus leading to an increase in γ-H2A accumulation. A similar genome wide study in *S. pombe* identified γ-H2A enriched loci that corresponded well with those observed in *S. cerevisiae,* including the mating-type locus (including the *RTS1* element, the region containing *MPS1* and the imprint, and the IR elements that flank the transcriptionally silenced donor loci), the rDNA loci (including the gene coding region and the replication barriers), and all heterochromatin regions, including the centromeres (at the *otr* elements, but not the *cnt* or *imr* elements nor at the flanking inverted repeats) and telomeres, both Tf2-type retrotransposons and wtf elements and finally in a subset of gene coding sequences that were characterized by the presence of repetitive sequences (Szilard, et al. 2010). Contrary to what was observed in *S. cerevisia* γ-H2A accumulation was almost exclusively dependent on Rad3 and only at the telomere (in the absence of Rad3) on Tel1. In the mating-type region (the *RTS1* element and *MPS1*), γ-H2A accumulation was dependent on Swi1 and Swi3 function in pausing and termination, while at the hetrochromatic regions γ-H2A accumulation is associated with the presence of Clr4-dependent heterochromatin and partially depends on Swi6. Several γ-H2A sites found in budding yeast were absent in fission yeast, including tRNA genes, *LTRs* (in the absence of the transposon) and replication origins. The absence of γ-H2A accumulation at tRNA genes and *LTRs* is interesting, as fork stalling is observed at these sites by 2D-gel analysis (see Section 5.), and might reflect that either different types of stalled fork exist or that the duration of the stall is important for γ-H2A accumulation.

12. Concluding remarks

It is evident that many types of replication barriers have been defined. Whilst there are differences between these elements, there are also similarities. At some barriers replication forks only pause and then restart again without fork collapse. However, at others the replication fork is stalled until an approaching fork arrives from the other side for mediation of replication termination. Different molecular responses and levels of genetic instability are observed at the barriers. What determines the fate of a stalled replication fork at a barrier is still generally unknown. However, it is evident that helicases, such as *S. cerevisiae* Rrm3 and *S. pombe* Srs2 promote replication through protein mediated barriers (Section 8. & 10.) and Tof1 and Mrc1 through barrier caused by "structure" in the template (Section 6.), while *S. pombe* Rtf2 acts to stabilize the stalled fork for replication termination (Section 8.). It is also evident, that many different proteins can act as replication impediments. Generally, these proteins do not promote barrier activity through the formation of "stable" complexes, although in the absence of *S. cerevisiae* Rrm3 barrier activity stalling at stable protein-DNA complexes can be observed (Section 9.). Barrier activity is most likely generated via direct interaction(s) with the progressing replisome. For example, most protein-mediated barriers are polar, only stalling replication forks when encountered from one side, while for *S. pombe* Sap1 acts as a barrier at some *cis*-acting sites but not others (Sections 8. & 3.6). It should be mentioned that strong replication barriers often consist of several closely spaced *cis*-acting sequences where one or more *trans*-acting factors mediate the replication barrier. Also, these *trans*-acting factors have the ability to dimerize or polymerize, potentially increasing the efficiency of interaction, but more likely providing additional topological constraints when the DNA is unwound by the replicative helicase. Also, it is common for known protein-mediated barrier activity to depend on the *trans*-acting factors Tof1/Csm3 (*S. cereviaise*) and Swi1/Swi3 (*S. pombe*), although there are some notable exceptions (for example, see Pryce et al. 2009). Putatively, the *S. cerevisiae* Tof1/Csm3 or *S. pombe* Swi1/Swi3 heteromeric complexes slide along the double-stranded DNA in front of the replicative helicase and senses the presence of barrier proteins. It has been shown earlier that in the absence of *S. cerevisiae* Tof1/Csm3 an uncoupling of the replicative helicase from the replicative polymerases can occur (Katou, et al. 2003; Nedelcheva, et al. 2005), thus Tof1/Csm3 (and phylogenetic related proteins) could directly inhibit MCM function when barrier proteins are encountered. Consistent with this model, the 3′ end of the leading-stand and the 5′ end of the lagging-strand have been mapped in close proximity about approximately 30-40 bp from the *cis*-acting sequences that mediate the barrier activity both at the *S. cerevisiae* rDNA barrier and at the *S. pombe MPS1* site (Figure 5A; Sections 3.6 & 8.1).

Interestingly, DNA structures in the template can also stall replication fork progression in a site-specific manner. These barrier signals most likely act on the lagging-strand as impediments to polymerase progression (Figure 5B). Interestingly, here *S. cerevisiae* Tof1 and Mrc1 are required for efficient replication through the elements (Mrc1 does not affect barrier activity at protein barriers), but not through the checkpoint activation function of these proteins. Still, the characteristics of these barriers suggest that the mechanism by which this

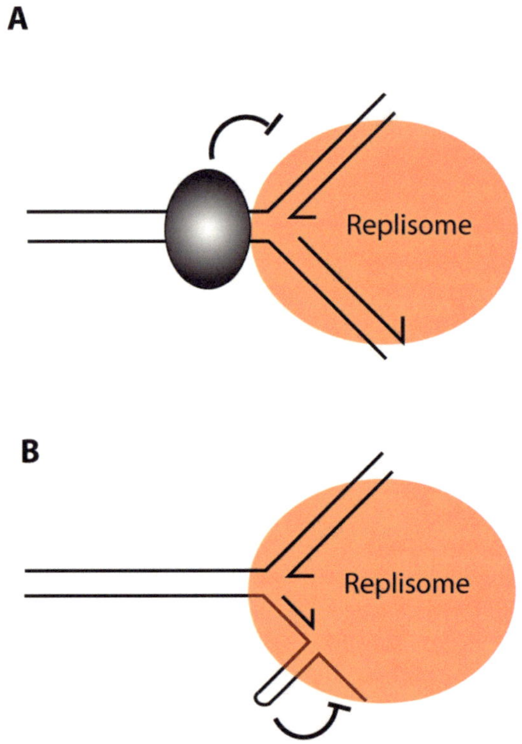

Fig. 5. The two types of replication barriers described. A) DNA bound factors can stall replisome progression, leading to a 3′ leading-strand end and 5′ lagging-strand end a certain distance from the barrier. B) Structure at the lagging-strand template leads to stalling of replisome progression.

type of barriers stalls replication forks is different from the one by which protein barriers act. Potentially, structures in the lagging-strand template strand could also explain by *S. pombe* tRNA genes mediate barrier activity in a Swi1 independent manner.

It is also evident from this comparison that replication barriers both prevent and cause genetic instability and a number of key points highlight this: I) Many of the described barriers have either been shown or are thought to prevent conflicts between progressing RNA polymerases I, II and III and replication forks, thus promoting genetic stability. II) Other barriers are thought to promote telomere addition for maintenance of genetic stability. III) Several barriers have been shown to cause genetic instability, including rDNA barriers (see Section 2.4), the *RTS1* element (Ahn, et al. 2005), transposons (Zaratiegui, et al. 2011), as well as DNA structure in the template (Section 7.). IV) Again others have specific roles in induction of recombination events, including genetic rearrangements important for contraction/expansions of rDNA arrays and cellular differentiation or development in *S. pombe* and *Tetrahymena* (Sections 3.2 & 8.).

It is highly likely that additional biological roles will be defined for replication barriers in the future. Here, research into such genetic elements' roles in cellular differentiation and development in higher eukaryotes would be important. In addition, it will be interesting to understand how replication barriers drive evolution through instability at the stalled forks. It is already evident from studies of fragile sites, genomic rearrangements, repeat expansion/contraction and mutations that underlie the genetic instability of cancer cells, that replication barriers are likely to have a profound role in disease formation. Thus, the importance of a better understanding of the molecular processes that lead to stalling of replication forks and that control the events at these forks, should not be underestimated.

13. References

Aguilera, A. & Gomez-Gonzalez, B. (2008). Genome instability: a mechanistic view of its causes and consequences. *Nature reviews. Genetics,* Vol. 9, No. 3, (Mar), pp. (204-217), 1471-0064 (Electronic) 1471-0056 (Linking)

Ahn, J.S., Osman, F. & Whitby, M.C. (2005). Replication fork blockage by RTS1 at an ectopic site promotes recombination in fission yeast. *The EMBO journal,* Vol. 24, No. 11, (Jun 1), pp. (2011-2023), 0261-4189 (Print) 0261-4189 (Linking)

Aiyar, A., Aras, S., Washington, A., Singh, G. & Luftig, R.B. (2009). Epstein-Barr Nuclear Antigen 1 modulates replication of oriP-plasmids by impeding replication and transcription fork migration through the family of repeats. *Virology journal,* Vol. 6, No. pp. (29), 1743-422X (Electronic) 1743-422X (Linking)

Ambinder, R.F., Shah, W.A., Rawlins, D.R., Hayward, G.S. & Hayward, S.D. (1990). Definition of the sequence requirements for binding of the EBNA-1 protein to its palindromic target sites in Epstein-Barr virus DNA. *Journal of virology,* Vol. 64, No. 5, (May), pp. (2369-2379), 0022-538X (Print) 0022-538X (Linking)

Arcangioli, B. & Klar, A.J. (1991). A novel switch-activating site (SAS1) and its cognate binding factor (SAP1) required for efficient mat1 switching in Schizosaccharomyces pombe. *The EMBO journal,* Vol. 10, No. 10, (Oct), pp. (3025-3032), 0261-4189 (Print) 0261-4189 (Linking)

Azvolinsky, A., Dunaway, S., Torres, J.Z., Bessler, J.B. & Zakian, V.A. (2006). The S. cerevisiae Rrm3p DNA helicase moves with the replication fork and affects replication of all yeast chromosomes. *Genes & development,* Vol. 20, No. 22, (Nov 15), pp. (3104-3116), 0890-9369 (Print) 0890-9369 (Linking)

Azvolinsky, A., Giresi, P.G., Lieb, J.D. & Zakian, V.A. (2009). Highly transcribed RNA polymerase II genes are impediments to replication fork progression in Saccharomyces cerevisiae. *Molecular cell,* Vol. 34, No. 6, (Jun 26), pp. (722-734), 1097-4164 (Electronic) 1097-2765 (Linking)

Bairwa, N.K., Mohanty, B.K., Stamenova, R., Curcio, M.J. & Bastia, D. (2011). The intra-S phase checkpoint protein Tof1 collaborates with the helicase Rrm3 and the F-box protein Dia2 to maintain genome stability in Saccharomyces cerevisiae. *The Journal of biological chemistry,* Vol. 286, No. 4, (Jan 28), pp. (2445-2454), 1083-351X (Electronic) 0021-9258 (Linking)

Bairwa, N.K., Zzaman, S., Mohanty, B.K. & Bastia, D. (2010). Replication fork arrest and rDNA silencing are two independent and separable functions of the replication terminator protein Fob1 of Saccharomyces cerevisiae. *The Journal of biological chemistry,* Vol. 285, No. 17, (Apr 23), pp. (12612-12619), 1083-351X (Electronic) 0021-9258 (Linking)

Biswas, S. & Bastia, D. (2008). Mechanistic insights into replication termination as revealed by investigations of the Reb1-Ter3 complex of Schizosaccharomyces pombe. *Molecular and cellular biology,* Vol. 28, No. 22, (Nov), pp. (6844-6857), 1098-5549 (Electronic) 0270-7306 (Linking)

Brewer, B.J. & Fangman, W.L. (1987). The localization of replication origins on ARS plasmids in S. cerevisiae. *Cell,* Vol. 51, No. 3, (Nov 6), pp. (463-471), 0092-8674 (Print) 0092-8674 (Linking)

Brewer, B.J., Lockshon, D. & Fangman, W.L. (1992). The arrest of replication forks in the rDNA of yeast occurs independently of transcription. *Cell,* Vol. 71, No. 2, (Oct 16), pp. (267-276), 0092-8674 (Print) 0092-8674 (Linking)

Burkhalter, M.D. & Sogo, J.M. (2004). rDNA enhancer affects replication initiation and mitotic recombination: Fob1 mediates nucleolytic processing independently of replication. *Molecular cell,* Vol. 15, No. 3, (Aug 13), pp. (409-421), 1097-2765 (Print) 1097-2765 (Linking)

Calzada, A., Hodgson, B., Kanemaki, M., Bueno, A. & Labib, K. (2005). Molecular anatomy and regulation of a stable replisome at a paused eukaryotic DNA replication fork. *Genes & development,* Vol. 19, No. 16, (Aug 15), pp. (1905-1919), 0890-9369 (Print) 0890-9369 (Linking)

Cha, R.S. & Kleckner, N. (2002). ATR homolog Mec1 promotes fork progression, thus averting breaks in replication slow zones. *Science,* Vol. 297, No. 5581, (Jul 26), pp. (602-606), 1095-9203 (Electronic) 0036-8075 (Linking)

Chen, X., Mariappan, S.V., Catasti, P., Ratliff, R., Moyzis, R.K., Laayoun, A., Smith, S.S., Bradbury, E.M. & Gupta, G. (1995). Hairpins are formed by the single DNA strands of the fragile X triplet repeats: structure and biological implications. *Proceedings of the National Academy of Sciences of the United States of America,* Vol. 92, No. 11, (May 23), pp. (5199-5203), 0027-8424 (Print) 0027-8424 (Linking)

Cobb, J.A., Schleker, T., Rojas, V., Bjergbaek, L., Tercero, J.A. & Gasser, S.M. (2005). Replisome instability, fork collapse, and gross chromosomal rearrangements arise synergistically from Mec1 kinase and RecQ helicase mutations. *Genes & development,* Vol. 19, No. 24, (Dec 15), pp. (3055-3069), 0890-9369 (Print) 0890-9369 (Linking)

Codlin, S. & Dalgaard, J.Z. (2003). Complex mechanism of site-specific DNA replication termination in fission yeast. *The EMBO journal,* Vol. 22, No. 13, (Jul 1), pp. (3431-3440), 0261-4189 (Print) 0261-4189 (Linking)

Dalgaard, J.Z. & Klar, A.J. (1999). Orientation of DNA replication establishes mating-type switching pattern in S. pombe. *Nature,* Vol. 400, No. 6740, (Jul 8), pp. (181-184), 0028-0836 (Print) 0028-0836 (Linking)

Dalgaard, J.Z. & Klar, A.J. (2000). swi1 and swi3 perform imprinting, pausing, and termination of DNA replication in S. pombe. *Cell,* Vol. 102, No. 6, (Sep 15), pp. (745-751), 0092-8674 (Print) 0092-8674 (Linking)

Dalgaard, J.Z. & Klar, A.J. (2001). A DNA replication-arrest site RTS1 regulates imprinting by determining the direction of replication at mat1 in S. pombe. *Genes & development,* Vol. 15, No. 16, (Aug 15), pp. (2060-2068), 0890-9369 (Print) 0890-9369 (Linking)

de Lahondes, R., Ribes, V. & Arcangioli, B. (2003). Fission yeast Sap1 protein is essential for chromosome stability. *Eukaryotic cell,* Vol. 2, No. 5, (Oct), pp. (910-921), 1535-9778 (Print) 1535-9786 (Linking)

Defossez, P.A., Prusty, R., Kaeberlein, M., Lin, S.J., Ferrigno, P., Silver, P.A., Keil, R.L. & Guarente, L. (1999). Elimination of replication block protein Fob1 extends the life span of yeast mother cells. *Molecular cell,* Vol. 3, No. 4, (Apr), pp. (447-455), 1097-2765 (Print) 1097-2765 (Linking)

Desany, B.A., Alcasabas, A.A., Bachant, J.B. & Elledge, S.J. (1998). Recovery from DNA replicational stress is the essential function of the S-phase checkpoint pathway. *Genes & development,* Vol. 12, No. 18, (Sep 15), pp. (2956-2970), 0890-9369 (Print) 0890-9369 (Linking)

Deshpande, A.M. & Newlon, C.S. (1996). DNA replication fork pause sites dependent on transcription. *Science,* Vol. 272, No. 5264, (May 17), pp. (1030-1033), 0036-8075 (Print) 0036-8075 (Linking)

Dhar, V. & Schildkraut, C.L. (1991). Role of EBNA-1 in arresting replication forks at the Epstein-Barr virus oriP family of tandem repeats. *Molecular and cellular biology,* Vol. 11, No. 12, (Dec), pp. (6268-6278), 0270-7306 (Print) 0270-7306 (Linking)

Di Felice, F., Cioci, F. & Camilloni, G. (2005). FOB1 affects DNA topoisomerase I in vivo cleavages in the enhancer region of the Saccharomyces cerevisiae ribosomal DNA locus. *Nucleic acids research,* Vol. 33, No. 19, pp. (6327-6337), 1362-4962 (Electronic) 0305-1048 (Linking)

Dlakic, M. (2002). A model of the replication fork blocking protein Fob1p based on the catalytic core domain of retroviral integrases. *Protein science : a publication of the Protein Society,* Vol. 11, No. 5, (May), pp. (1274-1277), 0961-8368 (Print) 0961-8368 (Linking)

Du, L.L., Nakamura, T.M. & Russell, P. (2006). Histone modification-dependent and -independent pathways for recruitment of checkpoint protein Crb2 to double-strand breaks. *Genes & development,* Vol. 20, No. 12, (Jun 15), pp. (1583-1596), 0890-9369 (Print) 0890-9369 (Linking)

Ermakova, O.V., Frappier, L. & Schildkraut, C.L. (1996). Role of the EBNA-1 protein in pausing of replication forks in the Epstein-Barr virus genome. *The Journal of biological chemistry,* Vol. 271, No. 51, (Dec 20), pp. (33009-33017), 0021-9258 (Print) 0021-9258 (Linking)

Evers, R. & Grummt, I. (1995). Molecular coevolution of mammalian ribosomal gene terminator sequences and the transcription termination factor TTF-I. *Proc Natl Acad Sci U S A,* Vol. 92, No. 13, (Jun 20), pp. (5827-5831), 0027-8424 (Print)

Eydmann, T., Sommariva, E., Inagawa, T., Mian, S., Klar, A.J. & Dalgaard, J.Z. (2008). Rtf1-mediated eukaryotic site-specific replication termination. *Genetics,* Vol. 180, No. 1, (Sep), pp. (27-39), 0016-6731 (Print) 0016-6731 (Linking)

Fritsch, O., Burkhalter, M.D., Kais, S., Sogo, J.M. & Schar, P. (2010). DNA ligase 4 stabilizes the ribosomal DNA array upon fork collapse at the replication fork barrier. *DNA repair,* Vol. 9, No. 8, (Aug 5), pp. (879-888), 1568-7856 (Electronic) 1568-7856 (Linking)

Gacy, A.M., Goellner, G., Juranic, N., Macura, S. & McMurray, C.T. (1995). Trinucleotide repeats that expand in human disease form hairpin structures in vitro. *Cell,* Vol. 81, No. 4, (May 19), pp. (533-540), 0092-8674 (Print) 0092-8674 (Linking)

Ganley, A.R., Hayashi, K., Horiuchi, T. & Kobayashi, T. (2005). Identifying gene-independent noncoding functional elements in the yeast ribosomal DNA by phylogenetic footprinting. *Proceedings of the National Academy of Sciences of the United States of America,* Vol. 102, No. 33, (Aug 16), pp. (11787-11792), 0027-8424 (Print) 0027-8424 (Linking)

Ganley, A.R., Ide, S., Saka, K. & Kobayashi, T. (2009). The effect of replication initiation on gene amplification in the rDNA and its relationship to aging. *Molecular cell,* Vol. 35, No. 5, (Sep 11), pp. (683-693), 1097-4164 (Electronic) 1097-2765 (Linking)

Gerber, J.K., Gogel, E., Berger, C., Wallisch, M., Muller, F., Grummt, I. & Grummt, F. (1997). Termination of mammalian rDNA replication: polar arrest of replication fork movement by transcription termination factor TTF-I. *Cell,* Vol. 90, No. 3, (Aug 8), pp. (559-567), 0092-8674 (Print) 0092-8674 (Linking)

Ghazvini, M., Ribes, V. & Arcangioli, B. (1995). The essential DNA-binding protein sap1 of Schizosaccharomyces pombe contains two independent oligomerization interfaces that dictate the relative orientation of the DNA-binding domain. *Molecular and cellular biology,* Vol. 15, No. 9, (Sep), pp. (4939-4946), 0270-7306 (Print) 0270-7306 (Linking)

Gonzalez-Aguilera, C., Tous, C., Gomez-Gonzalez, B., Huertas, P., Luna, R. & Aguilera, A. (2008). The THP1-SAC3-SUS1-CDC31 complex works in transcription elongation-mRNA export preventing RNA-mediated genome instability. *Molecular biology of the cell,* Vol. 19, No. 10, (Oct), pp. (4310-4318), 1939-4586 (Electronic) 1059-1524 (Linking)

Greenfeder, S.A. & Newlon, C.S. (1992). Replication forks pause at yeast centromeres. *Molecular and cellular biology,* Vol. 12, No. 9, (Sep), pp. (4056-4066), 0270-7306 (Print) 0270-7306 (Linking)

Gruber, M., Wellinger, R.E. & Sogo, J.M. (2000). Architecture of the replication fork stalled at the 3' end of yeast ribosomal genes. *Molecular and cellular biology,* Vol. 20, No. 15, (Aug), pp. (5777-5787), 0270-7306 (Print) 0270-7306 (Linking)

Grummt, I., Maier, U., Ohrlein, A., Hassouna, N. & Bachellerie, J.P. (1985a). Transcription of mouse rDNA terminates downstream of the 3' end of 28S RNA and involves interaction of factors with repeated sequences in the 3' spacer. *Cell,* Vol. 43, No. 3 Pt 2, (Dec), pp. (801-810), 0092-8674 (Print) 0092-8674 (Linking)

Grummt, I., Sorbaz, H., Hofmann, A. & Roth, E. (1985b). Spacer sequences downstream of the 28S RNA coding region are part of the mouse rDNA transcription unit. *Nucleic acids research,* Vol. 13, No. 7, (Apr 11), pp. (2293-2304), 0305-1048 (Print) 0305-1048 (Linking)

Hashash, N., Johnson, A.L. & Cha, R.S. (2011). Regulation of fragile sites expression in budding yeast by MEC1, RRM3 and hydroxyurea. *Journal of cell science,* Vol. 124, No. Pt 2, (Jan 15), pp. (181-185), 1477-9137 (Electronic) 0021-9533 (Linking)

Hernandez, P., Lamm, S.S., Bjerknes, C.A. & Hof, J.V. (1988). Replication termini in the rDNA of synchronized pea root cells (Pisum sativum). *The EMBO journal,* Vol. 7, No. 2, (Feb), pp. (303-308), 0261-4189 (Print) 0261-4189 (Linking)

Hernandez, P., Martin-Parras, L., Martinez-Robles, M.L. & Schvartzman, J.B. (1993). Conserved features in the mode of replication of eukaryotic ribosomal RNA genes. *The EMBO journal,* Vol. 12, No. 4, (Apr), pp. (1475-1485), 0261-4189 (Print) 0261-4189 (Linking)

Howe, J.G. & Shu, M.D. (1989). Epstein-Barr virus small RNA (EBER) genes: unique transcription units that combine RNA polymerase II and III promoter elements. *Cell,* Vol. 57, No. 5, (Jun 2), pp. (825-834), 0092-8674 (Print) 0092-8674 (Linking)

Howe, J.G. & Shu, M.D. (1993). Upstream basal promoter element important for exclusive RNA polymerase III transcription of the EBER 2 gene. *Molecular and cellular biology,* Vol. 13, No. 5, (May), pp. (2655-2665), 0270-7306 (Print) 0270-7306 (Linking)

Huang, J. & Moazed, D. (2003). Association of the RENT complex with nontranscribed and coding regions of rDNA and a regional requirement for the replication fork block protein Fob1 in rDNA silencing. *Genes & development,* Vol. 17, No. 17, (Sep 1), pp. (2162-2176), 0890-9369 (Print) 0890-9369 (Linking)

Huvet, M., Nicolay, S., Touchon, M., Audit, B., d'Aubenton-Carafa, Y., Arneodo, A. & Thermes, C. (2007). Human gene organization driven by the coordination of replication and transcription. *Genome research,* Vol. 17, No. 9, (Sep), pp. (1278-1285), 1088-9051 (Print) 1088-9051 (Linking)

Hyrien, O., Maric, C. & Mechali, M. (1995). Transition in specification of embryonic metazoan DNA replication origins. *Science,* Vol. 270, No. 5238, (Nov 10), pp. (994-997), 0036-8075 (Print) 0036-8075 (Linking)

Hyrien, O. & Mechali, M. (1993). Chromosomal replication initiates and terminates at random sequences but at regular intervals in the ribosomal DNA of Xenopus early embryos. *The EMBO journal,* Vol. 12, No. 12, (Dec), pp. (4511-4520), 0261-4189 (Print) 0261-4189 (Linking)

Inagawa, T., Yamada-Inagawa, T., Eydmann, T., Mian, I.S., Wang, T.S. & Dalgaard, J.Z. (2009). Schizosaccharomyces pombe Rtf2 mediates site-specific replication termination by inhibiting replication restart. *Proceedings of the National Academy of Sciences of the United States of America,* Vol. 106, No. 19, (May 12), pp. (7927-7932), 1091-6490 (Electronic) 0027-8424 (Linking)

Ivessa, A.S., Lenzmeier, B.A., Bessler, J.B., Goudsouzian, L.K., Schnakenberg, S.L. & Zakian, V.A. (2003). The Saccharomyces cerevisiae helicase Rrm3p facilitates replication past nonhistone protein-DNA complexes. *Molecular cell,* Vol. 12, No. 6, (Dec), pp. (1525-1536), 1097-2765 (Print) 1097-2765 (Linking)

Ivessa, A.S., Zhou, J.Q., Schulz, V.P., Monson, E.K. & Zakian, V.A. (2002). Saccharomyces Rrm3p, a 5' to 3' DNA helicase that promotes replication fork progression through telomeric and subtelomeric DNA. *Genes & development,* Vol. 16, No. 11, (Jun 1), pp. (1383-1396), 0890-9369 (Print) 0890-9369 (Linking)

Ivessa, A.S., Zhou, J.Q. & Zakian, V.A. (2000). The Saccharomyces Pif1p DNA helicase and the highly related Rrm3p have opposite effects on replication fork progression in ribosomal DNA. *Cell,* Vol. 100, No. 4, (Feb 18), pp. (479-489), 0092-8674 (Print) 0092-8674 (Linking)

Kadosh, D. & Struhl, K. (1997). Repression by Ume6 involves recruitment of a complex containing Sin3 corepressor and Rpd3 histone deacetylase to target promoters. *Cell,* Vol. 89, No. 3, (May 2), pp. (365-371), 0092-8674 (Print) 0092-8674 (Linking)

Katou, Y., Kanoh, Y., Bando, M., Noguchi, H., Tanaka, H., Ashikari, T., Sugimoto, K. & Shirahige, K. (2003). S-phase checkpoint proteins Tof1 and Mrc1 form a stable replication-pausing complex. *Nature,* Vol. 424, No. 6952, (Aug 28), pp. (1078-1083), 1476-4687 (Electronic) 0028-0836 (Linking)

Kaykov, A., Holmes, A.M. & Arcangioli, B. (2004). Formation, maintenance and consequences of the imprint at the mating-type locus in fission yeast. *The EMBO journal,* Vol. 23, No. 4, (Feb 25), pp. (930-938), 0261-4189 (Print) 0261-4189 (Linking)

Keil, R.L. & McWilliams, A.D. (1993). A gene with specific and global effects on recombination of sequences from tandemly repeated genes in Saccharomyces cerevisiae. *Genetics,* Vol. 135, No. 3, (Nov), pp. (711-718), 0016-6731 (Print) 0016-6731 (Linking)

Kim, H.M., Narayanan, V., Mieczkowski, P.A., Petes, T.D., Krasilnikova, M.M., Mirkin, S.M. & Lobachev, K.S. (2008). Chromosome fragility at GAA tracts in yeast depends on repeat orientation and requires mismatch repair. *The EMBO journal,* Vol. 27, No. 21, (Nov 5), pp. (2896-2906), 1460-2075 (Electronic)0261-4189 (Linking)

Kobayashi, T. (2003). The replication fork barrier site forms a unique structure with Fob1p and inhibits the replication fork. *Molecular and cellular biology,* Vol. 23, No. 24, (Dec), pp. (9178-9188), 0270-7306 (Print) 0270-7306 (Linking)

Kobayashi, T. & Ganley, A.R. (2005). Recombination regulation by transcription-induced cohesin dissociation in rDNA repeats. *Science,* Vol. 309, No. 5740, (Sep 2), pp. (1581-1584), 1095-9203 (Electronic) 0036-8075 (Linking)

Kobayashi, T., Heck, D.J., Nomura, M. & Horiuchi, T. (1998). Expansion and contraction of ribosomal DNA repeats in Saccharomyces cerevisiae: requirement of replication fork blocking (Fob1) protein and the role of RNA polymerase I. *Genes & development,* Vol. 12, No. 24, (Dec 15), pp. (3821-3830), 0890-9369 (Print) 0890-9369 (Linking)

Kobayashi, T. & Horiuchi, T. (1996). A yeast gene product, Fob1 protein, required for both replication fork blocking and recombinational hotspot activities. *Genes to cells : devoted to molecular & cellular mechanisms,* Vol. 1, No. 5, (May), pp. (465-474), 1356-9597 (Print) 1356-9597 (Linking)

Kobayashi, T., Horiuchi, T., Tongaonkar, P., Vu, L. & Nomura, M. (2004). SIR2 regulates recombination between different rDNA repeats, but not recombination within individual rRNA genes in yeast. *Cell,* Vol. 117, No. 4, (May 14), pp. (441-453), 0092-8674 (Print) 0092-8674 (Linking)

Krasilnikova, M.M. & Mirkin, S.M. (2004a). Analysis of triplet repeat replication by two-dimensional gel electrophoresis. *Methods in molecular biology,* Vol. 277, No. pp. (19-28), 1064-3745 (Print) 1064-3745 (Linking)

Krasilnikova, M.M. & Mirkin, S.M. (2004b). Replication stalling at Friedreich's ataxia (GAA)n repeats in vivo. *Molecular and cellular biology,* Vol. 24, No. 6, (Mar), pp. (2286-2295), 0270-7306 (Print) 0270-7306 (Linking)

Krejci, L., Van Komen, S., Li, Y., Villemain, J., Reddy, M.S., Klein, H., Ellenberger, T. & Sung, P. (2003). DNA helicase Srs2 disrupts the Rad51 presynaptic filament. *Nature,* Vol. 423, No. 6937, (May 15), pp. (305-309), 0028-0836 (Print) 0028-0836 (Linking)

Krings, G. & Bastia, D. (2004). swi1- and swi3-dependent and independent replication fork arrest at the ribosomal DNA of Schizosaccharomyces pombe. *Proceedings of the National Academy of Sciences of the United States of America,* Vol. 101, No. 39, (Sep 28), pp. (14085-14090), 0027-8424 (Print) 0027-8424 (Linking)

Krings, G. & Bastia, D. (2005). Sap1p binds to Ter1 at the ribosomal DNA of Schizosaccharomyces pombe and causes polar replication fork arrest. *The Journal of biological chemistry,* Vol. 280, No. 47, (Nov 25), pp. (39135-39142), 0021-9258 (Print) 0021-9258 (Linking)

Krings, G. & Bastia, D. (2006). Molecular architecture of a eukaryotic DNA replication terminus-terminator protein complex. *Molecular and cellular biology,* Vol. 26, No. 21, (Nov), pp. (8061-8074), 0270-7306 (Print) 0270-7306 (Linking)

Lang, W.H., Morrow, B.E., Ju, Q., Warner, J.R. & Reeder, R.H. (1994). A model for transcription termination by RNA polymerase I. *Cell,* Vol. 79, No. 3, (Nov 4), pp. (527-534), 0092-8674 (Print) 0092-8674 (Linking)

Langst, G., Becker, P.B. & Grummt, I. (1998). TTF-I determines the chromatin architecture of the active rDNA promoter. *Embo J,* Vol. 17, No. 11, (Jun 1), pp. (3135-3145), 0261-4189 (Print)

Lindstrom, D.L., Leverich, C.K., Henderson, K.A. & Gottschling, D.E. (2011). Replicative Age Induces Mitotic Recombination in the Ribosomal RNA Gene Cluster of Saccharomyces cerevisiae. *PLoS genetics,* Vol. 7, No. 3, (Mar), pp. (e1002015), 1553-7404 (Electronic) 1553-7390 (Linking)

Linskens, M.H. & Huberman, J.A. (1988). Organization of replication of ribosomal DNA in Saccharomyces cerevisiae. *Molecular and cellular biology,* Vol. 8, No. 11, (Nov), pp. (4927-4935), 0270-7306 (Print) 0270-7306 (Linking)

Little, R.D., Platt, T.H. & Schildkraut, C.L. (1993a). Initiation and termination of DNA replication in human rRNA genes. *Molecular and cellular biology,* Vol. 13, No. 10, (Oct), pp. (6600-6613), 0270-7306 (Print) 0270-7306 (Linking)

Little, R.D., Platt, T.H. & Schildkraut, C.L. (1993b). Initiation and termination of DNA replication in human rRNA genes. *Mol Cell Biol,* Vol. 13, No. 10, (Oct), pp. (6600-6613), 0270-7306 (Print)

Locovei, A.M., Spiga, M.G., Tanaka, K., Murakami, Y. & D'Urso, G. (2006). The CENP-B homolog, Abp1, interacts with the initiation protein Cdc23 (MCM10) and is required for efficient DNA replication in fission yeast. *Cell division,* Vol. 1, No. pp. (27), 1747-1028 (Electronic) 1747-1028 (Linking)

Lopes, M., Cotta-Ramusino, C., Pellicioli, A., Liberi, G., Plevani, P., Muzi-Falconi, M., Newlon, C.S. & Foiani, M. (2001). The DNA replication checkpoint response stabilizes stalled replication forks. *Nature,* Vol. 412, No. 6846, (Aug 2), pp. (557-561), 0028-0836 (Print) 0028-0836 (Linking)

Lopez-estrano, C., Schvartzman, J.B., Krimer, D.B. & Hernandez, P. (1998a). Co-localization of polar replication fork barriers and rRNA transcription terminators in mouse rDNA. *Journal of molecular biology,* Vol. 277, No. 2, (Mar 27), pp. (249-256), 0022-2836 (Print) 0022-2836 (Linking)

Lopez-estrano, C., Schvartzman, J.B., Krimer, D.B. & Hernandez, P. (1998b). Co-localization of polar replication fork barriers and rRNA transcription terminators in mouse rDNA. *J Mol Biol,* Vol. 277, No. 2, (Mar 27), pp. (249-256), 0022-2836 (Print)

Lopez-Estrano, C., Schvartzman, J.B., Krimer, D.B. & Hernandez, P. (1999). Characterization of the pea rDNA replication fork barrier: putative cis-acting and trans-acting factors. *Plant molecular biology,* Vol. 40, No. 1, (May), pp. (99-110), 0167-4412 (Print) 0167-4412 (Linking)

MacAlpine, D.M., Zhang, Z. & Kapler, G.M. (1997). Type I elements mediate replication fork pausing at conserved upstream sites in the Tetrahymena thermophila ribosomal DNA minichromosome. *Molecular and cellular biology,* Vol. 17, No. 8, (Aug), pp. (4517-4525), 0270-7306 (Print) 0270-7306 (Linking)

Makovets, S. (2009). Analysis of telomeric DNA replication using neutral-alkaline two-dimensional gel electrophoresis. *Methods in molecular biology,* Vol. 521, No. pp. (169-190), 1064-3745 (Print) 1064-3745 (Linking)

Makovets, S., Herskowitz, I. & Blackburn, E.H. (2004). Anatomy and dynamics of DNA replication fork movement in yeast telomeric regions. *Molecular and cellular biology,* Vol. 24, No. 9, (May), pp. (4019-4031), 0270-7306 (Print) 0270-7306 (Linking)

Malanga, M., Czubaty, A., Girstun, A., Staron, K. & Althaus, F.R. (2008). Poly(ADP-ribose) binds to the splicing factor ASF/SF2 and regulates its phosphorylation by DNA topoisomerase I. *The Journal of biological chemistry,* Vol. 283, No. 29, (Jul 18), pp. (19991-19998), 0021-9258 (Print) 0021-9258 (Linking)

Marechal, V., Dehee, A., Chikhi-Brachet, R., Piolot, T., Coppey-Moisan, M. & Nicolas, J.C. (1999). Mapping EBNA-1 domains involved in binding to metaphase chromosomes. *Journal of virology,* Vol. 73, No. 5, (May), pp. (4385-4392), 0022-538X (Print) 0022-538X (Linking)

Mariappan, S.V., Silks, L.A., 3rd, Chen, X., Springer, P.A., Wu, R., Moyzis, R.K., Bradbury, E.M., Garcia, A.E. & Gupta, G. (1998). Solution structures of the Huntington's disease DNA triplets, (CAG)n. *Journal of biomolecular structure & dynamics,* Vol. 15, No. 4, (Feb), pp. (723-744), 0739-1102 (Print) 0739-1102 (Linking)

Maric, C., Levacher, B. & Hyrien, O. (1999). Developmental regulation of replication fork pausing in Xenopus laevis ribosomal RNA genes. *Journal of molecular biology,* Vol. 291, No. 4, (Aug 27), pp. (775-788), 0022-2836 (Print) 0022-2836 (Linking)

Mayan-Santos, M.D., Martinez-Robles, M.L., Hernandez, P., Schvartzman, J.B. & Krimer, D.B. (2008). A redundancy of processes that cause replication fork stalling enhances recombination at two distinct sites in yeast rDNA. *Molecular microbiology,* Vol. 69, No. 2, (Jul), pp. (361-375), 1365-2958 (Electronic) 0950-382X (Linking)

McFarlane, R.J. & Whitehall, S.K. (2009). tRNA genes in eukaryotic genome organization and reorganization. *Cell cycle,* Vol. 8, No. 19, (Oct 1), pp. (3102-3106), 1551-4005 (Electronic) 1551-4005 (Linking)

Mejia-Ramirez, E., Sanchez-Gorostiaga, A., Krimer, D.B., Schvartzman, J.B. & Hernandez, P. (2005). The mating type switch-activating protein Sap1 Is required for replication fork arrest at the rRNA genes of fission yeast. *Molecular and cellular biology,* Vol. 25, No. 19, (Oct), pp. (8755-8761), 0270-7306 (Print) 0270-7306 (Linking)

Melekhovets, Y.F., Shwed, P.S. & Nazar, R.N. (1997). In vivo analyses of RNA polymerase I termination in Schizosaccharomyces pombe. *Nucleic acids research,* Vol. 25, No. 24, (Dec 15), pp. (5103-5109), 0305-1048 (Print) 0305-1048 (Linking)

Miller, K.M., Rog, O. & Cooper, J.P. (2006). Semi-conservative DNA replication through telomeres requires Taz1. *Nature,* Vol. 440, No. 7085, (Apr 6), pp. (824-828), 1476-4687 (Electronic) 0028-0836 (Linking)

Mimura, S., Komata, M., Kishi, T., Shirahige, K. & Kamura, T. (2009). SCF(Dia2) regulates DNA replication forks during S-phase in budding yeast. *The EMBO journal,* Vol. 28, No. 23, (Dec 2), pp. (3693-3705), 1460-2075 (Electronic) 0261-4189 (Linking)

Mirkin, E.V. & Mirkin, S.M. (2007). Replication fork stalling at natural impediments. *Microbiology and molecular biology reviews : MMBR,* Vol. 71, No. 1, (Mar), pp. (13-35), 1092-2172 (Print) 1092-2172 (Linking)

Mohanty, B.K., Bairwa, N.K. & Bastia, D. (2006). The Tof1p-Csm3p protein complex counteracts the Rrm3p helicase to control replication termination of Saccharomyces cerevisiae. *Proceedings of the National Academy of Sciences of the United States of America,* Vol. 103, No. 4, (Jan 24), pp. (897-902), 0027-8424 (Print) 0027-8424 (Linking)

Morohashi, H., Maculins, T. & Labib, K. (2009). The amino-terminal TPR domain of Dia2 tethers SCF(Dia2) to the replisome progression complex. *Current biology : CB,* Vol. 19, No. 22, (Dec 1), pp. (1943-1949), 1879-0445 (Electronic) 0960-9822 (Linking)

Nedelcheva, M.N., Roguev, A., Dolapchiev, L.B., Shevchenko, A., Taskov, H.B., Stewart, A.F. & Stoynov, S.S. (2005). Uncoupling of unwinding from DNA synthesis implies regulation of MCM helicase by Tof1/Mrc1/Csm3 checkpoint complex. *Journal of molecular biology,* Vol. 347, No. 3, (Apr 1), pp. (509-521), 0022-2836 (Print) 0022-2836 (Linking)

Nemeth, A., Guibert, S., Tiwari, V.K., Ohlsson, R. & Langst, G. (2008). Epigenetic regulation of TTF-I-mediated promoter-terminator interactions of rRNA genes. *The EMBO journal,* Vol. 27, No. 8, (Apr 23), pp. (1255-1265), 1460-2075 (Electronic) 0261-4189 (Linking)

Nemeth, A., Strohner, R., Grummt, I. & Langst, G. (2004). The chromatin remodeling complex NoRC and TTF-I cooperate in the regulation of the mammalian rRNA genes in vivo. *Nucleic acids research,* Vol. 32, No. 14, pp. (4091-4099), 1362-4962 (Electronic) 0305-1048 (Linking)

Nick McElhinny, S.A., Kumar, D., Clark, A.B., Watt, D.L., Watts, B.E., Lundstrom, E.B., Johansson, E., Chabes, A. & Kunkel, T.A. (2010a). Genome instability due to ribonucleotide incorporation into DNA. *Nature chemical biology,* Vol. 6, No. 10, (Oct), pp. (774-781), 1552-4469 (Electronic) 1552-4450 (Linking)

Nick McElhinny, S.A., Watts, B.E., Kumar, D., Watt, D.L., Lundstrom, E.B., Burgers, P.M., Johansson, E., Chabes, A. & Kunkel, T.A. (2010b). Abundant ribonucleotide incorporation into DNA by yeast replicative polymerases. *Proceedings of the National Academy of Sciences of the United States of America,* Vol. 107, No. 11, (Mar 16), pp. (4949-4954), 1091-6490 (Electronic) 0027-8424 (Linking)

Noguchi, C. & Noguchi, E. (2007). Sap1 promotes the association of the replication fork protection complex with chromatin and is involved in the replication checkpoint in Schizosaccharomyces pombe. *Genetics,* Vol. 175, No. 2, (Feb), pp. (553-566), 0016-6731 (Print) 0016-6731 (Linking)

Ohki, R. & Ishikawa, F. (2004). Telomere-bound TRF1 and TRF2 stall the replication fork at telomeric repeats. *Nucleic acids research,* Vol. 32, No. 5, pp. (1627-1637), 1362-4962 (Electronic) 0305-1048 (Linking)

Papamichos-Chronakis, M. & Peterson, C.L. (2008). The Ino80 chromatin-remodeling enzyme regulates replisome function and stability. *Nature structural & molecular biology,* Vol. 15, No. 4, (Apr), pp. (338-345), 1545-9985 (Electronic) 1545-9985 (Linking)

Pearson, C.E., Nichol Edamura, K. & Cleary, J.D. (2005). Repeat instability: mechanisms of dynamic mutations. *Nature reviews. Genetics,* Vol. 6, No. 10, (Oct), pp. (729-742), 1471-0056 (Print) 1471-0056 (Linking)

Pelletier, R., Krasilnikova, M.M., Samadashwily, G.M., Lahue, R. & Mirkin, S.M. (2003). Replication and expansion of trinucleotide repeats in yeast. *Molecular and cellular biology,* Vol. 23, No. 4, (Feb), pp. (1349-1357), 0270-7306 (Print) 0270-7306 (Linking)

Prado, F. & Aguilera, A. (2005). Impairment of replication fork progression mediates RNA polII transcription-associated recombination. *The EMBO journal,* Vol. 24, No. 6, (Mar 23), pp. (1267-1276), 0261-4189 (Print) 0261-4189 (Linking)

Pryce, D.W., Ramayah, S., Jaendling, A. & McFarlane, R.J. (2009). Recombination at DNA replication fork barriers is not universal and is differentially regulated by Swi1. *Proceedings of the National Academy of Sciences of the United States of America,* Vol. 106, No. 12, (Mar 24), pp. (4770-4775), 1091-6490 (Electronic) 0027-8424 (Linking)

Putter, V. & Grummt, F. (2002a). Transcription termination factor TTF-I exhibits contrahelicase activity during DNA replication. *EMBO Rep,* Vol. 3, No. 2, (Feb), pp. (147-152), 1469-221X (Print)

Putter, V. & Grummt, F. (2002b). Transcription termination factor TTF-I exhibits contrahelicase activity during DNA replication. *EMBO reports,* Vol. 3, No. 2, (Feb), pp. (147-152), 1469-221X (Print)

1469-221X (Linking)

Rawlins, D.R., Milman, G., Hayward, S.D. & Hayward, G.S. (1985). Sequence-specific DNA binding of the Epstein-Barr virus nuclear antigen (EBNA-1) to clustered sites in the plasmid maintenance region. *Cell,* Vol. 42, No. 3, (Oct), pp. (859-868), 0092-8674 (Print) 0092-8674 (Linking)

Reeder, R.H., Guevara, P. & Roan, J.G. (1999). Saccharomyces cerevisiae RNA polymerase I terminates transcription at the Reb1 terminator in vivo. *Molecular and cellular biology,* Vol. 19, No. 11, (Nov), pp. (7369-7376), 0270-7306 (Print) 0270-7306 (Linking)

Reeder, R.H. & Lang, W. (1994). The mechanism of transcription termination by RNA polymerase I. *Molecular microbiology,* Vol. 12, No. 1, (Apr), pp. (11-15), 0950-382X (Print) 0950-382X (Linking)

Robert, F., Pokholok, D.K., Hannett, N.M., Rinaldi, N.J., Chandy, M., Rolfe, A., Workman, J.L., Gifford, D.K. & Young, R.A. (2004). Global position and recruitment of HATs and HDACs in the yeast genome. *Molecular cell,* Vol. 16, No. 2, (Oct 22), pp. (199-209), 1097-2765 (Print) 1097-2765 (Linking)

Rodriguez-Sanchez, L., Rodriguez-Lopez, M., Garcia, Z., Tenorio-Gomez, M., Schvartzman, J.B., Krimer, D.B. & Hernandez, P. (2011). The fission yeast rDNA-binding protein Reb1 regulates G1 phase under nutritional stress. *Journal of cell science,* Vol. 124, No. Pt 1, (Jan 1), pp. (25-34), 1477-9137 (Electronic) 0021-9533 (Linking)

Rossi, F., Labourier, E., Forne, T., Divita, G., Derancourt, J., Riou, J.F., Antoine, E., Cathala, G., Brunel, C. & Tazi, J. (1996). Specific phosphorylation of SR proteins by mammalian DNA topoisomerase I. *Nature,* Vol. 381, No. 6577, (May 2), pp. (80-82), 0028-0836 (Print) 0028-0836 (Linking)

Rozenzhak, S., Mejia-Ramirez, E., Williams, J.S., Schaffer, L., Hammond, J.A., Head, S.R. & Russell, P. (2010). Rad3 decorates critical chromosomal domains with gammaH2A to protect genome integrity during S-Phase in fission yeast. *PLoS genetics,* Vol. 6, No. 7, (Jul), pp. (e1001032), 1553-7404 (Electronic) 1553-7390 (Linking)

Sanchez-Gorostiaga, A., Lopez-Estrano, C., Krimer, D.B., Schvartzman, J.B. & Hernandez, P. (2004). Transcription termination factor reb1p causes two replication fork barriers at its cognate sites in fission yeast ribosomal DNA in vivo. *Molecular and cellular biology,* Vol. 24, No. 1, (Jan), pp. (398-406), 0270-7306 (Print) 0270-7306 (Linking)

Sander, E.E. & Grummt, I. (1997). Oligomerization of the transcription termination factor TTF-I: implications for the structural organization of ribosomal transcription units. *Nucleic acids research,* Vol. 25, No. 6, (Mar 15), pp. (1142-1147), 0305-1048 (Print) 0305-1048 (Linking)

Sander, E.E., Mason, S.W., Munz, C. & Grummt, I. (1996a). The amino-terminal domain of the transcription termination factor TTF-I causes protein oligomerization and inhibition of DNA binding. *Nucleic acids research,* Vol. 24, No. 19, (Oct 1), pp. (3677-3684), 0305-1048 (Print) 0305-1048 (Linking)

Sander, E.E., Mason, S.W., Munz, C. & Grummt, I. (1996b). The amino-terminal domain of the transcription termination factor TTF-I causes protein oligomerization and inhibition of DNA binding. *Nucleic Acids Res,* Vol. 24, No. 19, (Oct 1), pp. (3677-3684), 0305-1048 (Print)

Sayrac, S., Vengrova, S., Godfrey, E.L. & Dalgaard, J.Z. (2011). Identification of a novel type of spacer element required for imprinting in fission yeast. *PLoS genetics,* Vol. 7, No. 3, (Mar), pp. (e1001328), 1553-7404 (Electronic) 1553-7390 (Linking)

Sears, J., Kolman, J., Wahl, G.M. & Aiyar, A. (2003). Metaphase chromosome tethering is necessary for the DNA synthesis and maintenance of oriP plasmids but is insufficient for transcription activation by Epstein-Barr nuclear antigen 1. *Journal of virology,* Vol. 77, No. 21, (Nov), pp. (11767-11780), 0022-538X (Print) 0022-538X (Linking)

Sears, J., Ujihara, M., Wong, S., Ott, C., Middeldorp, J. & Aiyar, A. (2004). The amino terminus of Epstein-Barr Virus (EBV) nuclear antigen 1 contains AT hooks that facilitate the replication and partitioning of latent EBV genomes by tethering them to cellular chromosomes. *Journal of virology,* Vol. 78, No. 21, (Nov), pp. (11487-11505), 0022-538X (Print) 0022-538X (Linking)

Singh, S.K., Sabatinos, S., Forsburg, S. & Bastia, D. (2010). Regulation of replication termination by Reb1 protein-mediated action at a distance. *Cell,* Vol. 142, No. 6, (Sep 17), pp. (868-878), 1097-4172 (Electronic) 0092-8674 (Linking)

Soret, J., Gabut, M., Dupon, C., Kohlhagen, G., Stevenin, J., Pommier, Y. & Tazi, J. (2003). Altered serine/arginine-rich protein phosphorylation and exonic enhancer-dependent splicing in Mammalian cells lacking topoisomerase I. *Cancer research,* Vol. 63, No. 23, (Dec 1), pp. (8203-8211), 0008-5472 (Print) 0008-5472 (Linking)

Stelter, P. & Ulrich, H.D. (2003). Control of spontaneous and damage-induced mutagenesis by SUMO and ubiquitin conjugation. *Nature,* Vol. 425, No. 6954, (Sep 11), pp. (188-191), 1476-4687 (Electronic) 0028-0836 (Linking)

Storici, F., Bebenek, K., Kunkel, T.A., Gordenin, D.A. & Resnick, M.A. (2007). RNA-templated DNA repair. *Nature,* Vol. 447, No. 7142, (May 17), pp. (338-341), 1476-4687 (Electronic) 0028-0836 (Linking)

Szilard, R.K., Jacques, P.E., Laramee, L., Cheng, B., Galicia, S., Bataille, A.R., Yeung, M., Mendez, M., Bergeron, M., Robert, F. & Durocher, D. (2010). Systematic identification of fragile sites via genome-wide location analysis of gamma-H2AX. *Nature structural & molecular biology,* Vol. 17, No. 3, (Mar), pp. (299-305), 1545-9985 (Electronic) 1545-9985 (Linking)

Takeuchi, Y., Horiuchi, T. & Kobayashi, T. (2003). Transcription-dependent recombination and the role of fork collision in yeast rDNA. *Genes & development,* Vol. 17, No. 12, (Jun 15), pp. (1497-1506), 0890-9369 (Print) 0890-9369 (Linking)

Tanaka, T., Yokoyama, M., Matsumoto, S., Fukatsu, R., You, Z. & Masai, H. (2010). Fission yeast Swi1-Swi3 complex facilitates DNA binding of Mrc1. *The Journal of biological chemistry*, Vol. 285, No. 51, (Dec 17), pp. (39609-39622), 1083-351X (Electronic) 0021-9258 (Linking)

Torres, J.Z., Bessler, J.B. & Zakian, V.A. (2004). Local chromatin structure at the ribosomal DNA causes replication fork pausing and genome instability in the absence of the S. cerevisiae DNA helicase Rrm3p. *Genes & development*, Vol. 18, No. 5, (Mar 1), pp. (498-503), 0890-9369 (Print) 0890-9369 (Linking)

Tower, J. (2004). Developmental gene amplification and origin regulation. *Annual review of genetics*, Vol. 38, No. pp. (273-304), 0066-4197 (Print) 0066-4197 (Linking)

Tuduri, S., Crabbe, L., Conti, C., Tourriere, H., Holtgreve-Grez, H., Jauch, A., Pantesco, V., De Vos, J., Thomas, A., Theillet, C., Pommier, Y., Tazi, J., Coquelle, A. & Pasero, P. (2009). Topoisomerase I suppresses genomic instability by preventing interference between replication and transcription. *Nature cell biology*, Vol. 11, No. 11, (Nov), pp. (1315-1324), 1476-4679 (Electronic) 1465-7392 (Linking)

Tuduri, S., Crabbe, L., Tourriere, H., Coquelle, A. & Pasero, P. (2010). Does interference between replication and transcription contribute to genomic instability in cancer cells? *Cell cycle*, Vol. 9, No. 10, (May 15), pp. (1886-1892), 1551-4005 (Electronic) 1551-4005 (Linking)

Veaute, X., Jeusset, J., Soustelle, C., Kowalczykowski, S.C., Le Cam, E. & Fabre, F. (2003). The Srs2 helicase prevents recombination by disrupting Rad51 nucleoprotein filaments. *Nature*, Vol. 423, No. 6937, (May 15), pp. (309-312), 0028-0836 (Print) 0028-0836 (Linking)

Vengrova, S. & Dalgaard, J.Z. (2004). RNase-sensitive DNA modification(s) initiates S. pombe mating-type switching. *Genes & development*, Vol. 18, No. 7, (Apr 1), pp. (794-804), 0890-9369 (Print) 0890-9369 (Linking)

Vengrova, S. & Dalgaard, J.Z. (2005). The Schizosaccharomyces pombe imprint--nick or ribonucleotide(s)? *Current biology : CB*, Vol. 15, No. 9, (May 10), pp. (R326-327; author reply R327), 0960-9822 (Print) 0960-9822 (Linking)

Vengrova, S. & Dalgaard, J.Z. (2006). The wild-type Schizosaccharomyces pombe mat1 imprint consists of two ribonucleotides. *EMBO reports*, Vol. 7, No. 1, (Jan), pp. (59-65), 1469-221X (Print) 1469-221X (Linking)

Voineagu, I., Narayanan, V., Lobachev, K.S. & Mirkin, S.M. (2008). Replication stalling at unstable inverted repeats: interplay between DNA hairpins and fork stabilizing proteins. *Proceedings of the National Academy of Sciences of the United States of America*, Vol. 105, No. 29, (Jul 22), pp. (9936-9941), 1091-6490 (Electronic) 0027-8424 (Linking)

Voineagu, I., Surka, C.F., Shishkin, A.A., Krasilnikova, M.M. & Mirkin, S.M. (2009). Replisome stalling and stabilization at CGG repeats, which are responsible for chromosomal fragility. *Nature structural & molecular biology*, Vol. 16, No. 2, (Feb), pp. (226-228), 1545-9985 (Electronic) 1545-9985 (Linking)

Wallisch, M., Kunkel, E., Hoehn, K. & Grummt, F. (2002). Ku antigen supports termination of mammalian rDNA replication by transcription termination factor TTF-I. *Biological chemistry*, Vol. 383, No. 5, (May), pp. (765-771), 1431-6730 (Print) 1431-6730 (Linking)

Wang, K.L. & Warner, J.R. (1998). Positive and negative autoregulation of REB1 transcription in Saccharomyces cerevisiae. *Mol Cell Biol,* Vol. 18, No. 7, (Jul), pp. (4368-4376), 0270-7306 (Print)

Ward, T.R., Hoang, M.L., Prusty, R., Lau, C.K., Keil, R.L., Fangman, W.L. & Brewer, B.J. (2000). Ribosomal DNA replication fork barrier and HOT1 recombination hot spot: shared sequences but independent activities. *Molecular and cellular biology,* Vol. 20, No. 13, (Jul), pp. (4948-4957), 0270-7306 (Print) 0270-7306 (Linking)

Watts, F.Z., Skilton, A., Ho, J.C., Boyd, L.K., Trickey, M.A., Gardner, L., Ogi, F.X. & Outwin, E.A. (2007). The role of Schizosaccharomyces pombe SUMO ligases in genome stability. *Biochemical Society transactions,* Vol. 35, No. Pt 6, (Dec), pp. (1379-1384), 0300-5127 (Print) 0300-5127 (Linking)

Weitao, T., Budd, M. & Campbell, J.L. (2003a). Evidence that yeast SGS1, DNA2, SRS2, and FOB1 interact to maintain rDNA stability. *Mutation research,* Vol. 532, No. 1-2, (Nov 27), pp. (157-172), 0027-5107 (Print) 0027-5107 (Linking)

Weitao, T., Budd, M., Hoopes, L.L. & Campbell, J.L. (2003b). Dna2 helicase/nuclease causes replicative fork stalling and double-strand breaks in the ribosomal DNA of Saccharomyces cerevisiae. *The Journal of biological chemistry,* Vol. 278, No. 25, (Jun 20), pp. (22513-22522), 0021-9258 (Print) 0021-9258 (Linking)

Wiesendanger, B., Lucchini, R., Koller, T. & Sogo, J.M. (1994). Replication fork barriers in the Xenopus rDNA. *Nucleic acids research,* Vol. 22, No. 23, (Nov 25), pp. (5038-5046), 0305-1048 (Print) 0305-1048 (Linking)

Williams, J.S., Williams, R.S., Dovey, C.L., Guenther, G., Tainer, J.A. & Russell, P. (2010). gammaH2A binds Brc1 to maintain genome integrity during S-phase. *The EMBO journal,* Vol. 29, No. 6, (Mar 17), pp. (1136-1148), 1460-2075 (Electronic) 0261-4189 (Linking)

Xie, J., Pierce, M., Gailus-Durner, V., Wagner, M., Winter, E. & Vershon, A.K. (1999). Sum1 and Hst1 repress middle sporulation-specific gene expression during mitosis in Saccharomyces cerevisiae. *The EMBO journal,* Vol. 18, No. 22, (Nov 15), pp. (6448-6454), 0261-4189 (Print) 0261-4189 (Linking)

Yakisich, J.S. & Kapler, G.M. (2006). Deletion of the Tetrahymena thermophila rDNA replication fork barrier region disrupts macronuclear rDNA excision and creates a fragile site in the micronuclear genome. *Nucleic acids research,* Vol. 34, No. 2, pp. (620-634), 1362-4962 (Electronic) 0305-1048 (Linking)

Yunus, A.A. & Lima, C.D. (2009). Structure of the Siz/PIAS SUMO E3 ligase Siz1 and determinants required for SUMO modification of PCNA. *Molecular cell,* Vol. 35, No. 5, (Sep 11), pp. (669-682), 1097-4164 (Electronic) 1097-2765 (Linking)

Zaratiegui, M., Vaughn, M.W., Irvine, D.V., Goto, D., Watt, S., Bahler, J., Arcangioli, B. & Martienssen, R.A. (2011). CENP-B preserves genome integrity at replication forks paused by retrotransposon LTR. *Nature,* Vol. 469, No. 7328, (Jan 6), pp. (112-115), 1476-4687 (Electronic) 0028-0836 (Linking)

Zhang, Z., Macalpine, D.M. & Kapler, G.M. (1997). Developmental regulation of DNA replication: replication fork barriers and programmed gene amplification in Tetrahymena thermophila. *Molecular and cellular biology,* Vol. 17, No. 10, (Oct), pp. (6147-6156), 0270-7306 (Print) 0270-7306 (Linking)

Zheng, M., Huang, X., Smith, G.K., Yang, X. & Gao, X. (1996). Genetically unstable CXG repeats are structurally dynamic and have a high propensity for folding. An NMR and UV spectroscopic study. *Journal of molecular biology,* Vol. 264, No. 2, (Nov 29), pp. (323-336), 0022-2836 (Print) 0022-2836 (Linking)

Zhou, J.Q., Qi, H., Schulz, V.P., Mateyak, M.K., Monson, E.K. & Zakian, V.A. (2002). Schizosaccharomyces pombe pfh1+ encodes an essential 5' to 3' DNA helicase that is a member of the PIF1 subfamily of DNA helicases. *Molecular biology of the cell,* Vol. 13, No. 6, (Jun), pp. (2180-2191), 1059-1524 (Print) 1059-1524 (Linking)

14

Control of Telomeric DNA Replication: Genetics, Molecular Biology, and Physiology

Akira Matsuura and Aiko Matsui
Graduate School of Advanced Integration Science, Chiba University
Japan

1. Introduction

Linear chromosome ends are capped with nucleoprotein complexes called telomeres. Telomeres are essential for the integrity of chromosomes, and loss of the capping function caused by telomere shortening or deficiency of a capping protein leads to detrimental consequences, including the formation of abnormal chromosomes, permanent cell cycle arrest (cellular senescence), and cell death (apoptosis). Telomeres are thought to play a major role in preventing normal chromosome ends from being recognized and processed as DNA double-strand breaks (DSBs).

The replication of linear eukaryotic chromosomes suffers from an intrinsic problem called the "end-replication problem", which in most cells is solved by the specialized enzyme telomerase. However, this telomerase-dependent mechanism is not the only solution to the end-replication problem in eukaryotic cells: a recombination-mediated mechanism has been found to participate in the maintenance of telomeres in several types of cells, including telomerase-defective yeast mutants, some immortalized tumor cells, and embryonic stem cells. Thus, it is now becoming clear that the regulation of telomere replication impacts on development and disease in higher eukaryotes.

In this chapter, we highlight recent topics in telomere biology, notably the regulation of telomere replication and the response to telomere dysfunction. We focus on the molecular regulation of telomere replication during both the mitotic cell cycle and development, and discuss cellular responses to defects in telomere replication and their relationships with human diseases.

2. The early days of telomere research

The physiological importance of the telomere for chromosome maintenance has been known since the 1920s, when the abnormal behavior of chromosomes lacking telomeres was described by two prominent cytogeneticists, Muller and Mclintock (Muller, 1938; Mclintock, 1941). Meanwhile, the significance of the telomere as a replication machinery of linear chromosomes became clear after the mechanism of DNA replication at the biochemical level was explained, around 1970. That the telomere solves the "end-replication problem"—the inability of the conventional DNA replication machinery to completely copy the ends of linear DNA—was independently proposed by Watson (1972) and Olovnikov (1973). However, the mechanism involved was still elusive at that time.

3. The structure of telomeric DNA

Various models to explain the solution of the end-replication problem in eukaryotic chromosomes were proposed in the 1970s and 1980s, but determination of the structure of the telomere and sequence of telomeric DNA sequence was necessary to determine which model was correct. Using the ciliate *Tetrahymena thermophila*, Blackburn and Gall (1978) found that the terminal portion of minichromosomes consisted of simple, tandem repeats of short DNA sequences (TTGGGG/AACCCC). Later, it was shown that similar sequences, with a signature of tandem repeats containing a cluster of G residues, were commonly found at the chromosomal termini in most eukaryotes.

The functional importance of the repeated sequence was proved in yeast by Szostak and Blackburn (1982). Usually, yeast plasmids replicate in a circular form; linearized plasmids cannot be maintained stably. However, when the terminal repeats of *Tetrahymena* were ligated to each end of a linear yeast plasmid, it was able to replicate in a linear form. This result indicated that the terminal fragments served a conserved function to protect the ends of linear DNA.

The G-rich strand of the telomere repeat is oriented 5′ to 3′ toward the chromosome terminus. Telomeric DNA consists of a double-stranded region of telomeric repeats, which terminates as a 3′ single-stranded overhang called the "G-overhang" (Wright et al., 1997; McElligott & Welllinger, 1997). The conserved nature of telomeric repeats, both as double-stranded DNA and single-stranded G-overhangs, is critical for the recruitment of proteins involved in the formation and function of telomeres.

Because of its specific sequence, telomeric DNA displays unusual properties. Single-stranded G-overhangs have the intrinsic ability to form a specialized structure called the "G-quadruplex" at physiological salt concentrations (Williamson et al., 1989). The G-quadruplex is a four-stranded helical structure composed of stacks of G-quartets that arise from the association of four guanines in a cyclic hydrogen-bonding arrangement. The existence of G-quadruplexes at telomeres has been confirmed *in vivo*, and their functional roles have begun to be explained (Smith et al., 2011).

The G-overhang also contributes to formation of a higher-order structure: the t-loop. The t-loop was first identified by electron microscopic analysis of *in vivo*-cross-linked human telomeric DNA, which was formed by the insertion of the G-overhang into the double-stranded region of telomeric DNA (Griffith et al., 1999). Subsequently, t-loop structures have been found in telomeres in other organisms, suggesting that it is the conserved feature of telomere structure.

4. The discovery of telomerase

The solution of the end-replication problem by the telomere was confirmed by the discovery of telomerase by Greider and Blackburn (1985). Telomerase was identified in *Tetrahymena* as a specialized enzyme that adds the telomeric G-rich sequence to the end of linear DNA. The addition of telomeric DNA by telomerase explained how the loss of terminal sequences caused by normal semi-conservative replication is counteracted. Telomerase is inactive in adult human cells, and telomere length gradually decreases during cellular senescence (de Lange et al., 1990). By contrast, telomerase is activated after immortalization (Counter et al., 1992).

The telomerase enzyme was co-purified with an RNA moiety, telomerase RNA (TERC), which specifies the sequence of telomeric repeats (Yu et al., 1990). Its catalytic subunit, identified by genetic screening in yeast (Lendvay et al., 1996) and biochemical purification from the ciliate *Euplotes aediculatus* (Lingner et al., 1996), contains the conserved motif for reverse transcriptase, and it was thus termed telomerase reverse transcriptase (TERT). Forced expression of *TERT* in mortal human cells can bypass senescence (Bodnar et al., 1998), proving that replicative senescence is caused by lack of *TERT* expression.

Other telomerase-associated proteins have been described. They are thought to be involved in the biogenesis of telomerase or to regulate the recruitment of telomerase to chromosome ends. For example, Est1 in budding yeast was identified as a protein whose deficiency reduced telomere length and cell viability after successive rounds of division (Lundblad & Szostak, 1989), and is now known to be involved in the loading of telomerase to telomeric DNA (Taggart et al., 2002).

5. Components of the telomere

5.1 Telomere binding proteins and the protein-counting model for telomere length control

In both mammals and yeast, telomerase-positive cells maintain telomeres at a constant length. Newly formed short telomeres are elongated such that they reach the length that is characteristic of the particular cell type, while over-elongated telomeres shorten until they reach the normal length (Negrini et al., 2007; Marcand et al., 1999). These observations indicate that telomerase activity is regulated at individual ends, and is regulated so as to counteract the loss of telomeric repeats due to the end-replication problem. Recent studies have elucidated the regulatory mechanism that ensures length homeostasis at every telomeric end: the protein complex that binds at double-stranded telomeric DNA exerts an inhibitory effect on telomerase activity.

In budding yeast, the telomere dsDNA-binding protein Rap1 serves to limit telomere length: the number of repeats at an individual telomere was reduced when hybrid proteins containing Rap1 were targeted there by a heterologous DNA-binding domain (Marcand et al., 1997). Through its C-terminal domain, Rap1 interacts with two proteins, Rif1 and Rif2. These two proteins act as telomerase inhibitors, andloss of either protein leads to telomere over-elongation (Hardy et al., 1992; Wotton and Shore, 1997). Thus, a model has been proposed to explain the regulation of telomere length: longer telomeres carrying numerous Rap1 binding sites, leading to the increased binding of telomerase inhibitors, which repress telomerase-dependent telomere elongation. Telomere length declines progressively with each replication cycle, causing the loss of telomere inhibitors at the ends of telomeres, allowing telomere repeat number to be restored by the action of telomerase. Consistent with this model, telomerase is not active at each telomere during every replication cycle, but is activated when the length of the repeat tract is reduced to a threshold level as a result of successive rounds of replication (Teixeira et al., 2004).

In fission yeast, the double-stranded DNA-binding protein Taz1 recruits Rif1 and Rap1 (Kanoh & Ishikawa, 2001; Chikashige & Hiraoka, 2001). Rap1 does not interact directly with Rif1 but, instead, interacts with Poz1, which serves as a negative regulator of telomere length (Miyoshi et al., 2008). In mammals, TRF1 and TRF2 bind to double-stranded telomeric DNA and exert *cis*-inhibitory effects on telomerase activity (Ancelin et al., 2002). They also recruit other proteins to assemble the six-protein shelterin complex (TRF1/TRF2/RAP1/TIN2/TPP1/POT1). All the components of shelterin have been shown to act as negative regulators of telomerase (Smogorzewska & de Lange, 2004)..

5.2 The CST complex

The proteins directly bound to the very ends of chromosomes are not only essential for protecting telomeres but are also involved in recruiting telomerase to chromosomes. A budding yeast *cdc13* mutant, originally isolated as a cell division cycle mutant, displays G_2 arrest after transfer to the restrictive temperature (Hartwell et al., 1973). Cdc13 forms a complex with Stn1 and Ten1 *in vivo* (Grandin et al., 1997; Grandin et al., 2001). Each component of the Cdc13-Stn1-Ten1 heterotrimeric complex (CST complex) has a single-stranded DNA binding motif, the OB-fold domain (Mitton-Fry et al., 2002). As a result, CST has a strong affinity for single stranded telomeric DNA, and thus localizes to the very ends of chromosomes (Taggart et al., 2002). Based on structural and functional similarities, CST has been proposed to be a telomere-specific replication protein A (RPA)-like complex (Gao et al., 2007). Cell cycle arrest in the *cdc13* mutant is due to loss of telomere protection: when CST function is disrupted, capping is dysfunctional and chromosome ends suffer the same fate as DSBs (Garvik et al., 1995). Moreover, the CST complex contributes to telomere replication by directly interacting with the telomerase-associated protein Est1 and DNA polymerase α (Qi and Zakian, 2000; Grossi et al., 2004). Cdc13 is phosphorylated at multiple sites by Cdk and Tel1 kinases (Li et al., 2009; Tseng et al., 2006). These modifications are thought to be important for recruitment of Est1 and telomerase to telomeres.

Although the organization of DNA ends is well conserved, mammalian telomere ends are primarily protected by a Pot1-Tpp1 complex, part of the larger shelterin complex (Wang et al., 2007). Components of shelterin have also been found in fission yeast and plants (Baumann & Cech, 2001; Miyoshi et al., 2008; Shakirov et al., 2005). Budding yeast CST and shelterin components do not have sequence similarity, suggesting that budding yeast may have a unique mode of telomere capping. However, recent studies have revealed that mammals and plants have Stn1 and Ten1 homologs, and that the two proteins form a complex with another protein called Ctc1 (Miyake et al., 2009; Surovtseva et al., 2009). The Ctc1-Stn1-Ten1 heterotrimeric complex associates with single-stranded DNA but with no sequence specificity. Human Ctc1 and Stn1 have been characterized as proteins that stimulate DNA polymerase α activity (Casteel et al., 2009) and appear to play a role in replication of "difficult" sites, including telomeric repeats.

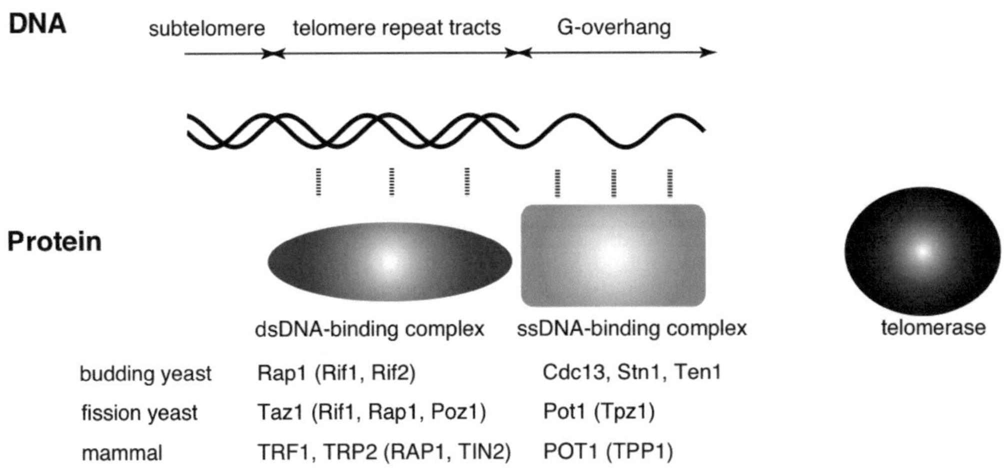

Fig. 1. Telomere DNA structure and the binding proteins in model organisms

5.3 Proteins involved in telomere replication

5.3.1 DNA repair proteins

One critical function of the telomere is assumed to be the prevention of normal chromosome ends being recognized as a damaged DNA ends. This is mediated by the formation of a specialized nucleoprotein complex. Paradoxically, however, telomere length is reduced by mutations in DSB-detection machineries such as Tel1 and the MRX (Mre11-Rad50-Xrs2) complex, indicating that proteins involved in the recognition and repair of DNA damage are important for telomere homeostasis (Greenwell et al., 1995; Nugent et al., 1998) . Epistasis analysis has established that MRX and Tel1 act in the telomerase pathway of telomere maintenance (Ritchie & Petes, 2000), and that Mre11 and Tel1 are required for the recruitment of telomerase to telomeres (Goudsouzian et al., 2006). Therefore, these proteins are involved in telomere length control as components of the telomerase-dependent telomere elongation pathway.

5.3.2 DNA polymerases

A DNA polymerase α/primase complex is responsible for initiating *de novo* lagging strand DNA synthesis. In budding yeast, mutations in Polα lead to telomerase-dependent telomere elongation and a telomerase-independent increase in G-overhang length during the S phase (Adams et al., 1996; Adams Martin et al., 2000). Moreover, Polα is essential for telomerase-dependent addition of telomeric DNA to DSBs (Diede & Gottschling, 1999).

The Polα complex physically interacts with the CST complex in budding yeast, while an analogous association between the lagging strand replication machinery and telomerase has been observed in ciliate and fission yeast. Polα is also implicated in telomere replication in higher eukaryotes: G-overhang length is increased in a mouse cell line with a temperature-sensitive Polα allele (Nakamura et al., 2005). As a mutation in replication protein C was also shown to lead to telomere elongation (Adams et al., 1996), it has been suggested that switching from polymerase α to replication factor C during lagging strand synthesis is critical for the regulation of telomerase activity.

5.3.3 Replication protein A

Replication protein A (RPA) is a heterotrimeric complex that binds to and stabilizes single-stranded DNA intermediates produced during various DNA metabolic processes, including DNA replication. RPA localizes to telomeres during the S phase (Schramke et al., 2004; Takata et al., 2005). Yeast cells harboring an RPA mutation were shown to have shortened telomeres (Ono et al., 2003).

5.3.4 DNA helicase

Telomeric DNA has the specialized structure described above, which may affect the progression of replication forks at the locus. Indeed, replication forks stall or pause at telomeres in yeast and human cells (Ivessa et al., 2002; Sfeir et al., 2009). Such difficulties seem to be overcome, at least partially, by some of the telomere-binding proteins. For example, in fission yeast, Taz1 contributes to the efficient replication of telomeres by preventing fork stalling (Miller et al., 2006). RecQ-type DNA helicases have been shown to facilitate telomere replication, probably by relieving the secondary DNA structure at telomeres (Sfeir et al., 2009).

6. Mechanism of telomerase recruitment during the cell cycle

Consistent with the requirement for a free 3′ single-stranded DNA end as a substrate for *in vitro* telomerase assay, a 3′ overhang in the G-rich strand at the end of chromosomes is critical for telomerase action. In budding yeast, the single-strand overhangs are present throughout the cell cycle, but are relatively short (10-15 nucleotides) for most of the cycle. The length of the overhangs increases transiently in the late S phase, during which telomere replication takes place (Marcand et al., 2000; Larrivee et al., 2004). The cell cycle-dependent formation of G-overhangs is mediated by the cyclin-dependent kinase Cdk1 (Cdc28-Clb in budding yeast), which is activated in the S and G_2/M phases (Frank et al., 2006; Vodenicharov & Wellinger, 2006).

Telomerase activity is indispensable for G-overhang formation during the S phase in yeast and mammals. Nucleolytic end processing activity also contributes to G-overhang formation (Wellinger et al., 1996). MRX in budding yeast and its mammalian ortholog, MRN (Mre11-Rad50-Nbs1), are important for G-overhang formation (Diede and Gottschling, 2001; Takata et al., 2005; Chai et al., 2006). Their activity is regulated by the associated protein Sae2, a target of Cdk1 (Huertas et al., 2008). However, at least in yeast, a redundant nucleolytic activity regulated by Sgs1 (RecQ) also controls end processing at telomeres (Bonetti et al., 2009). Interestingly, the MRX complex only binds to leading-strand telomeres, and this binding is critical for the binding of the CST complex and telomerase to leading-strand telomeres (Faure et al., 2010). As described above, genetic analysis has shown that MRX and telomerase act in the same pathway. This suggests that telomere elongation probably occurs mainly at leading-strand telomeres, at least in yeast. The leading strand polymerase Polε arrives at telomeres earlier than the lagging strand DNA polymerases Polα and Polδ (Moser et al., 2009). Thus, temporal regulation may contribute to the difference between the two strands. In mammalian cells, differences in the behaviors of leading- and lagging-strand telomeres have been also reported, such as the preferential occurrence of telomere-telomere fusions between leading-strand telomeres upon shelterin inactivation (Bailey et al., 2001).

7. Summary of telomeric DNA replication: an overview based on studies of budding yeast

Figure 2 presents a current model for telomere replication. In this model, telomere integrity is thought to be maintained by an elegant mechanism. The switch from a protected state to an accessible state allows telomerase recruitment. As discussed previously, this is achieved in both a cell cycle-dependent manner and a telomere length-regulated manner.

1. Replication fork progression. In yeast, telomeres replicate during the late S phase (Raghuraman et al., 2001). Replication is initiated from a replication origin located in the subtelomeric region, and the replication fork moves towards the chromosome terminus. In mammalian cells, the timing of telomere replication seems not to be restricted to the late S phase (Wright et al., 1999), and the direction of fork movement at telomeres is ambiguous.
2. End processing. After the replication fork reaches the terminus, C-strand-specific resection takes place to produce the G-overhang.
3. Recruitment of telomere proteins. Single-stranded DNA-binding complexes are recruited to the extended G-overhang. RPA may compete with CST or Pot1 for binding sites, but ultimately RPA is displaced by telomere-specific components. In mammalian

cells, telomeric repeat-containing RNA (TERRA) facilitates the RPA-to-Pot1 switch (Flynn et al., 2011).

4. Recruitment of telomerase. Usually, recruitment of Tel1 to telomeres is inhibited by Rif1 and Rif2 (Hirano et al., 2009). The conformation of short telomeres with reduced amounts of these two proteins changes to the accessible state, and Tel1 is thus recruited. Tel1 phosphorylates Cdc13 (and probably other proteins), thereby enabling it to interact with Est1 and permitting the telomerase to load to the ends of telomeres. It is not clear at present whether this regulatory mechanism is conserved among Tel1 orthologs in mammals and fission yeast.
5. Telomere elongation and C-strand filling. G-overhangs are elongated by the action of telomerase. Then, CST recruits the Polα complex to coordinate the synthesis of the complementary C-strand. The replicated telomere now returns to the protected state.

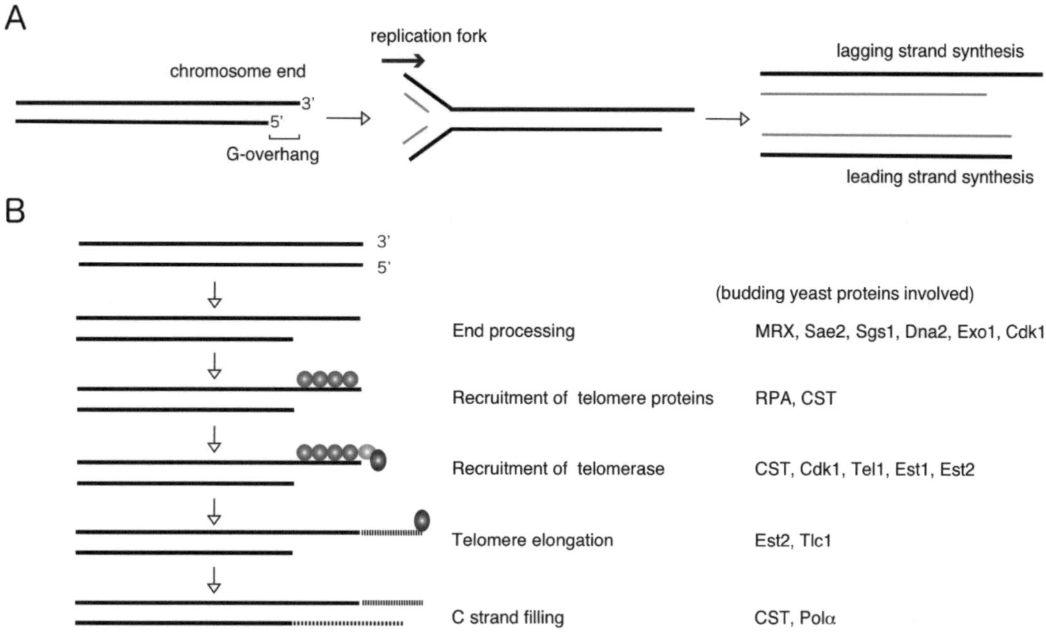

Fig. 2. Model for telomere replication in budding yeast. A: Fork movement towards the chromosome terminus. B: Telomerase-dependent telomere elongation.

8. Alternative mechanisms that bypasses telomerase deficiency

In budding yeast, telomerase-defective mutants gradually lose their proliferation capacity because of telomere shortening. However, a fraction of cells recovered viability without telomerase activity after prolonged periods of culturing. These "survivor" cells were found to acquire the potential to elongate chromosome ends through a recombination-mediated process (Lundblad & Blackburn, 1993). They are categorized as either type I or type II cells on the basis of their telomere composition and mode of maintenance (Teng & Zakian, 1999). Type I cells have a very short telomere repeat tract, but have amplified subtelomeric Y' sequences. By contrast, type II cells have long heterogeneous telomere repeats. Telomere maintenance in both cell types requires the homologous recombination gene *RAD52* (Le et al., 1999). The change in the survivor cells is likely to be epigenetic, and both types of telomerase-independent telomere maintenance are inherited as a non-Mendelian trait that is dominant over senescence (Makovets et al., 2008), although the exact mechanism remains unknown.

Similar mechanisms for escaping telomere dysfunction have also been observed in fission yeast. The genome of this organism consists of three chromosomes, and a population of cells can overcome the loss of telomerase by the recombination-mediated process (Nakamura et al., 1998). In addition, some survivor cells possess three circular chromosomes produced by end-to-end fusion between the arms of a chromosome. Cells harboring circular chromosomes can propagate normally by mitosis, but are unable to produce viable spores through meiosis (Naito et al., 1998; Nakamura et al., 1998). The requirement of chromosome linearity for normal chromosome segregation during meiosis has been discussed (Ishikawa & Naito, 1999).

Some cancer cell lines grow in spite of a lack of telomerase activity. Such cell lines show high heterogeneity in telomere length (Murnane et al., 1994) and are thought to elongate telomere sequences via a telomerase-independent, alternative lengthening of telomere (ALT) mechanism. Involvement of recombination in ALT was subsequently confirmed (Dunham et al., 2000), although its exact mechanism is still being debated.

9. Regulation of telomeres and telomerase during development and reprogramming

Telomerase activity is tightly regulated during vertebrate development, being high in male germ cells, low in mature oocytes and cleavage stage embryos, and high in blastocysts (Hiyama & Hiyama, 2007). In spite of the low telomerase activity during early cleavage development, telomeres in zygotes are remarkably long at the first cell division. Interestingly, telomere lengthening at this stage was observed in parthenote embryos derived from telomerase-null mice, indicating that it depends on factors of maternal origin and does not require telomerase (Liu et al., 2007). The recombination protein Rad50 is localized at telomeres during the early cleavage cycle, suggesting that telomere lengthening following fertilization is recombination-dependent. Recently, Zscan4, a protein that is expressed specifically in the two-cell stage embryo, was shown to be involved in this process (Zalzman et al., 2010). Activity of this alternative telomere maintenance mechanism decreases before the blastocyst stage, during which the telomerase-dependent mechanism is reestablished. Expression of telomerase is maintained in the stem cell compartment of several adult tissues, although telomerase levels in these tissues are not sufficient to prevent progressive telomere shortening with age in either humans or mice (Flores et al., 2008).

Embryonic stem (ES) cells and undifferentiated embryonal carcinoma (EC) cells display high levels of telomerase activity and *TERT* expression, both of which are rapidly downregulated during differentiation (Armstrong et al., 2005). Telomere length is elongated during the establishment of induced pluripotent stem (iPS) cells (Marion et al., 2009), which is associated with induction of the *TERT* gene. These observations suggest that acquisition of the capacity for indefinite self-renewal may be linked to the regulation of telomerase activity. Interestingly, in spite of their high telomerase activity, ES cells also express Zscan4. Knockdown of *Zscan4* in ES cells shortens telomeres, increases karyotype abnormalities, and consequently reduces cell proliferation (Zalzman et al., 2010). Thus, a unique mode of telomere maintenance may operate in ES cells.

10. Consequences of telomere shortening

During replicative senescence in human somatic cells, dysfunction caused by telomere shortening is sensed by DNA damage signals that induce cell cycle arrest via the p53 pathway (d'Adda di Fagagna et al., 2003). In cells in which p53 is mutated, dysfunctional telomeres promote genome instability and progression to cancer, indicating that replicative senescence contributes to the suppression of tumorigenesis (Chin et al., 1999). Moreover, increasing evidence implicates telomere dysfunction in age-related pathogenesis, such as progressive atrophy and functional decline in high-turnover tissues (Sahin and Depinho, 2010).

Although the hallmark of senescent cells is irreversible growth arrest, several responses besides those related to the cell cycle have been observed. Senescent cells develop an enlarged morphology, upregulate senescence-associated β-galactosidase (SA-βgal) activity, and show changes in metabolism, chromatin organization, and gene expression (Dimri et al., 1995; Funayama et al.,2006; Sahin et al., 2011). Moreover, senescent cells display a senescence-associated secretory phenotype (SASP), which is associated with increased secretion of cytokines and matrix metalloproteinases (Coppe et al., 2008). The mechanisms underlying the induction of these diverse phenotypes are largely unknown, although p38MAPK has been suggested to be involved (Freund et al., 2011).

Using telomerase-defective budding yeast cells as a model, mechanisms underlying the cellular responses to telomere shortening have been extensively studied. Genome-wide analysis of changes in gene expression showed that telomere-shortened cells have a unique transcriptional profile that shares features of DNA damage responses and environmental stress responses, and that is characterized by up-regulation of energy production genes (Nautiyal et al., 2002). Telomere shortening induces an increase in cell size, which is mediated by the DNA damage checkpoint kinase Mec1. Cell size expansion is associated with the enlargement of a vacuole that serves as a prominent lytic compartment in yeast. As a deficiency in vacuolar morphogenesis reduces the viability of telomere-shortened cells (Matsui & Matsuura, 2010), vacuolar function(s) may contribute to senescence-associated physiology.

11. The pathology of telomerase disorders

Several human disorders have been directly linked to reduced telomerase activity. Dyskeratosis congenita (DC) is an inherited disorder characterized by the degeneration of multiple tissues, including bone marrow. The mutations that cause DC have been implicated in telomere metabolism. X-chromosome-linked DC is caused by mutations in the *DKC1* gene, which encodes dyskerin, an RNA-binding protein that stabilizes TERC (Mitchell et al., 1999). Causative mutations for other DC subtypes of DC have been mapped to *TERT* and *TERC* itself. Cells from DC patients have shorter telomeres and display premature senescence (Westin et al., 2007). The pathology of DC demonstrates the critical importance of telomerase in humans, especially in the maintenance of stem cells (Kirwan & Dokal, 2009).

The Werner syndrome (WS) is a premature aging syndrome. Fibroblasts from WS patients show accelerated telomere attrition, while the gene responsible for WS, *WRN*, encodes a DNA helicase involved in DNA replication, especially at telomeres (Crabbe et al., 2004). Ataxia telangiectasia (AT) is another premature aging syndrome that is characterized by

marked telomere attrition. The gene responsible for AT, *ATM*, is the ortholog of the budding yeast gene *TEL1* and plays key roles in DNA damage signaling (Varizi, 1997).
The causal link between telomere shortening and the aging phenotype at the organism level was demonstrated in a series of genetic studies performed using mouse models. Experimental mice usually have extremely long telomeres, and *Wrn*- and *Atm*-knockout mice do not display a premature aging phenotype. However, if they are subjected to telomere-limiting conditions by crossing with telomerase-null mice, they exhibit an accelerated aging phenotype (Chang et al., 2004: Wong et al., 2003). This observation suggests that telomere shortening is rate-limiting for the pathogenesis of premature aging syndromes.

12. Extra-telomeric roles of telomerase

Mice with modifications in genes encoding telomerase components have demonstrated the role of telomere length in maintaining stem cells (Jaskelioff et al., 2011). In contrast, *Tert* overexpression has an anti-aging effect in mice. This effect is not seen in *Terc*-deficient mice (Tomas-Loba et al., 2008), indicating that telomerase activation is the main mechanism underlying it.
There is evidence that telomerase has extra-telomeric functions in stem cell maintenance, acting as a transcriptional modulator of the Wnt-β-catenin pathway (Park et al., 2009). It also exhibits RNA-dependent RNA polymerase activity as a complex with the RNA component of mitochondrial RNA processing ribonuclease (RMRP) (Maida et al., 2009). It is still not known whether these extra-telomeric functions are conserved in telomerase enzymes from other species.

13. Conclusion

Extensive studies using unicellular organisms have revealed that a wide variety of proteins are involved in telomere homeostasis, and it becomes evident that coordination between their actions contributes to the regulation of telomere replication. The emerging evidence now suggests that the regulatory mechanism is linked directly with development and pathogenesis of mammals. Further dissection of the regulatory network may shed light on novel strategies for the management of telomere-related physiologies such as aging and cancer.

14. Acknowledgments

We thank Textcheck for editing the manuscript. Work at Matsuura laboratory was supported by grants from MEXT.

15. References

Adams, A. K. & Holm, C. (1996) Specific DNA replication mutations affect telomere length in *Saccharomyces cerevisiae*. *Molecular and Cellular Biology*, Vol.16, pp. 4614-4620.

Adams Martin, A.; Dionne, I., Wellinger, R. J. & Holm, C. (2000) The function of DNA polymerase α at telomeric G tails is important for telomere homeostasis. *Molecular and Cellular Biology*, Vol.20, pp. 786-796.

Ancelin, K.; Brunori, M., Bauwens, S., Koering, C. E., Brun, C., Ricoul, M., Pommier, J. P., Sabatier, L. & Gilson, E. (2002) Targeting assay to study the *cis* functions of human telomeric proteins: evidence for inhibition of telomerase by TRF1 and for activation of telomere degradation by TRF2. *Molecular and Cellular Biology,* Vol.22, pp. 3474-3487.

Armstrong, L.; Saretzki, G., Peters, H., Wappler, I., Evans, J., Hole, N., von Zglinicki, T. & Lako, M. (2005) Overexpression of telomerase confers growth advantage, stress resistance, and enhanced differentiation of ESCs toward the hematopoietic lineage. *Stem Cells* Vol.23, pp. 516-529.

Bailey, S. M.; Cornforth, M. N., Kurimasa, A., Chen, D. J. and Goodwin, E. H. (2001) Strand-specific postreplicative processing of mammalian telomeres. *Science,* Vol.293, pp. 2462-2465.

Baumann, P. & Cech, T.R. (2001) Pot1, the putative telomere end-binding protein in fission yeast and humans. *Science*, Vol.292, pp. 1171-1175.

Blackburn, E. H. & Gall, J. G. (1978) A tandemly repeated sequence at the termini of the extrachromosomal ribosomal RNA genes in Tetrahymena. *Journal of Molecular Biology,* Vol.120, pp. 33-53.

Bodnar, A. G.; Ouellette, M., Frolkis, M., Holt, S. E., Chiu, C. P., Morin, G. B. Harley, C. B.; Shay, J. W., Lichtsteiner, S. & Wright, W. E. (1998) Extension of life-span by introduction of telomerase into normal human cells. *Science,* Vol. 279, pp. 349-352.

Bonetti, D.; Martina, M., Clerici, M., Lucchini, G. & Longhese, M. P. (2009) Multiple pathways regulate 3' overhang generation at *S. cerevisiae* telomeres. *Molecular Cell,* Vol.35, pp. 70-81.

Casteel, D. E.; Zhuang, S., Zeng, Y., Perrino, F. W., Boss, G. R., Goulian, M. & Pilz, R. B. (2009) A DNA polymerase-⟨·primase cofactor with homology to replication protein A-32 regulates DNA replication in mammalian cells. *Journal of Biological Chemistry,* Vol.284, pp. 5807-5818.

Chai, W.; Sfeir, A. J., Hoshiyama, H., Shay, J. W. & Wright, W. E. (2006) The involvement of the Mre11/Rad50/Nbs1 complex in the generation of G-overhangs at human telomeres. *EMBO Reports,* Vol.7, pp. 225-230.

Chang, S.; Multani, A. S., Cabrera, N. G., Naylor, M. L., Laud, P., Lombard, D., Pathak, S., Guarente, L. & DePinho, R. A. (2004) Essential role of limiting telomeres in the pathogenesis of Werner syndrome, *Nature Genetics,* Vol.36, pp. 877-882.

Chikashige, Y. & Hiraoka, Y. (2001) Telomere binding of the Rap1 protein is required for meiosis in fission yeast. *Current Biology*, Vol.11, pp. 1618-1623.

Chin, L.; Artandi, S. E., Shen, Q., Tam, A., Lee, S. L., Gottlieb, G. J., Greider, C. W. & DePinho, R. A. (1999) p53 deficiency rescues the adverse effects of telomere loss and cooperates with telomere dysfunction to accelerate carcinogenesis. Cell. Vol. 97, pp. 527-38.

Coppe, J. P.; Patil, C. K., Rodier, F., Sun, Y., Munoz, D. P., Goldstein, J., Nelson, P. S., Desprez, P. Y. & Campisi, J. (2008) Senescence-associated secretory phenotypes reveal cell-nonautonomous functions of oncogenic RAS and the p53 tumor suppressor. *PLoS Biology,* Vol.6, pp. 2853-2868.

Counter C. M.; Avilion, A. A. , LeFeuvre, C. E., Stewart, N.G., Greider, C.W., Harley, C. B. & Bacchetti, S. (1992) Telomere shortening associated with chromosome instability is arrested in immortal cells which express telomerase activity. *EMBO Journal,* Vol.11, pp. 1921-1929.

Crabbe, L.; Verdun, R. E., Haggblom, C. I. & Karlseder, J. (2004) Defective telomere lagging strand synthesis in cells lacking WRN helicase activity. *Science*, Vol.306, pp. 1951-1953.

de Lange, T.; Shiue, L., Myers, R. M., Cox, D. R., Naylor S. L., Killery, A. M. & Varmus, H. E. (1990) Structure and variability of human chromosome ends. *Molecular and Cellular Biology,* Vol.10, pp. 518-527.

d'Adda di Fagagna, F.; Reaper, P. M., Clay-Farrace, L., Fiegler, H., Carr, P., von Zglinicki, T., Saretzki, G., Carter, N. P. & Jackson, S. P. (2003) A DNA damage checkpoint response in telomere-initiated senescence. *Nature*, Vol.426, pp. 194-198.

Diede, S. J. & Gottschling, D. E. (1999) Telomerase-mediated telomere addition in vivo requires DNA primase and DNA polymerases α and δ. *Cell,* Vol.99, pp. 723-733.

Dimri, G. P.; Lee, X., Basile, G., Acosta, M., Scott, G., Roskelley, C., Medrano, E. E., Linskens, M., Rubelj, I., Pereira-Smith, O., Peacocke, M. & Campisi, J. (1995) A biomarker that identifies senescent human cells in culture and in aging skin *in vivo*. *Proceedings of the National Academy of Sciences of the United States of America,* Vol.92, pp.9363-9367.

Dunham, M. A.; Neumann, A. A., Fasching, C. L. & Reddel, R. R. (2000) Telomere maintenance by recombination in human cells. *Nature Genetics*, Vol.26, pp. 447-450.

Faure, V.; Coulon, S., Hardy, J. & Geli, V. (2010) Cdc13 and telomerase bind through different mechanisms at the lagging- and leading-strand telomeres. *Molecular Cell,* Vol.38, pp. 842-852.

Flores, I.; Canela, A., Vera, E., Tejera, A., Cotsarelis, G., Cotsarelis, G. & Blasco, M. A. (2008) The longest telomeres: a general signature of adult stem cell compartments. *Genes and Development*, Vol.22:, pp. 654-667.

Flynn, R.L.; Centore, R. C., O'Sullivan, R. J., Rai, R., Tse, A., Songyang, Z., Chang, S., Karlseder, J. & Zou, L. (2011) TERRA and hnRNPA1 orchestrate an RPA-to-POT1 switch on telomeric single-stranded DNA. *Nature,* Vol.471, pp. 532-536.

Frank, C. J.; Hyde, M. & Greider, C. W. (2006) Regulation of telomere elongation by the cyclin-dependent kinase CDK1. *Molecular Cell,* Vol.24, pp. 423-432.

Freund, A.; Patil, C. K. & Campisi, J. (2011) p38MAPK is a novel DNA damage response-independent regulator of the senescence-associated secretory phenotype. *EMBO Journal,* Vol.30, pp. 1536-1548

Funayama, R.; Saito, M., Tanobe, H. & Ishikawa, F. (2006) Loss of linker histone H1 in cellular senescence. *Journal of Cell Biology,* Vol. 175, pp. 869-880.

Gao, H.; Cervantes, R. B., Mandell, E. K., Otero, J. H. & Lundblad, V. (2007) RPA-like proteins mediate yeast telomere function. *Nature Structural and Molecular Biology,* Vol.14, pp. 208-214.

Goudsouzian, L. K.; Tuzon, C. T. & Zakian, V. A. (2006) *S. cerevisiae* Tel1p and Mre11p are required for normal levels of Est1p and Est2p telomere association. *Molecular Cell,* Vol.24, pp. 603-610.

Grandin, N.; Reed, S.I. & Charbonneau, M. (1997) Stn1, a new *Saccharomyces cerevisiae* protein, is implicated in telomere size regulation in association with Cdc13. *Genes and Development,* Vol.11, pp. 512-527.

Grandin, N.; Damon, C. & Charbonneau, M. (2001) Ten1 functions in telomere end protection and length regulation in association with Stn1 and Cdc13. *EMBO Journal,* Vol.20, pp. 1173-1183.

Greenwell, P.W.; Kronmal, S. L., Porter, S. E., Gassenhuber, J., Obermaier, B. & Petes, T. D. (1995) *TEL1,* a gene involved in controlling telomere length in S. cerevisiae, is homologous to the human ataxia telangiectasia gene. *Cell,* Vol.82, pp. 823-829.

Greider, C. W. & Blackburn, E. H. (1985) Identification of a specific telomere terminal transferase activity in *Tetrahymena* extracts. *Cell,* Vol.43, pp. 405-413.

Griffith, J. D.; Comeau, L., Rosenfield, S., Stansel, R. M., Bianchi, A., Moss, H. & de Lange, T. (1999) Mammalian telomeres end in a large duplex loop. *Cell,* Vol.97, pp. 503-514.

Grossi, S.; Puglisi, A., Dmitriev, P. V., Lopes, M. & Shore, D. (2004) Pol12, the B subunit of DNA polymerase α, functions in both telomere capping and length regulation. *Genes and Development,* Vol.18, pp. 992-1006.

Hardy, C. F.; Sussel, L. & Shore, D. (1992) A RAP1-interacting protein involved in transcriptional silencing and telomere length regulation. *Genes and Development,* Vol.6, pp. 801-814.

Hartwell, L. H.; Mortimer, R. K., Culotti, J. & Culotti, M. (1973) Genetic control of the cell division cycle in yeast: V. Genetic analysis of *cdc* mutants. *Genetics,* Vol.74, pp. 267-286.

Hirano, Y.; Fukunaga, K. & Sugimoto, K. (2009) Rif1 and Rif2 inhibit localization of Tel1 to DNA ends. *Molecular Cell,* Vol.33, pp. 312-322.

Hiyama, E. & Hiyama, K. (2007) Telomere and telomerase in stem cells. British Journal of Cancer. Vol.96, pp. 1020-1024.

Huertas, P.; Cortes-Ledesma, F., Sartori, A. A., Aguilera, A. & Jackson, S. P. (2008) CDK targets Sae2 to control DNA-end resection and homologous recombination. *Nature,* Vol.455, pp. 689-692.

Ishikawa, F. & Naito, T. (1999) Why do we have linear chromosomes? A matter of Adam and Eve. *Mutation Research,* Vol.434, pp. 99-107.

Ivessa, A. S., J. Q. Zhou, V. P. Schulz, E. K. Monson, and V. A. Zakian. (2002) *Saccharomyces* Rrm3p, a 5′ to 3′ DNA helicase that promotes replication fork progression through telomeric and subtelomeric DNA. *Genes and Development,* Vol.16, pp. 1383-1396.

Jaskelioff, M.; Muller, F. L., Paik, J. H., Thomas, E., Jiang, S., Adams, A. C., Sahin, E., Kost-Alimova, M., Protopopov, A., Cadiñanos, J., Horner, J. W., Maratos-Flier, E. & Depinho, R. A. (2011) Telomerase reactivation reverses tissue degeneration in aged telomerase-deficient mice. *Nature,* Vol.469, pp. 102-106.

Kanoh, J. & Ishikawa, F. (2001) spRap1 and spRif1, recruited to telomeres by Taz1, are essential for telomere function in fission yeast. *Current Biology,* Vol.11, pp. 1624-1630.

Kirwan, M. & Dokal, I. (2009) Dyskeratosis congenita, stem cells and telomeres. *Biochimica et Biophysica Acta,* Vol.1792, pp. 371-379.

Larrivee, M.; LeBel, C. & Wellinger, R. J. (2004) The generation of proper constitutive G-tails on yeast telomeres is dependent on the MRX complex. *Genes and Development,* Vol.18, pp. 1391-1396.

Le, S.; Moore, J. K., Haber, J. E. & Greider, C. W. (1999) *RAD50* and *RAD51* define two pathways that collaborate to maintain telomeres in the absence of telomerase. *Genetics*, Vol.152, pp. 143–152.

Lendvay, T. S.; Morris, D. K., Sah, J., Balasubramanian, B. & Lundblad, V. (1996) Senescence mutants of *Saccharomyces cerevisiae* with a defect in telomere replication identify three additional *EST* genes. *Genetics,* Vol.144, pp. 1399-1412.

Li, S.; Makovets, S., Matsuguchi, T., Blethrow, J. D., Shokat, K. M. & Blackburn, E. H. (2009) Cdk1-dependent phosphorylation of Cdc13 coordinates telomere elongation during cell-cycle progression. *Cell,* Vol.136, pp. 50-61.

Lingner, J. & Cech, T. R. (1996) Purification of telomerase from *Euplotes aediculatus*: requirement of a primer 3' overhang. *Proceedings of the National Academy of Sciences of the United States of America,* Vol. 93, pp. 10712-10717.

Liu, L.; Bailey, S. M., Okuka, M., Munoz, P., Li, C., Zhou, L., Wu, C., Czerwiec, E., Sandler, L., Seyfang, A., Blasco, M. A. & Keefe, D. L. (2007) Telomere lengthening early in development. *Nature Cell Biology,* Vol.9, pp. 1436-1441.

Lundblad, V. & Blackburn, E. H. (1993) An alternative pathway for yeast telomere maintenance rescues *est1*- senescence. *Cell,* Vol.73, pp. 347-360.

Lundblad, V. & Szostak, J. W. (1989) A mutant with a defect in telomere elongation leads to senescence in yeast. *Cell,* Vol.57, pp. 633-643.

Maida, Y.; Yasukawa, M., Furuuchi, M., Lassmann, T., Possemato, R., Okamoto, N., Kasim, V., Hayashizaki, Y., Hahn, W. C. & Masutomi, K. (2009) An RNA-dependent RNA polymerase formed by TERT and the RMRP RNA. *Nature,* Vol.461, pp. 230-235.

Makovets, S.; Williams, T. L. & Blackburn, E. H. (2008) The telotype defines the telomere state in *Saccharomyces cerevisiae* and is inherited as a dominant non-Mendelian characteristic in cells lacking telomerase. *Genetics,* Vol.178, pp. 245-257.

Marcand, S.; Brevet, V. & Gilson, E. (1999) Progressive cis-inhibition of telomerase upon telomere elongation. *EMBO Journal*, Vol.18, pp. 3509-3519.

Marcand, S.; Brevet, V., Mann, C. & Gilson, E. (2000) Cell cycle restriction of telomere elongation. *Current Biology,* Vol.10, pp. 487-490.

Marcand, S.; Gilson, E. & Shore, D. (1997) A protein-counting mechanism for telomere length regulation in yeast. *Science,* Vol.275, pp. 986-990.

Marion, R. M.; Strati, K., Li, H., Tejera, A., Schoeftner, S., Ortega, S., Serrano, M. & Blasco, M. A. (2009) Telomeres acquire embryonic stem cell characteristics in induced pluripotent stem cells. *Cell Stem Cell,* Vol.4, pp. 141-154.

Matsui, A. & Matsuura, A. (2010) Cell size regulation during telomere-directed senescence in *Saccharomyces cerevisiae. Bioscience, Biotechnology, and Biochemistry,* Vol.74, pp. 195-198.

McElligott, R & Wellinger, R. J. (1997) The terminal DNA structure of mammalian chromosomes. *EMBO Journal,* Vol.16, pp. 3705-3714.

Mclintock, B. (1941) The stability of broken ends of chromosomes in *Zea mays*. *Genetics,* Vol.26, pp. 234-282.

Miller, K. M.; Rog, O. & Cooper, J. P. (2006) Semi-conservative DNA replication through telomeres requires Taz1. *Nature*, Vol.440, pp. 824-828.

Mitchell, J. R.; Wood, E. & Collins, K. (1999) A telomerase component is defective in the human disease dyskeratosis congenita. *Nature*, Vol.402, pp. 551-515.

Mitton-Fry, R. M.; Anderson, E. M., Hughes, T. R., Lundblad, V. & Wuttke, D. S. (2002) Conserved structure for single-stranded telomeric DNA recognition. *Science*, Vol.296, pp. 145-147.

Miyake, Y.; Nakamura, M., Nabetani, A., Shimamura, S., Tamura, M., Yonehara, S., Saito, M. & Ishikawa, F. (2009) RPA-like mammalian Ctc1-Stn1-Ten1 complex binds to single-stranded DNA and protects telomeres independently of the Pot1 pathway. *Molecular Cell*, Vol.36, pp. 193-206.

Miyoshi, T.; Kanoh, J., Saito, M. & Ishikawa, F. (2008) Fission yeast Pot1-Tpp1 protects telomeres and regulates telomere length. *Science*, Vol.320, pp.1341-1344.

Moser, B. A.; Subramanian, L., Chang, Y. T., Noguchi, C., Noguchi, E., & Nakamura, T. M. (2009) Differential arrival of leading and lagging strand DNA polymerases at fission yeast telomeres. *EMBO Journal*, Vol.28, pp. 810-820.

Muller, H. J. (1938) The remaking of chromosomes. *Collecting Net*, Vol.8, pp. 182-198.

Murnane, J. P.; Sabatier, L., Marder, B. A. & Morgan, W. F. (1994) Telomere dynamics in an immortal human cell line. *EMBO Journal*, Vol.13, pp. 4953-4962.

Naito, T.; Matsuura, A. & Ishikawa, F. (1998) Circular chromosome formation in a fission yeast mutant defective in two *ATM* homologues. *Nature Genetics*, Vol.20, pp. 203-206.

Nakamura, M.; Nabetani, A., Mizuno, T., Hanaoka, F. & Ishikawa, F. (2005) Alterations of DNA and chromatin structures at telomeres and genetic instability in mouse cells defective in DNA polymerase α. *Molecular and Cellular Biology*, Vol.25, pp. 11073-11088.

Nakamura, T. M.; Cooper, J. P. & Cech, T. R. (1998) Two modes of survival of fission yeast without telomerase. *Science*, Vol.282, pp. 493-496.

Nautiyal, S.; DeRisi, J. L. & Blackburn, E. H. (2002) The genome-wide expression response to telomerase deletion in *Saccharomyces cerevisiae*. *Proceedings of the National Academy of Sciences of the United States of America*, Vol.99, pp. 9316-9321.

Negrini, S.; Ribaud, V., Bianchi, A. & Shore, D. (2007) DNA breaks are masked by multiple Rap1 binding in yeast: implications for telomere capping and telomerase regulation. *Genes and Development*, Vol. 21, pp. 292-302.

Nugent, C. I.; Bosco, G., Ross, L. O., Evans, S. K., Salinger, A. P., Moore, J. K., Haber, J. E. & Lundblad, V. (1998) Telomere maintenance is dependent on activities required for end repair of double-strand breaks. *Current Biology*, Vol.8, pp. 657-660.

Olovnikov, A. M. (1973). A theory of marginotomy. The incomplete copying of template margin in enzymic synthesis of polynucleotides and biological significance of the phenomenon. *Journal of Theoretical Biology*, Vol.41, pp. 181-190.

Ono, Y.; Tomita, K., Matsuura, A., Nakagawa, T., Masukata, H., Uritani, M., Ushimaru, T. & Ueno, M. (2003) A novel allele of fission yeast *rad11* that causes defects in DNA repair and telomere length regulation. *Nucleic Acids Research*, Vol.31, pp. 7141-7149.

Park, J. I.; Venteicher, A. S., Hong, J. Y., Choi, J., Jun, S., Shkreli, M., Chang, W., Meng, Z., Cheung, P., Ji, H., McLaughlin, M., Veenstra, T. D., Nusse, R., McCrea, P. D. & Artandi, S. E. (2009) Telomerase modulates Wnt signalling by association with target gene chromatin. *Nature,* Vol.460, pp. 66-72.

Qi, H. & Zakian, V. A. (2000) The *Saccharomyces* telomere-binding protein Cdc13p interacts with both the catalytic subunit of DNA polymerase α and the telomerase-associated Est1 protein. *Genes and Development,* Vol.14, pp. 1777-1788.

Raghuraman, M. K.; Winzeler, E. A., Collingwood, D., Hunt, S., Wodicka, L., Conway, A., Lockhart, D. J., Davis, R. W., Brewer, B. J. & Fangman, W. L.(2001) Replication dynamics of the yeast genome. *Science,* Vol.294, pp. 115-121.

Ritchie, K. B. & Petes, T. D. (2000) The Mre11p/Rad50p/Xrs2p complex and the Tel1p function in a single pathway for telomere maintenance in yeast. *Genetics,* Vol.155, pp. 475-479.

Sahin, E.; Colla, S., Liesa, M., Moslehi, J., Müller, F. L., Guo, M., Cooper, M., Kotton, D., Fabian, A. J., Walkey, C., Maser, R. S., Tonon, G., Foerster, F., Xiong, R., Wang, Y. A., Shukla, S. A., Jaskelioff, M., Martin, E. S., Heffernan, T. P., Protopopov, A., Ivanova, E., Mahoney, J. E., Kost-Alimova, M., Perry, S. R., Bronson, R., Liao, R., Mulligan, R., Shirihai, O. S., Chin, L. & DePinho, R. A. (2011) Telomere dysfunction induces metabolic and mitochondrial compromise. *Nature,* Vol.470, pp. 359-365.

Schramke, V.; Luciano, P., Brevet, V., Guillot, S., Corda, Y., Longhese, M. P., Gilson, E. & Géli, V. (2003) RPA regulates telomerase action by providing Est1p access to chromosome ends. *Nature Genetics,* Vol.36, pp. 46-54.

Shakirov, E. V.; Surovtseva, Y. V., Osbun, N. & Shippen, D. E. (2005) The *Arabidopsis* Pot1 and Pot2 proteins function in telomere length homeostasis and chromosome end protection. *Molecular and Cellular Biology,* Vol.25, pp. 7725-7733.

Sfeir, A.; Kosiyatrakul, S. T., Hockemeyer, D., MacRae, S. L., Karlseder, J., Schildkraut, C. L. & de Lange, T. (2009) Mammalian telomeres resemble fragile sites and require TRF1 for efficient replication. *Cell,* Vol.138, pp. 90-103.

Smith, J. S.; Chen, Q., Yatsunyk, L. A., Nicoludis, J. M., Garcia, M. S., Kranaster, R., Balasubramanian, S., Monchaud, D., Teulade-Fichou, M. P., Abramowitz, L., Schultz, D. C. & Johnson, F. B. (2011) Rudimentary G-quadruplex-based telomere capping in *Saccharomyces cerevisiae. Nature Structural & Molecular Biology,* Vol.18, pp. 478-485.

Smogorzewska, A. & de Lange, T. (2004) Regulation of telomerase by telomeric proteins. *Annual Review of Biochemistry,* Vol.73, pp. 177-208.

Surovtseva, Y. V.; Churikov, D., Boltz, K. A., Song, X., Lamb, J. C., Warrington, R., Leehy, K., Heacock, M., Price, C. M. & Shippen, D. E. (2009) Conserved telomere maintenance component 1 interacts with STN1 and maintains chromosome ends in higher eukaryotes. *Molecular Cell,* Vol.36, pp. 207-218.

Szostak, J. W. & Blackburn, E. H. (1982) Cloning yeast telomeres on linear plasmid vectors. *Cell,* Vol.29, pp. 245-255.

Taggart, A. K.; Teng, S. C, & Zakian, V. A. (2002) Est1p as a cell cycle-regulated activator of telomere-bound telomerase. *Science,* Vol.297, 1023-1026.

Takata, H.; Tanaka, Y. & Matsuura, A. (2005) Late S phase-specific recruitment of Mre11 complex triggers hierarchical assembly of telomere replication proteins in Saccharomyces cerevisiae. *Molecular Cell*, Vol.18, pp. 573-583.

Teixeira, M. T.; Arneric, M., Sperisen, P. & Lingner, J. (2004) Telomere length homeostasis is achieved via a switch between telomerase- extendible and -nonextendible states. *Cell*, Vol.117, pp. 323-335.

Teng, S. C. & Zakian, V. A. (1999) Telomere-telomere recombination is an efficient bypass pathway for telomere maintenance in *Saccharomyces cerevisiae. Molecular and Cellular Biology*, Vol.19, pp. 8083-8093.

Tomas-Loba, A.; Flores, I., Fernandez-Marcos, P. J., Cayuela, M. L., Maraver, A., Borras, C., Matheu, A., Klatt, P., Flores, J. M., Vina, J., Serrano, M. & Blasco, M. A. (2008) Telomerase reverse transcriptase delays aging in cancer-resistant mice. *Cell*, Vol.135, 609-622.

Tseng, S. F.; Lin, J. J. & Teng, S. C. (2006) The telomerase-recruitment domain of the telomere binding protein Cdc13 is regulated by Mec1p/Tel1p-dependent phosphorylation. *Nucleic Acids Research*, Vol.34, pp. 6327-6336.

Vaziri, H. (1997) Critical telomere shortening regulated by the ataxia-telangiectasia gene acts as a DNA damage signal leading to activation of p53 protein and limited life-span of human diploid fibroblasts. *Biochemistry*, Vol.62, pp. 1306-1310.

Vodenicharov, M.D. & Wellinger, R. J. (2006) DNA degradation at unprotected telomeres in yeast is regulated by the CDK1 (Cdc28/Clb) cell-cycle kinase. *Molecular Cell*, Vol.24, pp. 127-137.

Wang, F.; Podell, E. R., Zaug, A. J., Yang, Y., Baciu, P., Cech, T. R. & Lei, M. (2007) The POT1-TPP1 telomere complex is a telomerase processivity factor. *Nature*, Vol.445, pp. 506-510.

Watson, J. D. (1972) Origin of concatemeric T7 DNA. *Nature*, Vol.239, pp. 197-201.

Williamsom, J. R.; Raghuraman, M. K. & Cech, T. R. (1989) Monovalent cation-induced structure of telomeric DNA: The G-quartet model. *Cell*, Vol.59, pp. 871-880.

Wellinger, R. J.; Ethier, K., Labrecque, P. & Zakian, V. A. (1996) Evidence for a new step in telomere maintenance. *Cell*, Vol.85, pp. 423-433.

Westin, E. R.; Chavez, E., Lee, K. M., Gourronc, F. A., Riley, S., Lansdorp, P. M., Goldman, F. D. & Klingelhutz, A. J. (2007) Telomere restoration and extension of proliferative lifespan in dyskeratosis congenita fibroblasts. *Aging Cell*, Vol.6, pp. 383-394.

Wong, K. K.; Maser, R. S., Bachoo, R. M., Menon, J., Carrasco, D. R., Gu, Y., Alt, F. W., DePinho, R. A. (2003) Telomere dysfunction and *Atm* deficiency compromises organ homeostasis and accelerates ageing. *Nature*, Vol.421, pp. 643-648.

Wotton, D. & Shore, D. (1997) A novel Rap1p-interacting factor, Rif2p, cooperates with Rif1p to regulate telomere length in *Saccharomyces cerevisiae. Genes and Development*, Vol.11, pp. 748-760.

Wright, W. E.; Tesmer, V. M., Huffman, K. E., Levene, S. D. & Shay, J. W. (1997) Normal human chromosomes have long G-rich telomeric overhangs at one end. *Genes and Development*, Vol.11, pp. 2801-2809.

Wright, W. E.; Tesmer, V. M., Liao, M. L. & Shay, J. W. (1999) Normal human telomeres are not late replicating. *Experimental Cell Research*, Vol.251, pp. 492-499.Yu, G. L.;

Bradley, J. D., Attardi, L. D. & Blackburn, E. H. (1990) In vivo alteration of telomere sequences and senescence caused by mutated *Tetrahymena* telomerase RNAs. *Nature,* Vol.344, pp. 126-132.

Zalzman, M.; Falco, G., Sharova, L. V., Nishiyama, A., Thomas, M., Lee, S. L., Stagg, C. A., Hoang, H. G., Yang, H. T., Indig, F. E., Wersto, R. P. & Ko, M. S. (2010) Zscan4 regulates telomere elongation and genomic stability in ES cells. *Nature,* Vol.464, pp. 858-863.

15

Telomere Maintenance in Organisms without Telomerase

James M. Mason[1], Hemakumar M. Reddy[1] and Radmila Capkova Frydrychova[2]
[1]*National Institute of Environmental Health Sciences*
[2]*Institute of Entomology*
[1]*United States*
[2]*Czech Republic*

1. Introduction

Telomeres serve two vital functions to eukaryotes. They act as a protective chromosome cap to distinguish natural chromosome ends from double stranded DNA breaks and to avoid inappropriate fusions of telomeric sequences, and they maintain chromosome length by adding DNA to the ends of chromosomes. Telomeres thus balance the loss of terminal DNA due to the inability of the replication machinery to completely replicate linear DNA molecules (Olovnikov, 1973; Watson, 1972). In many cases the newly replicated chromosome ends are resected to allow for the formation of a t-loop that helps to hide the tip (Griffith et al., 1999; Wellinger et al., 1996). Most eukaryotes elongate chromosome ends with a special reverse transcriptase, telomerase, that carries a specific RNA template with telomeric sequence (Greider, 1996). The telomerase enzyme repeatedly adds copies of the short telomeric DNA sequence to the chromosome end. While there is strict conservation of telomeric sequence repeat in most species, the repeat unit has changed over evolutionary time. Holotrichous ciliates, e. g. *Tetrahymena,* use the sequence $(TTGGGG)_n$ (Blackburn & Gall, 1978), while hypotrichous ciliates, e. g. *Oxytricha,* use $(TTTTGGGG)_n$ (Klobutcher et al., 1981; Oka et al., 1980). The primary telomeric sequence in plants is $(TTTAGGG)_n$ (Richards & Ausubel, 1988; Zellinger & Riha, 2007), although the alga *Chlamydomonas* uses $(TTTTAGGG)_n$. In the yeasts the telomeric sequence has the same general motif, but is not as tightly controlled. *Saccharomyces* for example uses $(TG_{1\text{-}3})_n$ (Shampay et al., 1984; Wang & Zakian, 1990), while *Schizosaccharomyces* has $(TTACAG_{1\text{-}8})_n$ (Matsumoto et al., 1987). The sequence found at the telomeres of most metazoans is $(TTAGGG)_n$ (Meyne et al., 1989; Traut et al., 2007), although arthropods use $(TTAGG)_n$ (Okazaki et al., 1993).

Lack of the predominant telomeric sequence in a species does not, however, signify that telomerase-generated terminal sequences are missing. For example, the metazoan-type telomeric sequence is found in place of the plant sequence in *Aloe* species (Weiss & Scherthan, 2002). In order to establish that a telomerase- independent, chromosome maintenance system exists it is also necessary to show a lack of a telomerase gene and telomerase activity, and to identify the nature of the DNA sequence at the chromosome termini. Establishing the negative is always difficult, and confirming that a specific sequence is at, not merely near, the chromosome tip is not trivial. Conversely, the presence of a canonical telomeric sequence does not necessarily indicate telomerase as a telomere maintenance mechanism. Some species of Calcarea (sponges), Cnidaria (sea anemones and jellyfish) and Placozoa, which keep the metazoan telomeric sequence, display little or no telomerase activity (Traut et al., 2007).

Although telomerase may have been the mechanism of telomere maintenance of the last common eukaryotic ancestor, it is not the only mechanism used to maintain chromosome length. Telomerase has been lost a few times in the evolution of plants and animals. During insect evolution, for example, telomerase has been lost at least six times. Here, we discuss telomere maintenance mechanisms that replaced telomerase in telomere length maintenance. In most cases the nature of the chromosome ends in organisms lacking telomerase is not known. In some species the telomerase-generated short telomeric repeat arrays have been replaced by tandem arrays of DNA sequences that look much like heterochromatin and can be elongated by copying information from one chromosome end to another, i. e. gene conversion. A completely different mechanism has been found in *Drosophila*, where tandem arrays of non-long terminal repeat (LTR) retrotransposons are found. Newly synthesized copies of these retrotransposons target chromosome ends and can even transpose to unique sequence chromosome ends. Similar telomere-specific retrotransposons have been found in *Drosophila* species that diverged as long as 40 million years ago, suggesting that this mechanism is reasonably stable. Three families of retrotransposons are found at *Drosophila* telomeres; these elements may cooperate with each other during transposition to maintain all three in the *Drosophila* genome. Mutations are known that either increase or decrease the rate of addition to the chromosome ends, leading to longer or shorter terminal retrotransposon array lengths. While these mutations have not been well characterized, they suggest that telomere maintenance by retrotransposition is genetically regulated by the host.

2. Plants without telomerase

The plant telomeric sequence $(TTTAGGG)_n$ appears to be highly conserved in all phyla of the plant kingdom (Fuchs et al., 1995; Fuchs & Schubert, 1996; Richards & Ausubel, 1988). Nevertheless, in the order Asparagales the plant telomeric motif has been replaced with $(TTAGGG)_n$ but is still maintained by telomerase (Fajkus et al., 2005). In addition, three genera within the family Solanaceae appear to have lost both the canonical telomeric DNA motif as well as telomerase, which is required to maintain this motif.

2.1 The nightshade family

In the family Solanaceae the canonical plant telomeric repeat is replaced by a less conventional telomeric sequence that may be associated with a different compensation pathway. Detailed analysis of Solanaceae species revealed that although plant telomeric sequence is present in tobacco, tomato and other representatives of this family, the telomeric motif and telomerase activity are missing in the three closely related genera of *Cestrum*, *Vestia* and *Sessea*. The actual telomeric sequence and compensation mechanism in this group of plants, however, remain unknown (Fajkus et al., 1995; Peska et al., 2008; Sykorova et al., 2003; Watson & Riha, 2010).

2.2 The onion family

Chromosome termini of the onion, *Allium cepa*, and other Alliaceae species represent another known case of unusual telomeres lacking telomerase in plants. Telomeres of *A. cepa* consist of two tandemly organized repeats - a 375-bp satellite sequence and rDNA repeats (Barnes et al., 1985; Pich et al., 1996; Pich & Schubert, 1998). Besides this, the telomeres in *A. cepa* are enriched with *En/Spm* transposable element-like sequence and *Ty1-copia*-like retrotransposons. The *Ty1-copia* retroelements have been reported not only at telomeres of *A. cepa* but dispersed throughout its genome (Pearce et al., 1996; Pich & Schubert, 1998). Based on these findings it has been proposed that the telomeres of Alliaceae species are maintained through transposition of the mobile elements or through homologous recombination between the satellite sequences (Pich et al., 1996; Pich & Schubert, 1998).

3. Animals without telomerase

In the case of animals, the lack of a telomerase system has been reported in a few insect species. The $(TTAGG)_n$ sequence has been detected in most tested insect orders and is considered as the ancestral telomeric motif not only for insects but also for all arthropods (Vitkova et al., 2005). In some groups of arthropods, such as damselflies or spiders this telomeric motif was lost (Frydrychova et al., 2004; Vitkova et al., 2005), however in most cases it remains unknown if the sequence was replaced by another similar motif or a different type of sequence associated with a telomerase-independent elongation mechanism (Figure 1).

3.1 The silkworm

A highly interesting case of telomeres was revealed in another model organism, the silkworm, *Bombyx mori* (Lepidoptera). The telomeres of the silkworm consist of the insect telomeric repeats but harbor many types of non-LTR retrotransposons, designated *TRAS* and *SART* families (Fujiwara et al., 2005; Kubo et al., 2001; Okazaki et al., 1995). *TRAS* and *SART* are abundantly transcribed and actively transpose into TTAGG telomeric repeats in a highly sequence-specific manner. The silkworm genome contains a telomerase gene, but the telomerase itself displays little or no enzymatic activity. It is believed that compensation of telomeric loss in *B. mori* occurs almost exclusively by transposition of *TRAS* and *SART* elements to the chromosome ends (Fujiwara et al., 2005; Tatsuke et al., 2009). Nevertheless, in contrast to *Drosophila*, in which the telomerase system was completely lost and replaced by telomeric retrotransposition (see below), *B. mori* may be in transition from one telomere elongation pathway to another.

3.2 Lower diptera

Telomerase has not been found in any dipteran species (Figure 1). As fossils for this order date to the middle Triassic period, it is possible that telomerase may have been lost as much as 225 million years ago. Nevertheless, Diptera as a group are very successful, accounting for some 10% of known animal species. Thus, loss of telomerase does not seem to have been a major impediment to survival. Replacement of short telomerase-generated repeats with long satellite sequences is reported in lower dipteran species. Chromosome tips of non-biting midges (genus *Chironomus*) consist of large, 50-200 kb, blocks of complex, tandemly repeated sequences that are classified into subfamilies based on sequence similarities. Different telomeres display different sets of subfamilies, and the distribution of subfamilies differs between different individuals in a stock. The variation of the satellite sequences supports the proposal that telomeres in *Chironomus* are elongated by a homologous

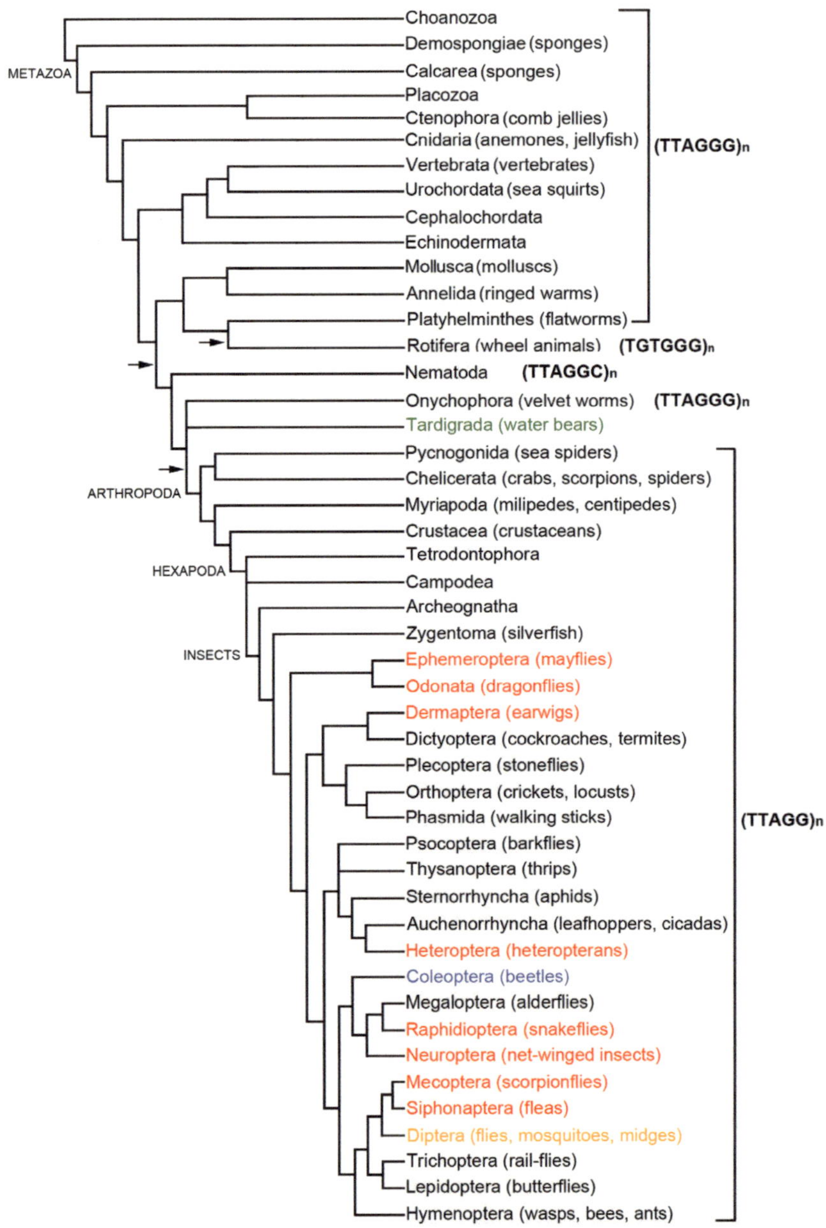

Fig. 1. Distribution of telomere repeat motifs in Metazoa. $(TTAGGG)_n$ is the ancestral telomeric sequence of Metazoa and its sister group, Choanozoa. The ancestral motif was replaced with $(TTAGG)_n$ and $(TTAGGC)_n$ in Arthropoda and Nematoda, respectively. Tardigrada (green) do not display either of these motifs. Insect orders in red do not exhibit the arthropod sequence. Coleoptera (blue) is heterogeneous for the arthropod motif. With a few exceptions among Diptera, Tardigrada and the insect orders in color have unknown telomeric sequences. Arrows mark the replacement of the metazoan motif with other motifs, as shown. The cladogram is based on Frydrychova et al., 2004; Vitkova et al., 2005; Traut et al., 2007.

recombination mechanism involving these long blocks of complex repeat units (Biessmann & Mason, 1997; Cohn & Edstrom, 1992; Cohn & Edström, 1992; Nielsen & Edstrom, 1993). A situation has been observed in *Anopheles gambiae* with a plasmid insertion into the complex satellite telomeric sequences at the tip of chromosome 2L. The plasmid sequence was used as a marker to follow the specific telomere, which was found to engage in frequent recombination events to extend the array length (Biessmann et al., 1998; Roth et al., 1997). Recently, a similar case was reported in *Rhynchosciara americana* (Madalena et al., 2010). Tandem arrays of short repeats, 16 and 22 bp in length, were found to extend to chromosome ends. Although telomere elongation could not be assayed in this case, it seems likely that the mechanism is similar to that seen in other dipterans. In many respects, these complex arrays resemble subtelomeric sequences (Pryde et al., 1997).

3.3 *Drosophila*

Most of our information on the structure and maintenance of telomeres in *Drosophila* is based on *D. melanogaster*, although some recent studies have been performed on other species, especially *D. virilis*. As in other dipterans, *Drosophila* telomeres do not posses a canonical telomeric sequence and are not maintained by a telomerase-dependent system. Instead, chromosome ends in *Drosophila* carry an array of retrotransposons. This unusual telomere structure is common among all drosophilids that have been studied (Casacuberta & Pardue, 2002, 2005), although species within this genus may have diverged as much as 40 million years ago (Russo et al., 1995).

3.3.1 *Drosophila melanogaster*

Three distinct telomeric regions have been identified in *Drosophila* (Andreyeva et al., 2005; Biessmann et al., 2005). At the extreme terminus is a proteinaceous chromosome cap that covers approximately 4 kb of terminal DNA sequence (Melnikova & Georgiev, 2005) and identifies the end as distinct from a chromosome break. The telomere-specific components of the cap in *Drosophila* are collectively termed 'terminin' by analogy to the shelterin protein complex at mammalian telomeres (Raffa et al., 2009). The terminin proteins differ from the shelterin proteins, in part because the TRF1 and TRF2 components of shelterin bind specifically to the canonical telomeric repeat, while the formation of the telomere cap in *Drosophila* is sequence independent, and in part because many of the terminin proteins are among the fastest evolving proteins in *Drosophila* (Gao et al., 2010; Raffa et al., 2010; Schmid & Tautz, 1997). There is no direct evidence that the cap in *Drosophila* plays a role in maintaining chromosome length. Most chromosome ends in *Drosophila* carry a tandem array of telomere-specific non-LTR retrotransposons (Mason & Biessmann, 1995; Pardue & DeBaryshe, 2003), although the length of this array can vary considerably. Located between the terminal retrotransposons and the unique sequence DNA of euchromatin is another repeat array. This array is often referred to as telomere associated sequences (TAS) or the subtelomere region (Karpen & Spradling, 1992; Walter et al., 1995). As in other eukaryotes TAS sequences in *Drosophila* include irregular arrays of relatively long repeat units that can vary from one chromosome end to another within the same organism (Pryde et al., 1997).

3.3.1.1 Telomeric retrotransposons

Studies on *D. melanogaster* revealed three telomere-specific retrotransposable elements, *HeT-A*, *TART* and *TAHRE* (collectively abbreviated HTT) present in multiple copies on each chromosome end. These retrotransposons are in the same family of elements as mammalian LINEs. Although the *D. melanogaster* genome has some 60 families of known retrotransposable elements, only these three are found at chromosome ends. Further, these three elements are present only in the telomere arrays. HTT elements are not found in euchromatic regions, although tandem arrays of short segments of the 3' noncoding region of *HeT-A* have been found in centric heterochromatin, especially in the *Y* chromosome (Abad et al., 2004a; Agudo et al., 1999; Berloco et al., 2005).

As a group the HTT elements have characteristics that distinguish them from other retrotransposons (Figure 2A). *HeT-A* is about 6 kb in length, has only a single open reading frame (ORF), encoding a Gag-like nucleic acid binding protein, but lacks an ORF for a

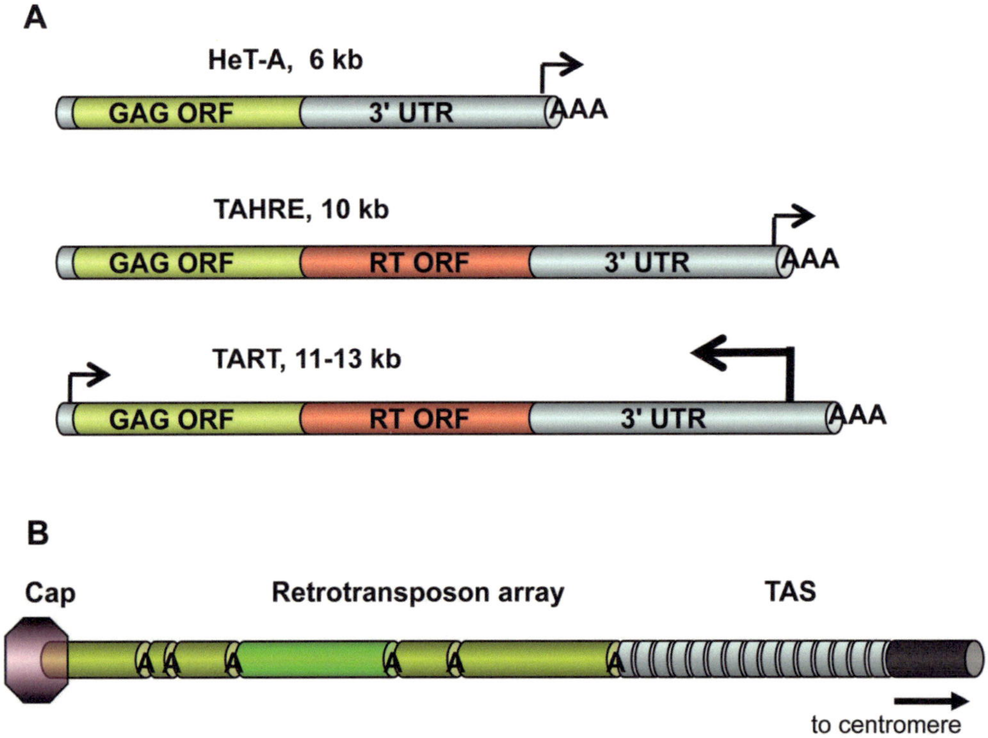

Fig. 2. Structure of Drosophila telomeres. (A) There are three families of telomeric non-LTR retrotransposons. The GAG open reading frame encodes a nucleic acid binding protein that helps to target chromosome ends. The RT open reading frame encodes a reverse transcriptase needed to copy the RNA intermediate onto the chromosome end. *HeT-A* does not carry a reverse transcriptase gene. All three elements carry relatively short 5' UTRs and very long 3' UTRs. Promoters are indicated by bent arrows. The 3' oligo(A) tail used to attach to chromosome ends is indicated by AAA. *TART* has a strong antisense promoter. (B) The Drosophila terminal array is composed of a tandem mixed array of variably 5' truncated transposons. At the distal end the chromosome carries a protein complex that binds to the end independently of DNA sequence and stabilizes the terminus. The "A" at each junction indicates the 3' oligo(A) tail. Proximal to the retrotransposons is a complex subterminal, telomere associated sequence (TAS) followed by unique sequence chromosomal DNA. Adapted from Capkova Frydrychova et al., 2008).

reverse transcriptase. *HeT-A* also has a 2.4 kb 3' untranslated region (UTR), which includes two to five imprecise 80 bp tandem repeats that may help establish chromatin structure. This region has a strong G-rich strand bias, which resembles the strand bias found in canonical telomeric motifs (Abad & Villasante, 1999; Biessmann et al., 1992b; Danilevskaya et al., 1998a), suggesting selection for their presence. Despite the fact that the sequence of the 3' UTR of *D. yakuba*, a sister species of *D. melanogaster*, has diverged by about 50%, these repeat features have been conserved (Danilevskaya et al., 1998b). The *TART* element is about 10 kb in length with two ORFs, which encode a Gag protein and a Pol protein with a reverse transcriptase domain. *TART* also carries a pair of perfect non-terminal repeats that may be important for its replication (Sheen & Levis, 1994; George et al., 2010). *TAHRE* is about 11-13 kb in length and has extensive sequence similarity to *HeT-A* along its entire length, except that it carries a second ORF for a reverse transcriptase (Abad et al., 2004b; Shpiz et al., 2007). As they all carry unusually long 3' UTRs of about 2-3 kb, the HTT retrotransposons are exceptions to the pattern that transposable elements usually have very little sequence that does not code for polypeptides involved in their own transposition (Abad et al., 2004b; Biessmann et al., 1992b; Sheen & Levis, 1994). It seems likely that this non-coding DNA is related to their role at the telomere (Villasante et al., 2007).

3.3.1.2 The terminal retrotransposon array

The three retrotransposons present in *Drosophila* telomeres are arranged in head-to-tail arrays of mixed complete and 5'-truncated elements with their 3' oligo-A tails oriented toward the centromere (Figure 2B). *HeT-A* is the most abundant of the three families, accounting for 80-90% of the telomeric array. *TART* elements occupy about 10%, while *TAHRE* elements occupy only 1-2% of the telomeric array. The 5' ends of many of these elements are truncated to varying extents, as might be expected from terminal erosion due to the end replication problem or incomplete reverse transcription (Mason & Biessmann, 1995). In one stock the HTT array length varied from about 20 to 150 kb for individual chromosome ends (Abad et al., 2004a). The length and composition of the telomeric retrotransposon arrays can also vary significantly between chromosomes and among fly stocks (Walter et al., 1995). In some mutants the terminal array may be several fold longer than found in standard laboratory strains (Melnikova & Georgiev, 2002; Savitsky et al., 2002; Siriaco et al., 2002). Conversely, not all chromosome ends in *Drosophila* have terminal retrotransposon arrays. Broken chromosomes with ends far from the original telomere have been found in a number of different circumstances (Capkova Frydrychova et al., 2008). It is important to note that these broken chromosome ends lack both the retrotransposon array and TAS but do not induce cell cycle arrest and are not subject to DNA repair or telomere fusions. These broken chromosome ends can be maintained *in vivo* for hundreds of generations without gaining new HTT sequences (Biessmann et al., 1990a; Cenci et al., 2003; Fanti et al., 1998). Thus, these broken chromosome ends have been 'healed' in the sense that McClintock (1941) described newly stabilized broken chromosome ends, and they are associated with a protein complex that includes a number of terminin proteins (Cenci et al., 2005; Ciapponi & Cenci, 2008). This suggests that chromosome caps in *Drosophila* are epigenetic and form independently of telomeric DNA sequence (Biessmann & Mason, 1988, 2003). These capped broken ends may eventually acquire retrotransposons by what appears to be a stochastic process (Biessmann et al., 1992a; Mikhailovsky et al., 1999).

As expected from the end replication problem, the broken chromosome ends recede. Erosion at these terminally deficient chromosomes was estimated at a constant rate of about 75 bp per sexual generation (Biessmann & Mason, 1988; Levis, 1989; Mikhailovsky et al., 1999). Considering the number of germline cell divisions, the rate of terminal erosion was estimated at 2-3 bp per chromosome end per cell cycle (Biessmann & Mason, 1988). This is formally equivalent to the degradation of an 8-12 nt RNA primer from the end of the lagging strand after each round of replication leaving a short 3' overhang (Biessmann et al., 1990a). In mammals telomere erosion is faster, in large part because chromosome ends are resected to produce relatively long 3' overhangs necessary for t-loop formation (Griffith et al., 1999; Wellinger et al., 1996). The slow rate of loss in *Drosophila* suggests that resection of the chromosome ends after replication is not extensive, and that t-loops are not required for telomere protection. It is possible that chromosome ends with telomeric retrotransposons behave differently from healed broken ends, but to date the evidence is lacking.

3.3.1.3 Transposition to elongate telomeres

To counter terminal erosion and maintain their length, telomeres must be elongated. The broken chromosome ends provide an entrée to study telomere elongation. Southern blots to monitor terminal fragment length at a broken chromosome end identified the addition of new sequence onto the terminal fragment at a frequency of about 1% per generation, with an average length for the added fragment of 6 kb (Biessmann et al., 1992a; Biessmann et al., 1990b). This averages out to an addition of 60 bp per generation, just enough to balance terminal erosion. It is important to note that the frequency of addition onto chromosome ends may be sensitive to different factors, including genetic background and possibly external conditions. Using genetic assays, two groups have identified stocks with much different frequencies of addition, possibly by as much as two orders of magnitude in either direction (Golubovsky et al., 2001; Savitsky et al., 2002; Savitsky et al., 2006). The new additions onto the receding chromosome ends were identified as *HeT-A* and *TART* elements, the same retrotransposons as found at natural telomeres. These elements were attached to the broken end by an oligo(A) tail, as would be expected from retrotransposition (Figure 3). Further, when broken chromosome ends that had gained a *HeT-A* element were used as a target they too acquired new *HeT-A* elements by transposition (Biessmann et al., 1992a). Thus, retrotransposition through target primed reverse transcription may be a mechanism for extending natural chromosome ends as well as broken ends.

3.3.1.3.1 The transcription step

The first step in the process of retrotransposition is transcription of the transposable element (Figure 3). All three telomeric elements have unusual transcription patterns. *TART* has active promoters at both the 5' and 3' ends that initiate in both the sense and antisense directions, although the major product seems to be a nearly full length antisense RNA (Danilevskaya et al., 1999; Maxwell et al., 2006). *TART* has a single promoter in the 5' UTR that drives transcription of the transposition intermediate (Maxwell et al., 2006). *HeT-A* and *TAHRE*, on the other hand, do not have promoters at the 5' end. Instead, they have a promoter in the 3' end that drives transcription of the adjacent downstream element (Danilevskaya et al., 1997; Shpiz et al., 2007). This literally means that *HeT-A* promotes its neighbor. The placement of this promoter is important for the long-term integrity of the telomeric array, because a promoter in the standard 5' position would be subject to erosion due to the end replication problem and lost immediately after transposition. A 3' promoter resurrects the element downstream. *HeT-A* transcription is developmentally regulated and occurs only in diploid cells of ovaries, testes, imaginal discs, and embryos (Capkova Frydrychova et al., 2007).

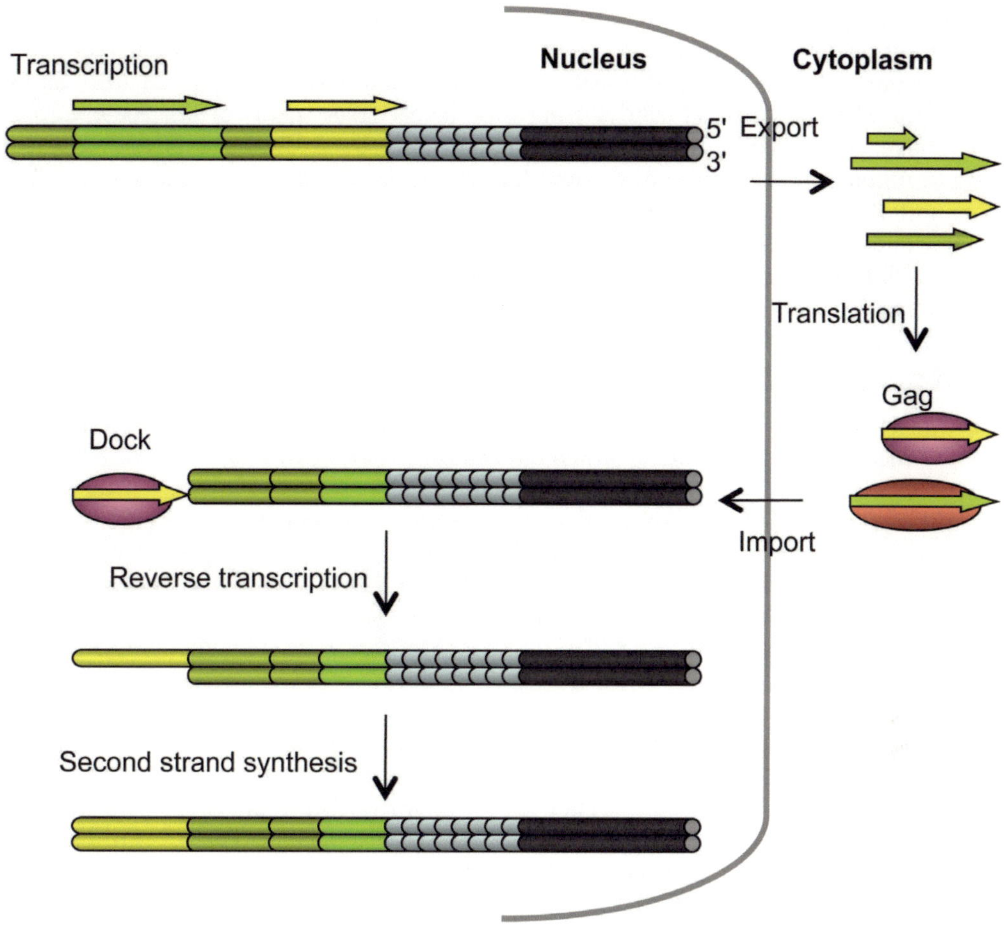

Fig. 3. Transposition as a mechanism for telomere elongation. The model proposes that transcripts (colored arrows) are generated from telomeric retrotransposons using promoter activity located in the 3' UTR of an upstream *HeT-A* or *TAHRE* element. Transcripts leave the nucleus to serve as mRNA for translation of the encoded Gag protein and possibly reverse transcriptase (ovals). Gag proteins bind the RNA, facilitate re-entry into the nucleus and target the chromosome end. After docking to a telomere a reverse transcriptase uses the free 3' hydroxyl group at the chromosome end as primer to copy the RNA intermediate into the first DNA strand. Second strand synthesis completes the addition of a new retrotransposon. Sequence analyses of recently transposed *HeT-A* elements and several in native telomeric arrays suggest that there is a selection for the incorporation of elements with a functional Gag ORF.

One appealing mechanism for controlling the length of the terminal retrotransposon array is to regulate transcription of these elements. Two forms of this mechanism have been proposed, but both have problems. First, it was noted that transgenes inserted into subtelomere regions are repressed and variegate (Cryderman et al., 1999; Roseman et al., 1995). In addition, TAS arrays can silence *in cis* the activity of a neighboring transgene as well as a *HeT-A* element when they are distal (telomeric) of TAS (Boivin et al., 2003;

Capkova Frydrychova et al., 2007; Kurenova et al., 1998), suggesting that TAS can control terminal retrotransposon array length by regulating transcription (Mason et al., 2003a). The TAS silencing effect, however, only extends a short distance into the terminal array and has little or no effect on overall *HeT-A* transcript levels (Biessmann et al., 2005; Capkova Frydrychova et al., 2007). Thus, silencing orchestrated by TAS arrays is not sufficiently strong to regulate transcription of the terminal retrotransposons. Second, it was noted that *HeT-A* and *TART* transcript levels are under the control of an RNA interference pathway (Savitsky et al., 2006; Shpiz et al., 2009). Transposition frequency and terminal array length, however, did not increase with increasing retrotransposon transcript levels (Capkova Frydrychova et al., 2008). It thus appears that the transcript levels of these retrotransposons are not the limiting factor in their transposition.

3.3.1.3.2 Telomere targeting

After transcription the RNA is transported into the cytoplasm and translated. The *HeT-A* RNA produces only a Gag protein, which binds a transcript, enters the nucleus and attaches to chromosome ends. Evidence supports the hypothesis that the Gag protein binds preferentially to the transcript that encoded it, because while many *HeT-A* elements in the terminal array are 5' truncated or otherwise lack an ORF, newly transposed *HeT-A* elements have a complete Gag ORF (Biessmann et al., 1994). Unlike Gag proteins for closely related parasitic retrotransposons, the *HeT-A* and *TART* Gag proteins are transported efficiently into the nucleus (Rashkova et al., 2002b). Unlike other non-LTR elements telomere specific elements do not require nicked DNA, because they are reverse transcribed directly onto the end of the chromosome. The *HeT-A* Gag can associate with telomeres on its own. The *TART* Gag, however, can only be seen to associate with telomeres in the presence of expressed *HeT-A* Gag protein (Rashkova et al., 2002a). Similarly, transport of the *TAHRE* Gag into the nucleus is facilitated by *HeT-A* and *TART* Gag proteins (Fuller et al., 2010). This presents a possible explanation for the presence of *HeT-A, TAHRE* and *TART* transposons in all *Drosophila* stocks. *HeT-A* does not encode a reverse transcriptase, which is required for retrotransposition, but may use the one encoded by either the *TART* or *TAHRE* elements. *TAHRE* and *TART*, on the other hand, cannot target chromosome ends without the aid of the *HeT-A* Gag protein.

3.3.1.3.3 Consequences of transposition on terminal array structure

Given the constant erosion of chromosome ends and the stochastic addition of transposon sequences to the same ends, one might expect that the terminal retrotransposon array would be very dynamic, constantly changing in length and composition. We have found this to be true using a genetic assay for the number of transposons at a specific telomere (Golubovsky et al., 2001; Mason et al., 2003b). One consequence of this turnover is that the transposon elements at the terminus are younger than those nearer to TAS. Virtually complete terminal arrays have been identified in overlapping BAC clones (Abad et al., 2004a). The age differential can be seen in the distribution of transposable elements that do not specifically target the chromosome end. These transposons are found primarily in the older, proximal portion of the terminal array (Pardue & DeBaryshe, 2008). Turnover in the younger, distal portion of array the removes evidence of these transposons. Newly transposed *P* elements have also been found inserted into the terminal array with reasonable frequency (Biessmann et al., 2005). Although the exact positions of these *P* elements in the terminal array could not be determined for most of the insertions, there is no evidence that any portion of the HTT array is refractory to insertion by non-telomere-specific elements.

HeT-A transcription start sites reside 31 and 62 bp upstream of the oligo-A tail (Danilevskaya et al., 1997). Thus, newly transposed transposons are slightly longer than the same elements before transposition, because they carry a tag at the 5' end identical to the 3' end of the previous upstream element (Traverse et al., 2010). Surprisingly, some of the elements carry multiple tags, suggesting that they have transposed several times without being subjected to terminal erosion. The simplest explanation is that multiple transposition events occur in rapid succession, possibly more than one per generation. Evidence of this has been found in measurements of transposition rate (Biessmann et al., 1992a), in which it was found that many of the new sequence additions were 12 kb or longer, and the 3' half of these long additions consisted of a (6 kb) *HeT-A* element. As these long addition events were shown to be the result of transposition, they could have resulted from either rapid multiple transposition events or transcriptional read-through to produce an RNA intermediate encompassing more than one element. The latter, however, have been found to be relatively rare (Capkova Frydrychova et al., 2007) and don't explain the presence of tandem tags. Rapid multiple transposition events may be the natural consequence of terminal transposition. When one retrotransposon attaches to the chromosome end, the old protective telomere cap must jump to the new terminus 6-12 kb away. If the cap is unstable during this transition, more transposons may have access to the new terminus, allowing for more transposition events to occur in rapid succession.

The 5' and 3' UTRs of *TART* carry perfect non-terminal repeats. These repeated regions vary among *TART* families and among individuals within a family but are identical at both ends of individual elements (Sheen & Levis, 1994). It has been proposed that the two repeated sequences evolve in concert by a mechanism of template switching during the reverse transcription step (George et al., 2010).

3.3.1.4 Recombination to elongate telomeres

Transposition is not the only mechanism for telomere elongation in *Drosophila*. Gene conversion allows genetic information to be transferred from one chromosome to another by homologous recombination (Figure 4). Georgiev and colleagues made use of broken chromosome ends with the *yellow* gene placed close to the terminus, such that the upstream controlling sequences were deleted, but the ORF was still present (Kahn et al., 2000; Mikhailovsky et al., 1999). Expression of the *yellow* gene was thus inactivated, but *HeT-A* transposition to the broken end could activate *yellow* expression via the promoter in its 3' UTR, while recombination with a wild type chromosome can reintroduce the *yellow* promoter and enhancers to their position on the broken end. Genetic assays were used to identify changes in *yellow* expression, then the length and sequence of the upstream region were characterized. Approximately 20-30% of the *yellow* reactivation events were the result of gene conversion. In one study the average length of the conversion track was estimated at 2.7 kb (Mikhailovsky et al., 1999), in another conversion tracks exceeding 20 kb were found (Kahn et al., 2000).

Although experiments using broken chromosome ends to monitor telomere elongation use an artificial system of telomere maintenance, it is assumed that the telomere elongation mechanisms identified in these experiments also work at the ends of long retrotransposon arrays. Extensions of long terminal arrays by individual transposition events or short gene conversion tracks cannot be monitored genetically or molecularly. If, however, genetic factors cause an imbalance between elongation and erosion, terminal retrotransposon arrays may grow or shrink. This can be measured cytologically by *in situ* hybridization on polytene chromosomes as changes in the terminal array length, or molecularly by quantitative PCR as changes in the genomic copy number of the telomere-specific retrotransposons.

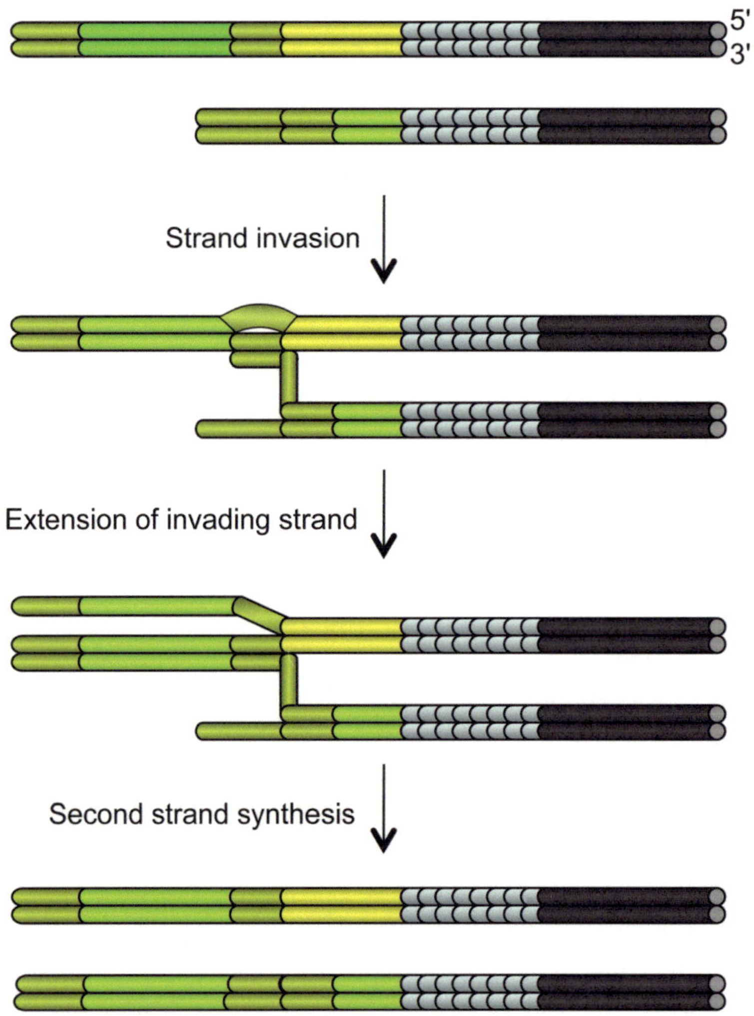

Fig. 4. Gene conversion as a mechanism for telomere elongation. The model proposes that the 3' strand of a chromosome end invades another chromosome, possibly a sister or homologue. The invading strand is extended using the host sequence as a template then is used as a template in second strand synthesis. Ligation of the newly replicated fragment results in an extended chromosome.

Mutations have been identified in three genes that cause terminal transposon array length to increase. Telomere length is sensitive to HP1 concentration, as mutations in the gene encoding this protein lead to an increase in *HeT-A* and *TART* transcript levels and a 100 fold increase in the frequency of new *HeT-A* and *TART* attachments (Savitsky et al., 2002). The increased rate of elongation resulted from both transposition and gene conversion, and was associated with extremely long terminal array length after several generations. As HP1 protein is enriched in the telomere cap, at least two possible hypotheses present themselves: (1) increased transcription increases transposition of the telomere-specific elements, and (2) disruption of the cap by decreasing one of its component proteins increases accessibility of the transposons. Our data (RCF and JMM, unpublished data), however, suggest that neither is true. Other mutations associated with increased *HeT-A* transcript levels are not associated with long telomeric arrays, and disruption of the cap by making heterozygous mutations in other genes encoding cap proteins does not increase telomeric array length. Two dominant mutations, *E(tc)* and *Tel* (Melnikova & Georgiev, 2002; Siriaco et al., 2002), exhibit abnormally long telomeres and are located in the same small genetic region in the middle of chromosome 3R. In the *Tel* mutant the copy number of *HeT-A* at telomeres is increased seven-fold, while *TART* and *TAHRE* copies are increased somewhat less (Siriaco et al., 2002; Walter et al., 2007). The mechanism of action of these mutations has not been elucidated, although one study indicated that the *Tel* mutation causes telomere elongation by transposition as well as gene conversion, while *E(tc)* causes mainly gene conversion (Proskuryakov & Melnikova, 2008).

3.3.2 *Drosophila virilis*

The DNA sequence of individual *HeT-A* and *TART* elements in *D. melanogaster* differ considerably throughout their lengths, but especially in the 3' UTR regions. Although it is possible to identify families of these elements, there is still some variation within each family. A comparison of telomeric retrotransposons between two sibling species of *Drosophila*, *D. melanogaster* and *D. yakuba*, shows substantial divergence in the *HeT-A* and *TART* UTRs but divergence in the ORFs that encode the Gag-like polypeptides (Casacuberta & Pardue, 2002; Danilevskaya et al., 1998b). These two elements have the most amino acid sequence conservation around the zinc knuckle motif typical of Gag proteins, and there are conserved islands scattered throughout the coding region. The overall structure of the elements, however, is well conserved. *HeT-A* in *D. yakuba* also lacks a *pol* ORF and has a very long 3' UTR. Although the high sequence divergence of the telomeric elements makes it difficult to find these elements in new species, it also increases the probability that the conserved features are of biological importance.

Searching for telomeric retrotransposons in more distantly related species presents a problem because of the extensive sequence divergence. Only the most conserved part of the *D. melanogaster TART pol* gene can cross-hybridize, even at low stringency, with *D. virilis* DNA. This hybridization, however, allowed the isolation of DNA fragments that provided entry into the *D. virilis* telomere arrays (Casacuberta & Pardue, 2003a). The *D. virilis TART* resembles its *D. melanogaster* homolog in several respects. They are both found in tandem arrays, but not in the euchromatic arms, and they both produce an excess of antisense transcripts. The *TART* in *D. virilis* is different in that it has a relatively short 3' UTR without perfect non-terminal repeats and a *pol* gene (ORF2) that encodes an additional 'X' domain 3' to the reverse transcriptase domain. A *HeT-A* element was found in the terminal array next to a *TART* from *D. virilis*. As with its homolog in *D. melanogaster*, the *HeT-A* element carried only a single ORF for a Gag protein and had a long 3' UTR (Casacuberta & Pardue, 2003b). Experiments to localize GFP-tagged Gag proteins indicated that the Gag encoded by the *D. virilis TART* element requires *HeT-A* Gag to target the telomeres, similar to the situation found in *D. melanogaster* (Casacuberta et al., 2007).

There are significant differences between the telomere specific elements in *D. melanogaster* and *D. virilis*. *HeT-A* in *D. virilis* has its promoter in the 5' UTR, similar to nontelomeric retrotransposons and thus produces transcripts that lack 5' tags. Even so, full length *HeT-A* elements persist in the array. The *D. virilis TART*, on the other hand, has a 3' promoter that generates 5' tags on its transcripts (George et al., 2010; Traverse et al., 2010). This arrangement is the reverse of that found in *D. melanogaster*. Unlike in *D. melanogaster*, the *HeT-A* 5' UTR in *D. virilis* is highly conserved. This suggests a different transposition mechanism for *HeT-A* in these two species. Unlike the situation in *D. melanogaster*, in which the retrotransposons attach to the chromosome terminus, it is possible that the *HeT-A* element in *D. virilis* inserts into the 5' UTR of other elements already in the array by making a sequence-specific nick followed by target primed reverse transcription. This proposed mechanism resembles that used by canonical non-LTR retrotransposons. The 'X' domain specific to the *D. virilis pol* gene may play a role in this endonuclease activity. If it is true that *HeT-A* elements behave differently in these two distantly related *Drosophila* species and that *HeT-A* in *D. virilis* uses a mechanism similar to nontelomeric retrotransposons, then retrotransposon telomeres may have arisen near the dawn of *Drosophila*. *HeT-A* transposons in the *Sophophora* subgenus, which includes *D. melanogaster*, may have lost the endonuclease needed to nick chromosomal DNA to initiate insertion, while *HeT-A* transposons in the *Drosophila* subgenus, which includes *D. virilis*, may have retained the endonuclease but made it sequence specific. Further, if telomeric retrotransposons arose in the *Drosophila* genus, it follows that other Dipteran species may have other means of controlling telomere length. This is consistent with the finding of complex tandem sequence arrays at the extreme chromosome ends in *Chironomus* and Sciaridae species (Cohn & Edstrom, 1992; Cohn & Edström, 1992; Madalena et al., 2010; Nielsen & Edstrom, 1993).

4. Conclusion

Although rare, telomerase has been lost several times in plants and animals. In some cases, such as Diptera, telomerase was lost in the distant past, and the descendents of this event have thrived and diversified. This raises the possibility that, once established, organisms with noncanonical mechanisms of telomere maintenance may not be at a severe selective disadvantage. How, then, do we account for the paucity of organisms lacking telomerase? One possibility is that there is a strong selective barrier to the loss of telomerase-generated DNA motifs. Binding of the shelterin protein complex necessary for the protection of chromosome ends depends on sequence-specific binding. The shelterin components TRF1 and TRF2 in particular recognize the double stranded telomeric motif, while POT1 recognizes the single stranded form (Palm & de Lange, 2008). Thus, in most cases loss of telomerase results in loss of the telomeric motif, followed by loss of the chromosome cap, massive chromosome rearrangement and death. If, however, telomeric attachment of the cap complex in some lineages does not depend strongly on a specific DNA sequence, loss of the telomeric motif might not have the same catastrophic consequences. This might explain why insects have lost telomerase and the canonical arthropod-type telomeric sequence multiple times (Figure 1). This hypothesis assumes the existence of an effective backup mechanism that can replace the canonical telomerase system. Alternatively, it may be misleading to suggest that loss of telomerase occurred only in the small number of organisms already reported. There may be, for example, cases similar to *B. mori*, in which an unconventional telomere structure maintained without telomerase is camouflaged by the presence of canonical telomeric sequences. Loss of telomerase in Solanaceae, Alliaceae and insects may thus represent the tip of the proverbial iceberg, and it is possible that many other groups will be found with unusual telomere structures.

Recombination seems like a ready backup mechanism for telomere maintenance by transferring information from one DNA strand to another, because it is widely used by eukaryotes both during meiotic recombination and as a means of repairing DNA damage (Heyer et al., 2010). Some organisms are known to use recombination to maintain the canonical telomeric DNA sequence in the absence of telomerase. In *Saccharomyces cerevisiae,* for example, loss of telomerase causes gradual loss of the terminal array and ultimately cell death. A few survivors, however, appear in a recombination-dependent manner (Lundblad & Blackburn, 1993). In mammals telomerase activity is reduced in most somatic tissues, thus limiting the growth of tumors. Most cancer cells overcome this obstacle by reactivating telomerase, but about 15% use an alternative lengthening of telomeres mechanism, which is recombination-dependent (Cesare & Reddel, 2010). Dysfunctional telomeres may actually stimulate telomeric recombination (Brault & Autexier, 2011). It is thus reasonable to hypothesize that a recombination-based gene conversion mechanism would be available if telomerase fails. As seen in yeast and human tumors, this pathway can maintain telomeric repeats. If the canonical motif is lost another DNA sequence, possibly related to the complex arrays of subtelomeric regions, could be maintained by the same mechanism. It is difficult to prove that organisms without telomerase use gene conversion to elongate their chromosome ends, in large part because many of these organisms lack the genetic tools to test the hypothesis. Recombination could be demonstrated in the malaria vector *Anopheles gambiae* because of the fortuitous transgene insertion into the telomeric array (Roth et al., 1997). In other cases it can be shown that a complex repeat array extends to, or close to, the chromosome end (Madalena et al., 2010; Nielsen & Edstrom, 1993). In these cases gene conversion was suggested as the default mechanism. Regardless of the mechanism, it is clear that a few well established lineages of both plants and animals lack telomerase and the canonical telomeric DNA motif it produces. Elucidation of these unusual telomeres will help us to understand what it means to be a telomere.

5. Acknowledgments

We thank František Marec, Jan Zrzavý and Sailesh Surapureddi for valuable comments on the manuscript. The authors were supported by the Intramural Research Program of the NIH, National Institute of Environmental Health Sciences, the MOBITAG project (Reg. No. 229518 of EU program FP7-REGPOT-2008-1) and the Institute of Entomology project Z50070508

6. References

Abad, J.P. & Villasante, A. (1999). The 3' Non-Coding Region of the *Drosophila melanogaster HeT-A* Telomeric Retrotransposon Contains Sequences with Propensity to Form G-Quadruplex DNA. *FEBS Letters,* Vol. 453, No. 1-2, (June 18, 1999), pp. 59-62, ISSN 0014-5793

Abad, J.P., de Pablos, B., Osoegawa, K., de Jong, P.J., Martin-Gallardo, A. & Villasante, A. (2004a). Genomic Analysis of *Drosophila melanogaster* Telomeres: Full-Length Copies of *HeT-A* and *TART* Elements at Telomeres. *Molecular Biology and Evolution,* Vol. 21, No. 9, (September 2004), pp. 1613-1619, ISSN 0737-4038

Abad, J.P., de Pablos, B., Osoegawa, K., de Jong, P.J., Martin-Gallardo, A. & Villasante, A. (2004b). *TAHRE,* a Novel Telomeric Retrotransposon from *Drosophila melanogaster,* Reveals the Origin of Drosophila Telomeres. *Molecular Biology and Evolution,* Vol. 21, No. 9, (September 2004), pp. 1620-1624, ISSN 0737-4038

Agudo, M., Losada, A., Abad, J.P., Pimpinelli, S., Ripoll, P. & Villasante, A. (1999). Centromeres from Telomeres? The Centromeric Region of the *Y* Chromosome of *Drosophila melanogaster* Contains a Tandem Array of Telomeric *HeT-A-* and *TART-*Related Sequences. *Nucleic Acids Research,* Vol. 27, No. 16, (August 1999), pp. 3318-3324, ISSN 0305-1048

Andreyeva, E.N., Belyaeva, E.S., Semeshin, V.F., Polkholkova, G.V. & Zhimulev, I.F. (2005). Three Distinct Chromatin Domains in Telomere Ends of Polytene Chromosomes in *Drosophila melanogaster Tel* Mutants. *Journal of Cell Science,* Vol. 118, No. 23, (December 1, 2005), pp. 5465-5477, ISSN 1477-9137

Barnes, S.R., James, A.M. & Jamieson, G. (1985). The Organization, Nucleotide Sequence, and Chromosomal Distribution of a Satellite DNA from *Allium Cepa. Chromosoma,* Vol. 92, No. 3, (June 1985), pp. 185-192, ISSN 0009-5915

Berloco, M., Fanti, L., Sheen, F., Levis, R.W. & Pimpinelli, S. (2005). Heterochromatic Distribution of *HeT-A-* and *TART-*Like Sequences in Several *Drosophila* Species. *Cytogenetic and Genome Research,* Vol. 110, No. 1-4, pp. 124-133, ISSN 1424-8581

Biessmann, H. & Mason, J.M. (1988). Progressive Loss of DNA Sequences from Terminal Chromosome Deficiencies in *Drosophila melanogaster. EMBO Journal,* Vol. 7, No. 4, (April 1998), pp. 1081-1086, ISSN 0261-4189

Biessmann, H., Carter, S.B. & Mason, J.M. (1990a). Chromosome Ends in *Drosophila* without Telomeric DNA Sequences. *Proceedings of the National Academy of Sciences of the United States of America,* Vol. 87, No. 5, (March 1990), pp. 1758-1761, ISSN 0027-8424

Biessmann, H., Mason, J.M., Ferry, K., d'Hulst, M., Valgeirsdottir, K., Traverse, K.L. & Pardue, M.L. (1990b). Addition of Telomere-Associated HeT DNA Sequences "Heals" Broken Chromosome Ends in *Drosophila. Cell,* Vol. 61, (May 18, 1990), No. 4, pp. 663-673, ISSN 0092-8674

Biessmann, H., Champion, L.E., O'Hair, M., Ikenaga, K., Kasravi, B. & Mason, J.M. (1992a). Frequent Transpositions of *Drosophila melanogaster HeT-A* Transposable Elements to Receding Chromosome Ends. *EMBO Journal,* Vol. 11, No. 12, pp. 4459-4469, ISSN 0261-4189

Biessmann, H., Valgeirsdottir, K., Lofsky, A., Chin, C., Ginther, B., Levis, R.W. & Pardue, M.L. (1992b). *HeT-A,* a Transposable Element Specifically Involved in Healing Broken Chromosome Ends in *Drosophila melanogaster. Molecular and Cellular Biology,* Vol. 12, No. 9, (September 1992), pp. 3910-3918, ISSN 0270-7306

Biessmann, H., Kasravi, B., Bui, T., Fujiwara, G., Champion, L.E. & Mason, J.M. (1994). Comparison of Two Active *HeT-A* Retroposons of *Drosophila melanogaster. Chromosoma,* Vol. 103, No. 2, (April 1994), pp. 90-98, ISSN 1432-0886

Biessmann, H. & Mason, J.M. (1997). Telomere Maintenance without Telomerase. *Chromosoma,* Vol. 106, No. 2, (July 1997), pp. 63-69, ISSN 1432-0886

Biessmann, H., Kobeski, F., Walter, M.F., Kasravi, A. & Roth, C.W. (1998). DNA Organization and Length Polymorphism at the 2L Telomeric Region of *Anopheles Gambiae. Insect Molecular Biology,* Vol. 7, No. 1, (February 1998), pp. 83-93, ISSN 1365-2583

Biessmann, H. & Mason, J.M. (2003). Telomerase-Independent Mechanisms of Telomere Elongation. *Cellular and Molecular Life Sciences*, Vol. 60, No. 11, (November 2003), pp. 2325-2333, ISSN 1420-682X

Biessmann, H., Prasad, S., Semeshin, V.E., Andreyeva, E.N., Nguyen, Q., Walter, M.F. & Mason, J.M. (2005). Two Distinct Domains in *Drosophila melanogaster* Telomeres. *Genetics*, Vol. 171, No. 4, (December 2005), pp. 1767-1777, ISSN 0016-6731

Blackburn, E.H. & Gall, J.G. (1978). A Tandemly Repeated Sequence at the Termini of the Extrachromosomal Ribosomal RNA Genes in *Tetrahymena*. *Journal of Molecular Biology*, Vol. 120, No. 1, (March 25, 1978), pp. 33-53, ISSN 0022-2836

Boivin, A., Gally, C., Netter, S., Anxolabehere, D. & Ronsseray, S. (2003). Telomeric Associated Sequences of *Drosophila* Recruit Polycomb-Group Proteins in Vivo and Can Induce Pairing-Sensitive Repression. *Genetics*, Vol. 164, No. 1, (May 2003), pp. 195-208, ISSN 0016-6731

Brault, M.E. & Autexier, C. (2011). Telomeric Recombination Induced by Dysfunctional Telomeres. *Molecular Biology of the Cell*, Vol. 22, No. 2, (January 2011), pp. 179-188, ISSN 1059-1524

Capkova Frydrychova, R., Biessmann, H., Konev, A.Y., Golubovsky, M.D., Johnson, J., Archer, T.K. & Mason, J.M. (2007). Transcriptional Activity of the Telomeric Retrotransposon *HeT-A* in *Drosophila melanogaster* Is Stimulated as a Consequence of Subterminal Deficiencies at Homologous and Nonhomologous Telomeres. *Molecular and Cellular Biology*, Vol. 27, No. 13, (July 2007), pp. 4991-5001, ISSN 0270-7306

Capkova Frydrychova, R., Biessmann, H. & Mason, J.M. (2008). Regulation of Telomere Length in *Drosophila*. *Cytogenetic and Genome Research*, Vol. 122, (February 2009), pp. 356-364, ISSN 1424-8581

Casacuberta, E. & Pardue, M.L. (2002). Coevolution of the Telomeric Retrotransposons across *Drosophila* Species. *Genetics*, Vol. 161, No. 3, (July 2002), pp. 1113-1124, ISSN 0016-6731

Casacuberta, E. & Pardue, M.L. (2003a). Transposon Telomeres Are Widely Distributed in the *Drosophila* Genus: *TART* Elements in the Virilis Group. *Proceedings of the National Academy of Sciences of the United States of America*, Vol. 100, No. 6, (March 18, 2003), pp. 3363-3368, ISSN 0027-8424

Casacuberta, E. & Pardue, M.L. (2003b). *HeT-A* Elements in *Drosophila virilis*: Retrotransposon Telomeres Are Conserved across the *Drosophila* Genus. *Proceedings of the National Academy of Sciences of the United States of America*, Vol. 100, No. 24, (November 25, 2003), pp. 14091-14096, ISSN 0027-8424

Casacuberta, E. & Pardue, M.L. (2005). *HeT-A* and *TART*, Two *Drosophila* Retrotransposons with a Bona Fide Role in Chromosome Structure for More Than 60 Million Years. *Cytogenetic and Genome Research*, Vol. 110, No. 1-4, pp. 152-159, ISSN 1424-8581

Casacuberta, E., Marin, F.A. & Pardue, M.L. (2007). Intracellular Targeting of Telomeric Retrotransposon Gag Proteins of Distantly Related *Drosophila* Species. *Proceedings of the National Academy of Sciences of the United States of America*, Vol. 104, No. 20, (May 15, 2007), pp. 8391-8396, ISSN 0027-8424

Cenci, G., Siriaco, G., Raffa, G.D., Kellum, R. & Gatti, M. (2003). The *Drosophila* HOAP Protein Is Required for Telomere Capping. *Nature Cell Biology*, Vol. 5, No. 1, (January 2003), pp. 82-84, ISSN 1465-7392

Cenci, G., Ciapponi, L. & Gatti, M. (2005). The Mechanism of Telomere Protection: A Comparison between *Drosophila* and Humans. *Chromosoma*, Vol. 114, No. 3, (August 2003), pp. 135-145, ISSN 1432-0886

Cesare, A.J. & Reddel, R.R. (2010). Alternative Lengthening of Telomeres: Models, Mechanisms and Implications. *Nature Reviews in Genetics*, Vol. 11, No. 5, (May 2010), pp. 319-330, ISSN 1471-0056

Ciapponi, L. & Cenci, G. (2008). Telomere Capping and Cellular Checkpoints: Clues from Fruit Flies. *Cytogenetic and Genome Research*, Vol. 122, No. 3-4, (February 2009), pp. 365-373, ISSN 1424-859X

Cohn, M. & Edstrom, J.E. (1992). Telomere-Associated Repeats in Chironomus Form Discrete Subfamilies Generated by Gene Conversion. *Journal of Molecular Evolution*, Vol. 35, No. 2, (August 1992), pp. 114-122, ISSN 0737-4038

Cohn, M. & Edström, J.E. (1992). Chromosome Ends in *Chironomus Pallidivittatus* Contain Different Subfamilies of Telomere-Associated Repeats. *Chromosoma*, Vol. 101, No. 10, (October 1992), pp. 634-640, ISSN 1432-0886

Cryderman, D.E., Morris, E.J., Biessmann, H., Elgin, S.C.R. & Wallrath, L.L. (1999). Silencing at *Drosophila* Telomeres: Nuclear Organization and Chromatin Structure Play Critical Roles. *EMBO Journal*, Vol. 18, No. 13, (July 1, 1999), pp. 3724-3735, ISSN 0261-4189

Danilevskaya, O.N., Arkhipova, I.R., Traverse, K.L. & Pardue, M.L. (1997). Promoting in Tandem: The Promoter for Telomere Transposon *HeT-A* and Implications for the Evolution of Retroviral LTRs. *Cell*, Vol. 88, No. 5, (March 7, 1997), pp. 647-655, ISSN 0092-8674

Danilevskaya, O.N., Lowenhaupt, K. & Pardue, M.L. (1998a). Conserved Subfamilies of the *Drosophila HeT-A* Telomere- Specific Retrotransposon. *Genetics*, Vol. 148, No. 1, (January 1998), pp. 233-242, ISSN 0016-6731

Danilevskaya, O.N., Tan, C., Wong, J., Alibhai, M. & Pardue, M.L. (1998b). Unusual Features of the *Drosophila melanogaster* Telomere Transposable Element *HeT-A* Are Conserved in *Drosophila yakuba* Telomere Elements. *Proceedings of the National Academy of Sciences of the United States of America*, Vol. 95, No. 7, (March 31, 1998), pp. 3770-3775, ISSN 0027-8424

Danilevskaya, O.N., Traverse, K.L., Hogan, N.C., Debaryshe, P.G. & Pardue, M.L. (1999). The Two *Drosophila* Telomeric Transposable Elements Have Very Different Patterns of Transcription. *Molecular and Cellular Biology*, Vol. 19, No. 1, (January 1999), pp. 873-881, ISSN 0270-7306

Fajkus, J., Kovarik, A., Kralovics, R. & Bezdek, M. (1995). Organization of Telomeric and Subtelomeric Chromatin in the Higher Plant *Nicotiana Tabacum*. *Molecular and General Genetics*, Vol. 247, No. 5, (September 1995), pp. 633-638, ISSN 1432-1874

Fajkus, J., Sykorova, E. & Leitch, A.R. (2005). Telomeres in Evolution and Evolution of Telomeres. *Chromosome Research*, Vol. 13, No. 5, (July 2005), pp. 469-479, ISSN 0967-3849

Fanti, L., Giovinazzo, G., Berloco, M. & Pimpinelli, S. (1998). The Heterochromatin Protein 1 Prevents Telomere Fusions in *Drosophila*. *Molecular Cell*, Vol. 2, No. 5, (November 1998), pp. 527-538, ISSN 1097-2765

Frydrychova, R., Grossmann, P., Trubac, P., Vitkova, M. & Marec, F.E. (2004). Phylogenetic Distribution of TTAGG Telomeric Repeats in Insects. *Genome*, Vol. 47, No. 1, (February 1, 2004), pp. 163-178, ISSN 1480-3321

Fuchs, J., Brandes, A. & Schubert, I. (1995). Telomere Sequence Localization and Karyotype Evolution in Higher Plants. *Plant Systematics and Evolution*, Vol. 196, No. 3-4, (September 1995), pp. 227-241, ISSN 0378-2697

Fuchs, J. & Schubert, I. (1996). *Arabidopsis*-Type Telomere Sequences on Chromosome Termini of Selaginella Martensii Spring (Pteridophyta). *Biologisches Zentralblatt*, Vol. 115, No. 4, pp. 260-265

Fujiwara, H., Osanai, M., Matsumoto, T. & Kojima, K.K. (2005). Telomere-Specific Non-LTR Retrotransposons and Telomere Maintenance in the Silkworm, *Bombyx mori*. *Chromosome Research*, Vol. 13, No. 5, (July 2005), pp. 455-467, ISSN 0967-3849

Fuller, A.M., Cook, E.G., Kelley, K.J. & Pardue, M.L. (2010). Gag Proteins of *Drosophila* Telomeric Retrotransposons: Collaborative Targeting to Chromosome Ends. *Genetics*, Vol. 184, No. 3, (March 2010), pp. 629-U637, ISSN 0016-6731

Gao, G.J., Walser, J.C., Beaucher, M.L., Morciano, P., Wesolowska, N., Chen, J. & Rong, Y.S. (2010). Hiphop Interacts with HOAP and HP1 to Protect *Drosophila* Telomeres in a Sequence-Independent Manner. *EMBO Journal*, Vol. 29, No. 4, (February 2010), pp. 819-829, ISSN 0261-4189

George, J.A., Traverse, K.L., DeBaryshe, P.G., Kelley, K.J. & Pardue, M.L. (2010). Evolution of Diverse Mechanisms for Protecting Chromosome Ends by *Drosophila TART* Telomere Retrotransposons. *Proceedings of the National Academy of Sciences of the United States of America*, Vol. 107, No. 49, (December 2010), pp. 21052-21057, ISSN 0027-8424

Golubovsky, M.D., Konev, A.Y., Walter, M.F., Biessmann, H. & Mason, J.M. (2001). Terminal Retrotransposons Activate a Subtelomeric *white* Transgene at the 2L Telomere in *Drosophila*. *Genetics*, Vol. 158, No. 3, (July 2001), pp. 1111-1123, ISSN 0016-6731

Greider, C.W. (1996). Telomere Length Regulation. *Annual Review of Biochemistry*, Vol. 65, pp. 337-365, ISSN 0066-4154

Griffith, J.D., Comeau, L., Rosenfield, S., Stansel, R.M., Bianchi, A., Moss, H. & de Lange, T. (1999). Mammalian Telomeres End in a Large Duplex Loop. *Cell*, Vol. 97, No. 4, (May 14, 1999), pp. 503-514, ISSN 0092-8674

Heyer, W.D., Ehmsen, K.T. & Liu, J. (2010). Regulation of Homologous Recombination in Eukaryotes. *Annual Review of Genetics*, Vol. 44, pp. 113-139, ISSN 1545-2948

Kahn, T., Savitsky, M. & Georgiev, P. (2000). Attachment of *HeT-A* Sequences to Chromosomal Termini in *Drosophila melanogaster* May Occur by Different Mechanisms. *Molecular and Cellular Biology*, Vol. 20, No. 20, (October 2000), pp. 7634-7642, ISSN 0270-7306

Karpen, G.H. & Spradling, A.C. (1992). Analysis of Subtelomeric Heterochromatin in the *Drosophila* Minichromosome *Dp1187* by Single-*P* Element Insertional Mutagenesis. *Genetics*, Vol. 132, No. 3, (November 1992), pp. 737-753, ISSN 0016-6731

Klobutcher, L.A., Swanton, M.T., Donini, P. & Prescott, D.M. (1981). All Gene-Sized DNA Molecules in Four Species of Hypotrichs Have the Same Terminal Sequence and an Unusual 3' Terminus. *Proceedings of the National Academy of Sciences of the United States of America*, Vol. 78, No. 5, (May 15, 1981), pp. 3015-3019, ISSN 0027-8424

Kubo, Y., Okazaki, S., Anzai, T. & Fujiwara, H. (2001). Structural and Phylogenetic Analysis of TRAS, Telomeric Repeat-Specific Non-LTR Retrotransposon Families in Lepidopteran Insects. *Molecular Biology and Evolution*, Vol. 18, No. 5, (May 2001), pp. 848-857, ISSN 0737-4038

Kurenova, E., Champion, L., Biessmann, H. & Mason, J.M. (1998). Directional Gene Silencing Induced by a Complex Subtelomeric Satellite from *Drosophila*. *Chromosoma*, Vol. 107, No. 5, (November 1998), pp. 311-320, ISSN 1432-0886

Levis, R.W. (1989). Viable Deletions of a Telomere from a *Drosophila* Chromosome. *Cell*, Vol. 58, No. 4, (August 25, 1989), pp. 791-801, ISSN 0092-8674

Lundblad, V. & Blackburn, E.H. (1993). An Alternative Pathway for Yeast Telomere Maintenance Rescues Est1- Senescence. *Cell*, Vol. 73, No. 2, (April 23, 1993), pp. 347-360, ISSN 0092-8674

Madalena, C.R.G., Amabis, J.M. & Gorab, E. (2010). Unusually Short Tandem Repeats Appear to Reach Chromosome Ends of *Rhynchosciara americana* (Diptera: Sciaridae). *Chromosoma*, Vol. 119, No. 6, (December 2010), pp. 613-623, ISSN 0009-5915

Mason, J.M. & Biessmann, H. (1995). The Unusual Telomeres of *Drosophila*. *Trends in Genetics*, Vol. 11, No. 2, (February 1995) pp. 58-62, ISSN 0168-9525

Mason, J.M., Konev, A.Y. & Biessmann, H. (2003a). Telomeric Position Effect in *Drosophila melanogaster* Reflects a Telomere Length Control Mechanism. *Genetica*, Vol. 117, No. 2, (March 2003), pp. 319-325, ISSN 0016-6707

Mason, J.M., Konev, A.Y., Golubovsky, M.D. & Biessmann, H. (2003b). *Cis*- and *Trans*-Acting Influences on Telomeric Position Effect in *Drosophila melanogaster* Detected with a Subterminal Transgene. *Genetics*, Vol. 163, No. 3, (March 2003), pp. 917-930, ISSN 0016-6731

Matsumoto, T., Fukui, K., Niwa, O., Sugawara, N., Szostak, J.W. & Yanagida, M. (1987). Identification of Healed Terminal DNA Fragments in Linear Minichromosomes of *Schizosaccharomyces pombe*. *Molecular and Cellular Biology*, Vol. 7, No. 12, (December 1987), pp. 4424-4430, ISSN 0270-7306

Maxwell, P.H., Belote, J.M. & Levis, R.W. (2006). Identification of Multiple Transcription Initiation, Polyadenylation, and Splice Sites in the *Drosophila melanogaster TART* Family of Telomeric Retrotransposons. *Nucleic Acids Research*, Vol. 34, No. 19, (November 2006), pp. 5498-5507, ISSN 0305-1048

McClintock, B. (1941). The Stability of Broken Ends of Chromosomes in *Zea Mays*. *Genetics*, Vol. 26, No. 2, (March 1941), pp. 234-282, ISSN 0016-6731

Melnikova, L. & Georgiev, P. (2002). Enhancer of Terminal Gene Conversion, a New Mutation in *Drosophila melanogaster* That Induces Telomere Elongation by Gene Conversion. *Genetics*, Vol. 162, No. 3, (November 2002), pp. 1301-1312, ISSN 0016-6731

Melnikova, L. & Georgiev, P. (2005). *Drosophila* Telomeres: The Non-Telomerase Alternative. *Chromosome Research*, Vol. 13, No. 5, (July 2005), pp. 431-441, ISSN 0967-3849

Meyne, J., Ratliff, R.L. & Moyzis, R.K. (1989). Conservation of the Human Telomere Sequence (TTAGGG)n among Vertebrates. *Proceedings of the National Academy of Sciences of the United States of America*, Vol. 86, No. 18, (September 15, 1989), pp. 7049-7053, ISSN 0027-8424

Mikhailovsky, S., Belenkaya, T. & Georgiev, P. (1999). Broken Chromosomal Ends Can Be Elongated by Conversion in *Drosophila melanogaster*. *Chromosoma*, Vol. 108, No. 2, (May 1999), pp. 114-120, ISSN 0009-5915

Nielsen, L. & Edstrom, J.E. (1993). Complex Telomere-Associated Repeat Units in Members of the Genus *Chironomus* Evolve from Sequences Similar to Simple Telomeric Repeats. *Molecular and Cellular Biology*, Vol. 13, No. 3, (March 1993), pp. 1583-1589, ISSN 0270-7306

Oka, Y., Shiota, S., Nakai, S., Nishida, Y. & Okubo, S. (1980). Inverted Terminal Repeat Sequence in the Macronuclear DNA of *Stylonychia pustulata*. *Gene*, Vol. 10, (September 1980), pp. 301-306, ISSN 0378-1119

Okazaki, S., Tsuchida, K., Maekawa, H., Ishikawa, H. & Fujiwara, H. (1993). Identification of a Pentanucleotide Telomeric Sequence, (TTAGG)n, in the Silkworm *Bombyx mori* and in Other Insects. *Molecular and Cellular Biology*, Vol. 13, No. 3, (March 1993), pp. 1424-1432, ISSN 0270-7306

Okazaki, S., Ishikawa, H. & Fujiwara, H. (1995). Structural Analysis of *TRAS1*, a Novel Family of Telomeric Repeat-Associated Retrotransposons in the Silkworm, *Bombyx mori*. *Molecular and Cellular Biology*, Vol. 15, No. 8, (August 1995), pp. 4545-4552, ISSN 0270-7306

Olovnikov, A.M. (1973). A Theory of Marginotomy. *Journal of Theoretical Biology*, Vol. 41, No. 1 (September 14, 1973) ,pp. 181-190, ISSN 0022-5193

Palm, W. & de Lange, T. (2008). How Shelterin Protects Mammalian Telomeres. *Annual Review of Genetics*, Vol. 42, pp. 301-334, ISSN 0066-4197

Pardue, M.L. & DeBaryshe, P.G. (2003). Retrotransposons Provide an Evolutionarily Robust Non-Telomerase Mechanism to Maintain Telomeres. *Annual Review of Genetics*, Vol. 37, pp. 485-511, ISSN 0066-4197

Pardue, M.L. & DeBaryshe, P.G. (2008). *Drosophila* Telomeres - a Variation on the Telomerase Theme. *Fly*, Vol. 2, No. 3, (May 2008), pp. 101-110, ISSN 1933-6934

Pearce, S.R., Pich, U., Harrison, G., Flavell, A.J., Heslop-Harrison, J.S.P., Schubert, I. & Kumar, A. (1996). The *Ty1-Copia* Group Retrotransposons of *Allium Cepa* Are Distributed Throughout the Chromosomes but Are Enriched in the Terminal Heterochromatin. *Chromosome Research.*, Vol. 4, No. 5, (November 1996), pp. 357-364, ISSN 0967-3849

Peska, V., Sykorova, E. & Fajkus, J. (2008). Two Faces of Solanaceae Telomeres: A Comparison between *Nicotiana* and *Cestrum* Telomeres and Telomere-Binding Proteins. *Cytogenetics and Genome Research*, Vol. 122, No. 3-4, (December 2008), pp. 380-387, ISSN 1424-8581

Pich, U., Fuchs, J. & Schubert, I. (1996). How Do Alliaceae Stabilize Their Chromosome Ends in the Absence of TTTAGGG Sequences? *Chromosome Research.*, Vol. 4, No. 3, (April 1996), pp. 207-213, ISSN 0967-3849

Pich, U. & Schubert, I. (1998). Terminal Heterochromatin and Alternative Telomeric Sequences in *Allium cepa*. *Chromosome Research*, Vol. 6, No. 4, (June 1998), pp. 315-321, ISSN 0967-3849

Proskuryakov, K.A. & Melnikova, L.S. (2008). Functional Separation of Genetic Factors *Telomere Elongation* (*Tel*) and *Enhancer of Terminal Gene Conversion* (*E(tc)*) Involved in Telomere Elongation in *Drosophila melanogaster*. *Doklady Biochemistry and Biophysics*, Vol. 421, No. 1, (August 2008), pp. 199-203, ISSN 1607-6729

Pryde, F.E., Gorham, H.C. & Louis, E.J. (1997). Chromosome Ends: All the Same under Their Caps. *Current Opinion in Genetics and Development*, Vol. 7, No. 6 (December 1997), pp. 822-828, ISSN 0959-437X

Raffa, G.D., Siriaco, G., Cugusi, S., Ciapponi, L., Cenci, G., Wojcik, E. & Gatti, M. (2009). The *Drosophila Modigliani* (*Moi*) Gene Encodes a HOAP-Interacting Protein Required for Telomere Protection. *Proceedings of the National Academy of Sciences of the United States of America*, Vol. 106, No. 7, (February 17, 2009), pp. 2271-2276, ISSN 0027-8424

Raffa, G.D., Raimondo, D., Sorino, C., Cugusi, S., Cenci, G., Cacchione, S., Gatti, M. & Ciapponi, L. (2010). Verrocchio, a *Drosophila* Ob Fold-Containing Protein, Is a Component of the Terminin Telomere-Capping Complex. *Genes and Development*, Vol. 24, No. 15, (August 2010), pp. 1596-1601, ISSN 0890-9369

Rashkova, S., Karam, S.E., Kellum, R. & Pardue, M.L. (2002a). Gag Proteins of the Two *Drosophila* Telomeric Retrotransposons Are Targeted to Chromosome Ends. *Journal of Cell Biology*, Vol. 159, No. 3, (November 11, 2002), pp. 397-402, ISSN 0021-9525

Rashkova, S., Karam, S.E. & Pardue, M.L. (2002b). Element-Specific Localization of *Drosophila* Retrotransposon Gag Proteins Occurs in Both Nucleus and Cytoplasm. *Proceedings of the National Academy of Sciences of the United States of America*, Vol. 99, No. 6, (March 19, 2002), pp. 3621-3626, ISSN 0027-8424

Richards, E.J. & Ausubel, F.M. (1988). Isolation of a Higher Eukaryotic Telomere from *Arabidopsis thaliana*. *Cell*, Vol. 53, No. 1, (April 8, 1988), pp. 127-136, ISSN 0092-8674

Roseman, R.R., Johnson, E.A., Rodesch, C.K., Bjerke, M., Nagoshi, R.N. & Geyer, P.K. (1995). A *P* Element Containing Suppressor of Hairy-Wing Binding Regions Has Novel Properties for Mutagenesis in *Drosophila melanogaster*. *Genetics*, Vol. 141, No. 3, (November 1995), pp. 1061-1074, ISSN 0016-6731

Roth, C.W., Kobeski, F., Walter, M.F. & Biessmann, H. (1997). Chromosome End Elongation by Recombination in the Mosquito *Anopheles gambiae*. *Molecular and Cellular Biology*, Vol. 17, No. 9, (September 1997), pp. 5176-5183, ISSN 0270-7306

Russo, C.A., Takezaki, N. & Nei, M. (1995). Molecular Phylogeny and Divergence Times of Drosophilid Species. *Molecular Biology and Evolution*, Vol. 12, No. 3, (May 1995), pp. 391-404, ISSN 0737-4038

Savitsky, M., Kravchuk, O., Melnikova, L. & Georgiev, P. (2002). Heterochromatin Protein 1 Is Involved in Control of Telomere Elongation in *Drosophila melanogaster*. *Molecular and Cellular Biology*, Vol. 22, No. 9, (May 2002), pp. 3204-3218, ISSN 0270-7306

Savitsky, M., Kwon, D., Georgiev, P., Kalmykova, A. & Gvozdev, V. (2006). Telomere Elongation Is under the Control of the RNAi-Based Mechanism in the *Drosophila* Germline. *Genes and Development*, Vol. 20, No. 3, (February 2006), pp. 345-354, ISSN 0890-9369

Schmid, K.J. & Tautz, D. (1997). A Screen for Fast Evolving Genes from *Drosophila*. *Proceedings of the National Academy of Sciences of the United States of America*, Vol. 94, No. 18, (September 2, 1997), pp. 9746-9750, ISSN 0027-8424

Shampay, J., Szostak, J.W. & Blackburn, E.H. (1984). DNA Sequences of Telomeres Maintained in Yeast. *Nature*, Vol. 310, No. 5973, (July 12, 1984), pp. 154-157, ISSN

Sheen, F.M. & Levis, R.W. (1994). Transposition of the Line-Like Retrotransposon *TART* to *Drosophila* Chromosome Termini. *Proceedings of the National Academy of Sciences of the United States of America*, Vol. 91, No. 26, (December 20, 1994), pp. 12510-12514, ISSN 0027-8424

Shpiz, S., Kwon, D., Uneva, A., Kim, M., Klenov, M., Rozovsky, Y., Georgiev, P., Savitsky, M. & Kalmykova, A. (2007). Characterization of *Drosophila* Telomeric Retroelement *TAHRE*: Transcription, Transpositions, and RNAi-Based Regulation of Expression. *Molecular Biology and Evolution*, Vol. 24, No. 11, (November 2007), pp. 2535-2545, ISSN 0737-4038

Shpiz, S., Kwon, D., Rozovsky, Y. & Kalmykova, A. (2009). rasiRNA Pathway Controls Antisense Expression of *Drosophila* Telomeric Retrotransposons in the Nucleus. *Nucleic Acids Research*, Vol. 37, No. 1, (January 2009), pp. 268-278, ISSN 0305-1048

Siriaco, G.M., Cenci, G., Haoudi, A., Champion, L.E., Zhou, C., Gatti, M. & Mason, J.M. (2002). *Telomere Elongation (Tel)*, a New Mutation in *Drosophila melanogaster* That Produces Long Telomeres. *Genetics*, Vol. 160, No. 1, (January 2002), pp. 235-245, ISSN 0016-6731

Sykorova, E., Lim, K.Y., Kunicka, Z., Chase, M.W., Bennett, M.D., Fajkus, J. & Leitch, A.R. (2003). Telomere Variability in the Monocotyledonous Plant Order Asparagales. *Proceedings. Biological Sciences/The Royal Society*, Vol. 270, No. 1527, (September 2003), pp. 1893-1904, ISSN 0962-8452

Tatsuke, T., Sakashita, K., Masaki, Y., Lee, J.M., Kawaguchi, Y. & Kusakabe, T. (2009). The Telomere-Specific Non-LTR Retrotransposons *SART1* and *TRAS1* Are Suppressed by Piwi Subfamily Proteins in the Silkworm, *Bombyx mori*. *Cellular & Molecular Biology Letters*, Vol. 15, No. 1, (March 2009), pp. 118-133, ISSN 1425-8153

Traut, W., Szczepanowski, M., Vitkova, M., Opitz, C., Marec, F. & Zrzavy, J. (2007). The Telomere Repeat Motif of Basal Metazoa. *Chromosome Research*, Vol. 15, No. 3, (April 2007), pp. 371-382, ISSN 0967-3849

Traverse, K.L., George, J.A., DeBaryshe, P.G. & Pardue, M.L. (2010). Evolution of Species-Specific Promoter-Associated Mechanisms for Protecting Chromosome Ends by *Drosophila* HeT-A Telomeric Transposons. *Proceedings of the National Academy of Sciences of the United States of America*, Vol. 107, No. 11, (March 16, 2010), pp. 5064-5069, ISSN 0027-8424

Villasante, A., Abad, J.P., Planello, R., Mendez-Lago, M., Celniker, S.E. & de Pablos, B. (2007). *Drosophila* Telomeric Retrotransposons Derived from an Ancestral Element That Was Recruited to Replace Telomerase. *Genome Research*, Vol. 17, No. 12, (December 2007), pp. 1909-1918, ISSN 1088-9051

Vitkova, M., Kral, J., Traut, W., Zrzavy, J. & Marec, F. (2005). The Evolutionary Origin of Insect Telomeric Repeats, (TTAGG)(n). *Chromosome Research*, Vol. 13, No. 2, (January 2005), pp. 145-156, ISSN 0967-3849

Walter, M.F., Jang, C., Kasravi, B., Donath, J., Mechler, B.M., Mason, J.M. & Biessmann, H. (1995). DNA Organization and Polymorphism of a Wild-Type *Drosophila* Telomere Region. *Chromosoma*, Vol. 104, No. 4, (December 1995), pp. 229-241, ISSN 1432-0886

Walter, M.F., Biessmann, M.R., Benitez, C., Török, T., Mason, J.M. & Biessmann, H. (2007). Effects of Telomere Length in *Drosophila melanogaster* on Life Span, Fecundity, and Fertility. *Chromosoma*, Vol. 116, No. 1, (February 2007), pp. 41-51, ISSN 1432-0886

Wang, S.S. & Zakian, V.A. (1990). Sequencing of *Saccharomyces* Telomeres Cloned Using T4 DNA Polymerase Reveals Two Domains. *Molecular and Cellular Biology*, Vol. 10, No. 8, (August 1990), pp. 4415-4419, ISSN 0270-7306

Watson, J.D. (1972). Origin of Concatameric T7 DNA. *Nature New Biology*, Vol. 239, No. 94, (October 18, 1972), pp. 197-201, ISSN : 0028-0836

Watson, J.M. & Riha, K. (2010). Comparative Biology of Telomeres: Where Plants Stand. *FEBS Letters*, Vol. 584, No. 17, (September 2010), pp. 3752-3759, ISSN 0014-5793

Weiss, H. & Scherthan, H. (2002). *Aloe* Spp. - Plants with Vertebrate-Like Telomeric Sequences. *Chromosome Research*, Vol. 10, No. 2, (March 2002), pp. 155-164, ISSN 0967-3849

Wellinger, R.J., Ethier, K., Labrecque, P. & Zakian, V.A. (1996). Evidence for a New Step in Telomere Maintenance. *Cell*, Vol. 85, No. 3, (May 3, 1996), pp. 423-433, ISSN 0092-8674

Zellinger, B. & Riha, K. (2007). Composition of Plant Telomeres. *Biochimica et Biophysica Acta-Gene Structure and Expression*, Vol. 1769, No. 5-6, (May 2007), pp. 399-409, ISSN 0167-4781

16

Eukaryote DNA Replication and Recombination: an Intimate Association

Ramsay J. McFarlane[1], Khalid Al-Zeer[1] and Jacob Z. Dalgaard[2]
[1]*North West Cancer Research Fund Institute, College of Natural Sciences, Brambell Building, Bangor University, Deiniol Road, Bangor, Gwynedd,*
[2]*Warwick Medical School, Clinical Science Research Institute, Gibbert Hill Campus, University of Warwick, Coventry, United Kingdom*

1. Introduction

When the anti-parallel duplex structure of DNA was first postulated it paved a logical pathway to the proposal of semi-conservative DNA replication in which the two parental strands are unwound to provide a template for *de novo* polynucleotide chain synthesis (Watson & Crick, 1953a; 1953b). Whilst the structure of DNA makes for a relatively simple model for the DNA replicative process this simplicity is counter balanced by the array of complex molecular pathways which must orchestrate the high fidelity duplication of chromosomes. These mechanisms need to cope with a variety of types of damage to the parental duplex, which must be processed in a relatively error free fashion. Failures to correct DNA damage associated with the progression of the DNA replicative machinery, the replisome, can render a cell unviable or diseased. Conversely, alterations to genomes, be they single base pair changes or more substantial structural rearrangements, are required to instil genetic change, which is essential for the evolution of living systems. One repair process associated with replication is genetic recombination, which serves to repair breakages in DNA strands and failed forks. Failures in recombinogenic processing of replication-associated lesions are linked to genome rearrangements and in humans these have been linked directly to genetic disease states, including cancers (Abeysinghe et al., 2006; Admire et al., 2006; Aguilera & Gómez-González, 2008; Bartek et al., 2007; Chen et al., 2010; Halazonetis et al., 2008; Lambert et al., 2005; Lemoine et al., 2005; Putnam et al., 2009a; Weinstock et al., 2006; Weinert et al., 2009; Moynahan & Jasin, 2010). Whilst recombination mechanisms serve other functions in genome dynamics, such as the programmed conjoining of homologous chromosomes during meiosis, it could be argued that the primary role of recombination is to mediate genome repair in close association with the replisome.

Here we will explore current understanding of the types of DNA replication-associated lesions which require recombination processing and the current models proposed for the various recombination mechanisms which ultimately repair and maintain genetic integrity during cellular duplication events. Replication-associated recombination also plays distinct functional roles in regulation of specific genomic events, such as mating type switching in fission yeast (Dalgaard & Klar, 1999), and it regulates some genomic regions via distinct mechanisms, such as the highly repetitive rDNA locus (Dalgaard et al., 2011; Eukaryotic Replication Barriers: How, Why and Where Forks Stall, this book). Whilst we will not consider these specific regulatory mechanisms here, this chapter will provide an understanding of the mechanistic basis of the role of recombination in preserving genome integrity in response to aberrations in the replicative process and will thus provide an enlightened platform for further reading relating to regulation of specific genomic events/regions.

2. The generation of replication-associated recombinogenic lesion

The process of DNA replication can result in unscheduled generation of recombinogenic DNA lesions which can take the form of single-stranded gaps within a duplex, one-sided DNA double-strand breaks (DSBs), two-sided DSBs or collapsed fork structures. Breaks in the DNA arise due to the replisome encountering an array of distinct problems. In this section we outline models which have been proposed for the generation of distinct classes of lesion.

2.1 The conversion of single-stranded nicks into DSBs

Nicks or short gaps can be generated in one strand of the duplex during normal cellular metabolism. They can be generated by a single broken bond in the sugar-phosphate backbone of one strand or by the excision of a nucleotides during excision repair processes, such as nucleotide excision repair (NER) (for example, see Moriel-Carretero & Aguilera, 2010a; 2010b); moreover, nicks in the duplex can be generated by internally or externally generated DNA damaging agents, such as highly reactive superoxide radicals or radiation.

When a nick is encountered in either the leading or the lagging strand template by a unidirectional DNA replication fork then a one-sided DSB can result (Figure 1A) (for example, see Harper et al., 2010). The generation of this break can be concomitant with the 'fill in' of the nick in the unbroken duplex, or the nick can remain in the duplex associated with the other parental strand. If a nick should be proximal to the point at which replication forks converge, or it stalls the progression of a unidirectional fork permitting time for the arrival of a converging fork to replicate from the opposite direction, then there is a chance that both forks will now encounter a template strand discontinuity, potentially resulting in a two-sided DSB (Figure 1B). The one-sided and two-sided DSBs differ considerably in that a one-sided DSB needs to undergo a repair mechanism which will ideally re-establish a functional DNA replication fork to permit the replicative process to continue; whereas a two-sided DSB needs to undergo post replication repair to produce a continuous duplex.

2.2 The generation of two-sided DSBs as a result of inter-strand cross linking

The Crick and Watson strands of a DNA duplex are held together by hydrogen bonds between the organic bases. Such hydrogen bonding is readily broken by the helicases associated with the replisome to expose the parental strands of a duplex to the template-dependent actions of the DNA polymerases. However, when covalent bonds are formed between two strands of a duplex, helicases can no longer dissociate the template strands and replication fork progression is halted. The prevalence of such covalent linkage in a cell not exposed to specific DNA damaging agents is unclear, although a number of anti-cancer

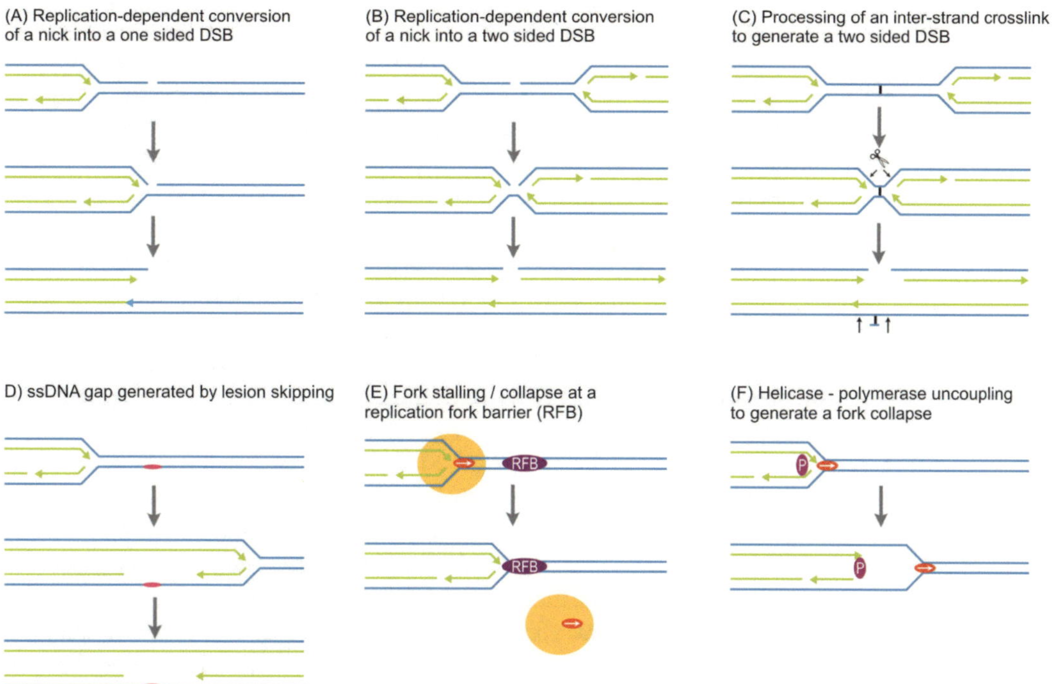

Fig. 1. Replication-associated recombinogenic lesions. (A) Generation of a one-sided DSB. A unidirectional replication fork approaches a nick (discontinuity in one of the parental duplexes), and a one-sided break is generated. (B) Generation of a two-sided DSB. Opposing forks converge on the side of a parental strand nick to generate a two-sided DSB. (C) Generation of a DSB from a inter-strand cross link (ICL). Replication forks converge on an ICL. This generates a structure which is cleaved by structure-specific nuclease activity, which in turn creates a two-sided DSB. The cross linked abduct remains associated with the unbroken duplex and translesion polymerase synthesise past the abduct generating a complete duplex with an abduct associated with one strand which can now undergo an excision repair (vertical black arrows). (D) single-stranded gap generated by lesion skipping. The replisome 'skips' a DNA damage abduct (purple oval) leaving a ssDNA gap behind the fork. (E) Replication fork collapse at a replication barrier. The replisome encounters a barrier to progression and fork stability becomes compromised. The replisome dissociates from the DNA leaving a fork-like branched structure which requires processing for repair / fork recovery. (F) Replication fork collapse due to uncoupling of the replicative helicase and the polymerase. The uncoupling of the helicase (red oval with white arrow) from the polymerases (purple oval) results in the helicases running ahead of new strand synthesis generating extensive regions of ssDNA and ultimately causing fork demise.

drugs, such as mitomycin C and cisplatin act through the generation of covalent inter-strand cross links (Vasquez, 2010). The proposed model for DSB generation in response to covalent cross links (and subsequent repair) is dependent upon additional factors mediating breakage in response to the stalling of the replication fork (Figure 1C) (Nakanishi et al., 2011). To generate a two-sided DSB it is proposed that forks travelling in opposing directions converge upon the site of the cross linkage. This triggers unknown nucleases, possibly the structure-specific endonuclease Mus81-Eme1(Mms4) (see below) to cleave one of the parental strands either side of the site of the cross link. This, in combination with the fact that leading and lagging strand synthesis for that template strand were not complete (due to the cross link) results in a two-sided DSB (Figure 1C). This results in a cross linked nucleotide (or nucleotides, dependent upon the position of the cleavage) being associated with the other, uncleaved template strand (Figure 1C, bottom). It is proposed that this cross linked entity has the ability to 'swing' out of the way of the DNA polymerases and that translesion polymerases replicate past the cross linked adduct; at this stage an inappropriate base may be inserted, and so this mechanism is potentially highly mutagenic. The cross linked adduct in the new daughter duplex is proposed to be recognised by the NER pathway (Wood, 2010), which will remove the adduct and use the strand which was newly synthesised via by translesion synthesis (TLS) as the template for repair. TLS is mediated by a number of distinct DNA polymerases (Prakash et al., 2005; Loeb & Monnat, 2008; Ho & Schärer, 2010), which are thought to be recruited to the sites of lesions via activity of proliferating-cell nuclear antigen (PCNA), a homotrimer which plays multiple roles at the replication fork during both normal and perturbed replication (Navadgi-Patil & Burgers, 2009; Stoimenov & Helleday, 2009). The repaired daughter template now becomes the homologous substrate for recombination-mediated DSB repair and so if a mutated DNA sequence is generated by a TLS it is transferred to the other duplex in a stable fashion, ensuring that this process results in two new duplexes, both with stably inherit cross linking agent-induced mutation.

2.3 The generation of recombinogenic single-stranded DNA gaps via lesion bypass

Whilst DSBs are one of the most potentially dangerous lesions in DNA due to the fact that they represent an un-tethering of covalent linkages, single-stranded DNA (ssDNA) gaps in DNA also represent significant biological problems, not only because they have the potential to mediate gross chromosomal rearrangements, but also because they represent the loss of one of the transcriptional templates (Lehmann & Fuchs, 2006). Also, if left unrepaired, gaps can be converted into DSBs in subsequent rounds of DNA replication (see above). Whilst ssDNA gaps can be generated by other means (for example, incomplete NER), they can be generated when the replisome encounters an adduct on the duplex (for example, see Lopes et al., 2006; Figure 1D). If the replisome can 'skip' the adduct, replication will progress leaving a ssDNA gap in the wake of the fork (Figure 1D). The nature of adducts capable of being 'skipped' and the prevalence of this route of gap generation is difficult to discern, but when generated, such lesions can trigger distinct repair pathways (see below).

2.4 The generation of dysfunctional fork structures

DNA replication forks can encounter blocks to their progression as a result of normal chromosome dynamics such as collisions between the replisome and RNA polymerases (Aguilera, 2002; Prado & Aguilera, 2005; Poveda et al., 2010; Tuduri et al., 2010) / nascent transcripts (Mischo et al., 2011), encounters with adducts on the DNA (for example, see Cordeiro-Stone et al., 1999) such as those which might be caused by DNA damaging agents (Mirkin & Mirkin, 2007) or encounters with unusual DNA structures (for example, see Narayanan et al., 2006). In some biological systems barriers to the progression of the DNA replication fork have evolved to play a programmed role in specific chromosomal regulatory pathways, such as the *RTS1* replication fork barrier which is required for efficient mating type switching in the fission yeast (Dalgaard & Klar, 2001; Dalgaard et al., 2009; Vengrova et al., 2002). Stalling of a fork can result in what is often referred to as 'fork collapse' where some or all of the proteins of the replisome dissociate from the fork leaving non-replicative fork structures (Figure 1E) (for example, see Weinert et al., 2009). Moreover, the replicative helicases, which unwind the DNA duplex to provide single-stranded template, can become uncoupled from the replicative polymerases (for example, see Pacek & Walter, 2004; Pagés & Fuchs, 2003; Lopes et al., 2006), this can result in fork collapse and more extensive regions of ssDNA become associated with the failed fork structure (Figure 1F). Nucleotide depletion is also thought to result in replication fork collapse; the ribonucleotide reductase inhibitor hydroxyl urea is frequently used to deplete nucleotide pools and so disrupt the progression of the S-phase. In these cases the fork failure does not result in strand breakage, but a structure is generated which is thought to require recombination-associated mechanisms to re-establish a functional fork structure. The replisome is associated with functions which serve to prevent fork collapse and these functions have intimate mechanistic links to the checkpoint signal transduction pathways which can be triggered in the event of a replication-associated lesion generating a significant initiator signal (most likely ssDNA). Moreover, there are factors associated with the repolisome known as the replication fork progression complex which serves to monitor the 'traffic' ahead of the DNA replication fork and mediate a stable and appropriate delay in the fork progression (presumably until the barrier is removed) and the so called 'sweepase' (for example, see Ivessa et al., 2003) which functions to remove barriers, such as RNA polymerases, to prevent them triggering a barrier response in the replisome thereby minimises the chance of a potential fork collapse scenario. This chapter will not review the function of these anti-collapse and fork stabilisation mechanisms, or their link to the cellular checkpoint systems and the reader is directed to a number of other excellent reviews which cover these subjects in more detail (Bartek et al., 2004; Branzei & Foiani, 2007a; 2007b; 2009; 2010; Grallert & Boye, 2008; Harrison & Haber, 2006; Lambert et al., 2007; Labib, 2008; Labib & Hodgson, 2007; McFarlane et al., 2010; Paulsen & Cimprich, 2007; Putnam et al., 2009b; Yao & O'Donnell, 2009).

3. Models for recombination-mediated recovery from replication-associated lesion damage

Homologous recombination requires the presence of a homologous duplex molecule which can be employed as a surrogate template for synthesis-dependent repair of breaks and gaps in duplex DNA molecules. During the repair of replication-generated two-sided DSBs or gaps the aim of recombination is to repair the lesions post replicatively. The aim of the repair process for other replication induced recombinogenic lesions is to re-engage a functional replication fork to permit the completion of genomic replication prior to cell division. Here we will consider the various models proposed for the repair of the recombinogenic lesions described above. For simplicity of understanding we will firstly outline the proposed models at the level of the DNA strands and then in subsequent sections we will consider the proteins which might mediate these repair mechanisms (see section 4).

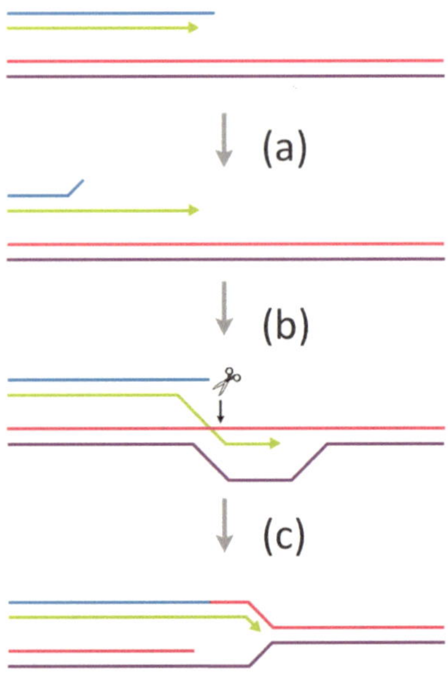

Fig. 2. Model for recombination mediated generation of a DNA replication fork from a one-sided DSB. (a) The one-sided break is processed to generate a single-stranded overhang with a free 3' end (arrow head). (b) The 3' single-stranded end invades the nascent sister chromatid to form a D-loop. (c) The D-loop undergoes nucleolytic processing and strand ligation to re-generate a functional DNA replication fork.

3.1 The processing of a one-sided DSB to re-establish a functional replication fork

On generation of a one-sided DNA break, it is likely that the broken nascent duplex remains associated with the other nascent duplex molecule. This association is primarily facilitated by cohesin, a complex of conserved proteins which serve to maintain inter-sister associations prior to sister chromatid segregation at the metaphase to anaphase transition (for reviews, see Merkenschlager, 2010; Nasmyth & Haering, 2009; Sherwood et al., 2010; Wood et al., 2010; Xiong & Gerton, 2010). The broken end will be exposed permitting association with recombination mediators and will undergo initial end processing. Given that homologous recombination repair of breaks is dependent upon one of the participating strands providing a substrate for new strand synthesis, a free 3′ ssDNA end must be generated during end processing. This processing is often referred to as end resection [Figure 2 step (a)] (see section 4.1). Following this, the free 3′ end of the ssDNA invades a homologous duplex, in this case the sister chromatid, to establish a so called D-loop (displacement loop) structure [Figure 2, step (b)]. This generates a structure which can be recognised by structure-specific endonucleases, such as the Mus81-Eme1 (Mms4) heterodimer (see section 4.), which cleaves the anti-parallel strand to which the invading strand is annealed; thus, following a one step strand ligation, a structure resembling a DNA replication fork is re-established and replication can proceed [Figure 2 step (c)]. This model is appealing as it is a relatively simple pathway to fork re-establishment and it is in essence similar to break-induced replication (for reviews, see McEachen & Haber, 2006; Llorente et al., 2008). It is dependent upon there being an intimate association between the recombination mediators and the factors required to re-build a functional replication fork, although little is known about this relationship at this proposed step.

3.2 Two-sided DSB repair

Two-sided DSBs provide a particular challenge for the cell as gaps in a DNA duplex must be 'filled' whilst maintaining the original DNA sequence, although, in the case of cross linking agent-induced DSBs, this can be mutagenic (see above). One of the major factors governing how a DSB is processed is the stage within the cell division cycle that the break is generated (Branzei & Foiani, 2008; Heyer et al., 2010). In G_1 of the cell division cycle homologous recombination repair of chromosomal breakage could have detrimental outcomes, such as a loss of heterozygocity through inter-homologue recombination events. Two-sided DSBs generated in G_1 are more likely to be processed by a non-homologous DNA end joining mechanism (for reviews, see Lieber, 2010; Mladenov & Iliakis, 2011). The lesions generated in G_1 are not likely to have a causal association with the DNA replication machinery and so will not be covered in this chapter.

Two-sided DSBs which arise in response to DNA replication-associated breakage will be produced in the presence of a sister chromatid (Figure 1B & C) which can provide an appropriate partner for homologous recombination-mediated DSB repair. The early stages of two-sided DSB processing are likely to have mechanistic commonalities with one-sided DSB repair. The ends will undergo processing to expose 3′ ssDNA ends [Figure 3(a)]. If end processing exposes regions of ssDNA which have short complimentary sequences, then these regions have the potential to anneal and form a stable intermediate which might then undergo processing, including endonucleolytic removal of the non-annealed flap (most likely by the XPF family endonucleases, Schwartz & Heyer, 2011), new strand synthesis and ligation, to seal the broken end [Figure 3(b)]. This process is referred to as single-strand annealing (SSA), and whilst it repairs the broken chromosome, it results in the deletion of DNA sequences between the short homology regions and this can be mutagenic.

Alternatively, processed breaks with 3′ single-stranded free ends can undergo recombination repair which entails the initial invasion of one of the free 3′ ends into an homologous sister duplex molecule, [Figure 3(c)]. Following strand invasion by the free 3′ end, repair DNA polymerases catalyse chain extension of the invading 3′ end using the anti-parallel strand of the invaded duplex as the template. This process generates new DNA which spans the position of the original break, and thus this repair pathway is replication-dependent. The structure at this point can be referred to as an extended D-loop, as the replicative extension of the invading strand has displaced the opposing strand in the invaded duplex to a greater extent [Figure 3(c)]. At this point one of two key pathways can ensue. Firstly, the extended invading strand can dissociate from the homologous duplex and dissolve the D-loop structure, with the invaded duplex remaining intact (see section 4.3). The dissociated broken end, and the now extended 3′ tail can anneal with the ssDNA of the 3′ tail of the other side of the DSB resulting in a hydrogen bond-dependent, end-to-end reconnecting of the DSB [Figure 3(d)]. Further DNA polymerase 'fill-in' and ligation result in a full repair of the DSB with no deletion of any DNA flanking the DSB site and provided the DNA sequence of the participating homologue was identical to that of the broken chromosome (which might not be the case for inter-strand crosslink-induced breaks), this is a non-mutagenic process, with the original sequence being faithfully restored [Figure 3(d)]. Moreover, this process does not involve the cross over exchange of duplexes between participating homologues and so, provided the polymerase steps of the process were faithful, no genetic change should arise from this pathway. This is referred to as synthesis-dependent strand annealing (SDSA) (for recent reviews of DSB repair see San Filippo et al., 2008; Heyer et al., 2010; Moynahan & Jasin, 2010).

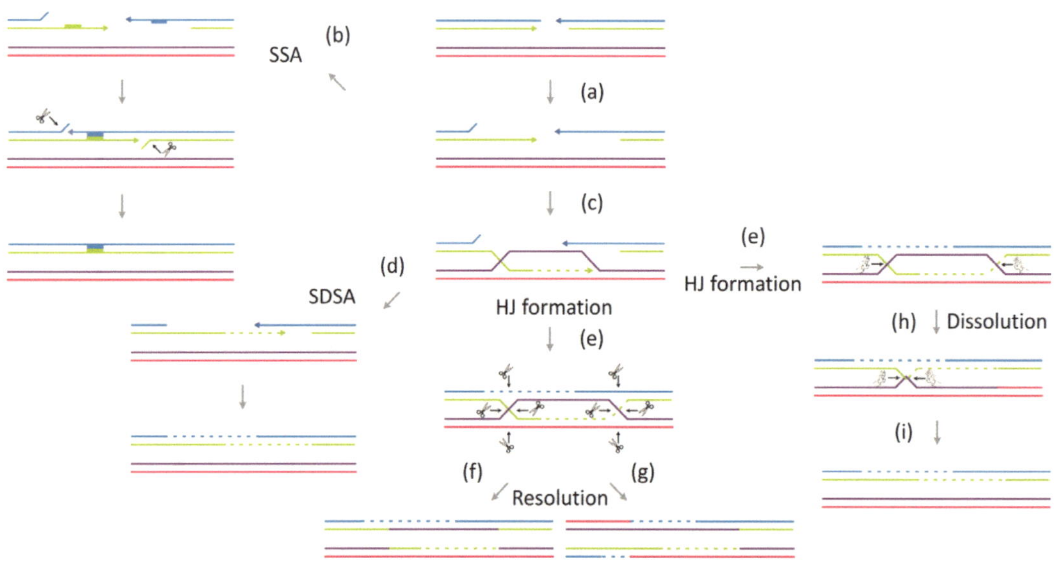

Fig. 3. Models for post replication DSB repair. (a) Following the generation of a DSB (Centre, top), the ends undergo processing by nuclease and/or helicase activity to generate single-stranded 3' ends (arrow heads). (b) Single-strand annealing (SSA): short regions of exposed complementary sequences within the single-stranded ends can anneal; this can result in an intermediate which is stable enough for repair polymerases and DNA ligase to seal the DSB, resulting in an unbroken duplex with an associated deletion of intervening DNA sequence. (c) D-loop formation: processed ends can also undergo a strand invasion reaction and displace a strand from an homologous DNA duplex to create a displacement-loop (D-loop) structure. The invading end forms the substrate for repair polymerase activity which uses the complementary strand for template-dependent chain elongation of the invading strand (dotted green line). (d) Synthesis-dependent strand annealing: the dissolving of the D-loop can result in the elongated 3' end of the invading single-stranded DNA annealing to the other 3' end of the DSB. This interaction is stable enough to permit repair polymerase and DNA ligase to 'fill-in' the gap and re-seal the duplex without cross over or deletion of break-associated sequence. (e) Double Holliday junction (dHJ) formation: the D-loop becomes extended by continuous polymerase activity at the 3' end of the invading strand. This stabilises the D-loop and second end capture occurs which results in a dHJ following further polymerase and DNA ligase activity. (f) & (g) dHJ resolution: Structure-specific nucleases cleave the dHJ resolving it, restoring two separate duplex molecules. This can be with (g) or without (f) crossing over of flanking chromatid arms, dependent upon the sites of cleavage within the two Holliday junctions. (h) & (i) dHJ dissolution: alternatively, branch migration activity mediated by helicases can 'push' the two Holliday junction together forming a hemicatenane structure; this is resolved by topoisomerase activity resulting in two separate duplexes without any associated crossing over of flanking chromatid arms.

At the D-loop stage [Figure 3(c)] a more extensive expansion of the D-loop (via polymerase activity or continued strand invasion) is thought to stabilise this structure, making its dissolution, and ultimately the SDSA pathway less likely. D-loop stabilisation results in the capture of the second 3′ end of the processed DSB; second end capture is mediated by the displaced strand of the D-loop which will have anti-parallel complementarity with the second end of the DSB (Nimonkar & Kowalczykowski, 2009). Second end capture and subsequent continued activity of repair polymerases and DNA ligase results in the formation of two adjacent Holliday junctions, often referred to as a double Holliday junction (dHJ) [Figure 3(e)]. dHJs are a covalent linkage between homologous duplexes, most likely formed between sister chromatids and have only recently been demonstrated to be recombination intermediates during DSB repair in mitotically dividing cells (Bzymek et al., 2010). For sister chromatids joined in this way to be properly segregated at anaphase the dHJ must be processed to restore two independent duplex molecules. This separation of conjoined duplexes can be mediated by one of two mechanisms. Firstly, the resolution of the dHJ by structure-specific endonucleases (see section 4.5), which can result in crossing over [Figure 3(g)] or non-cross over [Figure 3(f)] outcomes, dependent upon the position within the junction the resolving enzyme cleaves. Alternatively, the dHJ can be dissolved by helicase/translocase-like activities which branch migrates the two Holliday junctions toward each other, resulting in a structure known as a hemicatenane [Figure 3(h)]; this can then be resolved by topoisomerase activity to disconnect the duplexes [Figure 3(i)] (see Section 4.5).

3.3 Post replicative recombination-mediated repair of a single-stranded gap

The generation of gaps due to, for example, lesion skipping by the replisome, has the advantage that the replication process can largely continue without delay, leaving the gap to be repaired after the fork has passed [Figure 1D]. Such lesions are not as potentially harmful as DSBs as the covalent continuity of at least one of the strands ensures that the DNA molecule remains a continuous thread; this also has the advantage that the replication process will have produced a cohesin-dependent associated sister duplex; this ensures that there is an accessible homologous partner permitting a recombination-mediated mechanism to mediate the gap repair. Recombination mediated gap repair has some features in common with DSB repair, but also presents distinct challenges to the repair machineries of the cell. One commonality is that it needs to be initiated with a strand invasion reaction. In DSB repair this occurs after the broken ends have been processed to generate free 3' ends. In gap repair the substrates available to the recombination mediators provide some distinct options [Figure 4]. Firstly, the 3' end of the gapped strand can invade the intact replicated sister, generating a D-loop structure, thus providing a 3' ended substrate for polymerase-mediated strand extension, using the anti-parallel strand of the homologous duplex as a template [Figure 4 (a & b)]. As for the initial step in DSB repair, the D-loop can either be dissolved [Figure 4(c)] or can stabilise, permitting second strand capture, which in this case is the unreplicated strand from the parental duplex which the replisome skipped to form a dHJ [Figure 4(e)]. Dissolution of the D-loop following extension of the invading strand, results in a template-directed repair of the gap. This strand now re-anneals with the anti-parallel strand from the duplex from which it originated and following a final strand processing and re-ligation, the gap is filled [Figure 4(d)]. This processes results in any gap causing lesions to be transmitted to one of the new daughter duplexes, which can then be repaired (say by NER) [Figure 4(d)]. Alternatively, the second strand capture of by the displaced ssDNA of the stable D-loop can result in the formation of a dHJ, which can be resolved, resulting in either cross over or non-cross over products [Figure 4(f)], or dissolved [Figure 4(g)] in a similar fashion to the clearance of dHJs generated in DSB repair (see above) (Figure 3). An alternative possibility involves strand invasion of the intact sister

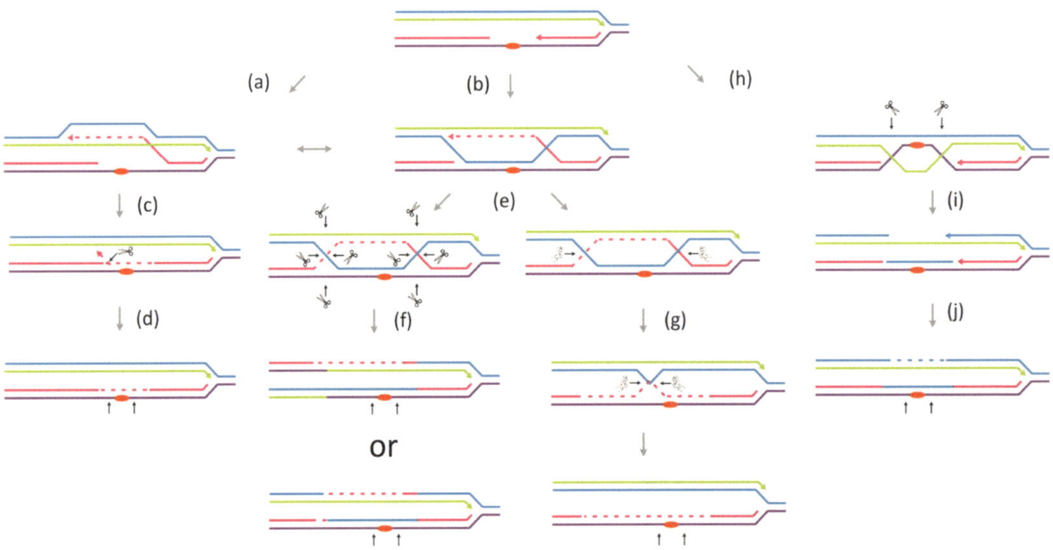

Fig. 4. Models for post replicative, recombination-mediated gap repair. Gaps may be generated by the replisome 'skipping' a lesion in one strand of the DNA (orange oval). (a & b) The 3' side of the gap (magenta arrow head) is converted to single-stranded DNA via helicase action. The single-stranded end invades the adjacent nascent sister chromatid to form a D-loop. The 3' end of the invading strand provides a substrate for DNA polymerase which extends the invading strand (dotted magenta line). The D-loop then either dissolves (a) or stabilises permitting second strand capture by the displaced D-loop (b). (c & d) If the D-loop is dissolved the newly elongated single-strand re-anneals with the single-stranded region filling the gap. Further processing by nucleases and ligase repair the gap; lesions associated with the gap remain in the new duplex and these can be acted on by other excision repair pathways (black vertical arrows flanking the lesion). (e) D-loop stabilisation associated with D-loop extension by continued DNA polymerase activity on the invading strand and second strand capture can result in a dHJ. The dHJ can be resolved by structure-specific nuclease digestion (f) or by dissolution (g). Resolution can potentially result in crossing over of the daughter duplexes, dependent upon the strand specificity of the dHJ cleavage reactions (f). Dissolution of the dHJ does not result in crossing over (g). (h-j) Strand invasion of the fully replicated duplex by the lesion-containing ssDNA gap results in a structure which provides a substrate for structure-specific nuclease attack (i). This results in a duplex at the site of the lesion and the gap is transferred to the undamaged daughter duplex and is subsequently filled by repair polymerases (j).

duplex by the ssDNA within the gap [Figure 4(h)]. Processing of this intermediate structure will result in a new duplex being generated at the previously gapped lesion site and a new lesion-free gap in the opposite duplex, which can now be filled by repair polymerase activity [Figure 4 (i & j)] (for recent reviews see San Filippo et al., 2008; Heyer et al., 2010; Moynahan & Jasin, 2010).

3.4 Recombination-mediated repair of collapsed DNA replication forks

When replication fork stabilisation mechanisms fail and forks collapse, there is a partial or full dissociation of the *trans*-acting factors required to continue the progression of DNA replication. This results in a fork structure which is stalled and incapable of re-associating with the factors needed for continued replication. The distinct events which can create collapsed forks (see above) are likely to provide failed replicative structures which present subtly distinct substrates to the recombination and replication re-start programs, however, the ultimate requirement will be to re-establish a functional DNA replication fork in all cases.

One way in which a failed fork can be processed is to convert it to a one-sided DSB [Figure 5(a)]. This could be via the action of structure-specific nucleases such as Mus81-Eme1 (see below). Such DSBs would then be acted upon by recombination factors to generate a new DNA replication fork (Section 3.1) [Figure 5(a)]. Alternatively, the failed fork can undergo a fork regression and the nascent strands of the daughter duplexes can anneal with one another to form a region of duplex DNA which protrudes away from the template duplex [Figure 5(b & c)] (Higgins et al., 1976; Sogo et al., 2000). This regressed fork structure is often referred to as a 'chicken foot' structure due to its passing resemblance to a three toed chicken's foot [Figure 5(b & c)]. The chicken foot structure can itself potentially be cleaved by nuclease activity to generate a one-sided DSB [Figure 5(d)], or it can undergo a number of distinct routes of processing; the processing of the structure can be dependent upon the

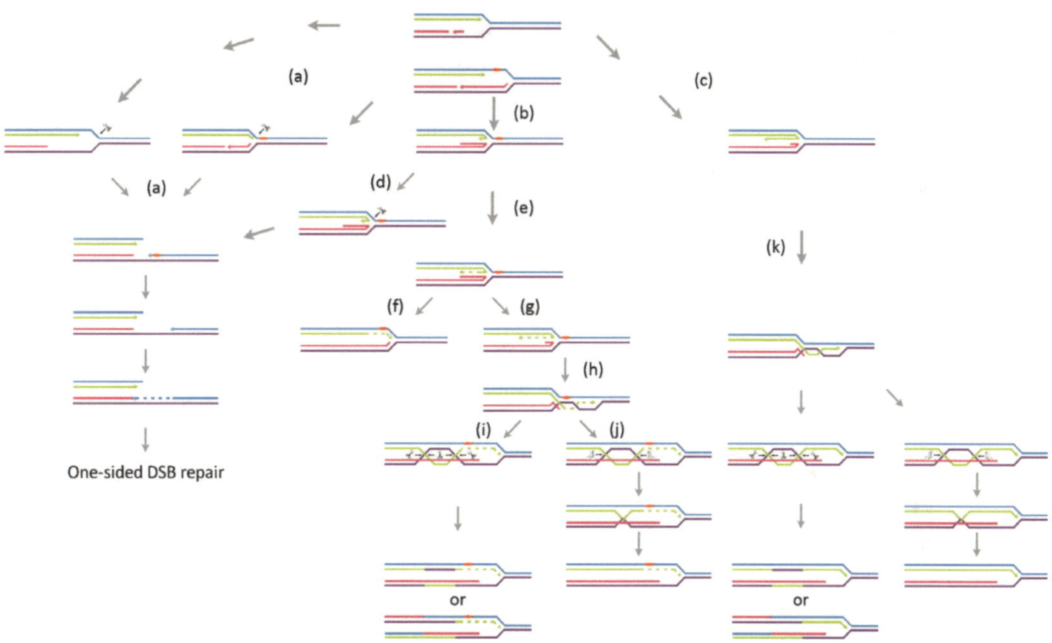

Fig. 5. Models for the recombinogenic repair of collapsed DNA replication forks. See the main text for full details (Section 3.4). The figure shows two distinct types of collapsed forks; these are schematically represented as the top two structures in the image. The top structure is a fork which has collapsed without encountering a DNA damage lesion (for example, another replication barrier or a helicase-polymerase uncoupling). The lower structure represents a fork which has collapsed due to a DNA damage abduct on one strand of the DNA (small red oval). The large grey arrows indicate the possible routes to repair / fork recovery. Holliday junction resolution is indicated by black arrows with a scissor symbol; Holliday junction dissolution is represented by black arrows with a pushing hand symbol.

structural configuration of the duplex generated by the re-annealing of the nascent daughter strands (the middle toe of the foot). This can have either a 5′ [Figure 5(b)] or 3′ [Figure 5(c)] ssDNA tail, depending upon how it was formed; for example, if lagging strand synthesis extends beyond the position reached by the leading strand, then a 5′ single-stranded tail can be generated on fork reversion [Figure 5(b)]; however, if the leading strand extended beyond the lagging strand at fork collapse the reversion will result in a tail with protruding single-stranded DNA with a free 3′ end [Figure 5(c)]. Duplex regions of nascent daughter strands which result in flush ends (no significant overhang of single-stranded DNA) can potentially be recognised as a DSB and processed to generate single-stranded 3' DNA ends [Figure 5(g)].

A reversed fork with a 5′ single-stranded overhang on the protruding nascent strand duplex [Figure 5(b)] can provide a substrate for polymerase mediated extension of the free 3′ end using the 5′ terminating strand as a template (sometimes referred to as template switching); this will result in a flush or near flush end to the nascent strand duplex [Figure 5(e)]. If the original fork collapse was caused by a lesion in leading strand template [Figure 5(b)], then re-reversal of the chicken foot following polymerase activity will result in the re-annealing of the leading strand with the 3' end now positioned beyond the lesion on the original leading strand template [Figure 5(f)]; thus the generation of a chicken foot intermediate provided a means to generate a new template (the nascent lagging strand) from which the leading strand could be extended to ultimately permit lesion bypass upon reversion of the chicken foot [Figure 5(f)]. Alternatively, if the flush ended duplex generated from annealed / filled in nascent strands is recognised by end processing factors, the 5' end can be resected exposing a 3' single-stranded tail in the nascent strands duplex [figure 5(g)]. This free 3' end now acts as a substrate for recombinases which mediate the invasion of this strand into the template duplex at a position ahead of the position at which the fork failed [Figure 5(h)]. Processing by DNA polymerase and ligase activities results in the formation of a dHJ structure behind the position of the strand invasion, which now becomes a newly established DNA replication fork [Figure 5(i &j)]. As for dHJ structures generated in gap repair or following two-sided DSB repair, the dHJ can be processed via a resolution (cross over or non-cross over) route [Figure 5(i)] or dissolution route [Figure 5(j)]. Either of these routes provides the fork the ability to bypass lesions on the original parental template which may have been an impediment to the progression of the fork.

If the original fork failed leaving a leading strand extended relative to the lagging strand, then reversion of the fork will directly generate a single-stranded tail to the duplex of nascent strand with a free 3' end [Figure 5(c)]. This provides a substrate directly for a recombinase-mediated strand invasion to ultimately re-establish a fork following dHJ processing. In this case, there is no template for further extension of the nascent leading strand prior to strand invasion from the chicken foot state, and so this is not a lesion bypass mechanism, rather a mechanism for re-establishment of a collapsed fork. Again, the dHJ structure can be resolved or dissolved, with the former potentially generating cross over products [Figure 5(k)] (for recent reviews of recombination-mediated fork recovery see Aguilera & Gómez-González, 2008; Allen et al., 2011; Branzei & Foiani, 2010; Petermann & Helleday, 2010).

4. Mediators of recombinational repair of failed DNA replication forks

The collapse of replication forks or the generation of recombinogenic lesions such as strand breakages can arise for a number of reasons and can generate a range of distinct substrates for subsequent recombinognic repair (Aguilera & Gómez-González, 2008; Budzowska & Kanaar, 2009; Branzei & Foiani, 2010; Peterman & Helleday, 2010; Allen et al., 2011). There are an array of factors which recognise these lesions, often with a strong substrate specificity, and there are also a number of distinct factors which can act upon processed substrates and the intermediates from which they form. Extensive studies have now started to shed light on this complexity and clear pictures are emerging for the role some of these factors may play in the models proposed for recombination-mediated repair of lesions generated during DNA replication (Section 3). Here we will overview some of the key factors which have been associated with these models.

4.1 DSBs: the first response

When DNA damage occurs, it is recognised by factors which signal to checkpoint pathways prompting the recruitment of other proteins which, in turn, initiate the repair process. In the case of DSBs one of the first responses is the alteration of the modification status of a histone variant known as H2AX (Fernandez-Capetillo et al., 2004; Ismail & Hendzel, 2008; Lukas & Bartek, 2009). This histone has a tyrosine residue (Y142) in the carboxy tail which, in the absence of DNA damage is phosphorylated by subunits of the H2AX interacting chromatin remodelling complex WICH (Poot et al., 2004; Bozhenok et al., 2002). On DNA damage this residue is de-phosphorylated by Eya1 and Eya3 phosphatases (Cook et al., 2009), permitting the phosphorylation of H2AX serine 139 (S139) by the ATM checkpoint kinase (Rogakou et al., 1998; Burma et al., 2001). This ATM-dependent modification is required for the binding of MDC1 a protein which recruits the MRN complex, one of the key mediators of DSB end resection (see below) (Stucki et al., 2005; Lukas et al., 2004; Stucki & Jackson, 2006). Recruitment of MDC1 is concomitant with the recruitment of RNF8, which functions in consort with the E3 ubiquitin conjugase Ubc13 to ubiquitinate histones H2A and H2B at break sites (Huen et al., 2007; Kolas et al., 2007; Mailand et al., 2007; Zhao et al., 2007; Wu et al., 2009a). These modified histones are recognised by RAP80, a co-constituent of a complex containing the breast cancer susceptibility gene BRCA1 (reviewed in Yun & Hiom, 2009b; Wu et al., 2010). The role of BRCA1 at broken ends remains unclear (Yun & Hiom, 2009b; Wu et al., 2010), but in combination with another protein, CtIP, it regulates the repair pathway choice between NHEJ and homologous recombination in a cell cycle-dependent fashion, possibly through the modulation of the MRN resection complex (see below; Yun & Hiom, 2009a). It has also been postulated to assist another breast cancer susceptibility gene, BRCA2, to stabilise the formation of filaments of the strand-exchange mediator Rad51 onto 3' ssDNA ends (see below; reviewed in Wu et al., 2010), as well as potentially modulating the activity of the MRN complex for end processing (see below; Greenberg et al., 2006).

Replication protein A (RPA) is a heterotrimer which is also recruited to ssDNA at break sites, although the order of recruitment of some of the *trans* acting factors to break sites remains uncertain. RPA plays central roles in a number of DNA processing pathways, including normal DNA replication (Oakley & Patrick, 2010). The role of RPA is thought to be to maintain ssDNA in a conformation which permits other factors to access ssDNA devoid of intra-strand hydrogen bonding, although RPA also seems to play a central role in recruiting and orchestrating the various factors capable of repair processing of ssDNA; moreover, RPA-ssDNA complexes at breaks are required for checkpoint activation (Zou & Elledge, 2003; Binz et al., 2004; Anantha & Borowiec, 2009; Oakley & Patrick, 2010). In response to DNA damage the mid-sized subunit of RPA, RPA2, undergoes phosphorylation by the checkpoint machinery and it is proposed that this phosphorylation switches the activity of RPA from one related to normal DNA replication to one in which it recruits DNA repair factors to ssDNA (Binz et al., 2004; Anantha & Borowiec, 2009; Oakley & Patrick, 2010). One of the factors RPA recruits is Rad52, which assists the loading of the strand invasion recombinase Rad51 (see below) to ssDNA (Park et al., 1996; Jackson et al., 2002; Plate et al., 2008). Rad51-mediated strand invasion and the correct association of Rad51 with ssDNA generated at broken ends is dependent upon the correct removal of RPA, which is dependent upon Rad52 and RPA phosphorylation (New et al., 1998; Wu et al., 2005; Anantha et al., 2007; Sleeth et al., 2007; Vassin et al., 2009; Deng et al., 2009; Sugiyama & Kantake, 2009). So, phosphorylated RPA plays a critical role in orchestrating the early events at break sites to ultimately favour a recombination-mediated repair pathway.

Homologous recombination-mediated repair of a broken end requires the resection of the 5' end (see above). This is mediated by a combination of helicase and nuclease activity and currently two pathways are proposed for extensive 5' end resection (Huertas, 2010; Mimitou & Symington, 2011). Both pathways are thought to be initiated by the heterotrimeric Mre11-Rad50-Nbs1(Xrs2 in *Saccharomyces cerevisiae*) (MRN / MRX) complex, along with its partner protein CtIP (also called RBBP8; Sae2 *in S. cerevisiae*), which are recruited to the ends by MDC1 (see above). The nuclease activity of Mre11 then mediates the removal of a short oligonucleotide from the 5' end (Neale et al., 2005; Zhu et al., 2008; Shim et al., 2010; Mimitou & Symington, 2008; 2011). This initial end processing makes the end refractory to the Ku proteins which mediate a non-homologous DNA end joining DSB repair pathway, which is more prevalent in G_1 and so is less relevant to replication-associated breakage (Mimitou & Symington, 2010); moreover, initial end processing paves a way for the two distinct and redundant pathways, in which the MRN(X) complex plays a structural role, to enhance the more extended processing of the 5' end. Indeed it has been postulated that MRN-CtIP recruits the mediators of the more extensive resection to the break sites (Mimitou & Symington, 2011). There appears to be species-specific distinctions for the importance of the initial short resection; in fission yeast and mouse cells this seems to play a more critical role than the primary resection event in *S. cerevisiae* (Limbo et al., 2007; Williams et al., 2008). Both pathways that mediate further extensive end processing are important to prevent unscheduled chromosomal changes, and it has been demonstrated that when both are compromised there are significant increases in *de novo* telomere generation at DSB sites (Chung et al., 2010; Lydeard et al., 2010). The first pathway for more extensive 5' resection involves the action of the 5'-3' exonuclease Exo1, whilst the second requires the action of the Sgs1-Top3-Rmi1 (STR) complex in concert with RPA (see above) and the endonuclease Dna2 (Mimitou & Symington, 2008; Zhu et al., 2008; Gravel et al., 2008; Nimonkar et al., 2011). Sgs1 is the *S. cerevisiae* orthologue of the mammalian RecQ-like helicase BLM (Chu & Hickson, 2009; Bernstein et al., 2010; Monnat, 2010). Reconstitution experiments appear to demonstrate that the RecQ-like helicase (Sgs1/BLM) is required to first unwind the duplex and the resection is then completed by the endonucleolytic activity of Dna2, with Top3-Rmi1 playing a non-essential stimulatory role (Gravel et al., 2008; Cejka et al., 2010a; 2010b; Nicolette et al., 2010; Niu et al., 2010; Nimonkar et al., 2011); in this case the role of Top3 differs from its role in Holliday junction dissolution function, where the Top3 catalytic activity is essential (Niu et al., 2010). In addition to driving the nucleolytic degradation of the 5' end, it has also been proposed that CtIP (Sae2) serves to bind to the 3' end to protect it from degradation (Hartsuiker et al., 2009; Nicolette et al., 2010; Mimitou & Symington, 2011).

Many of the studies which have resulted in delineating the pathways of events at DSBs for subsequent repair by homologous recombination have been carried out using ionizing radiation-induced DSBs or other means of generating DSBs. The relevance of these studies to the mechanisms of repair of DSBs which are generated by DNA replication associated events remains uncertain. Whilst it seems unlikely that these pathways will differ greatly, distinctions can be envisaged; for example, DSBs generated in non-replicating chromatin might present a chromatin substrate which is distinct from the chromatin in proximity to the replisome. Given the fact that many of the early signalling and recruitment events are linked directly to histone modifications (see above), then there may be unique replication-associated mechanisms which require elucidation.

4.2 Strand invasion

The repair of 3' ssDNA at ends of broken chromosomes or ssDNA regions generated via a replication discontinuity or fork regression by homologous recombination mechanisms need these ssDNA regions to undergo a strand invasion of a homologous duplex (Figures 2-4). This is mediated by the conserved Rad51 recombinase which is the eukaryote orthologue of the bacterial RecA protein (Sung, 1994; Baumann et al., 1996). Rad51 association with ssDNA involves a range of accessory factors which aid the removal of other ssDNA binding proteins such as RPA, which prevents ssDNA forming secondary structures which would inhibit Rad51 nucleation. Moreover, these accessory factors assist Rad51 in achieving ssDNA binding and nucleoprotein filament formation whilst competing with a range of other factors within an environment where many proteins are vying to access the ssDNA. The ordering and precise function of many of these accessory mediator proteins remains uncertain (San Filippo et al., 2008; Lisby & Rothstein, 2009; Heyer et al., 2010). There are many distinct classes of mediator function and how they intercalate with one another also remains unclear. The first of the mediators are the Rad51 paralogues, which form two distinct complexes. These proteins share core homology with Rad51, and whilst they can form functional dimers, they do not undergo nucleation into continuous filaments and they cannot independently mediate strand exchange. In humans there are five of these paralogues, RAD51B-D and XRCC2-3, and in budding yeast there are four which form two distinct complexes, Rad55-Rad57 and Shu1-Psy3 (Heyer et al., 2010). The fission yeast, *Schizosaccharomyces pombe,* also possesses multiple Rad51 (Rhp51 in *S. pombe*) paralogues, along with an additional Rad51 mediator, Sws1, suggesting that their mechanisms of action are likely to be highly conserved (Grishchuk & Kohli, 2003; Khasanov et al., 2004; Martin et al., 2006). In addition to these Rad51 paralogues, fission yeast and mammalian cells have another pair of Rad51 mediators, Swi5 and Sfr1 (Akamatsu et al., 2003; 2007; Haruta et al., 2006; Khasanov et al., 2008; Akamatsu & Jasin, 2010). *S. cerevisiae* also has orthologues of both of these proteins, but these appear to function in a meiosis-specific fashion (McKee & Kleckner, 1997; Tsubouchi & Roeder, 2004; Hayase et al., 2004).

A second mediator, Rad52 (Rad22 in *S. pombe*), oligomerises into a toroidal structure (Shinohara et al., 1998; Stasiak et al., 2000; Ranatunga et al., 2001) and interacts with Rad51. It is required for Rad51 loading onto ssDNA and for RPA removal (for review, see San Filippo et al., 2008; Mortensen et al., 2009). Much of the work to elucidate the role of Rad52 has come from budding yeast and the importance of Rad52 as a Rad51 mediator in mammalian cells remains unclear but it appears to have only a minor role as a mediator in more complex systems (Fujimori et al., 2001; Symington, 2002; San Filippo et al., 2008).

Rad52 also plays a critical role in SSA (Figure 3b), and break induced replication (for reviews, see McEachen & Haber, 2006; Llorente et al., 2008). During SSA it is postulated to mediate the stable formation of the SSA intermediate in a Rad51-independent fashion (Mortensen et al., 1996; Nimonkar et al., 2009; reviewed in Symington, 2002; San Filippo et al., 2008; Nimonkar & Kowalczykowski, 2009).

The third Rad51 mediator is the breast cancer susceptibility gene 2 (BRCA2; also called FANCD1). BRCA2 interacts with Rad51 (Scully et al., 1997; Sharan et al., 1997; Carreira & Kowalczykowski, 2009), which it does via 8 BRC domains, with some of the BRC domains preventing Rad51 nucleation on dsDNA and others aiding the loading on ssDNA; thus it is proposed that BRCA2 goes to the ds-ssDNA junctions preventing nucleation of Rad51 onto dsDNA whilst positively influencing ssDNA association (Yang et al., 2005; Carreira et al., 2009; Jensen et al., 2010). It has been demonstrated that this can occur at the 3' or 5' junctions with equal efficiency and thus it is postulated that BRCA2 plays an equal role in both end and gap repair as gapped DNA would have ss-dsDNA junctions with both 3' and 5' ends. Intriguingly, BRCA2 also appears to protect regions of ssDNA from MRN-mediated degradation at stalled replication forks. It is proposed that BRCA2 functions to inhibit the Mre11 destruction of the reversed forks which are intermediates in some stalled fork recovery pathways (Figure 5). This represents a novel function for BRCA2 in prevention of forming recombinogenic lesions, rather than mediating their repair (Schlacher et al., 2011).

An interacting partner of BRCA2 has recently been identified, partner and localizer of BRCA2 (PALB2; also called FANCN; Tischkowitz & Xia, 2010), which serves to assist BRCA2 localisation to the sites of DNA damage (Sy et al., 2009; Zhang et al., 2009a; 2009b). PALB2 also associates with BRCA1 and it is proposed that BRCA1 stabilises BRCA2, which in turn mediates Rad51 nucleation to ssDNA indicating a direct functional link between BRCA1and BRCA2 (Zhang et al., 2009a; 2009b; Moynahan & Jasin, 2010). BRCA1 seems to play an additional role as it associates with the BRIP1 helicase (also termed FANCJ / BACH1) which has a poorly defined role in homologous recombination, but has been proposed to dissolve non-canonical DNA structures such as G quadruplexes which may be refractory to normal replication and homologous recombination processing (Wu et al., 2008; Moynahan & Jasin, 2010). BRIP1 may play a key role in regulating levels of homologous recombination as it also has the potential to inhibit D-loop formation when over expressed and so could be an anti-recombinase (see below) (Sommers et al., 2009).

In addition to assisting BRCA2 in mediating Rad51 nucleation, PALB2 has also been demonstrated to enhance D-loop formation by Rad51 in conjunction with another Rad51 interacting protein, Rad51AP1 (Dray et al., 2010; Buisson et al., 2010). Whilst RAD51AP1 was first identified as a Rad51 interacting protein over ten years ago (Kovalenko et al, 1997; Mizuta et al., 1997), evidence has only more recently been put forward to demonstrate its function in enhancing Rad51-mediated strand invasion activity (Wiese et al., 2007; Modesti et al., 2007). PALB2 also interacts with MRG15, a component of a histone acteyltransferase-deacetylase complex implicated in both transcriptional regulation and DNA repair processes providing further clues as to how these proteins may interact with DNA in the context of chromatin (Hayakawa et al., 2010 and references therein).

The Rad54 motor protein is another conserved protein which assists in Rad51 function. However it plays a "Jack of all trades" role and seems to have other distinct functions in recombination (reviewed in Tan et al., 2003; Heyer et al., 2006; Symington & Heyer, 2006; Mazin et al., 2010). It has an ATP-dependent DNA translocase activity (with no measurable helicase activity) (Thomä et al., 2005; Amitani et al., 2006), and functionally interacts with

Rad51 to stimulate Rad51-mediated strand exchange and heteroduplex extension (Clever et al., 1997; Petukhova et al., 1998; Raschle et al., 2004; Solinger et al., 2001). Rad54 is a Snf2 family member and it has ATP-dependent chromatin remodelling activity which is thought to function to assist the Rad51 recombinase by either clearing recombinogenic lesions of histones, or remodelling the histones in the intact homologous duplex to be invaded and thereby assisting strand invasion / homology searching (Aleviadis & Kadonaga, 2002; Alexeev et al., 2003; Jaskelioff et al., 2003; Wolner & Peterson, 2005; Kwon et al., 2007; Zhang et al., 2007). Among its other activities Rad54 also has the ability to disrupt Rad51-generated D-loops via a structure branch migration activity (Burgreev et al., 2007), although this apparent paradox might simply relate to a requirement to switch from a D-loop intermediate to a preferred SDSA pathway to avoid crossover outcomes [Figure 3(d)] (Heyer et al., 2010). The switch between pro- to anti-recombinase may be regulated in a temporal fashion and may be regulated by distinct modifications / interactions associated with Rad54 (Mazin et al., 2010).

More recently, two new factors have been found to be essential for the proper loading of Rad51 to the sites of replication stress induced ssDNA in human cells. These factors are MMS22L (Mms22 in *S. cerevisiae*) and TONSL (NFKBIL2) (O'Donnell et al., 2010; Duro et al., 2010). Their depletion results in a failure to load Rad51 in response to replicative stress, despite end processing occurring, indicating that this dimeric factor works at the stage of regulating Rad51 activity, although the exact mechanism of their action remains unclear (O'Donnell et al., 2010; Duro et al., 2010). Consistent with a central role in delineating the homologous recombination pathway choice following replication fork stalling, both Mms22 and its binding partner Mms1 are required for recovery from genotoxic agents which perturb DNA replication in both fission and budding yeasts (Hryciw et al., 2002; Duro et al., 2008; Dovey et al., 2009; Vejrup-Hansen et al., 2011).

Rad51 forms a filament on ssDNA and this structure mediates the invasion of the homologous duplex in an ATP-dependent reaction (Holthausen et al. 2010). Stable nucleation progression requires an initial 4-5 Rad51 monomers to bind to the ssDNA; this process does not require the hydrolysis of ATP, but ATP binding does influence the reaction (van der Heijden et al., 2007). The exact mode of homologue searching remains unclear (for example, see Holthausen et al., 2010). Once D-loops are formed, they provide intermediates which can drive the synthesis-dependent repair of gapped or broken regions, paving the way for subsequent processing of the various intermediates that this key, initial event may have formed (Figures 2-5). Products of these events can be re-established forks, SDSA products, dHJs and break-induced replication initiating structures.

4.3 Anti-recombinase activities

Given the complexity of eukaryote genomes and the highly repetitive nature of some, there are instances where it is beneficial to the organism to avoid recombination pathways which might have potentially detrimental outcomes if it is permitted to proceed, or to proceed down a crossover proficient pathway. This is illustrated by Bloom's Syndrome patients who have a mutation in an anti-recombinase activity (BLM helicase), giving rise to measurably elevated levels of inter-sister chromatid exchange events and higher levels of genome instability (German et al., 1965). The recombination-mediated repair of breakage associated with replication is more likely to follow a non-crossover route via non-crossover resolution/dissolution of more complex recombination intermediates, such as dHJs and hemi-catanane-like structures, or via a SDSA pathway. A group of so called "anti-recombinase" proteins have been identified which can serve to prevent unwanted and ectopic recombination events and to direct recombination down specific, non-crossover lineages, such as SDSA [for example, see Figure3(d)]. Anti-recombinases are proposed to function at two key stages. Firstly they can disrupt the Rad51 presynaptic filament, thus preventing the generation of D-loop intermediates. Alternatively, they can serve to dissolve D-loop structures prior to them stabilising and generating more complex recombination intermediates capable of driving crossover events. These activities are largely mediated by a group of helicases and the study of their roles as anti-recombinases is made more complex by the fact that there is a high degree of functional redundancy and that they possess both pro- and anti-recombination activities, most likely linked to substrate and temporal specificity. The known anti-recombinase helicases are the Srs2 family (budding yeast and fission yeast), the RecQ family (conserved, but five family members have been identified in humans: BLM, WRN, RECQL1, RECQL4 and RECQL5), Fbh1 family (fission yeast and humans), FANCM family [fission yeast (Fml1/2), budding yeast (Mph1) and humans] and RTEL and BRIP1 (FANCJ) (humans; XPD family helicases) (for reviews, see Branzei & Foiani, 2007c; Chu & Hickson, 2009; Whitby, 2010; White, 2009; Wu et al., 2009; Bernstein et al., 2010;Marini & Krejci, 2010; Monnat, 2010; Yusufzai & Kadonaga, 2011). In addition to the helicases, the Rad54 translocase also has the ability to dissolve recombination intermediates and has potential anti-recombinase activity (see above; Bugreev et al., 2007).

How these multiple factors are co-ordinated /uniquely specified to distinct damage sites is poorly understood; however, SUMOylation of the replisome component PCNA is known to be required for the recruitment of at least one anti-recombinase, Srs2, indicating an intimate link between residual replication mediators and regulators of replication recovery pathways (Stelter & Ultrich, 2003; Papouli et al., 2005; Pfander et al., 2005)

4.4 Regression of stalled / damaged forks

A number of the pathways postulated for the recovery of a DNA replication fork from a terminal breakdown or for lesion bypass require the regression of the replication fork to make a four way structure, the chicken foot, which has structural similarities to a Holliday junction (Figure 5; see above). As for anti-recombination activities a number of potential players have been posited to mediate fork regression. Firstly, the human RecQ orthologue, BLM, which is also proposed to function in Holliday junction dissolution (see below), has been demonstrated to possess fork regression activity (Ralf et al., 2006), although the physiological relevance of this is difficult to discern.

Secondly, extensive studies have indicated that the FANCM helicase/translocase has the ability to regress stalled forks into the four way structure (Gari et al, 2008a; 2008b; Sun et al., 2008). Intriguingly, FANCM has been demonstrated to form a functional bridging role between the BLM pathway and FANC pathways, suggesting that distinct potential fork reversion activities have a close association in response to stalled replication forks (Deans & West, 2009). The histone-fold protein dimer MHF1-MHF2 has recently been identified as a co-factor for FANCM (Thompson & Jones, 2010; Singh et al., 2010; Yan et al., 2010); this factor has been implicated in centromere kinetochore function (Amano et al., 2009) which has lead to the suggestion that FANMC activity is required to prevent functional genomic regions, made up of repeat sequences which may be highly refractory to DNA replication, from becoming highly unstable (Yan et al., 2010). However, a recent model has been proposed in which recombination triggered by modulation of the progression of a DNA replication fork may play a functional role in centromere dynamics and may also account for the specific requirement for the FANCM co-factors to associate with centromereic regions (McFarlane & Humphreys, 2010).

The third pathway proposed to play a role in fork regression is mediated by another Snf2 family helicase/translocase of *S. cerevisiae*, Rad5, which has previously been implicated in translesion synthesis (for review, see Unk et al., 2010). Rad5 has E3 ubiquitin ligase activity, which is mediated through a RING finger domain (Ulrich & Jentsch, 2000). Rad5 can mediate fork regression (Blastyák et al., 2007) and four way structures observed in wild-type *S. cerevisae* cells, in response to fork stalling agents, do not accumulate in Rad5-deficient cells (Minca & Kowalski, 2010). It has been proposed that Rad5 may regress a stalled fork and that this provides a substrate for recombination-mediated processing to re-establish a functional fork (Figure 5) (Yusufzai & Kadonaga, 2011). Mammalian cells have two putative Rad5 orthologues, the helices-like transcription factor (HLTF) and SNF2 histone linker PHD RING helicase (SHPRH) (Unk et al., 2010). To date fork regression activity has been demonstrated for HLTF, but not SHRPH (Blastyák et al., 2010). Both HLTF and SHRPH possess E3 ubiquitin ligase activity and they mediate the polyubiquitination of PCNA at stalled forks, indicating a role for these proteins in modulation of replisome factors in response to stalled forks (Motegi et al., 2008), although another, independent PCNA ubiquitination pathway has also been demonstrated indicating possible functional redundancy (Krijger et al., 2011). Additionally, this paralogue pair has been demonstrated to have distinct ubiquitination activities to regulate unique mutation avoidance mechanisms (Lin et al., 2011).

Recently, the ATP-dependent annealing helicase SMARCAL1 (SWI/SNF-related, matrix-associated, actin-dependent regulator of chromatin, sub-family a-like 1) / HARP (HepA-related protein) (Yusufzai & Kadonaga, 2008), which is associated with Human Schimke Immune-osseous Dysplasia (SIOD) (Boerkoel et al., 2002), has been implicated as a potential fork regression helicase (Bansbach et al., 2009; Ciccia et al., 2009; Driscoll & Cimprich, 2009; Yuan et al., 2009; Yusufzai et al., 2009). It is proposed that SMARCAL1/HARP is recruited to stalled forks via an active direct recruitment interaction with RPA where it serves to reduce the levels of potentially deleterious ssDNA via a strand annealing mechanism (Driscoll & Cimprich, 2009; Yusufzai & Kadonaga, 2011). A second strand annealing helicase activity has recently been identified, AH2 (annealing helicase 2) suggesting there could be a family of annealing helicases which play a role in genome stability regulation, although no direct link between AH2 and replication fork protection / regression has yet been demonstrated (Yusufzai & Kadonaga, 2010).

In addition to the above factors the Rad54 translocase can mediate branch migration of Holliday junction-like structures (Mazin et al., 2010). It has been proposed that, in combination with Rad51, it is capable of mediating a fork regression (Bugreev et al., 2011). Interestingly, Rad54 also exhibits interactions with the structure-specific nuclease Mus81 (reviewed in Mazin et al., 2010), which has been postulated to cleave regressed forks (see below), this might point to failed forks being highly dynamic and promiscuous for which pathway is ultimately 'chosen' for fork repair (Figure 5). Rad54 is likely to lie at the centre of such fluidity, as it can serve at multiple stages of the recombination processes associated with stalled fork recovery possessing both pro- and anti-recombination activities (Tan et al., 2003; Heyer et al., 2006; Mazin et al, 2010).

Whilst these various helicase/translocase activities have been associated with the regression of forks, to date no activity has been proposed to revert the regressed four way structure to reform the replication fork, although this role could be mediated by the Rad54 protein

(Bugreev et al., 2011). It is assumed that such activity is required, but it is also postulated that the regressed fork, the chicken foot, can provide a substrate for structure-specific nucleases. Such nucleases could cleave the regressed fork forming a substrate for further recombination-mediated fork restoration / repair pathways (Figures 5). One conserved candidate for this cleavage is the Mus81-Eme1(Mms4) dimer, which has nucleolytic activity on a range of structures which could be generated by fork regression (Osman & Whitby, 2007). However, there are other structure-specific nucleases, namely the Slx1-Slx4 (SLX4-BTBD12) and Gen1 (Yen1) nucleases which have been demonstrated to have the ability to cleave structures which may be generated by stalled or regressed forks (reviewed in Svendsen & Harper, 2010; Schwartz & Heyer, 2011).

4.5 Holliday junction resolution / dissolution

Whilst Holliday junction resolution in bacteria is mediated by a relatively simple single protein mechanism, identifying the activities which are responsible for the processing of Holliday junctions in eukaryotes has revealed a significantly more complex picture. However, from this complexity key players are starting to emerge which are capable of mediating Holliday junction resolution or dissolution (Mankouri & Hickson, 2007; Schwartz & Heyer, 2011; Svendsen & Harper, 2010). As for other mechanisms in the repair of replication-associated damage, it is clear there is a degree of functional redundancy between these pathways (for example, see Weschsler et al., 2011). dHJs can undergo classical endonucleolytic resolution, or they can alternatively undergo dissolution (Figures 3-5); however, single Holliday junctions, are incapable of being processed down the dissolution route. Unlike resolution, dissolution cannot result in crossing over and dissolution does not require a classical Holliday junction resolvase activity.

The first of the potential Holliday junction resolution activities is provided by the Mus81 structure-specific endonuclease. This works in concert with a partner protein Eme1 (Mms4) (Osman & Whitby, 2007; Ciccia et al., 2008). It is required for the recovery from replicative stress and Mus81-deficient cells are sensitive to agents which cause replication-associated DNA damage (for examples, see Boddy et al., 2001; Roseeaulin et al., 2008; Svendsen et al., 2009) and exhibit high levels of chromosomal re-arrangements during normal mitotic proliferation (for example, see Dendouga et al., 2005). Mus81 has been demonstrated to have Holliday junction resolution activity, possibly via a nick and counter nick mechanism (Boddy et al., 2000; Gaillard et al., 2003), but conclusive evidence that this activity is responsible for its role in maintaining genome stability in response to replication fork failures is difficult to discern for two reasons. Firstly, Mus81 has the ability to cleave other, non- Holliday junction structures during the processing of substrates generated by replication-associated DNA damage (Ciccia et al., 2003; Osman et al., 2003; Whitby et al., 2003; Fricke et al., 2005). Secondly, Mus81 does not show a particularly strong preference for Holliday junctions with continuous strands and favours structures which resemble nicked Holliday junctions (for example, see Fricke et al., 2005), although Mus81 modifications / interaction might favour Holliday junction specificity *in vivo* (Osman & Whitby, 2007; Schwartz & Heyer, 2011). Interestingly, Mus81 has been demonstrated to interact with Rad54, which has Holliday junction branch migrating capabilities; this might serve to indicate that targeting of Mus81 specifically to Holliday structures can be linked to early events within the repair process via the central regulator Rad54 (Interthal & Heyer, 2000).

The second Holliday junction resolvase activity is the Slx1-Slx4 complex (Fekairi et al., 2009; Svendsen et al,. 2009), which has been demonstrated to mediate the repair of failed replication forks (Frickle & Brill, 2003; Deng et al., 2005) and, as for many replciation repair factor genes, is implicated in the cancer predisposition disorder Fanconia anemia (Crossan et al., 2011). As for Mus81, Slx1-4 has structure-specific endonucelase activity which does not favour fixed Holliday junctions, leading to early suggestions that they played no role in Holliday junction resolution (Fricke & Brill, 2003). Later work has now demonstrated the ability of Slx1-4 complex to cleave Holliday junctions (Fekairi et al., 2009; Munoz et al., 2009; Svendsen et al,. 2009), although the physiological significance of these studies remains controversial (Schwartz & Heyer, 2011).

Thirdly, Gen1 (Yen1) was identified as a *bona fide* Holliday junction resolvease (Ip et al., 2008; Rass et al., 2010), although it too cleaves model replication fork intermediates (Ip et al., 2008; Rass et al., 2010). Human and yeast cells dysfunctional for Gen1(Yen1) do not have measurable phenotypes indicating a role in genome maintenance (for example, see Svendsen et al., 2009), but further analysis demonstrates a degree of redundancy with other proposed Holliday junction processing pathways (Blanco et al., 2010; Tay & Wu, 2010; Ho et al., 2010; Weschsler et al., 2011). The failure of Gen1(Yen1)-deficient cells to exhibit any significant defect in genome stability pathways, and the complete absence of a Gen1 orthologue in the fission yeast, has lead to the suggestion that Holliday junctions do not play a major role in DNA damage processing pathways, including the responses to failed replication forks (Schwartz & Heyer, 2011). This argument is further supported by the findings that other Holliday junction resolving nucleases have a very low preference for *bona fide* Holliday junctions (see above). However, the presence of measurable dHJs in mitotic cells at least demonstrates that these structures are present and so play some role in at least one DNA damage recovery pathway during mitotic proliferation (Bzymek et al., 2010).

Finally, many of the models described above which involve a dHJ as a recombination intermediate indicate that these intermediates can be dissolved to form hemicatanene structures (see above; Figures 3-5). In Section 4.1 we describe the STR complex (Sgs1-Top3-Rmi1) which plays an enhancer role during extensive end resection of DSBs (see above). This complex also has the ability to serve as a "dissolvasome" for dHJs (Mankouri & Hickson, 2007). Dissolvasome activity involves Sgs1 (BLM) helicase mediating the convergent migration of the two Holliday junctions to form the hemincatanane and Top3 activity then resolves the catanated strands (Chang et al., 2005; Mullen et al., 2005; Yin et al., 2005; Raynard et al., 2006; Wu et al., 2006; Bussen et al., 2007; Yang et al., 2010). The role of Rmi1 is to stimulate the final Top3-mediated de-catenation reaction (Cejka et al., 2010). Mammalian cells have an additional factor, Rmi2, which also serves as an essential component of the dissolvasome complex (BLM-Top3α-Rmi1-Rmi2) (Singh et al., 2008). Given that sister chromatid exchanges are rare events in cells with a fully functional dissolvasome, and that these become elevated when dissolvasome components are perturbed (for example, German et al., 1965), it is likely that this is a major route for dHJ processing, although there is considerable overlap and redundancy with other dHJ resolution factors (see above; for example, Weschler et al., 2011), although Holliday junction containing structures do persist in *S. cerevisiae* cells following DNA damage in the absence of Sgs1 and Top3 function (Mankouri et al., 2011).

5. Closing remarks

DNA replication is at the very center of the regulation of life on earth. Perturbation of replicative processes can generate an array of highly distinct lesions which require processing to ensure that the biological requirements associated with genome duplication are met in full. This has resulted in the evolution of multiple complexes and competing pathways, each capable of acting on specific substrates. These pathways share common players and parsimony has driven the development of distinct and in some cases opposing roles for central regulators. Moreover, the complexity of distinct pathways requires the temporal modification of specific regulators, which must be co-ordinately timed to allow step-wise progression of a given process. Here we have presented some of the models proposed for the repair and processing of replication-associated lesions. We have demonstrated the many possible routes a specific substrate can follow and we have provided a basic overview of the key *trans* factors and their functional capabilities. It is clear that many of these factors have overlapping roles and that the many pathways in which they serve make elucidation of the exact mechanisms difficult and many key questions remain open to experimental scrutiny.

6. Acknowledgements

We would like to thank Dr. Jane Wakeman for helpful comments on the manuscript. We would like to apologise to those people whose work we have not had space to cite.

7. References

Abeysinghe, S.S.; Chuzhanova, N. & Cooper, D.N. (2006). Gross deletions and translocations in human genetic disease. *Genome Dynamics* Vol.1, (2006), pp. 17-34. ISSN 1660-9263

Admire, A.; Shanks, L.; Danzl, N.; Wang, M.; Weier, U.; Stevens, W.; Hunt, E. & Weinert, T. (2006). Cycles of chromosome instability are associated with a fragile site and are increased by defects in DNA replication and checkpoint controls in yeast. *Genes and Development* Vol.20, No.2, (January 2006), pp.159-173 ISSN 0890-9369

Aguilera, A. (2002). The connection between transcription and genomic instability. *EMBO Journal* Vol.21, No.3, (February 2002), pp.195-201 ISSN 0261-4189

Aguilera, A. & Gómez-González, B. (2008). Genome instability: a mechanistic view of its causes and consequences. *Nature Reviews Genetics* Vol.9, No.3, (March 2008), pp.204-217 ISSN 1471-0056

Akamatsu, Y; Dziadkowiec, D.; Ikequchi, M.; Shinagawa, H. & Iwasaki, H. (2003). Two different Swi5-containing protein complexes are involved in mating-type switching and recombination repair in fission yeast. *Proceedings of the National Academy of Science of the United States of America* Vol.100, No.26, (December 2003), pp.15770-15775 ISSN 0027-8424

Akamatsu, Y.; Tsutsui, Y.; Morishita, T.; Siddique, M.S.; Kurokawa, Y.; Ikequchi, M.; Yamao, F.; Arcangioli, B. & Iwasaki, H. (2007). Fission yeast Swi5/Sfr1 and Rhp55/Rhp57 differentially regulate Rhp51-dependent recombination outcomes. *EMBO Journal* Vol.26, No.5, (March 2007), pp.1352-1362 ISSN 0261-4189

Akamatsu, Y. & Jasin, M. (2010). Role for the mammalian Swi5-Sfr1 complex in DNA strand break repair through homologous recombination. *PLoS Genetics* Vol.6, No.10, (October 2010), pp.e1001160 ISSN 1553-7390

Alexeev, A.; Mazin, A. & Kowalczykowski, S.C. (2003). Rad54 protein possesses chromatin-remodeling activity stimulated by the Rad51-ssDNA nucleoprotein filament. *Nature Structural Biology* Vol.10, No.3, (March 2003), pp.182-186 ISSN 1072-8368

Alexiadis, V. & Kadonaga, J.T. (2002). Strand pairing by Rad54 and Rad51 is enhanced by chromatin. *Genes and Development* Vol.16, No.21, (November 2002), pp.2767-2771 ISSN 0890-9369

Allen, C.; Ashley, A.K.; Hromas, R. & Nickoloff, J.A. (2011). More forks on the road to replication stress recovery. *Journal of Molecular Cell Biology* Vol.3, No.1, (February 2011), pp.4-12 ISSN 1759-4685

Amano, M.; Suzuki, A.; Hori, T.; Backer, C.; Okawa, K.; Cheeseman, I.M. & Fukagawa, T. (2009). The CENP-S complex is essential for the stable assembly of outer kinetochore structure. *Journal of Cell Biology* Vol.186, No.2, (July 2009), pp.173-182 ISSN 0021-9525

Amitani, I.; Baskin, R.J. & Kowalczykowski, S.C. (2006). Visualization of Rad54, a chromatin remodelling protein, translocating on single DNA molecules. *Molecular Cell* Vol.23, No.1, (July 2006), pp.143-148 ISSN 1097-2765

Anantha, R.W. & Borowiec, J.A. (2009). Mitotic crisis: the unmasking of a novel role for RPA. *Cell Cycle* Vol.8,No.3, (February 2009), pp.357-361 ISSN 1551-4004

Anantha, R.W.; Vassin, V.M. & Borowiec, J.A. (2007). Sequential nand synergistic modification of human RPA stimulates chromosomal DNA repair. *Journal of Biological Chemistry* Vol.282, No.49, (December 2007), pp.35910-35923 ISSN 0021-9258

Bansbach, C.E.; Bétous, R.; Lovejoy, C.A.; Glick, G.G. & Cortez, D. (2009). The annealing helicase SMARCAL1 maintains genome integrity at stalled replication forks. *Genes and Development* Vol.23, No.20, (September 2009), pp.2405-2414 ISSN 0890-9369

Bartek, J.; Lukas, C. & Lukas, J. (2004). Checking on DNA damage in S phase. *Nature Reviews in Cell Biology* Vol.5, No.10, (October 2004), pp.792-804 ISSN 1471-0072

Bartek, J.; Bartkova, J. & Lukas, J. (2007). DNA damage signalling guards against activated oncogenes and tumour progression. *Oncogene* Vol.26, No.56, (December 2007), pp.7773-7779 ISSN 0950-9232

Baumann, P.; Benson, F.E. & West, S.C. (1996). Human Rad51 protein promotes ATP-dependent homologous pairing and strand transfer reactions in vitro. *Cell* Vol.87, No.4, (November 1996), pp.757-766 ISSN 0092-8674

Bernstein, K.A., Gangloff, S. & Rothstein, R. (2010). The RecQ DNA helicases in DNA repair. *Annual Reviews of Genetics* Vol.44, (2010), pp.393-417 ISSN 0066-4197

Binz, S.K.; Sheehan, A.M. & Wold, M.S. (2004). Replication protein A phosphorylation and the cellular response to DNA damage. *DNA Repair* Vol.3, No.2-9, (August-September 2004), pp.1015-1024 ISSN 1568-7856

Blanco, M.G.; Matos, J.; Rass, U.; Ip, S.C. & West, S.C. (2010). Functional overlap between the structure-specific nucleases Yen1 and Mus81-Mms4 for DNA damage repair in S. cerevisiae. *DNA Repair* Vol.9, No.4, (April 2010), pp.394-402 ISSN 1568-7856

Blastyák, A.; Pintér, L.; Unk, I.; Prakash, L.; Prakash, S. & Haracska, L. (2007). Yeast Rad5 protein required for postreplication repair has a DNA helicase activity specific for replication fork regression. *Molecular Cell* Vol.28, No.2, (October 2007), pp.181-183 ISSN 1097-2765

Blastyák, A.; Hajdú, I.; Unk, I. & Haracska, L. (2010). Role of double-strand DNA translocase activity of human HLTF in replication of damaged DNA. *Molecular and Cellular Biology* Vol.30, No.3, (February 2010), pp.684-693 ISSN 1098-5549

Boddy, M.N.; Gaillard, P.H.; McDonald, W.H.; Shanahan, P.; Yates, J.R. 3rd. & Russell, P. (2001). Mus81-Eme1 are essential components of a Holliday junction resolvase. *Cell* Vol.107, No.4, (November 2001), pp.537-548 ISSN 0092-8674

Boerkoel, C.F.; Takashima, H.; John, J.; Stankiewicz, P.; Rosenbarker, L.; André, J.L.; Bogdanovic, R.; Burquet, A.; Cockfield, S.; Cordeiro, I.; Fründ, S.; Illies, F.; Joseph, M.; Kaitila, I.; Lama, G.; Loirat, C.; McLeod, D.R.; Milford, D.V.; Petty, E.M.; Rodrigo, F.; Saraiva, J.M.; Schmidt, B.; Smith, G.C.; Spranger, J.; Stein, A.; Thiele, H.; Tizard, J.; Weksberg, R.; Lupski, J.R. & Stockton, D.W. (2002). Mutant chromatin remodelling protein SMARCAL1 causes Schimke immune-osseous dysplasia. *Nature Genetics* Vol.30, No.2, (February 2002), pp.215-220 ISSN 1061-4036

Bozhenok, L.; Wade, P.A. & Varga-Weisz, P. (2002). WSTF-ISWI chromatin remodelling complex targets heterochromatic replication foci. *EMBO Journal* Vol.21, No.9, (May 2002), pp.2231-2241 ISSN 0261-4189

Branzei, D. & Foiani, M. (2007a). Interplay of replication checkpoints and repair proteins at stalled replication forks. *DNA Repair* Vol.6, No.7, (July 2007), pp.994-1003 ISSN 1568-7856

Branzei, D. & Foiani, M. (2007b). Template switching: from replication fork repair to genome rearrangements. *Cell* Vol.131, No.7, (December 2007), pp.1228-1230 ISSN 0092-8674

Branzei, D. & Foiani, M. (2007c). RecQ helicases queuing with Srs2 to disrupt Rad51 filament and suppress recombination. *Genes and Development* Vol. 21, No.23, (December 2007), pp.3019-3026 ISSN 0890-9369

Branzei, D. & Foiani, M. (2008). Regulation of DNA repair throughout the cell cycle. *Nature Reviews in Molecular Cell Biology* Vol.9, no.4, (April 2008), pp.297-308 ISSN 1471-0072

Branzei, D. & Foiani, M. (2009). The checkpoint response to replication stress. *DNA Repair* Vol. 8. No.9, (September 2009), pp.1038-1046 ISSN 1568-7856

Branzei, D. & Foiani, M. (2010). Maintaining genome stability at the replication fork. *Nature Reviews in Molecular Cell Biology* Vol.11, No.3, (March 2010), pp.208-219 ISSN 1471-0072

Budzowska, M. & Kanaar, R. (2009). Mechanisms of dealing with DNA damage-induced replication problems. *Cell Biochemistry and Biophysics* Vol.53, No.1, (November 2009), pp.17-31 ISSN 1085-9195

Bugreev, D.V.; Hanaoka, F. & Mazin, A.V. (2007). Rad54 dissociates homologous recombination intermediates by branch migration. *Nature Structural and Molecular Biology* Vol.14, No.8, (July 2007), pp.746-753 ISSN 1545-9985

Bugreev, D.V.; Rossi, M.J. & Mazin, A.V. (2011). Cooperation of RAD51 and RAD54 in regression of a model replication fork. *Nucleic Acids Research* Vol.39, No.6, (March 2011), pp.2153-2164 ISSN 0305-1048

Buisson, R.; Dion-Côté, A.M.; Coulombe, Y.; Launag, H.; Cai, H.; Stasiak, A.Z.; Stasiak, A.; Xia, B. & Masson, J.Y. (2010). Cooperation of breast cancer proteins PALB2 and piccolo BRCA2 in stimulating homologous recombination. *Nature Structural and Molecular Biology* Vol.17, No.10, (October 2010), pp1247-1254 ISSN 1545-9985

Burma, S.; Chen, B.P.; Murphy, M.; Kurimasa, A. & Chen, D.J. (2001). ATM phosphorylates histone H2AX in response to DNA double-strand breaks. *Journal of Biological Chemistry* Vol.276, No.45, (November 2001), pp.42462-42467 ISSN 0021-9258

Bussen, W.; Raynard, S.; Busygina, V.; Singh, A.K. & Sung, P. (2007). Holliday junction processing activity of the BLM-Topo IIIα-BLAP75 complex. *Journal of Biological Chemistry* Vol.282, No.43, (October 2007), pp.31484-31892 ISSN 0021-9258

Bzymek, M.; Thayer, N.H.; Oh, S.D.; Kleckner, N. & Hunter, N. (2010). Double Holliday junctions are intermediates of DNA break repair. *Nature* Vol.464, No.7290, (April 2010), pp.937-941 ISSN 0028-0836

Carreira, A.; Hilario, J.; Amitani, I.; Baskin, R.J.; Shivji, M.K.; Venkitaraman, A.R. & Kowalczykowski, S.C. (2009). The BRC repeats of BRCA2 modualte the DNA-binding selectivity of RAD51. *Cell* Vol.136, No.6, (March 2009), pp.1032-1043 ISSN 0092-8674

Carreira, A. & Kowalczykowski, S.C. (2009). BRCA2: shining light on the regulation of DNA-binding selectivity by RAD51. *Cell Cycle* Vol.8, No.21, (November 2009), pp.3445-3447 ISSN 1551-4005

Cejka, P.; Plank, J.L.; Bachrati, C.Z.; Hickson, I.D. & Kowalczykowski, S.C. (2010). Rmi1 stimulates decatenation of double Holliday junctions during dissolution by Sgs1-Top3. *Nature Structural and Molecular Biology* Vol.17, No.11, (November 2010), pp.1377-1382 ISSN 1545-9985

Cejka, P.; Cannavo, E.; Polaczek, P.; Masuda-Sasa, T.; Pokharel, S.; Campbell, J.L. & Kowalczykowski, S.C. (2010). DNA end resection by Dna2-Sgs1-RPA and its stimulation by Top3-Rmi1 and Mre11-Rad50-Xrs2. *Nature* Vol.467, No.7311, (September 2010), pp.112-116 ISSN 0028-0836

Chang, M.; Bellaoui, M.; Zhang, C.; Desai, R.; Morozov, P.; Delgado-Cruzata, L.; Rothstein, R.; Freyer, G.A.; Boone, C. & Brown, G.W. (2005). RMI1/NCE4, a suppressor of genome instability, encodes a member of the RecQ helicase/Topo III complex. *EMBO Journal* Vol.24, No.11, (June 2005), pp.2024-2033 ISSN 0261-4189

Chen, J.M.; Cooper, D.N.; Férec, C.; Kehrer-Sawatzki, H. & Patrinos, G.P. (2010). Genomic rearrangements in inherited disease and cancer. *Seminars in Cancer Biology* Vol.20, No.4, (August 2010), pp. 222-233 ISSN 1044-579X

Chung, W.H.; Zhu, Z.; Papusha, A.; Malkova, A. & Ira, G. (2010). Defective resection at DNA double-strand breaks leads to de novo telomere formation and enhances gene targeting. *PLoS Genetics* Vol.6, No.5, (May 2010), pp.e1000948 ISSN 1553-7390

Chu, W.K. & Hickson, I.D. (2009). RecQ helicases: multifunctional genome caretakers. *Nature Reviews Cancer* Vol.9, No.9, (September 2009), pp.644-654 ISSN 1474-175X

Ciccia, A.; Constantinou, A. & West, S.C. (2003). Identification and characterisation of the human mus81-eme1 endonuclease. *Journal of Biological Chemistry* Vol.278, no.27, (July 2003), pp.25172-25178 ISSN 0021-9258

Ciccia, A.; Bredemeyer, A.L.; Sowa, M.E.; Terret, M.E.; Jallepalli, P.V.; Harper, J.W. & Elledge, S.J. (2009). The SIOD disorder protein SMARCAL1 is an RPA-interacting protein involved in replication fork restart. *Genes and Development* Vol.23, No.20, (September 2009), pp.2415-2425 ISSN 0890-9369

Ciccia, A.; McDonald, N. & West, S.C. (2008). Structural and functional relationships of the XPF/MUS81 family of proteins. *Annual Review of Biochemistry* Vol.77, (2008), pp.259-287 ISSN 006-4154

Clever, B.; Interthal, H.; Schmuckli-Maurer, J.; King, J.; Sigrist, M. & Heyer, W.D. (1997). Recombinational repair in yeast: functional interactions between Rad51 and Rad54 proteins. *EMBO Journal* Vol.16, No.9, (May 1997), pp.2535-2544 ISSN 0261-4189

Cook, P.J.; Ju, B.G.; Telese, F.; Wang, X.; Glass, C.K. & Rosenfeld, M.G. (2009). Tyrosine dephosphorylation of H2AX modulates apoptosis and survival decisions. *Nature* Vol.458, No.7238, (April 2009), pp.591-596 ISSN 0028-0836

Cordeiro-Stone, M.; Makhov, A.M.; Zaritskaya, L.S. & Griffith, J.D. (1999). Analysis of DNA replication forks encountering a pyrimidine dimer in the template to the leading strand. *Journal of Molecular Biology* Vol.289, No.5, (June 1999), pp.1207-1218 ISSN 022-2836

Crossan, G.P.; van de Weyden, L.; Rosado, I.V.; Langevin, F.; Gaillard, P.H.; McIntyre, R.E.; Sanger mouse Genetics Project; Gallagher, F.; Kettunen, M.I.; Lewis, D.Y.; Brindle, K.; Arends, M.J.; Adams, D.J. & Patel, K.J. (2011). Disruption of mouse Slx4, a regulator of structure-specific nucelases, phenocopies Fanconia anemia. *Nature Genetics* Vol.43, no.2, (February 2011), pp.147-152 ISSN 1061-4036

Dalgaard, J.Z.; Eydmann, T.; Koulintchenko, M.; Sayrac, S.; Vengrova, S. & Yamada-Inagawa, T. (2009). Random and site-specific replication termination. *Methods in Molecular Biology* Vol.521, (2009), pp.35-53 ISSN 1064-3745

Dalgaard, J.Z. & Klar, A.J. (1999). Orientation of DNA replication establishes mating-type switching pattern in S. pombe. *Nature* Vol.400, No.6740, (July 1999), pp.181-184 ISSN 0028-0836

Dalgaard, J.Z. & Klar, A.J. (2001). Does S. pombe exploit the intrinsic asymmetry of DNA synthesis to imprint daughter cells for mating-type switching? *Trends in Genetics* Vol.17, No.3, (March 2001), pp.153-157 ISSN 0168-9525

Deans, A.J. & West, S.C. (2009). FANCM connects the genome instability disorder Bloom's Syndrome and Fanconia Anemia. *Molecular Cell* Vol.36, No.6, (December 2009), pp.943-953 ISSN 1097-2765

Dendouga, N.; Gao, H.; Moechars, D.; Janicot, M.; Vialard, J. & McGowan, C.H. (2005). Disruption of murine Mus81 increases genomic instability and DNA damage sensitivity but does not promote tumorigenesis. *Molecular and Cellular Biology* Vol.25, No.17, (September 2005), pp.7569-7579 ISSN 0270-7306

Deng, C.; Brown, J.A.; You, D. & Brown, J.M. (2005). Multiple endonucleases function to repair covalent topoisomerase I complexes in Saccharomyces cerevisiae. *Genetics* Vol.170, No.2, (June 2005), pp.591-600 ISSN 0016-6731

Deng, X.; Prakash, A.; Dhar, K.; Baia, G.S.; Kolar, C.; Oakley, G.G. & Borqstahl, G.E. (2009). Human replication protein A-Rad52-single-stranded DNA complex: stoichiometry and evidence for strand transfer regulation by phosphorylation. *Biochemistry* Vol.48, No.28, (July 2009), pp.6633-6643 ISSN 0006-2960

Dovey, C.L.; Aslanian, A.; Sofueva, S.; Yates, J.R. 3rd & Russell, P. (2009). Mms1-Mms22 complex protects genome integrity in Schizosaccharomyces pombe. *DNA Repair* Vol.8, No.13, (December 2009), pp.1390-1399 ISSN 1568-7856

Dray, E.; Etchin, J.; Wiese, C.; Saro, D.; Williams, G.J.; Hammel, M.; Yu, X.; Galkin, V.E.; Liu, D.; Tsai, M.S.; Sy, S.M.; Schild, D.; Egelman, E.; Chen, J. & Sung, P. (2010). Enhancement of RAD51 recombinase activity by the tumour suppressor PALB2. *Nature Structural and Molecular Biology* Vol.17, No.10, (October 2010), pp.1255-1259 ISSN 1545-9985

Driscoll, R. & Cimprich, K.A. (2009). HARPing on about the DNA damage response during replication. *Genes and Development* Vol.23, No.20, (September 2009), pp.2359-2365 ISSN 0890-9369

Duro, E.; Lundin, C.; Ask, K.; Sanchez-Pulido, L.; MacArtney, T.J.; Toth, R.; Ponting, C.P.; Groth, A.; Helleday, T. & Rouse, J. (2010). Identification of the MMS22L-TONSL complex that promotes homologous recombination. *Molecular Cell* Vol.40, No.4, (November 2010), pp.632-644 ISSN 1097-2765

Duro, E.; Vaisica, J.A.; Brown, G.W. & Rouse, J. (2008). Budding yeast Mms22 and Mms1 regulate homologous recombination induced by replisome blockage. *DNA Repair* Vol.7, No.5, (May 2008), pp.811-818 ISSN 1568-7856

Fekairi, S.; Scaglione, S.; Chahwan, C.; Taylor, E.R.; Tissier, A.; Coulson, S.; Dong, M.Q.; Ruse, C.; Yates, J.R. 3rd.; Russell, P.; Fuchs, R.P.; McGowan, C.H. & Gaillard, P.H. (2009). Human SLX4 is a Holliday junction resolvase subunit that binds multiple DNA repair/recombination endonucleases. *Cell* Vol.138, No.1, (July 2009), pp.78-89 ISSN 0092-8674

Fernandez-Capetillo, O.; Lee, A.; Nussenweig, M. & Nussenzweig, A. (2004). H2AX: the histone guardian of the genome. *DNA Repair* Vol.3, No.8-9, (August-September 2004), pp.959-967 ISSN 1568-7856

Fricke, W.M. & Brill, S.J. (2003). Slx1-Slx4 is a second structure-specific endonuclease functionally redundant with Sgs1-Top3. *Genes and Development* Vol.17, No.14, (July 2003), pp.1768-1778 ISSN 0890-9369

Fricke, W.M.; Bastin-Shanower, S.A. & Brill, S.J. (2005). Substrate specificity of the Saccharomyces cerevisiae Mus81-Mms4 endonuclease. *DNA Repair* Vol.4, No.2, (February 2005), pp.243-251 ISSN 1568-7856

Fujimori, A.; Tachiiri, S.; Sonoda, E.; Thompson, L.H.; Dhar, P.K.; Hiraoka, M.; Takeda, S.; Zhang, Y.; Reth, M. & Takata, M. (2001). Rad52 partially substitutes for the Rad51 paralog XRCC3 in maintaining chromosomal integrity in vertebrate cells. *EMBO Journal* Vol.20, No.19, (October 2001), pp.5513-5520 ISSN 0261-4189

Gaillard, P.H.; Noguchi, E.; Shanahan, P. & Russell, P. (2003). The endogenous Mus81-Eme1 complex resolves Holliday junctions by a nick and counternick mechanism. *Molecular Cell* Vol.12, No.3, (September 2003), pp.747-759 ISSN 1097-2765

Gari, K.; Décaillet, C.; Delannoy, M.; Wu, L. & Constantinou, A. (2008a). Remodeling of DNA replication structures by the branch point translocase FANCM. *Proceedings of the National Academy of Science or the United States of America* Vol.105, No.42, (October 2008), pp.16107-16112 ISSN 0027-8424

Gari, K.; Décaillet, C.; Stasiak, A.Z.; Stasiak, A. & Constantinou, A. (2008b). The Fanconia anemia protein FANCM can promote branch migration of Holliday junctions and replication forks. *Molecular Cell* Vol.29, No.1, (January 2008), pp.141-148 ISSN 1097-2765

German, J.; Archibald, R. & Bloom, D. (1965). Chromosomal breakage in a rare and probably genetically determined syndrome of man. *Science* Vol.148, (April 1965), pp.506-507 ISSN 0036-8075

Grallert, B. & Boye, E. (2008). The multiple facets of the intra-S checkpoint. *Cell Cycle* Vol.7, No.15, (August 2008), pp.2315-2320 ISSN 1551-4005

Gravel, S.; Chapman, J.R.; Magill, C. & Jackson, S.P. (2008). DNA helicases Sgs1 and BLM promote DNA double-strand break resection. *Genes and Development* Vol.22, No.20, (October 2002), pp.2767-2772 ISSN 0890-9369

Greenberg, R.A.; Sobhian, B.; Pathania, S.; Cantor, S.B.; Nakatani, Y. & Livingston, D.M. (2006). Multifactorial contributions to an acute DNA damage response by BRCA1/BARD1-containing complexes. *Genes and Development* Vol.20, No.1, (January 2006), pp.34-46 ISSN 0890-9369

Grishchuk, A.L. & Kohli, J. (2003). Five RecA-like proteins of Schizosaccharomyces pombe are involved in meiotic recombination. *Genetics* Vol.165, No.3, (November 2003), pp.1031-1043 ISSN 0016-6731

Halazonetis, T.D.; Gorgoulis, V.G. & Bartek, J. (2008) An oncogene-induced DNA damage model for cancer development. *Science* Vol.319, No.5868, (March 2008), pp.1352-1355 ISSN 0036-8075

Harper, J.V.; Anderson, J.A. & O'Neill, P. (2010). Radiation induced DNA DSBs: contribution from stalled replication forks? *DNA Repair* Vol.8, No.8, (August 2010), pp.907-913 ISSN 1568-7856

Harrison, J.C. & Haber, J.E. (2006). Surviving the breakup: the DNA damage checkpoint. *Annual Reviews in Genetics* Vol.40, (2006), pp. 209-235, ISSN 0066-4197

Hartsuiker, E.; Neale, M.J. & Carr, A.M. (2009). Distinct requirements for the Rad32(Mre11) nuclease and Ctp1(CtIP) in the removal of covalently bound topoisomerase I and II from DNA. *Molecular Cell* Vol.33, No.1, (January 2009), pp.117-123 ISSN 1097-2765

Haruta, N.; Kurokawa, Y.; Murayama, Y.; Akamatsu, Y.; Unzai, S.; Tsutsui, Y. & Iwasaki, H. (2006). The Swi5-Sfr1 complex stimulates Rhp51/Rad51- and Dmc1-mediated DNA strand exchange in vitro. *Nature Structural and Molecular Biology* Vol.13, No.9, (September 2006), pp.823-830 ISSN 1545-9985

Hayakawa, T.; Zhang, F.; Hayakawa, Y.; Ohtani, Y.; Shinmyozu, K.; Nakayama, J. & Andreassen, P.R. (2010). MRG15 binds directly to PALB2 and stimulates homology-directed repair of chromosomal breaks. *Journal of Cell Science* Vol.123, No.7, (April 2010), pp.1124-1130 ISSN 0021-9533

Hayase, A.; Takaqi, M.; Miyazaki, T.; Oshiumi, H.; Shinohara, M. & Shinohara, A. (2004). A protein complex containing Mei5 and Sae3 promotes the assembly of the meiosis-specific RecA homolog Dmc1. *Cell* Vol.119, No.7, (December 2004), pp.927-940 ISSN 0092-8674

Heyer, W.D.; Ehmsen, K.T. & Liu, J. (2010) Regulation of homologous recombination. *Annual Reviews of Genetics* Vol.44, (2010), pp.113-139 ISSN 0066-4197

Heyer, W.D.; Li, X.; Rolfsmeier, M. & Zhang, X.P. (2006). Rad54: the Swiss Army knife of homologous recombination? *Nucleic Acids Research* Vol. 34, No.15, (August 2006), pp.4115-4125 ISSN 0305-1048

Higgins, N.P.; Kato, K. & Strauss, B. (1976). A model for replication repair in mammalian cells. *Journal of Molecular Biology* Vol.101, No.3, (March 1976), pp.417-425 ISSN 0022-2836

Ho, C.K.; Mazón, G.; Lam, A.F. & Symington, L.S. (2010). Mus81 and Yen1 promote reciprocal exchange during mitotic recombination to maintain genome integrity in budding yeast. *Molecular Cell* Vol.40, No.6, (December 2010), pp.988-1000 ISSN 1097-2765

Ho, T.V. & Schärer, O.D. (2010). Translesion DNA synthesis polymerases in DNA interstrand crosslink repair. *Environmental and Molecular Mutagenesis* Vol.51, No.6, (July 2010), pp.552-566 ISSN 0893-6692

Holthausen, J.T.; Wyman, C. & Kanaar, R. (2010). Regulation of DNA strand exchange in homologous recombination. *DNA Repair* Vol.9, no.12, (December 2010), pp.1264-1274 ISSN 1568-7856

Hryciw, T.; Tang, M.; Fontanie, T. & Xiao, W. (2002). MMS1 protects against replication-dependent DNA damage in Saccharomyces cerevisiae. *Molecular Genetics and Genomics* Vol.266, No.5, (January 2002), pp.848-857 ISSN 1617-4623

Huen, M.S.; Grant, R.; Manke, I.; Minn, K.; Yu, X.; Yaffe, M.B. & Chen, J. (2007). RNF8 transduces the DNA-damage signal via histone ubiquitylation and checkpoint assembly. *Cell* Vol.131, No.5, (November 2007), pp.901-914 ISSN 0092-8674

Huertas, P. (2010). DNA resection in eukaryotes: deciding how to fix the break. *Nature Structural and Molecular Biology* Vol.17, No.1, (January 2010), pp.11-16 ISSN 1545-9985

Interthal, H. & Heyer, W.D. (2000). MUS81 encodes a novel helix-hairpin-helix protein involved in the response to UV-and methylation-induced DNA damage in Saccharomyces cerevisiae. *Molecular and General Genetics* Vol.263, No.5, (Jun 2000), pp.812-827 ISSN 0026-8925

Ip, S.C.; Rass, U.; Blanco, M.G.; Flynn, H.R.; Skehel, J.M. & West, S.C. (2008). Identification of Holliday junction resolvases from humans and yeast. *Nature* Vol.456, No.7220, (November 2008), 357-361 ISSN 0028-0836

Ismail, I.H. & Hendzel, M.J. (2008). The γH2AX: is it just a surrogate marker of double-strand breaks or much more? *Environmental and Molecular Mutagenesis* Vol.49, no.1, (January 2008), pp.73-82 ISSN 0893-6692

Ivessa, A.S.; Lenzmeier, B.A.; Bessler, J.B.; Goudsouzian, L.K.; Schnakenberg, S.L. & Zakian, V.A. (2003). The Saccharomyces cerevisiae helicase Rrm3p facilitates replication past non-histone protein-DNA complexes. *Molecular Cell* Vol.12, No.6, (December 2003), pp.1525-1536 ISSN 1097-2765

Jackson, D.; Dhar, K.; Wahl, J.K.; Wold, M.S. & Borgstahl, G.E. (2002). Analysis of the human replication protein A:Rad52 complex: evidence for crosstalk between RPA32, RPA70, Rad52 and DNA. *Journal of Molecular Biology* Vol.32, No.1, (August 2002), pp.133-148 ISSN 0022-2836

Jaskelioff, M.; van Komen, S.; Krebs, J.E.; Sung, P. & Peterson, C.L. (2003). Rad54p is a chromatin remodelling enzyme required for heteroduplex DNA joint formation with chromatin. *Journal of Biological Chemistry* Vol.278, No.11, (January 2003), pp.9212-9218 ISSN 0021-9258

Jensen, R.B.; Carreira, A. & Kowalczykowski, S.C. (2010). Purified human BRCA2 stimulates RAD51-mediated recombination. *Nature* Vol.467, No.7316, (October 2010), pp.678-683 ISSN 0028-0836

Khasanov, F.K.; Salakhova, A.F.; Chepurnaja, O.V.; Korolev, V.G. & Bashkirov, V.I. (2004). Identification and characterization of the rlp1+, the novel Rad51 paralog in the fission yeast Schizosaccharomyces pombe. *DNA Repair* Vol.3, No.10, (October 2004), pp.1363-1374 ISSN 1568-7856

Khasanov, F.K.; Salakhova, A.F.; Khasanova, O.S.; Grishchuk, A.L.; Chepurnaja, O.V.; Korolev, V.G.; Kohli, J. & Bashkirov, V.I. (2008). Genetic analysis reveals different roles of Schizosaccharomyces pombe sfr1/dds20 in meiotic and mitotic DNA recombination and repair. *Current Genetics* Vol.54, No.4, (October 2008), pp.197-221 ISSN 0172-8083

Kolas, N.K.; Chapman, J.R.; Nakada, S.; Ylanko, J.; Chahwan, R.; Sweeney, F.D.; Panier, S.; Mendez, M.; Wildenhain, J.; Thomson, T.M.; Pelletier, L.; Jackson, S.P. & Durocher, D. (2007). Orchestration of the DNA-damage response by the RNF8 ubiquitin ligase. *Science* Vol.318, No.5856, (December 2007), pp.1637-1640 ISSN 0036-8075

Kovalenko, O.V.; Golub, E.I.; Bray-Ward, P.; Ward, D.C. & Radding, C.M. (1997). A novel nucleic acid-binding protein that interacts with human Rad51 recombinase. *Nucleic Acids Research* Vol.25, No.24, (December 1997), pp.4946-4953 ISN 0305-1048

Krijger, P.H.; Lee, K.Y.; Wit, N.; van der Berk, P.C.; Wu, X.; Roest, H.P.; Maas, A.; Ding, H.; Hoeijmaker, J.H.; Myung, K. & Jacobs, H. (2011). HLTF and SHPRH are not essential for PCNA polyubiquitination, survival and somatic hypermutation: existence of an alternative E3 ligase. *DNA Repair* Vol. 10, No.4, (January 2011), pp.438-444 ISSN 1568-7856

Kwon, Y.; Chi, P., Roh, D.H.; Klein, H. & Sung, P. (2007). Synergistic action of the Saccharomyces cerevisae homologous recombination factors Rad54 and Rad51 in chromatin remodeling. *DNA Repair* Vol.6, No.10, (June 2007), pp.1496-1506 ISSN 1568-7856

Labib, K. (2008). Making connections at DNA replication forks: Mrc1 takes the lead. *Molecular Cell* Vol.32, No.2, (October 2008), pp.116-168 ISSN 1097-2765

Labib, K. & Hodgson, B. (2007) Replication fork barriers: pause for a break or stalling for time? *EMBO Reports* Vol.8, No.4, (April 2007), pp.346-353 ISSN 1469-221X

Lambert, S.; Watson, A.; Sheedy, D.M.; Martin, B. & Carr, A.M. (2005). Gross chromosomal rearrangements and elevated recombination at an inducible site-specific replication fork barrier. *Cell* Vol.121, No.5, (June 2005), pp.689-702 ISSN 0092-8674

Lambert, S.; Froget, B. & Carr, A.M. (2007). Arrested replication fork processing: interplay between checkpoints and recombination. *DNA Repair* Vol.6, No.7, (July 2007), pp.1042-1061 ISSN 1568-7856

Lehmann, A.R. & Fuchs, R.P. (2006). Gaps and forks in DNA replication: rediscovering old models. *DNA Repair* Vol.5, No.12, (December 2006), pp.1495-1498 ISSN 1568-7856

Lemoine, F.J.; Degtyareva, N.P.; Lobachev, K. & Petes, T.D. (2005). Chromosomal translocations in yeast induced by low levels of DNA polymerase: a model for chromosome fragile sites. *Cell* Vol.120, No.5, (March 2005), pp.587-598 ISSN 0092-8674

Lieber, M.R. (2010). The mechanisms of double-strand break repair by the nonhomologous DNA end-joining pathway. *Annual Reviews of Biochemistry* Vol.79, (2010), pp.181-211 ISSN 0066-4154

Limbo, O.; Chahwan, C.; Yamada, Y.; de Bruin, R.A.; Wittenberg, C. & Russell, P. (2007). Ctp1 is a cell-cycle-regulated protein that functions with Mre11 complex to control double-strand break repair by homologous recombination. *Molecular Cell* Vol.28, No.1, (October 2007), pp.134-146 ISSN 1097-2765

Lin, J.R.; Zeman, M.K.; Chen, J.Y.; Yee, M.C. & Cimprich, K.A. (2011). SHPRH and HLTF act in a damage-specific manner to coordinate different forms of postreplication repair and prevent mutagenesis. *Molecular Cell* Vol.42, No.2, (April 2011), pp.237-249 ISSN 1097-2765

Lisby, M. & Rothstein, R. (2009). Choreography of recombination proteins during the DNA damage response. *DNA Repair* Vol.8, No.9, (September 2009), pp.1068-1076 ISSN 1568-7856

Loeb, L.A. & Monnat, R.J. Jr. (2008). DNA polymerases and human disease. *Nature Reviews Genetics* Vol.9, No.8, (August 2008), pp.594-604 ISSN 1471-0056

Lopes, M.; Foiani, M., & Sogo, J.M. (2006). Multiple mechanisms control chromosome integrity after replication fork uncoupling and restart at irreparable UV lesions. *Molecular Cell* Vol.21, No.1, (January 2006), pp.15-27 ISSN 1097-2765

Llorente, B.; Smith, C.E. & Symington, L.S. (2008). Break-induced replication: what is it and what is it for? *Cell Cycle* Vol.7, No.7. (January 2008), 859-864 ISSN 1551-4005

Lukas, J. & Bartek, J. (2009). DNA repair: new tales of an old tail. *Nature* Vol.458, No.7238, (April 2009), pp.581-583 ISSN 0028-0836

Lukas, C.; Melander, F.; Stucji, M.; Falck, J.; Bekker-Jensen, S.; Goldberg, M.; Lerenthal, Y.; Jackson, S.P.; Bartek, J. & Lukas, J. (2004). Mdc1 couples DNA double-strand break recognition by Nbs1 with its H2AX-dependent chromatin retention. *EMBO Journal* Vol.23, No.13, (July 2004), pp.2674-2683 ISSN 0261-4189

Lydeard, J.R.; Lipkin-Moore, Z.; Jain, S.; Eapen, W. & Haber, J.E. (2010). Sgs1 and Exo1 redundantly inhibit break-induced replication and de novo telomere addition at broken chromosome ends. *PLoS Genetics* Vol.6, No.5, (May 2010), pp.e1000973

Mailand, N.; Bekker-Jensen, S.; Faustrup, H.; Melander, F.; Bartek, J.; Lukas, C. & Lukas, J. (2007). RNF8 ubiquitylates histones at DNA double-strand breaks and promotes assembly of repair proteins. *Cell* Vol.131, No.5, (November 2007), pp.887-900 ISSN 0092-8674

Mankouri, H.W.; Ashton, T.M. & Hickson, I.D. (2011). Holliday junction-containing structures persist in cells lacking Sgs1 or Top3 following exposure to DNA damage. *Proceedings of the National Academy of Science of the United States of America* Vol.108, No.12, (March 2011), pp.4944-4949 ISSN 0027-8424

Mankouri, H.W. & Hickson, I.D. (2007). The RecQ helicase-topoisomerase III-Rmi1 complex: a DNA structure-specific 'dissolvasome'? *Trends in Biochemical Sciences* Vol.32, no.12, (December 2007), pp.538-546 ISSN 0968-0004

Marini, V. & Krejci, L. (2010). Srs2: The "odd-job man" in DNA repair. *DNA Repair* Vol.9, No.3, (February 2010), pp.268-275 ISSN 1568-7856

Martín, V.; Chahwan, C.; Gao, H.; Blais, V.; Wohlschlegel, J.; Yates, J.R. 3rd.; McGowan, C.H. & Russell, P. (2006). Sws1 is a conserved regulator of homologous recombination in eukaryotic cells. *EMBO Journal* Vol.25, No.11, (May 2006), pp.2564-2574 ISSN 0261-4189

Mazin, A.V.; Mazina, O.M.; Bugreev, D.V. & Rossi, M.J. (2010). Rad54, the motor of homologous recombination. *DNA Repair* Vol.9, No.3, (January 2010), pp.286-302 ISSN 1568-7856

McEachern, M.J. & Haber, J.E. (2006). Break-induced replication and recombinational telomere elongation in yeast. *Annual Reviews of Biochemistry* Vol.75, (2006), pp.111-135 ISSN 0066-4154

McFarlane, R.J. & Humphrey, T.C. (2010). A role for recombination in centromere function. *Trends in Genetics* Vol.26, No.5, (May 2010), pp.209-213 ISSN 0168-9525

McFarlane, R.J.; Mian, S. & Dalgaard, J.Z. (2010). The many facets of the Tim-Tipin protein families' roles in chromosome biology. *Cell Cycle* Vol.9, No.4, (February 2010), pp.700-705 ISSN 1551-4005

McKee, A.H. & Kleckner, N. (1997). Mutations in Saccharomyces cerevisiae that block meiotic prophase chromosome metabolism and confer cell cycle arrest at pachytene indentify two new meiosis-specific genes SAE1 and SAE3. *Genetics* Vol.146, No.3, (July 1997), pp.817-834 ISSN 0016-6731

Merkenschlager, M. (2010). Cohesin: a global player in chromosome biology with local ties to the gene regulation. *Current Opinion in Genetics and Development* Vol20, No.5, (October 2010), pp.555-561 ISSN 0959-437X

Mimitou, E.P. & Symington, L.S. (2008). Sae2, Exo1 and Sgs1 collaborate in DNA double-strand break processing. *Nature* Vol.455, No.7214, (October 2008), pp.770-774 ISSN 0028-0836

Mimitou, E.P. & Symington, L.S. (2010). Ku prevents Exo1 and Sgs1-dependent resection of DNA ends in the absence of a functional MRX complex or Sae2. *EMBO Journ*al Vol.29, No.6, (October 2010), pp.3358-3369 ISSN 0261-4189

Mimitou, E.P. & Symington, L.S. (2011). DNA end resection-unraveling the tail. *DNA Repair* Vol.10, No.3, (March 2011), pp.344-348 ISSN 1568-7856

Minca, E.C. & Kowalski, D. (2010). Multiple Rad5 activities mediate sister chromatid recombination to bypass DNA damage at stalled replication forks. *Molecular Cell* Vol.38, No.5, (June 2010), pp.649-661 ISSN 1097-2765

Mirkin, E.V. & Mirkin, S.M. (2007). Replication fork stalling at natural impediments. *Microbiology and Molecular Biology Reviews* Vol.71, No.1, (March 2007), pp.13-35 ISSN 1092-2172

Mischo, H.E.; Gómez-González, B.; Grechnik, P.; Rondón, A.G.; Wei, W.; Steinmetz, L.; Aguilera, A. & Proudfoot, N. (2011). Yeast Sen1 helicase protects the genome from transcription-associated instability. *Molecular Cell*, Vol.41, No.1, (January 2011), pp. 21-32, ISSN 1097-276

Mizuta, R.; La Salle, J.M.; Cheng, H.L.; Shinohara, A.; Ogawa, H.; Copeland, N.; Jenkins, N.A., Lalande, M. & Alt, F.W. (1997). RAB22 and RAB163/mouse BRCA2: proteins that specifically interact with RAD51 protein. *Proceedings of the National Academy of Science of the United States of America* Vol.94, No.13, (June 1997), pp.6927-6932 ISSN 0027-8424

Mladenov, E. & Iliakis, G. (2011). Induction and repair of DNA double-strand breaks: the increasing spectrum of non-homologous end joining pathways. *Mutation Research* In press ISSN 00275107

Modesti, M.; Budzowska, M.; Baldeyron, C.; Demmers, J.A.; Ghirlando, R. & Kanaar, R. (2007). RAD51AP1 is a structure-specific DNA binding protein that stimulates joint molecule formation during RAD51-mediated homologous recombination. *Molecular Cell* Vol.28, No.3, (November 2007), pp.468-481 ISSN 1097-2765

Monnat, R.J. Jr. (2010). Human RecQ helicases: roles in DNA metabolism, mutagenesis and cancer biology. *Seminars in Cancer Biology* Vol.20, No.5, (October 2010), pp.329-339 ISSN 1044-579X

Moriel-Carratero, M. & Aguilera, A. (2010a). A postincision-deficient TFIIH causes replication fork breakage and uncovers alternative Rad51- or Pol32-mediated restart mechanisms. *Molecular Cell,* Vol.37, No.5, (March 2010), pp. 690-701, ISSN 1097-2765

Moriel-Carratero, M. & Aguilera, A. (2010b). Replication fork breakage and re-start: new insight into Rad3/XPD-associated deficiencies. *Cell Cycle,* Vol.9, No.15, (August 2010), pp.2958-2962, ISSN 1551-4005

Mortensen, U.H.; Bendixen, C.; Sunjevaric, I. & Rothstein, R. (1996). DNA strand annealing is promoted by the yeast Rad52 protein. *Proceedings of the National Academy of Science of the United States of America* Vol.93, No.20, (October 1996), pp.10729-10734 ISSN 0027-8424

Mortensen, U.H.; Lisby, M. & Rothstein, R. (2009). Rad52. *Current Biology* Vol.19, No.16, (August 2009), pp.R676-R677 ISSN 0960-9822

Motegi, A.; Liaw, H.J.; Lee, K.Y.; Roest, H.P.; Maas, A.; Wu, X.; Moinova, H.; Markowitz, S.D.; Ding, H.; Hoeijmaker, J.H. & Myung, K. (2008). Polyubiquitination of proliferating cell nuclear antigen by HLTF and SHPRH prevents genomic instability from stalled replication forks. *Proceedings of the National Academy of Science of the United States of America* Vol.105, No.34, (August 2008), pp.12411-12416 ISSN 0027-8424

Moynahan, M.E. & Jasin, M. (2010). Mitotic homologous recombination maintains genomic stability and suppresses tumorigenesis. *Nature Reviews Molecular Cell Biology* Vol.11, No.3, (March 2010), pp.196-207 ISSN 1471-0072

Mullen, J.R.; Nallaseth, F.S.; Lan, Y.Q.; Slagle, C.E. & Brill, S.J. (2005). Yeast Rmi1/Nce4 controls genome stability as a subunit of the Sgs1-Top3 complex. *Molecular and Cellular Biology* Vol.25, No.11, (June 2005), pp.4476-4487 ISSN 0270-7306

Munoz, I.M.; Hain, K.; Déclais, A.C.; Gardiner, M.; Toh, G.W.; Sanchez-Pulido, L.; Heuckmann, J.M.; Toth, R.; Macartney, T.; Eppink, B.; Kanaar, R.; Ponting, C.P.; Lilley, D.M. & Rouse, J. (2009). Coordination of structure-specific nucleases by human SLX4/BTBD12 is required for DNA repair. *Molecular Cell* Vol.35, No.1, (July 2009), pp.116-127 ISSN 1097-2765

Neale, M.J.; Pan, J. & Keeney, S. (2005). Endonucleolytic processing of covalent protein-linked DNA double –strand breaks. *Nature* Vol.436, No.7053, (August 2005), pp.1053-1057 ISSN 0028-0836

Nakanishi, K.; Cavallo, F.; Perrouault, L.; Giovannangeli, C.; Moynahan, M.E., Barchi, M.; Brunet, E. & Jasin, M. (2011). Homology-directed Fanconi anemia pathway crosslink repair is dependent on DNA replication. *Nature Structural and Molecular Biology* Vol.18, No.4, (April 2011), pp.500-503 ISSN 1545-9985

Narayanan, V.; Mieczkowski, P.A.; Kim, H.M.; Petes, T.D. & Lobachev, K.S. (2006). The pattern of gene amplification is determined by the chromosomal location of hairpin-capped breaks. *Cell* Vol.125, No.7, (June 2006), pp.1283-1296 ISSN 0092-8674

Nasmyth, K. & Haering, C.H. (2009). Cohesin: its roles and mechanisms. *Annual Reviews of Genetics* Vol.43, (2009), pp.525-558 ISSN 0066-4197

Navadgi-Patil, V.M. & Burgers, P.M. (2009). A tale of two tails: activation of DNA damage checkpoint kinase Mec1/ATR by the 9-1-1 clamp and by Dpb11/TopBP1. *DNA Repair* Vol.8, No.9, (September 2009), pp.996-1003 ISSN 1568-7856

New, J.H.; Sugiyama, T.; Zaitseva, E. & Kowalczykowski, S.C. (1998). Rad52 protein stimulates DNA strand exchange by Rad51 and replication protein A. *Nature* Vol.391, No.6665, (January 1998), pp.407-410 ISSN 0028-0836

Nicolette, M.L.; Lee, K.; Guo, Z.; Rani, M.; Chow, J.M.; Lee, S.E. & Paull, T.T. (2010). Mre11-Rad50-Xrs2 and Sae2 promote 5′ strand resection of DNA double-strand breaks. *Nature Structural and Molecular Biology* Vol.17, No.12, (December 2010), pp.1478-1485 ISSN 1545-9985

Nimonkar, A.V.; Genschel, J.; Kinoshita, E.; Polaczek, P.; Campbell, J.L.; Wyman, C.; Modrich, P. & Kowalczykowski, S.C. (2011). BLM-DNA2-RPA-MRN and EXO1-BLM-RPA-MRN constitute two DNA end resection machineries for human DNA break repair. *Genes and Development* Vol.25, No.4, (February 2011), pp.350-362 ISSN 0890-9369

Nimonkar, A.V. & Kowalczykowski, S.C. (2009). Second-end capture in double-strand break repair: how to catch a DNA by its tail. *Cell Cycle* Vol.8, No.12, (June 2009), pp.1816-1817 ISSN 1551-4005

Nimonkar, A.V.; Sica, R.A. & Kowalczykowski, S.C. (2009). Rad52 promotes second-end capture in double strand break repair to form complement-stabilized joint molecules. *Proceedings of the National Academy of Science of the United States of America* Vol.106, No.9, (March 2009), pp.3077-3082 ISSN 0027-8424

Niu, H.; Chung, W.H.; Zhu, Z.; Kwon, Y.; Zhao, W.; Chi, P.; Prakash, R.; Seong, C.; Liu, L.; Ira, G. & Sung, P. (2010). Mechanism of the ATP-dependent DNA end-resection machinery from Saccharomyces cerevisiase. *Nature* Vol.467, No.7311, (September 2010), pp.108-111 ISSN 0028-0836

Oakley, G.G. & Patrick, S.M. (2010). Replication protein A: directing traffic at the intersection of replication and repair. *Frontiers in Bioscience* Vol.15, No.1, (June 2010), pp.883-900 ISSN 1093-4715

O'Donnell, L.; Panier, S.; Wildenhain, J.; Tkach, J.M.; Al-Hakim, A.; Landry, M.C.; Escribano-Diaz, C.; Szilard, R.K.; Young, J.T.; Munro, M.; Canny, M.D.; Kolas, N.K.; Zhang, W.; Harding, S.M.; Ylanko, J.; Mendez, M.; Mullin, M.; Sun, T.; Habermann, B.; Datti, A.; Bristow, R.G., Gingras, A.C.; Tyers, M.D.; Brown, G.W. & Durocher, D. (2010). The MMS22L-TONSL complex mediates recovery from replication stress and homologous recombination. *Molecular Cell* Vol.40, No.4, (November 2010), pp.619-631 ISSN 1097-2765

Osman, F.; Dixon, J.; Doe, C.L. & Whitby, M.C. (2003). Generating crossovers by resolution of nicked Holliday junctions: a role for Mus81-Eme1 in meiosis. *Molecular Cell* Vol.12, No.3, (September 2003), pp.761-774 ISSN 1097-2765

Osman, F. & Whitby, M.C. (2007). Exploring the roles of Mus81-Eme1/Mms4 at perturbed replication forks. *DNA Repair* Vol.6, No.7, (July 2007), pp.1004-1017 ISSN 1568-7856

Pacek, M. & Walter, J.C. (2004). A requirement for MCM7 and Cdc45 in chromosome unwinding during eukaryotic DNA replication. *EMBO Journal* Vol.23, No.18, (August 2004), pp.3667-3676 ISSN 0261-4189

Pagés, V. & Fuchs, R.P. (2003). Uncoupling of leading- and lagging-strand DNA replication during lesion bypass in vivo. *Science* Vol.300, No.5623, (May 2003), pp.1300-1303 ISSN 1095-8075

Papouli, E.; Chen, S.; Davies, A.A.; Huttner, D.; Krejci, L.; Sung, P. & Ulrich, H.D. (2005). Crosstalk between SUMO and ubiquitin on PCNA is mediated by recruitment of the helicase Srs2. *Molecular Cell* Vol.19, No.1, (July 2005), pp.123-133 ISSN 1097-2765

Park, M.S.; Ludwig, D.L.; Stigger, E. & Lee, S.H. (1996). Physical interaction between human RAD52 and RPA is required for homologous recombination in mammalian cells. *Journal of Biological Chemistry* Vol.271, No.31, (August 1996), pp.18996-19000 ISSN 0021-9258

Paulsen, R.D. & Cimprich, K.A. (2007). The ATR pathway: fine-tuning the fork. *DNA Repair* Vol.6, No.7, (July 2007), pp.953-966 ISSN 1568-7856

Petermann, E. & Helleday, T. (2010). Pathways of mammalian replication fork restart. *Nature Reviews Molecular Cell Biology* Vol.11, No.10, (October 2010), pp.683-687 ISSN 1471-0072

Petukhova, G.; Stratton, S. & Sung, P. (1998). Catalysis of homologous DNA pairing by yeast Rad51 and Rad54 proteins. *Nature* Vol.393, No.6680, (May 1998), pp.91-94 ISSN 0028-0836

Pfander, B.; Moldovan, G.L.; Sacher, M.; Hoege, C. & Jentsch, S. (2005). SUMO-modified PCNA recruits Srs2 to prevent recombination during S phase. *Nature* Vol.436, No.7049, (June 2005), pp.428-433 ISSN 0028-0836

Plate, I.; Hallwyl, S.C.; Shi, I.; Krejci, L.; Müller, C.; Albertsen, L.; Sung, P. & Mortensen, U.H. (2008). Interaction with RPA is necessary for Rad52 repair center formation and for its mediator activity. *Journal of Biological Chemistry* Vol.283, No.43, (October 2008), pp.29077-29085 ISSN 0021-9258

Poot, R.A.; Bozhenok, L.; van den Berg, D.L.; Steffensen, S.; Ferreira, F.; Grimaldi, M.; Gilbert, N.; Ferreira, J. & Varga-Weisz, P.D. (2004). The Williams syndrome transcription factor interacts with PCNA to target chromatin by ISWI to replication foci. *Nature Cell Biology* Vol.6, No.12, (December 2004), pp.1236-1244 ISSN 1465-7392

Poveda, A.M.; Le Clech, M. & Pasero, P. (2010). Transcription and replication: breaking the rules of the road causes genomic instability. *Transcription* Vol.1, No.2, (September 2010), pp.99-102 ISSN 2154-1272

Prado, F. & Aguilera, A. (2005). Impairment of replication fork progression mediates RNA polII transcription-associated recombination. *EMBO Journal* Vol.24, No.6, (March 2005), pp.1267-1276 ISSN 0261-4189

Prakash, S.; Johnson, R.E. & Prakash, L. (2005). Eukaryotic translesion synthesis DNA polymerases: specificity of structure and function. *Annual Reviews in Biochemistry* Vol. 74, (2005), pp.317-353 ISSN 0066-4154

Putnam, C.D.; Hayes, T.K. & Kolodner, R.D. (2009a). Specific pathways prevent duplication-mediated genome rearrangements. *Nature* Vol.460, No.7258, (August 2009), pp.984-989 ISSN 0028-0836

Putnam, C.D.; Jaehnig, E.J. & Kolodner, R.D. (2009b). Perspectives on the DNA damage and replication checkpoint response in Saccharomyces cerevisiae. *DNA Repair* Vol.8, No.9, (September 2009), pp.974-982 ISSN 1568-7856

Ralf, C.; Hickson, I.D. & Wu, L. (2006). The Bloom's syndrome helicase can promote the regression of a model replication fork. *Journal of Biological Chemistry* Vol.281, No.32, (August 2006), pp.22839-22846 ISSN 0021-9258

Ranatunga, W.; Jackson, D.; Lloyd, J.A.; Forget, A.L.; Knight, K.L. & Borgstahl, G.E. (2001). Human Rad52 exhibits two modes of self-association. *Journal of Biological Chemistry* Vol.276, No.19, (February 2001), pp.15876-15880 ISSN 0021-9258

Raschle, M.; van Komen, S.; Chi, P.; Ellenberger, T. & Sung, P. (2004). Multiple interactions with Rad51 recombinase govern the homologous recombination function of Rad54. *Journal of Biological Chemistry* Vol.279, No.50, (September 2004), pp.1973-1980 ISSN 0021-9258

Rass, U.; Compton, S.A.; Matos, J.; Singleton, M.R.; Ip, S.C.; Blanco, M.G.; Griffith, J.D. & West, S.C. (2010). Mechanism of Holliday junction resolution by the human GEN1 protein. *Genes and Development* Vol.24, No.14, (July 2010), pp.1559-1569 ISSN 1549-5477

Raynard, S.; Bussen, W. & Sung, P. (2006). A double Holliday junction dissolvasome compromising BLM, topoisomerase IIIα, and BLAP75. *Journal of Biological Chemistry* Vol.281, No.20, (May 2006), pp.13861-13864 ISSN 0021-9258

Rogakou, E.P.; Pilch, D.R.; Orr, A.H.; Ivanova, V.S. & Bonner, W.M. (1998). DNA double-strand breaks induce histone H2AX phosphorylation on serine 139. *Journal of Biological Chemistry* Vol.6, No.273, (March 1998), pp.5858-5868 ISSN 0021-9258

Roseaulin, L.; Yamada, Y.; Tsutsui, Y.; Russell, P.; Iwasaki, H. & Arcangioli, B. (2008). Mus81 is essential for sister chromatid recombination at broken replication forks. *EMBO Journal* Vol.27, No.9, (April 2008), pp.1378-1387 ISSN 0261-4189

San Filippo, J.; Sung, P. & Klein, H. (2008). Mechanism of eukaryotic homologous recombination. *Annual Reviews of Biochemistry* Vol.77, (2008), pp.229-257 ISSN 0066-4154

Schlacher, K.; Christ, N.; Siaud, N.; Egashira, A.; Wu, H. & Jasin, M. (2011). Homologous recombination-independent role for BRCA2 in blocking stalled replication fork degradation by MRE11. *Cell* Vol.144, No.10, (May 2011), pp. ISSN 0092-8674

Schwartz, E.K. & Heyer, W.D. (2011). Processing of joint molecule intermediates by structure-selective endonucleases during homologous recombination in eukaryotes. *Chromosoma* Vol.120, No.2, (April 2011), pp.109-127 ISSN 0009-5915

Scully, R.; Chen, J.; Ochs, R.L.; Keegan, K.; Hoekstra, M.; Feunteun, J. & Livingston, D.M. (1997). Dynamic changes of BRCA1 subnuclear location and phosphorylation state are initiated by DNA damage. *Cell* Vol.90, No.3, (August 1997), pp.425-435 ISSN 0092-8674

Sharan, S.K.; Morimatsu, M.; Albrecht, U.; Lim, D.S.; Reqel, E.; Dinh, C.; Sands, A.; Eichele, G.; Hasty, P. & Bradley, A. (1997). Embryonic lethality and radiation hypersensitivity mediated by Rad51 in mice lacking BRCA2. *Nature* Vol.386, No.6627, (April 1997), pp.804-810 ISSN 0028-0836

Sherwood, R.; Takahashi, T.S. & Jallepalli, P.V. (2010). Sister acts: coordinating DNA replication and cohesion establishment. *Genes and Development* Vol24, No.24, (December 2010), pp.2723-2731 ISSN0890-9369

Shim, E.Y.; Chung, W.H.; Nicolette, M.L.; Zhang, Y.; Davis, M.; Zhu, Z.; Paull, T.T.; Ira, G. & Lee, S.E. (2010). Saccharomyces cerevisiae Mre11/Rad50/Xrs2 and Ku proteins regulate association of Exo1 and Dna2 with DNA breaks. *EMBO Journal* Vol.29, No.19, (October 2010), pp.3370-3380 ISSN 0261-4189

Shinohara, A.; Shinohara, M.; Ohta, T.; Matsuda, S. & Ogawa, T. (1998). Rad52 forms ring structures and co-operates with RPA in single-strand annealing. *Genes to Cells* Vol.3, No.3, (March 1998), pp.145-156 ISSN 1356-9597

Singh, T.R.; Ali, A.M.; Busygina, V.; Raynard, S.; Fan, Q.; Du, C.H.; Andreassen, P.R.; Sung, P. & Meetei, A.R. (2008). BLAP18/RMI2, a novel OB-fold –containing protein, is an essential component of the Bloom helicase-double Holliday junction dissolvasome. *Genes and Development* Vol.22, No.20, (October 2008), pp.2856-2868 ISSN 0890-9369

Singh, T.R.; Saro, D.; Ali, A.M.; Zheng, X.F.; Du, C.H.; Killen, M.W.; Sachpatzidis, A.; Wahengbam, K.; Pierce, A.J.; Xiong, Y.; Sung, P. & Meetei, A.R. (2010). MHF1-MHF2, a histone-fold-containing protein complex, participates in the Fanconia anemia pathway via FANCM. *Molecular Cell* Vol.37, No.6, (March 2010), pp.879-886 ISSN 1097-2765

Sleeth, K.M.; Sørensen, C.S.; Issaeva, N.; Dziegielewski, J.; Bartek, J. & Helleday, T. (2007). RPA mediates recombination repair during replication stress and is displaced from DNA by checkpoint signalling in human cells. *Journal of Molecular Biology* Vol.373, No.1, (October 2007), pp.38-47 ISSN 0022-2836

Sogo, J.M.; Lopes, M. & Foiani, M. (2000). Fork reversal and ssDNA accumulation at stalled replication forks owing to checkpoint defects. *Science* Vol.297, No.5581, (July 2000), pp.599-602 ISSN 0036-8075

Solinger, J.A.; Lutz, G.; Sugiyama, T.; Kowalczykowski, S.C. & Heyer, W.D. (2001). Rad54 protein stimulates heteroduplex DNA formation in the synaptic phase of DNA strand exchenge via specific interactions with the presynaptic Rad51 nucleoprotein filament. *Journal of Molecular Biology* Vol.307, No.5, (April 2001), 1207-1221 ISSN 0022-2836

Sommers, J.A.; Rawtani, N.; Gupta, R.; Bugreev, D.V.; Mazin, A.V.; Cantor, S.B. & Brosh, R.M. Jr. (2009). FANCJ uses its motor ATPase to destabilize protein-DNA complexes, unwind triplexes, and inhibit RAD51 strand exchange. *Journal of Biological Chemistry* Vol.284, No.12, (March 2009), pp.7505-7517 ISSN 0021-9258

Stasiak, A.Z.; Larquet, E.; Stasiak, A.; Müller, S.; Engel, A.; van Dyck, E.; West, S.C. & Egelman, E.H. (2000). The human Rad52 protein exists as a heptameric ring. *Current Biology* Vol.10, No.6, (March 2000), pp.337-340 ISSN 0960-9822

Stelter, P. & Ulrich, H.D. (2003). Control of spontaneous and damage-induced mutagenesis by SUMO and ubiquitin conjugation. *Nature* Vol.425, No.6954, (September 2003), pp.188-191 ISSN 0028-0836

Stoimenov, I. & Helleday, T. (2009). PCNA on the crossroad of cancer. *Biochemical Society Transactions* Vol.37, No.3, (June 2009), pp.605-613 ISSN 0300-5127

Stucki, M.; Clapperton, J.A.; Mohammad, D.; Yaffe, M.B.; Smerdon, S.J. & Jackson, S.P. (2005). MCD1 directly binds phosphorylated histone H2AX to regulate cellular responses to DNA double-strand breaks. *Cell* Vol.123, No.7, (December 2005), pp.1213-1226 ISSN 0092-8674

Stucki, M. & Jackson, S.P. (2006). γH2AX and MDC1: anchoring the DNA-damage-response machinery to broken chromosomes. *DNA Repair* Vol.5, No.5, (May 2006), pp.534-543 ISSN 1568-7856

Sugiyama, T. & Kantake, N. (2009). Dynamic regulatory interactions of rad51, rad52, and replication protein-A in recombination intermediates. *Journal of Molecular Biology* Vol.390, No.1, (June 2009), pp.45-55 ISSN 0022-2836

Sun, W.; Nandi, S.; Osman, F.; Ahn, J.S.; Jakovleska, J.; Lorenz, A. & Whitby, M.C. (2008). The FANCM ortholog Fml1 promotes recombination at stalled replication forks and limits crossing over during DNA doiuble-strand break repair. *Molecular Cell* Vol.32, No.1, (October 2008), pp.118-128 ISSN 1097-2765

Sung, P. (1994). Catalysis of ATP-dependent homologous DNA pairing and strand exchange by yeast RAD51 protein. *Science* Vol.265, No.5176, (August 1994), pp.1241-1243 ISSN 0036-8075

Svendsen, J.M & Harper, J.W. (2010). GEN1/Yen1 and the SLX4 complex: solutions to the problem of Holliday junction resolution. *Genes and Development* Vol.24, No.6, (March 2010), pp.521-536 ISSN 0890-9369

Svendsen, J.M.; Smogorzewska, A.; Sowa, M.E.; O'connell, B.C.; Gygi, S.P.; Elledge, S.J. & Harper, J.W. (2009). Mammalian BTBD12/SLX4 assembles a Holliday junction resolvase and is required for DNA repair. *Cell* Vol.138, No.1, (July 2009), pp.63-77 ISSN 0092-8674

Sy, S.M.; Huen, M.S. & Chen, J. (2009). PALB2 is an integral component of the BRCA complex required for homologous recombination repair. *Proceedings of the National Academy of Science of the United States of America* Vol.106, No.17, (April 2009), pp.7155-7160 ISSN 0027-8424

Symington, L.S. (2002). Role of Rad52 epistasis group genes in homologous recombination and double-strand break repair. *Microbiology and Molecular Biology Reviews* Vol.66, No.4, (December 2002), pp.630-670 ISSN 1092-2172

Symington, L.S. & Heyer, W.D. (2006). Some disassembly required: role of DNA translocases in the disruption of recombination intermediates and dead-end complexes. *Genes and Development* Vol.20, No.18, (September 2006), pp.2479-2486 ISSN 0890-9369

Tan, T.L.; Kanaar, R. & Wyman, C. (2003). Rad54, a Jack of all trades in homologous recombination. *DNA Repair* Vol.2, No.7, (July 2003), pp.787-794 ISSN 1568-7856

Tay, Y.D. & Wu, L. (2010). Overlapping roles for Yen1 and Mus81 in cellular Holliday junction processing. *Journal of Biological Chemistry* Vol285, No.15, (April 2010), pp11427-11432 ISSN 0021-9258

Thomä, N.H.; Czyzewski, B.K.; Alexeev, A.A.; Mazin, A.V.; Kowalczykowski, S.C. & Pavletich, N.P. (2005). Structure of teh SWI2/SNF2 chromatin-remodeling domain of eukaryotic Rad54. *Nature Structural and Molecular Biology* Vol.12, No.4, (April 2005), pp.350-356 ISSN 1545-9985

Thompson, L.H. & Jones, N.J. (2010). Stabilizing and remodeling the blocked DNA replication fork: anchoring FANCM and the Fanconia anemia damage response. *Molecular Cell* Vol.37, No.6, (March 2010), pp.749-751 ISSN 1097-2765

Tischlowitz, M. & Xia, B. (2010). PALB2/FANCN: recombining cancer and Fanconia anemia. *Cancer Research* Vol.70, No.19, (September 2010), pp.7353-7359 ISSN 0008-5472

Tsubouchi, H. & Roeder, G.S. (2004). The budding yeast mei5 and sae3 proteins act together with dmc1 during meiotic recombination. *Genetics* Vol.168, No.3, (November 2004), pp.1219-1230 ISSN 0016-6731

Tuduri, S.; Crabbe, L.; Tourrière, H.; Coquelle, A. & Pasero, P. (2010). Does interference between replication and transcription contribute to genomic instability in cancer cells? *Cell Cycle* Vol.9, No.10, (May 2010), pp.1886-1892 ISSN 1551-4005

Ulrich, H.D. & Jentsch, S. (2000). Two RING finger proteins mediate cooperation between ubiquitin-conjugating enzymes in DNA repair. *EMBO Journal* Vol.19, no.13, (July 2000), pp.3388-3397 ISSN 0261-4189

Unk, I.; Hajdú, I.; Blastyák, A. & Haracska, L. (2010). Role of yeast Rad5 and its human orthologs, HLTF and SHPRH in DNA damage tolerance. *DNA Repair* Vol.9, No.3, (March 2010), pp.257-267 ISSN 1568-7856

Van der Heijden, T.; Seidel, R.; Modesti, M.; Kanaar, R.; Wyman, C. & Dekker, C. (2007). Real-time assembly and disassembly of human RAD51 filaments on individual DNA molecules. *Nucleic Acids Research* Vol.35, No.17, (August 2007), pp.5646-5657 ISSN 0305-1048

Vasquez, K.M. (2010). Targeting and processing of site-specific DNA interstrand crosslinks. *Environmental and Molecular Mutagenesis* Vol.51, No.6, (July 2010), pp.527-539 ISSN 0893-6692

Vassin, V.M.; Anantha, R.W.; Sokolova, E.; Kanner, S. & Borowies, J.A. (2009). Human RPA phosphorylation by ATR stimulates DNA synthesis and prevents ssDNA accumulation during DNA-replication stress. *Journal of Cell Science* Vol.122, No.22, (November 2009), pp.4070-4080 ISSN 0021-9533

Vejrup-Hansen, R.; Mizuno, K.; Miyabe, I.; Fleck, O.; Holmberg, C.; Murray, J.M.; Carr, A.M. & Nielsen, O. (2011). Schizosaccharomyces pombe Mms1 channels repair of perturbed replication into Rhp51 independent homologous recombination. *DNA Repair* Vol.10, No.3, (March 2011), pp.283-295 ISSN 1568-7856

Vengrova, S.; Codlin, S. & Dalgaard, J.Z. (2002). RTS1-an eukaryotic terminator or replication. *The International Journal of Biochemistry and Cell Biology* Vol.34, No.9, (September 2002), pp.1031-1034 ISSN 1357-2725

Watson, J.D. & Crick, F.H. (1953a). Molecular structure of nucleic acids; a structure for deoxyribose nucleic acid. *Nature* Vol.171, No.4356, (April 1953), pp.737-738 ISSN 0028-0836

Watson, J.D. & Crick, F.H. (1953b). Genetic implications of the structure of deoxyribonucleic acid. *Nature* Vol.171, No.4361, (May 1953), pp.964-967 ISSN 0028-0836

Weschsler, T.; Newman, S. & West, S.C. (2011). Aberrant chromosome morphology in human cells defective for Holliday junction resolution. *Nature* Vol.471, No.7340, (March 2011), pp.642-646 ISSN 0028-0836

Weinert, T.; Kaochar, S.; Jones, H.; Paek, A. & Clarke, A.J. (2009). The replication fork's five degrees of freedom, their failure and genome rearrangements. *Current Opinions in Cell Biology* Vol.21, No.6, (December 2009), pp.778-784 ISSN 0955-0674

Weinstock, D.M.; Richardson, C.A.; Elliot, B. & Jasin, M. (2006) Modeling oncogenic translocations: distinct roles for double-strand break repair pathways in translocation formation in mammalian cells. *DNA Repair* Vol.5, No.9-10, (September 2006), pp.1065-1074 ISSN 1568-7856

Whitby, M.C. (2010). The FANCM family of DNA helicases/translocases. *DNA Repair* Vol.9, No.3, (February 2010), pp.224-236 ISSN 1568-7856

Whitby, M.C.; Osman, F. & Dixon, J. (2003). Cleavage of model replication forks by fission yeast Mus81-Eme1 and budding yeast Mus81-Mms4. *Journal of Biological Chemistry* Vol.278, No.9, (February 2003), pp.6928-6935 ISSN 0021-9258

White, M.F. (2009). Structure, function and evolution of the XPD family of iron-sulfur-containing 5' to 3' DNA helicases. *Biochemical Society Transaction* Vol.37, No.3, (June 2009), pp.547-551 ISSN 0300-5127

Wiese, C.; Dray, E.; Groesser, T.; San Filippo, J.; Shi, I.; Collins, D.W.; Tsai, M.S.; Williams, G.J.; Rydberg, B.; Sung, P. & Schild, D. (2007). Promotion of homologous recombination and genomic stability by RAD51AP1 via RAD51 recombinase enhancement. *Molecular Cell* Vol.28, No.3, (November 2007), pp.482-490 ISSN 1097-2765

Williams, R.S.; Moncalian, G.; Williams, J.S.; Yamada, Y.; Limbo, O.; Shin, D.S.; Groocock, L.M.; Cahill, D.; Hitomi, C.; Guenther, G.; Moiani, D.; Carney, J.P.; Russell, P. & Tainer, J.A. (2008). Mre11 dimers coordinate DNA bridging and nuclease processing in double-strand break repair. *Cell* Vol.135, No.1, (October 2008), pp.97-109 ISSN 0092-8674

Wolner, B. & Peterson, C.L. (2005). ATP-dependent and ATP-independent roles for the Rad54 chromatin remodelling enzyme during recombination repair of a DNA double strand break. *Journal of Biological Chemistry* Vol.280, No.11, (January 2005), pp.10855-10860 ISSN 0021-9258

Wood, R.D. (2010) Mammalian nucleotide excision repair proteins and interstrand crosslink repair. *Environmental Molecular Mutagenesis* Vol.51, No.6, (July 2010) pp.520-526 ISSN 0893-6692

Wood, A.J.; Severson, A.F. & Meyer, B.J. (2010). Condensin and cohesion complexity: the expanding repertoire of functions. *Nature Reviews Genetics* Vol.11, No.6; (May 2010), pp.391-404 ISSN 1471-0056

Wu, L.; Barchrati, C.Z.; Ou, J.; Xu, C.; Yin, J.; Chang, M.; Wang, W.; Li, L.; Brown, G.W. & Hickson, I.D. (2006). BLAP75/RMI1 promotes the BLM-dependent dissolution of homologous recombination intermediates. *Proceedings of the National Academy of Science of the United States of America* Vol.103, No.11, (March 2006), pp.4068-4073 ISSN 0027-8424

Wu, J.; Huen, M.S.; Lu, L.Y.; Dou, Y.; Ljungman, M.; Chen, J. & Yu, X. (2009a). Histone ubiquitination associates with BRCA1-dependent DNA damage response. *Molecular and Cellular Biology* Vol.29, No.3, (February 2009), pp.849-860 ISSN 0270-7306

Wu, X.; Yang, Z.; Liu, Y. & Zou, Y. (2005). Preferential localization of hyperphosphorylation replication protein A to double-strand break repair and checkpoint complexes upon DNA damage. *Biochemical Journal* Vol.391, No.3, (November 2005), pp.473-480 ISSN 0264-6021

Wu, J.; Lu, L.Y. & Yu, X. (2010). The role of BRCA1 in DNA damage response. *Protein and Cell* Vol.1, No.2, (February 2010), pp.117-123 ISSN 1674-8018

Wu, Y.; Suhasini, A.N. & Brosh, R.M. Jr. (2009b). Welcome the family of FANCJ-like helicases to the block of genome stability maintenance proteins. *Cellular and Molecular Life Sciences* Vol.66, No.7, (April 2009), pp.1209-1222 ISSN 1420-682X

Wu, Y.; Shin-ya, K. & Brosh, R.M. Jr. (2008). FANCJ helicase defective in Fanconia anemia and breast cancer unwinds G-quadruplex DNA to defend genomic stability. *Molecular and Cellular Biology* Vol.28, No.12, (June 2008), 4116-4128 ISSN 0270-7306

Xiong, B. & Gerton, J.L. (2010). Regulators of the cohesion network. *Annual Reviews of Biochemistry* Vol.79, (2020), pp.131-153 ISSN 0066-4154

Yao, N.Y. & O'Donnell, M. (2009). Replisome structure and conformational dynamics underlie fork progression past obstacles. *Current Opinions in Cell Biology* Vol.21, No.3, (June 2009), pp.336-343 ISSN 0955-0674

Yan, Z.; Delannoy, M.; Ling, C.; Daee, D.; Osman, F.; Muniandy, P.A.; Shen, X.; Oostra, A.B.; Du, H.; Steltenpool, J.; Lin, T.; Schuster, B.; Décaillet, C.; Stasiak, A.; Stasiak, A.Z.; Stone, S.; Hoatlin, M.E.; Schindler, D.; Woodcock, C.L.; Joenje, H.; Sen, R.; de Winter, J.P.; Li, L.; Seidman, M.M.; Whitby, M.C.; Myung, K.; Constantinou, A. & Wang, W. (2010). A histone-fold complex and FANCM form a conserved DNA-remodeling complex to maintain genome stability. *Molecular Cell* Vol.37, No.6, (March 2010), pp.865-878 ISSN 1097-2765

Yang, H.; Li, Q.; Fan, J.; Holloman, W.K. & Pavletich, N.P. (2005). The BRCA2 homologue Brh2 nucelates RAD51 filament formation at a dsDNA-ssDNA junction. *Nature* Vol.433, No.7026, (February 2005), pp.653-657 ISSN 0028-0836

Yang, J.; Bachrati, C.Z.; Ou, J.; Hickson, I.D. & Brown, G.W. (2010). Human topoisomerase IIIα is a single-stranded DNA decatenase that is stimulated by BLM and RMI1. *Journal of Biological Chemistry* Vol.285, No.28, (July 2010), pp.21426-21436 ISSN 0021-9258

Yin, J.; Sobeck, A.; Xu, C.; Meetei, A.R.; Hoatlin, M.; Li, L. & Wang, W. (2005). BLAP75, an essential component of Bloom's syndrome protein complexes that maintain genome integrity. *EMBO Journal* Vol.24, No.7, (April 2005), pp.1465-1476 ISSN 0261-4189

Yuan, J.; Ghosal, G. & Chen, J. (2009). The annealing helicase HARP protects stalled replication forks. *Genes and Development* Vol.23, No.20, (September 2009), pp.2394-2399 ISSN 0890-9369

Yun, M.H. & Hiom, K. (2009a). CtIP-BRCA1 modulates the choice of DNA double-strand break repair pathway throughout the cell cycle. *Nature* Vol.459, No.7245, (May 2009), pp.460-463 ISSN 0028-0836

Yun, M.H. & Hiom, K. (2009b). Understanding the functions of BRCA1 in the DNA-damage response. *Biochemical Society Transactions* Vol.37, No.3, (June 2009), pp.597-604 ISSN 0300-5127

Yusufzai, T. & Kadonaga, J.T. (2008). HARP is an ATP-driven annealing helicase. *Science* Vol.322, No.5902, (October 2008), pp.748-750 ISSN 0036-8075

Yusufzai, T. & Kadonaga, J.T. (2010). Annealing helicase 2 (AH2), a DNA-rewinding motor with an HNH motif. *Proceedings of the National Academy of Science of the United States of America* Vol.107, No.49, (November 2010), pp.20970-20973 ISSN 0027-8424

Yusufzai, T. & Kadonaga, J.T. (2011). Branching out with DNA helicases. *Current Opinions in Genetics and Development* Vol.21, No.2, (February 2011), pp.214-218 ISSN 0959-437X

Yusufzai, T.; Kong, X.; Yokomori, K. & Kadonaga, J.T. (2009). The annealing helicase HARP is recruited to DNA repair sites via an interaction with RPA. *Genes and Development* Vol.23, No.20, (September 2009), pp.2400-2404 ISSN 0890-9369

Zhang, Z.; Fan, H.Y.; Goldman, J.A. & Kingston, R.E. (2007). Homology-driven chromatin remodeling by human RAD54. *Nature Structural and Molecular Biology* Vol.14, No.5, (May 2007), pp.397-405 ISSN 1545-9985

Zhang, F.; Fan, Q., Ren, K. & Andreassen, P.R. (2009a). PALB2 functionally connects the breast cancer susceptibility proteins BRCA1 and BRCA2. *Molecular Cancer Research* Vol.7, No.7, (July 2009), pp.1110-1118 ISSN 1541-7786

Zhang, F.; Ma, J.; Wu, J.; Ye, L.; Cai, H.; Xia, B. & Yu, X. (2009b). PALB2 links BRCA1 and BRCA2 in the DNA-damage response. *Current Biology* Vol.19, No.6, (March 2009), pp.524-529 ISSN 0960-9822

Zhao, G.Y.; Sonada, E.; Barber, L.J.; Oka, H.; Murakawa, Y.; Yamada, K.; Ikura, T.; Wang, X.; Kobayashi, M.; Yamamoto, K.; Boulton, S.J. & Takeda, S. (2007). A critical role for the ubiquitin-conjugating enzyme Ubc13 in initiating homologous recombination. *Molecular Cell* Vol.25, No.5, (March 2007), pp.663-675 ISSN 1097-2765

Zhu, Z.; Chung, W.H.; Shim, E.Y.; Lee, S.E. & Ira, G. (2008). Sgs1 helicase and two nucelases Dna2 and Exo1 resect DNA double-strand break ends. *Cell* Vol.134, No.6, (September 2008), pp.981-994 ISSN 0092-8674

Zou, L. & Elledge, S.J (2003). Sensing DNA damage through ATRIP recognition of RPA-ssDNA complexes. *Science* Vol.300, No.5625, (June 2003), pp.1542-1548 ISSN 0036-8075

Part 4

The Cell Cycle and Replication

17

Cell Cycle Regulation of DNA Replication in *S. cerevisiae*

Jorrit M. Enserink
Centre for Molecular Biology and Neuroscience (CMBN)
Oslo University Hospital, Oslo
Norway

1. Introduction

Cell duplication is a strictly regulated process that underlies growth and development of all organisms. The ordered series of events that lead to the duplication of a cell is commonly referred to as the cell cycle. The purpose of the cell cycle is to transmit an intact and complete copy of the genome from one generation to the next. Although certain highly specialized cell types undergo multiple rounds of replication per cell cycle in a developmentally coordinated process termed endoreplication, like for example megakaryocytes, plant endosperm, *Drosophila* follicle and nurse cells, and rodent trophoblasts (Lee, Davidson et al. 2009), the vast majority of cells in an organism replicate their DNA only once per cell cycle. Endoreplication differs from the aberrant process of re-replication in that it is highly regulated, and DNA content increases by clearly delineated genome doublings, whereas re-replication results from unscheduled activation of the DNA replication process (Lee, Davidson et al. 2009). Re-replication can result in genome instability that can have adverse effects on the well-being of the organism. Multiple mechanisms have evolved that prevent re-replication by restricting DNA replication to one specific phase of the cell cycle. Several protein complexes required for the various steps of DNA replication are separated in time and space during the cell cycle, and are only active during brief phases of the cell cycle. In this chapter I will discuss regulation of DNA replication by the cell cycle.

2. The cell cycle

2.1 Regulation of the cell cycle by cyclin dependent kinases

The cell cycle is generally divided into four specific phases: G1 phase, during which the cell grows and prepares for cell cycle entry; S phase, during which DNA synthesis takes place; G2 phase, during which cells prepare for M phase; and M phase, in which chromosomes segregate and cells divide. In eukaryotic cells, the cell cycle is controlled by cyclin dependent kinases (CDKs; Figure 1). CDKs have been highly conserved during evolution; even to such a degree that vertebrate CDK1 can substitute for *Saccharomyces cerevisiae* Cdk1. A single CDK, Cdk1 (also known as Cdc28) is necessary and sufficient for cell cycle control in *S. cerevisiae* (Enserink and Kolodner 2010). Nine different cyclins form complexes with Cdk1 throughout the cell cycle to regulate efficient cell cycle progression. In higher

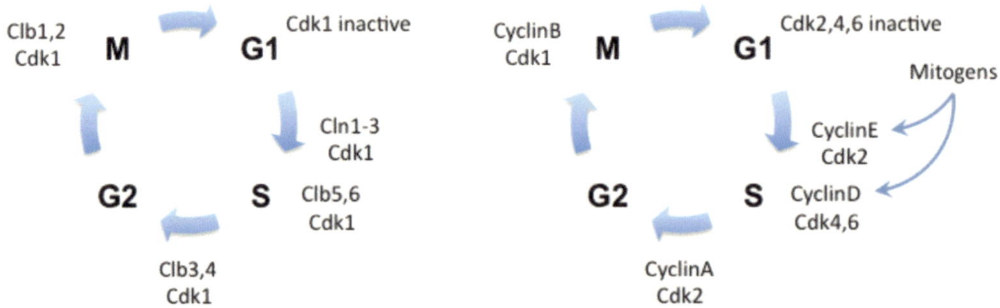

Fig. 1. Regulation of the cell cycle by CDKs. Cell cycle regulation by CDKs is highly conserved throughout evolution. A single CDK regulates the cell cycle in *S. cerevisiae*, while multiple CDKs have been associated with cell cycle control in higher eukaryotes. Nonetheless, a single CDK suffices for cell cycle control in higher eukaryotes, except during embryogenesis.

eukaryotes, several CDKs are involved in cell cycle regulation, i.e. Cdk1, Cdk2, Cdk4 and Cdk6 (Satyanarayana and Kaldis 2009). Mitogens induce transcription of cyclin D and cyclin E, which form complexes with Cdk4/6 and Cdk2, respectively, to induce entry into the cell cycle. Cdk1 is traditionally thought of as a mitotic CDK that is only involved in regulation of mitosis (Satyanarayana and Kaldis 2009). However, mouse knockout models have changed this paradigm; only Cdk1 was shown to be necessary and sufficient for cell cycle control, while Cdk2/4/6 do not suffice to regulate the cell cycle (Malumbres and Barbacid 2009). Instead, Cdk2/4/6 are important for development of the organism by controlling the cell cycle in cells of specialized tissues (Malumbres and Barbacid 2009). Note that this single-CDK model is very similar to the yeast cell cycle model in which a single CDK suffices for cell cycle regulation.

2.2 Regulation of cyclin dependent kinases

CDK activity is controlled at multiple levels (Figure 2). CDKs are inactive during G1 phase because cyclin levels are low (Pines 1994). As the cell progresses through G1 phase, cyclin levels increase, and binding of cyclin to CDK increases the catalytic activity of the kinase (Jeffrey, Russo et al. 1995). CDKs, like other kinases, have a two-lobed structure. In absence of cyclins the catalytic cleft is blocked by a large, flexible structure called the T loop, and the phosphates of the ATP molecule are improperly aligned (Pavletich 1999). When cyclins bind, the T loop moves away from the catalytic cleft, and the phosphates of the ATP molecule realign, allowing phosphorylation of substrate proteins. In addition, phosphorylation of the T loop increases the affinity of the CDK for cyclins and further exposes the catalytic cleft (Russo, Jeffrey et al. 1996). CDK activity is negatively regulated by cyclin dependent kinase inhibitors (CKIs), such as $p21^{WAF}$, $p27^{CIP}$ and $p16^{INK4}$. CKIs directly bind cyclin-CDK complexes, and inhibit binding of ATP to the kinase ($p27^{CIP}$) or prevent binding of the cyclin ($p16^{INK4}$) (Pavletich 1999). Furthermore, CDKs can be phosphorylated on residues in the N-terminus by Wee1 kinases, leading to inhibition of CDK activity . For instance, *S. cerevisiae* Cdk1 is phosphorylated on Y19 by Swe1, which prevents entry into M phase (Booher, Deshaies et al. 1993). Phosphatases of the Cdc25 family (Mih1 in *S. cerevisiae*) dephosphorylate these N-terminal residues to alleviate inhibition of Cdk1, thereby allowing the cell to resume the cell cycle (Russell and Nurse 1986).

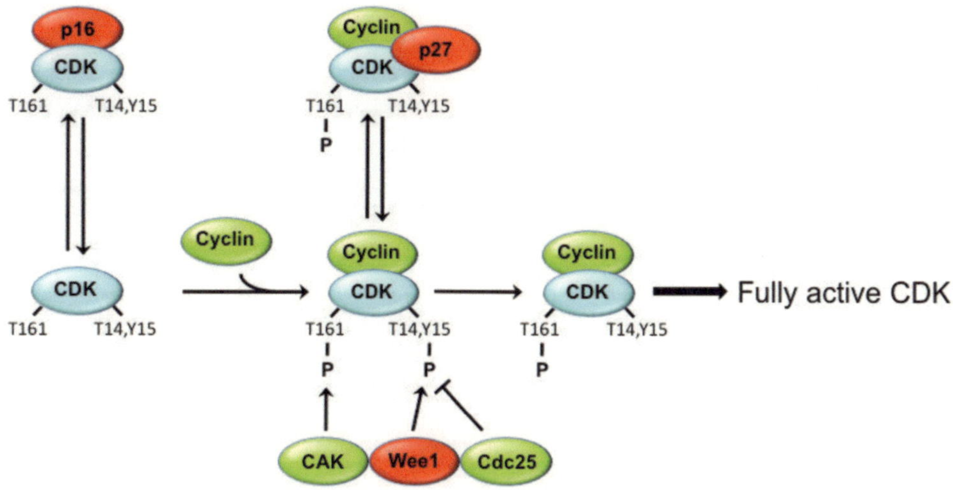

Fig. 2. Regulation of CDK activity. CAK is composed of three subunits in higher eukaryotes and consists of Cdk7, cyclin H and MAT1, while in *S. cerevisiae* the kinase Cak1 provides CAK activity. T161 is similar to T163 in *S. cerevisiae*, and T14 and Y15 correspond to *S. cerevisiae* Y19. See text for details.

2.3 Positive feedback induces entry into S phase

A notable feature of cell cycle regulation is the abundant use of feedback loops, which make cell cycle transitions particularly switch-like (Ferrell, Tsai et al. 2011). One example is the transition from G1 to S phase (Fig. 3A). During G1 phase, CDKs are inactive due to low cyclin levels and the presence of CKIs. However, as the cell progresses through G1, cyclin levels (Cln3 in *S. cerevisiae*) gradually increase. Cln3-Cdk1 complexes then phosphorylate a protein called Whi5 (Costanzo, Nishikawa et al. 2004; de Bruin, McDonald et al. 2004). Whi5 is a transcriptional suppressor that interacts with SBF, a transcription factor complex required for transcription of genes involved in cell cycle entry and DNA replication (the so-called G1 transcriptional program). Whi5 also recruits histone deacetylases (HDACs) that maintain the chromatin surrounding the SBF-Whi5 complex in a repressive state (Huang, Kaluarachchi et al. 2009; Wang, Carey et al. 2009). Thus, as long as Whi5 is bound to SBF, the cell cannot enter the cell cycle. However, phosphorylation of Whi5 by Cln3-Cdk1 induces the release of Whi5 and HDACs from SBF (Costanzo, Nishikawa et al. 2004; de Bruin, McDonald et al. 2004; Huang, Kaluarachchi et al. 2009; Wang, Carey et al. 2009). SBF then activates transcription of the G1 transcriptional program. Importantly, several cyclins (e.g. Cln1 and Cln2) are part of this transcriptional program, and in a positive feedback loop the newly synthesized cyclins will further activate Cdk1 to phosphorylate more Whi5, leading to further activation of SBF (Charvin, Oikonomou et al. 2010). This positive feedback loop makes cell cycle entry behave like a switch, ensuring coherent cell cycle entry. Cell cycle entry also requires destruction of the CKI Sic1, which inhibits Clb5-Cdk1 and Clb6-Cdk1 (Schwob, Bohm et al. 1994). Clb5,6-Cdk1, as we will see below, activate DNA replication. Sic1 is phosphorylated by Cln-Cdk1 complexes, which targets it for destruction by the SCF (Nash, Tang et al. 2001). Thus, both Whi5 and Sic1 need to be inhibited for efficient cell cycle entry.

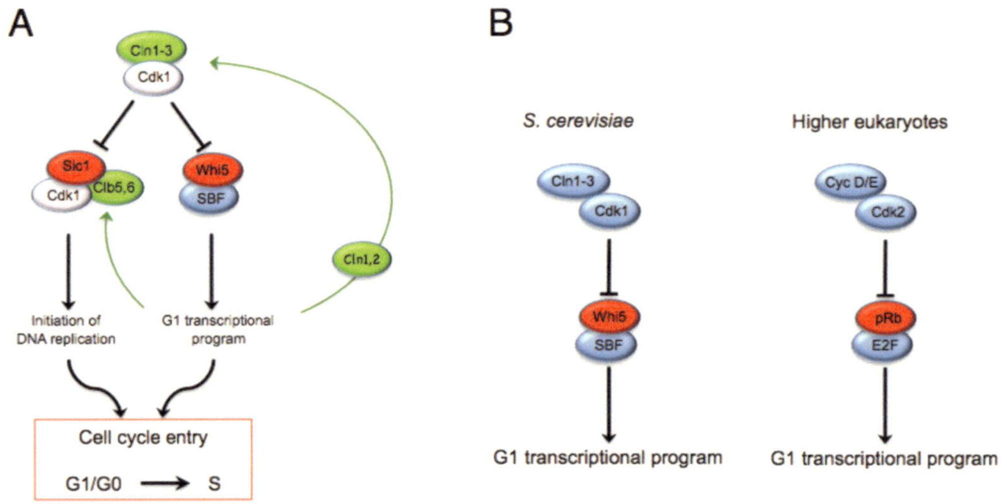

Fig. 3. Regulation of cell cycle entry in *S. cerevisiae*. A, Efficient cell cycle entry requires feedback mechanisms. Cln3-Cdk1 initially phosphorylates a small amount of Whi5, leading to minor activation of the G1 transcriptional program. Cyclins *CLN1*, *CLN2*, *CLB5* and *CLB6* are part of this program, and in a positive feedback loop, Cln1 and Cln2 will bind and activate Cdk1, leading to phosphorylation of more Whi5. DNA replication will not start before the CKI Sic1, which inhibits Clb5-Cdk1 and Clb6-Cdk1 complexes, is degraded. Sic1 degradation is initiated by phosphorylation by Cln1,2-Cdk1 complexes, resulting in degradation of Sic1 by the SCF. B, The mechanism of cell cycle control is highly conserved between eukaryotes.

The mechanism of cell cycle entry is highly conserved between *S. cerevisiae* and higher eukaryotes (Fig. 3B). For instance, in vertebrates the retinoblastoma protein, pRB, binds and thereby inhibits the transcription factor E2F. pRB also recruits HDAC complexes to keep the surrounding chromatin in a repressed state. Upon phosphorylation by cyclin D-Cdk4,6 and cyclin E-Cdk2 complexes, pRB and the HDACs dissociate from E2F (van den Heuvel and Dyson 2008). E2F then activates a transcriptional program that mediates expression of proteins involved in cell cycle entry and DNA replication.

Once the cell has successfully entered the cell cycle, it shuts off the G1 transcriptional program. This is important for proper cell cycle progression and promotes unidirectionality of the cell cycle. In *S. cerevisiae,* one important mechanism of shutting off the G1 transcriptional program involves the transcriptional repressor Nrm1 (de Bruin, Kalashnikova et al. 2006). Nrm1 inhibits transcription of the G1 transcriptional program. In addition, the G1 cyclins Cln1 and Cln2 are degraded, leading to dephosphorylation of Whi5, thereby allowing it to re-enter the nucleus to inhibit the G1 transcriptional program. Finally, the G1 transcriptional program is inhibited by Clb-Cdk1 complexes, which phosphorylate and inhibit the SBF transcription factor complex (Koch, Schleiffer et al. 1996).

3. CDKs control DNA replication at multiple levels

The purpose of the cell cycle is to faithfully transmit a complete copy of the genome from one generation to the next. Two events are fundamental to this process: DNA replication, and segregation of the replicated chromosomes into the daughter cells. It is important that chromosome segregation does not occur before DNA replication is complete, otherwise the cell would experience massive genome instability. Therefore, these two processes are separated in time; chromosome segregation (which takes place in M phase) does not occur until DNA replication (which occurs in S phase) has finished (Murray and Kirschner 1989). Furthermore, as I will discuss below, several mechanisms have evolved that make sure that DNA replication only takes place during S phase and just once per cell cycle.

3.1 Licensing of origins of replication is restricted to G1 phase

DNA replication is a multi-step process. It starts with origin licensing, a process in which a specific protein-DNA complex called the prereplicative complex (pre-RC) is formed at origins in G1 phase, when Cdk1 is inactive (Fig. 4 and Fig. 5). In *S. cerevisiae*, origins were first identified by their capability to sustain replication of mini-chromosomes and plasmids, and therefore these sequences are commonly referred to as Autonomously Replicating Sequences (ARSs) (Stinchcomb, Struhl et al. 1979). ARSs typically are 100-200 bp in length with little sequence conservation, except for an 11 bp ARS consensus sequence (5'-WTTTAYRTTTW-3'), and mutations in this sequence abolish the function of the ARS (Theis and Newlon 1997; Newlon and Theis 2002). The ARS consensus sequence is recognized by the Origin of Replication Complex (ORC), which consists of Orc1, Orc2, Orc3, Orc4, Orc5 and Orc6 (Bell and Stillman 1992). The ORC is constitutively associated with the ARS throughout the cell cycle. The ORC recruits the ATPase Cdc6, the DNA replication licensing factor Cdt1 and the Mcm2-7 helicase complex (Araki 2010). Loading of the Mcm2-7 complex is what defines pre-RC formation; it confers DNA replication competence to the cell and is the first regulated step of DNA replication before actual DNA synthesis. At this stage, the Mcm2-7 helicase complex is associated with the ORC but still inactive; pre-RC formation is followed by initiation of DNA replication, during which Mcm2-7 is activated.

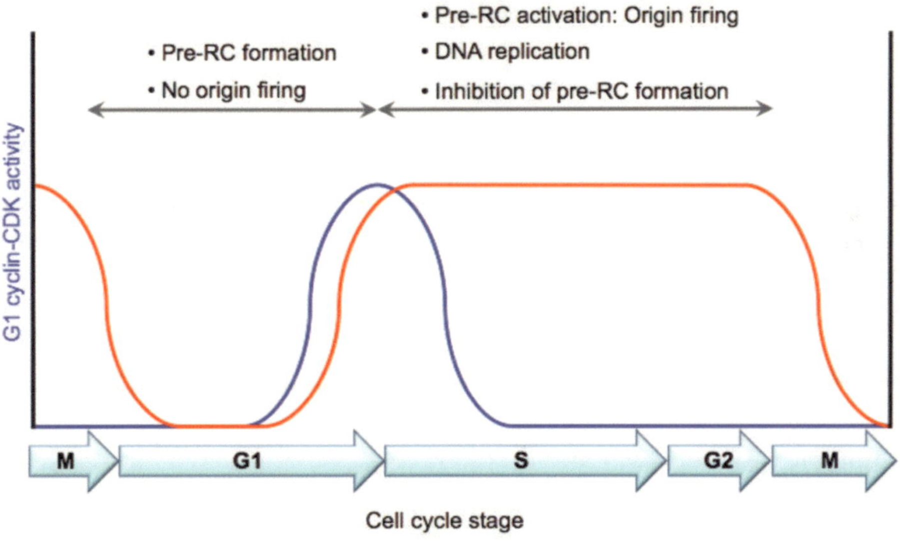

Fig. 4. Licensing of origins of replication can only take place in G1 phase when Cdk1 is inactive, while origin activation only occurs during S phase when Cdk1 is active. See text for details.

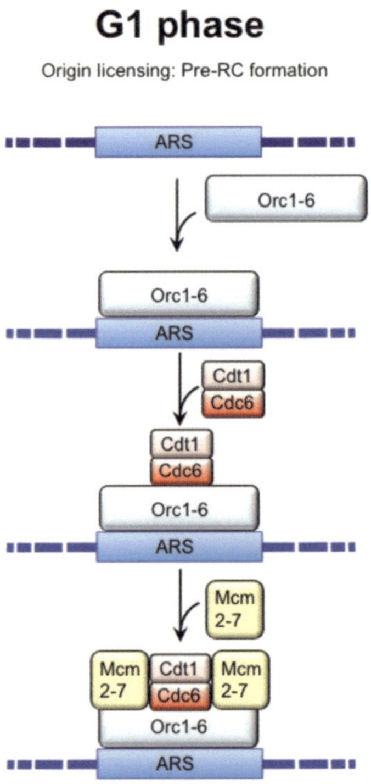

Fig. 5. Regulation of DNA replication by the cell cycle: Origin licensing. Origin licensing takes place during G1 phase, when Cdk1 activity is low. The ORC becomes associated with ARS DNA directly after DNA replication and stays associated with DNA throughout the cell cycle. The ORC serves as a platform for Cdt1 and Cdc6 recruitment to the origin. Finally, an origin is replication competent when the MCM2-7 complex arrives.

3.2 Phosphorylation of DNA replication factors induces firing of origins of replication during S phase

Clb5-Cdk1 and Clb6-Cdk1 complexes are responsible for inducing DNA replication (Schwob and Nasmyth 1993). The activity of these complexes is restricted to S phase because the Clb5,6 cyclin genes are part of the G1 transcriptional program, and therefore expression of Clb5,6 peaks at the G1-S transition. However, Clb5,6-Cdk1 complexes are still maintained in an inactive state by the CKI Sic1 until the cell is ready to initiate DNA replication (Schwob, Bohm et al. 1994). Cln1,2-Cdk1 complexes then phosphorylate Sic1, which leads to ubiquitination of Sic1 by the Skp1-Cullin-F-box (SCF) complex, targeting it for degradation by the proteasome (Nash, Tang et al. 2001). This then results in activation of Clb5,6-Cdk1 complexes.

Clb5,6-Cdk1 complexes induce DNA replication by phosphorylating Sld2 and Sld3 (Fig. 6) (Araki 2010). Phosphorylation of Sld2 and Sld3 increases their affinity for Dpb11 (Araki 2010). Dpb11 has two pairs of tandem BRCT domains, which are known to be phosphopeptide binding domains; the N-terminal pair of BRCT domains interact with Sld3, while the C-terminal pair preferentially bind Sld2 (Araki 2010). The interaction between Dpb11, Sld2 and Sld3 is necessary and sufficient for initiation of DNA replication, although the exact molecular mechanism remains obscure (Araki 2010).

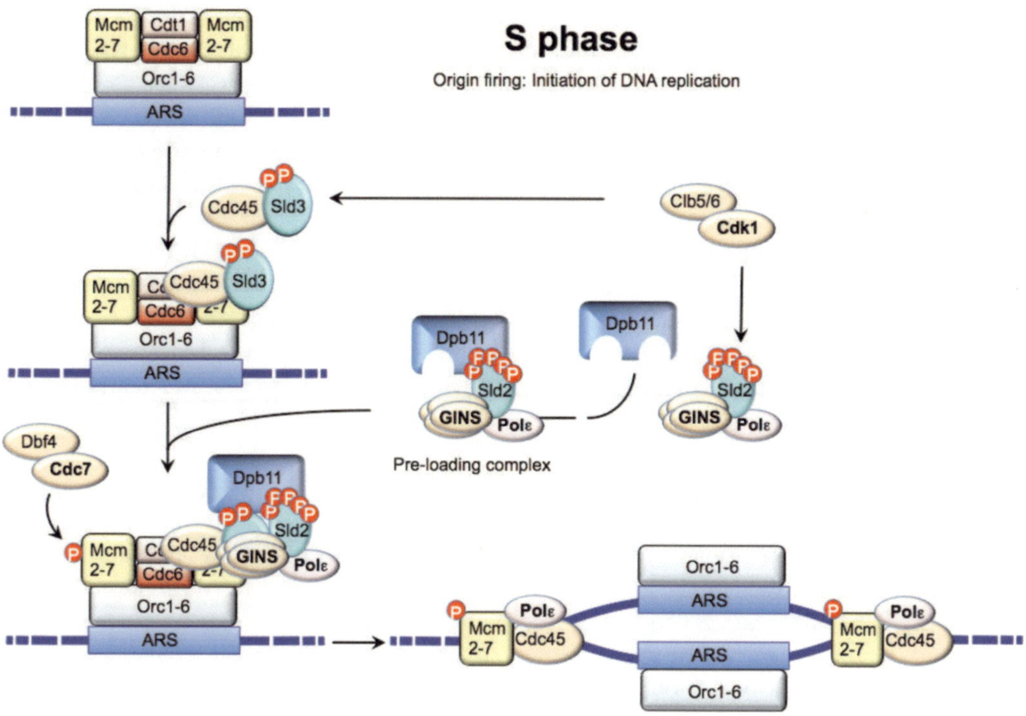

Fig. 6. Regulation of DNA replication by the cell cycle: Origin firing. At the end of G1 phase, cyclin-Cdk1 complexes phosphorylate Sld2 and Sld3, leading to recruitment of GINS and Polε to the origin. The additional phosphorylation of MCM2-7 by DDK results in formation of a complex between Cdc45, GINS and MCM2-7, which then induces unwinding of DNA and initiation of DNA replication.

It was recently reported that phosphorylation of Sld2 may promote formation of the pre-loading complex (pre-LC), which consists of Sld2, Dpb11, GINS and Polε (Muramatsu, Hirai et al. 2010). GINS and Polε form a subcomplex throughout the cell cycle, which associates with Sld2-Dpb11 upon phosphorylation of Sld2 by Cdk1 (Muramatsu, Hirai et al. 2010). One proposed function for formation of the pre-LC is that the pre-LC serves to bring the GINS complex to the pre-RC complex through the interaction of Dpb11 with the pre-RC-associated, Cdk1-phosphorylated Sld3 (Araki 2010). Arrival of GINS at the pre-RC would then result in formation of the Cdc45-MCM2-7-GINS (CMG) complex, which represents the active helicase that unwinds DNA to mediate DNA replication (Araki 2010).

In addition to Clb5,6-Cdk1, a second kinase complex termed Dbf4-dependent kinase (DDK), which consists of the regulatory subunit Dbf4 and the catalytic subunit Cdc7, controls initiation of DNA replication (Araki 2010). DDK is only active during S phase, because Dbf4 is only expressed in late G1, and because Dbf4 is degraded by the APC (Tanaka and Araki 2010). Because Cdk1 phosphorylates and inactivates components of the APC (Jaspersen, Charles et al. 1999; Ostapenko, Burton et al. 2008), Dbf4 is stabilized when Cdk1 becomes active, i.e. at the G1/S transition (Tanaka and Araki 2010). DDK is recruited to origins independently of the pre-LC complex, probably through its interaction with the MCM2-7. DDK directly phosphorylates the MCM2-7 complex, which is thought to increase its affinity for Cdc45 and GINS, thus leading to formation of the CMG complex (Tanaka and Araki 2010). DNA polε extends the leading strand at each replication fork, while DNA Polα/primase synthesizes Okazaki fragments that are extended by DNA Polδ on the lagging strand.

The requirement for Cdk1 can be bypassed to induce DNA replication outside of S phase. To circumvent the requirement for Cdk1, both Sld2 and Sld3 phosphorylation must be bypassed (Araki 2010). The requirement for Sld2 phosphorylation can be bypassed by expressing a phospho-mimetic form of Sld2, either Sld2-T84D or Sld2-11D. The requirement for Sld3 can be bypassed by expressing an Sld3-Dpb11 fusion protein. However, cells that express phospho-mimetic Sld2 and Sld3-Dpb11 still depend on DDK1 activity to induce DNA replication (Araki 2010). Dbf4 is normally unstable in G1 phase, but overexpressing Dbf4 in combination with expressing Sld2-T84D/Sld2-11D and Sld3-Dpb11 leads to DNA replication in G1 phase.

3.3 Expression of most DNA replication factors is limited to a specific phase of the cell cycle

Importantly, the expression of many genes that encode DNA replication factors is confined to a specific phase of the cell cycle (Table 1). In general, genes that have functions in early stages of the DNA replication process (i.e. licensing of origins of replication) are transcribed in G2 and M phase, such that their protein levels are highest in G1 phase. Genes that function later in the DNA replication process (e.g. proteins that are part of the DNA replication complex) peak during late G1, such that their levels are highest in S phase when DNA replication takes place. The confined expression of DNA replication factors to specific phases of the cell cycle plays an important role in restricting DNA replication to S phase (Enserink and Kolodner 2010).

Gene	Description	Maximum expression	Function in DNA replication
ORC3	Subunit of the origin recognition complex	Late S	Pre-RC complex
ORC1	Subunit of the origin recognition complex	G2	Pre-RC complex
ORC4	Subunit of the origin recognition complex	G2	Pre-RC complex
ORC6	Subunit of the origin recognition complex	G2	Pre-RC complex
CDT1	DNA replication licensing factor	G2	Pre-RC complex
MCM2	Helicase	Late M	Replicative helicase
MCM3	Helicase	Late M	Replicative helicase
MCM4	Helicase	Late M	Replicative helicase
MCM5	Helicase	Late M	Replicative helicase
MCM6	Helicase	Late M	Replicative helicase
MCM7	Helicase	Late M	Replicative helicase
CDC6	Component of the pre-RC complex	Late M	Pre-RC complex
SLD2	Required for initiation of DNA replication	Late G1	Origin firing
CLB5	Cyclin involved in Sld2 phosphorylation	Late G1	Origin firing
CLB6	Cyclin involved in Sld2 phosphorylation	Late G1	Origin firing
CSM3	Required for stable replication fork pausing	Late G1	Replication fork

Gene	Description	Maximum expression	Function in DNA replication
TOF1	Required for stable replication fork pausing	Late G1	Replication fork
PSF1	GINS complex	Late G1	Replicative helicase
PSF2	GINS complex	Late G1	Replicative helicase
DBF4	Regulatory subunit of Cdc7-Dbf4 kinase complex	Late G1	Origin firing
DPB11	Loads DNA polε onto pre-RCs	Late G1	Origin firing
RFA1	Replication factor A complex	Late G1	Replication fork
RFA2	Replication factor A complex	Late G1	Replication fork
RFA3	Replication factor A complex	Early S	Replication fork
POL30	PCNA	Late G1	Replication fork
CDC45	DNA replication initiation factor; recruited to MCM pre-RC complexes	Late G1	Replicative helicase
MRC1	DNA replication and checkpoint signaling	Late G1	Replication fork
POL2	DNA polymerase ε catalytic subunit	Late G1	Replication fork
POL3	DNA polymerase δ catalytic subunit	Late G1	Replication fork
POL31	DNA polymerase δ subunit	Late G1	Replication fork
POL32	DNA polymerase δ subunit	Late G1	Replication fork
POL12	DNA polymerase α primase subunit	Late G1	Replication fork
CDC9	Ligase that joins Okazaki fragments	Late G1	Replication fork
RNH201	RNase H2, degrades Okazaki fragments	Late G1	Replication fork
RNH202	RNase H2, degrades Okazaki fragments	Late G1	Replication fork
RAD27	Flap Endonuclease	Late G1	Replication fork
ELG1	Alternative RFC complex component	Late G1	Replication fork
RNR1	Ribonucleotide reductase, dNTP synthesis	Late G1	dNTP synthesis
RFC3	Replication factor C complex	Late G1	PCNA loading
RFC4	Replication factor C complex	Late G1	PCNA loading
RFC5	Replication factor C complex	Late G1	PCNA loading
SLD5	GINS complex	G1/S border	Replicative helicase
RNR2	Ribonucleotide reductase, dNTP synthesis	G1/S border	dNTP synthesis
RNR3	Ribonucleotide reductase, dNTP synthesis	G1/S border	dNTP synthesis
CDC7	Catalytic subunit of Cdc7-Dbf4 kinase complex	G1/S border	Origin firing
DPB2	DNA polymerase ε subunit	G1	Replication fork
DPB3	DNA polymerase ε subunit	G1	Replication fork
POL1	DNA polymerase α primase catalytic subunit	Late G1	Replication fork

Table 1. Periodic expression of *S. cerevisiae* genes involved in DNA replication. Source: Cyclebase.org (Gauthier, Jensen et al. 2010)

3.4 Preventing re-replication

A major challenge to the cell is to make sure that its genetic material does not get copied more than once. Several mechanisms are in place to prevent that firing of origins takes place outside of S phase, and that origins do not fire more than once per cell cycle (Fig. 7). One major mechanism that prevents re-replication focuses on Cdc6 (Remus and Diffley 2009), and Cdc6 is inhibited at three levels. First, transcription of Cdc6 is limited to G1-S phase (Moll, Tebb et al. 1991). Second, phosphorylation of Cdc6 by Cdk1 targets it for degradation by the SCF (Drury, Perkins et al. 1997). Third, any remaining free Cdc6 is 'mopped up' through phosphorylation by Cdk1, which induces the binding of Cdc6 to Clb2-Cdk1, thereby preventing Cdc6 from licensing origins (Mimura, Seki et al. 2004). Although depletion of Cdc6 efficiently inhibits re-firing or origins, additional mechanisms exist to prevent re-replication. For instance, the MCM2-7 complex and the associated Cdt1 are shuttled out of the nucleus in a Cdk1-dependent manner (Labib, Diffley et al. 1999; Nguyen, Co et al. 2000; Liku, Nguyen et al. 2005). Finally, the ORC complex is inhibited through phosphorylation by Cdk1 (Nguyen, Co et al. 2001).

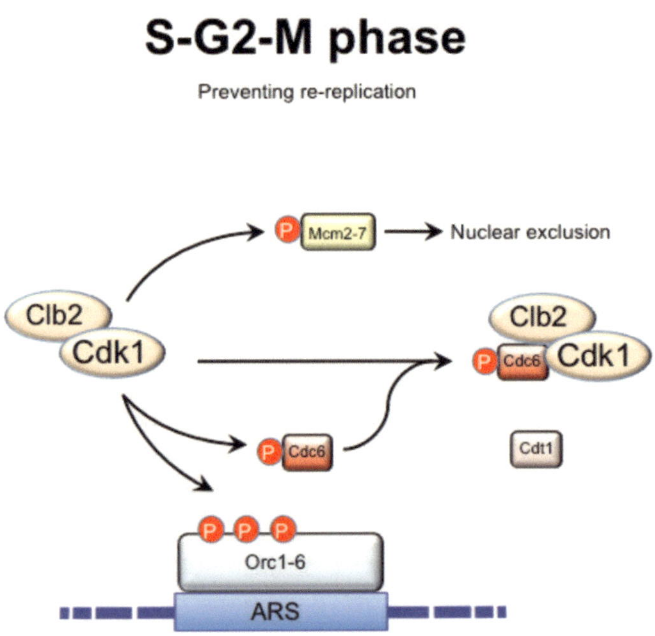

Fig. 7. Mechanisms that prevent re-replication. The Clb2-Cdk1 complex phosphorylates ORC, which prevents ORC from recruiting Cdc6 and Cdt1. Phosphorylation of the Mcm2-7 complex may lead to nuclear export of the helicase complex, as well as the associated Cdt1. Phosphorylation of Cdc6 induces its destruction by the SCF, but also leads to sequestration of Cdc6 by the Clb2-Cdk1, thus preventing Cdc6 from localizing to the ORC.

3.5 Precocious activation of Cdk1 leads to DNA damage during S phase

A key feature of tumor cells is uncontrolled entry into the cell cycle, which is nearly always the result of defects in the pRB pathway. Studies in yeast have shown that this is highly detrimental to genome stability (Lengronne and Schwob 2002; Tanaka and Diffley 2002; Enserink, Hombauer et al. 2009). Precocious activation of Cdk1, either through overexpression of *CLN2-1* (Tanaka and Diffley 2002), encoding a dominant, activated cyclin, or deletion of the CKI *SIC1* (Lengronne and Schwob 2002), leads to unscheduled entry into S phase. The cell now enters S phase when it has not yet finished licensing the origins of replication, and leads to initiation of DNA replication from fewer origins. As a result, the cell experiences increased numbers of DNA double strand breaks, which give rise to genome rearrangements. Interestingly, these adverse effects of precocious S phase entry on genome stability can be suppressed by increasing the number of origins from which cells initiate DNA replication (Lengronne and Schwob 2002; Tanaka and Diffley 2002). Thus, genome instability that results from precocious Cdk1 activation and unscheduled S phase entry is almost entirely the consequence of inefficient activation of DNA replication.

4. Checkpoints monitor DNA replication stress and DNA damage

Stalled replication forks are a threat to the cell's genome because they could collapse, leaving the cell with partially unreplicated, broken chromosomal DNA. Therefore, cells have developed elaborate systems that sense DNA damage and stalling of DNA replication forks to arrest the cell cycle and to induce DNA repair (Fig. 8) (Hartwell and Weinert 1989).

Cells respond to DNA replication blocks and to damaged DNA by activating checkpoints that arrest or slow the cell cycle and then help activate DNA repair pathways (Hartwell and Weinert 1989). The DNA damage checkpoint acts at the G1/S and G2/M borders in the presence of damaged DNA. In addition, two types of checkpoints have been described in S phase: the DNA replication checkpoint, which arrests cell cycle progression and inhibits firing of late replication origins in response to replication stress; and the intra-S checkpoint, which slows DNA replication and cell cycle progression in response to DNA damage (Putnam, Jaehnig et al. 2009). Here I will focus mainly on the DNA replication checkpoint.

Typically, checkpoints are thought to function in a signalling hierarchy: Damage signals -> damage sensors -> signal transducers -> effectors (Fig. 8) (Putnam, Jaehnig et al. 2009). However, several damage sensors are part of the DNA replication fork, and they are themselves targets of these signalling pathways (Putnam, Jaehnig et al. 2009). Therefore, these pathways are not strictly linear.

The DNA replication checkpoint plays a major role in maintenance of genome stability. It is activated when DNA replication forks stall, for instance due to a lesion in the DNA or due to depletion of dNTPs (Branzei and Foiani 2010). Exactly how this is sensed remains unclear, but likely involves exposure of single-stranded DNA (ssDNA) (Byun, Pacek et al. 2005). ssDNA may be generated because the CMG complex keeps unwinding double-stranded DNA, even though it is uncoupled from DNA replication because the replication fork has stalled (Byun, Pacek et al. 2005). The ssDNA binding complex RPA, a heterotrimeric protein complex consisting of Rfa1, Rfa2 and Rfa3, may have a function in sensing ssDNA (Zou and Elledge 2003). Other proteins that have been proposed to act as sensors include Rfc5, PCNA, Dpb11, Pol2 and Sgs1 (Kolodner, Putnam et al. 2002). How these proteins relay the signal to activate the checkpoint is not very clear. Two phosphatidyl inositol 3' kinase-related kinases (PIKK) family kinases, Mec1 and Tel1, play a central role in checkpoint activation in *S. cerevisiae* (Kolodner, Putnam et al. 2002). Mec1 is thought to be activated primarily by stalled replication forks, while Tel1 typically responds to damaged DNA (Kolodner, Putnam et al. 2002). As mentioned above, ssDNA is generated upon stalling of replication forks, which is bound by RPA. RPA may recruit the kinase Mec1 and its binding partner Ddc2, leading to activation of Ddc2-Mec1. Mrc1, which is part of the replication fork, becomes phosphorylated by Mec1, which leads to recruitment of Rad53 (Alcasabas, Osborn et al. 2001). Rad53 is phosphorylated by Mec1, but also by itself, leading to its activation. Because Mrc1 mediates the signal to downstream kinases it is often referred to as a mediator. Another mediator is Rad9, which also activates Rad53 (Gilbert, Green et al. 2001) but is thought to function mainly downstream of Tel1.

In addition to Rad53, another kinase, Chk1, becomes activated by the checkpoint, while the kinase Dun1 is thought to function downstream of Rad53 (Putnam, Jaehnig et al. 2009). Together, these kinases phosphorylate a large number of substrates involved in cell cycle control, DNA repair and nucleotide metabolism (Fig. 8).

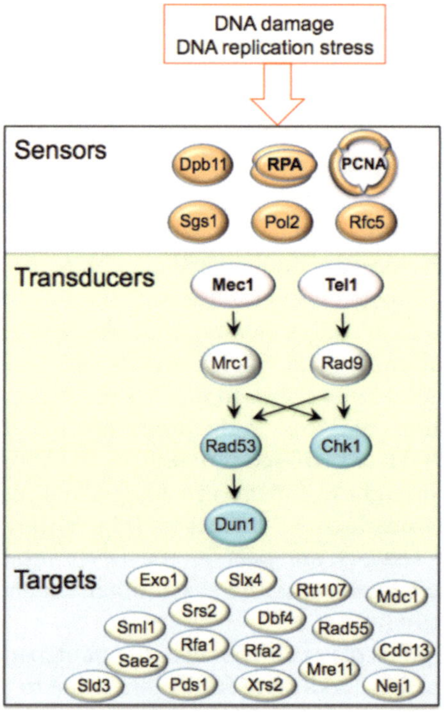

Fig. 8. Overview of the DNA damage and DNA replication checkpoints. DNA damage and DNA replication stress is sensed by a number of proteins, although the exact mechanism remains unclear and additional sensors likely exist. Two central kinases, Mec1 and Tel1, amplify and transmit the signal to downstream kinases Rad53, Dun1, and Chk1. Many targets of these kinases exist and only a selection is shown here.

4.1 Cdk1 activity remains high during activation of the replication checkpoint in *S. cerevisiae*

The replication checkpoint has several important functions that help maintain cell viability during DNA replication stress. The best known function of the checkpoint is to induce cell cycle arrest (Hartwell and Weinert 1989). In contrast to higher eukaryotes, Cdk1 activity remains high during checkpoint arrest (Sorger and Murray 1992). One reason for maintaining high Cdk1 activity during S phase arrest is that Cdk1 activity, as described above, prevents re-licensing of origins that have already fired (Zegerman and Diffley 2010).

Thereby, the cell will not activate additional origins of replication in the face of replication stress, which could further threaten genome stability. Another reason for maintaining Cdk1 activity is that Cdk1 is important for repair of DNA double strand break (DSBs) that may have arisen as a result from collapsed DNA replication forks (Ira, Pellicioli et al. 2004). Here, Cdk1 phosphorylates and activates the nuclease Sae2 (Huertas, Cortes-Ledesma et al. 2008), which is required for resection of DNA double strand breaks, the first step of homologous recombination (HR). At the same time, Cdk1 actively suppresses the recruitment of proteins involved in non-homologous end-joining (NHEJ) (Zhang, Shim et al. 2009). This mechanism ensures that in G1 (when there is only one copy of the genome present in the cell and therefore no template for HR) NHEJ is the preferred mechanism of repair of DSBs, while during the cell cycle stages that Cdk1 is active (S-G2-M) HR is the preferred repair pathway.

4.2 The DNA replication checkpoint enforces cell cycle arrest

If Cdk1 remains active during activation of the DNA replication checkpoint, how then is cell cycle arrest enforced? One main mechanism of preventing cell cycle progression is the inhibition of firing of late origins of replication by Rad53 through phosphorylation of Sld3 and Dbf4 (Lopez-Mosqueda, Maas et al. 2010; Zegerman and Diffley 2010) (Fig. 9). Rad53-mediated Sld3 phosphorylation may prevent the interaction of Sld3 with Cdc45 and Dpb11, thus preventing origins from firing. However, the mechanism whereby Rad53-mediated Dbf4 phosphorylation prevents DDK from activating origins remains unknown (Lopez-Mosqueda, Maas et al. 2010; Zegerman and Diffley 2010). Rad53, in conjunction with Pds1, also prevents cell cycle progression by stabilizing Pds1 (Sanchez, Bachant et al. 1999; Agarwal, Tang et al. 2003). Pds1 is the yeast version of securin, an inhibitor of the separase Esp1. Esp1 is important for activating anaphase by cleaving cohesin, a protein complex that keeps sister chromatids together after DNA replication. Thus, stabilization of Pds1 by Rad53 and Chk1 helps prevent anaphase onset.

4.3 The DNA replication checkpoint stabilizes replication forks

A major function of the replication checkpoint is to stabilize replication forks. Stalled replication forks are at risk of collapse, which would result in partially unreplicated DNA and DNA double strand breaks, often leading to genome instability. Mec1 and Rad53 are the main players in stabilizing replication forks, while Chk1 appears to have a more redundant function (Segurado and Diffley 2008). The exact molecular mechanism remains unclear. Many substrates of Mec1 and Rad53 have been suggested (Segurado and Tercero 2009). A main target of Rad53 may be Exo1 (Segurado and Diffley 2008), although the exact molecular mechanism is not very clear. The targets of Mec1 and Chk1 in replication fork stabilization remain unknown. After the problems leading to DNA replication stress and activation of the checkpoint have been rectified, the replication forks need to restart. This process requires the activity of Rad53 and may also involve HR-dependent mechanisms (Petermann and Helleday 2010).

4.4 Other processes controlled by the DNA replication checkpoint

Although I will not go into great detail, it is worth mentioning that activation of the replication checkpoint has several other consequences. One important target of the checkpoint is Sml1, which is an inhibitor of ribonucleotide reductase, which synthesizes

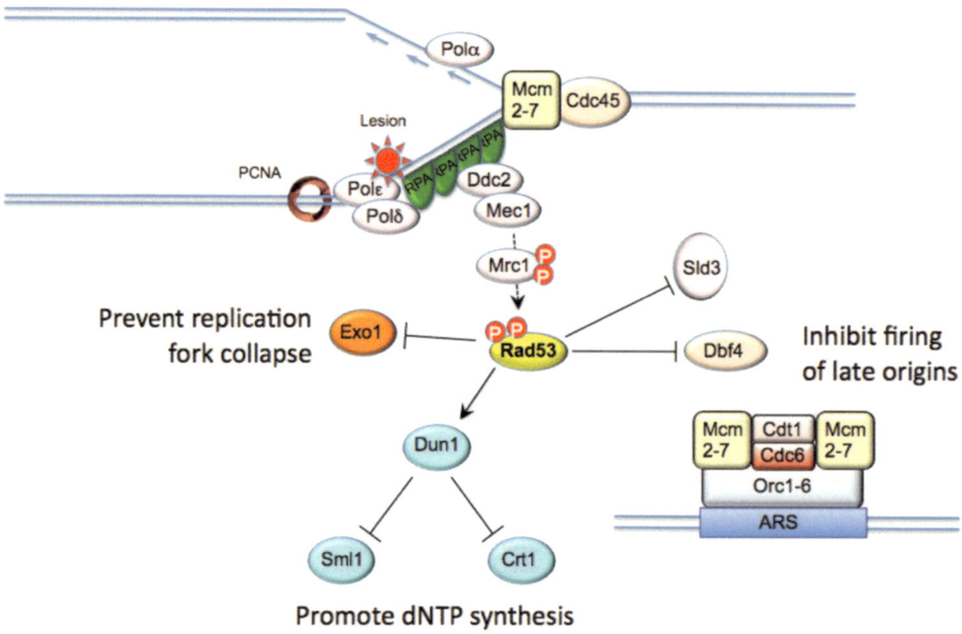

Fig. 9. Effects of the DNA replication checkpoint. When a DNA replication fork stalls due to a lesion in the DNA, the MCM2-7 helicase may continue unwinding DNA. The resulting ssDNA is bound by RPA (shown in green), which may recruit and activate Mec1. Mec1, through the replication fork-associated adaptor protein Mrc1, activates Rad53. Rad53 then inhibits firing of late origins of replication through phosphorylation and inhibition of Sld3 and Dbf4. Rad53 also protects replication fork collapse by inhibiting Exo1, and it promotes dNTP synthesis through Dun1, which phosphorylates and inhibits Sml1, which inhibits ribonucleotide reductase, and Crt1. Dun1 also inhibits Crt1, a transcriptional repressor of genes that encode ribonucleotide reductase.

dNTPs. Sml1 is phosphorylated by the checkpoint kinase Dun1, leading to destruction of Sml1 and thus increased activity of ribonucleotide reductase, which is important for sustaining cellular dNTP levels (Zhao and Rothstein 2002). Another process controlled by the checkpoint is transcription. Activation of the DNA replication checkpoint by chemicals such as MMS, which methylates DNA leading to replication fork stalling, broadly alters transcription of a large number of genes (Putnam, Jaehnig et al. 2009). Many of these genes do not confer resistance to agents that induce DNA replication stress (Putnam, Jaehnig et al. 2009). Nonetheless, there also exist specific pathways that activate transcription of genes that have important functions in maintaining cell viability during DNA replication stress. For example, Dun1 phosphorylates and inhibits the transcriptional repressor Crt1, which leads to increased transcription of the ribonucleotide reductase encoding genes *RNR1-4* (Putnam, Jaehnig et al. 2009). Finally, the replication checkpoint is important for preventing chromosome separation by targeting the mitotic spindle (Krishnan, Nirantar et al. 2004), it ensures proper cell morphogenesis during DNA replication stress (Enserink, Smolka et al. 2006; Smolka, Chen et al. 2006), maintains cellular histone levels (Gunjan and Verreault 2003), and affects migration of the nucleus (Dotiwala, Haase et al. 2007). Additional functions likely exist to maintain cell viability during DNA replication stress.

5. Concluding remarks

DNA replication and cell cycle control are tightly connected. The cyclin dependent kinase Cdk1 is involved both in initiation of DNA replication and in safeguarding that replication takes place once per cell cycle. Deregulated Cdk1 activity leads to inefficient DNA replication and genome instability, and checkpoints have evolved that monitor DNA replication and chromosomal integrity. While the past decade has strongly increased our understanding of the processes that control DNA replication, the details of the molecular mechanisms often remain shrouded, and it will be exciting to see this field develop.

6. References

Agarwal, R., Z. Tang, et al. (2003). "Two distinct pathways for inhibiting pds1 ubiquitination in response to DNA damage." J Biol Chem 278(45): 45027-33.

Alcasabas, A. A., A. J. Osborn, et al. (2001). "Mrc1 transduces signals of DNA replication stress to activate Rad53." Nat Cell Biol 3(11): 958-65.

Araki, H. (2010). "Cyclin-dependent kinase-dependent initiation of chromosomal DNA replication." Curr Opin Cell Biol 22(6): 766-71.

Bell, S. P. and B. Stillman (1992). "ATP-dependent recognition of eukaryotic origins of DNA replication by a multiprotein complex." Nature 357(6374): 128-34.

Booher, R. N., R. J. Deshaies, et al. (1993). "Properties of Saccharomyces cerevisiae wee1 and its differential regulation of p34CDC28 in response to G1 and G2 cyclins." Embo J 12(9): 3417-26.

Branzei, D. and M. Foiani (2010). "Maintaining genome stability at the replication fork." Nat Rev Mol Cell Biol 11(3): 208-19.

Byun, T. S., M. Pacek, et al. (2005). "Functional uncoupling of MCM helicase and DNA polymerase activities activates the ATR-dependent checkpoint." Genes Dev 19(9): 1040-52.

Charvin, G., C. Oikonomou, et al. (2010). "Origin of irreversibility of cell cycle start in budding yeast." PLoS Biol 8(1): e1000284.

Costanzo, M., J. L. Nishikawa, et al. (2004). "CDK activity antagonizes Whi5, an inhibitor of G1/S transcription in yeast." Cell 117(7): 899-913.

de Bruin, R. A., T. I. Kalashnikova, et al. (2006). "Constraining G1-specific transcription to late G1 phase: the MBF-associated corepressor Nrm1 acts via negative feedback." Mol Cell 23(4): 483-96.

de Bruin, R. A., W. H. McDonald, et al. (2004). "Cln3 activates G1-specific transcription via phosphorylation of the SBF bound repressor Whi5." Cell 117(7): 887-98.

Dotiwala, F., J. Haase, et al. (2007). "The yeast DNA damage checkpoint proteins control a cytoplasmic response to DNA damage." Proc Natl Acad Sci U S A 104(27): 11358-63.

Drury, L. S., G. Perkins, et al. (1997). "The Cdc4/34/53 pathway targets Cdc6p for proteolysis in budding yeast." EMBO J 16(19): 5966-76.

Enserink, J. M., H. Hombauer, et al. (2009). "Cdc28/Cdk1 positively and negatively affects genome stability in S. cerevisiae." J Cell Biol 185(3): 423-37.

Enserink, J. M. and R. D. Kolodner (2010). "An overview of Cdk1-controlled targets and processes." Cell Div 5: 11.

Enserink, J. M., M. B. Smolka, et al. (2006). "Checkpoint proteins control morphogenetic events during DNA replication stress in Saccharomyces cerevisiae." J Cell Biol 175(5): 729-41.

Ferrell, J. E., Jr., T. Y. Tsai, et al. (2011). "Modeling the cell cycle: why do certain circuits oscillate?" Cell 144(6): 874-85.

Gilbert, C. S., C. M. Green, et al. (2001). "Budding yeast Rad9 is an ATP-dependent Rad53 activating machine." Mol Cell 8(1): 129-36.

Gunjan, A. and A. Verreault (2003). "A Rad53 kinase-dependent surveillance mechanism that regulates histone protein levels in S. cerevisiae." Cell 115(5): 537-49.

Hartwell, L. H. and T. A. Weinert (1989). "Checkpoints: controls that ensure the order of cell cycle events." Science 246(4930): 629-34.

Huang, D., S. Kaluarachchi, et al. (2009). "Dual regulation by pairs of cyclin-dependent protein kinases and histone deacetylases controls G1 transcription in budding yeast." PLoS Biol 7(9): e1000188.

Huertas, P., F. Cortes-Ledesma, et al. (2008). "CDK targets Sae2 to control DNA-end resection and homologous recombination." Nature 455(7213): 689-92.

Ira, G., A. Pellicioli, et al. (2004). "DNA end resection, homologous recombination and DNA damage checkpoint activation require CDK1." Nature 431(7011): 1011-7.

Jaspersen, S. L., J. F. Charles, et al. (1999). "Inhibitory phosphorylation of the APC regulator Hct1 is controlled by the kinase Cdc28 and the phosphatase Cdc14." Curr Biol 9(5): 227-36.

Jeffrey, P. D., A. A. Russo, et al. (1995). "Mechanism of CDK activation revealed by the structure of a cyclinA-CDK2 complex." Nature 376(6538): 313-20.

Koch, C., A. Schleiffer, et al. (1996). "Switching transcription on and off during the yeast cell cycle: Cln/Cdc28 kinases activate bound transcription factor SBF (Swi4/Swi6) at start, whereas Clb/Cdc28 kinases displace it from the promoter in G2." Genes Dev 10(2): 129-41.

Kolodner, R. D., C. D. Putnam, et al. (2002). "Maintenance of genome stability in Saccharomyces cerevisiae." Science 297(5581): 552-7.

Krishnan, V., S. Nirantar, et al. (2004). "DNA replication checkpoint prevents precocious chromosome segregation by regulating spindle behavior." Mol Cell 16(5): 687-700.

Labib, K., J. F. Diffley, et al. (1999). "G1-phase and B-type cyclins exclude the DNA-replication factor Mcm4 from the nucleus." Nat Cell Biol 1(7): 415-22.

Lee, H. O., J. M. Davidson, et al. (2009). "Endoreplication: polyploidy with purpose." Genes Dev 23(21): 2461-77.

Lengronne, A. and E. Schwob (2002). "The yeast CDK inhibitor Sic1 prevents genomic instability by promoting replication origin licensing in late G(1)." Mol Cell 9(5): 1067-78.

Liku, M. E., V. Q. Nguyen, et al. (2005). "CDK phosphorylation of a novel NLS-NES module distributed between two subunits of the Mcm2-7 complex prevents chromosomal rereplication." Mol Biol Cell 16(10): 5026-39.

Lopez-Mosqueda, J., N. L. Maas, et al. (2010). "Damage-induced phosphorylation of Sld3 is important to block late origin firing." Nature 467(7314): 479-83.

Malumbres, M. and M. Barbacid (2009). "Cell cycle, CDKs and cancer: a changing paradigm." Nat Rev Cancer 9(3): 153-66.

Mimura, S., T. Seki, et al. (2004). "Phosphorylation-dependent binding of mitotic cyclins to Cdc6 contributes to DNA replication control." Nature 431(7012): 1118-23.
Moll, T., G. Tebb, et al. (1991). "The role of phosphorylation and the CDC28 protein kinase in cell cycle-regulated nuclear import of the S. cerevisiae transcription factor SWI5." Cell 66(4): 743-58.
Muramatsu, S., K. Hirai, et al. (2010). "CDK-dependent complex formation between replication proteins Dpb11, Sld2, Pol (epsilon}, and GINS in budding yeast." Genes Dev 24(6): 602-12.
Murray, A. W. and M. W. Kirschner (1989). "Dominoes and clocks: the union of two views of the cell cycle." Science 246(4930): 614-21.
Nash, P., X. Tang, et al. (2001). "Multisite phosphorylation of a CDK inhibitor sets a threshold for the onset of DNA replication." Nature 414(6863): 514-21.
Newlon, C. S. and J. F. Theis (2002). "DNA replication joins the revolution: whole-genome views of DNA replication in budding yeast." Bioessays 24(4): 300-4.
Nguyen, V. Q., C. Co, et al. (2000). "Clb/Cdc28 kinases promote nuclear export of the replication initiator proteins Mcm2-7." Curr Biol 10(4): 195-205.
Nguyen, V. Q., C. Co, et al. (2001). "Cyclin-dependent kinases prevent DNA re-replication through multiple mechanisms." Nature 411(6841): 1068-73.
Ostapenko, D., J. L. Burton, et al. (2008). "Pseudosubstrate inhibition of the anaphase-promoting complex by Acm1: regulation by proteolysis and Cdc28 phosphorylation." Mol Cell Biol 28(15): 4653-64.
Pavletich, N. P. (1999). "Mechanisms of cyclin-dependent kinase regulation: structures of Cdks, their cyclin activators, and Cip and INK4 inhibitors." J Mol Biol 287(5): 821-8.
Petermann, E. and T. Helleday (2010). "Pathways of mammalian replication fork restart." Nat Rev Mol Cell Biol 11(10): 683-7.
Pines, J. (1994). "The cell cycle kinases." Semin Cancer Biol 5(4): 305-13.
Putnam, C. D., E. J. Jaehnig, et al. (2009). "Perspectives on the DNA damage and replication checkpoint responses in Saccharomyces cerevisiae." DNA Repair (Amst).
Remus, D. and J. F. Diffley (2009). "Eukaryotic DNA replication control: lock and load, then fire." Curr Opin Cell Biol 21(6): 771-7.
Russell, P. and P. Nurse (1986). "cdc25+ functions as an inducer in the mitotic control of fission yeast." Cell 45(1): 145-53.
Russo, A. A., P. D. Jeffrey, et al. (1996). "Structural basis of cyclin-dependent kinase activation by phosphorylation." Nat Struct Biol 3(8): 696-700.
Sanchez, Y., J. Bachant, et al. (1999). "Control of the DNA damage checkpoint by chk1 and rad53 protein kinases through distinct mechanisms." Science 286(5442): 1166-71.
Satyanarayana, A. and P. Kaldis (2009). "Mammalian cell-cycle regulation: several Cdks, numerous cyclins and diverse compensatory mechanisms." Oncogene 28(33): 2925-39.
Schwob, E., T. Bohm, et al. (1994). "The B-type cyclin kinase inhibitor p40SIC1 controls the G1 to S transition in S. cerevisiae." Cell 79(2): 233-44.
Schwob, E. and K. Nasmyth (1993). "CLB5 and CLB6, a new pair of B cyclins involved in DNA replication in Saccharomyces cerevisiae." Genes Dev 7(7A): 1160-75.
Segurado, M. and J. F. Diffley (2008). "Separate roles for the DNA damage checkpoint protein kinases in stabilizing DNA replication forks." Genes Dev 22(13): 1816-27.

Segurado, M. and J. A. Tercero (2009). "The S-phase checkpoint: targeting the replication fork." Biol Cell 101(11): 617-27.

Smolka, M. B., S. H. Chen, et al. (2006). "An FHA domain-mediated protein interaction network of Rad53 reveals its role in polarized cell growth." J Cell Biol 175(5): 743-53.

Sorger, P. K. and A. W. Murray (1992). "S-phase feedback control in budding yeast independent of tyrosine phosphorylation of p34cdc28." Nature 355(6358): 365-8.

Stinchcomb, D. T., K. Struhl, et al. (1979). "Isolation and characterisation of a yeast chromosomal replicator." Nature 282(5734): 39-43.

Tanaka, S. and H. Araki (2010). "Regulation of the initiation step of DNA replication by cyclin-dependent kinases." Chromosoma 119(6): 565-74.

Tanaka, S. and J. F. Diffley (2002). "Deregulated G1-cyclin expression induces genomic instability by preventing efficient pre-RC formation." Genes Dev 16(20): 2639-49.

Theis, J. F. and C. S. Newlon (1997). "The ARS309 chromosomal replicator of Saccharomyces cerevisiae depends on an exceptional ARS consensus sequence." Proc Natl Acad Sci U S A 94(20): 10786-91.

van den Heuvel, S. and N. J. Dyson (2008). "Conserved functions of the pRB and E2F families." Nat Rev Mol Cell Biol 9(9): 713-24.

Wang, H., L. B. Carey, et al. (2009). "Recruitment of Cln3 cyclin to promoters controls cell cycle entry via histone deacetylase and other targets." PLoS Biol 7(9): e1000189.

Zegerman, P. and J. F. Diffley (2010). "Checkpoint-dependent inhibition of DNA replication initiation by Sld3 and Dbf4 phosphorylation." Nature 467(7314): 474-8.

Zhang, Y., E. Y. Shim, et al. (2009). "Regulation of repair choice: Cdk1 suppresses recruitment of end joining factors at DNA breaks." DNA Repair (Amst) 8(10): 1235-41.

Zhao, X. and R. Rothstein (2002). "The Dun1 checkpoint kinase phosphorylates and regulates the ribonucleotide reductase inhibitor Sml1." Proc Natl Acad Sci U S A 99(6): 3746-51.

Zou, L. and S. J. Elledge (2003). "Sensing DNA damage through ATRIP recognition of RPA-ssDNA complexes." Science 300(5625): 1542-8.

18

Free Histones and the Cell Cycle

Douglas Maya, Macarena Morillo-Huesca,
Sebastián Chávez and Mari-Cruz Muñoz-Centeno*
University of Seville
Spain

1. Introduction

DNA replication, the basis of biological inheritance, is a fundamental process occurring during the S-phase of the cell cycle in all eukaryotes. In the nucleus, DNA is associated with histones, basic proteins that help package the lengthy genome to form nucleoprotein filaments called chromatin. Histones are essential for viability as they pack DNA into the nucleus and regulate access to the genetic information contained within the DNA. Due to their strong positive charge, non-chromatin-bound histones can bind non-specifically to negatively charged molecules in the cell, including nucleic acids such as DNA and RNA, as well as negatively charged proteins. Therefore, histone levels are tightly regulated to prevent harmful effects of free histone accumulation: this regulation takes place transcriptionally, posttranscriptionally, translationally and posttranslationally (reviewed in Gunjan et al., 2005). Despite this regulation, different situations can induce an accumulation of non-chromatin-bound histones, called "free" or "excess" histones (Gunjan & Verreault, 2003). In the budding yeast *Saccharomyces cerevisiae*, elevated free histones levels lead to increased DNA damage sensitivity and genomic instability in the form of enhanced mitotic chromosome loss (Gunjan & Verreault, 2003; Singh et al., 2009; Meeks-Wagner & Hartwell, 1986).

A delicate balance between histone and DNA synthesis during the package of the genome into chromatin is essential for cell viability. For this reason, a key regulatory event during the G1/S transition is the induction of histone genes, which allows the coupling of bulk histone synthesis to ongoing DNA replication. In proliferating cells, the synthesis of the vast majority of histones occurs during the S-phase of the cell cycle (Osley, 1991). Moreover in recent years, a novel surveillance mechanism has been described in budding yeast that monitors the accumulation of non-chromatin-bound histones and promotes their rapid degradation by the proteasome in a Rad53 kinase-dependent manner (Gunjan & Verrault, 2003).

In this chapter, we will focus on the model yeast *Sacharomyces cerevisiae* to review how an excess of free histones may be generated in the cell and the different regulatory mechanisms, preventing free histones accumulation in proliferating cells. An overview of the field would be useful to better understand and discuss how essential processes such as chromatin reassembly, transcription elongation, DNA replication and the cell cycle can be coupled through free histone levels. A putative role for Rad53 as a super-integrator of different signals will be discussed.

---

* Corresponding author

2. DNA replication: a crucial event integrated in the cell cycle

DNA replication takes place during the S-phase of the cell cycle. To transmit genetic information over generations, DNA must be precisely replicated before chromosomal segregation takes place. For this purpose, the eukaryotic cell has regulatory mechanisms to limit chromosomal DNA duplication to once per cell cycle, to decide the onset of a new round of DNA replication and to respond to situations in which the genome is at risk.

2.1 Early events in chromosome replication

Accurate and complete DNA replication in each cell cycle and repair of DNA lesions are critical for the maintenance of genetic stability (Aguilera & Gomez-Gonzalez, 2008; Branzei & Foiani, 2008). Failures in this process reduce cell survival and lead to cancer and other diseases in higher metazoans (Hoeijmakers, 2001; Friedberg, 2003). Chromosomal DNA replication in eukaryotes initiates from multiple specific regions of chromosome DNA, known as origins of replication. Therefore, it is crucial to understand how each individual origin is regulated during the cell cycle.

In the budding yeast *S. cerevisiae,* as in higher eukaryotics, activation of multiple replication origins occurs as a two-step reaction (for reviews, see Diffley, 1996, 2004; Bell & Dutta, 2002; Tanaka & Araki, 2010). In the first reaction, called "licensing", a specific protein-DNA complex, known as the pre-replicative complex (pre-RC), is loaded onto origins in the G1 phase. The pre-RC comprises an ORC (origin recognition complex), Cdc6, Cdt1, and the replicative helicase Mcm2-7, which is inactive at this stage. In the second reaction, licensed origins fire at different times during the S-phase to each initiate a pair of replication forks. This origin "firing", or initiation, requires the action of two kinases: cyclin-dependent kinases (CDKs) and Cdc7/Dbf4 (DDK). At the mitotic exit through the G1 phase, CDKs and DDK activities are low, so the replicative helicase Mcm2-7 remains inactive. S-phase-CDKs and DDK activities become more intense during late G1 and promote the assembly of the active replicative helicase. S-CDKs phosphorylate Sld2 and Sld3, enabling them to bind to Dpb11 (Tanaka et al., 2007; Zegerman & Diffley, 2007), whereas DDK acts by phosphorylating subunits of the Mcm2-7 helicase (Sheu & Stillman, 2010). Once the active helicase is assembled, replication origin DNA is unwound and replication forks are formed to synthesise DNA.

In order to coordinate these processes, a regulatory link between DNA replication and cell cycle progression must exist. Firstly, faithful inheritance of the genetic material requires DNA replication to be precisely controlled so that it occurs once per cell cycle. If not, the pre-RC would be reassembled at origins that have already fired, resulting in an over-replication of some parts of the genome. The key to this regulation lies in the initiation of DNA replication and regulatory cell cycle elements control during the M/G1 and G1/S transitions. CDKs play an important role in separating these two reactions (Arias & Walter, 2007). During the mitotic exit and G1, CDK activity is reduced by two different mechanisms: down-regulation in the level of these cyclins and accumulation of the CDK inhibitor Sic1 (Stegmeier & Amon, 2004). Under these conditions, the pre-RCs are assembled at replication origins, but initiation does not occur because CDK activity is low. In the following S phase, S-CDK is activated and DNA replication initiates. At the same time, and very importantly, reassembly of the pre-RC at origins is blocked by CDK to inhibit re-replication (Diffley, 2004; Tanaka et al., 2007): CDK can phosphorylate all the pre-RC components, ORC, Cdc6, Cdt1, and Mcm2-7, to down-regulate their activities for the pre-RC formation (reviewed in

Tanaka & Araki, 2010). Less is known, however, about the dephosphorylation of initiation proteins, whether it is necessary for replication origin resetting and the acting phosphatase(s) that might control this process and, therefore, replication licensing. Recently it has been demonstrated that Cdc14p resets the competency of replication licensing by dephosphorylating multiple initiation proteins during the mitotic exit in budding yeast (Zhai et al., 2010).

2.2 The importance of the G1/S transition

In *S. cerevisiae*, commitment to a new round of cell division takes place towards the end of the G1 phase of the cell cycle, a process called START (Hartwell & Kastan, 1994). This is the main regulatory event of the G1 phase of the cell cycle, and involves an extensive transcriptional programme driven by transcription factors SBF (Swi4-Swi6) and MBF (Mbp1-Swi6) (Costanzo et al., 2004; de Bruin et al., 2004). Activation of these factors depends ultimately on G1 cyclin Cln3.

There are three G1 cyclins in *S. cerevisiae*: *CLN1*, *CLN2* and *CLN3*. MBF and SBF activation in START depends on the cyclin/cyclin-dependent-kinase (CDK) complex Cln3-Cdc28 which phosphorylates the negative regulator of START, Whi5, by promoting its release from SBF (Swi4-Swi6) (Costanzo et al., 2004; de Bruin et al., 2004). Activation of the MBF-dependent transcription by Cln3-Cdc28 is thought to act through a mechanism that is independent of Whi5 which involves the phosphorylation of Mbp1. Accordingly, a recent work has determined the transcriptional targets of Cln3 and their dependence on the SBF or MBF factors (Ferrezuelo et al., 2010). This analysis has produced more than 200 transcription factor-target assignments validated by ChiP assays and by functional enrichment, and supports a model whereby Cln3 differentially activates SBF and MBF. Activation leads to the modification and recruitment of the factors involved in transcription initiation and, therefore, to transcription activation (Costanzo et al., 2004; de Bruin et al., 2004; Takahata et al., 2009). Activation of these factors results in the accumulation of G1 and S-phase cyclins, which promotes S-phase entry (reviewed in Wittenberg, 2005). The kinase activity of Cln1,2-Cdc28 notably triggers the degradation of cyclin-dependent kinase inhibitor Sic1, which no longer inhibits the S phase-promoting complex Clb5,6-Cdc28 (Schneider et al., 1996; Schwob et al., 1994). In addition, a positive feedback mechanism involving Cln1 and Cln2 has been proposed to operate under physiological conditions in SBF/MBF activation (Skotheim et al., 2008). The main events in the *S. cerevisiae* G1-to-S transition are schematised in Figure 1.

Cells tightly regulate the different cell cycle transitions to ensure the correct transmission of genetic information. Checkpoints are surveillance mechanisms that prevent one cell cycle stage from starting if a previous cell cycle stage has not been successfully completed. Checkpoints can be considered as signal transduction cascades with three components: sensors to detect incomplete or aberrant cell cycle events; transducers of the checkpoint signal; and targets that are modified by transducers to cause cell cycle arrest (Elledge, 1996). As the G1-to S phase transition (START) signifies a commitment to complete cell division, eukaryotic cells are capable of undergoing transient arrest during the G1/S transition if conditions which would be unfavourable for cell division, such as nutrient limitation (Gallego et al., 1997), environmental toxins (Philpott et al., 1998) or damaged DNA, are encountered. Impaired ability to either initiate the arrest or to subsequently recover from the arrest and to resume cell division appears to be detrimental (Hartwell & Kastan, 1994; Lydall & Weinert, 1995; Shaulian et al., 2000). In recent years, the way different DNA-damage situations can trigger cell cycle checkpoint machinery has been studied in great detail. DNA damage or replicative stress, depending on where the cell happens to be in the cell cycle, can cause cell cycle arrest via the "G1/S" checkpoint, the "intra-S" checkpoint or the "G2/M" checkpoint (Jares et al., 2000; Segurado & Tercero, 2009).

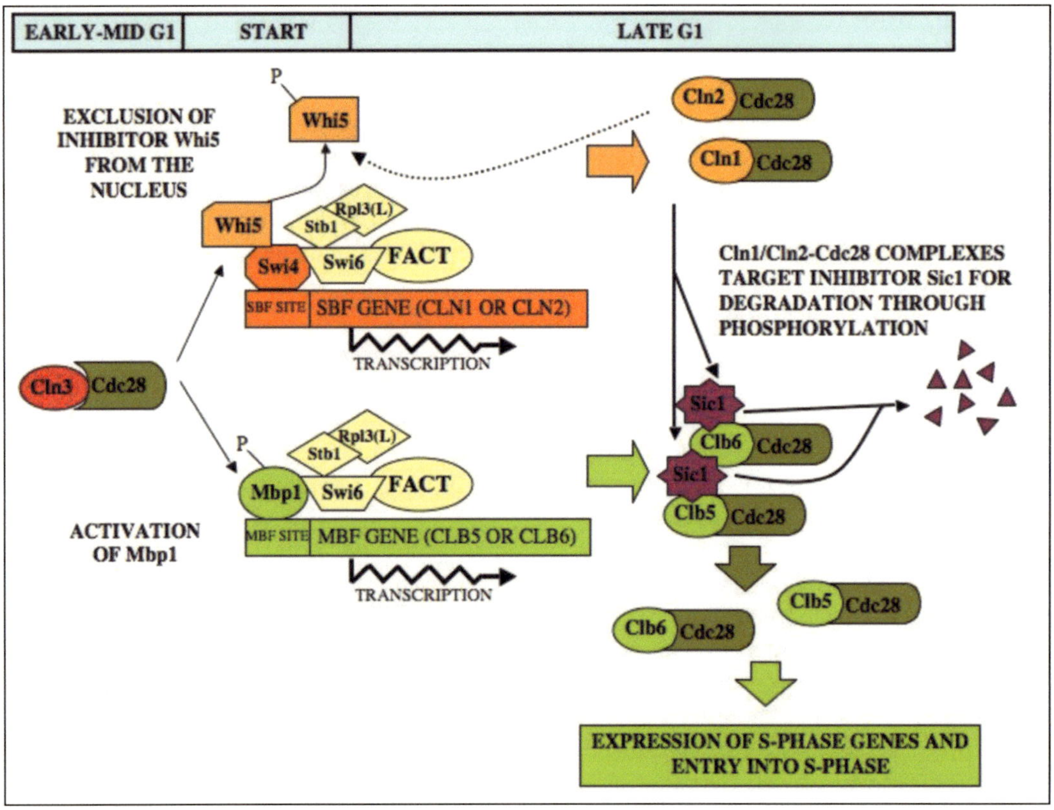

Fig. 1. The G1/S transition in *S. cerevisiae*

2.3 The "intra-S-phase" checkpoint response

The DNA-damage signalling pathway is highly conserved throughout eukaryotes (Lydall & Weinert, 1996). Under DNA damage situations, kinase Mec1 in *S. cerevisiae* is phosphorylated (Morrow et al., 1995; Siede et al., 1996) and causes the phosphorylation of the kinase encoded by *RAD53* (Sanchez et al., 1996; Sun et al., 1996). Then Rad53p phosphorylates the transcription factor Swi6p, causing a delay in the accumulation of mRNA for G1 cyclins and, thus, transient cell cycle arrest (Sidorova & Breeden, 1997). Below we will discuss the function of Rad53 if a DNA-damage situation is detected after START. An essential role for DEAD-Box Helicase DHH1 in G1/S DNA-damage checkpoint recovery has been proposed (Bergkessel & Reese, 2004).

Another relevant response to cope with situations where the genome is at risk, owing to DNA damage or replicative stress, takes place during DNA replication, this being the so-called S-phase or replication checkpoint pathway (also called "intra-S-phase", which refers to cells that have already passed START and begun replication) (Nyberg et al., 2002; Osborn et al., 2002; Paulovich & Hartwell, 1995; Segurado & Tercero, 2009). Two central players in this checkpoint in budding yeast are the aforementioned kinases Mec1 and Rad53. They are homologues of Rad3 and Cds1, respectively, in the fission yeast *Schizosaccharomyces pombe*, or ATR and Chk2 in mammalian cells, which are deficient in many cancer cells.

In budding yeast, the signalling cascade triggered under replication stress culminates with the phosphorylation of Rad53 (Branzei & Foiani, 2009). This kinase is essential for the activation of the molecular mechanisms required to cope with replication arrest: (1) it promotes the stabilisation of stalled replication forks and allows DNA replication restart after removal of the blocking agent (Santocanale & Diffley, 1998; Tercero & Diffley, 2001); (2) it is also responsible for inducing the transcription factors of ribonucleotide reductase genes or DNA damage response genes (Allen et al., 1994; Huang et al., 1998; Zhao et al., 2001); (3) finally, Rad53 prevents the firing of late replication origins (Duch et al., 2011; Zegerman & Diffley, 2010) and restrains spindle elongation, thus preventing mitosis (Allen et al., 1994; Bachant et al., 2005; Weinert et al., 1994). Kinase Cdc7/Dbf4 is a target of the intra-S-phase checkpoint (Jares et al., 2000).

3. Replicating chromatin: DNA is associated with histones

The DNA of eukaryotic cells fits the confines of the nucleus by a hierarchical scheme of folding and compaction into chromatin. Nucleosomes, the repeating structural units of chromatin, consist in an octameric histone core comprising two copies each of H2A, H2B, H3 and H4, around which 147 bp of DNA are wrapped in 1.65 superhelical turns (Andrews & Luger, 2011; Luger et al., 1997). A linker or H1 histone molecule then associates with the nucleosome core particle (Brown, 2003). Thus nucleosomes are formed into regularly spaced arrays along DNA and can be mobilised by different ATP-dependent remodelling complexes, such as SWI/SNF or RSC, or ATP-independent ones, like the FACT complex. Histones are essential for viability as they pack DNA into the nucleus and regulate access to the genetic information contained within it.

The chromatin structure plays a central role in gene regulation and other nuclear processes, including DNA replication (Groth et al., 2007). During replication, the cell must replicate not only its DNA, but also its chromatin. Accordingly, another regulatory process during the G1/S transition is the induction of histone genes, which allows the coupling of bulk histone synthesis with ongoing DNA replication. In proliferating cells, the synthesis of the vast majority of histones occurs during the S-phase of the cell cycle. Inhibition of DNA synthesis results in a rapid repression of histone genes, indicating that it is tightly coupled with DNA replication.

An interesting question underlying this close coupling between DNA replication and histones expression is: *Why are histone protein levels subject to such a high degree of regulation?* Insufficiency of histones has been seen to be nonviable for the cell (Han et al., 1987). Interestingly, excess histones have also proved deleterious for cell growth, and they provoke genomic instability (Meeks-Wagner & Hartwell, 1986), increased DNA damage sensitivity and cytotoxicity (Gunjan & Verreault, 2003; Singh, Kabbaj, et al., 2009). These effects could be due to the strong positive charge of histones. Non-chromatin-bound histones, named "excess" or "free" histones, could bind non-specifically to negatively charged molecules in the cell, including nucleic acids such as DNA and RNA, as well as to negatively charged proteins. Recently in-depth research has been done into the mechanisms via which excess or free histones exert their deleterious effects *in vivo* (Singh et al., 2010). Using microarray analysis, the authors of this work found that excess histones mediate their deleterious effects via multiple mechanisms in budding yeast, largely by inappropriate electrostatic interactions with the cellular macromolecules carrying the opposite charge. This analysis also revealed that around 240 genes were either up- or down-regulated by 2-fold, or more, overexpression of the histone gene pair H3/H4. After considering all this information, it is easy to think that cells need to have a very tight regulation of histone protein levels to maintain genomic stability and cell viability.

4. Avoiding free histones in yeast: controlling histones levels

To prevent deleterious effects of free histone accumulation, histone proteins are regulated transcriptionally, posttranscriptionally, translationally and posttranslationally (reviewed in Gunjan et al., 2005).

4.1 Transcriptional regulation

Cells must replicate not only their DNA during the S-phase, but also their chromatin. Accordingly, the transcription of histone genes is activated at the beginning of the S-phase to provide sufficient core histones to assemble replicated DNA. Correspondingly, inhibition of DNA synthesis results in a rapid repression of histone genes, indicating that it is tightly coupled with DNA replication (Osley, 1991; Breeden, 2003; reviewed in Gunjan et al., 2005).

The major core histone genes in *S. cerevisiae* are organised into four loci, each containing two histones genes that are divergently transcribed from a central promoter: two loci encode H2A and H2B (*HTA1-HTB1* and *HTA2-HTB2*) (Hereford et al., 1979), while the other two encode H3 and H4 (*HHT1-HHF1* and *HHT2-HHF2*) (Sutton et al., 2001). The tight cell cycle regulation of the histone genes results from their transcriptional repression in phases G1 and G2, their transcriptional activation just before the S-phase and the posttranscriptional regulation of their mRNAs. During the S-phase, histone genes can also respond to changes; for instance, accumulation of histones in response to the genotoxic agents interfering with DNA replication induces their repression (reviewed by Gunjan et al., 2005).

Three of the four divergent histone gene promoters (the two gene pairs that encode H3/H4, and *HTA1-HTB1*, one of the two gene pairs encoding H2A/H2B) are repressed by Hir proteins: Hir1, Hir2, Hir3 and Hpc2. Thus, the *S. cerevisiae* cells lacking any of the four Hir proteins are incapable of efficiently repressing these histone genes outside the S-phase or by following the replication arrest during this phase (Osley & Lycan, 1987; Xu et al., 1992; Sherwood et al., 1993). This repression is mediated through a negative *cis*-acting sequence (*NEG*) present in the histone promoters, except in *HTA2-HTB2* (Osley et al., 1986). The fourth histone gene pair (*HTA2-HTB2*) shows a similar regulation pattern to the other three, but its repression is independent of the Hir proteins. It is also important to highlight that the SBF transcription factor, a regulator of the aforementioned G1/S-specific genes, also plays a role in *HTA1-HTB1* regulation. Evidence for this role includes, among others, that SBF mutants exhibit modestly reduced HTA1 and HTB1 mRNA levels (Hess & Winston, 2005), and that Swi4 has been detected by chromatin immunoprecipitation at *HTA1-HTB1* (ChiP) (Simon et al., 2001).

4.2 Posttranscriptional regulation

The increase in histone mRNAs during the S-phase is not only due to a cell cycle-regulated promoter in histone genes, but also to a regulated stability of histone messengers: histone mRNAs accumulate in the S-phase and are rapidly degraded as cells progress to the G2 phase of the cell cycle. This regulation mode is better understood in higher eukaryotes (Marzluff & Duronio, 2002), although the mechanisms to modulate the stability of histone RNAs differ among eukaryotic organisms. In *S. cerevisiae,* histone mRNA abundance oscillates and clearly peaks during the S-phase, even when histones are expressed from a constitutive promoter (Lycan et al., 1987; Xu et al., 1990; Campbell et al., 2002). This stability is regulated through the 3′ elements of the genes. Moreover, loss of Trf4 and Trf5 (polyA polymerases), or of Rrp6 (a component of the nuclear exosome), results in elevated levels of the transcripts encoding DNA replication-dependent histones. *TRF4, TRF5* and *RRP6* have been identified as new players in the regulation of histones mRNA levels in yeast (Reis & Campbell, 2007).

4.3 Controlling histone protein levels by proteolysis

In recent years, a novel mechanism to prevent the accumulation of free histones, which is superimposed upon the regulation of histone gene transcription and mRNA stability, has been described in budding yeast (Gunjan & Verreault, 2003; reviewed in Gunjan et al., 2006). The authors demonstrated that Rad53, but not Mec1, is required for the degradation of the excess histones that are not packaged into chromatin. Consequently, *rad53* mutants accumulate abnormally large amounts of soluble histones and are sensitive to histone overexpression. Remarkably, DNA damage sensitivity, slow growth and chromosome loss of *rad53* mutants, can be significantly suppressed by a disruption of one of the two loci encoding histones H3/H4; thus it may be argued that these phenotypes are partially due to the presence of excess histones. This relevant work also demonstrated that Rad53 associates with histones *in vivo* and that this interaction is modulated by its kinase activity. In summary, this new surveillance mechanism not only monitors the accumulation of excess histones, but also induces their degradation. Excess histones associate with Rad53 *in vivo* and undergo modifications such as tyrosine phosphorylation and polyubiquitination before their proteolysis by the proteasome. A tyrosine 99 residue of H3 has been identified as being critical for the proficient ubiquitylation and degradation of this histone. Finally, different proteins have been identified as enzymes involved in the ubiquitylation of free or excess histones like the E2 proteins Ubc4 and Ubc5, as well as E3 ubiquitin ligase Tom1 (Singh, Kabbaj, et al., 2009; reviewed in Singh & Gunjan, 2011).

5. Generating free histones during the cell cycle

So far we have discussed how cells tightly regulate histone levels to prevent harmful effects of free histones from binding non-specifically to nucleic acids and from interfering with processes that require access to genetic information. Firstly, delicate transcriptional and posttranscriptional regulations of histone genes, coupled with DNA replication during the S-phase of the cell cycle, efficiently avoid an accumulation of non-chromatin-bound histones. This kind of mechanisms is evolutionarily conserved (Osley, 1991; Marzluff & Duronio, 2002). Secondly, despite this regulation, situations where free histones appear exist and a posttranslational mechanism mediated by Rad53 induces the proteolysis of excess histones. Finally, therefore, it is interesting to wonder about the processes generating excess histones during the cell cycle (reviewed in Singh et al., 2009).

Firstly, it has been well-established that all eukaryotes have multiple genes encoding each histone protein. Histones are primarily synthesised in the S-phase and deposited by chromatin assembly factors or histone chaperones on replicating DNA to form chromatin in a process known as chromatin assembly (Gunjan et al., 2005). Different hypotheses have attempted to explain why eukaryotic cells carry such a large number of histone genes. The most simple explanation seems to be that the high demand of histones for chromatin assembly on newly replicated DNA can only be achieved by multiple histone genes. However, it has been shown that *S. cerevisiae* only requires half its complement of histone genes for viability (Osley, 1991). Moreover, the full complement of histones genes in budding yeast synthesises excess histones which are deleterious to cells, making them more sensitive to a variety of DNA damaging agents (Gunjan & Verreault, 2003). Even if it may be a challenge to comprehensively integrate all this information, it is clear that yeast cells synthesise histones in excess in accordance requirements for chromatin assembly during the S-phase. Thus, yeast cells ensure that all the genome is fully packaged into chromatin following the DNA replication that synthesises excess histones during the S-phase by degrading unincorporated histones at the end of DNA replication.

Secondly, rigorously coupling histone synthesis with DNA replication (Stein & Stein, 1984) ensures the rapid incorporation of histones into newly synthesised DNA to form chromatin. However, different situations can generate DNA replication slow down or arrest, resulting in an accumulation of unincorporated newly synthesised histones (Bonner et al., 1988). To better illustrate these situations, replication inhibitors bring about a drastic drop in DNA synthesis and chromatin assembly. Moreover, DNA damage results in DNA replication slowing down or stalling, which is due to either the physical impediment posed by DNA lesions or, more likely, the activation of the intra-S-phase DNA damage checkpoint that prevents new origins from firing (Paulovich & Hartwell, 1995; Tercero & Diffley, 2001).

A third source of excess histones (non-chromatin-bound ones) may be those histones removed during DNA damage, repair and recombination. When DNA damage occurs in the chromatin context, repair factors have to gain access to the damaged site to carry out necessary repairs. In this sense, there is evidence suggesting that histones may be evicted locally from a DNA double strand break (DSB) site to allow access to the repair machinery (Tsukuda et al., 2005). A minor contribution of this last process to free histone accumulation may be expected.

6. A novel source of excess free histones: evicted from transcription

DNA is tightly packed into chromatin. Nucleosomes need to be disassembled and reassembled to allow efficient transcription by RNA polymerases. There are many different factors relating to this process. One very well described essential factor involved in RNA pol II transcription is the FACT complex (reviewed by Reinberg & Sims, 2006; Formosa, 2008). This complex is the only factor known to date that stimulates RNA Pol II-dependent transcription elongation through chromatin in a highly purified system (Orphanides et al., 1998; Pavri et al., 2006) and also *in vivo* (Jimeno-Gonzalez et al., 2006; Biswas et al., 2006; Formosa, 2003; Mason & Struhl, 2003; Saunders et al., 2003). In the budding yeast *S. cerevisiae*, the FACT complex is composed of two essential proteins: Spt16/Cdc68/Ssf1 (hereafter referred to as Spt16) and Pob3 (Stuwe et al., 2008; Orphanides et al., 1999). yFACT and the HMG-box protein Nhp6 form a heterodimer that is capable of binding nucleosomes (Formosa et al., 2001) and of recognising them *in vitro* (Rhoades et al., 2004; Xin et al., 2009). Both Spt16 and Pob3 are able to bind H3/H4 tetramers and H2A/H2B dimers, sometimes in a functionally redundant manner (Stuwe et al., 2008; VanDemark et al., 2008). These interactions are thought to destabilise nucleosomes during transcription (Belotserkovskaya & Reinberg, 2004; Xin et al., 2009). Thus, yFACT plays a role in maintaining the integrity of the chromatin structure during transcription (Mason & Struhl, 2003; Kaplan et al., 2003; Cheung et al., 2008; Vanti et al., 2009; Jamai et al., 2009). In addition to transcription defects, defects on Spt16 can also lead to cell cycle defects. *SPT16* was originally identified during a screening looking for *cdc* (cell division cycle) mutants (Malone et al., 1991; Rowley et al., 1991). Mutant *cdc68* (also named *spt16-197* and *spt16G132D*) is a thermosensitive mutant with a very clear accumulation of G1 cells.

Our group, in collaboration with the labs of Geli and Gunjan, has recently demonstrated that a dysfunction in chromatin reassembly during active Pol II transcription through defects on the Spt16 protein can generate an accumulation of free histones. We have shown that a strong genetic interaction takes place between the *spt16-197* mutant and those mutants affected in the kinase activity of Rad53. This interaction does not seem to relate to the DNA damage response since other very well-established proteins involved in this response, like Mec1 or Rad9, show no interaction. Since Rad53, but not Mec1 or Rad9, is involved in the detection and subsequent degradation of excess histones, we hypothesised that a dysfunction of Spt16 might lead to an increase in free histones, which would need to be targeted for degradation via Rad53. According to this model, we observed that deleting the *HTA2-HTB2* locus can partially suppress the *ts* phenotype of *spt16-197*. Using co-immunoprecipitation assays to detect free non-chromatin-bound histones, we demonstrated that Pol II-dependent transcription in the absence of active FACT causes an accumulation of evicted histones, which could become toxic for the cell if not targeted for degradation by Rad53 (Morillo-Huesca et al., 2010).

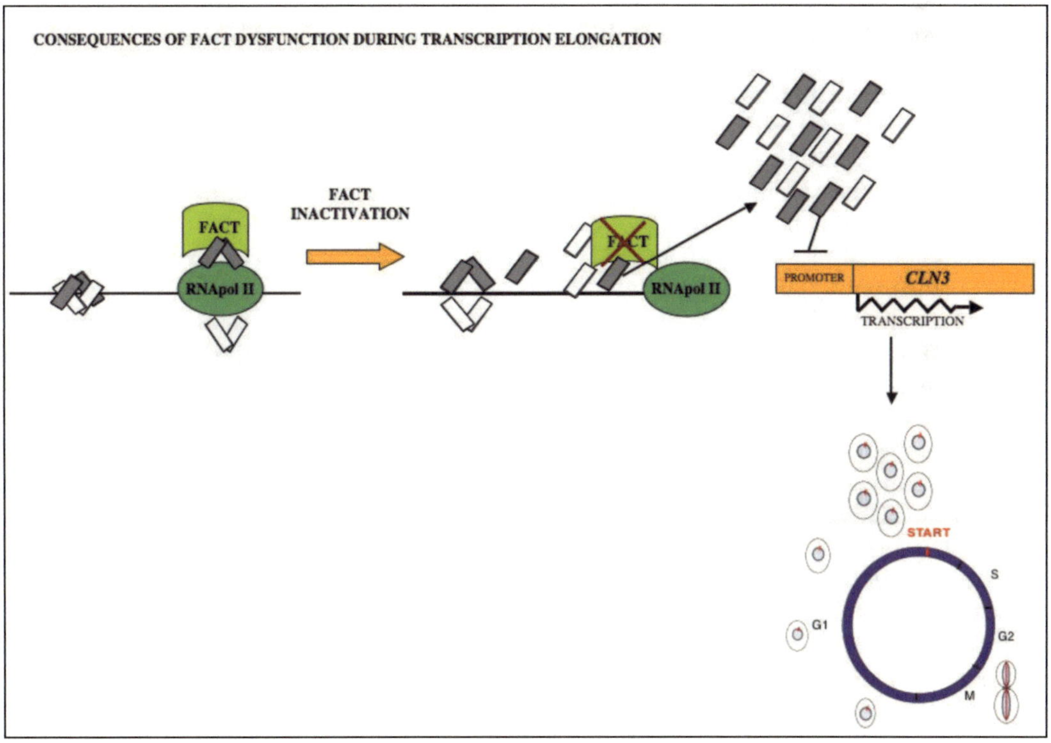

Fig. 2. FACT inactivation causes accumulation of free histones and a subsequent G1 delay.

Beyond the S-phase, transcribed chromatin is probably the main source of free histones in yeast cells, presumably due to the minor imbalances between histone supply and demand during chromatin reassembly. Our results indicate a novel and important role for FACT in yeast, that of a protective factor against the toxic risk represented by evicted histones. This model agrees with a recent publication which reports how Spt16 promotes the redeposition of the original H3 and H4 histones evicted by elongating Pol II (Jamai et al., 2009). The protective role against evicted histones is probably not an exclusive function of FACT, but a function of the other factors that cooperate during chromatin reassembly, like Spt6, for which we have also provided some evidence (Morillo-Huesca et al., 2010).

7. A novel signal regulating the G1/S transition: free histone levels

Our work has allowed us to propose that a dysfunction of chromatin reassembly factors, like FACT and Spt6, generates an accumulation of the excess histones evicted from transcription. In addition to this, we have found an interesting connection between free histone levels and cell cycle defects in the G1/S transition. We postulate that free or non-chromatin-bound histones can trigger the down-regulation of *CLN3*, thereby arresting cells at G1 (START) and contributing to control free histone levels before starting DNA replication (Morillo-Huesca et al., 2010). Our results indicate a so far unknown connection between chromatin dynamics and cell cycle regulation. Firstly, genetic and molecular evidence indicates that, in the absence of FACT or the Spt6 function, the expression of *CLN3* is down-regulated by a mechanism that specifically represses its transcriptional promoter. Secondly, and significantly, the G1 delay studied was not mediated by the DNA-damage checkpoint, although a *rad53* mutant enhances both the thermosensitivity of the *spt16* mutant and its G1 phenotype. This result, in combination with the lack of phosphorylation of Rad53 after FACT inactivation, indicates that excess histones are involved in this phenomenon. This conclusion is strengthened by the results of the experiments that manipulate *in vivo* histone levels: (i) deletion of one of the two loci encoding H2A and H2B partially suppressed the *ts* phenotype and the accumulation of G1 cells of the *spt16* mutant, indicating that a reduction in histone levels can alleviate the *cdc* phenotype due to a FACT dysfunction; (ii) overproduction of histone levels in wild-type cells leads to a clear accumulation of the cells in G1 (asynchronous culture) and a more marked delay in the entry of synchronised cells in the S-phase (Morillo-Huesca et al., 2010). This delay in the G1/S transition also correlates with *CLN3* down-regulation. These results, obtained in wild-type cells, demonstrate that a histone-mediated G1 delay can be obtained in a background with no possible indirect effects mediated by either the role of FACT in the expression of the G1-S regulators or the function of Rad53 in the control of early replication events.

In mammalian cells, histone overexpression slows down entry into and progression through the S-phase (Groth et al., 2007). Interestingly, depletion of human Spt16 leads to the repression of H1, H2A and H2B genes (Li et al., 2007), which could be the result of the accumulation of the free histones in human cells after FACT dysfunction. Given the analogy between the G1-S regulators in yeast (Cln3-SBF-Whi5-Rpd3) and mammals (CyclinD1-E2F-Rb-HDAC1) (Wang et al., 2009; Takahata et al., 2009), the functional link between the accumulation of free histones and the regulation of the G1-S transition may be evolutionarily conserved.

This chapter emphasises that excess free histones may have serious implications for the normal progression of DNA replication when the toxicity of free histones is maximal in the

S-phase (Gunjan & Verreault, 2003). According to this scenario, a G1 delay in response to excess histones favours cell viability. In our model, represented in Figure 2, the G1 delay should allow cells to reduce the free histones levels through the Rad53/Tom1-mediated histone degradation pathway before entering the S-phase. It is interesting to note that Rad53 participates in different linked functions, such as the DNA damage checkpoint, the excess histone degradation pathway, and at the initiation of DNA replication. A model has been recently proposed in which Rad53 acts as a "nucleosome buffer" by interacting with origins of replication to prevent excess histones from binding to origins and to maintain a proper chromatin configuration (Holzen & Sclafani, 2010). For this reason, we propose the term *chromatin repair* to denote a combination of DNA repair, chromatin reassembly and excess histone degradation. An attractive role for Rad53 as a super-integrator of all chromatin repair functions can be presumed.

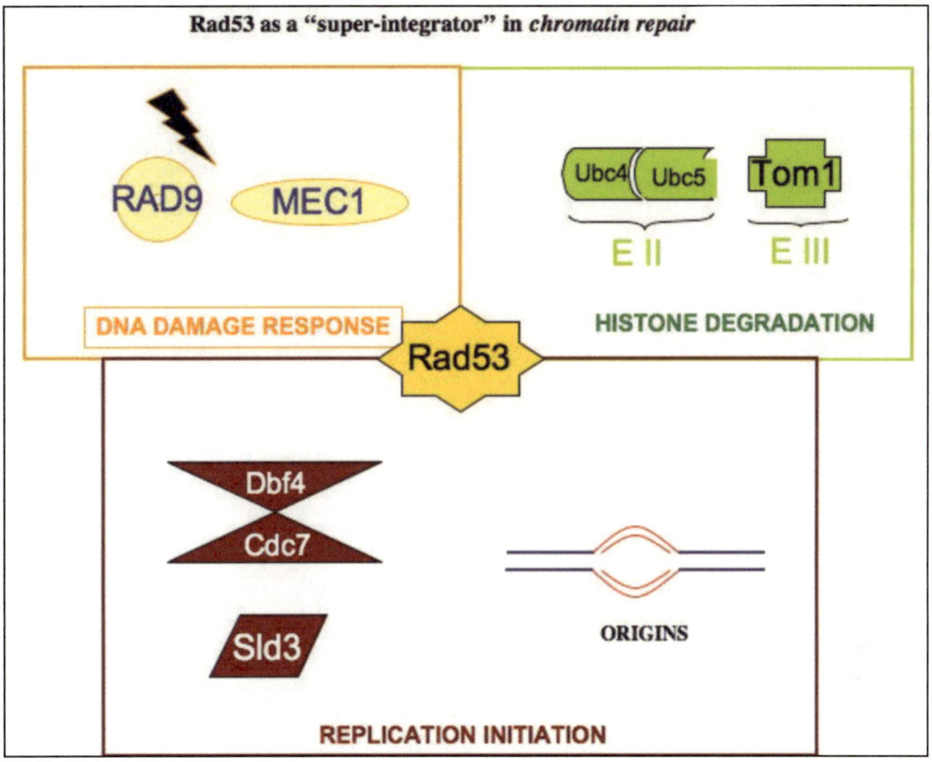

Fig. 3. Rad53 functions

8. Conclusion

In this chapter we have reviewed the contribution of transcription to the levels of free histones and their influence on the cell cycle and DNA replication. Nucleosomes need to be disassembled to allow DNA transcription by RNA polymerases. An essential factor for disassembly/reassembly process during DNA transcription is the FACT complex. We concluded, using loss-of-function FACT mutants, that FACT dysfunction provokes downregulation of *CLN3*, one of the cyclins that plays a key role in the control of the G1/S transition. FACT dysfunction increases the level of the free histones released from chromatin during transcription, and the G1 delay of the FACT mutant is enhanced by a second mutation affecting Rad53, a protein that regulates DNA repair and excess histone degradation. The overexpression of histones in wild type cells also causes a cell cycle delay before DNA replication. All this experimental evidence points out to a so-far unknown connection between chromatin dynamics and the regulation of the cell cycle, mediated by free histones.

Finally, we propose an attractive overall concept, *chromatin repair*, to signify the combination of DNA repair, chromatin reassembly and excess histone degradation. An attractive role for Rad53 as a super-integrator of all chromatin repair functions can be presumed as this protein plays key roles in the mentioned linked functions.

9. Acknowledgment

We thank Akash Gunjan´s and Vincent Geli´s labs for their fruitful collaboration. This work has been supported by the Spanish Ministry of Education and Science (grant BFU2007-67575-C03-02/BMC), by the Andalusian Government (grant P07-CVI02623) and by the European Union (FEDER). D.M. was covered by a F.P.I. fellowship from the Regional Andalusian Government and M. M-H. by a fellowship from the Spanish Ministry of Education and Science. We thank Helen Warburton for English corrections.

10. References

Aguilera, A., and B. Gomez-Gonzalez. (2008). Genome instability: a mechanistic view of its causes and consequences. Nat Rev Genet, Vol. 9, No. 3, pp. (204-17).

Allen, J. B., Z. Zhou, W. Siede, E. C. Friedberg, and S. J. Elledge. (1994). The SAD1/RAD53 protein kinase controls multiple checkpoints and DNA damage-induced transcription in yeast. Genes Dev, Vol. 8, No. 20, pp. (2401-15).

Andrews, AJ., and K. Luger. (2011). Nucleosome Structure(s) and Stability: Variations on a Theme. Annu Rev Biophys, Vol. 40, No., pp. (99-117).

Arias, E. E., and J. C. Walter. (2007). Strength in numbers: preventing rereplication via multiple mechanisms in eukaryotic cells. Genes Dev, Vol. 21, No. 5, pp. (497-518).

Bachant, J., S. R. Jessen, S. E. Kavanaugh, and C. S. Fielding. (2005). The yeast S phase checkpoint enables replicating chromosomes to bi-orient and restrain spindle extension during S phase distress. J Cell Biol, Vol. 168, No. 7, pp. (999-1012).

Bell, S. P., and A. Dutta. (2002). DNA replication in eukaryotic cells. Annu Rev Biochem, Vol. 71, No., pp. (333-74).

Belotserkovskaya, R., and D. Reinberg. (2004). Facts about FACT and transcript elongation through chromatin. Curr Opin Genet Dev, Vol. 14, No. 2, pp. (139-46).

Bergkessel, M., and J. C. Reese. (2004). An essential role for the Saccharomyces cerevisiae DEAD-box helicase DHH1 in G1/S DNA-damage checkpoint recovery. Genetics, Vol. 167, No. 1, pp. (21-33).

Biswas, D., R. Dutta-Biswas, D. Mitra, Y. Shibata, B. D. Strahl, T. Formosa, and D. J. Stillman. (2006). Opposing roles for Set2 and yFACT in regulating TBP binding at promoters. Embo J, Vol. 25, No. 19, pp. (4479-89).

Bonner, W. M., R. S. Wu, H. T. Panusz, and C. Muneses. (1988). Kinetics of accumulation and depletion of soluble newly synthesized histone in the reciprocal regulation of histone and DNA synthesis. Biochemistry, Vol. 27, No. 17, pp. (6542-50).

Branzei, D., and M. Foiani. (2008). Regulation of DNA repair throughout the cell cycle. Nat Rev Mol Cell Biol, Vol. 9, No. 4, pp. (297-308).

Branzei, D., and M. Foiani. (2009). The checkpoint response to replication stress. DNA Repair (Amst), Vol. 8, No. 9, pp. (1038-46).

Breeden, L. L. (2003). Periodic transcription: a cycle within a cycle. Curr Biol, Vol. 13, No. 1, pp. (R31-8).

Brown, D. T. (2003). Histone H1 and the dynamic regulation of chromatin function. Biochem Cell Biol, Vol. 81, No. 3, pp. (221-7).

Campbell, S. G., M. Li Del Olmo, P. Beglan, and U. Bond. (2002). A sequence element downstream of the yeast HTB1 gene contributes to mRNA 3' processing and cell cycle regulation. Mol Cell Biol, Vol. 22, No. 24, pp. (8415-25).

Cheung, V., G. Chua, N. N. Batada, C. R. Landry, S. W. Michnick, T. R. Hughes, and F. Winston. (2008). Chromatin- and transcription-related factors repress transcription from within coding regions throughout the Saccharomyces cerevisiae genome. PLoS Biol, Vol. 6, No. 11, pp. (e277).

Costanzo, M., J. L. Nishikawa, X. Tang, J. S. Millman, O. Schub, K. Breitkreuz, D. Dewar, I. Rupes, B. Andrews, and M. Tyers. (2004). CDK activity antagonizes Whi5, an inhibitor of G1/S transcription in yeast. Cell, Vol. 117, No. 7, pp. (899-913).

de Bruin, R. A., W. H. McDonald, T. I. Kalashnikova, J. Yates, 3rd, and C. Wittenberg. (2004). Cln3 activates G1-specific transcription via phosphorylation of the SBF bound repressor Whi5. Cell, Vol. 117, No. 7, pp. (887-98).

Diffley, J. F. (1996). Once and only once upon a time: specifying and regulating origins of DNA replication in eukaryotic cells. Genes Dev, Vol. 10, No. 22, pp. (2819-30).

Diffley, J.F. (2004). Regulation of early events in chromosome replication. Curr Biol, Vol. 14, No. 18, pp. (R778-86).

Duch, A., G. Palou, Z. O. Jonsson, R. Palou, E. Calvo, J. Wohlschlegel, and D. G. Quintana. (2011). A Dbf4 mutant contributes to bypassing the Rad53-mediated block of origins of replication in response to genotoxic stress. J Biol Chem, Vol. 286, No. 4, pp. (2486-91).

Elledge, S. J. (1996). Cell cycle checkpoints: preventing an identity crisis. Science, Vol. 274, No. 5293, pp. (1664-72).

Ferrezuelo, F., N. Colomina, B. Futcher, and M. Aldea. (2010). The transcriptional network activated by Cln3 cyclin at the G1-to-S transition of the yeast cell cycle. Genome Biol, Vol. 11, No. 6, pp. (R67).

Formosa, T. (2003). Changing the DNA landscape: putting a SPN on chromatin. Curr Top Microbiol Immunol, Vol. 274, No., pp. (171-201).

Formosa, T. (2008). FACT and the reorganized nucleosome. Mol Biosyst, Vol. 4, No. 11, pp. (1085-93).

Formosa, T., P. Eriksson, J. Wittmeyer, J. Ginn, Y. Yu, and D. J. Stillman. (2001). Spt16-Pob3 and the HMG protein Nhp6 combine to form the nucleosome-binding factor SPN. Embo J, Vol. 20, No. 13, pp. (3506-17).

Friedberg, E. C. (2003). DNA damage and repair. Nature, Vol. 421, No. 6921, pp. (436-40).

Gallego, C., E. Gari, N. Colomina, E. Herrero, and M. Aldea. (1997). The Cln3 cyclin is down-regulated by translational repression and degradation during the G1 arrest caused by nitrogen deprivation in budding yeast. Embo J, Vol. 16, No. 23, pp. (7196-206).

Groth, A., A. Corpet, A. J. Cook, D. Roche, J. Bartek, J. Lukas, and G. Almouzni. (2007). Regulation of replication fork progression through histone supply and demand. Science, Vol. 318, No. 5858, pp. (1928-31).

Gunjan, A., J. Paik, and A. Verreault. (2005). Regulation of histone synthesis and nucleosome assembly. Biochimie, Vol. 87, No. 7, pp. (625-35).

Gunjan, A., J. Paik, and A. Verreault. (2006). The emergence of regulated histone proteolysis. Curr Opin Genet Dev, Vol. 16, No. 2, pp. (112-8).

Gunjan, A., and A. Verreault. (2003). A Rad53 kinase-dependent surveillance mechanism that regulates histone protein levels in S. cerevisiae. Cell, Vol. 115, No. 5, pp. (537-49).

Han, M., M. Chang, U. J. Kim, and M. Grunstein. (1987). Histone H2B repression causes cell-cycle-specific arrest in yeast: effects on chromosomal segregation, replication, and transcription. Cell, Vol. 48, No. 4, pp. (589-97).

Hartwell, L. H., and M. B. Kastan. (1994). Cell cycle control and cancer. Science, Vol. 266, No. 5192, pp. (1821-8).

Hereford, L., K. Fahrner, J. Woolford, Jr., M. Rosbash, and D. B. Kaback. (1979). Isolation of yeast histone genes H2A and H2B. Cell, Vol. 18, No. 4, pp. (1261-71).

Hess, D., and F. Winston. (2005). Evidence that Spt10 and Spt21 of Saccharomyces cerevisiae play distinct roles in vivo and functionally interact with MCB-binding factor, SCB-binding factor and Snf1. Genetics, Vol. 170, No. 1, pp. (87-94).

Hoeijmakers, J. H. (2001). Genome maintenance mechanisms for preventing cancer. Nature, Vol. 411, No. 6835, pp. (366-74).

Holzen, T. M., and R. Sclafani. (2010). Genetic interaction of RAD53 protein kinase with histones is important for DNA replication. Cell Cycle, Vol. 9, No. 23, pp. (4735-47).

Huang, M., Z. Zhou, and S. J. Elledge. (1998). The DNA replication and damage checkpoint pathways induce transcription by inhibition of the Crt1 repressor. Cell, Vol. 94, No. 5, pp. (595-605).

Jamai, A., A. Puglisi, and M. Strubin. (2009). Histone chaperone spt16 promotes redeposition of the original h3-h4 histones evicted by elongating RNA polymerase. Mol Cell, Vol. 35, No. 3, pp. (377-83).

Jares, P., A. Donaldson, and J. J. Blow. (2000). The Cdc7/Dbf4 protein kinase: target of the S phase checkpoint? EMBO Rep, Vol. 1, No. 4, pp. (319-22).

Jimeno-Gonzalez, S., F. Gomez-Herreros, P. M. Alepuz, and S. Chavez. (2006). A gene-specific requirement for FACT during transcription is related to the chromatin organization of the transcribed region. Mol Cell Biol, Vol. 26, No. 23, pp. (8710-21).

Kaplan, C. D., L. Laprade, and F. Winston. (2003). Transcription elongation factors repress transcription initiation from cryptic sites. Science, Vol. 301, No. 5636, pp. (1096-9).

Li, Y., S. X. Zeng, I. Landais, and H. Lu. (2007). Human SSRP1 has Spt16-dependent and -independent roles in gene transcription. J Biol Chem, Vol. 282, No. 10, pp. (6936-45).

Luger, K., T. J. Rechsteiner, A. J. Flaus, M. M. Waye, and T. J. Richmond. (1997). Characterization of nucleosome core particles containing histone proteins made in bacteria. J Mol Biol, Vol. 272, No. 3, pp. (301-11).

Lycan, D. E., M. A. Osley, and L. M. Hereford. (1987). Role of transcriptional and posttranscriptional regulation in expression of histone genes in Saccharomyces cerevisiae. Mol Cell Biol, Vol. 7, No. 2, pp. (614-21).

Lydall, D., and T. Weinert. (1995). Yeast checkpoint genes in DNA damage processing: implications for repair and arrest. Science, Vol. 270, No. 5241, pp. (1488-91).

Lydall, D., and T. Weinert. (1996). From DNA damage to cell cycle arrest and suicide: a budding yeast perspective. Curr Opin Genet Dev, Vol. 6, No. 1, pp. (4-11).

Malone, E. A., C. D. Clark, A. Chiang, and F. Winston. (1991). Mutations in SPT16/CDC68 suppress cis- and trans-acting mutations that affect promoter function in Saccharomyces cerevisiae. Mol Cell Biol, Vol. 11, No. 11, pp. (5710-7).

Marzluff, W. F., and R. J. Duronio. (2002). Histone mRNA expression: multiple levels of cell cycle regulation and important developmental consequences. Curr Opin Cell Biol, Vol. 14, No. 6, pp. (692-9).

Mason, P. B., and K. Struhl. (2003). The FACT complex travels with elongating RNA polymerase II and is important for the fidelity of transcriptional initiation in vivo. Mol Cell Biol, Vol. 23, No. 22, pp. (8323-33).

Meeks-Wagner, D., and L. H. Hartwell. (1986). Normal stoichiometry of histone dimer sets is necessary for high fidelity of mitotic chromosome transmission. Cell, Vol. 44, No. 1, pp. (43-52).

Morillo-Huesca, M., D. Maya, M. C. Munoz-Centeno, R. K. Singh, V. Oreal, G. U. Reddy, D. Liang, V. Geli, A. Gunjan, and S. Chavez. (2010). FACT prevents the accumulation of free histones evicted from transcribed chromatin and a subsequent cell cycle delay in G1. PLoS Genet, Vol. 6, No. 5, pp. (e1000964).

Morrow, D. M., D. A. Tagle, Y. Shiloh, F. S. Collins, and P. Hieter. (1995). TEL1, an S. cerevisiae homolog of the human gene mutated in ataxia telangiectasia, is functionally related to the yeast checkpoint gene MEC1. Cell, Vol. 82, No. 5, pp. (831-40).

Nyberg, K. A., R. J. Michelson, C. W. Putnam, and T. A. Weinert. (2002). Toward maintaining the genome: DNA damage and replication checkpoints. Annu Rev Genet, Vol. 36, No., pp. (617-56).

Orphanides, G., G. LeRoy, C. H. Chang, D. S. Luse, and D. Reinberg. (1998). FACT, a factor that facilitates transcript elongation through nucleosomes. Cell, Vol. 92, No. 1, pp. (105-16).

Orphanides, G., W. H. Wu, W. S. Lane, M. Hampsey, and D. Reinberg. (1999). The chromatin-specific transcription elongation factor FACT comprises human SPT16 and SSRP1 proteins. Nature, Vol. 400, No. 6741, pp. (284-8).

Osborn, A. J., S. J. Elledge, and L. Zou. (2002). Checking on the fork: the DNA-replication stress-response pathway. Trends Cell Biol, Vol. 12, No. 11, pp. (509-16).

Osley, M. A. (1991). The regulation of histone synthesis in the cell cycle. Annu Rev Biochem, Vol. 60, No., pp. (827-61).

Osley, M. A., J. Gould, S. Kim, M. Y. Kane, and L. Hereford. (1986). Identification of sequences in a yeast histone promoter involved in periodic transcription. Cell, Vol. 45, No. 4, pp. (537-44).

Osley, M. A., and D. Lycan. (1987). Trans-acting regulatory mutations that alter transcription of Saccharomyces cerevisiae histone genes. Mol Cell Biol, Vol. 7, No. 12, pp. (4204-10).

Paulovich, A. G., and L. H. Hartwell. (1995). A checkpoint regulates the rate of progression through S phase in S. cerevisiae in response to DNA damage. Cell, Vol. 82, No. 5, pp. (841-7).

Pavri, R., B. Zhu, G. Li, P. Trojer, S. Mandal, A. Shilatifard, and D. Reinberg. (2006). Histone H2B monoubiquitination functions cooperatively with FACT to regulate elongation by RNA polymerase II. Cell, Vol. 125, No. 4, pp. (703-17).

Philpott, C. C., J. Rashford, Y. Yamaguchi-Iwai, T. A. Rouault, A. Dancis, and R. D. Klausner. (1998). Cell-cycle arrest and inhibition of G1 cyclin translation by iron in AFT1-1(up) yeast. Embo J, Vol. 17, No. 17, pp. (5026-36).

Reinberg, D., and R. J. Sims, 3rd. (2006). de FACTo nucleosome dynamics. J Biol Chem, Vol. 281, No. 33, pp. (23297-301).

Reis, C. C., and J. L. Campbell. (2007). Contribution of Trf4/5 and the nuclear exosome to genome stability through regulation of histone mRNA levels in Saccharomyces cerevisiae. Genetics, Vol. 175, No. 3, pp. (993-1010).

Rhoades, A. R., S. Ruone, and T. Formosa. (2004). Structural features of nucleosomes reorganized by yeast FACT and its HMG box component, Nhp6. Mol Cell Biol, Vol. 24, No. 9, pp. (3907-17).

Rowley, A., R. A. Singer, and G. C. Johnston. (1991). CDC68, a yeast gene that affects regulation of cell proliferation and transcription, encodes a protein with a highly acidic carboxyl terminus. Mol Cell Biol, Vol. 11, No. 11, pp. (5718-26).

Sanchez, Y., B. A. Desany, W. J. Jones, Q. Liu, B. Wang, and S. J. Elledge. (1996). Regulation of RAD53 by the ATM-like kinases MEC1 and TEL1 in yeast cell cycle checkpoint pathways. Science, Vol. 271, No. 5247, pp. (357-60).

Santocanale, C., and J. F. Diffley. (1998). A Mec1- and Rad53-dependent checkpoint controls late-firing origins of DNA replication. Nature, Vol. 395, No. 6702, pp. (615-8).

Saunders, A., J. Werner, E. D. Andrulis, T. Nakayama, S. Hirose, D. Reinberg, and J. T. Lis. (2003). Tracking FACT and the RNA polymerase II elongation complex through chromatin in vivo. Science, Vol. 301, No. 5636, pp. (1094-6).

Schneider, B. L., Q. H. Yang, and A. B. Futcher. (1996). Linkage of replication to start by the Cdk inhibitor Sic1. Science, Vol. 272, No. 5261, pp. (560-2).

Schwob, E., T. Bohm, M. D. Mendenhall, and K. Nasmyth. (1994). The B-type cyclin kinase inhibitor p40SIC1 controls the G1 to S transition in S. cerevisiae. Cell, Vol. 79, No. 2, pp. (233-44).

Segurado, M., and JA. Tercero. (2009). The S-phase checkpoint: targeting the replication fork. Biol Cell, Vol. 19, No. 101(11), pp. (617-27).

Shaulian, E., M. Schreiber, F. Piu, M. Beeche, E. F. Wagner, and M. Karin. (2000). The mammalian UV response: c-Jun induction is required for exit from p53-imposed growth arrest. Cell, Vol. 103, No. 6, pp. (897-907).

Sherwood, P. W., S. V. Tsang, and M. A. Osley. (1993). Characterization of HIR1 and HIR2, two genes required for regulation of histone gene transcription in Saccharomyces cerevisiae. Mol Cell Biol, Vol. 13, No. 1, pp. (28-38).

Sheu, Y. J., and B. Stillman. (2010). The Dbf4-Cdc7 kinase promotes S phase by alleviating an inhibitory activity in Mcm4. Nature, Vol. 463, No. 7277, pp. (113-7).

Sidorova, J. M., and L. L. Breeden. (1997). Rad53-dependent phosphorylation of Swi6 and down-regulation of CLN1 and CLN2 transcription occur in response to DNA damage in Saccharomyces cerevisiae. Genes Dev, Vol. 11, No. 22, pp. (3032-45).

Siede, W., J. B. Allen, S. J. Elledge, and E. C. Friedberg. (1996). The Saccharomyces cerevisiae MEC1 gene, which encodes a homolog of the human ATM gene product, is required for G1 arrest following radiation treatment. J Bacteriol, Vol. 178, No. 19, pp. (5841-3).

Simon, I., J. Barnett, N. Hannett, C. T. Harbison, N. J. Rinaldi, T. L. Volkert, J. J. Wyrick, J. Zeitlinger, D. K. Gifford, T. S. Jaakkola, and R. A. Young. (2001). Serial regulation of transcriptional regulators in the yeast cell cycle. Cell, Vol. 106, No. 6, pp. (697-708).

Singh, R. K., and A. Gunjan. (2011). Histone tyrosine phosphorylation comes of age. Epigenetics, Vol. 6, No. 2, pp. (153-60).

Singh, R. K., M. H. Kabbaj, J. Paik, and A. Gunjan. (2009). Histone levels are regulated by phosphorylation and ubiquitylation-dependent proteolysis. Nat Cell Biol, Vol. 11, No. 8, pp. (925-33).

Singh, R. K., D. Liang, U. R. Gajjalaiahvari, M. H. Kabbaj, J. Paik, and A. Gunjan. (2010). Excess histone levels mediate cytotoxicity via multiple mechanisms. Cell Cycle, Vol. 9, No. 20, pp. (4236-44).

Singh, R. K., J. Paik, and A. Gunjan. (2009). Generation and management of excess histones during the cell cycle. Front Biosci, Vol. 14, No., pp. (3145-58).

Skotheim, J. M., S. Di Talia, E. D. Siggia, and F. R. Cross. (2008). Positive feedback of G1 cyclins ensures coherent cell cycle entry. Nature, Vol. 454, No. 7202, pp. (291-6).

Stegmeier, F. , and A. Amon. (2004). Closing mitosis: the functions of the Cdc14 phosphatase and its regulation. Annu Rev Genet, Vol. 38, No., pp. (203-232).

Stein, G. S., and J. L. Stein. (1984). Is human histone gene expression autogenously regulated? Mol Cell Biochem, Vol. 64, No. 2, pp. (105-10).

Stuwe, T., M. Hothorn, E. Lejeune, V. Rybin, M. Bortfeld, K. Scheffzek, and A. G. Ladurner. (2008). The FACT Spt16 "peptidase" domain is a histone H3-H4 binding module. Proc Natl Acad Sci U S A, Vol. 105, No. 26, pp. (8884-9).

Sun, Z., D. S. Fay, F. Marini, M. Foiani, and D. F. Stern. (1996). Spk1/Rad53 is regulated by Mec1-dependent protein phosphorylation in DNA replication and damage checkpoint pathways. Genes Dev, Vol. 10, No. 4, pp. (395-406).

Sutton, A., J. Bucaria, M. A. Osley, and R. Sternglanz. (2001). Yeast ASF1 protein is required for cell cycle regulation of histone gene transcription. Genetics, Vol. 158, No. 2, pp. (587-96).

Takahata, S., Y. Yu, and D. J. Stillman. (2009). The E2F functional analogue SBF recruits the Rpd3(L) HDAC, via Whi5 and Stb1, and the FACT chromatin reorganizer, to yeast G1 cyclin promoters. Embo J, Vol. 28, No. 21, pp. (3378-89).

Tanaka, S., and H. Araki. (2010). Regulation of the initiation step of DNA replication by cyclin-dependent kinases. Chromosoma, Vol. 119, No. 6, pp. (565-74).

Tanaka, S., Y.S. Tak, and H. Araki. (2007). The role of CDK in the initiation step of DNA replication in eukaryotes. Cell Div., Vol. 5, No. Jun, pp. (2-16).

Tercero, J. A., and J. F. Diffley. (2001). Regulation of DNA replication fork progression through damaged DNA by the Mec1/Rad53 checkpoint. Nature, Vol. 412, No. 6846, pp. (553-7).

Tsukuda, T., A. B. Fleming, J. A. Nickoloff, and M. A. Osley. (2005). Chromatin remodelling at a DNA double-strand break site in Saccharomyces cerevisiae. Nature, Vol. 438, No. 7066, pp. (379-83).

VanDemark, A. P., H. Xin, L. McCullough, R. Rawlins, S. Bentley, A. Heroux, D. J. Stillman, C. P. Hill, and T. Formosa. (2008). Structural and functional analysis of the Spt16p N-terminal domain reveals overlapping roles of yFACT subunits. J Biol Chem, Vol. 283, No. 8, pp. (5058-68).

Vanti, M., E. Gallastegui, I. Respaldiza, A. Rodriguez-Gil, F. Gomez-Herreros, S. Jimeno-Gonzalez, A. Jordan, and S. Chavez. (2009). Yeast genetic analysis reveals the involvement of chromatin reassembly factors in repressing HIV-1 basal transcription. PLoS Genet, Vol. 5, No. 1, pp. (e1000339).

Wang, H., L. B. Carey, Y. Cai, H. Wijnen, and B. Futcher. (2009). Recruitment of Cln3 cyclin to promoters controls cell cycle entry via histone deacetylase and other targets. PLoS Biol, Vol. 7, No. 9, pp. (e1000189).

Weinert, T. A., G. L. Kiser, and L. H. Hartwell. (1994). Mitotic checkpoint genes in budding yeast and the dependence of mitosis on DNA replication and repair. Genes Dev, Vol. 8, No. 6, pp. (652-65).

Wittenberg, C. (2005). Cell cycle: cyclin guides the way. Nature, Vol. 434, No. 7029, pp. (34-5).

Xin, H., S. Takahata, M. Blanksma, L. McCullough, D. J. Stillman, and T. Formosa. (2009). yFACT induces global accessibility of nucleosomal DNA without H2A-H2B displacement. Mol Cell, Vol. 35, No. 3, pp. (365-76).

Xu, H., U. J. Kim, T. Schuster, and M. Grunstein. (1992). Identification of a new set of cell cycle-regulatory genes that regulate S-phase transcription of histone genes in Saccharomyces cerevisiae. Mol Cell Biol, Vol. 12, No. 11, pp. (5249-59).

Xu, H. X., L. Johnson, and M. Grunstein. (1990). Coding and noncoding sequences at the 3' end of yeast histone H2B mRNA confer cell cycle regulation. Mol Cell Biol, Vol. 10, No. 6, pp. (2687-94).

Zegerman, P., and J. F. Diffley. (2007). Phosphorylation of Sld2 and Sld3 by cyclin-dependent kinases promotes DNA replication in budding yeast. Nature, Vol. 445, No. 7125, pp. (281-5).

Zegerman, P., and J.F. Diffley. (2010). Checkpoint-dependent inhibition of DNA replication initiation by Sld3 and Dbf4 phosphorylation. Nature, Vol. 467, No. 7314, pp. (474-8).

Zhai, Y., P. Y. Yung, L. Huo, and C. Liang. (2010). Cdc14p resets the competency of replication licensing by dephosphorylating multiple initiation proteins during mitotic exit in budding yeast. J Cell Sci, Vol. 123, No. Pt 22, pp. (3933-43).

Zhao, X., A. Chabes, V. Domkin, L. Thelander, and R. Rothstein. (2001). The ribonucleotide reductase inhibitor Sml1 is a new target of the Mec1/Rad53 kinase cascade during growth and in response to DNA damage. Embo J, Vol. 20, No. 13, pp. (3544-53).

19

Involvement of Linker Histones in the Regulation of Replication Timing

Christophe Thiriet, Gwenola Auda-Boucher and Yvonnick Chéraud
University of Nantes/CNRS-UMR 6204
Chromatin dynamics and Epigenetics
France

1. Introduction

In eukaryotic cells, genomic DNA is associated with proteins to form chromatin, wherein the basic subunit is the nucleosome (van Holde 1989; Luger et al. 1997). The histones that compose the nucleosome can undergo posttranslational modifications, which are believed to generate an epigenetic code involved in chromatin activity regulation (Jenuwein and Allis 2001). Like other chromatin activities, replication has been correlated with histone modification. However unlike other activities, such as transcription or repair, wherein core histones are specifically modified, the histone posttranslational modifications that have been shown involved in replication regulation also interest the linker histone. While the linker histone has been shown mobile within the nucleus, the way the linker histone can be associated with replication timing regulation is of general interest. The present chapter reviews structural features of chromatin and the function of linker histone in higher order of chromatin. As replication implies the accessibility of the replication machinery to DNA, the modalities that are associated with a release of compact structure involving the linker histone will be discussed as well as the function of protein kinases in this process. This will lead to a model proposing how chromatin structure can switch from a non-permissive structure to a replication competent chromatin structure. Finally, with regard to our knowledge of chromatin replication requirements and the mobility of chromatin structures, the concluding remarks point out concerns that are not yet addressed in the timely regulated process of replication.

2. Replication of eukaryotic genomes

Genomes of eukaryotic cells are compartmentalized within the nucleus during the interphase during which DNA is organized in chromatin. Although chromatin structure is far to be fully understood, clearly the association of proteins to DNA adds a substantial level of complexity compared to bacteria in all cellular processes that require DNA as substrate (van Holde 1989; Wolffe 1998). DNA replication does not make exception to this rule, even if it is required for faithful inheritance of the genome at each cell division and takes place only once every cell cycle.

Despite specificities of eukaryotic genome replication, notable features of DNA duplication are shared between eukaryotes and bacteria (Mechali 2001). For instance, to be duplicated, double stranded DNA must open to make possible the access of each strand of the double helix to the DNA synthesis machineries. The initiation of the opening of DNA is performed at specific sites, named replication origins which reveal different degrees of elaboration. In *Escherichia coli*, DNA replication is initiated from a unique site and replication proceeds within two directions from this site. In contrast, in eukaryotes, the replication origins are multiple as it has been estimated in Chinese hamster cells that 30,000 to 50,000 origins are activated during each cell cycle (Huberman and Riggs 1966). Furthermore, among eukaryotes the actual nature and the number of replication origins are variable. Unlike higher eukaryotes, in *S. cerevisiae* a consensus sequence found ~300 times through the genome functions as replication origin (Nieduszynski et al. 2006). However, during the genome duplication phase of the cell cycle, not all replication origins are activated at the same time and even only a subset of the replication origins are mobilized during a considered cell cycle. The firing of replication origin is timely regulated during the S-phase. The association of DNA with proteins to form chromatin impedes the access to DNA and in a such repressive environment how DNA replication proceeds and is coordinated in space and in time across the entire genome within the living is an important question.

2.1 The genome is structured into chromatin

In the nucleus, the most abundant proteins associated with genomic DNA are the histone proteins. The arrangement of the histones and DNA in chromatin is highly structured and allows to the genetic information to be ordered. The packaging of DNA in eukaryotes is commonly perceived at different levels (Woodcock and Dimitrov 2001; Luger and Hansen 2005). The primary organization level of the eukaryotic genome is the nucleosome core particle. The nucleosome core particle is composed of 147 pb DNA wrapped around the histone octamer, which contains two copies each of the four core histone proteins H2A, H2B, H3 and H4. The histones H3 and H4 form a central tetramer associated with two heterodimers of H2A/H2B on each side composing therefore a tripartite wherein the diad axis is the symmetry axis (Arents et al. 1991; Luger et al. 1997).

Although the nucleosome core particle is defined at the atomic level and is conserved through evolution, the link between only two nucleosome core particles is more variable as the linker DNA length separating them varies between species, but also between tissues of the same organism and within a single nucleus (van Holde 1989). Furthermore, in vitro analysis of a dinucleosomal template exhibited mobility of the core histone within the template constituted of two tandem 5S RNA genes, although this sequence is known for its ability to position the nucleosome (Ura et al. 1995). Importantly, the addition of the linker histones within the dinucleosome template revealed an inhibition of nucleosome mobility (Ura et al. 1995; Ura et al. 1996). Therefore, it has been proposed that the linker histone might stabilize the nucleosomal structure by restricting the core histone mobility (Ura et al. 1995). It is clear that genome organization into a succession of nucleosomes corresponding to the beads-on-a-string results in a complex arrangement that is called higher-order chromatin structure which is still poorly understood.

Despite the striking absence of a model for higher-order chromatin structure, experiments using reconstituted nucleosomal arrays have been quite informative. Experiments analyzing the chromatin array folding showed that core histone tail domains contribute to higher-order formation (Tse and Hansen 1997). Similarly, core histone tail acetylation has been proposed to disrupt the higher order chromatin structure (Tse et al. 1998; Wang and Hayes 2008). In addition to the critical function of the core histones in the folding of chromatin, the linker histone has been shown to stabilize the folding of nucleosomal arrays (Carruthers et al. 1998). Indeed, extensive analyses using analytical ultracentrifugation, quantitative agarose gel electrophoresis, electron cryomicroscopy, and nuclease digestion revealed that the presence of the linker histone within nucleosomal arrays results in structures that are indistinguishable from native chicken erythrocyte chromatin (Carruthers et al. 1998).

2.2 Linker histone acts like a genome organizer

Although in vitro experiments using reconstituted model systems suggested an important function of linker histone (H1) in high-order chromatin structure, in vivo analyses were not as conclusive. While in the protozoan *Tetrahymena* the genetic depletion of the unique linker histone did not exhibit a striking phenotype (Shen et al. 1995), but a lost in transcription regulation in a gene subset and reduction in the nucleosome repeat length (Shen and Gorovsky 1996), the knock-out of this histone class in mouse cannot be achieved (Fan et al. 2003). Indeed, gene inactivation studies in the murine model exhibited a compensation effect when lacking one subtype of linker histone among the six existing in somatic cells (Fan et al. 2001). However, depletion of three subtypes led to embryonic lethality whereby developmental defects appeared as early as mid-gestation with a broad range of aberrations (Fan et al. 2003). Interestingly, similar results were observed in Drosophila suggesting that the linker histone might play a critical function in metazoans (Lu et al. 2009). Furthermore, Drosophila experiments showed that chromatin organization is impaired in absence of the linker histone and affects pericentric heterochromatin transcription (Lu et al. 2009). Clearly, even if these results demonstrate a critical function of the linker histone, whether the defects appeared within individual cells missing linker histone during their lifespan or the result of epigenetic inheritance from progenitor cells remains elusive.

Surprisingly, while the linker histone exhibits a primary function in metazoan development and organization of the genome, the analyses of H1 binding in living cells revealed that its binding into chromatin is dynamic. Indeed, FRAP experiments using fusion linker histone-GFP revealed that following photobleaching, GFP fluorescent signal is recovered within a few minutes (Lever et al. 2000; Misteli et al. 2000). Furthermore, only minor differences in the photobleaching recovery were noticed between heterochromatin and euchromatin. However, the treatment of cells with phosphatase inhibitor, which leads to an increase of phosphorylation of the H1 C-terminal domain, resulted in a greater mobility of H1 (Lever et al. 2000). The observations of living cells provided interesting features of linker histones like their mobility in different chromatin structures. Nonetheless, whether the linker histone stability within chromatin is affected by the cell cycle stage was not addressed. Using the original methodology of incorporation of exogenous proteins within the slime mold *Physarum polycephalum*, allowing the analyses at specific cell cycle stages, it has been shown that the stability of linker histone binding depended upon the cell cycle stage (Thiriet and Hayes 2001). Indeed, although the efficiency of the spontaneous incorporation of exogenous linker histone was similar throughout the cell cycle, the analyses of linker histone binding to chromatin revealed a lower affinity in S-phase chromatin compared to G2-phase chromatin. Interestingly, these results suggest that chromatin activity might affect the linker histone characteristics. Noteworthy, whereas the incorporation of different linker histones revealed a role of different linker histone subtypes in transcription, any of the reported effects were only transiently observed (Thiriet and Hayes 1999). It has been shown that exogenous core histones incorporated into *Physarum* were stable throughout the cell cycle (Prior et al. 1980; Prior et al. 1983; Thiriet and Hayes 2005), the instability of linker histones in this organism points out the issue of the half life of cellular linker histones. Indeed, to date we note a critical absence of studies determining the half-life of histone proteins.

2.3 Learning linker histone mechanism from transcription

Genetic depletion of linker histones in the unicellular *Tetrahymena* did not exhibit a striking phenotype of the cells, although nuclear volume was enlarged and evidenced the involvement of linker histones in chromatin packaging (Shen et al. 1995). Despite the global structural effect of linker histones in the folding of genetic information, chromatin activity analyses of the *Tetrahymena* H1 knocked-out strain showed effects on transcriptional activities both positively and negatively of specific genes (Shen and Gorovsky 1996). Importantly, the specific transcription profiles determined within the knocked-out strain was recapitulated in the strain wherein linker histone phosphorylation sites were mutated to glutamic acid, mimicking the fully phosphorylated state of the histone (Dou et al. 1999). Further investigations of the mechanism by which linker histone phosphorylation affects transcription activity revealed the generation of mutant strains wherein the charge resembled that of the phosphorylated state without mimicking the structure of the phosphorylation induced transcription defects (Dou and Gorovsky 2000). Therefore, it was concluded that H1 phosphorylation acts by changing the overall charge within the histone domain, rather than by direct recognition of the phosphate added by the post-translational modification.

The potential lack of physical recognition of the added phosphate in the carboxy-terminal domain of H1 associated with transcription is consistent with the idea that this unstructured domain of the linker histone is intrinsically disordered (Hansen et al. 2006). Unlike other histone classes, the linker histones comprise a family presenting variability between members. Interestingly, six isoforms of H1 have been identified in most higher eukaryotes, and several isoforms can localize within a single cell (Alami et al. 2003). Although the actual function of the variability of linker histones is undetermined, most linker histones share an identical structure composed of an unstructured amino-terminal domain, a globular domain defined by a three α-helix and an unstructured carboxy-terminal domain that can be subjected to phosphorylation. Conversely, the amino-acid composition of the carboxy-terminal domain of linker histones is amazingly similar between isoforms, although the sequences diverge. These remarkable properties led to propose that the carboxy-terminal domain of linker histones might function as an intrinsically disordered region, wherein the global amino-acid composition rather than the actual primary sequence would provide the chromatin binding properties (Hansen et al. 2006).

2.4 Linker histone function in replication

In contrast to transcription, replication of the genome takes place only once per cell cycle during the S-phase. The infrequency of the replication activity at determined genome location significantly complicates chromatin replication mechanisms. This experimental difficulty can be over-ruled using systems that exhibited synchronous nuclear activities either induced artificially with blocking reagents followed by cell released, or with cellular models exhibiting naturally synchronous activities within a population of nuclei. The powerful model system *Physarum polycephalum* enables to examine chromatin replication mechanisms, as at the plasmodial stage of the life cycle of this organism grows by successive cell cycles and forms a syncytium with a large of nuclei (estimated to ~ 5 10^8 in a usually used 5-7cm diameter macroplasmodium) in a unique cytoplasm conferring to the nucleus population a perfect synchrony (Thiriet and Hayes 1999). These specific characteristics have been useful for performing analyses of replication using biochemical approaches, such as the determination of the replication timing of specific genes during S-phase, the mapping of replication origins in absence of a consensus sequence and recently the relationship between chromatin structure and replication timing (Thiriet and Hayes 2009).

It has been shown that the incorporation of exogenous linker histones was stably associated with chromatin only in the G2-phase and exhibit significant inhibition of transcription in correlation with the linker histone subtype that was introduced into the cell (Thiriet and Hayes 2001). This inhibitory effect of the linker histone seemed controversial with the absence of global effect of linker histones observed in *Tetrahymena* (Shen and Gorovsky 1996). Nevertheless, it is important to note that the experimental designs in both analyses were somehow opposite as genetic depletion was carried out in *Tetrahymena* while in the *Physarum* experiments additional linker histones were added. Therefore, it was of special interest to examine the effects of linker histone depletion in the *Physarum* model system. This was achieved by knocking-down the expression of linker histones (Thiriet and Hayes 2009). Interestingly, as the nuclei are perfectly synchronous throughout the cell cycle, siRNA can be incorporated and analyzed at specific cell cycle stages. Unexpectedly, the observation of *Physarum* cells revealed a faster cellular growth in the early S-phase under linker histone depletion. The cell cycle stage specificity of the H1 depletion led to determine whether replication was affected by the absence of linker histones. By carrying out pulses of incorporation of radiolabelled DNA precursor during the duration of the S-phase followed by the determination of specific activity of the genomic DNA, it was observed that the maximum of radioactivity was reached faster in H1-depleted cells than in controls. Importantly, as the maximum of radioelement contained in DNA was similar in both experimental conditions and reached a plateau corresponding to replication completion, the genome was thus duplicated only once in presence and in absence of the linker histones. Therefore, the linker histones did not initiate multiple rounds of replication of chromatin regions, but affect the rate of chromatin duplication.

While these experiments revealed a global function in the control of the ubiquitous activity of genome replication, consistently with the deleterious effects of partial depletion in metazoan development, the mechanism by which H1 acts on replication needed to be clarified. Indeed, two distinct mechanisms could account for the acceleration of genome duplication. Following initiation, the fork of replication might progress faster through chromatin. Alternatively, the linker histone might directly act on the firing of replication origins. It has been shown in metazoans that the setting up of replication origins is performed by a multi-step process prior to the cell cycle dedicated to genome replication. These steps should be tightly controlled as only a subset of the potential replication origins are activated at each cell cycle and any origin is activated only once in the S-phase. Therefore, labelling of the replication origins is required and this involves their recognition by factors that associate with DNA to form a pre-replication complex wherein the upgrade will raise to the initiation complex. Throughout the S-phase, the initiation complex is temporally coordinated for firing at specific times during the duplication stage of the cell cycle (Maric and Prioleau 2010). The choice of the timing of the replication origin firing is not harmless for the cell, as replication timing has been correlated with the transcriptional activity of genes. Unambiguous demonstration of this correlation was performed in *Physarum*, wherein two distinct copies of the developmentally regulated genes encoding for profilin exhibited a reprogramming of their timing of replication linked to transcriptional activity specific to each profiling gene (Maric et al. 2003). Consistently, analyses in mouse embryonic stem cells exhibited changes in the replication program during cell differentiation (Hiratani et al. 2008).

The molecular mechanism leading to faster replication in conjunction with the absence of linker histone was elucidated by pulse labelling experiments of replicating chromatin with a thymidine analogue. Microscopic observations of the incorporation of the analogue into genomic DNA revealed that the number of distinguishable foci almost double in absence of H1, whereas the intensity of the foci which reflected the amount of incorporated precursor remains statistically unchanged (Thiriet and Hayes 2009). It was therefore concluded that depletion of linker histones has merely disturbed replication timing regulation and not the velocity of the replication fork progression through chromatin. These results were in agreement with the determination of the replication timing of specific replicons. The early establishment of the usage of the replication origins and the temporal coordination that is associated to their activation suggested the existence of an epigenetic control. Remarkably, the abolishment of the replication epigenetic control coincides with the depletion of linker histones. It is therefore reasonable to propose that linker histones are involved in the epigenetic regulation of chromatin replication.

2.5 Epigenetic repression abolishment by H1 phosphorylation

The studies of H1 function during transcription showed that the mimics of H1 phosphorylation exhibit transcription defects closely related to genetic depletion of the linker histone (Dou et al. 1999; Dou and Gorovsky 2000). Accordingly, it was proposed that the phosphorylation of H1 facilitates the mobility of the linker histone (Lever et al. 2000). Hence, to verify whether this post-translational modification of H1 might also affect replication, inhibition of phosphatase activity was performed and replication effects were determined. The analysis of a lately replicated locus revealed incorporation of thymidine analogue in early S-phase concomitantly with hyperphosphorylation of the linker histone (Thiriet and Hayes 2009). Although H1 has been shown in vitro to be an excellent substrate for many kinases (Ducommun et al. 1990), the complex containing the kinase Cdk2 and Cdc45 displays the characteristics of a good candidate to accomplish this task in S-phase. Indeed, transfection of Cdc45 promotes chromatin decondensation and co-localized phosphorylated H1 in culture (Alexandrow and Hamlin 2005). Co-immunoprecipitation experiments revealed the formation of a complex containing at least Cdc45 and Cdk2. Furthermore, determination of the sequential deposition to chromatin revealed that Cdc45 associates with chromatin prior to Cdk2 suggesting that Cdc45 recruits Cdk2 to chromatin targets. Interestingly, the same study showed that the Cyclin A kinase associated with chromatin with kinetics nearly identical to those of Cdk2, and suggested that the H1 kinase activity might be redundant in the S-phase (Alexandrow and Hamlin 2005).

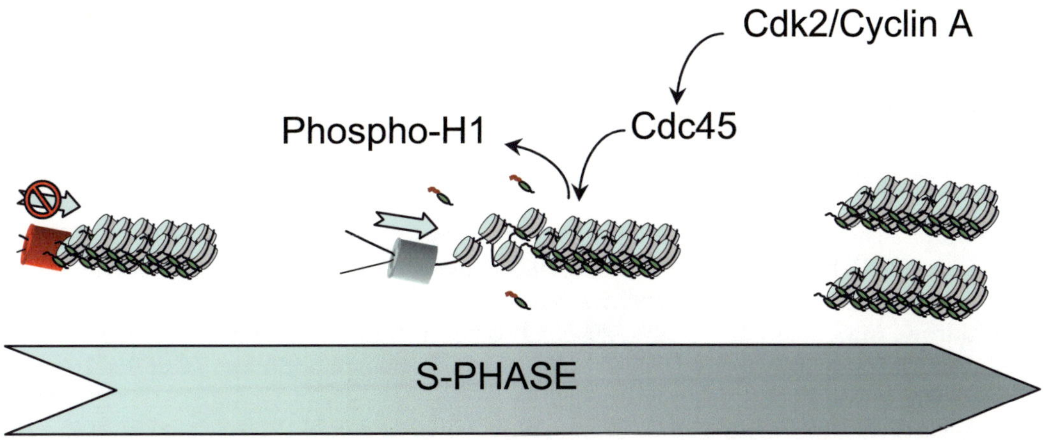

Fig. 1. Model of replication origin firing induced by H1 phosphorylation. The repressive chromatin structure for replication proceeding (left) becomes permissive after the release of the linker histone induced by H1 phosphorylation (middle) and leads the duplication of chromatin (right).

3. Conclusion

Despite the ubiquitous composition of chromatin, among histone classes, the linker histone presents the greatest variability through evolution and between subtypes from a single organism. On the basis of in vitro analyses of linker histones, their function has been associated with chromatin folding and higher order structure. However, the biochemical features that are common to all linker histone subtypes, do not provide satisfactory explanations to the embryonic lethality observed in mouse when three from the six somatic isoforms are depleted, whereas the depletion of only one isoform exhibits compensation effects (Fan et al. 2001). Therefore, understanding the biological function of linker histones within eukaryotic cells is a major task. Surprisingly, while metazoans showed essential roles of linker histones in early development, the lack of H1 in protozoans did not exhibit drastic phenotypes and was even depicted like a transcription regulator in a subset of genes (Fan et al. 2003). One issue in these observations was the rational between the contrasted effects of H1. It was unlikely that the result of evolution was to generate divergent function with no alteration of biochemical properties. Thus, the linker histone function possibly required to act on a global chromatin activity that needs to be tightly coordinated during development. Unexpectedly, it was shown in the slime mold *Physarum polycephalum* that cells lacking linker histone exhibited a lost in the regulation of the replication origin firing, which was also associated with an increase of DNA accessibility (Thiriet and Hayes 2009). These experiments led to propose that linker histones might have a critical role in replication timing regulation (Fig.1). Although these experiments were the first demonstration of a global effect of linker histones, they are consistent with the genome regulation requirement observed during development and differentiation. Nonetheless, if linker histone function has been proposed to temporally regulation replication of chromatin, the issue of variety of the linker histone isoforms is not yet addressed in the replication context.

4. Acknowledgements

We are grateful to members of the Thiriet's lab for valuable discussions. Our group is funded by "La ligue contre le cancer" (Committees 41, 44 and 86), ANR, Cancéropôle Grand-Ouest, CNRS, and University of Nantes.

5. References

Alami, R., Y. Fan, S. Pack, T.M. Sonbuchner, A. Besse, Q. Lin, J.M. Greally, A.I. Skoultchi, and E.E. Bouhassira. 2003. Mammalian linker-histone subtypes differentially affect gene expression in vivo. *Proc Natl Acad Sci U S A* 100: 5920-5.

Alexandrow, M.G. and J.L. Hamlin. 2005. Chromatin decondensation in S-phase involves recruitment of Cdk2 by Cdc45 and histone H1 phosphorylation. *J Cell Biol* 168: 875-86.

Arents, G., R.W. Burlingame, B.C. Wang, W.E. Love, and E.N. Moudrianakis. 1991. The nucleosomal core histone octamer at 3.1 A resolution: a tripartite protein assembly and a left-handed superhelix. *Proc Natl Acad Sci U S A* 88: 10148-52.

Carruthers, L.M., J. Bednar, C.L. Woodcock, and J.C. Hansen. 1998. Linker histones stabilize the intrinsic salt-dependent folding of nucleosomal arrays: mechanistic ramifications for higher-order chromatin folding. *Biochemistry* 37: 14776-87.

Dou, Y. and M.A. Gorovsky. 2000. Phosphorylation of linker histone H1 regulates gene expression in vivo by creating a charge patch. *Mol Cell* 6: 225-31.

Dou, Y., C.A. Mizzen, M. Abrams, C.D. Allis, and M.A. Gorovsky. 1999. Phosphorylation of linker histone H1 regulates gene expression in vivo by mimicking H1 removal. *Mol Cell* 4: 641-7.

Ducommun, B., Y. Tollon, M. Gares, D. Beach, and M. Wright. 1990. Cell cycle regulation of p34cdc2 kinase activity in Physarum polycephalum. *J Cell Sci* 96 (Pt 4): 683-9.

Fan, Y., T. Nikitina, E.M. Morin-Kensicki, J. Zhao, T.R. Magnuson, C.L. Woodcock, and A.I. Skoultchi. 2003. H1 linker histones are essential for mouse development and affect nucleosome spacing in vivo. *Mol Cell Biol* 23: 4559-72.

Fan, Y., A. Sirotkin, R.G. Russell, J. Ayala, and A.I. Skoultchi. 2001. Individual somatic H1 subtypes are dispensable for mouse development even in mice lacking the H1(0) replacement subtype. *Mol Cell Biol* 21: 7933-43.

Hansen, J.C., X. Lu, E.D. Ross, and R.W. Woody. 2006. Intrinsic protein disorder, amino acid composition, and histone terminal domains. *J Biol Chem* 281: 1853-6.

Hiratani, I., T. Ryba, M. Itoh, T. Yokochi, M. Schwaiger, C.W. Chang, Y. Lyou, T.M. Townes, D. Schubeler, and D.M. Gilbert. 2008. Global reorganization of replication domains during embryonic stem cell differentiation. *PLoS Biol* 6: e245.

Huberman, J.A. and A.D. Riggs. 1966. Autoradiography of chromosomal DNA fibers from Chinese hamster cells. *Proc Natl Acad Sci U S A* 55: 599-606.

Jenuwein, T. and C.D. Allis. 2001. Translating the histone code. *Science* 293: 1074-80.

Lever, M.A., J.P. Th'ng, X. Sun, and M.J. Hendzel. 2000. Rapid exchange of histone H1.1 on chromatin in living human cells. *Nature* 408: 873-6.

Lu, X., S.N. Wontakal, A.V. Emelyanov, P. Morcillo, A.Y. Konev, D.V. Fyodorov, and A.I. Skoultchi. 2009. Linker histone H1 is essential for Drosophila development, the establishment of pericentric heterochromatin, and a normal polytene chromosome structure. *Genes Dev* 23: 452-65.

Luger, K. and J.C. Hansen. 2005. Nucleosome and chromatin fiber dynamics. *Curr Opin Struct Biol* 15: 188-96.

Luger, K., A.W. Mader, R.K. Richmond, D.F. Sargent, and T.J. Richmond. 1997. Crystal structure of the nucleosome core particle at 2.8 A resolution. *Nature* 389: 251-60.

Maric, C., M. Benard, and G. Pierron. 2003. Developmentally regulated usage of Physarum DNA replication origins. *EMBO Rep* 4: 474-8.

Maric, C. and M.N. Prioleau. 2010. Interplay between DNA replication and gene expression: a harmonious coexistence. *Curr Opin Cell Biol* 22: 277-83.

Mechali, M. 2001. DNA replication origins: from sequence specificity to epigenetics. *Nat Rev Genet* 2: 640-5.

Misteli, T., A. Gunjan, R. Hock, M. Bustin, and D.T. Brown. 2000. Dynamic binding of histone H1 to chromatin in living cells. *Nature* 408: 877-81.

Nieduszynski, C.A., Y. Knox, and A.D. Donaldson. 2006. Genome-wide identification of replication origins in yeast by comparative genomics. *Genes Dev* 20: 1874-9.

Prior, C.P., C.R. Cantor, E.M. Johnson, and V.G. Allfrey. 1980. Incorporation of exogenous pyrene-labeled histone into Physarum chromatin: a system for studying changes in nucleosomes assembled in vivo. *Cell* 20: 597-608.

Prior, C.P., C.R. Cantor, E.M. Johnson, V.C. Littau, and V.G. Allfrey. 1983. Reversible changes in nucleosome structure and histone H3 accessibility in transcriptionally active and inactive states of rDNA chromatin. *Cell* 34: 1033-42.

Shen, X. and M.A. Gorovsky. 1996. Linker histone H1 regulates specific gene expression but not global transcription in vivo. *Cell* 86: 475-83.

Shen, X., L. Yu, J.W. Weir, and M.A. Gorovsky. 1995. Linker histones are not essential and affect chromatin condensation in vivo. *Cell* 82: 47-56.

Thiriet, C. and J.J. Hayes. 1999. Histone proteins in vivo: cell-cycle-dependent physiological effects of exogenous linker histones incorporated into Physarum polycephalum. *Methods* 17: 140-50.

-. 2001. Assembly into chromatin and subtype-specific transcriptional effects of exogenous linker histones directly introduced into a living Physarum cell. *J Cell Sci* 114: 965-73.

-. 2005. Replication-independent core histone dynamics at transcriptionally active loci in vivo. *Genes Dev* 19: 677-82.

-. 2009. Linker histone phosphorylation regulates global timing of replication origin firing. *J Biol Chem* 284: 2823-9.

Tse, C. and J.C. Hansen. 1997. Hybrid trypsinized nucleosomal arrays: identification of multiple functional roles of the H2A/H2B and H3/H4 N-termini in chromatin fiber compaction. *Biochemistry* 36: 11381-8.

Tse, C., T. Sera, A.P. Wolffe, and J.C. Hansen. 1998. Disruption of higher-order folding by core histone acetylation dramatically enhances transcription of nucleosomal arrays by RNA polymerase III. *Mol Cell Biol* 18: 4629-38.

Ura, K., J.J. Hayes, and A.P. Wolffe. 1995. A positive role for nucleosome mobility in the transcriptional activity of chromatin templates: restriction by linker histones. *Embo J* 14: 3752-65.

Ura, K., K. Nightingale, and A.P. Wolffe. 1996. Differential association of HMG1 and linker histones B4 and H1 with dinucleosomal DNA: structural transitions and transcriptional repression. *Embo J* 15: 4959-69.

van Holde, K.E. 1989. *Chromatin*. Springer-Verlag, New-York.

Wang, X. and J.J. Hayes. 2008. Acetylation mimics within individual core histone tail domains indicate distinct roles in regulating the stability of higher-order chromatin structure. *Mol Cell Biol* 28: 227-36.

Wolffe, A.P. 1998. *Chromatin: Structure and Function*. Academic Press, San Diego.

Woodcock, C.L. and S. Dimitrov. 2001. Higher-order structure of chromatin and chromosomes. *Curr Opin Genet Dev* 11: 130-5.

20

Replication Timing: Evolution, Nuclear Organization and Relevance for Human Disease

Megan Lynne Wright and Frank Grützner
The Robinson Institute, School of Molecular & Biomedical Sciences, University of Adelaide, Adelaide Australia

1. Introduction

DNA replication in eukaryotes is multifaceted, dynamic and highly organised. In contrast to bacterial cells, which replicate from single origins of replication, complex eukaryote genomes replicate from thousands of origins of replication. Although we know that the timing of replication depends on the chromatin environment, the function and evolution of mechanisms controlling replication timing are unclear. Many studies in species ranging from yeast to humans have demonstrated how replication timing depends on proximity to certain sequences such as telomeres and centromeres (Ferguson and Fangman, 1992; Friedman et al., 1996; Heun et al., 2001), chromatin status (euchromatin and heterochromatin) and is linked to gene function and expression (housekeeping genes versus tissue specific genes and monoallelically expressed genes) (Hiratani and Gilbert, 2009; Hiratani et al., 2009). Replication timing has been linked to fundamental epigenetic regulatory mechanisms including genomic imprinting (Kitsberg et al., 1993; Knoll et al., 1994), X chromosome inactivation (Gilbert, 2002; Takagi et al., 1982; Wutz and Jaenisch, 2000), interchromosomal interactions (Ryba et al. 2010) and is increasingly recognised to be important in human disease (DePamphilis, 2006).
This chapter integrates established knowledge with recent scientific breakthroughs, using genome-wide approaches linking different aspects of epigenetic control with replication timing, to provide a state-of-the-art overview and perspective for future work in this area of research. Despite detailed knowledge on replication timing in a select number of model organisms (e.g. yeast, drosophila, mouse) we are only beginning to understand how replication timing evolved in relation to other epigenetic mechanisms (e.g. genomic imprinting, X inactivation, and long-range chromatin interaction). The evolution of these epigenetic mechanisms will be presented together with novel ideas about how cytological and genome-wide approaches and methodologies can be combined to provide a comprehensive picture of spatial and temporal organization, the evolution of replication timing in eukaryotic genomes, and their relevance in human disease.

2. Background

2.1 Replication initiation

The complete and accurate replication of DNA during the S-phase is of fundamental importance for all organisms. The mechanism of replication is highly conserved across evolution, whereby a cell must gather the proteins to initiate replication at specific origins of replication (OR)s, unwind the DNA, move the replication fork bi-directionally away from the OR in such a manner as to allow the replication of the new daughter strand of DNA using the old parental DNA strand, and then cease replication. However whilst the replication process is highly conserved, different eukaryotes use different proteins and forms of control over replication (Gilbert, 2010).

Whilst general similarities exist in the type of machinery required to copy and create a new DNA strand across organisms, some areas of genome replication remain elusive. One such area in eukaryotes is replication initiation and timeline. Linear eukaryotic chromosomes replicate from many ORs which are spread out along their structure and are recognized by the origin recognition complex (ORC) (reviewed in Masai et al., 2010). These OR sites are where replication forks form and move bi-directionally away from the OR, replicating the DNA sequence as they move, then terminating when they meet another fork approaching from the opposite direction. The ORCs recognize almost all ORs, and will assemble at these regions in a highly conserved manner across eukaryotes. However, whilst ORCs bind specific sequence motifs in some eukaryotes, such as in budding yeast (Bell and Stillman, 1992), in other eukaryotes specificity is not well defined through sequence. Fission yeast and *Drosophila* have ORCs that recognize AT-rich sequences (Austin et al., 1999; Chuang and Kelly, 1999), rather than specific motifs. Moreover, human ORCs, which are chosen as initiators of replication, have also been shown to require AT-rich sequences as well as various other features, including matrix attachment region sequences, dinucleotide repeats and asymmetrical purine-pyrimidine sequences (Altman and Fanning, 2004; Debatisse et al., 2004; Paixao et al., 2004; Schaarschmidt et al., 2004; Wang et al., 2004). Other factors that may affect the initiation of replication at certain ORs also include DNA topology, transcription factors, and elements of the pre-replicative complex (pre-RC) (reviewed in Masai et al., 2010).

During late mitosis and G1, the chromatin-bound ORCs are loaded with minichromosome maintenance (MCM) complex, and thus become pre-RCs, with the ability to gather the required components to start replication. The pre-RCs assemble at most of the OR regions, however only a few of these complexes start replication in their region. The cell's choice to start replication at some ORs as opposed to others is unclear; whilst it is thought that the assembly of the pre-RCs at most ORs is used as backup in case the cell runs into trouble during replication, the choice as to whether a Pre-RC becomes an active replication initiator is not well understood (Doksani et al., 2009; Ibarra et al., 2008; Koren et al., 2010; Woodward et al., 2006).

There are, however, some known factors that may contribute to a pre-RC site becoming an active OR (reviewed in Masai et al., 2010). Firstly, the selection of replication initiation sites may be controlled by both the existence of a pre-RC and its assembly in combination with events that actually cause initiation. For example, the firing of an OR appears to affect the firing of adjacent ORs, as shown in the example of budding yeast, where active ORs suppress the initiation of replication at adjacent ORs (Brewer and Fangman, 1993). In this example, the suppression of adjacent potential ORs may be caused by the disruption of pre-RC complexes at these sites by the replication process initiated at the active OR (reviewed in Masai et al., 2010). Also, read-through transcription may affect the firing of downstream ORs (Haase et al., 1994; Saha et al., 2004). Furthermore chromatin structure, which refers to the chemical characteristics of the chromatin strand, may influence the initiation of replication by affecting the pre-RC assembly. There is evidence to show that histone acetylases and deacetylases play roles in the assembly of pre-RCs by interacting with, or disturbing the loading of, pre-RC elements such as the MCM complex (Burke et al., 2001; Iizuka et al., 2006; Pappas et al., 2004; Pasero et al., 2002).

Finally, distal elements, such as locus control regions (LCRs) are known to affect initiation (Hayashida et al., 2006; Kalejta et al., 1998), with the initiation of replication at regions such as the human *β-globin* locus being controlled by a 5′ LCR (Aladjem et al., 1995).

2.2 Temporal programmes of ORs in eukaryotic chromosomes

Replication of eukaryotic genomes follows a defined temporal program, whereby the firing of ORs occurs in a predetermined but tissue specific manner. Hence this process is dynamic in terms of the selection of OR activation, as the cellular environment also plays a role in the temporal regulation of replication across the genome. Experiments have shown that a reduction in cellular thymidine caused a reduction in replication fork speed. This caused more intermediate ORs to be activated in order to compensate for the reduction in replication speed (Anglana et al., 2003; Taylor, 1977), and showed that cellular environments indeed affect the dynamics of OR firing. This shows that a cell is able to change its pre-determined temporal replication program if it undergoes replication stress, with the most relevant aspect of OR activation being the genomic context and how it impacts the replication program.

Factors that are involved in OR firing include chromatin loops, dormant and active pre-RC complexes and fork replication rate, and finally nuclear organisation. Firstly, there is some evidence to suggest that chromatin loops affect replication firing. Studies in *Xenopus* egg extracts transferred with erythrocyte nuclei showed that cells that entered into M-phase instantly after somatic transfer took longer to replicate than cells which were held in mitosis and allowed to undergo a single mitosis event. This was due to the influence of the single round of mitosis on the chromatin structure; the round of mitosis supported the formation of smaller chromatin loops which correlated with higher ORC protein recruitment and more efficient genome replication (Lemaitre et al., 2005). Another study showed that the ORs closer to regions of chromatin loop anchorage in G1 initiated replication in the following S-phase earlier than ORs located further away from anchorage regions, indicating that loop-formation was part of the control mechanism for OR firing (Courbet et al., 2008).

Fork replication rate also appears to have a role in the temporal organization of OR firing. Genomic integrity may be aided by the presence of dormant origins of replication, as MCMs are often present in much greater amounts than those needed at pre-RCs, and the reduced presence or loss of pre-RCs result in genomic instability, S-phase arrest, and cell death (Edwards et al., 2002; Hyrien et al., 2003; Lengronne and Schwob, 2002; Shreeram et al., 2002; Tanaka and Diffley, 2002). Dormant ORs have been shown to activate when forks are stalled, with one model hypothesizing that OR activation occurs stochastically, whereby the presence of a stalled fork increases the chances of adjacent dormant ORs being activated (Blow and Ge, 2009; Ibarra et al., 2008). Other models propose that the presence of a stalled fork changes the topology of the DNA strand and the chromatin structure within the region, thus causing nearby and usually dormant ORs to activate (Ibarra et al., 2008).

Finally, nuclear organisation has a role to play in a cell's replication program. Distinct chromosome territories exist as separate nuclear architecture compartments in interphase cells. Within these territories, a higher order of chromatin structure exists, where domains containing specific chromosomal arms and bands have been found to be located in the nucleus in similar regions of certain cell types (Dietzel et al., 1998). It has also been proposed that these chromatin-rich chromosome territories (CTs) are separated by chromatin-poor areas called 'interchromatin compartments', which contain transcriptional and splicing machinery, as well as DNA replication and damage-repair machinery (reviewed in Aten and Kanaar, 2006; Cremer and Cremer, 2001; Misteli, 2001). However recent work showed extensive intermingling of CTs contradicting the existence of the interchomatin compartment (reviewed in Aten and Kanaar, 2006; Branco and Pombo, 2006; reviewed in Cremer and Cremer, 2010). Within separate chromosome territories there are many replication foci, whereby early and late replicating DNA can be found in spatially separate and distinct regions (Zink et al., 1999). Overall late replicating DNA (including the late replicating inactive X chromosome) is often located at the nuclear periphery or around the nucleolus organizing region (Sadoni et al., 1999).

3. Asynchronous replication

Asynchronous replication is another variation in the eukaryotic temporal replication repertoire. Asynchronous replication occurs when the ORs present in the same regions on two homologous chromosomes, initiate replication at different times. This results in one of the alleles replicating earlier than the allele on the other homologue. Notably, the alleles of asynchronously replicating genes are also observed to locate to separate discrete foci in a nucleus. This form of replication is a feature of monoallelically expressed genes, including genes that undergo allelic exclusion, imprinted genes, and genes from the X-chromosome in female somatic cells.

3.1 Approaches to measuring asynchronous replication and its effects on genome biology and disease

3.1.1 Chromosome banding

Chromosome banding techniques gave the first insights into the epigenetics behind replication, and more specifically, asynchronous replication. It is now well established that replication timing is not uniform across eukaryotic genomes, with select chromosomal regions showing early or late replication in the S-phase. This phenomenon has been observed in distinct banding regions along condensed metaphase chromosomes.

The discovery of early and late replication banding on metaphase chromosomes using the Bromodeoxyuridine (BrdU) incorporation technique, can be attributed to Latt (1973). Latt discovered that the differential incorporation of BrdU, a thymidine replacement, during the S-phase between early and late replicating regions of DNA, could be measured using 33258 Hoechst fluorescence. An efficiency reduction of the Hoechst dye fluorescence occurs when it is bound to the incorporated poly(dA-BrdU) compared to the poly(dA-dT). Incorporation of BrdU into either the late or early replicating DNA can be adjusted by culturing cells in BrdU for different time periods; specifically early replication stage BrdU incorporation was achieved by first culturing in BrdU with the addition of a terminal pulse of [3H]-dT, whilst late replication BrdU incorporation was achieved by culturing in medium containing thymidine to which BrdU was only added 6 hours before harvest. This allowed identification of 5-10 megabasepair regions on chromosomes replicating either early or late in the S-phase.

Latt's early research defined a fundamental relationship between chromosome organisation and replication timing; eukaryotic chromosomes do not undergo equivalent amounts of replication both within a chromosome and across a karyotype, whereby a distinct non-equivalence of replication is represented by the presence of discrete bands for early and late replicating regions on a chromosome. Furthermore, the late-replicating inactive X chromosome in human females, which is noted to have a slightly more condensed karyotype, showed distinctly opposing fluorescence to the less-condensed active-X chromosome.

Higher-resolution replication banding has since been established in humans and numerous vertebrate species (Biederman and Lin, 1979; Costantini and Bernardi, 2008; Drets et al., 1978). Currently, there are three tiers of replication resolution: 1) low-resolution banding (e.g. De Latt's BrdU bands, and Giemsa and Quinacrine bands); 2) higher resolution banding (GC content in grouped isochore regions); and 3) individual isochores (Costantini and Bernardi, 2008). Isochores are regions of DNA, above 300 kb (on average around 0.9 Mb in size in the human genome), that have a similar GC content, and also have similar gene content (Costantini and Bernardi, 2008; Costantini et al., 2006; Costantini et al., 2007). Specifically, there are five groups of isochores, whereby lower GC content is classed with the isochore groups L1 and L2 (less than 40% GC-content, and few genes), intermediate groups are H1 and H2 (with around 47% and 52% GC-content, and intermediate amounts of genes), and finally the highest group is H3 (with above 52% GC-content, and high amounts of genes) (Bernardi, 1995). A replicon is a genomic region around 50-400 kb in size, that replicates from a single origin of replication. It has been shown that replicons that exist within a certain isochore region, all undergo similar replication timing, with clusters of early replicating replicons being found next to each other, and clusters of late-replicating replicons being grouped as well (Watanabe et al., 2002). Through the comparisons of the three tiers of resolution, it was found that groups of early and late replicating isochores corresponded to, and approached the same size of, high-resolution replication banding regions (4-7 Mb).

The results of the highest-replication isochore banding when compared to the other banding techniques has indicated that in mammalian chromosomes there are three nested structures important to replication (Figure 1). The first structure is that of the replicon (50-450 kb), whereby individual replicons undergo dynamic firing of their ORs. These replicons however usually exist in clusters of 10 or more, and every replicon in the cluster will usually undergo replication at the same time during the S-phase. The second is that of the isochore (> 300 kb) which is a region that exists as a combination of replicons all with similar early or late replication status and GC content, which can undergo early or late replication in the cell cycle. The third structure is that of the cytogenetic bands, which indicates large regions on a chromosome undergoing early or late replication, and corresponds well to groups of all-early or all-late replicating isochores (Costantini and Bernardi, 2008). This shows that the arrangement of mitotic chromosome structure is closely related to replication timing, from the chromosome banding level, all the way through to the level of organisation of the individual replicons. This pattern is maintained in interphase, where chromosome territories in the S-phase have clusters of early and late replicating foci, which correspond to the R- and G/C bands observed in mitotic chromosomes respectively (Sadoni et al., 1999).

Replication banding techniques have allowed early and late timing replication zones to be delineated along metaphase chromosomes, where areas of similarly replicating replicons are grouped making larger replicon clusters (Watanabe et al., 2002). However, the large genomic regions that bridge the transition of an early-replicating replicon cluster to a late-replicating replicon cluster appear to lack any ORs, and rely on the continuous movement of

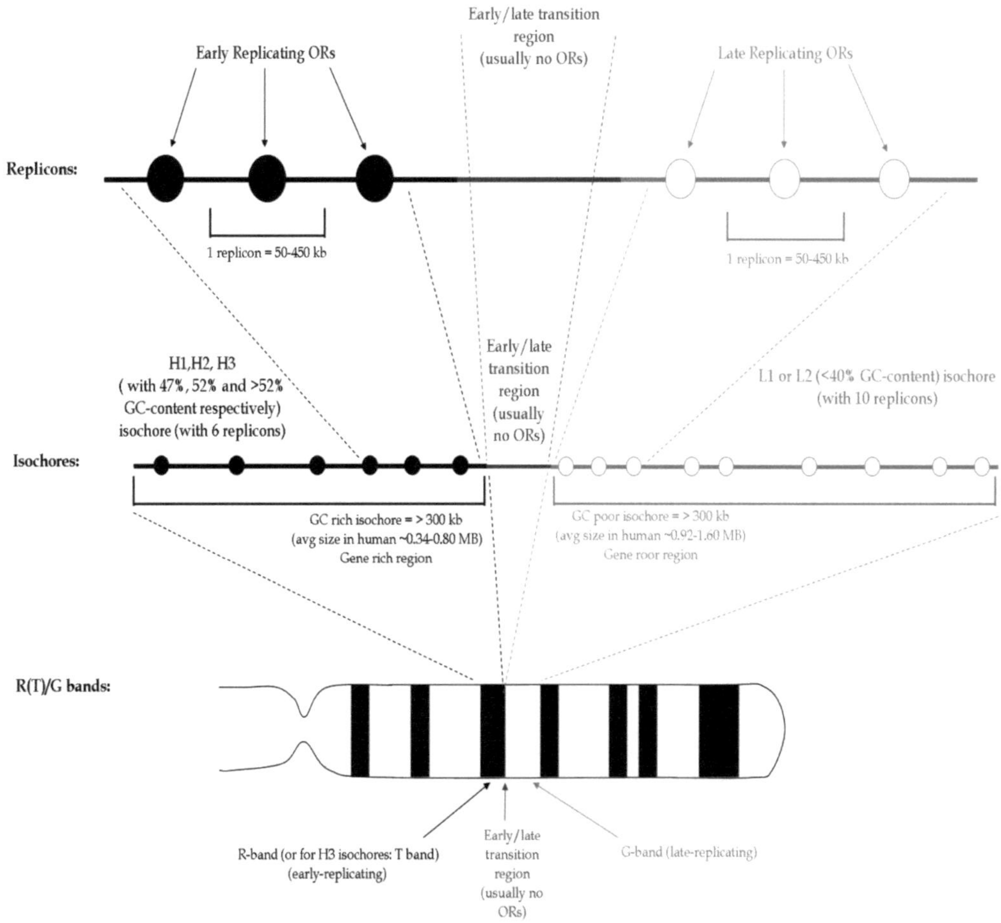

Fig. 1. The three nested structures of replication (see text for explanation).

forks from adjacent replicon-clusters/isochore regions for replication to occur in their region (reviewed in Farkash-Amar et al., 2008; Hiratani et al., 2008; Watanabe and Maekawa, 2010). This means that the fork from the earlier firing OR will have to move across the replication transition region, until it meets another fork from the late-replicating region. This will often pause replication in these early to late transition zones, which can cause genomic instability in the form of DNA breaks and rearrangements (Raghuraman et al., 2001; Rothstein et al., 2000). Furthermore, common genomic fragile sites frequently reside in early to late replication transition regions, and also lack backup ORs (Debatisse et al., 2006; Ge et al., 2007; Ibarra et al., 2008).

In addition to the increased genomic instability there is also an increase in the number of non-B-form DNA structures in replication transition regions (reviewed in Watanabe and Maekawa, 2010). Replication switch points (from early to late) are often associated with purine/pyrimidine rich areas, as these DNA regions can form structures called triplexes (H-DNA) that are known stop replication forks (Baran et al., 1991; Brinton et al., 1991; Ohno et al., 2000). The non-B-form structures however also have mutagenic properties, causing somatic recombination events (Kalish and Glazer, 2005; Knauert et al., 2006). It has thus been proposed that these replication transition regions, which correspond to the regions between R/G bands, are subject to more genomic instability due to the increased presence of non-B-DNA structures in these genomic areas (Watanabe and Maekawa, 2010).

Replication timing is affected in regions of the human genome involved in disease. Generally it has been proposed that regions of the human genome that reside in areas where replication timing switches (early to late) would be unstable and more prone to DNA damage (reviewed in Watanabe and Maekawa, 2010). Notably, these regions of replication timing transition are also associated with many human diseases, including cancer (Watanabe et al., 2009; Watanabe et al., 2002; Watanabe et al., 2004). Regions or genes associated with other diseases, such as familial Alzheimer's, familial amyotrophic lateral sclerosis and phenylketonuria, are also found in these replication timing transition regions. Furthermore, there are over 70 human diseases associated with non-B DNA structures, including neurological and psychiatric diseases, and many genomic disorders, indicating that the increase of these structures in replication timing transition regions may be a first step in the mutational process associated with these diseases (reviewed in Watanabe and Maekawa, 2010).

3.1.2 Measuring asynchronous replication with the dot assay technique

Molecular cytogenetic techniques like Fluorescence *in situ* Hybridization (FISH) and an explosion of available genomic clones and whole chromosome probes has let to huge refinement of physical maps on metaphase and interphase chromosomes. This also enabled replication timing to be investigated on the single gene level. In these experiments, DNA probes designed to hybridise to a specific gene allowed the replication status to be observed in three states in a nucleus; two signals (single-single (SS) dot) represents an unreplicated status, whilst a three signal status (single-double (SD) dot) represents a locus undergoing

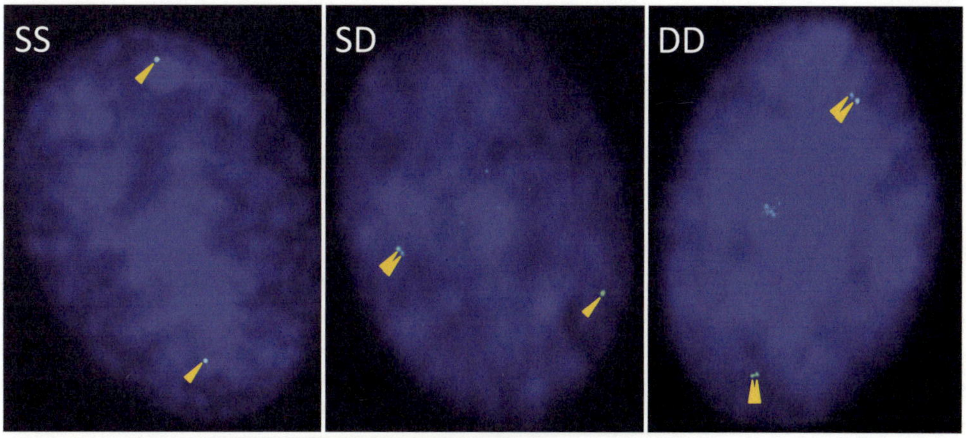

Fig. 2. Cytogenetic FISH dot assay
Mammalian interphase nuclei stained with DAPI (blue). Yellow arrows point to allele copies (green FISH signals) observed in each nucleus. The SS panel has two clearly defined green signals representing the two allele copies present in the nucleus, meaning the locus has not replicated. The SD panel shows three green signals, indicating that one allele has undergone replication, whilst the other allele is lagging behind and not yet replicated. The DD panel shows 4 green signals, indicating that both the alleles have replicated, and the locus has finished replicating.

replication, where one allele has replicated and the other is lagging, and finally a four signal status (double-double (DD) dot) represents a locus that is fully replicated (Selig et al., 1992). Asynchrony in this case is measured by the frequency of three-signal (SD dot) status observed in a cell line. However, the classification of asynchronous replication varies in the literature, with an asynchronously replicating state being assigned for loci with anywhere between 30-50% SD signal, and a non-asynchronously replicating locus generally having below 30% SD signal (Baumer et al., 2004; Wilson et al., 2007).

4. Replication timing in heteromorphic sex chromosomes

Replication banding and FISH dot assay techniques have not only shed light on how chromosome structure can affect replication, they have also allowed new insights into how replication timing of single genes has evolved. Changes in replication banding specific to one homolog in a karyotype have been used to identify early stage cytologically "homomorphic" sex chromosomes in various vertebrates (Nishida-Umehara et al., 1999; Schempp and Schmid, 1981). Heteromorphic sex chromosomes evolved from a pair of autosomes by a combination of suppression of recombination and accumulation of sexual antagonist genes (Ohno, 1967). The isolation of one of the sex chromosomes in one sex (Y chromosomes in mammals and some fish, the W chromosome in birds and many non-mammal vertebrates) has led to degeneration and massive gene loss. The evolution of heteromorphic sex chromosomes has been indicated to lead to a gene dosage difference between the sexes. In mammals this has resulted in the inactivation of one of the X chromosomes in female somatic cells.

X chromosome inactivation is a unique example where the status of chromatin can be changed from active to inactive (facultative heterochromatin) on a chromosome-wide level. In therian female mammals (marsupials and placental mammals), one of the X chromosomes in somatic cells is heterochromatic and late replicating (Holmquist, 1987; Lyon, 1961; Ohno et al., 1963; Schweizer et al., 1987; Takagi, 1974). This transcriptionally silenced and condensed X-chromosome is visible as a Barr body in somatic cells. In the third major group of mammals, the egg laying monotremes (platypuses and echidnas), it is less clear if X inactivation and late replication occurs. Earlier replication banding did not reveal obvious asynchronously replicating X chromosomes (Wrigley and Graves, 1988). More recently molecular cytological data suggests the platypus X-chromosomes display partial and gene specific forms of inactivation, but still undergo some level of asynchronous replication of X-specific genes (Deakin et al., 2008a; Ho et al., 2009). Furthermore, a wholesale shift in replication timing for the avian Z-chromosome, which shares extensive homology with the extraordinary ten sex chromosome system in monotremes, is not observed in male homogametic birds, indicating that this process is only present in therian mammals (Arnold et al., 2008; Grutzner et al., 2004; Rens et al., 2007; Veyrunes et al., 2008).

4.1 Chromatin marks behind X-inactivation

The X-inactivation process results in monoallelic expression of the vast majority of X-linked genes in humans and mice. Its process is dependent on critical elements which reside in the X-inactivation centre (XIC) on each X-chromosome, particularly the imprinted *Xist* and *Tsix* genes, and long-range chromatin elements (Boumil and Lee, 2001; Brockdorff et al., 1991; Brown et al., 1991; Clerc and Avner, 2003). The *Tsix* gene appears to regulate chromatin structure at the *Xist* locus, causing its expression to be upregulated. This upregulation of Xist RNA corresponds to chromatin changes in the inactive X, most of which are associated with silencing (Heard, 2005). These *Xist*-induced marks on the inactive X include methylation of CpG dinucleotides in gene promoters, and histone modifications such as hypomethylation of H3K4 and hypoacetylation of H3K9 and H4, also monomethylation of H4K20 and trimethylation of H3K27, and finally H2AK119 ubiquitination (reviewed in Zakharova et al., 2009). Furthermore, the chromatin from the inactivated-X chromosome is enriched for the histone variant macroH2A1, and the final epigenetic mark is the late replication status of the inactive-X during the S-phase (reviewed in Zakharova et al., 2009). This inactivated state facilitates a change in the expression potential of the inactive X, and thus provides gene dosage compensation in female therian mammals (Hellman and Chess, 2007). It has also been observed that the active human X-chromosome is hypomethylated at gene-rich areas compared to the inactive X-chromosome, which displays hypermethylation (Hellman and Chess, 2007).

In placental mammals X inactivation of the maternal or paternal X chromosome is random, in marsupials and mouse extra-embryonic tissues only the paternal X is inactivated (reviewed in Lee, 2003). The epigenetic marks associated with marsupial X-inactivation include the loss or reduction of active histone marks on the inactive-X including H3K4 dimethylation, H4 acetylation, H3K9 acetylation marks (Koina et al., 2009; Wakefield et al., 1997). However, the absence of inactivating histone marks in marsupials, as observed on the inactive-X in placental mammals, may be due to the absence of a XIC region in marsupials (Duret et al., 2006; Hore et al., 2007; Koina et al., 2009). The evolution of the *Xist* non-coding RNA gene involves the pseudogenization of a protein-coding gene in the placental mammalian genome. As such, this gene is not present in marsupial and monotreme mammals, and cannot be found in the regions orthologous to the XIC in these mammalian clades. In marsupials and monotremes, the orthologous flanking genes to the placental mammal XIC region map to different ends of the X-chromosome and chromosome 6 respectively (Davidow et al., 2007; Deakin et al., 2008b; Duret et al., 2006; Hore et al., 2007; Shevchenko et al., 2007).

The FISH based dot assay was utilized to measure replication timing of genes from X-specific regions within the five platypus X-chromosomes. This did not reveal a clear cut replication asynchrony on X specific regions but one of the homologous pairs, namely the X3 chromosomes, showed significantly differential condensation, indicative of wholesale chromatin silencing (Ho et al., 2009). The other four sex chromosome pairs in platypus females, however, show no significant difference in condensation between homologs indicating that the X-inactivation process in monotremes may be region specific (Ho et al., 2009). In male homogametic birds (with ZZ sex chromosomes), studies have shown that whilst the entire chicken Z-chromosome replicates synchronously, the inactivation process appears to be partial and gene-specific, with dosage-compensation occurring stochastically, and in a stage and tissue-specific manner (Arnold et al., 2008; Deakin et al., 2008a; Ho et al., 2009; Kuroda et al., 2001; Kuroiwa et al., 2002; Mank and Ellegren, 2009). Moreover, there is evidence that dosage compensation in monotreme mammals operates in a similar manner as in birds, with platypus females showing stochastic transcriptional inhibition of genes from X-chromosomes (Deakin et al., 2008a). In this case, some X-genes were shown not to be dosage compensated, whilst monoallelic expression was observed at other X-chromosome loci (Deakin et al., 2008a).

5. Asynchronous replication in genes subject to genomic imprinting and allelic exclusion

Genomic imprinting refers to the parent of origin dependent monoallelic expression of an autosomal gene, engendered by the inheritance of parental-specific methylation at an allele. To date, imprinting mechanisms have only been found in therian mammals, which rely on extensive intrauterine foetal-maternal exchange during early development. The 'parental conflict hypothesis' proposed that imprinting is a way of parental genomes counteracting the effects of each other during foetal development, particularly in foetal-maternal placental nutrient exchange (Moore and Haig, 1991). Monotremes, unlike therian mammals, have a brief intrauterine foetal-maternal exchange and there is no competition of the parental genomes over maternal resources. In line with the 'parental conflict hypothesis' to date no imprinting has been discovered in this basal mammalian lineage, suggesting that imprinting evolved after their divergence from therian mammals (Renfree et al., 2009).

5.1 Imprinted genes

Imprinted genes are asynchronously replicated (Table 1), where the replication of one allele lags behind the other in the S-phase, even though the two alleles should be controlled by similarly situated ORs. Traditionally, imprinting involves DNA methylation at only one allele of a gene (i.e. the copy from just one parent is methylated) (Delcuve et al., 2009). In most cases the imprinted allele is methylated and transcriptionally silent. The active or silenced transcriptional state of an allele appears to go hand in hand with replication timing, whereby the expressed allele is early replicated, whilst the silenced allele undergoes late replication in the S-phase (reviewed in Zakharova et al., 2009).

Imprinting control regions (ICRs) are the elements which control the imprinting status of an allele (Bartolomei, 2009). The parentally inherited methylation status, which is established during gametogenesis, of an ICR dictates its control over an allele, meaning that maternal and paternal ICRs at a locus will interact differently with transcriptional control elements, due to their dissimilar methylation status (Bartolomei, 2009). Notably, maternally-imprinted ICRs are often found in the promoters for antisense transcripts, whilst paternally-imprinted ICRs usually reside in intergenic regions (reviewed in Edwards and Ferguson-Smith, 2007). Moreover, the formation of large imprinted gene clusters, where regions of maternally and paternally expressed genes are interspersed with non-imprinted genes, allows many imprinted genes to share regulatory elements, such as ICRs (reviewed in Bartolomei, 2009).

The asynchronously replicating status of imprinted loci has been linked to DNA methylation and other epigenetic marks associated with imprinted gene silencing (Dünzinger et al., 2005). However in birds, which have no fetal-maternal exchange and display no form of genomic imprinting, there are several conserved regions of mammalian imprinted gene orthologs that are asynchronously replicated (Dünzinger et al., 2005). These asynchronously replicating regions are found on chicken macrochromosomes which, compared to their microchromosome counterparts, are hypoacetylated, hypomethylated, late replicating, and display a lower recombination rate during meiosis (Consortium, 2004; Grutzner et al., 2001; McQueen et al., 1998; Schmid et al., 1989). This indicates that asynchronous replication predates imprinting, and that the common vertebrate ancestor of mammals and birds had genomic regions with a 'pre-imprinted' status, whereby asynchronous replication still occurred (Dünzinger et al., 2005). It will be interesting to see whether monotreme orthologs of imprinted genes also replicate asynchronously, as observed in birds (Dünzinger et al., 2005).

5.2 Allelic exclusion genes

Allelic exclusion is a process whereby the future expression from one allele of a locus is chosen in a cell, resulting in monoallelic expression at the locus. Allelic exclusion is a feature of many multigene families, with olfactory gene clusters and immunoglobulin gene clusters being two classic groups of genes utilizing this form of epigenetic control. However there are also other groups of genes which utilize allelic exclusion, including interleukins and the p120 catenin (Gimelbrant et al., 2005; Hollander et al., 1998). Many epigenetic elements control the cell's choice over which allele will be active, including cis and trans-acting DNA sequences, long-range interactions, and chromatin modification (reviewed in Zakharova et al., 2009).

5.2.1 Olfactory genes

Whilst some olfactory receptor (ORc) genes are dispersed in the mammalian genome, many exist in clusters (Kambere and Lane, 2007). The largest cluster in mouse consists of 244 ORc genes, whilst in human the largest cluster contains 116 genes (Godfrey et al., 2004; Malnic et al., 2004). Both species have individual ORc genes and ORc clusters spread across many different chromosomes, with a few chromosomes containing large clusters of ORcs (Glusman et al., 2001; Kambere and Lane, 2007). However, even though the eutherian genome contains around 1000 ORc genes, only a single ORc gene will be expressed in a single olfactory neuron, meaning that that neuron will only express one type of odorant receptor (Malnic et al., 1999). Furthermore in a process known as allelic inactivation, the locus that is being expressed undergoes differential epigenetic processes at each allele that cause one allele to be inactivated, and thus monoallelic expression of the gene (Chess et al., 1994).

Chromosome conformation capture (3C) assays have given an insight into the mechanisms surrounding the selection of a single ORc gene (Lomvardas et al., 2006; Serizawa et al., 2003). The recently developed 3C technique has become invaluable to studies on nuclear architecture, as it is able to detect and quantify long-range DNA interactions *in vivo*, at high resolution, between sequences in close nuclear proximity. The technique relies on the cross-linking of proteins using formaldehyde in intact nuclei or cells (Dekker et al., 2002). The result is that proteins are cross-linked to other proteins and to adjacent chromatin (Orlando et al., 1997). DNA regions that are actually touching at the time of fixation will be held together via the cross-linking of their DNA bound proteins. The cross-linked genomic DNA is then digested with DNA restriction enzymes and the resulting DNA segments are then ligated. Finally, PCR across these ligation sites detects long-range interacting regions at the DNA sequence level (Dekker et al., 2002).

The 3C experiments on olfactory neurons indicated that ORcs undergo an interaction with a long-range interacting region called the "H element", located within the mouse ORc gene cluster *MOR28*, and perhaps do so in a competitive manner in order to become the activated ORc gene (Fuss et al., 2007; Lomvardas et al., 2006; Serizawa et al., 2003) so that only one gene will be chosen and actively expressed (Lomvardas et al., 2006; Serizawa et al., 2003). However another study showed that deletion of the H element only affected proximal genes within its *MOR28* cluster, with no effect on genes outside this cluster, indicating that it cannot be the only factor involved in terms of activating ORc genes in long-range *cis* and *trans* conformations (Fuss et al., 2007).

ORc genes are observed to undergo asynchronous replication (Table 1), with different clusters and individual ORc genes on the same chromosome undergoing replication at the same time in the S-phase, and the establishment of this form of replication occurring in early embryogenesis (Chess et al., 1994; Mostoslavsky et al., 2001; Singh et al., 2003). The asynchronous replication of ORc loci is believed to be controlled in part by the Polycomb group methyltransferase *Eed*, as ORc genes lose their asynchronously replicating status in its absence (Alexander et al., 2007). This could explain how ORc genes located on the same chromosome are observed to undergo asynchronous replication, with *Eed* being a requirement for asynchronous replication, regardless of position on a chromosome (Alexander et al., 2007; Singh et al., 2003).

5.2.2 Immunoglobulin gene loci

It has been suggested that asynchronous replication plays an important role in the selection of which parental allele will undergo V(D)J rearrangement. The allelic exclusion process in mouse occurs for the genes which do not undergo intrachromosomal recombination, and thus are silenced. The rearrangement process of the immunoglobulin genes in mouse requires crosstalk between two loci from two different chromosomes, namely the IgH locus (containing V, D and J gene segments), and Igκ locus (containing V and J segments). The *de novo* methylation of all the VDJ alleles occurs at the implantation stage, and this is also when asynchronous replication is established (Table 1) (Mostoslavsky et al., 2001). However, the selection of one allele at each locus to undergo early replication puts this allele down a demethylation and chromatin opening pathway, allowing it to be rearranged and to become a functional gene (Goldmit et al., 2002). The other late replicating allele however, remains methylated and cannot be rearranged, and is therefore functionally silenced (Goldmit et al., 2002). The two alleles also have different histone marks with the inactive allele binding the heterochromatin specific protein HP1, and the active allele displaying active histone marks such as di- or trimethylated H3K4, and H3 and H4 acetylation (reviewed in Zakharova et al., 2009).

Asynchronous replication and monoallelic expression are hallmarks of genes which undergo imprinting, X-inactivation, and allelic exclusion. Whilst each might come with its own epigenetic makeup, there are also similarities in the types of epigenetic marks observed to differentiate the active allele (with active histone marks) from the inactive allele (with silencing histone marks). Furthermore, the very fact that asynchronous replication occurs together with different forms of epigenetic monoallelic expression suggests that asynchronous replication may have evolved as a mechanism to control the expression of underlying genes, helping to establish the correct epigenetic marks for monoallelic expression.

6. The CTCF protein and the interactome

The CCCTC-binding factor (CTCF) is a renowned genome organiser, and has roles in regulating long-range chromatin interactions (both intrachromsomal and interchromosomal), but also has roles in other processes such as transcriptional insulation, activation/repression, imprinting control, and X-inactivation (Ling et al., 2006; Murrell et al., 2004; Phillips and Corces, 2009). It is also implicated to have roles in sister chromatid cohesion during DNA replication, as CTCF has been shown to interact with the STAG1

<table>
<tr><th colspan="2"></th><th colspan="3">Placentals</th><th colspan="3">Monotremes (Platypus)</th><th colspan="3">Birds (Chicken)</th></tr>
<tr><th></th><th>Gene/ Region</th><th>% SD</th><th>N</th><th>Reference</th><th>% SD</th><th>N</th><th>Reference</th><th>% SD</th><th>N</th><th>Reference</th></tr>
<tr><td rowspan="5">Sex chromosome specific regions</td><td>Xist</td><td>39% Mus</td><td>138</td><td>(Gribnau et al., 2005)</td><td colspan="3" rowspan="3">NA</td><td colspan="3" rowspan="5">NA</td></tr>
<tr><td>Mecp2</td><td>33% Mus</td><td>108</td><td>(Gribnau et al., 2005)</td></tr>
<tr><td>Smcx</td><td>38% Mus</td><td>157</td><td>(Gribnau et al., 2005)</td></tr>
<tr><td>OGN</td><td colspan="3" rowspan="2">NA</td><td>22%</td><td>587</td><td>(Ho et al., 2009)</td></tr>
<tr><td>APC</td><td>29%</td><td>420</td><td>(Ho et al., 2009)</td></tr>
<tr><td rowspan="3">Imprinted genes (in eutherians)</td><td>Igf2</td><td>23% Mus</td><td>>100</td><td>(Kitsberg et al., 1993)</td><td colspan="3" rowspan="7">NA</td><td>25%*</td><td>258</td><td>(Dünzinger et al., 2005)</td></tr>
<tr><td>Igf2R</td><td>35% Mus</td><td>>100</td><td>(Kitsberg et al., 1993)</td><td>22%</td><td>279</td><td>(Dünzinger et al., 2005)</td></tr>
<tr><td>Mest/Copg2</td><td>25% HSA</td><td>>200</td><td>(Bentley et al., 2003)</td><td>18%</td><td>299</td><td>(Dünzinger et al., 2005)</td></tr>
<tr><td rowspan="4">Allelic exclusion</td><td>TCRβ</td><td>46% Mus</td><td>100-300</td><td>(Mostoslavsky et al., 2001)</td><td colspan="3" rowspan="4">NA</td></tr>
<tr><td>B-cell receptor (κ)</td><td>48% Mus</td><td>100-300</td><td>(Mostoslavsky et al., 2001)</td></tr>
<tr><td>IL-2</td><td>68% Mus</td><td>100</td><td>(Hollander et al., 1998)</td></tr>
<tr><td>Olfactory receptor</td><td>31% Mus</td><td>> 99</td><td>(Simon et al., 1999)</td></tr>
</table>

Table 1. A subset of the asynchronous replication data that exists for genes/genomic regions which are sex chromosome specific, imprinted (in eutherians), or undergo allelic exclusion.

subunit of cohesin and localize cohesin to specific CTCF binding sites on chromosome arms (Parelho et al., 2008; Rubio et al., 2008). Important in this context is that the CTCF protein has been shown to mediate asynchronous replication and imprinting control for the *Igf2-H19* cluster (Bergstrom et al., 2007).

6.1 The evolution of CTCF

The CTCF protein is highly conserved across higher eukaryotes, and the active site shows close to 100% homology between mouse, human and chicken suggesting that the protein has a highly conserved role (Ohlsson et al., 2001). A *CTCF* gene duplication event is believed to have occurred in the amniote ancestor preceding the divergence of reptiles and birds, as they both have functional CTCF, but not its gene paralogue, *BORIS* (brother of regulator of imprinted sites) (Hore et al., 2008). BORIS has similar DNA binding capabilities to CTCF, but shows antagonistc epigenetic regulation to *CTCF*, as well as gonad-specific expression in placental and marsupial mammals (Hore et al., 2008). Conversely, BORIS appears to be widely expressed in monotremes and reptiles, indicating that the gene underwent a functional change after the divergence of therian mammals, which is interesting because as yet, there is no evidence that CTCF binding sites exist in the genomes of earlier diverged monotreme mammals (Hore et al., 2008; Weidman et al., 2004). However, CTCF sites have been observed in the chicken genome which is an earlier-split vertebrate than the monotreme clade, and tied with the evidence that CTCF binding occurs in therian genomes (Baniahmad et al., 1990; Lobanenkov et al., 1990), it is likely that CTCF sites exist in the montreme genome.

6.2 CTCF and genome organization

It is hypothesised that although chromatin fibres are subjected to random contacts, and thus will always inhabit slightly different positions in the nucleus, the characteristics of the interacting regions on chromosomes allow interactions to occur (de Laat and Grosveld, 2007). Furthermore, it has been argued that genomic regions preferentially interact with other genomic regions that have similar characteristics to their own, such as regions that share CTCF binding (de Laat and Grosveld, 2007). It has been hypothesised that regions of a chromosome which undergo similar replication timing, like asynchronously replicating genes, may be pulled into similar replication domains (Ryba et al., 2010; Singh et al., 2003). Within the mammalian cell nucleus, chromatin from separate chromosomes is organised into the aforementioned chromosome territories. Within these CTs, a higher order of chromatin structure exists, where domains containing specific chromosomal arms and bands have been found to be located in the nucleus in similar regions of certain cell types (Dietzel et al., 1998). Genes are readily transcribed when they reside on the periphery of chromosome territories, and can even loop out of the territories. Furthermore, genes that are late-replicating and inactivated are often seen to reside on the outer regions of chromosome territories near the nuclear periphery. Looping of the chromatin fibres allows genes to easily interact with the transcriptional machinery residing in the interchromatin compartments (Cremer and Cremer, 2001; Osborne et al., 2004). Imprinted and allelic exclusion genes often 'loop out' and undergo long-range interactions for regulatory purposes (Ling and Hoffman, 2007; Lomvardas et al., 2006).

A good example of CTCF controlling some of the discussed epigenetic, replication, and transcriptional mechanisms occurs at the imprinted *Igf2/H19* domain. The ICR for this imprinted cluster lies between these two genes, in the 5' flanking sequence of *H19*, and the maternal allele interacts with CTCF (Kurukuti et al., 2006). CTCF regulates and insulates imprinted gene transcription for the *Igf2/H19* region by controlling the intrachromosomal interactions of the maternal and paternal alleles (Murrell et al., 2004). When endogenous CTCF is knocked-down in mice, loss of *Igf2* imprinting is observed, whilst deletion of the ICR leads to biallelic expression of *H19* (Ling et al., 2006). In mouse, the paternal chromosome forms a DNA loop between the differentially methylated region (DMR) 2, present in the *Igf2* gene, and the methylated ICR, aided by putative binding factors (Murrell et al., 2004). When the paternal *Igf2* allele promoter comes into close proximity with the *H19* enhancer elements, *Igf2* transcription occurs (Murrell et al., 2004). The DMR1 on the maternal chromosome interacts with the unmethylated ICR, which causes the maternal *Igf2* allele to be sequestered into a transcriptional silencing loop. This causes the maternal *H19* allele to become proximal to its enhancers, allowing it to be expressed (Murrell et al., 2004).

Conversely, CTCF also facilitates an interchromosomal interaction in mouse between the *Igf2/H19* domain, and the *Wsb1/Nf1* region on a different chromosome (Ling et al., 2006).

Specifically, the ICR in the imprinted *Igf2/H19* domain, which contains CTCF binding sites, has been found to interact with another region with CTCF binding sites between the *Wsb1* (WD repeat and SOCS box-containing 1) and *Nf1* (Neurofibromin 1) genes (Ling et al., 2006). Whilst the *Wsb1* and *Nf1* do not appear to be imprinted, as their expression is biallelic, only the paternal copy of the *Wsb1/Nf1* region interacts with CTCF (Krueger and Osborne, 2006; Ling et al., 2006). As explained before, CTCF only binds the maternal copy of the ICR region (flanked by *Igf2* and *H19*). It is consequently hypothesized that the long-range interaction observed between the ICR and *Wsb1/Nf1* region occurs between the maternal and paternal copies respectively, and is mediated by the genome-organizing protein CTCF (Ling et al., 2006).

6.3 Replication timing and CTCF

The specific binding of CTCF at the maternal ICR in the mouse *Igf2/H19* domain has been shown to mediate asynchronous replication in this imprinted region (Bergstrom et al., 2007). The inheritance of a mutated maternal ICR, which lacks CTCF binding, caused the usually late replicating maternal *Igf2/H19* domain to become early replicating (Bergstrom et al., 2007) showing that CTCF binding is required for asynchronous replication of these loci. The mechanism by which CTCF might regulate asynchronous replication at this domain, however, is still unclear. In addition to replication CTCF is involved in other epigenetic effects, including long-range interactions (both intrachromosomal and interchromosomal), insulator activity and transcriptional activation (Kurukuti et al., 2006; Ohlsson et al., 2001; Zhao et al., 2006). Notably, it has been shown that regions which undergo greater amounts of long-range chromatin interaction are subject to late replication timing (Ryba et al., 2010).
Another example of the close relationship between replication, CTCF, and methylation occurs at the differentially methylated silencer region controlling the expression of the *AWT1/ WT1-AS* genes (Hancock et al., 2007). The CTCF protein can only bind the late-replicating unmethylated paternal silencer region within the *AWT1/WT1-AS* cluster, allowing expression of the paternal alleles. The homologous early-replicating maternal region however, has a methylated silencer which does not facilitate CTCF binding and so the maternal *AWT1/WT1-AS* alleles are not expressed (Hancock et al., 2007). It is interesting to speculate as to whether CTCF also controls the asynchronous replication observed at the *WT1* locus in human, and perhaps even in birds (Bickmore and Carothers, 1995; Dünzinger et al., 2005). It is also interesting to note that in both cases the late-replicating allele at these imprinted loci, namely in the maternal *Igf2/H19* allele and the paternal *AWT1/WT1-AS* allele, is the allele which binds CTCF (Bergstrom et al., 2007; Bickmore and Carothers, 1995; Hancock et al., 2007). Whilst CTCF is observed to mediate asynchronous replication and imprinting at the *Igf2/H19* domain in eutherian mammals, the fact that the imprinted orthologs of *Igf2/H19* and *AWT1/WT1-AS* still asynchronously replicate could suggest that CTCF binding in these regions evolved before establishment of genomic imprinting.

6.4 The role of CTCF in replication timing changes in cancer

CTCF may also play a role in the progression of cancer and has many of the characteristics of a tumour suppressor gene; in the human genome it maps to a small region, 16q22.1, which characteristically undergoes loss of heterozygosity in many solid tumours (reviewed in Filippova et al., 1998). Furthermore, changes in DNA consensus sites and DNA methylation patterns in cancers are known to cause loss of CTCF binding, which could result in the loss of functional control of these regions (Filippova et al., 2002; Ohlsson et al., 2001). The regions required for zinc-finger formation, and their corresponding DNA binding sites are often mutated in tumours, changing the CTCF binding-landscape of a genome (Filippova et al., 2002). Specifically, the presence of these mutations in tumours was observed to abolish CTCF's association with the *Igf2/H19* growth regulating genes, whilst not changing its association with non-growth regulating genes (Filippova et al., 2002; Ohlsson et al., 2001). The loss of CTCF association with the *Igf2/H19* region in tumours could be associated with a shift in replication asynchrony. As mentioned in the previous section, when CTCF binding is abolished in the maternal *Igf2/H19* region it results in the loss of asynchronous replication at the locus (Bergstrom et al., 2007). Furthermore, omission of CTCF binding to the maternal *Igf2/H19* ICR has also been observed to abrogate inter-chromosomal interactions for this region (Ling et al., 2006). These results all indicate that the loss of CTCF binding for specific genomic regions in tumours has downstream epigenetic effects, such as loss of replication asynchrony and chromatin interaction, for the genes usually involved in CTCF-interaction.

7. Evolution of replication timing and epigenetic control

7.1 The evolution of replication timing

At the genome level, recent work shows that asynchronous replication pre-dates the establishment of monoallelic expression and genomic imprinting (Zechner et al. 2006, Wright et al. in preparation). The bird genome, which lacks genomic imprinting, contains conserved regions of mammalian imprinted gene orthologs that are asynchronously replicated (Dünzinger et al., 2005). This indicates that asynchronous replication most likely predates imprinting, and that the common vertebrate ancestor of mammals and birds had genomic regions with a 'pre-imprinted' status which still underwent asynchronous replication without any form of traditional imprinting (Dünzinger et al., 2005). It is interesting to note that a recent genome-wide study has indicated that regions with conserved synteny also have conserved replication profiles among human and mouse (e.g. Ryba et al., 2010). Imprinted clusters are renowned for having conserved synteny, and it has been suggested that the selection of highly conserved arrays of imprinted gene orthologs occured during vertebrate evolution, however why these regions were selected for syntenic conservation has been difficult to explain (Dünzinger et al., 2005).

At the replicon level, there has been a model proposing that spatiotemporal properties of mammalian ORs contribute to a combination of pre-determined and stochastic DNA replication (Takahashi, 1987). This mechanism is echoed in budding yeast, which also shows OR activation in a combined chronological and stochastic manner (Barberis et al., 2010; Spiesser et al., 2009). This model, combined with the finding that conserved syntenic regions in human and mouse have very similar replication profiles, indicates that there is a conservation of the temporal programme controlling replicon firing. Furthermore there appears to be a highly conserved order in which amniote imprinted genes or imprinted gene orthologs replicate; with individual imprinted genes following similar temporal patterns when entering replication in birds, monotremes, and eutherians (Wright et al. in preparation). This indicates that in closer related clades of eukaryotes, this temporal replication program may be highly conserved.

7.2 The chromatin interactome and replication profiling

Developing molecular technologies are allowing greater insights into the many interactions occurring in a genome, but also showing how spatial organisation can affect other processes in a genome, such as replication timing. Extensions of the previously discussed 3C molecular interaction technology include Associative Chromosome Trap (ACT), Circular Chromosome Conformation Capture or Chromosome Conformation Capture-on-Chip (4C), and Carbon-Copy Chromosome Conformation Capture (5C), all of which can measure more than a single to single region interaction (Dekker et al., 2002; Dostie et al., 2006; Ling et al., 2006; Simonis et al., 2006; Zhao et al., 2006). In addition to these technologies, new techniques are allowing interactions to be measured across entire genomes, resulting in the mapping of an "interactome", whereby all the long-range interactions occurring in a genome are measured (Fullwood et al., 2009; Lieberman-Aiden et al., 2009). Specifically, there are two techniques that have been developed to do this, Chromatin Interaction Analysis by Paired-End Tag sequencing (ChIA-PET) and Hi-C (which measures the three-dimensional architecture of a genome by coupling proximity-based ligation with parallel sequencing) (Fullwood et al., 2009; Lieberman-Aiden et al., 2009). These experiments, in conjunction with replication-timing profiling by microarrays, have indicated that the interactome of a genome is very closely aligned with replication timing (Ryba et al., 2010).

The chromatin "interactome" is now understood to play a critical part in genome organisation; allowing complex regulatory networks of interactions to occur, each of which with functional significance, all of which highly dynamic and organised within a nucleus by proteins such as CTCF and the Estrogen-receptor alpha (Botta et al., 2010; Fullwood et al., 2009). These interactions also appear to be conserved in similar cell types across mammalian evolution, suggesting that perhaps these long-range interactions are part of an evolutionary conserved mechanism of spatial organisation (Ryba et al., 2010). Furthermore, initiation of replication appears to be an evolutionarily conserved process across eukaryotic evolution, and the overlay of entire genome replication timing profiles with interactome maps have shown that late-replicating regions are often undergoing greater amounts of long-range interaction (Ryba et al., 2010). These findings, in conjunction with asynchronous replication data, could indicate that long-range interactions which occur in abundance at imprinted and monoallelically expressed loci, are affecting asynchronous replication. Specifically, there is data supporting the argument that the allele undergoing long-range interaction could also be the allele which undergoes late-replication. Firstly, it has been observed that asynchronously replicated alleles often localize to spatially distinct regions in a nucleus (Gribnau et al., 2003; Sadoni et al., 1999). Secondly, as mentioned previously, the late-replicating maternal *Igf2/H19* allele and the paternal *AWT1/WT1-AS* allele, are also the alleles which bind CTCF, in an imprinting dependent manner. It could be that the binding of proteins which mediate long-range chromatin interaction at these alleles is facilitating greater amounts of interaction, which is reflected in their late replicating status, and also in the asynchronous replication of these genes (Bergstrom et al., 2007; Bickmore and Carothers, 1995; Hancock et al., 2007).

7.3 Measuring replication to combat cancer

It has been proposed that measuring changes in replication profiles may be a way of detecting abnormalities associated with cancer, not observed through usual techniques (reviewed in Watanabe and Maekawa, 2010). Epigenetic reprogramming in diseased cells is often observed to occur with changes in replication timing patterns, with changes in replication being observed with chromosomal rearrangements in cancer cell lines (D'Antoni et al., 2004; Gondor and Ohlsson, 2009; State et al., 2003). Better detection of prostate cancer may come in the form of measuring replication timing changes observed in peripheral blood lymphocytes undergoing aneuploidy (Dotan et al., 2004). In terms of protein detection of cancer, measuring the function of the tumour suppressor gene p53, may be a good determinant in the progression of cancer. P53 is the most commonly mutated gene in human cancers, and is a G1/S-phase and S-phase checkpoint regulator during DNA replication. Loss of its function is observed to affect the replication timing of human colon carcinoma cells (Watanabe et al., 2007).

Changes in replication timing may also be affected by altered function of CTCF in cancer. As mentioned previously, it has been observed that mutation of CTCF binding sites near growth factor genes, such as in the *Igf2/H19* region, occurs in many tumours (Filippova et al., 2002). These mutations may cause a loss of CTCF binding in the region, which has been observed to abolish asynchronous replication of the *Igf2* locus, and changes the replication timing of the gene (Bergstrom et al., 2007). However the mutation of CTCF binding sites would also change the interactome profile of a cell. Loss of CTCF-binding through mutation around genes like *Igf2* and *H19* would result in them no longer undergoing their "normal" chromatin interactions, perhaps causing different spatial organization of these loci in the nucleus of a cancerous cell.

7.4 The chromatin interactome: controlling eukaryotic replication timing

To date there is a lack of data that could provide insight about the evolution of an interactome. It has been observed that many long-range interacting regions share many of the same (but not necessarily all) epigenetic characteristics, such as asynchronous replication, monoallelic expression, differentially methylated regions and histone modifications and variants, imprinting, and CTCF binding. It is currently unknown how these epigenetic events evolved and investigating those epigenetic features in a range of vertebrate genomes could tease apart the sequence of events that has led to a complex network of epigenetic regulation.

Chromatin interactions may have evolved in many genomic control processes, but it is the binding of master genome regulators, like CTCF, which dictate where these interactions can occur. The CTCF protein is highly conserved among amniotes, conserved in vertebrates, and exists in *Drosophila* and subsets of nematodes (Heger et al., 2009; Ohlsson et al., 2001). Furthermore, there is evidence to suggest that CTCF binding and function are conserved in humans, mouse, and chicken, in genes such as β-globin, whereby CTCF binding at this locus allows cell-type specific intrachromosomal interactions to occur (Bell et al., 1999; Yusufzai et al., 2004). CTCF binding and chromatin interaction in this region suggest that CTCF spatial control of chromatin, at least in this region, was present in the common ancestor of amniotes. The evolutionary conservation of replication timing and the strikingly similar genomic interactome in similar cell types among human and mouse suggests that replication timing is intrinsically tied to long-range interaction. Moreover, there is evidence to suggest that replication timing relies on the presence of long-range interactions at specific loci, with the knockdown of long-range mediator proteins causing interactions to be abolished, and also causing replication asynchrony to cease (Bergstrom et al., 2007; Fullwood et al., 2009; Ling et al., 2006). The loss of replication asynchrony in this case could be due to ectopic spatial organisation of the alleles, whereby the loss of the interaction mediator protein causes the allele of a locus to reside in an atypical subnuclear domain. This irregular replication domain would not have the correct molecular and chemical characteristics to allow the ORs of the spatially ectopic allele to fire in the normal temporal order. This could cause the erroneous firing of ORs in such a way as to abolish replication asynchrony at the locus.

8. Conclusion

Replication timing of DNA at S-phase is tightly regulated and affects gene activity, nuclear organisation, as well as other aspects of genome biology. Differences in replication timing have been used to identify individual chromosomes and differentiated sex chromosomes for several decades. Since then, an increasing number of proteins have been identified as important for regulating replication timing and genome-wide approaches are now used to study replication timing. A fascinating variation of the replication-timing theme is asynchronous replication, which appears to be closely aligned with other epigenetic mechanisms involved in long-range interaction, genomic imprinting and X chromosome inactivation. Whilst previous research has stipulated that asynchronous replication and long range interactions have evolved as a result of epigenetic control of (eg. monoallelic expression), there is emerging evidence that both predate the presence of other epigenetic processes. We suggest that the interactome has played a role in the evolution of spatial nuclear organisation. In addition, mutations in sequences important for long-range interaction and replication timing, and also changes in the replication timing program itself, are important factors influencing a diverse array of human diseases, including cancer. The study of replication timing in different organisms and in human disease will reveal the full extent to which replication timing contributes to the epigenetic landscape in normal and abnormal cells.

9. Acknowledgements

Megan L. Wright is funded by an Australian Postgraduate Award. Frank Grutzner is an ARC Senior Research Fellow.

10. References

Aladjem, M. I., Groudine, M., Brody, L. L., Dieken, E. S., Fournier, R. E., Wahl, G. M. and Epner, E. M. (1995). Participation of the human beta-globin locus control region in initiation of DNA replication. *Science* 270, 815-9.

Alexander, M. K., Mlynarczyk-Evans, S., Royce-Tolland, M., Plocik, A., Kalantry, S., Magnuson, T. and Panning, B. (2007). Differences between homologous alleles of olfactory receptor genes require the Polycomb Group protein Eed. *J Cell Biol* 179, 269-76.

Altman, A. L. and Fanning, E. (2004). Defined sequence modules and an architectural element cooperate to promote initiation at an ectopic mammalian chromosomal replication origin. *Mol Cell Biol* 24, 4138-50.

Anglana, M., Apiou, F., Bensimon, A. and Debatisse, M. (2003). Dynamics of DNA replication in mammalian somatic cells: nucleotide pool modulates origin choice and interorigin spacing. *Cell* 114, 385-94.

Arnold, A. P., Itoh, Y. and Melamed, E. (2008). A bird's-eye view of sex chromosome dosage compensation. *Annu Rev Genomics Hum Genet* 9, 109-27.

Aten, J. A. and Kanaar, R. (2006). Chromosomal organization: mingling with the neighbors. *PLoS Biol* 4, e155.

Austin, R. J., Orr-Weaver, T. L. and Bell, S. P. (1999). Drosophila ORC specifically binds to ACE3, an origin of DNA replication control element. *Genes Dev* 13, 2639-49.

Baniahmad, A., Steiner, C., Kohne, A. C. and Renkawitz, R. (1990). Modular structure of a chicken lysozyme silencer: involvement of an unusual thyroid hormone receptor binding site. *Cell* 61, 505-14.

Baran, N., Lapidot, A. and Manor, H. (1991). Formation of DNA triplexes accounts for arrests of DNA synthesis at d(TC)n and d(GA)n tracts. *Proceedings of the National Academy of Sciences* 88, 507-511.

Barberis, M., Spiesser, T. W. and Klipp, E. (2010). Replication origins and timing of temporal replication in budding yeast: how to solve the conundrum? *Curr Genomics* 11, 199-211.

Bartolomei, M. S. (2009). Genomic imprinting: employing and avoiding epigenetic processes. *Genes Dev* 23, 2124-33.

Baumer, A., Riegel, M. and Schinzel, A. (2004). Non-random asynchronous replication at 22q11.2 favours unequal meiotic crossovers leading to the human 22q11.2 deletion. *Journal of Medical Genetics* 41, 413-420.

Bell, A. C., West, A. G. and Felsenfeld, G. (1999). The Protein CTCF Is Required for the Enhancer Blocking Activity of Vertebrate Insulators. *Cell* 98, 387-396.

Bell, S. P. and Stillman, B. (1992). ATP-dependent recognition of eukaryotic origins of DNA replication by a multiprotein complex. *Nature* 357, 128-34.

Bentley, L., Nakabayashi, K., Monk, D., Beechey, C., Peters, J., Birjandi, Z., Khayat, F. E., Patel, M., Preece, M. A., Stanier, P. et al. (2003). The imprinted region on human chromosome 7q32 extends to the carboxypeptidase A gene cluster: an imprinted candidate for Silver-Russell syndrome. *J Med Genet* 40, 249-56.

Bergstrom, R., Whitehead, J., Kurukuti, S. and Ohlsson, R. (2007). CTCF regulates asynchronous replication of the imprinted H19/Igf2 domain. *Cell Cycle* 6, 450-4.

Bernardi, G. (1995). The human genome: organization and evolutionary history. *Annu Rev Genet* 29, 445-76.

Bickmore, W. A. and Carothers, A. D. (1995). Factors affecting the timing and imprinting of replication on a mammalian chromosome. *J Cell Sci* 108 (Pt 8), 2801-9.

Biederman, B. and Lin, C. C. (1979). R-banding methods for chromosome identification using acridine orange following heat denaturation (RFA) and bromodeoxyuridine labeling (RBA). *Methods in Cell Science* 5, 1189-1192.

Blow, J. J. and Ge, X. Q. (2009). A model for DNA replication showing how dormant origins safeguard against replication fork failure. *EMBO Rep* 10, 406-12.

Botta, M., Haider, S., Leung, I. X. Y., Lio, P. and Mozziconacci, J. (2010). Intra- and inter-chromosomal interactions correlate with CTCF binding genome wide. *Mol Syst Biol* 6.

Boumil, R. M. and Lee, J. T. (2001). Forty years of decoding the silence in X-chromosome inactivation. *Hum Mol Genet* 10, 2225-32.

Branco, M. R. and Pombo, A. (2006). Intermingling of chromosome territories in interphase suggests role in translocations and transcription-dependent associations. *PLoS Biol* 4, e138.

Brewer, B. J. and Fangman, W. L. (1993). Initiation at closely spaced replication origins in a yeast chromosome. *Science* 262, 1728-31.

Brinton, B. T., Caddle, M. S. and Heintz, N. H. (1991). Position and orientation-dependent effects of a eukaryotic Z-triplex DNA motif on episomal DNA replication in COS-7 cells. *Journal of Biological Chemistry* 266, 5153-5161.

Brockdorff, N., Ashworth, A., Kay, G. F., Cooper, P., Smith, S., McCabe, V. M., Norris, D. P., Penny, G. D., Patel, D. and Rastan, S. (1991). Conservation of position and exclusive expression of mouse Xist from the inactive X chromosome. *Nature* 351, 329-31.

Brown, C. J., Ballabio, A., Rupert, J. L., Lafreniere, R. G., Grompe, M., Tonlorenzi, R. and Willard, H. F. (1991). A gene from the region of the human X inactivation centre is expressed exclusively from the inactive X chromosome. *Nature* 349, 38-44.

Burke, T. W., Cook, J. G., Asano, M. and Nevins, J. R. (2001). Replication factors MCM2 and ORC1 interact with the histone acetyltransferase HBO1. *J Biol Chem* 276, 15397-408.

Chess, A., Simon, I., Cedar, H. and Axel, R. (1994). Allelic inactivation regulates olfactory receptor gene expression. *Cell* 78, 823-34.

Chuang, R. Y. and Kelly, T. J. (1999). The fission yeast homologue of Orc4p binds to replication origin DNA via multiple AT-hooks. *Proc Natl Acad Sci U S A* 96, 2656-61.

Clerc, P. and Avner, P. (2003). Multiple elements within the Xic regulate random X inactivation in mice. *Semin Cell Dev Biol* 14, 85-92.

Consortium, I. C. G. S. (2004). Sequence and comparative analysis of the chicken genome provide unique perspectives on vertebrate evolution. *Nature* 432, 695-716.

Costantini, M. and Bernardi, G. (2008). Replication timing, chromosomal bands, and isochores. *Proc Natl Acad Sci U S A* 105, 3433-7.

Costantini, M., Clay, O., Auletta, F. and Bernardi, G. (2006). An isochore map of human chromosomes. *Genome Res* 16, 536-41.

Costantini, M., Clay, O., Federico, C., Saccone, S., Auletta, F. and Bernardi, G. (2007). Human chromosomal bands: nested structure, high-definition map and molecular basis. *Chromosoma* 116, 29-40.

Courbet, S., Gay, S., Arnoult, N., Wronka, G., Anglana, M., Brison, O. and Debatisse, M. (2008). Replication fork movement sets chromatin loop size and origin choice in mammalian cells. *Nature* 455, 557-60.

Cremer, T. and Cremer, C. (2001). Chromosome territories, nuclear architecture and gene regulation in mammalian cells. *Nat Rev Genet* 2, 292-301.

Cremer, T. and Cremer, M. (2010). Chromosome territories. *Cold Spring Harb Perspect Biol* 2, a003889.

D'Antoni, S., Mattina, T., Di Mare, P., Federico, C., Motta, S. and Saccone, S. (2004). Altered replication timing of the HIRA/Tuple1 locus in the DiGeorge and Velocardiofacial syndromes. *Gene* 333, 111-119.

Davidow, L. S., Breen, M., Duke, S. E., Samollow, P. B., McCarrey, J. R. and Lee, J. T. (2007). The search for a marsupial XIC reveals a break with vertebrate synteny. *Chromosome Res* 15, 137-46.

de Laat, W. and Grosveld, F. (2007). Inter-chromosomal gene regulation in the mammalian cell nucleus. *Curr Opin Genet Dev* 17, 456-64.

Deakin, J. E., Hore, T. A., Koina, E. and Marshall Graves, J. A. (2008a). The status of dosage compensation in the multiple X chromosomes of the platypus. *PLoS Genet* 4, e1000140.

Deakin, J. E., Koina, E., Waters, P. D., Doherty, R., Patel, V. S., Delbridge, M. L., Dobson, B., Fong, J., Hu, Y., van den Hurk, C. et al. (2008b). Physical map of two tammar wallaby chromosomes: a strategy for mapping in non-model mammals. *Chromosome Res* 16, 1159-75.

Debatisse, M., El Achkar, E. and Dutrillaux, B. (2006). Common fragile sites nested at the interfaces of early and late-replicating chromosome bands: cis acting components of the G2/M checkpoint? *Cell Cycle* 5, 578-81.

Debatisse, M., Toledo, F. and Anglana, M. (2004). Replication initiation in mammalian cells: changing preferences. *Cell Cycle* 3, 19-21.

Dekker, J., Rippe, K., Dekker, M. and Kleckner, N. (2002). Capturing chromosome conformation. *Science* 295, 1306-11.

Delcuve, G. P., Rastegar, M. and Davie, J. R. (2009). Epigenetic control. *Journal of Cellular Physiology* 219, 243-250.

DePamphilis, M. L. (2006). DNA replication and human disease. New York: Cold Spring Harbor Laboratory Press.

Dietzel, S., Jauch, A., Kienle, D., Qu, G., Holtgreve-Grez, H., Eils, R., Munkel, C., Bittner, M., Meltzer, P. S., Trent, J. M. et al. (1998). Separate and variably shaped chromosome arm domains are disclosed by chromosome arm painting in human cell nuclei. *Chromosome Res* 6, 25-33.

Doksani, Y., Bermejo, R., Fiorani, S., Haber, J. E. and Foiani, M. (2009). Replicon dynamics, dormant origin firing, and terminal fork integrity after double-strand break formation. *Cell* 137, 247-58.

Dostie, J. e., Richmond, T. A., Arnaout, R. A., Selzer, R. R., Lee, W. L., Honan, T. A., Rubio, E. D., Krumm, A., Lamb, J., Nusbaum, C. et al. (2006). Chromosome Conformation Capture Carbon Copy (5C): A massively parallel solution for mapping interactions between genomic elements. *Genome Research* 16, 1299-1309.

Dotan, Z. A., Dotan, A., Ramon, J. and Avivi, L. (2004). Altered mode of allelic replication accompanied by aneuploidy in peripheral blood lymphocytes of prostate cancer patients, vol. 111 (ed., pp. 60-66: Wiley Subscription Services, Inc., A Wiley Company.

Drets, M. E., Folle, G. A. and Comings, D. E. (1978). Mechanisms of chromosome banding. X. Chromosome and nuclear changes induced by photo-oxidation and their relation to R-banding with anti-C antibodies. *Chromosoma* 69, 101-12.

Dünzinger, U., Nanda, I., Schmid, M., Haaf, T. and Zechner, U. (2005). Chicken orthologues of mammalian imprinted genes are clustered on macrochromosomes and replicate asynchronously. *Trends in Genetics* 21, 488-492.

Duret, L., Chureau, C., Samain, S., Weissenbach, J. and Avner, P. (2006). The Xist RNA gene evolved in eutherians by pseudogenization of a protein-coding gene. *Science* 312, 1653-5.

Edwards, C. A. and Ferguson-Smith, A. C. (2007). Mechanisms regulating imprinted genes in clusters. *Current Opinion in Cell Biology* 19, 281-289.

Edwards, M. C., Tutter, A. V., Cvetic, C., Gilbert, C. H., Prokhorova, T. A. and Walter, J. C. (2002). MCM2-7 complexes bind chromatin in a distributed pattern surrounding the origin recognition complex in Xenopus egg extracts. *J Biol Chem* 277, 33049-57.

Farkash-Amar, S., Lipson, D., Polten, A., Goren, A., Helmstetter, C., Yakhini, Z. and Simon, I. (2008). Global organization of replication time zones of the mouse genome. *Genome Res* 18, 1562-70.

Ferguson, B. M. and Fangman, W. L. (1992). A position effect on the time of replication origin activation in yeast. *Cell* 68, 333-9.

Filippova, G. N., Lindblom, A., Meincke, L. J., Klenova, E. M., Neiman, P. E., Collins, S. J., Doggett, N. A. and Lobanenkov, V. V. (1998). A widely expressed transcription factor with multiple DNA sequence specificity, CTCF, is localized at chromosome segment 16q22.1 within one of the smallest regions of overlap for common deletions in breast and prostate cancers. *Genes Chromosomes Cancer* 22, 26-36.

Filippova, G. N., Qi, C. F., Ulmer, J. E., Moore, J. M., Ward, M. D., Hu, Y. J., Loukinov, D. I., Pugacheva, E. M., Klenova, E. M., Grundy, P. E. et al. (2002). Tumor-associated zinc finger mutations in the CTCF transcription factor selectively alter tts DNA-binding specificity. *Cancer Res* 62, 48-52.

Friedman, K. L., Diller, J. D., Ferguson, B. M., Nyland, S. V., Brewer, B. J. and Fangman, W. L. (1996). Multiple determinants controlling activation of yeast replication origins late in S phase. *Genes Dev* 10, 1595-607.

Fullwood, M. J., Liu, M. H., Pan, Y. F., Liu, J., Xu, H., Mohamed, Y. B., Orlov, Y. L., Velkov, S., Ho, A., Mei, P. H. et al. (2009). An oestrogen-receptor-[agr]-bound human chromatin interactome. *Nature* 462, 58-64.

Fuss, S. H., Omura, M. and Mombaerts, P. (2007). Local and cis effects of the H element on expression of odorant receptor genes in mouse. *Cell* 130, 373-84.

Ge, X. Q., Jackson, D. A. and Blow, J. J. (2007). Dormant origins licensed by excess Mcm2-7 are required for human cells to survive replicative stress. *Genes Dev* 21, 3331-41.

Gilbert, D. M. (2002). Replication timing and transcriptional control: beyond cause and effect. *Curr Opin Cell Biol* 14, 377-83.

Gilbert, D. M. (2010). Evaluating genome-scale approaches to eukaryotic DNA replication. *Nat Rev Genet* 11, 673-84.

Gimelbrant, A. A., Ensminger, A. W., Qi, P., Zucker, J. and Chess, A. (2005). Monoallelic expression and asynchronous replication of p120 catenin in mouse and human cells. *J Biol Chem* 280, 1354-9.

Glusman, G., Yanai, I., Rubin, I. and Lancet, D. (2001). The complete human olfactory subgenome. *Genome Res* 11, 685-702.

Godfrey, P. A., Malnic, B. and Buck, L. B. (2004). The mouse olfactory receptor gene family. *Proc Natl Acad Sci U S A* 101, 2156-61.

Goldmit, M., Schlissel, M., Cedar, H. and Bergman, Y. (2002). Differential accessibility at the kappa chain locus plays a role in allelic exclusion. *EMBO J* 21, 5255-61.

Gondor, A. and Ohlsson, R. (2009). Replication timing and epigenetic reprogramming of gene expression: a two-way relationship? *Nat Rev Genet* 10, 269-276.

Gribnau, J., Hochedlinger, K., Hata, K., Li, E. and Jaenisch, R. (2003). Asynchronous replication timing of imprinted loci is independent of DNA methylation, but consistent with differential subnuclear localization. *Genes Dev* 17, 759-73.

Gribnau, J., Luikenhuis, S., Hochedlinger, K., Monkhorst, K. and Jaenisch, R. (2005). X chromosome choice occurs independently of asynchronous replication timing. *J Cell Biol* 168, 365-73.

Grutzner, F., Rens, W., Tsend-Ayush, E., El-Mogharbel, N., O'Brien, P. C., Jones, R. C., Ferguson-Smith, M. A. and Marshall Graves, J. A. (2004). In the platypus a meiotic chain of ten sex chromosomes shares genes with the bird Z and mammal X chromosomes. *Nature* 432, 913-7.

Grutzner, F., Zend-Ajusch, E., Stout, K., Munsche, S., Niveleau, A., Nanda, I., Schmid, M. and Haaf, T. (2001). Chicken microchromosomes are hypermethylated and can be identified by specific painting probes. *Cytogenet Cell Genet* 93, 265-9.

Haase, S. B., Heinzel, S. S. and Calos, M. P. (1994). Transcription inhibits the replication of autonomously replicating plasmids in human cells. *Mol Cell Biol* 14, 2516-24.

Hancock, A. L., Brown, K. W., Moorwood, K., Moon, H., Holmgren, C., Mardikar, S. H., Dallosso, A. R., Klenova, E., Loukinov, D., Ohlsson, R. et al. (2007). A CTCF-binding silencer regulates the imprinted genes AWT1 and WT1-AS and exhibits sequential epigenetic defects during Wilms' tumourigenesis. *Hum Mol Genet* 16, 343-54.

Hayashida, T., Oda, M., Ohsawa, K., Yamaguchi, A., Hosozawa, T., Locksley, R. M., Giacca, M., Masai, H. and Miyatake, S. (2006). Replication initiation from a novel origin identified in the Th2 cytokine cluster locus requires a distant conserved noncoding sequence. *J Immunol* 176, 5446-54.

Heard, E. (2005). Delving into the diversity of facultative heterochromatin: the epigenetics of the inactive X chromosome. *Curr Opin Genet Dev* 15, 482-9.

Heger, P., Marin, B. and Schierenberg, E. (2009). Loss of the insulator protein CTCF during nematode evolution. *BMC Molecular Biology* 10, 84.

Hellman, A. and Chess, A. (2007). Gene body-specific methylation on the active X chromosome. *Science* 315, 1141-3.

Heun, P., Laroche, T., Raghuraman, M. K. and Gasser, S. M. (2001). The positioning and dynamics of origins of replication in the budding yeast nucleus. *J Cell Biol* 152, 385-400.

Hiratani, I. and Gilbert, D. M. (2009). Replication timing as an epigenetic mark. *Epigenetics* 4, 93-7.

Hiratani, I., Ryba, T., Itoh, M., Yokochi, T., Schwaiger, M., Chang, C. W., Lyou, Y., Townes, T. M., Schubeler, D. and Gilbert, D. M. (2008). Global reorganization of replication domains during embryonic stem cell differentiation. *PLoS Biol* 6, e245.

Hiratani, I., Takebayashi, S., Lu, J. and Gilbert, D. M. (2009). Replication timing and transcriptional control: beyond cause and effect--part II. *Curr Opin Genet Dev* 19, 142-9.

Ho, K. K. K., Deakin, J. E., Wright, M. L., Graves, J. A. M. and GrÃ¼tzner, F. (2009). Replication asynchrony and differential condensation of X chromosomes in female platypus (Ornithorhynchus anatinus). *Reproduction, Fertility and Development* 21, 952-963.

Hollander, G. A., Zuklys, S., Morel, C., Mizoguchi, E., Mobisson, K., Simpson, S., Terhorst, C., Wishart, W., Golan, D. E., Bhan, A. K. et al. (1998). Monoallelic expression of the interleukin-2 locus. *Science* 279, 2118-21.

Holmquist, G. P. (1987). Role of replication time in the control of tissue-specific gene expression. *Am J Hum Genet* 40, 151-73.

Hore, T. A., Deakin, J. E. and Marshall Graves, J. A. (2008). The evolution of epigenetic regulators CTCF and BORIS/CTCFL in amniotes. *PLoS Genet* 4, e1000169.

Hore, T. A., Koina, E., Wakefield, M. J. and Marshall Graves, J. A. (2007). The region homologous to the X-chromosome inactivation centre has been disrupted in marsupial and monotreme mammals. *Chromosome Res* 15, 147-61.

Hyrien, O., Marheineke, K. and Goldar, A. (2003). Paradoxes of eukaryotic DNA replication: MCM proteins and the random completion problem. *Bioessays* 25, 116-25.

Ibarra, A., Schwob, E. and Mendez, J. (2008). Excess MCM proteins protect human cells from replicative stress by licensing backup origins of replication. *Proc Natl Acad Sci U S A* 105, 8956-61.

Iizuka, M., Matsui, T., Takisawa, H. and Smith, M. M. (2006). Regulation of replication licensing by acetyltransferase Hbo1. *Mol Cell Biol* 26, 1098-108.

Kalejta, R. F., Li, X., Mesner, L. D., Dijkwel, P. A., Lin, H. B. and Hamlin, J. L. (1998). Distal sequences, but not ori-beta/OBR-1, are essential for initiation of DNA replication in the Chinese hamster DHFR origin. *Mol Cell* 2, 797-806.

Kalish, J. M. and Glazer, P. M. (2005). Targeted genome modification via triple helix formation. *Ann N Y Acad Sci* 1058, 151-61.

Kambere, M. B. and Lane, R. P. (2007). Co-regulation of a large and rapidly evolving repertoire of odorant receptor genes. *BMC Neurosci* 8 Suppl 3, S2.

Kitsberg, D., Selig, S., Brandeis, M., Simon, I., Keshet, I., Driscoll, D. J., Nicholls, R. D. and Cedar, H. (1993). Allele-specific replication timing of imprinted gene regions. *Nature* 364, 459-63.

Knauert, M. P., Kalish, J. M., Hegan, D. C. and Glazer, P. M. (2006). Triplex-stimulated intermolecular recombination at a single-copy genomic target. *Mol Ther* 14, 392-400.

Knoll, J. H., Cheng, S. D. and Lalande, M. (1994). Allele specificity of DNA replication timing in the Angelman/Prader-Willi syndrome imprinted chromosomal region. *Nat Genet* 6, 41-6.

Koina, E., Chaumeil, J., Greaves, I. K., Tremethick, D. J. and Graves, J. A. (2009). Specific patterns of histone marks accompany X chromosome inactivation in a marsupial. *Chromosome Res* 17, 115-26.

Koren, A., Soifer, I. and Barkai, N. (2010). MRC1-dependent scaling of the budding yeast DNA replication timing program. *Genome Res* 20, 781-90.

Krueger, C. and Osborne, C. S. (2006). Raising the curtains on interchromosomal interactions. *Trends in Genetics* 22, 637-639.

Kuroda, Y., Arai, N., Arita, M., Teranishi, M., Hori, T., Harata, M. and Mizuno, S. (2001). Absence of Z-chromosome inactivation for five genes in male chickens. *Chromosome Res* 9, 457-68.

Kuroiwa, A., Yokomine, T., Sasaki, H., Tsudzuki, M., Tanaka, K., Namikawa, T. and Matsuda, Y. (2002). Biallelic expression of Z-linked genes in male chickens. *Cytogenet Genome Res* 99, 310-4.

Kurukuti, S., Tiwari, V. K., Tavoosidana, G., Pugacheva, E., Murrell, A., Zhao, Z., Lobanenkov, V., Reik, W. and Ohlsson, R. (2006). CTCF binding at the H19 imprinting control region mediates maternally inherited higher-order chromatin conformation to restrict enhancer access to Igf2. *Proc Natl Acad Sci U S A* 103, 10684-9.

Lee, J. T. (2003). Molecular links between X-inactivation and autosomal imprinting: X-inactivation as a driving force for the evolution of imprinting? *Curr Biol* 13, R242-54.

Lemaitre, J. M., Danis, E., Pasero, P., Vassetzky, Y. and Mechali, M. (2005). Mitotic remodeling of the replicon and chromosome structure. *Cell* 123, 787-801.

Lengronne, A. and Schwob, E. (2002). The yeast CDK inhibitor Sic1 prevents genomic instability by promoting replication origin licensing in late G(1). *Mol Cell* 9, 1067-78.

Lieberman-Aiden, E., van Berkum, N. L., Williams, L., Imakaev, M., Ragoczy, T., Telling, A., Amit, I., Lajoie, B. R., Sabo, P. J., Dorschner, M. O. et al. (2009). Comprehensive mapping of long-range interactions reveals folding principles of the human genome. *Science* 326, 289-93.

Ling, J. Q. and Hoffman, A. R. (2007). Epigenetics of Long-Range Chromatin Interactions. *Pediatric Research* 61, 11R-16R 10.1203/pdr.0b013e31804575db.

Ling, J. Q., Li, T., Hu, J. F., Vu, T. H., Chen, H. L., Qiu, X. W., Cherry, A. M. and Hoffman, A. R. (2006). CTCF mediates interchromosomal colocalization between Igf2/H19 and Wsb1/Nf1. *Science* 312, 269-72.

Lobanenkov, V. V., Nicolas, R. H., Adler, V. V., Paterson, H., Klenova, E. M., Polotskaja, A. V. and Goodwin, G. H. (1990). A novel sequence-specific DNA binding protein which interacts with three regularly spaced direct repeats of the CCCTC-motif in the 5'-flanking sequence of the chicken c-myc gene. *Oncogene* 5, 1743-53.

Lomvardas, S., Barnea, G., Pisapia, D. J., Mendelsohn, M., Kirkland, J. and Axel, R. (2006). Interchromosomal interactions and olfactory receptor choice. *Cell* 126, 403-13.

Lyon, M. F. (1961). Gene action in the X-chromosome of the mouse (Mus musculus L.). *Nature* 190, 372-3.

Malnic, B., Godfrey, P. A. and Buck, L. B. (2004). The human olfactory receptor gene family. *Proc Natl Acad Sci U S A* 101, 2584-9.

Malnic, B., Hirono, J., Sato, T. and Buck, L. B. (1999). Combinatorial receptor codes for odors. *Cell* 96, 713-23.

Mank, J. E. and Ellegren, H. (2009). All dosage compensation is local: gene-by-gene regulation of sex-biased expression on the chicken Z chromosome. *Heredity* 102, 312-320.

Masai, H., Matsumoto, S., You, Z., Yoshizawa-Sugata, N. and Oda, M. (2010). Eukaryotic chromosome DNA replication: where, when, and how? *Annu Rev Biochem* 79, 89-130.

McQueen, H. A., Siriaco, G. and Bird, A. P. (1998). Chicken microchromosomes are hyperacetylated, early replicating, and gene rich. *Genome Res* 8, 621-30.

Misteli, T. (2001). Protein dynamics: implications for nuclear architecture and gene expression. *Science* 291, 843-7.

Moore, T. and Haig, D. (1991). Genomic imprinting in mammalian development: a parental tug-of-war. *Trends in Genetics* 7, 45-49.

Mostoslavsky, R., Singh, N., Tenzen, T., Goldmit, M., Gabay, C., Elizur, S., Qi, P., Reubinoff, B. E., Chess, A., Cedar, H. et al. (2001). Asynchronous replication and allelic exclusion in the immune system. *Nature* 414, 221-5.

Murrell, A., Heeson, S. and Reik, W. (2004). Interaction between differentially methylated regions partitions the imprinted genes Igf2 and H19 into parent-specific chromatin loops. *Nat Genet* 36, 889-93.

Nishida-Umehara, C., Fujiwara, A., Ogawa, A., Mizuno, S., Abe, S. and Yoshida, M. C. (1999). Differentiation of Z and W Chromosomes Revealed by Replication Banding

and FISH Mapping of Sex-chromosome-linked DNA Markers in the Cassowary (Aves, Ratitae). *Chromosome Research* 7, 635-640.
Ohlsson, R., Renkawitz, R. and Lobanenkov, V. (2001). CTCF is a uniquely versatile transcription regulator linked to epigenetics and disease. *Trends Genet* 17, 520-7.
Ohno, M., Tenzen, T., Watanabe, Y., Yamagata, T., Kanaya, S. and Ikemura, T. (2000). Non-B DNA structures spatially and sequence-specifically associated with individual centromeres in the human interphase nuleus. In *Chromosomes Today*, vol. 13 (ed. E. Olmo and C. A. Redi), pp. 57-69. Berlin: Birkhauser.
Ohno, S. (1967). Sex Chromosomes and sex-linked genes. Berlin: Springer-Verlag
Ohno, S., Jainchill, J. and Stenius, C. (1963). The Creeping Vole (Microtus Oregoni) as a Gonosomic Mosaic. I. The Oy/Xy Constitution of the Male. *Cytogenetics* 14, 232-9.
Orlando, V., Strutt, H. and Paro, R. (1997). Analysis of chromatin structure by in vivo formaldehyde cross-linking. *Methods* 11, 205-14.
Osborne, C. S., Chakalova, L., Brown, K. E., Carter, D., Horton, A., Debrand, E., Goyenechea, B., Mitchell, J. A., Lopes, S., Reik, W. et al. (2004). Active genes dynamically colocalize to shared sites of ongoing transcription. *Nat Genet* 36, 1065-71.
Paixao, S., Colaluca, I. N., Cubells, M., Peverali, F. A., Destro, A., Giadrossi, S., Giacca, M., Falaschi, A., Riva, S. and Biamonti, G. (2004). Modular structure of the human lamin B2 replicator. *Mol Cell Biol* 24, 2958-67.
Pappas, D. L., Jr., Frisch, R. and Weinreich, M. (2004). The NAD(+)-dependent Sir2p histone deacetylase is a negative regulator of chromosomal DNA replication. *Genes Dev* 18, 769-81.
Parelho, V., Hadjur, S., Spivakov, M., Leleu, M., Sauer, S., Gregson, H. C., Jarmuz, A., Canzonetta, C., Webster, Z., Nesterova, T. et al. (2008). Cohesins functionally associate with CTCF on mammalian chromosome arms. *Cell* 132, 422-33.
Pasero, P., Bensimon, A. and Schwob, E. (2002). Single-molecule analysis reveals clustering and epigenetic regulation of replication origins at the yeast rDNA locus. *Genes Dev* 16, 2479-84.
Phillips, J. E. and Corces, V. G. (2009). CTCF: master weaver of the genome. *Cell* 137, 1194-211.
Raghuraman, M. K., Winzeler, E. A., Collingwood, D., Hunt, S., Wodicka, L., Conway, A., Lockhart, D. J., Davis, R. W., Brewer, B. J. and Fangman, W. L. (2001). Replication dynamics of the yeast genome. *Science* 294, 115-21.
Renfree, M. B., Papenfuss, A. T., Shaw, G. and Pask, A. J. (2009). Eggs, embryos and the evolution of imprinting: insights from the platypus genome. *Reproduction, Fertility and Development* 21, 935-942.
Rens, W., O'Brien, P. C., Grutzner, F., Clarke, O., Graphodatskaya, D., Tsend-Ayush, E., Trifonov, V. A., Skelton, H., Wallis, M. C., Johnston, S. et al. (2007). The multiple sex chromosomes of platypus and echidna are not completely identical and several share homology with the avian Z. *Genome Biol* 8, R243.
Rothstein, R., Michel, B. and Gangloff, S. (2000). Replication fork pausing and recombination or "gimme a break". *Genes Dev* 14, 1-10.
Rubio, E. D., Reiss, D. J., Welcsh, P. L., Disteche, C. M., Filippova, G. N., Baliga, N. S., Aebersold, R., Ranish, J. A. and Krumm, A. (2008). CTCF physically links cohesin to chromatin. *Proc Natl Acad Sci U S A* 105, 8309-14.

Ryba, T., Hiratani, I., Lu, J., Itoh, M., Kulik, M., Zhang, J., Schulz, T. C., Robins, A. J., Dalton, S. and Gilbert, D. M. (2010). Evolutionarily conserved replication timing profiles predict long-range chromatin interactions and distinguish closely related cell types. *Genome Res* 20, 761-70.

Sadoni, N., Langer, S., Fauth, C., Bernardi, G., Cremer, T., Turner, B. M. and Zink, D. (1999). Nuclear organization of mammalian genomes. Polar chromosome territories build up functionally distinct higher order compartments. *J Cell Biol* 146, 1211-26.

Saha, S., Shan, Y., Mesner, L. D. and Hamlin, J. L. (2004). The promoter of the Chinese hamster ovary dihydrofolate reductase gene regulates the activity of the local origin and helps define its boundaries. *Genes Dev* 18, 397-410.

Schaarschmidt, D., Baltin, J., Stehle, I. M., Lipps, H. J. and Knippers, R. (2004). An episomal mammalian replicon: sequence-independent binding of the origin recognition complex. *EMBO J* 23, 191-201.

Schempp, W. and Schmid, M. (1981). Chromosome banding in Amphibia. VI. BrdU-replication patterns in anura and demonstration of XX/XY sex chromosomes in Rana esculenta. *Chromosoma* 83, 697-710.

Schmid, M., Enderle, E., Schindler, D. and Schempp, W. (1989). Chromosome banding and DNA replication patterns in bird karyotypes. *Cytogenet Cell Genet* 52, 139-46.

Schweizer, D., Loidl, J. and Hamilton, B. (1987). Heterochromatin and the phenomenon of chromosome banding. *Results Probl Cell Differ* 14, 235-54.

Selig, S., Okumura, K., Ward, D. C. and Cedar, H. (1992). Delineation of DNA replication time zones by fluorescence in situ hybridization. *EMBO J* 11, 1217-25.

Serizawa, S., Miyamichi, K., Nakatani, H., Suzuki, M., Saito, M., Yoshihara, Y. and Sakano, H. (2003). Negative feedback regulation ensures the one receptor-one olfactory neuron rule in mouse. *Science* 302, 2088-94.

Shevchenko, A. I., Zakharova, I. S., Elisaphenko, E. A., Kolesnikov, N. N., Whitehead, S., Bird, C., Ross, M., Weidman, J. R., Jirtle, R. L., Karamysheva, T. V. et al. (2007). Genes flanking Xist in mouse and human are separated on the X chromosome in American marsupials. *Chromosome Res* 15, 127-36.

Shreeram, S., Sparks, A., Lane, D. P. and Blow, J. J. (2002). Cell type-specific responses of human cells to inhibition of replication licensing. *Oncogene* 21, 6624-32.

Simon, I., Tenzen, T., Reubinoff, B. E., Hillman, D., McCarrey, J. R. and Cedar, H. (1999). Asynchronous replication of imprinted genes is established in the gametes and maintained during development. *Nature* 401, 929-32.

Simonis, M., Klous, P., Splinter, E., Moshkin, Y., Willemsen, R., de Wit, E., van Steensel, B. and de Laat, W. (2006). Nuclear organization of active and inactive chromatin domains uncovered by chromosome conformation capture-on-chip (4C). *Nat Genet* 38, 1348-54.

Singh, N., Ebrahimi, F. A., Gimelbrant, A. A., Ensminger, A. W., Tackett, M. R., Qi, P., Gribnau, J. and Chess, A. (2003). Coordination of the random asynchronous replication of autosomal loci. *Nat Genet* 33, 339-41.

Spiesser, T., Klipp, E. and Barberis, M. (2009). A model for the spatiotemporal organization of DNA replication in <i>Saccharomyces cerevisiae</i>. *Molecular Genetics and Genomics* 282, 25-35.

State, M. W., Greally, J. M., Cuker, A., Bowers, P. N., Henegariu, O., Morgan, T. M., Gunel, M., DiLuna, M., King, R. A., Nelson, C. et al. (2003). Epigenetic abnormalities associated with a chromosome 18(q21-q22) inversion and a Gilles de la Tourette syndrome phenotype. *Proc Natl Acad Sci U S A* 100, 4684-9.

Takagi, N. (1974). Differentiation of X chromosomes in early female mouse embryos. *Exp Cell Res* 86, 127-35.

Takagi, N., Sugawara, O. and Sasaki, M. (1982). Regional and temporal changes in the pattern of X-chromosome replication during the early post-implantation development of the female mouse. *Chromosoma* 85, 275-86.

Takahashi, M. (1987). A model for the spatio-temporal organization of DNA replication in mammalian cells. *J Theor Biol* 129, 91-115.

Tanaka, S. and Diffley, J. F. (2002). Deregulated G1-cyclin expression induces genomic instability by preventing efficient pre-RC formation. *Genes Dev* 16, 2639-49.

Taylor, J. H. (1977). Increase in DNA replication sites in cells held at the beginning of S phase. *Chromosoma* 62, 291-300.

Veyrunes, F., Waters, P. D., Miethke, P., Rens, W., McMillan, D., Alsop, A. E., Grutzner, F., Deakin, J. E., Whittington, C. M., Schatzkamer, K. et al. (2008). Bird-like sex chromosomes of platypus imply recent origin of mammal sex chromosomes. *Genome Res* 18, 965-73.

Wakefield, M. J., Keohane, A. M., Turner, B. M. and Graves, J. A. (1997). Histone underacetylation is an ancient component of mammalian X chromosome inactivation. *Proc Natl Acad Sci U S A* 94, 9665-8.

Wang, L., Lin, C. M., Brooks, S., Cimbora, D., Groudine, M. and Aladjem, M. I. (2004). The human beta-globin replication initiation region consists of two modular independent replicators. *Mol Cell Biol* 24, 3373-86.

Watanabe, Y., Abe, T., Ikemura, T. and Maekawa, M. (2009). Relationships between replication timing and GC content of cancer-related genes on human chromosomes 11q and 21q. *Gene* 433, 26-31.

Watanabe, Y., Fujiyama, A., Ichiba, Y., Hattori, M., Yada, T., Sakaki, Y. and Ikemura, T. (2002). Chromosome-wide assessment of replication timing for human chromosomes 11q and 21q: disease-related genes in timing-switch regions. *Hum Mol Genet* 11, 13-21.

Watanabe, Y., Ikemura, T. and Sugimura, H. (2004). Amplicons on human chromosome 11q are located in the early/late-switch regions of replication timing. *Genomics* 84, 796-805.

Watanabe, Y. and Maekawa, M. (2010). Spatiotemporal regulation of DNA replication in the human genome and its association with genomic instability and disease. *Curr Med Chem* 17, 222-33.

Watanabe, Y., Shibata, K., Sugimura, H. and Maekawa, M. (2007). p53-Dependent change in replication timing of the human genome. *Biochemical and Biophysical Research Communications* 364, 289-293.

Weidman, J. R., Murphy, S. K., Nolan, C. M., Dietrich, F. S. and Jirtle, R. L. (2004). Phylogenetic footprint analysis of IGF2 in extant mammals. *Genome Res* 14, 1726-32.

Wilson, N. D., Ross, L. J., Close, J., Mott, R., Crow, T. J. and Volpi, E. V. (2007). Replication profile of PCDH11X and PCDH11Y, a gene pair located in the non-pseudoautosomal homologous region Xq21.3/Yp11.2. *Chromosome Res* 15, 485-98.

Woodward, A. M., Gohler, T., Luciani, M. G., Oehlmann, M., Ge, X., Gartner, A., Jackson, D. A. and Blow, J. J. (2006). Excess Mcm2-7 license dormant origins of replication that can be used under conditions of replicative stress. *J Cell Biol* 173, 673-83.

Wrigley, J. M. and Graves, J. A. (1988). Sex chromosome homology and incomplete, tissue-specific X-inactivation suggest that monotremes represent an intermediate stage of mammalian sex chromosome evolution. *J Hered* 79, 115-8.

Wutz, A. and Jaenisch, R. (2000). A shift from reversible to irreversible X inactivation is triggered during ES cell differentiation. *Mol Cell* 5, 695-705.

Yusufzai, T. M., Tagami, H., Nakatani, Y. and Felsenfeld, G. (2004). CTCF Tethers an Insulator to Subnuclear Sites, Suggesting Shared Insulator Mechanisms across Species. *Molecular Cell* 13, 291-298.

Zakharova, I. S., Shevchenko, A. I. and Zakian, S. M. (2009). Monoallelic gene expression in mammals. *Chromosoma* 118, 279-90.

Zhao, Z., Tavoosidana, G., Sjolinder, M., Gondor, A., Mariano, P., Wang, S., Kanduri, C., Lezcano, M., Sandhu, K. S., Singh, U. et al. (2006). Circular chromosome conformation capture (4C) uncovers extensive networks of epigenetically regulated intra- and interchromosomal interactions. *Nat Genet* 38, 1341-7.

Zink, D., Bornfleth, H., Visser, A., Cremer, C. and Cremer, T. (1999). Organization of early and late replicating DNA in human chromosome territories. *Exp Cell Res* 247, 176-88.

21

The Silencing Face of DNA Replication: Gene Repression Mediated by DNA Replication Factors

Patricia Chisamore-Robert, Daniel Jeffery and Krassimir Yankulov
Department of Molecular and Cellular Biology, University of Guelph
Canada

1. Introduction

DNA replication in eukaryotes initiates at multiple origins. The activation of these origins is a critically important event in the life of each cell and is tightly regulated by numerous highly conserved trans-factors.

Saccharomyces cerevisiae origins (called Autonomously Replicating Sequences, *ARSs*) contain a core *A* element called *ACS* (*ARS* Consensus Sequence), plus an array of auxiliary *B* elements. Most *ARSs* fire at their chromosomal positions, but there are numerous dormant *ARSs* as well. Instead of being origins, these dormant *ARSs* serve as *silencer* elements, which function in the epigenetic repression of nearby genes. Even more, many DNA replication trans-factors have also been reported to affect gene silencing. This puzzling functional duality of *ARS* and DNA replication factors has attracted significant interest. Evidence from other species has suggested that the overlap between gene silencing and DNA replication operates in other eukaryotes. In this chapter we will review in detail the activity of *ARSs* as origins of replication and as silencers. We will focus on sequence dissimilarities between silencer and origin *ARSs* and will propose a model for the functional duality of DNA replication factors.

1.1 Origins of DNA replication in *S.cerevisiae*

Eukaryotic origins of DNA replication display a significant inter-species diversity. In higher eukaryotes this diversity reaches a point where origin locations are difficult to identify by homology search (Mechali, 2010). A remarkable exception of this diversity occurs in the yeast *S.cerevisiae.* In this organism the first functional origins have been identified by screens for DNA elements which confer DNA replication on plasmids (Stinchcomb *et al.*, 1979; Chan & Tye, 1980; Kearsey, 1983). Comparison between these autonomously replicating sequences (*ARSs*) have shown that they encompass approximately 200bp of DNA and contain perfect or one-base mismatches to the 11 bp *ARS* consensus sequence (*ACS*) 5'-WTTAYRTTTW-3' (where W=A/T; Y=C/T; R=A/G). Linker scanning substitutions in several *ARSs* have determined that the *ACS* is the sole essential element for DNA replication (Marahrens & Stillman, 1992; Rao *et al.*, 1994; Lin & Kowalski, 1997; Chang *et al.*, 2008). However, auxiliary *B* elements (*B1-B4*) within *ARSs* are also necessary for full origin activity (Marahrens & Stillman, 1992; Lin & Kowalski, 1997). The *B2*, *B3* and *B4* elements are not present in all *ARSs*. *B2* is a site for the unwinding of DNA while *B3* is a binding site for Abf1p (*ARS*-binding factor 1), which is a protein involved in numerous chromatin-associated functions including DNA replication, gene silencing, transcriptional activation and DNA repair (Rehman & Yankulov, 2009). The function of *B4* is unknown, but its mutation reduces replicator activity (Lin & Kowalski, 1997). Interestingly, the destruction of more than one of the *B* elements substantially reduces origin firing activity (Marahrens & Stillman, 1992) and *ACS* alone is not sufficient to confer replicator activity at natural yeast chromosomes (Raghuraman *et al.*, 2001).

The *B1* element, along with the *ACS*, is found in all known *ARSs* and forms a bipartite binding site for the Origin Recognition Complex (ORC) (Rao & Stillman, 1995). However, the *B1* sequence is not nearly as conserved as *ACS*. The cross-*ARS* homology at the putative position of *B1* has been identified as a WTW motif found 17-19 bp upstream of the *ACS* (Chang *et al.*, 2008) or an AWnY (W=A/T; Y=C/T; n=any nucleotide) motif 16 bases upstream of *ACS* (Palacios DeBeer *et al.*, 2003). Even more, the whole region upstream of *ACS* is A/T rich thus providing multiple nearby WTW/AWnY motifs. Ultimately, the precise position of *B1* and its significance remains somewhat elusive.

1.2 *ARSs* initiate replication

A wealth of information has been accumulated on the mechanisms by which *ARSs* initiate DNA replication (Fig. 1). ORC, which is built of six different Orc proteins, binds the *ACS-B1* elements to nucleate the formation of the pre-replicative complexes (Blow & Dutta, 2005; Labib, 2010). Shortly after mitosis, Cdt1p and Cdc6p recruit the heterohexameric MCM complex to the *ARS*-bound ORC. Thus, *ARSs* are poised to initiate DNA replication upon receiving a regulatory stimulus. This stimulus is provided in S-phase by two protein kinases, DDK and CDK2 (Labib, 2010). It seems that the critical event in the stimulation of origins is the phosphorylation of Mcm4p (Sheu & Stillman, 2010) by DDK. However, other components of the pre-initiation complex are also phosphorylated with similar timing (Labib, 2010). These events culminate in the activation of the MCM helicase, in the unwinding of origin DNA and in the assembly of the DNA replication machinery.

There are about 12 000 matches or near-matches to *ACS* in the genome of *S. cerevisiae* (Nieduszynski *et al.*, 2006). Of these, only 500-700 are loaded with ORC and MCM proteins (Wyrick *et al.*, 2001) and only about 400 initiate DNA replication (Raghuraman *et al.*, 2001). In general, the early firing origins are located in the central portion of the chromosomes, while the later firing origins are found at the periphery (Raghuraman *et al.*, 2001). It is believed that the same initiation events take place at all origins of DNA replication, but at different times throughout S-phase. Interestingly, the dormant origins positioned in the immediate subtelomeric regions or at the mating type loci (see below) also recruit the ORC and the MCM complexes (Wyrick *et al.*, 2001; Rehman *et al.*, 2006), but seldom if at all fire. It is not known how DDK, CDK2 and other initiation factors are regulated to confer the temporal pattern of origin firing, how they discriminate dormant origins or how all these events are coordinated.

The disparity between loading and firing of *ARSs* in *S.cerevisiae* is reminiscent to the situation in metazoans, where tens of thousands of genomic positions are primed as origins, but only a small subset actually fire. It is believed that this excess of available origins can accommodate the significant differences in growth conditions during metazoan development as well as the substantial variation in chromatin structure in different cell types (Mechali, 2010). For example, local chromatin structure, transcription and/or different environmental and physiological conditions will contribute to the selection of the most suitable origins. In this way, unnecessary interference with gene expression or the disturbance of established heterochromatin domains will be avoided.

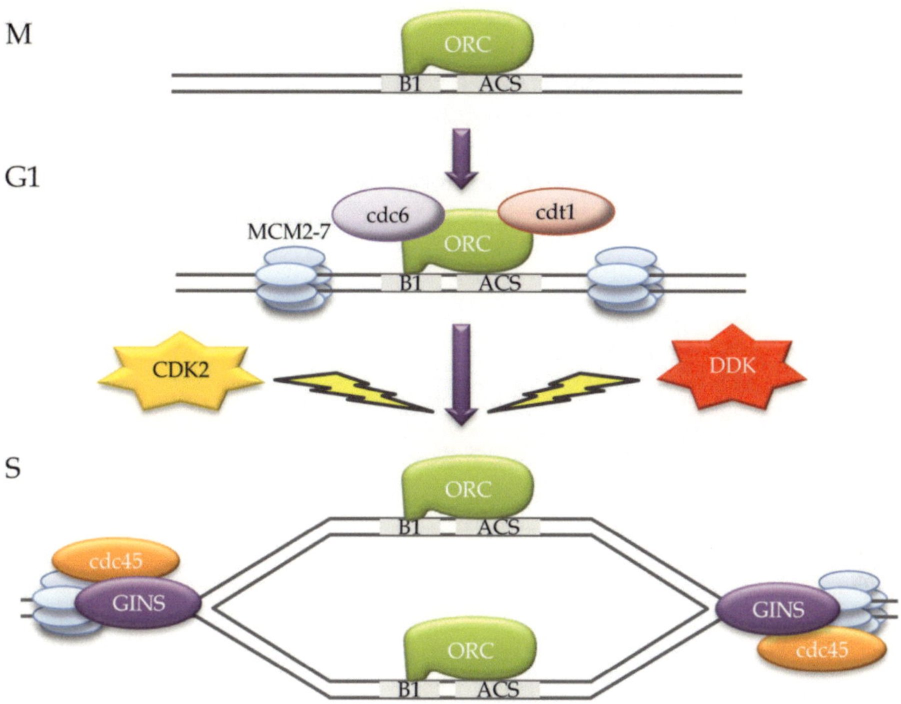

Fig. 1. Origin activation in *S.cerevisiae* - ORC binds the *ACS-B1* elements. In early G1 phase, ORC recruits Cdc6p and Cdt1p. In turn, Cdc6p and Cdt1p load the hexameric helicase complex MCM2-7. In the G1/S transition, the Dbf4-dependent kinase DDK (also known as Cdc7p) and the Clb5-dependent kinase CDK2 (Cdc28p) phosphorylate the MCM2-7 complexes to trigger their helicase activity. DDK also phosphorylates Cdc45p, which is then able to recruit the GINS and other elongation factors for the progression of DNA replication.

The so-called Jesuit model ("For many are called, but few are chosen" (Matthew 22:14, the Bible)) has been proposed to explain the limited firing of origins. This model implicates that the considerable flexibility of DNA replication programs is most likely controlled by the abundance of pre-replicative complex factors (such as ORC and MCM2-7) and a corresponding limitation of initiation factors (such as Cdc45, Cdc7p and CDK2) (DePamphilis, 1993). Budding yeast provides an interesting twist to this model. Not only are certain origins chosen to fire while others are not, but some of the non-firing origins aqcuire a completely new role and contribute to the local silencing of genes.

1.3 *ARSs* act as silencers

Eukaryotic genes are regulated by a variety of mechanisms including complete silencing *via* condensed heterochromatin structure. The condensed/relaxed chromatin structures are faithfully transmitted to daughter cells thus ensuring the continuity of gene expression programs. This intriguing epigenetic phenomenon has been extensively studied at the mating type (*HMR***a** and *HMLα*) (Fig. 2) and at the telomeric loci (Fig. 3) of *S.cerevisiae.* At all these loci the critical role in gene silencing is played by the SIR (Silent Information Regulator) proteins (Rusche *et al.*, 2003). Through contacts with DNA-binding proteins, Sir1p, Sir3p and Sir4p recruit the Histone-Deacetylase Sir2p. In turn, Sir2p deacetylates the tails of H3/H4 histones on the nearby nucleosome. Additional Sir3p and Sir4p then associate with the deacetylated histone tails to recruit more Sir2p and expand the domain of deacetylated nucleosomes. Ultimately, the deacetylation of histones culminates in the establishment of compacted heterochromatin, which suppresses gene expression. The spreading of SIR proteins is countered by Histone-Acetyl-Transferases and other factors, whose identity and modes of action are not so well understood (Lafon *et al.*, 2007; Ehrentraut *et al.*, 2010).

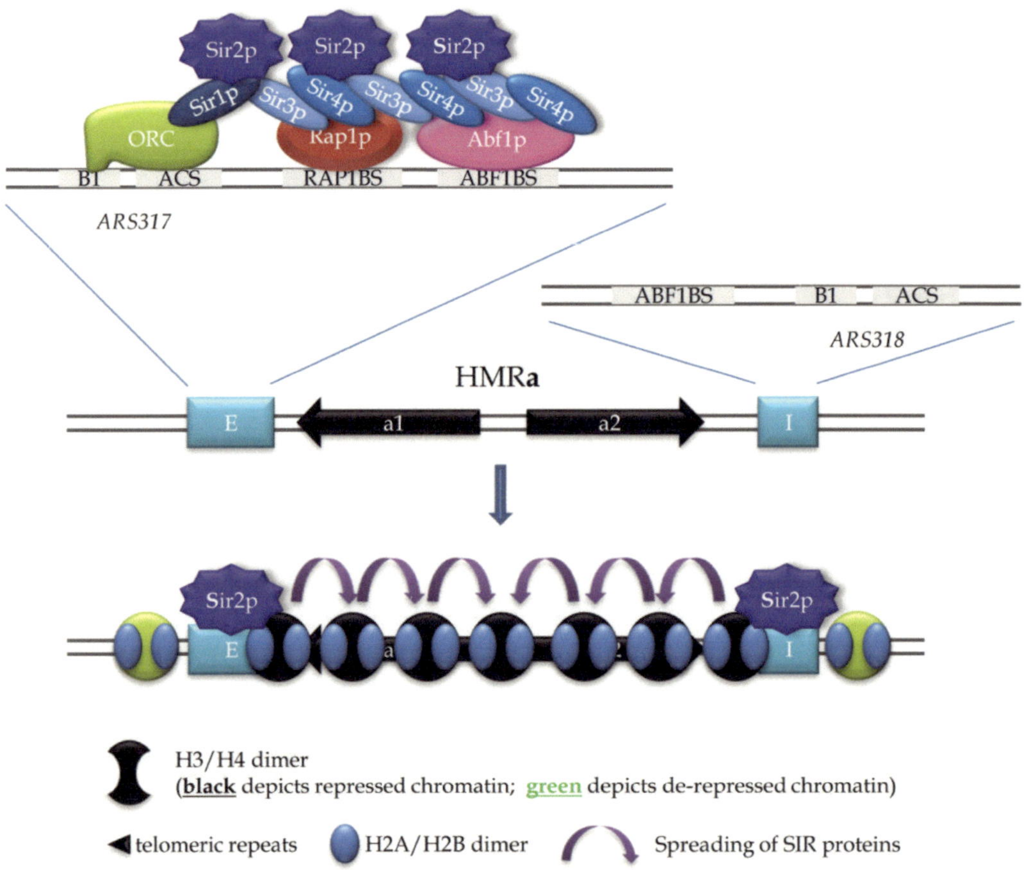

Fig. 2. Gene silencing at the *HMR***a** locus - *ARS317* and *ARS318* recruit ORC (only recruitment by *ARS317* is shown), which in turn recruits Sir1p. Both Rap1p and Abf1p recruit Sir3p and Sir4p. The tethering of Sir1,3,4p confers the nucleation of the silenced domain and recruits Sir2p. Sir2p deacetylates adjacent histone tails, which recruit more Sir3p/Sir4p and contribute to the spreading of SIR proteins, as demonstrated (blue arrow).

The silent mating type loci, *HMR***a** and *HMLα*, are constitutively and completely repressed by robust heterochromatin structure. The genes encoded by these loci are expressed only when translocated to the *MAT* locus (Rusche *et al.*, 2003). In turn, the *MAT* locus can accomodate and express only the **a** or the α genes. In this way, it is gauranteed that no erraneous expression of the two opposing mating types occurs.

*HMR***a** and *HMLα* are each flanked by *E* and *I* silencers (Fig. 2). Remarkably, *ARSs* have been identified as essential elements in all four silencers of the these loci (Abraham *et al.*, 1983; Broach *et al.*, 1983; Rusche *et al.*, 2003). For example, the *HMR***a**-*E* silencer contains *ARS317* as well as binding sites for Rap1p and Abf1p, whereas the *HMR***a**-*I* silencer contains *ARS318* and an Abf1p binding site (Fig. 2). Depending on the genomic context, both Abf1p and Rap1p bind to gene silencers or activator elements (Shore & Nasmyth, 1987; Shore *et al.*, 1987). Just as in replication origins, ORC binds to the bipartite *ACS-B1* of the *ARSs* in the mating type loci silencers. However, instead of recruiting replication machinery, the Orc1p subunit of ORC recruits Sir1p, while Rap1p and Abf1p bind and recruit Sir3p and Sir4p. As shown in Fig. 2, Sir1p, Sir3p and Sir4p recruit Sir2p to establish a focal point of silencing and initiate the spreading of the SIR proteins. Similar events take place at *ARS318* in the *HMR***a**-*I* silencer.

It is important to note that the *ARSs* of the mating type loci are not substantially different from replicator *ARSs*. Both types of *ARS* bind to ORC *in vivo* and *in vitro* (Palacios DeBeer *et al.*, 2003). If placed on a plasmid, the silencer *ARSs* act as perfectly good origins of DNA replication (Chan & Tye, 1980). The opposite is also true; replicator *ARSs* can acquire silencer activity when inserted in the mating type loci (McNally & Rine, 1991; Weinreich *et al.*, 2004; Casey *et al.*, 2008).

1.4 *ARSs* act as proto-silencers

ARSs also play a somewhat similar silencing role at the telomeres (Fig. 3). At these loci, the telomeric repeats act as the principal silencers while *ARSs* have a silencer-enhancing role (Fourel *et al.*, 2002). The telomeric $TG_{1\text{-}3}$ repeats provide multiple binding sites for Rap1p. Similar to the mating type loci, Rap1p recruits Sir3p and Sir4p to establish the initiation point for the SIR protein spreading (Fourel *et al.*, 2002; Rusche *et al.*, 2003). *ARSs* and Sir1p are not required for this step. However, the absence of subtelomeric *ARSs* or Sir1p significantly reduces the span of the silenced domain and its stability while the artificial tethering of Sir1p to the telomere boosts the silencing of nearby genes (Chien *et al.*, 1993). Thus, subtelomeric *ARSs* and their ability to recruit Sir1p through Orc1p play an important, yet secondary role in gene silencing at the telomeres. At other locations, isolated *ARSs* do not induce gene repression, but can boost the activity of an existing silencer. For this reason they were classified as proto-silencers (Fourel *et al.*, 2002).

The complexity of telomeric silencing does not end there. Besides *ARSs*, the repetitive *Core X* and *Y'* elements in the sub-telomere also contain isolated Rap1p and Abf1p binding sites. All these act as weak multiple proto-silencers. In addition, the *Core X* and *Y'* elements harbour anti-silencer modules called sub-telomeric anti-silencing regions (STARs) (Fourel *et al.*, 1999; Fourel *et al.*, 2004; Power, 2011). The combined assembly of proto-silencers and weak anti-silencers produces a multitude of variations in the strength, stability and spreading of telomeric silencing (Fourel *et al.*, 2004). Even more, *Core X* and *Y'* elements contain isolated clusters of telomeric $TG_{1\text{-}3}$ repeats and are able to interact with the telomeres forming t-loop and D-loop structures. The folding back of telomeric DNA brings the SIR

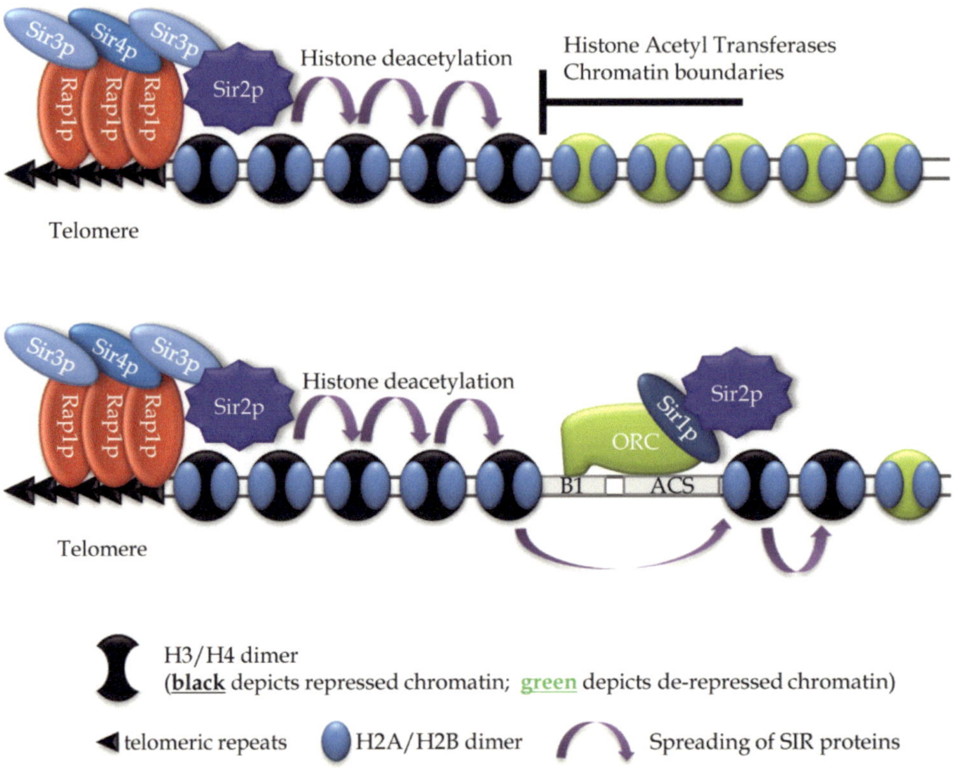

Fig. 3. Gene silencing at the telomeres - Rap1p binds to the telomere and recruits Sir3p and Sir4p. The recruitment of Sir2p and the spreading of SIR proteins is as explained in the text. Subtelomeric *ARSs* recruit ORC and Sir1p and enhance the spreading of SIR proteins and histone deacetylation away from the telomeres. This spreading is countered by Histone-Acetyl-Transferases and is limited by chromatin boundaries and insulators. Repressed chromatin acts to silence any genes wrapped within it while genes within de-repressed chromatin remain active.

proteins bound to the telomeric repeats into close proximity with those bound to the subtelomeric *Core X* element. This interaction creates a highly condensed heterochromatic structure in a specific region of the sub-telomere while the stretch of DNA between the *Core X* and the telomere may actually be euchromatic. The formation of these fold-back structures generates discontinuous telomeric silencing and strong silencing domains can be formed many kilobases away from the telomere (Pryde & Louis, 1999; Fourel *et al.*, 2004). Importantly, as any other *ARSs*, telomeric proto-silencer *ARSs* also contain a normal *ACS-B1* module, bind ORC and act as origins when placed on mini-chromosomes (Wyrick *et al.*, 2001; Rusche *et al.*, 2003; Chan & Tye, 1980).

2. Results

2.1 What determines the activity of *ARSs*?

As mentioned earlier, replicator and silencer *ARSs* are almost completely interchangeable. For example, *ARSs* derived from origins can recapture the silencer activity in *HMR***a** and the proto-silencer activity at the telomere when transferred to these positions (Palacios DeBeer *et al.*, 2003; Weinreich *et al.*, 2004; Casey *et al.*, 2008; Rehman *et al.*, 2009). Telomeric and silencer *ARSs* also act as replicators when moved to a plasmid (Chan & Tye, 1983). Even more, many *bona fide* DNA replication factors have also been identified as silencing factors and mutations in them affect both the efficiency of origins and the epigenetic silencing at telomeres and the mating type loci (Axelrod & Rine, 1991; Ehrenhofer-Murray *et al.*, 1999; Rehman *et al.*, 2006).

So, what confers the functional plasticity of *ARSs*? The fair answer is that we do not really know. Many studies have correlated the efficiency of origins to their proximity to heterochromatin (Weinreich *et al.*, 2004; Field *et al.*, 2008; Mechali, 2010). Indeed, origins in compact chromatin tend to fire less frequently than origins in open chromatin. It is conceivable that open chromatin is necessary for the assembly of the pre-replicative complexes (Doyon *et al.*, 2006; Espinosa *et al.*, 2010). However, chromatin structure is not the only regulator of origin activity. For example, in the mini-chromosome maintenance assay, (which involves the transfer of different origins to a plasmid and examining their efficiency under the same genetic context), it was found that different *ARSs* fire at different rates and support different levels of DNA replication (Chan & Tye, 1980; Chang *et al.*, 2008). These observations immediately suggest that variation in the sequence of *ARSs* must also play a role in the fine tuning of *ARS* function.

The next step was to take highly efficient *ARSs* from euchromatic regions and insert them into heterochromatic regions known to have poor replication initiation efficiency. Consequently, the high efficiency of the *ARSs* was lost, showing that the genomic context was powerful enough to overcome the effects of the sequence variation (Weinreich *et al.*, 2004). However, a parallel change in the activity of *ARSs* has been discovered. Not only were the relocated *ARSs* showing reduced replication and late firing, they were now boosting the epigenetic silencing of the nearby genes, contrary to their activities in their native chromosomal locations. A fine twist to these phenomena is that the replicator *ARSs* did not make perfect silencers (Casey *et al.*, 2008) or proto-silencers (Rehman *et al.*, 2009), reflecting the fact that silencer *ARSs* sometimes do not make perfect replicators (Chang *et al.*, 2008; Palacios DeBeer *et al.*, 2003). It is not clear how the new chromatin environment of the relocated *ARSs* has contributed to their functional conversions.

This leads us to the question: is there any feature of an *ARS* that determines its predisposition to act as a silencer or a replicator? We and others have recently aligned a number of *ARSs* in search for some correlation between sequence and function. It was possible to delineate a *B1* element consensus (WTW) from the origins on chromosome III (Chang *et al.*, 2008). However, silencer and telomeric *ARSs* showed even lower conservation of this *B1* element compared to other *ARSs* (Rehman & Yankulov, 2009). Another line of evidence has previously shown that *B1* can modulate the affinity of *ACS-B1* to ORC *in vitro* and that silencer *ACS-B1* have higher affinity to ORC (Palacios DeBeer *et al.*, 2003).

We have hypothesised that the mode of ORC association to *ACS-B1* can ultimately influence how well an *ARS* will act as an origin or a silencer. If this is the case, variations in the *B1* element and its flanking sequences can potentially contribute to the functional conversions of *ARSs*. For example, if *B1* causes ORC to acquire a specific conformation and higher affinity, ORC could end up recruiting the silencing machinery through the Orc1p-Sir1p interaction. In addition, it is also possible that the orientation of *ACS-B1* towards another silencer could have an impact on the conformation of ORC, again promoting epigenetic silencing rather than replicator function. In both situations, *ACS-B1* should provide for a significant level of flexibility of ORC, which in turn should allow the acquisition of silencer/replicator function depending on the chromatin context. In the following sections we will present our on-going studies that are testing these models.

2.2 Destruction of *B1* has different effects in silencer and replicator *ARSs*

Initial assessment of the role of the *B1* element has been performed on two well characterised *ARSs*, the replicator *ARS1* and the telomeric proto-silencer *ARS319* (Fig. 4). We inserted these origins with an adjacent *URA3* reporter in the left telomere of chromosome *VII* and assessed the level of repression by a routine assay for the sensitivity of cells to FOA (5-Fluoro-Orotic Acid). FOA is a neutral substance, which is turned into a toxin by the *URA3*-encoded Orotidine-5'-phosphate-decarboxylase. Hence, cells with repressed *URA3* will grow in the presence of FOA, while cells expressing *URA3* will be sensitive to FOA. After transforming with the integrating constructs, cells were selected on media without uracil (SC-ura) and telomeric integration was confirmed by PCR. The transformed cells were then grown in non-selective media for 15-20 generations to reach equilibrium of epigenetically repressed and transcribed *URA3* and then plated on non-selective plates and plates containing FOA. The proportion of cells with repressed *URA3* (%FOA^R) was assessed as the number of colonies on plates containing FOA (SC+FOA) divided by the number of colonies on non-selective plates. The difference in %FOA^R values is indicative of the difference in the levels of silencing at the analysed locus.

These analyses revealed that the destruction of the *B1* element (TTT→ccT) in *ARS1* moderately reduced the %FOA^R values suggesting that this *B1* element contributes to the overall gene silencing at telomeres (Fig. 4). Exactly the same mutation has also significantly reduced the replicator activity of *ARS1* (Marahrens & Stillman, 1992). Surprisingly, the destruction of the putative *B1* element (ATT→ccT) of *ARS319* had very little effect on telomeric silencing (Fig. 4) and only moderately reduced the replicator activity of *ARS319* (Chang *et al.*, 2008). These puzzling results suggest that *ARS319* does not possess an ordinary *B1* element. It is possible that *B1* in *ARS319* is offset from the customary position found in other *ARSs*. Alternatively, *ARS319* has a broader *B1* element that is not affected by the replacement of only two nucleotides.

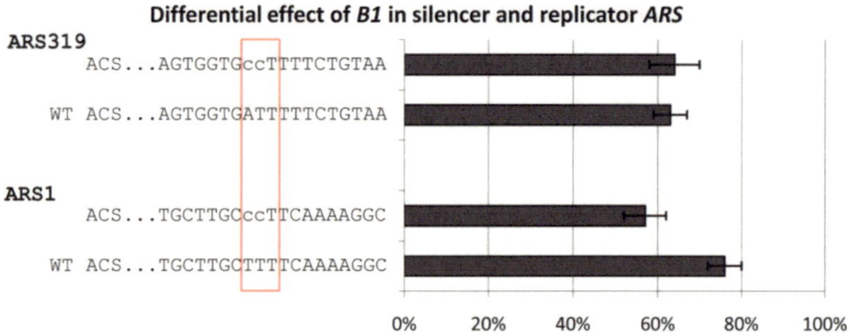

Fig. 4. Differential effect of *B1* in silencers and replicators – FOA sensitivity assays were performed to assess the level of silencing in mutant and *wild type* proto-silencer (*ARS319*) and replicator (*ARS1*) *ARSs* at the *VII-L* telomere in *S.cerevisiae*. Average %FOA^R with standard errors are shown. The hypothesized *B1* WTW motif is indicated by the red rectangle. Site-directed mutations are indicated by lower-case letters above the *wild type* (WT) sequences.

2.3 Scanning mutations of the *B1* element in a silencer *ARS* show little effect on its silencing and replicator activity

ARS317 is a well-characterised core component of the *HMR***a**-*E* silencer. Similar to the proto-silencer *ARS319*, mutations in the putative *B1* element (TTA→Tcc) of *ARS317* have little effect on its replicator activity (Chang *et al.*, 2008). In order to assess the role of the *ARS317-B1* element in gene silencing, we performed a two-nucleotide substitution scanning mutagenesis of the region encompassing its putative *B1* (Fig. 5). All *ACS-b1* mutants were cloned next to *URA3* and inserted in the left telomere of chromosome *VII* as before. The level of repression of *URA3* was assessed by the FOA sensitivity assay as described in the previous section. The results indicated that the destruction of the WTW motif (TTA→ccA or TTA→TTc) did not reduce, but actually slightly increased the silencing of *URA3* (Fig. 5). The only moderate decrease in silencing was observed in the construct 1.5, where a GC pair proximal to *ACS* was replaced with an AA (GC→aa). This result is somewhat surprising as G/C bases do not conform to the general A/T rich nature of this region. In conclusion, the canonical *B1* elements of both *ARS317* and *ARS319* seemed dispensable for silencer function (Fig. 4 and Fig. 5) and had little or no effect on the replicator activity of these *ARSs* (Chang *et al.*, 2008).

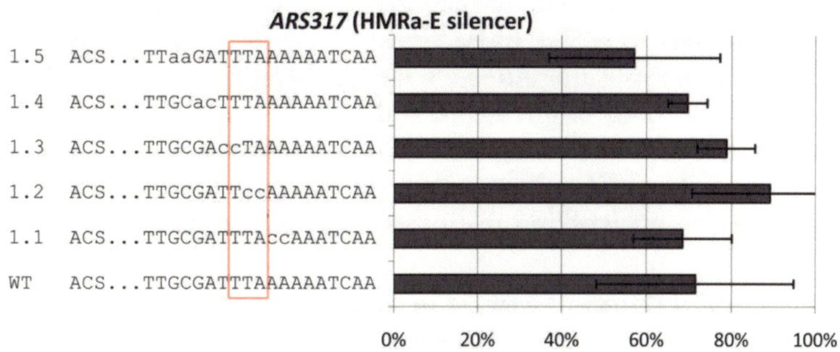

Fig. 5. FOA sensitivity of scanning mutations in *B1* in *ARS317* - FOA sensitivity assays were performed to assess the level of silencing in five mutants (1.1-1.5) and *wild type* (WT) *ARS317* at the *VII-L* telomere in *S.cerevisiae*. Average %FOA^R with standard errors are shown. The hypothesized *B1* WTW motif is indicated by the red rectangle. Site-directed substitution constructs are indicated by lower-case letters above the *wild type* (WT) sequence.

2.4 Scanning mutations of the *B1* element of a replicator *ARS* affect both silencer and replicator function

We conducted a similar scanning mutagenesis analysis of the *B1* element in one of the most active origins of DNA replication in the genome of *S.cerevisiae, ARS305* (Huang & Kowalski, 1996). Two-nucleotide substitutions were introduced at the positions shown in Fig. 6 and the mutant *ACS-b1* constructs were attached to *URA3*. These reporter cassettes were inserted in the left telomere of chromosome *VII* and analysed for the levels of *URA3* repression. The analysis showed that, similar to *ARS1*, the destruction of *B1* in *ARS305* reduced the levels of gene silencing at the *VII-L* telomere (Fig. 6). In Fig. 6, it is interesting to note that the 1.1 construct (substitution of one base from the WTW motif and one adjacent base) did not reduce the silencing ability while the 1.2 construct (substitution of two bases in the WTW motif) caused silencing ability to decrease by approximately 15%. Also, it is curious that mutations in the WTW flanking sequences (constructs 1.3 and 1.5) showed the greatest

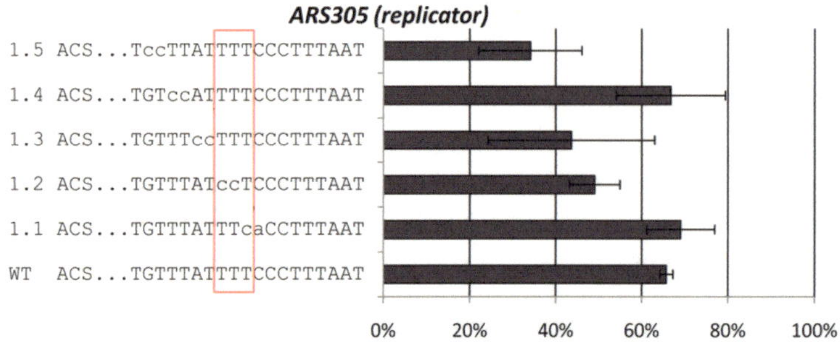

Fig. 6. FOA sensitivity of scanning mutations in *B1* in *ARS305* - FOA sensitivity assays were performed to assess the level of silencing in five scanning mutants (1.1-1.5) and *wild type* (WT) *ARS305* at the *VII-L* telomere in *S.cerevisiae*. Average %FOA^R with standard errors are shown. The hypothesized *B1* WTW motif is indicated by the red rectangle. Site-directed substitution constructs are indicated by lower-case letters above the *wild type* (WT) sequence.

reductions in silencing (30% and 20% reductions of %FOA^R respectively). Very similar mutations have been shown to affect the activity of *ARS305* as a replicator (Huang & Kowalski, 1996). So, the two replicator *ARSs* we have analysed possess a well preserved *B1* element, which functions in both origin firing and in epigenetic silencing. Also, scanning substitutions of the *ARS305 B1* element revealed that mutations in the *B1* flanking sequences have significant effects on gene silencing as well. In contrast, the two silencer *ARSs* were unaffected by any of the two-nucleotide substitutions in the *B1* region.

2.5 Is there any substantial difference to *B1* in replicators and silencers?

The subtle differences in the activities of *B1* elements in select replicator and silencer *ARSs* prompted us to perform extensive sequence alignments of multiple *ARSs* according to their function and/or location in the genome. *ARSs* were grouped as replicators (*ARSs* that are located away from the telomeres and the silencer loci, which confer autonomous replication when moved to a plasmid), silencers (*ARSs* from the *HM* loci and the *rDNA* locus) and *ARSs* within 5 kb of the telomeres. We note that the latter category contains *ARSs* that are imbedded in the repetitive *Core X* and *Y'* subtelomeric elements (Chan & Tye, 1983; Walmsley *et al.*, 1984) and that they share higher homology in the sequences outside the *ACS*. All sequences were imported in WebLogo (www.weblogo.berkeley.edu) and analysed for similarities (Fig. 7).

These analyses confirmed the higher sequence conservation in the vicinity of replicator *B1* elements that was reported earlier (Chang *et al.*, 2008). Nevertheless, telomeric proto-silencer and silencer *ARSs* seem to contain broader WTTTTT and WTTT consensus sequences, respectively, as compared to the WTW consensus of the replicators. These slight variations corroborate the differences observed in the scanning mutation analyses of *ARS305* (replicator) and *ARS317* (silencer). It is quite possible that the broader A/T rich stretch in *B1* of the silencer *ARSs* contribute to the lower effect of the two-nucleotide substitutions in *ARS317* as compared to *ARS305* (Figs. 5 and 6). However, we need to stress that both the effects in the silencing assays and the difference in the *B1* sequence are subtle and do not really reveal a major feature that can distinguish between the two types of *ARS*.

2.6 The orientation of *ACS-B1* determines the levels of telomeric gene silencing

Previous studies have indicated that the orientation of the *HMR***a** and *HMLα* silencers impose directional repression of genes (Zou *et al.*, 2006a; Zou *et al.*, 2006b). In particular, the *HML-I* and the *HMR-E* silencers were found to more efficiently repress *URA3* reporters if oriented *B1-ACS-Rap1-Abf1-URA3* (Fig. 2) (Zou *et al.*, 2006b). These effects were linked to the ability of *ACS* (and supposedly ORC) to robustly position a nucleosome towards the *Abf1* side of the silencer (Zou *et al.*, 2006a). Towards the *B1* side of *ACS* there is no stably positioned nucleosome and the silencing of *URA3* is significantly weaker. Interestingly, the replicator *ARS1* has a stably positioned nucleosome at both the *B1* and the *Abf1* sides of *ACS* (Lipford & Bell, 2001; Zou *et al.*, 2006a).

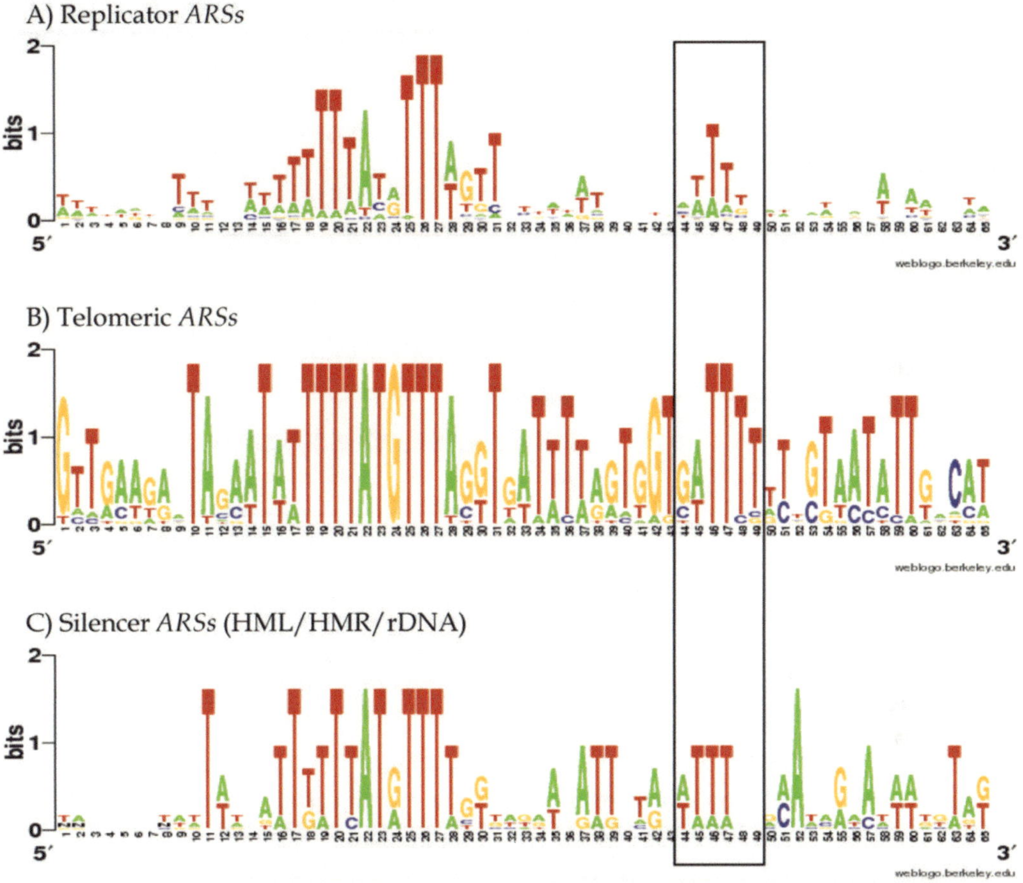

Fig. 7. Sequence alignments of replicator, proto-silencer and silencer *ARSs* - WebLogo alignments were performed using *ARS* sequences from *SGD* (www.yeastgenome.org). Sequences were aligned along the *ACS* (5'-WTTTAYRTTTW-3') and include 17 bp upstream and 37 bp downstream of *ACS*. The *B1* element is indicated by the black rectangle. *ARSs* were chosen based on: A) non-telomeric location with known replicator activity (25 *ARSs* included); B) proximity to telomere (within 5kb) and confirmed autonomous replication on a mini-chromosome (13 *ARSs* included); C) non-telomeric location and confirmed silencer or proto-silencer activity (HML/HMR/rDNA, 6 *ARSs* included).

It is not entirely clear what determines the directional effects of the *HML-I* and *HMR-E* silencers. For example, do Abf1p and Rap1p (and presumably other proto-silencers) facilitate the rigorous control of the nucleosome positions or does *ACS-B1*/ORC work independently? In this line of thought, many origins (such as *ARS305, ARS307, ARS605*) do not contain Abf1p or Rap1p binding sites, while in others (*ARS1, ARS319*) *B1* and the Abf1p binding site reside on the same side of *ACS* (Marahrens & Stillman, 1992; Rao *et al.*, 1994; Huang & Kowalski, 1996; Rehman *et al.*, 2009). Invariably, all these *ARSs* improve gene silencing when inserted at the telomere ((Rehman *et al.*, 2009) this article). We decided to test if these *ARSs* also display directional silencing.

Initial experiments were conducted using *ARS605* and *ARS319*. As mentioned earlier, *ARS605* has no apparent Abf1p binding site, while in *ARS319* both *B1* and the Abf1p binding sites are at the same side of *ACS*. We have cloned these origins in both orientations relative to *URA3* and the telomere to produce the *URA3-ACS605-B1-tel, URA3-B1-ACS605-tel, URA3-ACS319-B1-tel* and *URA3-B1-ACS319-tel* constructs. These constructs were inserted in the left telomere of chromosome *VII* and the levels of *URA3* repression were assessed as before (Fig. 8).

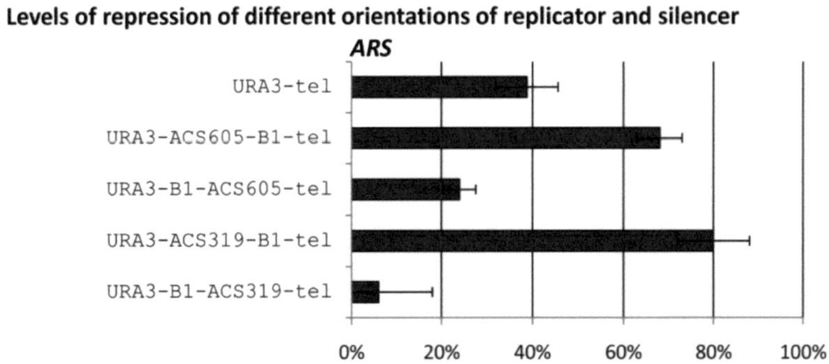

Fig. 8. Effect of the orientation of *ACS-B1* on telomeric silencing - FOA sensitivity assays were performed to assess the level of silencing in two *ACS-B1* orientations for *ARS605* and *ARS319* at the *VII-L* telomere in *S.cerevisiae*. *URA3*-tel acted as a control showing level of silencing when no proto-silencer is present. Average %FOA^R with standard errors are shown.

Our results indicate that both *ARS319* and *ARS605* boost the repression of *URA3* in the *URA3-ACS-B1-tel* orientation. These results are in tune with earlier observations (Zou *et al.*, 2006a; Zou *et al.*, 2006b). Very interestingly, in the opposite direction these *ARSs* markedly reduced the repression of *URA3* (Fig. 8). So, similar to *HML-I (ARS302)* and *HMR-E (ARS317), ARS605* and *ARS319* display directional silencing, but also act as anti-silencers in the opposite direction. Assuming that a similar robustly positioned nucleosome next to *ACS* determines the direction of silencing of *ARS605* and *ARS319*, we argue that the lack of a stable nucleosome at the *B1* side of these *ACSs* can serve as an insulator against the spreading of SIR proteins from the telomere and dampen silencing. We also suggest that other *ARSs* including *ARS302* and *ARS317* will have a similar insulating activity. Together, our results indicate that the orientation of ORC towards a nearby silencing domain (such as the telomere or the *HM* loci) has a significant impact on the strength of silencing.

3. Discussion

3.1 Role of the *B1* element in *ARS* duality

The central topic of the presented studies is the enigmatic dual function of *ARSs* as replicators and as silencers. Because earlier studies have shown distinct affinity of ORC to *ARSs* in silencers and replicators and because *B1* has been proposed to affect ORC affinity (Palacios DeBeer *et al.*, 2003), we have focused on the role of this element on gene silencing at the telomeres. We have compared our results to similar analyses on the role of *B1* in origin activity.

We have found that mutations in the *B1* elements of replicator *ARSs* reduce their activity in telomeric silencing (Figs. 4 and 6). Similar mutations have also reduced the replicator activity of these *ARSs* (Chang *et al.*, 2008; Marahrens & Stillman, 1992). So, replicator *ARSs* seem to have a well defined *B1* that is important, but not required, for both replication and silencing. However, mutations in the *B1* elements of silencer *ARSs* seem not to affect silencing (Figs. 4-5). Similarly, mutations in the *B1* of these *ARSs* have a lesser effect on replication activity than the effects seen in replicator *ARSs* (Chang *et al.*, 2008; Marahrens & Stillman, 1992). This leads us to the hypothesis that silencer *ARSs* have a special type of *B1* element. In this line of thought, we have also noticed that mutations in the sequences flanking the WTW motif in replicator *ARSs* affect silencing to a greater extent than silencer *ARSs* (Fig. 6). This observation suggests that the sequences flanking WTW are more important for silencing than for replication and argue in favour of a broader *B1* element in silencer *ARSs*.

We propose that the subtle functional differences between silencer and replicator *ARSs* is due to the broader *B1* consensus sequence in silencers. We suggest that silencer *ARSs* contain more A/T base pairs around the WTW motif. Support for this hypothesis was provided by the alignment of different types of *ARSs*. In Fig. 7, we introduced the notion of wider *B1* elements, where a consensus of WTTTTT was found for proto-silencer *ARSs* and WTTT was found for silencer *ARSs*. Replicator *ARSs* showed only the previously described WTW motif (Chang *et al.*, 2008). It is possible that *ARSs* with broad *B1* elements would be more accommodating to mutations within the consensus because the adjacent bases would still resemble a WTW motif. The adjacent WTW sites may be able to act as alternative sites for the attachment of ORC (Fig. 9). It is also possible that these *ARSs* possess additional *B1* elements that render the mutations in WTW insignificant.

Earlier structure-function analyses of the association of ORC to *ARS1* (Rao & Stillman, 1995) have indicated that ORC binds to both *ACS* and *B1* (Fig. 9). Through cross-linking studies, a third minor position of ORC contact with DNA (depicted by "*nnn*" in Fig. 9) has also been revealed in-between *ACS* and *B1* (Rao & Stillman, 1995). This third site has never been shown to influence the activity of *ARS1*, but could be important for fine conformational variations in ORC. On the other hand, the small effects of *B1* in replicator and silencer assays stress its auxiliary nature. Whereas *ACS* is required for interaction with ORC, the precise roles of *B1* and the "*nnn*" sequences remain elusive. It is possible that these auxiliary sequences are adaptor elements, which modulate alternative structures of ORC (Fig. 9).

We can imagine that some of these alternative structures would not expose Orc1p, reducing its interaction with Sir1p, and thus promoting replicator activity instead of silencing. Other conformations of ORC, which expose Orc1p, would stimulate its interaction with Sir1p and increase the *ARS's* silencer activity. The broader *B1* element present in proto-silencer and silencer *ARSs* may allow ORC more binding flexibility than the narrower WTW in replicator *ARSs*. This increased flexibility may result in greater variations in ORC conformation, thus providing more opportunities for Orc1p to be exposed. A broader *B1* can also provide additional sites for the attachment of ORC and in turn increase the affinity of ORC to *ACS-B1*. Such a scenario can explain the previous observations on the link between ORC affinity and stronger silencing. In particular, it has been discovered that strong ORC-DNA interaction at *HMR***a** increased heterochromatin formation and decreased and delayed the initiation of DNA replication. Conversely, weak ORC-DNA interaction caused earlier and increased replication initiation and decreased the formation of heterochromatin (Palacios DeBeer *et al.*, 2003).

Very importantly, alterations in *B1* by no means eliminate the dual nature of *ARS*. Whereas broad *B1* elements seem to prevail in silencer and proto-silencer *ARSs* (Fig. 7), many replicator *B1* elements reside in an A/T rich environment as well. This environment can also supply alternative sites for ORC binding. In summary, the *B1* elements seem to unveil a minor difference between replicators and silencers, but this difference is not strong enough on its own to determine the function of an *ARS*.

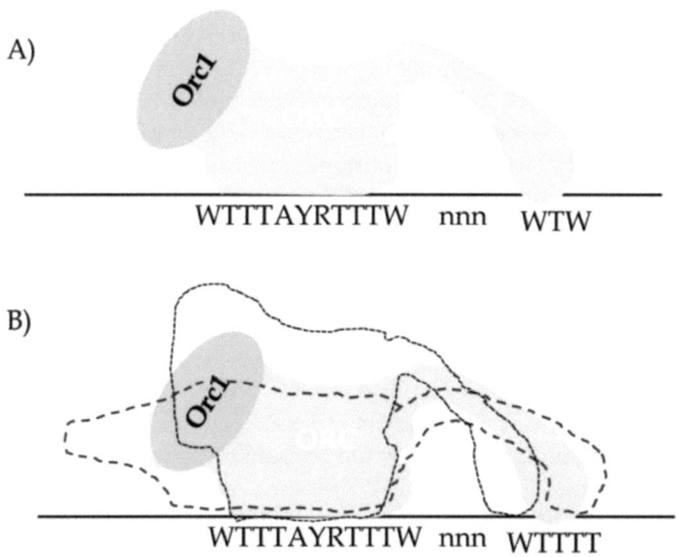

Fig. 9. ORC conformations as dictated by the *ACS-B1* elements - ORC binds the bipartite *ACS-B1* site. The ACS (WTTTAYRTTTW) is essential for ORC binding while *B1* (WTW) and a third minor position of interaction (nnn) are auxiliary. A) Depiction of the conformation of ORC when bound to an *ARS* with a distinct WTW *B1* element. B) Depiction of the flexibility of ORC to adjust its conformation when the *B1* consensus is broader (WTTTT), showing that it is possible that some conformations may hide or further expose the Orc1p subunit.

3.2 Flexibility of ORC and the role of chromatin in *ARS* duality

The orientation of *ACS-B1* towards a potent silencer seems to be more important than the nature of *B1*. In support, we (Fig. 8) and others (Zou *et al.*, 2006a; Zou *et al.*, 2006b) have found that the orientation of *ARSs* towards a powerful silencer such as the telomere or the *HM* loci can significantly contribute to gene silencing. These effects suggest that ORC is highly flexible since a simple switch of direction contributes so significantly to silencing and anti-silencing. An interesting experiment would be to test how the replicator activity of *ARSs* is affected based on its orientation towards a silencer.

It is well known that the origin activity of an *ARS* is governed by chromatin structure (Weinreich *et al.*, 2004). As mentioned previously, both replicator and silencer *ARSs* act as functional origins of replication when placed on plasmids (Chan & Tye, 1980). Similarly, both replicator and silencer *ARSs* act as functional silencers and proto-silencers in the *HM* loci and at the subtelomeres, respectively (Casey *et al.*, 2008; McNally & Rine, 1991; Weinreich *et al.*, 2004). Since an *ARS's* location within the genome determines its function regardless of its original silencer/replicator classification, it appears that the sequence of the *ARSs* is of lesser importance than the genomic context. Hence, it seems that the communication of ORC with heterochromatin is more important than the way ORC interacts with *ACS-B1*. Again, ORC is posing as a highly flexible complex, this time in regards to its interaction with chromatin.

Our ideas that the flexibility of ORC can be influenced by chromatin feed some thought on how origins are chosen as per the Jesuit model. In metazoans, the positions of potential origins and origins that actually fire will vary depending on the epigenetic state of the genome. It makes sense not to fire origins that will disturb heterochromatin. One of the ways to ensure that this does not happen is to force the key regulatory factor for origin activation (this being ORC) to function in a different mode. This way, though ORC interacts with all of the potential origins, it will recruit replication machinery only if it is in a euchromatic region. If ORC is bound to DNA that lies within a heterochromatic region, the heterochromatin dictates that ORC will only recruit silencing machinery and maintain the heterochromatic state instead of stimulating replication.

4. Conclusion

Despite our extensive efforts, we have not identified a clear and strong distinctive feature for the replicator or the silencer *ARSs*. This brings us back to the idea that *ARS*, together with the associated ORC and other DNA replication factors, is a flexible bi-functional module that can be remoulded depending on the chromosomal context and perhaps by additional factors such as the need of the cell to divide or to modulate its gene expression. In other eukaryotes we see no readily identifiable consensus sequence in origins of DNA replication (Mechali, 2010). Even so, strong links of ORC to gene silencing and heterochromatin have been identified by many studies in *Schizosaccharomyces pombe* and in higher eukaryotes (Pak *et al.*, 1997; Auth *et al.*, 2006; Deng *et al.*, 2007; Stuermer *et al.*, 2007; Kato *et al.*, 2008; Deng *et al.*, 2009; Prasanth *et al.*, 2010). Perhaps ORC has evolved to lose its stringent sequence requirements for binding to DNA, but the origin-ORC module has maintained its flexibility and the ability to accommodate varying conformations.

It is somewhat anecdotal that while looking for updates on the Jesuit model for the firing of metazoan origins (DePamphilis, 1993) we came across this citation dealing with the duality of the universe: "...Light and Darkness, Life and Death, Right and Left.... are inseparable.... For this reason each one will dissolve into its earliest Origin..." (The Gospel of Philip, New Testament Apocrypha). It seems that duality has been encripted in the earliest origin and then preserved through evolution.

5. Acknowldegements

The studies in this article have been supported by grants to K.Yankulov from NSERC. D. Jeffery has been supported by studentships from OGSST and from NSERC. P. Chisamore-Robert is supported through stipend from the University of Guelph and NSERC.

6. References

Abraham, J., Feldman, J., Nasmyth, K.A., Strathern, J.N., Klar, A.J., Broach, J.R., & Hicks, J.B. (1983). Sites required for position-effect regulation of mating-type information in yeast. Cold Spring Harb Symp Quant Biol *47 Pt 2*, 989-998.

Auth, T., Kunkel, E., & Grummt, F. (2006). Interaction between HP1alpha and replication proteins in mammalian cells. Exp Cell Res *312*, 3349-3359.

Axelrod, A., & Rine, J. (1991). A role for CDC7 in repression of transcription at the silent mating-type locus HMR in Saccharomyces cerevisiae. Mol Cell Biol *11*, 1080-1091.

Blow, J.J., & Dutta, A. (2005). Preventing re-replication of chromosomal DNA. Nat Rev Mol Cell Biol *6*, 476-486.

Broach, J.R., Li, Y.Y., Feldman, J., Jayaram, M., Abraham, J., Nasmyth, K.A., & Hicks, J.B. (1983). Localization and sequence analysis of yeast origins of DNA replication. Cold Spring Harb Symp Quant Biol *47 Pt 2*, 1165-1173.

Casey, L., Patterson, E.E., Muller, U., & Fox, C.A. (2008). Conversion of a replication origin to a silencer through a pathway shared by a Forkhead transcription factor and an S phase cyclin. Mol Biol Cell *19*, 608-622.

Chan, C.S., & Tye, B.K. (1980). Autonomously replicating sequences in Saccharomyces cerevisiae. Proc Natl Acad Sci U S A *77*, 6329-6333.

Chan, C.S., & Tye, B.K. (1983). Organization of DNA sequences and replication origins at yeast telomeres. Cell *33*, 563-573.

Chang, F., Theis, J.F., Miller, J., Nieduszynski, C.A., Newlon, C.S., & Weinreich, M. (2008). Analysis of chromosome III replicators reveals an unusual structure for the ARS318 silencer origin and a conserved WTW sequence within the origin recognition complex binding site. Mol Cell Biol *28*, 5071-5081.

Chien, C.T., Buck, S., Sternglanz, R., & Shore, D. (1993). Targeting of SIR1 protein establishes transcriptional silencing at HM loci and telomeres in yeast. Cell *75*, 531-541.

Deng, Z., Dheekollu, J., Broccoli, D., Dutta, A., & Lieberman, P.M. (2007). The origin recognition complex localizes to telomere repeats and prevents telomere-circle formation. Curr Biol *17*, 1989-1995.

Deng, Z., Norseen, J., Wiedmer, A., Riethman, H., & Lieberman, P.M. (2009). TERRA RNA binding to TRF2 facilitates heterochromatin formation and ORC recruitment at telomeres. Mol Cell *35*, 403-413.

DePamphilis, M.L. (1993). Eukaryotic DNA replication: anatomy of an origin. Annu Rev Biochem *62*, 29-63.

Doyon, Y., Cayrou, C., Ullah, M., Landry, A.J., Cote, V., Selleck, W., Lane, W.S., Tan, S., Yang, X.J., & Cote, J. (2006). ING tumor suppressor proteins are critical regulators of chromatin acetylation required for genome expression and perpetuation. Mol Cell *21*, 51-64.

Ehrenhofer-Murray, A.E., Kamakaka, R.T., & Rine, J. (1999). A role for the replication proteins PCNA, RF-C, polymerase epsilon and Cdc45 in transcriptional silencing in Saccharomyces cerevisiae. Genetics *153*, 1171-1182.

Ehrentraut, S., Weber, J.M., Dybowski, J.N., Hoffmann, D., & Ehrenhofer-Murray, A.E. (2010). Rpd3-dependent boundary formation at telomeres by removal of Sir2 substrate. Proc Natl Acad Sci U S A *107*, 5522-5527.

Espinosa, M.C., Rehman, M.A., Chisamore-Robert, P., Jeffery, D., & Yankulov, K. (2010). GCN5 is a positive regulator of origins of DNA replication in Saccharomyces cerevisiae. PLoS One *5*, e8964.

Field, Y., Kaplan, N., Fondufe-Mittendorf, Y., Moore, I.K., Sharon, E., Lubling, Y., Widom, J., & Segal, E. (2008). Distinct modes of regulation by chromatin encoded through nucleosome positioning signals. PLoS Comput Biol *4*, e1000216.

Fourel, G., Lebrun, E., & Gilson, E. (2002). Protosilencers as building blocks for heterochromatin. Bioessays *24*, 828-835.

Fourel, G., Magdinier, F., & Gilson, E. (2004). Insulator dynamics and the setting of chromatin domains. Bioessays *26*, 523-532.

Fourel, G., Revardel, E., Koering, C.E., & Gilson, E. (1999). Cohabitation of insulators and silencing elements in yeast subtelomeric regions. EMBO J *18*, 2522-2537.

Huang, R.Y., & Kowalski, D. (1996). Multiple DNA elements in ARS305 determine replication origin activity in a yeast chromosome. Nucleic Acids Res *24*, 816-823.

Kato, H., Matsunaga, F., Miyazaki, S., Yin, L., D'Urso, G., Tanaka, K., & Murakami, Y. (2008). Schizosaccharomyces pombe Orc5 plays multiple roles in the maintenance of genome stability throughout the cell cycle. Cell Cycle *7*, 1085-1096.

Kearsey, S. (1983). Analysis of sequences conferring autonomous replication in baker's yeast. EMBO J *2*, 1571-1575.

Labib, K. (2010). How do Cdc7 and cyclin-dependent kinases trigger the initiation of chromosome replication in eukaryotic cells? Genes Dev *24*, 1208-1219.

Lafon, A., Chang, C.S., Scott, E.M., Jacobson, S.J., & Pillus, L. (2007). MYST opportunities for growth control: yeast genes illuminate human cancer gene functions. Oncogene *26*, 5373-5384.

Lin, S., & Kowalski, D. (1997). Functional equivalency and diversity of cis-acting elements among yeast replication origins. Mol Cell Biol *17*, 5473-5484.

Lipford, J.R., & Bell, S.P. (2001). Nucleosomes positioned by ORC facilitate the initiation of DNA replication. Mol Cell *7*, 21-30.

Marahrens, Y., & Stillman, B. (1992). A yeast chromosomal origin of DNA replication defined by multiple functional elements. Science *255*, 817-823.

McNally, F.J., & Rine, J. (1991). A synthetic silencer mediates SIR-dependent functions in Saccharomyces cerevisiae. Mol Cell Biol *11*, 5648-5659.

Mechali, M. (2010). Eukaryotic DNA replication origins: many choices for appropriate answers. Nat Rev Mol Cell Biol *11*, 728-738.

Nieduszynski, C.A., Knox, Y., & Donaldson A.D. (2006). Genome-wide identification of replication origins in yeast by comparative genomics. *Genes Dev.* Vol. 20, 14, pp. (1874-1879)

Pak, D.T., Pflumm, M., Chesnokov, I., Huang, D.W., Kellum, R., Marr, J., Romanowski, P., & Botchan, M.R. (1997). Association of the origin recognition complex with heterochromatin and HP1 in higher eukaryotes. Cell *91*, 311-323.

Palacios DeBeer, M.A., Muller, U., & Fox, C.A. (2003). Differential DNA affinity specifies roles for the origin recognition complex in budding yeast heterochromatin. Genes Dev *17*, 1817-1822.

Power, P., Jeffery, D., Rehman, M.A., Chatarji, A, & K. Yankulov. (2011). Sub-Telomeric core X and Y' Elements in S.cerevisiae Suppress Extreme Variations in Gene Silencing PLoS One *6(3)*, e17523.

Prasanth, S.G., Shen, Z., Prasanth, K.V., & Stillman, B. (2010). Human origin recognition complex is essential for HP1 binding to chromatin and heterochromatin organization. Proc Natl Acad Sci U S A *107*, 15093-15098.

Pryde, F.E., & Louis, E.J. (1999). Limitations of silencing at native yeast telomeres. EMBO J *18*, 2538-2550.

Raghuraman, M.K., Winzeler, E.A., Collingwood, D., Hunt, S., Wodicka, L., Conway, A., Lockhart, D.J., Davis, R.W., Brewer, B.J., & Fangman, W.L. (2001). Replication dynamics of the yeast genome. Science *294*, 115-121.

Rao, H., Marahrens, Y., & Stillman, B. (1994). Functional conservation of multiple elements in yeast chromosomal replicators. Mol Cell Biol *14*, 7643-7651.

Rao, H., & Stillman, B. (1995). The origin recognition complex interacts with a bipartite DNA binding site within yeast replicators. Proc Natl Acad Sci U S A *92*, 2224-2228.

Rehman, M.A., Fourel, G., Mathews, A., Ramdin, D., Espinosa, M., Gilson, E., & Yankulov, K. (2006). Differential requirement of DNA replication factors for subtelomeric ARS consensus sequence protosilencers in Saccharomyces cerevisiae. Genetics *174*, 1801-1810.

Rehman, M.A., Wang, D., Fourel, G., Gilson, E., & Yankulov, K. (2009). Subtelomeric ACS-containing proto-silencers act as antisilencers in replication factors mutants in Saccharomyces cerevisiae. Mol Biol Cell *20*, 631-641.

Rehman, M.A., & Yankulov, K. (2009). The dual role of autonomously replicating sequences as origins of replication and as silencers. Curr Genet *55*, 357-363.

Rusche, L.N., Kirchmaier, A.L., & Rine, J. (2003). The establishment, inheritance, and function of silenced chromatin in Saccharomyces cerevisiae. Annu Rev Biochem *72*, 481-516.

Sheu, Y.J., & Stillman, B. (2010). The Dbf4-Cdc7 kinase promotes S phase by alleviating an inhibitory activity in Mcm4. Nature *463*, 113-117.

Shore, D., & Nasmyth, K. (1987). Purification and cloning of a DNA binding protein from yeast that binds to both silencer and activator elements. Cell *51*, 721-732.

Shore, D., Stillman, D.J., Brand, A.H., & Nasmyth, K.A. (1987). Identification of silencer binding proteins from yeast: possible roles in SIR control and DNA replication. EMBO J *6*, 461-467.

Stinchcomb, D.T., Struhl, K., & Davis, R.W. (1979). Isolation and characterisation of a yeast chromosomal replicator. Nature *282*, 39-43.

Stuermer, A., Hoehn, K., Faul, T., Auth, T., Brand, N., Kneissl, M., Putter, V., & Grummt, F. (2007). Mouse pre-replicative complex proteins colocalise and interact with the centrosome. Eur J Cell Biol *86*, 37-50.

Walmsley, R.W., Chan, C.S., Tye, B.K., & Petes, T.D. (1984). Unusual DNA sequences associated with the ends of yeast chromosomes. Nature *310*, 157-160.

Weinreich, M., Palacios DeBeer, M.A., & Fox, C.A. (2004). The activities of eukaryotic replication origins in chromatin. Biochim Biophys Acta *1677*, 142-157.

Wyrick, J.J., Aparicio, J.G., Chen, T., Barnett, J.D., Jennings, E.G., Young, R.A., Bell, S.P., & Aparicio, O.M. (2001). Genome-wide distribution of ORC and MCM proteins in S. cerevisiae: high-resolution mapping of replication origins. Science *294*, 2357-2360.

Zou, Y., Yu, Q., & Bi, X. (2006a). Asymmetric positioning of nucleosomes and directional establishment of transcriptionally silent chromatin by Saccharomyces cerevisiae silencers. Mol Cell Biol *26*, 7806-7819.

Zou, Y., Yu, Q., Chiu, Y.H., & Bi, X. (2006b). Position effect on the directionality of silencer function in Saccharomyces cerevisiae. Genetics *174*, 203-213.

Part 5

Proteins in Replication

22

Faithful DNA Replication Requires Regulation of CDK Activity by Checkpoint Kinases

Claus Storgaard Sørensen[1], Halfdan Beck[1],
Viola Nähse-Kumpf[2] and Randi G. Syljuåsen[2]
[1]Biotech Research and Innovation Centre (BRIC), University of Copenhagen,
[2]Department of Radiation Biology, Institute for Cancer Research, Norwegian Radium Hospital, Oslo University Hospital, Oslo,
[1]Denmark
[2]Norway

1. Introduction

The most fundamental aspect of cell division is the precise transfer of genetic material to daughter cells. In order to maintain genome stability the daughter cells need to receive an exact copy of the genetic material from the original cell. This is achieved mainly through two processes. First, the genetic material is carefully copied during the process of DNA replication in S phase of the cell cycle, and thereafter it is precisely segregated into two identical daughter cells during mitosis (M phase). Additional control and preparation for DNA replication occurs in G1 phase, which is the gap phase between M and S phases, and DNA repair processes and preparation for mitosis occurs in G2 phase, which is the gap phase between S and M phases.

A major obstacle for genome stability is endogenous sources of DNA damage during S phase, which can lead to mutations or chromosome rearrangements if left unrepaired. Such mutations and chromosome rearrangements can again cause cell death or lead to the development of diseases associated with genomic instability such as cancer and neurodegenerative disorders (Jackson and Bartek, 2009). The cellular mechanisms that protect against induction of endogenous DNA damage during S phase are therefore particularly important.

DNA replication is tightly regulated by a number of signaling pathways including regulators of Cyclin-Dependent Kinase (CDK) activity. Following exposure to external sources of DNA damage CDK activity is restrained due to activation of the checkpoint kinases Ataxia Telangiactasia-like Rad3 kinase (ATR), Checkpoint kinase 1 (CHK1) and WEE1 kinase (Cliby et al., 1998; Rowley et al., 1992; Sørensen et al., 2003). Importantly, recent work have suggested that proper control of CDK activity by these checkpoint kinases is also required during normal S phase to protect cells against the induction of harmful DNA lesions (Beck et al., 2010; Lam et al., 2004; Syljuåsen et al., 2005). In this chapter we review the roles of ATR, CHK1, and WEE1 during normal DNA replication, and discuss their critical function in maintaining genome stability by preventing induction of harmful DNA lesions in S phase. We also discuss the links of ATR, CHK1, and WEE1 with cancer.

2. Regulation of key cellular processes by ATR, CHK1, and WEE1 kinases

2.1 Regulation of ATR and its biological roles

Human ATR is a Ser/Thr kinase first cloned as a member of the phosphatidylinositol-3-kinase related kinases (PIKK) family (Cimprich et al., 1996). Other family members are ATM and DNA-PKcs, which are all regulating DNA damage responses. Whereas ATM and DNA-PK are activated by DNA double strand breaks (DSBs), ATR is activated upon the generation of lesions containing single stranded DNA (ssDNA) (Lopez-Contreras and Fernandez-Capetillo, 2010).

ssDNA can evolve during normal replication, at stalled replication forks, and following DSB processing such as the DNA end resection required in the initial step of homologous recombination (HR) repair (Mimitou and Symington, 2011; Zou and Elledge, 2003). Coating of ssDNA by RPA helps loading of ATR to DNA damage sites (Bochkarev et al., 1997; Fanning et al., 2006; Zhou and Elledge, 2000). ATR recognition of RPA-coated ssDNA is dependent on the ATR-interacting protein (ATRIP) (Cortez et al., 2001), which binds RPA directly (Ball et al., 2007). ATR and ATRIP are constitutively associated, it is assumed that none of them exists freely (Cortez et al., 2001). However, the binding of ATR/ATRIP to RPA is not sufficient for ATR activation (Byun et al., 2005; MacDougall et al., 2007; Stokes et al., 2002). It also needs to be activated by TOPBP1, and this occurs via an independent mechanism dependent on the RAD17 clamp loader and the 9-1-1 (RAD9-RAD1-HUS1) complex. RAD17 is recruited by RPA-coated ssDNA and loads the 9-1-1 complex, which subsequently recruits TOPBP1 and brings it in close proximity to ATR so that TOPBP1 can activate ATR (Kumagai et al., 2006). ssDNA may in itself not elicit strong ATR activation as evidenced from recent work in *Xenopus* extracts. High level ATR activation were observed at areas of ssDNA with 5′-primed ends, which greatly exceeded activation by naked ssDNA pieces (MacDougall et al., 2007). It has been suggested that these ends may be the loading site for the 9-1-1 complex (Majka et al., 2006) which can ensure that small pieces of ssDNA generated during replication does not lead to high levels of checkpoint activation.

Activated ATR regulates a plethora of cellular responses among DNA repair and cell cycle effects, and deletion of ATR in mice causes embryonic lethality (Brown and Baltimore, 2000; de Klein et al., 2000). ATR plays a major role in maintaining genome stability during S phase where it is essential for stabilizing stalled replication forks (Paulsen and Cimprich, 2007) and prevents excessive origin firing (Friedel et al., 2009). Consistent with these findings, deletion of ATR in mice causes embryonic lethality associated with loss of genome integrity (Brown and Baltimore, 2000; de Klein et al., 2000). In response to DNA damaging agents ATR regulates the S and G2/M checkpoints (Cliby et al., 1998). ATR also controls postreplicative DNA repair (Gohler et al., 2011) and homologous recombination repair (Wang et al., 2004), and contributes to promote telomere maintenance (McNees et al., 2010; Pennarun et al., 2010).

In a large scale proteomic analysis more than 700 ATM/ATR targets have been identified; most of the targets can be recognized by both ATM and ATR (Matsuoka et al., 2007). The major target of ATR activation is CHK1, which couples the recognition of ssDNA with cell cycle effects in S and G2/M phases (Liu et al., 2000). Among other regulators of DNA damage signaling, ATR also phosphorylates histone H2AX (Ward and Chen, 2001), the Bloom's syndrome helicase (BLM) (Davies et al., 2007) and p53 (Tibbetts et al., 1999).

2.2 Regulation of CHK1 and its biological roles

CHK1 is a Ser/Thr kinase and was first discovered in fission yeast (Walworth et al., 1993). Human and murine CHK1 was identified to by Sanchez et al. (1997) and Flaggs et al. (1997).

CHK1 is a constitutively active kinase that is further phosphorylated by ATR upon several stimuli like replication stress, DSBs, UV and other DNA damaging agents. Upon the generation of ssDNA containing lesions, active ATR further phosphorylates CHK1 on Ser 317 and Ser345 and stimulates its function (Guo et al., 2000; Liu et al., 2000; Zhao and Piwnica-Worms, 2001). Claspin is required for the CHK1 phosphorylation by ATR (Kumagai and Dunphy, 2000). After the ATR induced phosphorylation, CHK1 undergoes autophosphorylation at Ser296 (Clarke and Clarke, 2005; Kasahara et al., 2010). Only a few CHK1 molecules are phosphorylated simultaneously on the ATR sites and on Ser296. CHK1-pSer296 was found only in the soluble fraction, whereas CHK1-pSer317 and CHK1-pSer345 were found both on chromatin and in the soluble fraction. It is likely that the autophosphorylation leads to dephosphorylation at the ATR sites (Kasahara et al., 2010). Given that CHK1 is a constitutively active kinase, the DNA damage induced ATR phosphorylation likely does not upregulate CHK1 kinase activity per se. Rather, it was reported that phosphorylated CHK1 dissociates from chromatin (Smits et al., 2006; Zhang et al., 2005) and ATR regulation of CHK1 may thereby control transition of DNA damage signals from chromatin to its targets.

CHK1 deficiency is embryonic lethal in mice (Liu et al., 2000; Takai et al., 2000) demonstrating that CHK1 is an essential kinase. Similar to ATR, CHK1 is essential for maintaining genome integrity during S phase. CHK1 controls S phase progression both in the absence and presence of DNA damaging agents (Sørensen et al., 2003) and inhibition of CHK1 in normal S phase causes DNA damage (Syljuåsen et al., 2005). CHK1 controls replication initiation and is required for normal replication fork progression (Petermann et al., 2006; Petermann et al., 2010) and stabilizes stalled replication forks (Feijoo et al., 2001). When DNA synthesis is blocked, a fraction of CHK1 depleted cells enter mitosis prematurely with incompletely replicated DNA (Zachos et al., 2005). CHK1 also controls mitotic entry in unperturbed cells (Kramer et al., 2004) and the G2/M checkpoint after DNA damage (Sanchez et al., 1997) as well as homologous recombination repair (Sørensen et al., 2005). Moreover, CHK1 is also involved in control of transcription (Shimada et al., 2008) and was reported to play a role in mitotic spindle checkpoint function (Zachos et al., 2007). The cell cycle regulatory role of ATR/CHK1 in S and G2 phases is thought to be largely due to CHK1-mediated control of the CDC25 phosphatases (Beck et al., 2010). Among other substrates of CHK1 are RAD51 (Sørensen et al., 2005) and FANCE (Wang et al., 2007).

CHK1 is constitutively targeted by ATR in S-phase, and the cell cycle regulatory role of CHK1 in S phase is largely to restrain the activity of the CDC25A phosphatase. CDC25A dephosphorylates the tyrosine 15 residue of CDK1 and CDK2 and thereby activates CDK1 and CDK2. Following CHK1 activation, CHK1 phosphorylation of CDC25A, facilitated by 14-3-3γ (Kasahara et al., 2010) leads to ubiquitin dependent degradation of CDC25A. The NEK11 kinase is also activated by CHK1, and NEK11-mediated phosphorylation of CDC25A promotes its degradation (Melixetian et al., 2009). The degradation of CDC25A leads to increased phosphorylation of the tyrosine 15 residue and inhibition of CDK activity, thus inducing cell cycle arrest (Bartek and Lukas, 2003; Zhou and Elledge, 2000). CHK1 can also phosphorylate CDC25B and CDC25C (Sanchez et al., 1997; Schmitt et al., 2006) which may also contribute to restrain CDK activity, although CDC25C is dispensable for activation of the G2 checkpoint (Chen et al., 2001). Interestingly, CHK1 constitutively phosphorylates CDC25B (Schmitt et al., 2006) and the effects of CDC25B overexpression seems to resemble those of CHK1-inhibition, as CDC25B overexpression also results in increased recruitment of CDC45 to chromatin and subsequent DNA damage in S phase cells (Bugler et al., 2010).

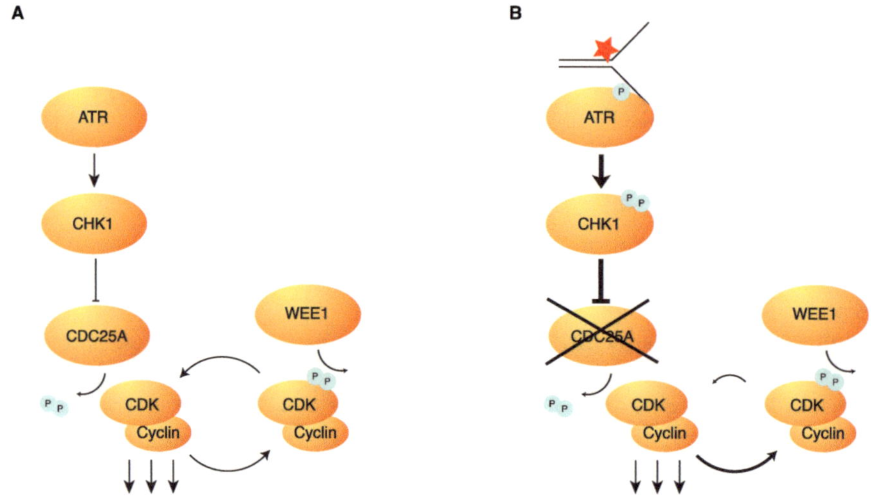

Fig. 1. Regulation of CDK activity by ATR, CHK1 and WEE1. (A) CDK activity is regulated by phosphorylation and dephosphorylation. WEE1 kinase inhibits CDK activity by phosphorylating Tyrosine 15, and WEE1 activity is counteracted by the CDC25A phosphatase. During replication in unperturbed S phase CHK1 controls CDC25A levels by a phosphorylation that signals proteolytic degradation. (B) Replication stress is sensed by ATR, which in turn stimulates CHK1. This mediates CDC25A degradation and inhibits CDK activity by shifting the equilibrium towards phosphorylated CDK.

2.3 Regulation of WEE1 and its biological roles

Wee1 was first discovered in fission yeast. Wee1 deficiency led to the 'wee' phenotype because premature mitosis was induced which led to a smaller cell size (Russell and Nurse, 1987). Wee1 is a Ser/Thr and Tyr protein kinase which negatively regulates cell cycle progression by phosphorylating and inhibiting CDKs thereby enabling the completion of DNA replication and the timely entry into mitosis (Heald et al., 1993). WEE1 kinase catalyzes the inhibitory Tyrosine 15 phosphorylation of CDK1 and CDK2 and thereby inhibits CDK activity (Parker and Piwnica-Worms, 1992; Watanabe et al., 1995). At entry into mitosis WEE1 is inhibited by phosphorylation as well as degraded by ubiquitin-dependent proteolysis, thus boosting CDK activity to promote mitosis. CDK phosphorylation primes WEE1 for ubiquitylation via the beta-TRCP SCF type of ubiquitin ligase, and this activity may be further supported by the Tome-1 SCF ubiquitin ligase (Ayad et al., 2003). In *Xenopus*, activated XCHK1 also phosphorylates the XWee1 kinase, contributing to increased Tyrosine 15 phosphorylation and inhibition of CDK activity upon CHK1 activation (Lee et al., 2001).

In mice Wee1 is essential for embryonic survival. Wee1 deficient MEFs display growth defects, chromosome aneuploidy, gamma-H2AX foci formation and CHK2 activation (Tominaga et al., 2006). Most previous reports suggest that human WEE1 mainly functions in the G2 phase to restrain mitotic entry. However, recent data revealed that inhibition of WEE1 in S phase leads to induction of DNA damage in a manner dependent on CDK1 and CDK2 and the replication proteins MCM2 and CDT1 (Beck et al., 2010). These data suggest that human WEE1 also has an important function in regulation of normal S phase progression.

3. Regulation of DNA replication by CDKs

3.1 Replication initiation

DNA replication is a tightly regulated process, where cells must secure that all parts of the genome are replicated precisely once during S-phase. Cells initiate replication from a large number of chromosomal loci known as replication origins. The activation of origins constitutes a very important means of replication control, because cells cannot regulate the speed of the DNA polymerases. In the budding yeast replication origins are specific DNA sequences, which are recognized by ORC (origin recognition complex) and additional series of protein recruitment. However, in metazoans the origins have no consensus sequence and the licensing appears to be a more stochastic event (Goren and Cedar, 2003; Zink, 2006). Activation of each replication origin leads to the assembly of a bi-directional replication fork (Bell and Dutta, 2002). Replication is further organized into clusters of origins that fire in near-synchrony (Goren and Cedar, 2003; Pope et al., 2010). These clusters are organized in replication factories, which contain between 5-50 forks (Berezney et al., 2000), and can be visualized as replication foci. After the initiation process, the protein complex at each origin changes to a post-replication state, thereby preventing further initiation events from the same origins for the rest of the cell cycle (Bell and Dutta, 2002; Blow and Dutta, 2005).

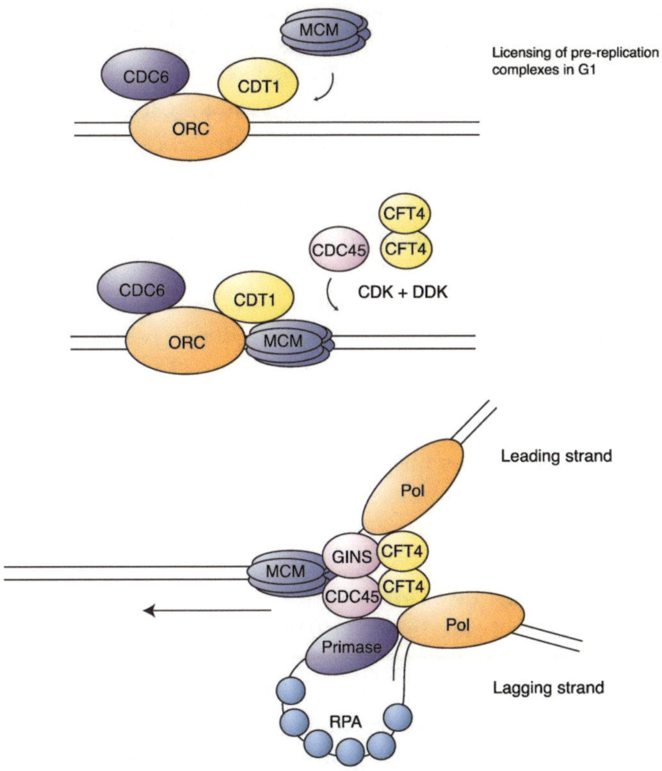

Fig. 2. Replication initiation. Origin licensing occurs in G1 by the MCM2-7 complex being recruited to ORC by CDT1 and CDC6. Loading of CDC45-GINS is crucial for replication initiation and is facilitated by AND-1/CTF4 in a CDK2 dependent manner. This allows the assembly of a replication fork with primase and polymerases onto the leading and lagging strand.

The formation of a replication fork occurs by the ordered assembly of several replication proteins during exit from mitosis and in G1 phase of the cell cycle. Binding of the ORC protein complex provides a molecular landing pad for the sequential assembly of pre-replication complexes consisting of CDC6, CDT1, and the MCM2-7 helicase complex (Bochman and Schwacha, 2009; Remus and Diffley, 2009). Initiation of DNA replication is then triggered sequentially by the action of at least two sets of protein kinase activities: the CDKs and DBF4-CDC7 (DDK) (Labib, 2010; Sclafani and Holzen, 2007). CDK2 is considered the most important CDK in regulation of DNA replication. However, CDK1 clearly also plays a role, as CDK1 can compensate for loss of CDK2 in regulation of DNA replication in CDK2 knockout mice (Aleem et al., 2005). Furthermore, CDK1 appears to regulate replication of hepatocytes, which contain higher CDK1 levels in S phase than many other cell types (Garnier et al., 2009).

The targets of CDK and DDK activity have received much attention, and the MCM helicase has been shown to be phosphorylated by the kinases, however, the functional role is not yet fully elucidated (Labib, 2010). Two major processes controlled by CDK activity are the loading of CDC45 and AND-1/CTF4 at origins (Zhu et al., 2007). In addition novel CDK targets are emerging with a role in DNA replication, such as TopBP1, Treslin and GEMC1. Once phosphorylated by CDK2, TopBP1 collaborates with the recently discovered Treslin to load CDC45 (Kumagai et al., 2010). Similarly, another CDK target, GEMC1, was recently found to be essential for replication initiation. It also associates with TopBP1 and CDC45 and is required for CDC45 and GINS loading (Balestrini et al., 2010).

The CDC45 protein is a key factor required for initiation, and it associates with the MCM helicase at origins of replication and is dependent on the presence of the GINS complex (Go-Ichi-Ni-San) (Kubota et al., 2003; Moyer et al., 2006; Takayama et al., 2003). MCM unwinding of the DNA duplex generates regions of single-stranded DNA (ssDNA) and this is closely coupled with replication. However, the isolated MCM complex appears rather inactive as a DNA helicase and its activation is likely to involve posttranslational modifications and association with other factors, such as CDC45 and GINS. Further binding of MCM10 leads to the recruitment of AND-1/CTF4 to support origin unwinding and binding of the primase DNA polymerase (Pol) α to initiate replication (Zhu et al., 2007). The first RNA primer is synthesized by the primase activity of Pol α and elongated by its DNA polymerase activity. The RNA–DNA hybrid is recognized by replication factor C (RFC), which loads PCNA, the replicative sliding clamp that mediates the polymerase switch from Pol α to the processive polymerases Pol δ and ε, allowing continuous DNA synthesis (Nasheuer et al., 2002; Takeda and Dutta, 2005).

3.2 CDK-dependent control of origin firing through S phase

Thousands of origins in the genome are fired at distinct times through the S-phase. Usually, euchromatin, with active gene transcription, is replicated early, whereas heterochromatin is replicated late. As many more origins are licensed than are ever used in a normal S-phase most origins are replicated passively (Woodward et al., 2006). Besides being required for firing of origins, CDK activity seems to be required for activation of individual replication clusters/factories as well as driving progress through the replication-timing program (Gillespie and Blow, 2010; Goren and Cedar, 2003; Hiratani et al., 2008; Thomson et al., 2010). These mechanisms are, however, poorly understood. In case of replication fork stalling or replication stress, local dormant origins will fire to compensate for the lack of replication. Under conditions of exogenous DNA damage, checkpoint pathways block the activation of origins that normally fire in late S phase, which constitutes the basis for the S phase checkpoint (Karnani and Dutta, 2011; Santocanale and Diffley, 1998; Woodward et al., 2006).

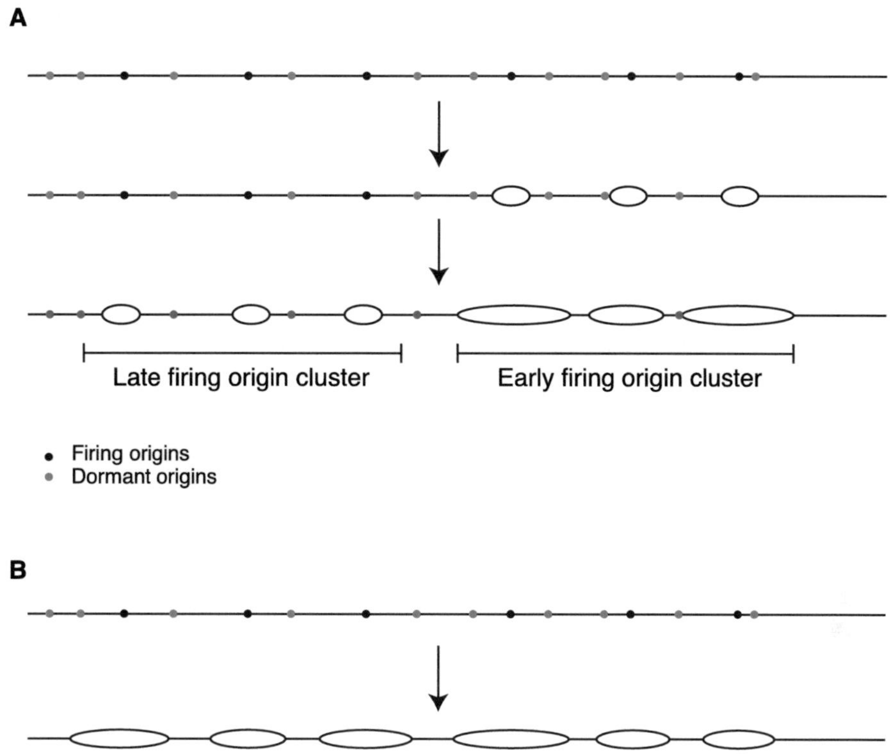

Fig. 3. (A) Many more origins than used are licensed in G1 phase. In S phase a replication program is initiated, where origins are organized into replication clusters that can be divided into early and late firing origins. (B) Under circumstances where CDK activity is deregulated and unusually high the late origins will fire inappropriately.

4. ATR, CHK1 and WEE1 are required for genomic integrity during S phase

4.1 ATR/CHK1 regulate genome integrity during unperturbed S phase

Even though CHK1's involvement in the ATR-CHK1-CDC25A regulation of CDKs to enforce a DNA damage checkpoint has been the major focus, recent discoveries are revealing a critical role of the tight regulation of CDK activity to secure DNA replication. Recent data uncovered that CHK1-mediated control of CDK activity is critical to maintain coordinated duplication of the genome and preventing a catastrophic outcome of the sensitive replication process. When DNA replication is out of control, the genome is destabilized and accumulates a massive amount of DNA double strand breaks (Syljuåsen et al., 2005). These results are consistent with a study in mice where conditional CHK1 heterozygosity caused accumulation of DNA damage during DNA replication (Lam et al., 2004). The occurrence of this DNA damage is still elusive but is clearly replication dependent and directly related to replication forks.

4.2 WEE1 emerges as a regulator of genome integrity in S phase

Until recently, WEE1 was thought to mainly regulate the entry into mitosis. However, WEE1 was recently identified as another central regulator of genome integrity in S phase (Beck et al., 2010). WEE1 depletion rapidly induced DNA damage in S phase in newly replicated DNA, which is accompanied by a marked increase in ssDNA (Beck et al., 2010). This DNA damage is dependent on CDK1 and CDK2 as well as the replication proteins MCM2 and CDT1. This is remarkably similar to the phenotype observed after ablation of CHK1, however, DNA damage after CHK1 inhibition is highly dependent on CDC25A (Beck et al., 2010). It is apparent that the mitotic kinase WEE1 and CHK1 jointly maintain balanced cellular control of CDK activity during normal DNA replication.

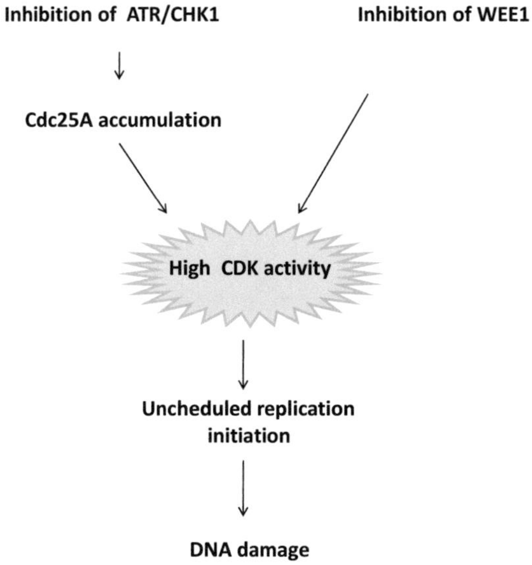

Fig. 4. Model describing induction of DNA damage in S phase following inhibition of the ATR, CHK1 or WEE1 kinases. Inhibition of ATR or CHK1 leads to accumulation of CDC25A and thereby increases CDK activity, while inhibition of WEE1 increases CDK activity directly due to loss of WEE1-mediated inhibitory phosphorylation on CDK. The high CDK activity causes unscheduled firing of replication origins, which subsequently leads to induction of DNA breaks.

4.3 Loss of genome integrity is associated with unscheduled replication of late origins

CHK1 has recently emerged as an important component in the maintenance of genomic integrity because it blocks the appearance of aberrant replication-associated lesions (Syljuåsen et al., 2005). When CHK1 activity is lost CDC25A is stabilized and accumulates. The accompanying hyper-activation of CDK activity results in a loss of control of the replication program. This leads to an increased loading of replication factor CDC45 onto chromatin, as well as a dramatic replication initiation (Syljuåsen et al., 2005). This is accompanied by a subsequent increase in ssDNA at replication forks and association of RPA indicating replication stress (Syljuåsen et al., 2005). In addition, slower replication fork speeds are observed when CHK1 is inhibited (Petermann et al., 2010). This is likely not directly due to the elevated CDK activity operating at existing forks. The fork slowing may be the consequence of high numbers of initiated replication forks, which can have a major impact on functional replication, for example by titrating out factors that are rate-limiting for replication elongation. Similarly to CHK1, WEE1 depletion also causes increased ssDNA and RPA foci formation indicative of replication stress (Beck et al., 2010), and WEE1 inhibition can also induce a marked increase in origin firing (our unpublished observations). Based on our previous data and the common regulation of CDK activity, we hypothesize that the major cellular defect following depletion of ATR/CHK or WEE1 is unscheduled replication of late origins.

How unscheduled replication leads to induction of DNA breaks is not well understood. DNA breaks can arise in several ways during replication (Lambert and Carr, 2005). The replication process in itself creates sensitive DNA structures since replication forks contain unwound, single-stranded DNA. The template strands on each arm of replication forks are no longer base-paired to their original complementary strands, and they are instead base-paired to newly synthesized DNA. Consequently, single-strand lesions within unwound DNA at replication forks cause double-strand breaks when the replication fork reaches such lesions. Furthermore, stalled replication forks with exposed ssDNA stretches are recombinogenic. Homologous recombination is known to salvage stalled forks but is also thought to generate structures that are resolved by endonuclease Mus81/Eme1 thereby leading to double-strand breaks (Hanada et al., 2007). Nucleases may target the replication forks in a deregulated and excessive manner when CDK activity is deregulated. Based on these observations, it is apparent that the replicating DNA molecules have conformations that facilitate the progression from replication stress to DNA breaks and loss of genome integrity.

4.4 ATR, CHK1 and WEE1 are required to prevent breakage at the replication fork

The occurrence of high level CDK-mediated DNA damage was initially surprising since this is not observed in yeast in a similar manner. The lesions in mammalian cells have been linked directly to replication forks and are dependent on replication factors like CDC45 and CDT1 (Beck et al., 2010; Syljuåsen et al., 2005). However, the generation of the double strand breaks is not understood. In addition to the over-initiation of origins, additional possible explanations also exist that more directly explain the occurrence of double strand breaks. CHK1 may negatively regulate endonucleases, such as MUS81/EME1. MUS81 generates breaks at stalled forks to support their repair by homologous recombination repair, which also re-establishes the replication fork (Hanada et al., 2007). If CHK1 negatively regulates such endonucleases during normal DNA replication, loss of CHK1 will lead to activation of the endonucleases and potentially excessive induction of DNA breaks. Given that WEE1 inhibition leads to a similar phenotype, it would be expected that it is the deregulated CDK activity that is the causative effect in activating such a DNA processing activity.

ATR and CHK1 are also known to directly support fork stability (Bartek et al., 2004; Lambert and Carr, 2005). Another possibility would thus be that lack of ATR/CHK1-mediated support of stalled forks will lead to fork collapse and DNA breaks. It is however not clear if WEE1 has a similar role, in addition, the role of CHK1 effects appears largely through the CDC25A-CDK pathway (Beck et al., 2010). A major and direct contribution of fork stability issues to the phenotype is therefore not very likely. Unbalanced or depleted nucleotide pools could also cause fork stalling and eventual collapse similar to that observed in cells treated with hydroxyurea (Katou et al., 2003), an inhibitor of nucleotide metabolism.

However, this would likely not occur with the rapid kinetics observed after CHK1 and WEE1 depletion, where inhibitors induce DNA damage within 2 hours of treatment. Hence, it appears more likely that CDK targets with enzymatic activity, i.e. a nuclease exhibiting aberrant activity, could cause the DNA damage. It remains to be determined to what extent such activities control genome integrity as well as the nature of the deregulated enzymes.

5. The disease links of ATR, CHK1, and WEE1 and their potential as targets for treatment of cancer

5.1 Cancer-associated ATR/CHK1 mutations

An important issue is whether genomic instability arising from replicative problems caused by ATR, CHK1 and WEE1 disruption may contribute to the development of human disease such as cancer. Heterozygous ATR and CHK1 mutations have been reported in a subset of endometrial, colon, and stomach cancers (Bertoni et al., 1999; Kim et al., 2007; Lewis et al., 2005; Menoyo et al., 2001; Vassileva et al., 2002; Zighelboim et al., 2009), and CHK1 mutations were also found in malignant melanoma (Kumar et al., 2005). Supporting that such mutations are likely of functional importance, is expression of truncating mutations of ATR in human cell lines abrogated CHK1 phosphorylation and topotecan-induced S phase arrest (Lewis et al., 2005). On the other hand, ATR and CHK1 mutations were not found in other types of cancer such as hereditary breast and ovarian cancers (Heikkinen et al., 2005; Marsh et al., 2007; Solyom et al., 2010) or in families with the cancer prone Li-Fraumeni syndrome (Vahteristo et al., 2001). It is important to note that in addition to inactivating mutations, suppression of ATR/CHK1 signaling in human cancer might potentially occur in many other different ways, and in vivo assessment of ATR and CHK1 kinase activities would be required in order to exclude that defects in the function of these kinases occur during tumor progression. Interestingly, a recent report suggested that as opposed to mutations, CHK1 deletions may contribute to breast cancer progression (Mu et al., 2011). Further evidence that heterozygous mutations of ATR and CHK1 might contribute to tumor progression stems from studies of ATR and CHK1 heterozogosity in mice. In one report ATR heterozygous (+/-) mice showed a modest increase in late tumor development (Brown and Baltimore, 2000) although increased tumorigenesis was not observed in other cases (Murga et al., 2009; Ruzankina et al., 2007). However, ATR heterozygozity caused a significant increase in tumorigenesis on a mismatch repair-deficient (Mlh1 -/-) background (Fang et al., 2004). CHK1 heterozygous (+/-) mice were prone to tumorigenesis on a WNT-1 transgenic background (Liu et al., 2000) and CHK1 heterozygosity induced in mouse mammary glands using a Cre/loxP system caused induction of mammary tumors in a p53 heterozygous background (Fishler et al., 2010).

The roles of ATR and CHK1 in control of DNA replication likely contribute to their tumor suppression function. Supporting that the extent of downregulation by hypomorphic mutations is sufficient to cause harmful DNA lesions associated with deregulated replication, conditional CHK1 heterozygosity in mice caused spontaneous DNA damage in S phase (Lam et al., 2004). Also, a mouse model for the human Seckel syndrome based on a mutation in the ATR gene revealed high incidence of cells showing pan-nuclear staining of gamma-H2AX in cultured MEFs *in vitro* as well as in embryos *in vivo* (Murga et al., 2009). The strong gamma-H2AX staining occurred only in Cyclin A positive cells and was attributed to increased replication stress occurring as a consequence of reduced ATR function. However, no tumors were found in these mice even in the absence of p53, which may suggest that the induced replication stress in these mice had reached a level of severity that rather caused cell death (Murga et al., 2009). Another mouse model hypomorphic for ATR also displayed increased DNA damage as assayed by gamma-H2AX levels, which could likely be due to replicative problems, although analysis of cell cycle was not included (Ragland et al., 2009). Altogether, it seems plausible that replication associated DNA damage due to insufficient CHK1 or ATR levels in S phase caused by hypomorphic mutations in these genes could contribute to promote genomic instability and tumor progression. Analogous, it was proposed that oncogene-induced DNA damage due to increased CDK activity and replication stress promotes tumor progression at early stages (Bartkova et al., 2010; Bartkova et al., 2005; Gorgoulis et al., 2005; Halazonetis et al., 2008).

In addition to its role in cancer, ATR hypomorphic mutations have also been associated with the Seckel syndrome, which is characterized by severe microcephaly, dwarfism and dysmorphic facial features (O'Driscoll et al., 2003). In addition, a deletion in ATR was found in one patient with the Blepharophimosis-ptosis-epicanthus inversus syndrome showing microcephaly and growth retardation (O'Driscoll et al., 2007). It remains to be investigated whether replication associated DNA damage are involved in the development of these syndromes.

5.2 Cancer-associated downregulation of WEE1

Mutations of WEE1 have not yet been reported in human cancer. However, several reports suggest that WEE1 function may be sometimes compromised due to other types of cancer-associated alterations. Expression of microRNA-155 (miR-155) is elevated in several human cancers and was recently shown to cause downregulation of WEE1 (Tili et al., 2011). Downregulation of the WEE1 protein was also observed in pituitary adenomas, and this was also associated with miRNA expression (Butz et al., 2010). Moreover, prostate epithelium, which is prone to prostate cancer development, also expressed very low levels of WEE1 (Kiviharju-af Hallstrom et al., 2007). Based on our studies (Beck et al., 2010), low levels of WEE1 during human tumorigenesis would likely lead to deregulated replication with subsequent spontaneous DNA damage in S phase. We propose that prevention of such damage might contribute to the tumor suppressor function of WEE1 in some cases.

5.3 Overexpression of WEE1 and CHK1 in human cancer

On the other hand, WEE1 is overexpressed in human glioblastoma and a subset of breast cancers (Iorns et al., 2009; Mir et al., 2010), and CHK1 mRNA expression was elevated in MYC-amplified neuroblastoma (Cole et al., 2010). The mechanism behind upregulation of CHK1 in MYC-amplified neuroblastoma is not known (Cole et al., 2010). However, the high WEE1 expression in gliomas may be due to low levels of microRNA mir-128 as high WEE1 expression correlated with low expression of mir-128 in gliomas, and forced overexpression of mir-128 in glioma cells resulted in downregulation of WEE1 (Wuchty et al., 2011). High levels of WEE1 and CHK1 would be expected to suppress rather than to promote cell growth, and at first glance it may be difficult to reconcile how high levels of CHK1 or WEE1 would be consistent with a selective pressure during tumorigenesis towards genetic alterations allowing uncontrolled growth. An explanation may be that other alterations in these tumors exist that promote increased replication stress, and if the CDK activity was too high, the replication associated damage would reach a level of severity resulting in cell death. The elevated expression of WEE1 or CHK1 could thus likely be needed for cell survival following other genetic alterations that have occurred during tumorigenesis. In line with this hypothesis, inhibition of WEE1 led to induction of DNA damage and cell death in tumors expressing high WEE1 levels (Mir et al., 2010). Furthermore, MYC is known to cause replication stress and elevated CHK1 expression was found selectively in MYC-amplified neuroblastoma (Cimprich et al., 1996).

5.4 CHK1-inhibition as a strategy for cancer treatment

ATR, CHK1 and WEE1 have been suggested as targets for cancer treatment. Indeed, several inhibitors of CHK1 are currently in clinical trials (Dai and Grant, 2010; Ma et al., 2010). When used in combination with chemotherapeutic agents or radiation, CHK1-inhibitors can cause selective sensitization of p53 negative cells (Ashwell and Zabludoff, 2008; Dixon and Norbury, 2002; Petersen et al., 2010). It was proposed that p53-negative cancer cells are particularly sensitive to CHK1-inhibitors in combination with DNA damaging agents because they lack the p53-dependent G1 checkpoint and therefore may depend more on the G2 checkpoint for DNA damage repair (Russell et al., 1995). However, CHK1-inhibiton also sensitizes p53 positive cells (Hirose et al., 2001; Tse et al., 2007), and p53-status does not always predict responses to CHK1-inhibition (Petersen et al., 2010; Zenvirt et al., 2010).

In addition to G2 checkpoint abrogation, other effects of CHK1-inhibition likely contribute to cause cell death, including inhibition of homologous recombination repair (Morgan et al., 2010; Sørensen et al., 2005) as well as induction of DNA damage in S phase due to replication problems (Cole et al., 2010; McNeely et al., 2010; Syljuåsen et al., 2005). The cytotoxic effects of CHK1-inhibition associated with increased CDK activity and induction

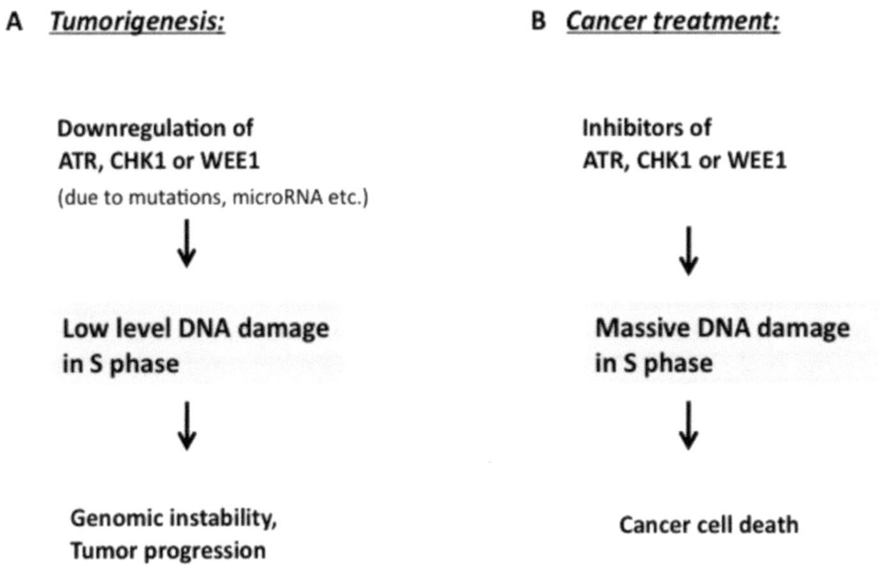

Fig. 5. Possible implications of loss of ATR, CHK1 and WEE1–mediated control of S phase events for malignant progression and cancer treatment. (A) Reduced expression or activity of ATR, CHK1 and WEE1 during tumorigenesis may cause DNA replication failures leading to DNA damage in S phase and subsequent genomic instability and tumor progression. (B) During cancer treatment with inhibitors of ATR, CHK1 or WEE1, massive induction of DNA damage in S phase due to deregulated replication may induce marked cancer cell death.

of DNA damage are expected to occur in S phase cells of cancerous as well as normal tissues, and would thus likely contribute to normal tissue damage following treatment with CHK1-inhibitors. However, the tumors would often contain a higher fraction of cycling cells than the surrounding normal tissue, resulting in tumor selective effects. In addition, tumor cells with elevated replication stress due to other genetic alterations (Bartkova et al., 2010; Halazonetis et al., 2008) may be more dependent on CHK1-mediated control of CDK activity in S phase, which would likely further promote the selective killing of tumor cells compared to normal tissue (Gilad et al., 2010).

5.5 Inhibition of WEE1 and ATR for cancer treatment

Similar to CHK1-inhibitors, inhibitors of WEE1 kinase are also in clinical trials and were reported to selectively sensitize p53-deficient tumor cells to DNA damaging agents (Hirai et al., 2010; Hirai et al., 2009; Leijen et al., 2010; Rajeshkumar et al., 2011). Furthermore, a non-transformed mammary epithelial cell line was less affected by WEE1 silencing compared to breast cancer cell lines, suggesting that WEE1-inhibition would not be toxic to normal cells (Murrow et al., 2010). Inhibition of ATR can also sensitize cancer cells and ATR has also been suggested as a therapeutic target, although small-molecule ATR-inhibitors are not yet available (Wagner and Kaufmann, 2010). Based on the roles of WEE1 and ATR in restraining CDK activity and thereby preventing unscheduled DNA replication, we propose that induction of DNA damage in S phase will contribute to the cytotoxic effects of WEE1 and ATR -inhibitors and potentially affect both tumor and normal cells in a similar manner as discussed above for CHK1-inhibitors.

6. Conclusion

It is essential for living organisms to secure that the genetic material is passed faithfully to daughter cells. Defects compromise genetic integrity and can ultimately lead to cancer and additional diseases. The duplication of the human genome in the S-phase of the cell cycle is therefore highly regulated with a large number of control mechanisms securing correct timing and quality of the process. Recent work has revealed that the checkpoint kinases ATR, CHK1 and WEE1 are constitutively active during normal S phase progression in the absence of exogenous DNA damage, and this function is critical to maintain genome integrity. These checkpoint kinases control genome integrity by restraining CDK activity. Loss of checkpoint kinase -mediated control of CDK activity will cause unscheduled firing of replication origins in S phase and thereby lead to the induction of DNA breaks in a not yet fully understood mechanism. Such replication-associated DNA lesions may contribute to promote loss of genome integrity and cancer progression following heterozygous mutations or other ways of inactivation of ATR, CHK1 or WEE1 during tumorigenesis. Furthermore, replication-associated DNA damage occurring in response to small-molecule inhibitors of ATR, CHK1 and WEE1 should be taken into account when such inhibitors are considered for cancer treatment.

7. Acknowledgements

The authors acknowledge support from The Danish Cancer Society, The Novo Foundation, The Lundbeck Foundation, The Danish Medical Research Council, The Norwegian Cancer Society, The Norwegian Research Council and South-Eastern Norway Health Authority.

8. References

Aleem, E., Kiyokawa, H., and Kaldis, P. (2005). Cdc2-cyclin E complexes regulate the G1/S phase transition. *Nat Cell Biol.* Vol. 7, pp. 831-836.

Ashwell, S., and Zabludoff, S. (2008). DNA damage detection and repair pathways--recent advances with inhibitors of checkpoint kinases in cancer therapy. *Clin Cancer Res.* Vol. 14, pp. 4032-4037.

Ayad, N.G., Rankin, S., Murakami, M., Jebanathirajah, J., Gygi, S., and Kirschner, M.W. (2003). Tome-1, a trigger of mitotic entry, is degraded during G1 via the APC. *Cell.* Vol. 113, pp. 101-113.

Balestrini, A., Cosentino, C., Errico, A., Garner, E., and Costanzo, V. (2010). GEMC1 is a TopBP1-interacting protein required for chromosomal DNA replication. *Nature Cell Biology.* Vol. 12, pp. 484-491.

Ball, H.L., Ehrhardt, M.R., Mordes, D.A., Glick, G.G., Chazin, W.J., and Cortez, D. (2007). Function of a conserved checkpoint recruitment domain in ATRIP proteins. *Mol Cell Biol.* Vol. 27, pp. 3367-3377.

Bartek, J., Lukas, C., and Lukas, J. (2004). Checking on DNA damage in S phase. *Nature reviews. Molecular cell biology.* Vol. 5, pp. 792-804.

Bartek, J., and Lukas, J. (2003). Chk1 and Chk2 kinases in checkpoint control and cancer. *Cancer cell.* Vol. 3, pp. 421-429.

Bartkova, J., Hamerlik, P., Stockhausen, M.T., Ehrmann, J., Hlobilkova, A., Laursen, H., Kalita, O., Kolar, Z., Poulsen, H.S., Broholm, H., Lukas, J., and Bartek, J. (2010). Replication stress and oxidative damage contribute to aberrant constitutive activation of DNA damage signalling in human gliomas. *Oncogene.* Vol. 29, pp. 5095-5102.

Bartkova, J., Horejsi, Z., Koed, K., Kramer, A., Tort, F., Zieger, K., Guldberg, P., Sehested, M., Nesland, J.M., Lukas, C., Orntoft, T., Lukas, J., and Bartek, J. (2005). DNA damage response as a candidate anti-cancer barrier in early human tumorigenesis. *Nature.* Vol. 434, pp. 864-870.

Beck, H., Nähse, V., Larsen, M.S., Groth, P., Clancy, T., Lees, M., Jørgensen, M., Helleday, T., Syljuåsen, R.G., and Sørensen, C.S. (2010). Regulators of cyclin-dependent kinases are crucial for maintaining genome integrity in S phase. *The Journal of cell biology.* Vol. 188, pp. 629-638.

Bell, S.P., and Dutta, A. (2002). DNA replication in eukaryotic cells. *Annual review of biochemistry.* Vol. 71, pp. 333-374.

Berezney, R., Dubey, D.D., and Huberman, J.A. (2000). Heterogeneity of eukaryotic replicons, replicon clusters, and replication foci. *Chromosoma.* Vol. 108, pp. 471-484.

Bertoni, F., Codegoni, A.M., Furlan, D., Tibiletti, M.G., Capella, C., and Broggini, M. (1999). CHK1 frameshift mutations in genetically unstable colorectal and endometrial cancers. *Genes Chromosomes Cancer.* Vol. 26, pp. 176-180.

Blow, J.J., and Dutta, A. (2005). Preventing re-replication of chromosomal DNA. *Nature reviews. Molecular cell biology.* Vol. 6, pp. 476-486.

Bochkarev, A., Pfuetzner, R.A., Edwards, A.M., and Frappier, L. (1997). Structure of the single-stranded-DNA-binding domain of replication protein A bound to DNA. *Nature.* Vol. 385, pp. 176-181.

Bochman, M.L., and Schwacha, A. (2009). The Mcm complex: unwinding the mechanism of a replicative helicase. *Microbiol Mol Biol Rev*. Vol. 73, pp. 652-683.

Brown, E.J., and Baltimore, D. (2000). ATR disruption leads to chromosomal fragmentation and early embryonic lethality. *Genes & development*. Vol. 14, pp. 397-402.

Bugler, B., Schmitt, E., Aressy, B., and Ducommun, B. (2010). Unscheduled expression of CDC25B in S-phase leads to replicative stress and DNA damage. *Mol Cancer*. Vol. 9, pp. 29.

Butz, H., Liko, I., Czirjak, S., Igaz, P., Khan, M.M., Zivkovic, V., Balint, K., Korbonits, M., Racz, K., and Patocs, A. (2010). Down-regulation of Wee1 kinase by a specific subset of microRNA in human sporadic pituitary adenomas. *J Clin Endocrinol Metab*. Vol. 95, pp. E181-191.

Byun, T.S., Pacek, M., Yee, M.C., Walter, J.C., and Cimprich, K.A. (2005). Functional uncoupling of MCM helicase and DNA polymerase activities activates the ATR-dependent checkpoint. *Genes & development*. Vol. 19, pp. 1040-1052.

Chen, M.S., Hurov, J., White, L.S., Woodford-Thomas, T., and Piwnica-Worms, H. (2001). Absence of apparent phenotype in mice lacking Cdc25C protein phosphatase. *Mol Cell Biol*. Vol. 21, pp. 3853-3861.

Cimprich, K.A., Shin, T.B., Keith, C.T., and Schreiber, S.L. (1996). cDNA cloning and gene mapping of a candidate human cell cycle checkpoint protein. *Proceedings of the National Academy of Sciences of the United States of America*. Vol. 93, pp. 2850-2855.

Clarke, C.A., and Clarke, P.R. (2005). DNA-dependent phosphorylation of Chk1 and Claspin in a human cell-free system. *Biochem J*. Vol. 388, pp. 705-712.

Cliby, W.A., Roberts, C.J., Cimprich, K.A., Stringer, C.M., Lamb, J.R., Schreiber, S.L., and Friend, S.H. (1998). Overexpression of a kinase-inactive ATR protein causes sensitivity to DNA-damaging agents and defects in cell cycle checkpoints. *Embo J*. Vol. 17, pp. 159-169.

Cole, K.A., Huggins, J., Laquaglia, M., Hulderman, C.E., Russell, M.R., Bosse, K., Diskin, S.J., Attiyeh, E.F., Sennett, R., Norris, G., Laudenslager, M., Wood, A.C., Mayes, P.A., Jagannathan, J., Winter, C., Mosse, Y.P., and Maris, J.M. (2010). RNAi screen of the protein kinome identifies checkpoint kinase 1 (CHK1) as a therapeutic target in neuroblastoma. *Proceedings of the National Academy of Sciences of the United States of America*. Vol. 108, pp. 3336-3341.

Cortez, D., Guntuku, S., Qin, J., and Elledge, S.J. (2001). ATR and ATRIP: partners in checkpoint signaling. *Science*. Vol. 294, pp. 1713-1716.

Dai, Y., and Grant, S. (2010). New insights into checkpoint kinase 1 in the DNA damage response signaling network. *Clin Cancer Res*. Vol. 16, pp. 376-383.

Davies, S.L., North, P.S., and Hickson, I.D. (2007). Role for BLM in replication-fork restart and suppression of origin firing after replicative stress. *Nature structural & molecular biology*. Vol. 14, pp. 677-679.

de Klein, A., Muijtjens, M., van Os, R., Verhoeven, Y., Smit, B., Carr, A.M., Lehmann, A.R., and Hoeijmakers, J.H. (2000). Targeted disruption of the cell-cycle checkpoint gene ATR leads to early embryonic lethality in mice. *Curr Biol*. Vol. 10, pp. 479-482.

Dixon, H., and Norbury, C.J. (2002). Therapeutic exploitation of checkpoint defects in cancer cells lacking p53 function. *Cell Cycle*. Vol. 1, pp. 362-368.

Fang, Y., Tsao, C.C., Goodman, B.K., Furumai, R., Tirado, C.A., Abraham, R.T., and Wang, X.F. (2004). ATR functions as a gene dosage-dependent tumor suppressor on a mismatch repair-deficient background. *Embo J.* Vol. 23, pp. 3164-3174.

Fanning, E., Klimovich, V., and Nager, A.R. (2006). A dynamic model for replication protein A (RPA) function in DNA processing pathways. *Nucleic Acids Res.* Vol. 34, pp. 4126-4137.

Feijoo, C., Hall-Jackson, C., Wu, R., Jenkins, D., Leitch, J., Gilbert, D.M., and Smythe, C. (2001). Activation of mammalian Chk1 during DNA replication arrest: a role for Chk1 in the intra-S phase checkpoint monitoring replication origin firing. *The Journal of cell biology.* Vol. 154, pp. 913-923.

Fishler, T., Li, Y.Y., Wang, R.H., Kim, H.S., Sengupta, K., Vassilopoulos, A., Lahusen, T., Xu, X., Lee, M.H., Liu, Q., Elledge, S.J., Ried, T., and Deng, C.X. (2010). Genetic instability and mammary tumor formation in mice carrying mammary-specific disruption of Chk1 and p53. *Oncogene.* Vol. 29, pp. 4007-4017.

Flaggs, G., Plug, A.W., Dunks, K.M., Mundt, K.E., Ford, J.C., Quiggle, M.R., Taylor, E.M., Westphal, C.H., Ashley, T., Hoekstra, M.F., and Carr, A.M. (1997). Atm-dependent interactions of a mammalian chk1 homolog with meiotic chromosomes. *Curr Biol.* Vol. 7, pp. 977-986.

Friedel, A.M., Pike, B.L., and Gasser, S.M. (2009). ATR/Mec1: coordinating fork stability and repair. *Curr Opin Cell Biol.* Vol. 21, pp. 237-244.

Garnier, D., Loyer, P., Ribault, C., Guguen-Guillouzo, C., and Corlu, A. (2009). Cyclin-dependent kinase 1 plays a critical role in DNA replication control during rat liver regeneration. *Hepatology.* Vol. 50, pp. 1946-1956.

Gilad, O., Nabet, B.Y., Ragland, R.L., Schoppy, D.W., Smith, K.D., Durham, A.C., and Brown, E.J. (2010). Combining ATR suppression with oncogenic Ras synergistically increases genomic instability, causing synthetic lethality or tumorigenesis in a dosage-dependent manner. *Cancer Res.* Vol. 70, pp. 9693-9702.

Gillespie, P.J., and Blow, J.J. (2010). Clusters, factories and domains: The complex structure of S-phase comes into focus. *Cell Cycle.* Vol. 9, pp. 3218-3226.

Gohler, T., Sabbioneda, S., Green, C.M., and Lehmann, A.R. (2011). ATR-mediated phosphorylation of DNA polymerase eta is needed for efficient recovery from UV damage. *The Journal of cell biology.* Vol. 192, pp. 219-227.

Goren, A., and Cedar, H. (2003). Replicating by the clock. *Nature reviews. Molecular cell biology.* Vol. 4, pp. 25-32.

Gorgoulis, V.G., Vassiliou, L.V., Karakaidos, P., Zacharatos, P., Kotsinas, A., Liloglou, T., Venere, M., Ditullio, R.A., Jr., Kastrinakis, N.G., Levy, B., Kletsas, D., Yoneta, A., Herlyn, M., Kittas, C., and Halazonetis, T.D. (2005). Activation of the DNA damage checkpoint and genomic instability in human precancerous lesions. *Nature.* Vol. 434, pp. 907-913.

Guo, Z., Kumagai, A., Wang, S.X., and Dunphy, W.G. (2000). Requirement for Atr in phosphorylation of Chk1 and cell cycle regulation in response to DNA replication blocks and UV-damaged DNA in Xenopus egg extracts. *Genes & development.* Vol. 14, pp. 2745-2756.

Halazonetis, T.D., Gorgoulis, V.G., and Bartek, J. (2008). An oncogene-induced DNA damage model for cancer development. *Science.* Vol. 319, pp. 1352-1355.

Hanada, K., Budzowska, M., Davies, S.L., van Drunen, E., Onizawa, H., Beverloo, H.B., Maas, A., Essers, J., Hickson, I.D., and Kanaar, R. (2007). The structure-specific endonuclease Mus81 contributes to replication restart by generating double-strand DNA breaks. *Nature structural & molecular biology*. Vol. 14, pp. 1096-1104.

Heald, R., McLoughlin, M., and McKeon, F. (1993). Human wee1 maintains mitotic timing by protecting the nucleus from cytoplasmically activated Cdc2 kinase. *Cell*. Vol. 74, pp. 463-474.

Heikkinen, K., Mansikka, V., Karppinen, S.M., Rapakko, K., and Winqvist, R. (2005). Mutation analysis of the ATR gene in breast and ovarian cancer families. *Breast Cancer Res*. Vol. 7, pp. R495-501.

Hirai, H., Arai, T., Okada, M., Nishibata, T., Kobayashi, M., Sakai, N., Imagaki, K., Ohtani, J., Sakai, T., Yoshizumi, T., Mizuarai, S., Iwasawa, Y., and Kotani, H. (2010). MK-1775, a small molecule Wee1 inhibitor, enhances anti-tumor efficacy of various DNA-damaging agents, including 5-fluorouracil. *Cancer Biol Ther*. Vol. 9, pp. 514-522.

Hirai, H., Iwasawa, Y., Okada, M., Arai, T., Nishibata, T., Kobayashi, M., Kimura, T., Kaneko, N., Ohtani, J., Yamanaka, K., Itadani, H., Takahashi-Suzuki, I., Fukasawa, K., Oki, H., Nambu, T., Jiang, J., Sakai, T., Arakawa, H., Sakamoto, T., Sagara, T., Yoshizumi, T., Mizuarai, S., and Kotani, H. (2009). Small-molecule inhibition of Wee1 kinase by MK-1775 selectively sensitizes p53-deficient tumor cells to DNA-damaging agents. *Mol Cancer Ther*. Vol. 8, pp. 2992-3000.

Hiratani, I., Ryba, T., Itoh, M., Yokochi, T., Schwaiger, M., Chang, C.W., Lyou, Y., Townes, T.M., Schubeler, D., and Gilbert, D.M. (2008). Global reorganization of replication domains during embryonic stem cell differentiation. *PLoS biology*. Vol. 6, pp. e245.

Hirose, Y., Berger, M.S., and Pieper, R.O. (2001). Abrogation of the Chk1-mediated G(2) checkpoint pathway potentiates temozolomide-induced toxicity in a p53-independent manner in human glioblastoma cells. *Cancer Res*. Vol. 61, pp. 5843-5849.

Iorns, E., Lord, C.J., Grigoriadis, A., McDonald, S., Fenwick, K., Mackay, A., Mein, C.A., Natrajan, R., Savage, K., Tamber, N., Reis-Filho, J.S., Turner, N.C., and Ashworth, A. (2009). Integrated functional, gene expression and genomic analysis for the identification of cancer targets. *PLoS One*. Vol. 4, pp. e5120.

Jackson, S.P., and Bartek, J. (2009). The DNA-damage response in human biology and disease. *Nature*. Vol. 461, pp. 1071-1078.

Karnani, N., and Dutta, A. (2011). The effect of the intra-S-phase checkpoint on origins of replication in human cells. *Genes & development*. Vol. 25, pp. 621-633.

Kasahara, K., Goto, H., Enomoto, M., Tomono, Y., Kiyono, T., and Inagaki, M. (2010). 14-3-3gamma mediates Cdc25A proteolysis to block premature mitotic entry after DNA damage. *Embo J*. Vol. 29, pp. 2802-2812.

Katou, Y., Kanoh, Y., Bando, M., Noguchi, H., Tanaka, H., Ashikari, T., Sugimoto, K., and Shirahige, K. (2003). S-phase checkpoint proteins Tof1 and Mrc1 form a stable replication-pausing complex. *Nature*. Vol. 424, pp. 1078-1083.

Kim, C.J., Lee, J.H., Song, J.W., Cho, Y.G., Kim, S.Y., Nam, S.W., Yoo, N.J., Park, W.S., and Lee, J.Y. (2007). Chk1 frameshift mutation in sporadic and hereditary non-polyposis colorectal cancers with microsatellite instability. *Eur J Surg Oncol*. Vol. 33, pp. 580-585.

Kiviharju-af Hallstrom, T.M., Jaamaa, S., Monkkonen, M., Peltonen, K., Andersson, L.C., Medema, R.H., Peehl, D.M., and Laiho, M. (2007). Human prostate epithelium lacks Wee1A-mediated DNA damage-induced checkpoint enforcement. *Proceedings of the National Academy of Sciences of the United States of America*. Vol. 104, pp. 7211-7216.

Kramer, A., Mailand, N., Lukas, C., Syljuasen, R.G., Wilkinson, C.J., Nigg, E.A., Bartek, J., and Lukas, J. (2004). Centrosome-associated Chk1 prevents premature activation of cyclin-B-Cdk1 kinase. *Nat Cell Biol*. Vol. 6, pp. 884-891.

Kubota, Y., Takase, Y., Komori, Y., Hashimoto, Y., Arata, T., Kamimura, Y., Araki, H., and Takisawa, H. (2003). A novel ring-like complex of Xenopus proteins essential for the initiation of DNA replication. *Genes & development*. Vol. 17, pp. 1141-1152.

Kumagai, A., and Dunphy, W.G. (2000). Claspin, a novel protein required for the activation of Chk1 during a DNA replication checkpoint response in Xenopus egg extracts. *Mol Cell*. Vol. 6, pp. 839-849.

Kumagai, A., Lee, J., Yoo, H.Y., and Dunphy, W.G. (2006). TopBP1 activates the ATR-ATRIP complex. *Cell*. Vol. 124, pp. 943-955.

Kumagai, A., Shevchenko, A., Shevchenko, A., and Dunphy, W.G. (2010). Treslin Collaborates with TopBP1 in Triggering the Initiation of DNA Replication. *Cell*. Vol. 140, pp. 349-359.

Kumar, K., Rahman, Q., Schipper, H., Matschegewski, C., Schiffmann, D., and Papp, T. (2005). Mutational analysis of 9 different tumour-associated genes in human malignant mesothelioma cell lines. *Oncol Rep*. Vol. 14, pp. 743-750.

Labib, K. (2010). How do Cdc7 and cyclin-dependent kinases trigger the initiation of chromosome replication in eukaryotic cells? *Genes & development*. Vol. 24, pp. 1208-1219.

Lam, M.H., Liu, Q., Elledge, S.J., and Rosen, J.M. (2004). Chk1 is haploinsufficient for multiple functions critical to tumor suppression. *Cancer cell*. Vol. 6, pp. 45-59.

Lambert, S., and Carr, A.M. (2005). Checkpoint responses to replication fork barriers. *Biochimie*. Vol. 87, pp. 591-602.

Lee, J., Kumagai, A., and Dunphy, W.G. (2001). Positive regulation of Wee1 by Chk1 and 14-3-3 proteins. *Mol Biol Cell*. Vol. 12, pp. 551-563.

Leijen, S., Beijnen, J.H., and Schellens, J.H. (2010). Abrogation of the G2 checkpoint by inhibition of Wee-1 kinase results in sensitization of p53-deficient tumor cells to DNA-damaging agents. *Curr Clin Pharmacol*. Vol. 5, pp. 186-191.

Lewis, K.A., Mullany, S., Thomas, B., Chien, J., Loewen, R., Shridhar, V., and Cliby, W.A. (2005). Heterozygous ATR mutations in mismatch repair-deficient cancer cells have functional significance. *Cancer Res*. Vol. 65, pp. 7091-7095.

Liu, Q., Guntuku, S., Cui, X.S., Matsuoka, S., Cortez, D., Tamai, K., Luo, G., Carattini-Rivera, S., DeMayo, F., Bradley, A., Donehower, L.A., and Elledge, S.J. (2000). Chk1 is an essential kinase that is regulated by Atr and required for the G(2)/M DNA damage checkpoint. *Genes Dev*. Vol. 14, pp. 1448-1459.

Lopez-Contreras, A.J., and Fernandez-Capetillo, O. (2010). The ATR barrier to replication-born DNA damage. *DNA Repair (Amst)*. Vol. 9, pp. 1249-1255.

Ma, C.X., Janetka, J.W., and Piwnica-Worms, H. (2010). Death by releasing the breaks: CHK1 inhibitors as cancer therapeutics. *Trends Mol Med*. Vol. 17, pp. 88-96.

MacDougall, C.A., Byun, T.S., Van, C., Yee, M.C., and Cimprich, K.A. (2007). The structural determinants of checkpoint activation. *Genes Dev*. Vol. 21, pp. 898-903.

Majka, J., Binz, S.K., Wold, M.S., and Burgers, P.M. (2006). Replication protein A directs loading of the DNA damage checkpoint clamp to 5'-DNA junctions. *The Journal of biological chemistry*. Vol. 281, pp. 27855-27861.

Marsh, A., Healey, S., Lewis, A., Spurdle, A.B., Kedda, M.A., Khanna, K.K., Mann, G.J., Pupo, G.M., Lakhani, S.R., and Chenevix-Trench, G. (2007). Mutation analysis of five candidate genes in familial breast cancer. *Breast Cancer Res Treat*. Vol. 105, pp. 377-389.

Matsuoka, S., Ballif, B.A., Smogorzewska, A., McDonald, E.R., 3rd, Hurov, K.E., Luo, J., Bakalarski, C.E., Zhao, Z., Solimini, N., Lerenthal, Y., Shiloh, Y., Gygi, S.P., and Elledge, S.J. (2007). ATM and ATR substrate analysis reveals extensive protein networks responsive to DNA damage. *Science*. Vol. 316, pp. 1160-1166.

McNeely, S., Conti, C., Sheikh, T., Patel, H., Zabludoff, S., Pommier, Y., Schwartz, G., and Tse, A. (2010). Chk1 inhibition after replicative stress activates a double strand break response mediated by ATM and DNA-dependent protein kinase. *Cell Cycle*. Vol. 9, pp. 995-1004.

McNees, C.J., Tejera, A.M., Martinez, P., Murga, M., Mulero, F., Fernandez-Capetillo, O., and Blasco, M.A. (2010). ATR suppresses telomere fragility and recombination but is dispensable for elongation of short telomeres by telomerase. *The Journal of cell biology*. Vol. 188, pp. 639-652.

Melixetian, M., Klein, D.K., Sorensen, C.S., and Helin, K. (2009). NEK11 regulates CDC25A degradation and the IR-induced G2/M checkpoint. *Nat Cell Biol*. Vol. 11, pp. 1247-1253.

Menoyo, A., Alazzouzi, H., Espin, E., Armengol, M., Yamamoto, H., and Schwartz, S., Jr. (2001). Somatic mutations in the DNA damage-response genes ATR and CHK1 in sporadic stomach tumors with microsatellite instability. *Cancer Res*. Vol. 61, pp. 7727-7730.

Mimitou, E.P., and Symington, L.S. (2011). DNA end resection--unraveling the tail. *DNA Repair (Amst)*. Vol. 10, pp. 344-348.

Mir, S.E., De Witt Hamer, P.C., Krawczyk, P.M., Balaj, L., Claes, A., Niers, J.M., Van Tilborg, A.A., Zwinderman, A.H., Geerts, D., Kaspers, G.J., Peter Vandertop, W., Cloos, J., Tannous, B.A., Wesseling, P., Aten, J.A., Noske, D.P., Van Noorden, C.J., and Wurdinger, T. (2010). In silico analysis of kinase expression identifies WEE1 as a gatekeeper against mitotic catastrophe in glioblastoma. *Cancer cell*. Vol. 18, pp. 244-257.

Morgan, M.A., Parsels, L.A., Zhao, L., Parsels, J.D., Davis, M.A., Hassan, M.C., Arumugarajah, S., Hylander-Gans, L., Morosini, D., Simeone, D.M., Canman, C.E., Normolle, D.P., Zabludoff, S.D., Maybaum, J., and Lawrence, T.S. (2010). Mechanism of radiosensitization by the Chk1/2 inhibitor AZD7762 involves abrogation of the G2 checkpoint and inhibition of homologous recombinational DNA repair. *Cancer Res*. Vol. 70, pp. 4972-4981.

Moyer, S.E., Lewis, P.W., and Botchan, M.R. (2006). Isolation of the Cdc45/Mcm2-7/GINS (CMG) complex, a candidate for the eukaryotic DNA replication fork helicase.

Proceedings of the National Academy of Sciences of the United States of America. Vol. 103, pp. 10236-10241.
Mu, K., Li, L., Yang, Q., Zhang, T., Gao, P., Meng, B., Liu, Z., Wang, Y., and Zhou, G. (2011). Detection of CHK1 and CCND1 gene copy number changes in breast cancer with dual-colour fluorescence in-situ hybridization. *Histopathology*. Vol. 58, pp. 601-607.
Murga, M., Bunting, S., Montana, M.F., Soria, R., Mulero, F., Canamero, M., Lee, Y., McKinnon, P.J., Nussenzweig, A., and Fernandez-Capetillo, O. (2009). A mouse model of ATR-Seckel shows embryonic replicative stress and accelerated aging. *Nat Genet*. Vol. 41, pp. 891-898.
Murrow, L.M., Garimella, S.V., Jones, T.L., Caplen, N.J., and Lipkowitz, S. (2010). Identification of WEE1 as a potential molecular target in cancer cells by RNAi screening of the human tyrosine kinome. *Breast Cancer Res Treat*. Vol. 122, pp. 347-357.
Nasheuer, H.P., Smith, R., Bauerschmidt, C., Grosse, F., and Weisshart, K. (2002). Initiation of eukaryotic DNA replication: regulation and mechanisms. *Progress in nucleic acid research and molecular biology*. Vol. 72, pp. 41-94.
O'Driscoll, M., Dobyns, W.B., van Hagen, J.M., and Jeggo, P.A. (2007). Cellular and clinical impact of haploinsufficiency for genes involved in ATR signaling. *Am J Hum Genet*. Vol. 81, pp. 77-86.
O'Driscoll, M., Ruiz-Perez, V.L., Woods, C.G., Jeggo, P.A., and Goodship, J.A. (2003). A splicing mutation affecting expression of ataxia-telangiectasia and Rad3-related protein (ATR) results in Seckel syndrome. *Nat Genet*. Vol. 33, pp. 497-501.
Parker, L.L., and Piwnica-Worms, H. (1992). Inactivation of the p34cdc2-cyclin B complex by the human WEE1 tyrosine kinase. *Science*. Vol. 257, pp. 1955-1957.
Paulsen, R.D., and Cimprich, K.A. (2007). The ATR pathway: fine-tuning the fork. *DNA Repair (Amst)*. Vol. 6, pp. 953-966.
Pennarun, G., Hoffschir, F., Revaud, D., Granotier, C., Gauthier, L.R., Mailliet, P., Biard, D.S., and Boussin, F.D. (2010). ATR contributes to telomere maintenance in human cells. *Nucleic Acids Res*. Vol. 38, pp. 2955-2963.
Petermann, E., Maya-Mendoza, A., Zachos, G., Gillespie, D.A., Jackson, D.A., and Caldecott, K.W. (2006). Chk1 requirement for high global rates of replication fork progression during normal vertebrate S phase. *Mol Cell Biol*. Vol. 26, pp. 3319-3326.
Petermann, E., Woodcock, M., and Helleday, T. (2010). Chk1 promotes replication fork progression by controlling replication initiation. *Proceedings of the National Academy of Sciences of the United States of America*. Vol. 107, pp. 16090-16095.
Petersen, L., Hasvold, G., Lukas, J., Bartek, J., and Syljuasen, R.G. (2010). p53-dependent G(1) arrest in 1st or 2nd cell cycle may protect human cancer cells from cell death after treatment with ionizing radiation and Chk1 inhibitors. *Cell Prolif*. Vol. 43, pp. 365-371.
Pope, B.D., Hiratani, I., and Gilbert, D.M. (2010). Domain-wide regulation of DNA replication timing during mammalian development. *Chromosome research : an international journal on the molecular, supramolecular and evolutionary aspects of chromosome biology*. Vol. 18, pp. 127-136.

Ragland, R.L., Arlt, M.F., Hughes, E.D., Saunders, T.L., and Glover, T.W. (2009). Mice hypomorphic for Atr have increased DNA damage and abnormal checkpoint response. *Mamm Genome*. Vol. 20, pp. 375-385.

Rajeshkumar, N.V., De Oliveira, E., Ottenhof, N., Watters, J.W., Brooks, D., Demuth, T., Shumway, S.D., Mizuarai, S., Hirai, H., Maitra, A., and Hidalgo, M. (2011). MK-1775, a potent Wee1 inhibitor, synergizes with gemcitabine to achieve tumor regressions, selectively in p53-deficient pancreatic cancer xenografts. *Clin Cancer Res*. Vol., pp.

Remus, D., and Diffley, J.F. (2009). Eukaryotic DNA replication control: lock and load, then fire. *Curr Opin Cell Biol*. Vol. 21, pp. 771-777.

Rowley, R., Hudson, J., and Young, P.G. (1992). The wee1 protein kinase is required for radiation-induced mitotic delay. *Nature*. Vol. 356, pp. 353-355.

Russell, K.J., Wiens, L.W., Demers, G.W., Galloway, D.A., Plon, S.E., and Groudine, M. (1995). Abrogation of the G2 checkpoint results in differential radiosensitization of G1 checkpoint-deficient and G1 checkpoint-competent cells. *Cancer Res*. Vol. 55, pp. 1639-1642.

Russell, P., and Nurse, P. (1987). Negative regulation of mitosis by wee1+, a gene encoding a protein kinase homolog. *Cell*. Vol. 49, pp. 559-567.

Ruzankina, Y., Pinzon-Guzman, C., Asare, A., Ong, T., Pontano, L., Cotsarelis, G., Zediak, V.P., Velez, M., Bhandoola, A., and Brown, E.J. (2007). Deletion of the developmentally essential gene ATR in adult mice leads to age-related phenotypes and stem cell loss. *Cell Stem Cell*. Vol. 1, pp. 113-126.

Sanchez, Y., Wong, C., Thoma, R.S., Richman, R., Wu, Z., Piwnica-Worms, H., and Elledge, S.J. (1997). Conservation of the Chk1 checkpoint pathway in mammals: linkage of DNA damage to Cdk regulation through Cdc25. *Science*. Vol. 277, pp. 1497-1501.

Santocanale, C., and Diffley, J.F. (1998). A Mec1- and Rad53-dependent checkpoint controls late-firing origins of DNA replication. *Nature*. Vol. 395, pp. 615-618.

Schmitt, E., Boutros, R., Froment, C., Monsarrat, B., Ducommun, B., and Dozier, C. (2006). CHK1 phosphorylates CDC25B during the cell cycle in the absence of DNA damage. *J Cell Sci*. Vol. 119, pp. 4269-4275.

Sclafani, R.A., and Holzen, T.M. (2007). Cell Cycle Regulation of DNA Replication. *Annual Review of Genetics*. Vol. 41, pp. 237-280.

Shimada, M., Niida, H., Zineldeen, D.H., Tagami, H., Tanaka, M., Saito, H., and Nakanishi, M. (2008). Chk1 is a histone H3 threonine 11 kinase that regulates DNA damage-induced transcriptional repression. *Cell*. Vol. 132, pp. 221-232.

Smits, V.A., Reaper, P.M., and Jackson, S.P. (2006). Rapid PIKK-dependent release of Chk1 from chromatin promotes the DNA-damage checkpoint response. *Curr Biol*. Vol. 16, pp. 150-159.

Solyom, S., Pylkas, K., and Winqvist, R. (2010). Screening for large genomic rearrangements of the BRIP1 and CHK1 genes in Finnish breast cancer families. *Fam Cancer*. Vol. 9, pp. 537-540.

Sørensen, C.S., Hansen, L.T., Dziegielewski, J., Syljuåsen, R.G., Lundin, C., Bartek, J., and Helleday, T. (2005). The cell-cycle checkpoint kinase Chk1 is required for mammalian homologous recombination repair. *Nat Cell Biol*. Vol. 7, pp. 195-201.

Sørensen, C.S., Syljuåsen, R.G., Falck, J., Schroeder, T., Ronnstrand, L., Khanna, K.K., Zhou, B.B., Bartek, J., and Lukas, J. (2003). Chk1 regulates the S phase checkpoint by coupling the physiological turnover and ionizing radiation-induced accelerated proteolysis of Cdc25A. *Cancer cell*. Vol. 3, pp. 247-258.

Stokes, M.P., Van Hatten, R., Lindsay, H.D., and Michael, W.M. (2002). DNA replication is required for the checkpoint response to damaged DNA in Xenopus egg extracts. *The Journal of cell biology*. Vol. 158, pp. 863-872.

Syljuåsen, R.G., Sørensen, C.S., Hansen, L.T., Fugger, K., Lundin, C., Johansson, F., Helleday, T., Sehested, M., Lukas, J., and Bartek, J. (2005). Inhibition of human Chk1 causes increased initiation of DNA replication, phosphorylation of ATR targets, and DNA breakage. *Mol Cell Biol*. Vol. 25, pp. 3553-3562.

Takai, H., Tominaga, K., Motoyama, N., Minamishima, Y.A., Nagahama, H., Tsukiyama, T., Ikeda, K., Nakayama, K., Nakanishi, M., and Nakayama, K. (2000). Aberrant cell cycle checkpoint function and early embryonic death in Chk1(-/-) mice. *Genes Dev*. Vol. 14, pp. 1439-1447.

Takayama, Y., Kamimura, Y., Okawa, M., Muramatsu, S., Sugino, A., and Araki, H. (2003). GINS, a novel multiprotein complex required for chromosomal DNA replication in budding yeast. *Genes & development*. Vol. 17, pp. 1153-1165.

Takeda, D.Y., and Dutta, A. (2005). DNA replication and progression through S phase. *Oncogene*. Vol. 24, pp. 2827-2843.

Thomson, A.M., Gillespie, P.J., and Blow, J.J. (2010). Replication factory activation can be decoupled from the replication timing program by modulating Cdk levels. *The Journal of cell biology*. Vol. 188, pp. 209-221.

Tibbetts, R.S., Brumbaugh, K.M., Williams, J.M., Sarkaria, J.N., Cliby, W.A., Shieh, S.Y., Taya, Y., Prives, C., and Abraham, R.T. (1999). A role for ATR in the DNA damage-induced phosphorylation of p53. *Genes Dev*. Vol. 13, pp. 152-157.

Tili, E., Michaille, J.J., Wernicke, D., Alder, H., Costinean, S., Volinia, S., and Croce, C.M. (2011). Mutator activity induced by microRNA-155 (miR-155) links inflammation and cancer. *Proceedings of the National Academy of Sciences of the United States of America*. Vol. 108, pp. 4908-4913.

Tominaga, Y., Li, C., Wang, R.H., and Deng, C.X. (2006). Murine Wee1 plays a critical role in cell cycle regulation and pre-implantation stages of embryonic development. *Int J Biol Sci*. Vol. 2, pp. 161-170.

Tse, A.N., Carvajal, R., and Schwartz, G.K. (2007). Targeting checkpoint kinase 1 in cancer therapeutics. *Clin Cancer Res*. Vol. 13, pp. 1955-1960.

Vahteristo, P., Tamminen, A., Karvinen, P., Eerola, H., Eklund, C., Aaltonen, L.A., Blomqvist, C., Aittomaki, K., and Nevanlinna, H. (2001). p53, CHK2, and CHK1 genes in Finnish families with Li-Fraumeni syndrome: further evidence of CHK2 in inherited cancer predisposition. *Cancer Res*. Vol. 61, pp. 5718-5722.

Vassileva, V., Millar, A., Briollais, L., Chapman, W., and Bapat, B. (2002). Genes involved in DNA repair are mutational targets in endometrial cancers with microsatellite instability. *Cancer Res*. Vol. 62, pp. 4095-4099.

Wagner, J.M., and Kaufmann, S.H. (2010). Prospects for the Use of ATR Inhibitors to Treat Cancer. *Pharmaceuticals*. Vol. 3, pp. 1311-1334.

Walworth, N., Davey, S., and Beach, D. (1993). Fission yeast chk1 protein kinase links the rad checkpoint pathway to cdc2. *Nature*. Vol. 363, pp. 368-371.

Wang, H., Wang, H., Powell, S.N., Iliakis, G., and Wang, Y. (2004). ATR affecting cell radiosensitivity is dependent on homologous recombination repair but independent of nonhomologous end joining. *Cancer Res*. Vol. 64, pp. 7139-7143.

Wang, X., Kennedy, R.D., Ray, K., Stuckert, P., Ellenberger, T., and D'Andrea, A.D. (2007). Chk1-mediated phosphorylation of FANCE is required for the Fanconi anemia/BRCA pathway. *Mol Cell Biol*. Vol. 27, pp. 3098-3108.

Ward, I.M., and Chen, J. (2001). Histone H2AX is phosphorylated in an ATR-dependent manner in response to replicational stress. *The Journal of biological chemistry*. Vol. 276, pp. 47759-47762.

Watanabe, N., Broome, M., and Hunter, T. (1995). Regulation of the human WEE1Hu CDK tyrosine 15-kinase during the cell cycle. *Embo J*. Vol. 14, pp. 1878-1891.

Woodward, A.M., Gohler, T., Luciani, M.G., Oehlmann, M., Ge, X., Gartner, A., Jackson, D.A., and Blow, J.J. (2006). Excess Mcm2-7 license dormant origins of replication that can be used under conditions of replicative stress. *The Journal of cell biology*. Vol. 173, pp. 673-683.

Wuchty, S., Arjona, D., Li, A., Kotliarov, Y., Walling, J., Ahn, S., Zhang, A., Maric, D., Anolik, R., Zenklusen, J.C., and Fine, H.A. (2011). Prediction of Associations between microRNAs and Gene Expression in Glioma Biology. *PLoS One*. Vol. 6, pp. e14681.

Zachos, G., Black, E.J., Walker, M., Scott, M.T., Vagnarelli, P., Earnshaw, W.C., and Gillespie, D.A. (2007). Chk1 is required for spindle checkpoint function. *Dev Cell*. Vol. 12, pp. 247-260.

Zachos, G., Rainey, M.D., and Gillespie, D.A. (2005). Chk1-dependent S-M checkpoint delay in vertebrate cells is linked to maintenance of viable replication structures. *Mol Cell Biol*. Vol. 25, pp. 563-574.

Zenvirt, S., Kravchenko-Balasha, N., and Levitzki, A. (2010). Status of p53 in human cancer cells does not predict efficacy of CHK1 kinase inhibitors combined with chemotherapeutic agents. *Oncogene*. Vol. 29, pp. 6149-6159.

Zhang, Y.W., Otterness, D.M., Chiang, G.G., Xie, W., Liu, Y.C., Mercurio, F., and Abraham, R.T. (2005). Genotoxic stress targets human Chk1 for degradation by the ubiquitin-proteasome pathway. *Mol Cell*. Vol. 19, pp. 607-618.

Zhao, H., and Piwnica-Worms, H. (2001). ATR-mediated checkpoint pathways regulate phosphorylation and activation of human Chk1. *Mol Cell Biol*. Vol. 21, pp. 4129-4139.

Zhou, B.B., and Elledge, S.J. (2000). The DNA damage response: putting checkpoints in perspective. *Nature*. Vol. 408, pp. 433-439.

Zhu, W., Ukomadu, C., Jha, S., Senga, T., Dhar, S.K., Wohlschlegel, J.A., Nutt, L.K., Kornbluth, S., and Dutta, A. (2007). Mcm10 and And-1/CTF4 recruit DNA polymerase α to chromatin for initiation of DNA replication. *Genes & development*. Vol. 21, pp. 2288-2299.

Zighelboim, I., Schmidt, A.P., Gao, F., Thaker, P.H., Powell, M.A., Rader, J.S., Gibb, R.K., Mutch, D.G., and Goodfellow, P.J. (2009). ATR mutation in endometrioid

endometrial cancer is associated with poor clinical outcomes. *J Clin Oncol*. Vol. 27, pp. 3091-3096.
Zink, D. (2006). The temporal program of DNA replication: new insights into old questions. *Chromosoma*. Vol. 115, pp. 273-287.
Zou, L., and Elledge, S.J. (2003). Sensing DNA damage through ATRIP recognition of RPA-ssDNA complexes. *Science*. Vol. 300, pp. 1542-1548.

Regulation of the G1/S Transition in Adult Liver: Expression and Activation of the Cyclin Dependent Kinase Cdk1 in Differentiated Hepatocytes is Controlled by Extracellular Signals and is Crucial for Commitment to DNA Replication

Loyer Pascal and Corlu Anne
Inserm, UMR 991, Liver Metabolisms and Cancer, Université de Rennes 1, CHU Rennes, F-35033 Cedex, France

1. Introduction

In eukaryotic cells, DNA replication and mitosis are the two processes allowing cell division and generation of two identical daughter cells without loss or alterations of genetic information. These two crucial steps are separated by the G1 and G2 (the acronym for gap) phases that are essential for metabolic adaptation and checking genome integrity before DNA replication and mitosis. Progression of eukaryotic cells through the cell cycle is regulated by the sequential formation, activation, and subsequent inactivation of structurally related serine/threonine protein kinases, the Cyclin-Dependent Kinase or Cdks (Malumbres et al., 2009). Cdks become active upon binding to their regulatory and periodically expressed subunits, namely, the cyclins. Timing of activation of these complexes is determined by a variety of mechanisms including transcriptional regulation, formation of complexes between Cdks, cyclins and other regulatory partners such as Cdk inhibitors (Cdki). In addition, phosphorylation, subcellular localization and selective proteolysis regulate the catalytic activity of these complexes. The first Cdk to be identified, cdc2, was initially discovered as the protein kinase in complex with several cyclins controlling both G1/S and G2/M transitions of the cell cycle in the yeast *Schyzosaccharomyces pombe* (Nurse and Thuriaux, 1980). In contrast to the yeast in which cdc2 is "the" master cell cycle regulator, in mammalian cells at least 20 Cdks, 5 Cdk-like protein kinases (Malumbres et al., 2009) and more than 30 cyclins have been identified that form multiple Cdk/cyclin complexes controlling the cell cycle progression (Malumbres and Barbacid, 2005) and regulating gene transcription and RNA processing (Loyer et al., 2005). Over the last two decades, it has become apparent that these multiple Cdk/cyclin complexes play specific roles in the regulation of a subset of events in the different phases of the cell cycle. A broadly accepted view of the mammalian cell cycle considers that cyclin D1-bound to either Cdk4 or Cdk6 controls progression in late G1 phase through phosphorylation of the retinoblastoma protein (Rb) allowing activation of the E2F transcription factors and downstream transcriptional activation of genes involved in G1/S transition and S phase (Sherr, 1994). Cdk2 successively associates with cyclin E and A, completes the hyperphosphorylation of Rb, phosphorylates components of the DNA replication machinery and governs centrosome duplication at the G1/S transition and in S phase. Finally, activity of Cdk1 associated with both A- and B-type cyclins is required for entry and progression through M phase. In this model of mammalian cell cycle, Cdk2 and Cdk1 are thought to function independently at two distinct periods, respectively the G1 to S and G2 to M transitions, without functional redundancy (Bashir and Pagano, 2005).

This model of cell cycle control has first been challenged by the finding that some cancer cells proliferate despite Cdk2 inhibition (Tetsu and McCormick, 2003). Independently, the demonstration was brought that knock-out mice for Cdk2 as well as E-type cyclins are viable and that cell cycle of cultured Cdk2$^{-/-}$ mouse embryonic fibroblasts (MEFs) do not show major alterations besides a delayed commitment to S phase (Berthet et al., 2003; Ortega et al., 2003). These data indicated that Cdk2/cyclin E complexes are dispensable for commitment to S phase and/or that other Cdk(s) would compensate for the loss of Cdk2. In contrast, Cdk1$^{-/-}$ mouse embryo's development is arrested at a very early stage and knock-down of Cdk1 expression by shRNA in synchronized Cdk2$^{-/-}$ MEFs strongly reduces S phase entry (Aleem et al., 2004) demonstrating that other Cdks cannot compensate for Cdk1 ablation. A revisited model of cell cycle regulation in which Cdk1 would compensate for Cdk2 ablation by controlling the G1/S transition and initiation of DNA replication was proposed (Kaldis and Aleem, 2005). Consequently, several new questions have been raised: Does Cdk1 initiate the G1/S transition only in Cdk2$^{-/-}$ cells isolated from genetically modified mice or does Cdk1 generally act as the predominant Cdk in somatic cells? Alternatively, Cdk1 and Cdk2 may act in synergy or redundantly to promote both DNA replication and centrosome duplication during the G1/S transition. It has been proposed that the role of Cdk1 at the G1/S transition may have been overlooked in higher eukaryotic cells since Cdk2 activity appeared higher to that of CDK1 at the onset of DNA replication and because this Cdk1 activity was negligible compared to the peak of Cdk1 activity at the G2/M transition (Bashir and Pagano, 2005). Interestingly, it was also demonstrated that both Cdk1 and Cdk2 were required for efficient DNA replication in *Xenopus* egg extracts (Krasinska et al., 2008) suggesting that at least in some non genetically modified cell types, Cdk1 could contribute to S phase initiation and/or DNA replication. It is clear that Cdks play a pivotal role in orchestrating commitment to S phase and DNA replication but from the most recent publications studying the function of Cdk1 and Cdk2 throughout the cell cycle a large of body of data evidences qualitative and quantitative differences in expression of Cdk/cyclin complexes between mammalian cell types leading to the emerging picture of slightly distinct Cdk-dependent molecular mechanisms during G1 phase that all, however, trigger G1/S transition.

In this review, we briefly discuss some general knowledge of the growth factor dependent entry into and progression through the cell cycle in mammalian cells and the differences observed in the Cdk and cyclin expression between cell types. However, the main goal of this chapter is to highlight the role of Cdk1 in the G1/S transition in differentiated adult hepatocyte. In normal liver, hepatocytes are quiescent differentiated cells that keep the ability to re-enter the cell cycle when liver tissue integrity is challenged. This model has been widely used to study the cell cycle. We will present the *in vivo* and *in vitro* models of normal proliferating hepatocytes and our data showing the involvement of Cdk1 in the G1/S transition in these cells. In addition, our recent data unveiling an unexpected link between extracellular signals (cytokines, growth factors and extracellular matrix components) and the control of the G1/S transition via the induction of Cdk1 will be developed in this chapter.

2. The cell cycle: a universal cell division process with a large diversity of cell signaling pathways controlling entry into and progression through G1 phase in mammalian cells

The molecular pathways controlling the progression throughout the cell cycle and both DNA replication and mitosis are remarkably conserved among eukaryotic cells (Araki, 2011). Although mammalian cells show a higher degree of complexity, at least some of the molecular mechanisms remain conserved from yeast to humans. A good example of these conserved pathways through evolution is the protein kinase Cdk1: invalidation of Cdk1 also called CDC28 in budding yeast *Saccharomyces cerevisiae* using a thermo-sensitive mutant can be rescued (complementation) by its human homolog Cdk1 (Ninomiya-Tsuji et al., 1991). The most conserved aspects of the cell cycle are probably DNA replication and major check-points for DNA integrity and mitosis. In contrast with these conserved mechanisms, multicellular organisms developed during evolution specific pathways to control the transition from quiescence to DNA replication. In mammalian cells, specific combinations of extracellular signal stimuli for each cell type promote the exit from quiescence, progression throughout G1 phase and commitment to DNA replication. Proliferation stimuli are constituted by a vast panel of growth factors and cytokines activating downstream intracellular signalling pathways after binding to membrane receptors mainly through a cascade of phosphorylation and dephosphorylation events that ultimately triggers changes in gene expression in order to induce the proteins absolutely required for duplication of cellular components including DNA and the subsequent mitosis (Iyer et al., 1999). In this picture, there is a striking contrast between the diversity of proliferation stimuli and early steps of proliferation signalling pathways and, on the other side, the limited number of proteins that control G1/S transition and DNA replication. In another word, cell cycle entry begins with proteins differentially expressed among cell types, which activate the ubiquitous machinery of DNA replication present in all dividing cells. During their journey towards DNA replication and mitosis, cells initially quiescent or exiting mitosis will sequentially activate less and less specific protein complexes throughout the G1 phase to eventually fire the DNA replication machinery identical between cell types. A crucial question, which is currently actively investigated, is how so many distinct proliferation stimuli and signalling pathways can lead to the activation of a limited number of proteins controlling commitment to and progression through DNA replication. To address this question, we will come back on the basis of progression throughout the G1 phase of the cell cycle and how the overall proliferation signalling pathway "narrows down" to activate the DNA replication at the G1/S transition.

2.1 The G1 phase and the mitogen dependent cell cycle progression

Most studies regarding cell cycle are conducted using synchronized cell models in which cells progress synchronously through the different phases of the cell cycle in order to analyze expression and activation of regulators at each step of the cell cycle. Yeasts and ovocytes from amphibians, especially *Xenopus*, and marine organisms such as star fish and sea urchin have provided cell models that proliferate spontaneously in a highly

synchronized manner to investigate cell cycle regulation. In addition, the genesis of thermo-sensitive yeast mutants for the cell cycle progression constituted an extremely powerful technical approach to isolate genes playing crucial roles in the cell cycle regulation. From the mid 70's to the late 80's, the burst of data obtained in these eukaryotic cells lead to the identification of major cell cycle regulators including the cyclins (Sherr, 1995) and their catalytic subunit partners the Cdks (Malumbres et al., 2009). Mammalian homologs of these cell cycle regulators were subsequently isolated and by the mid-90's a network of Cdk/cyclin complexes emerged. Pioneers in this field of investigation, Drs L. Hartwell, P. Nurse and T. Hunt who deciphered the cell cycle regulation in yeast and ovocytes were awarded with the 2001 Nobel Prize of medicine not only for the identification of new pathways regulating cell division (Nurse, 2002) but also for opening a complete new field in cancer research since many of these cell cycle regulators are altered during oncogenesis and/or are potential therapeutic targets for cancer treatments (Knockaert et al., 2002).
In mammals, synchronized cell proliferation *in vivo* is restricted to very few cell types among which proliferation of hepatocytes during liver regeneration following partial hepatectomy has probably been the most used model. Sections 2 and 3 in this chapter will focus on the major findings reported by our groups and others regarding regulation of the G1/S transition in hepatocytes. *In vivo*, cell renewal is mainly achieved through the proliferation of adult stem and progenitor cells that proliferate actively although these cells can probably arrest in G0 before additional rounds of division or entering a program of differentiation. Because stem/progenitor cells are rare cells and cannot be easily purified, there are few data regarding cell cycle regulation in these cell types. There are, however, adult differentiated cell types that remain arrested in G0, which can re-enter the cell cycle for several rounds of division upon appropriate proliferation stimuli including lymphocytes (Ajchenbaum et al., 1993), monocytes (Tushinski and Stanley, 1985) and fibroblasts (Iyer et al., 1999) which can be isolated relatively easily from blood or skin, respectively, plated in culture and used for cell cycle studies. Although these cell types are suitable models for conducting cell cycle studies there have been a limited number of publications reporting cell cycle data using lymphocytes and monocytes mainly because these primary cells need to be renewed for each experiment. The most widely used cell models in the field of cell cycle regulation are the immortalized or transformed cell lines artificially synchronized by drug treatments arresting the cells in G1/S or G2/M transitions and the primary fibroblasts arrested by serum starvation in a G0-like state (Figure 1). Although the scoop of this chapter is to focus on the progression in late G1 and the G1/S transition, it is important to point out that the comparison between these *in vitro* models of G0-like or early G1 arrest and *in vivo* G0 arrested cells were poorly documented for many years. However, recent reports evidenced differences between "arrested" cells in various conditions (Coller et al., 2006; Sang et al., 2008). For instance, the serum starvation of fibroblasts plated at low density obviously provides an experimental condition completely different from G0-arrested cells *in vivo*, which stop dividing for other reasons than the lack of growth factors or nutrients. Nevertheless, these *in vitro* synchronized mammalian cells provided powerful models to investigate cell cycle in mammalian cells and allowed to collect crucial data on the progression from early G1 to the commitment to DNA synthesis.
In the mid-70's, the *in vitro* synchronized mammalian cells allowed to define the concept of "restriction point" during the G1 phase (Pardee, 1974). A major feature of the G1 phase is that cells need a mitogenic stimulation to enter into and progress through G1 phase until

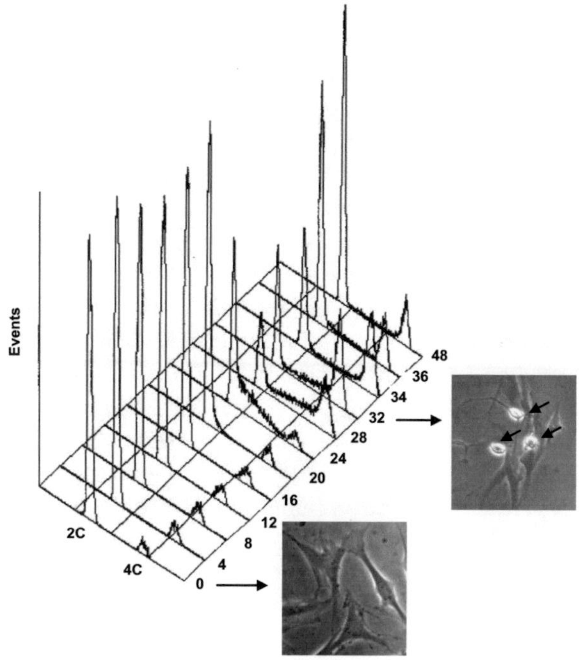

Fig. 1. Flow cytometry analysi of the DNA content in human foreskin fibroblasts plated at low cell density and synchronized by serum starvation. Cells were arrested in G0-like stage by serum starvation for 3 days and cell cycle was re-induced by adding back serum to culture medium. A time-course analysis of the DNA content was performed using propidium iodide staining by flow cytometry. Over 95% of arrested cells (0) in G0-like and cells progressing in G1 phase (from 4 to 20 hours after stimulation) showed a "2C" DNA content. At 24 hours, the number of cells with "2C" decreases as initiation of DNA replication begins (2C< cells<4C). At 24 hours, the peak of replications takes place and the percentage of cells reaching G2/M increases (cells with "4C" DNA content; mitosis : arrows). By 34 hours, cell cycle has been completed and cells initiate a new cell cycle by re-entering G1 phase.

they reach the so-called "mitogen dependent restriction point" in late G1 beyond which completion of the cell cycle becomes independent from extracellular stimuli. A. Pardee and co-workers evidenced this restriction point by using serum-starved fibroblasts stimulated to re-enter the cell cycle by adding back the serum (Pardee, 1974). They were able to show that a minimal period of stimulation was required to reach the late G1 and that, beyond this point, the cell cycle would be completed even after removing growth factors. This restriction point is very similar to the Start point in yeast that controls the commitment to S phase (Reed, 1992). Data from this group and others showed that the G1 phase is the longest phase of the cell cycle in all mammalian cells but the timing varies considerably between cell types. It is essential to distinguish the G1 progression between cells that proliferate actively and enter G1 after completion of mitosis and cells re-entering the cell cycle after a prolonged quiescence or G0. It is now well established that the transition from G0 to G1 is characterized by a profound modification of the expressed gene profile (Iyer et al., 1999) required for metabolic adaptation to cell proliferation and resulting in a longer period of time for the cells to initiate progression in late G1 compared to the cells exiting mitosis. Following the discovery of the mitogen-dependent restriction point, it was demonstrated that progression through the G1 phase can be divided in several periods. Using purified priming and growth factors to stimulate progression of fibroblasts arrested in G0-like state by serum starvation, it was reported that progression of fibroblasts throughout G1 could be divided in 4 periods: competence, entry, progression and assembly (Figure 2). Stimulation of starved fibroblasts by PDGF is able to promote progression in early G1 in arrested cells until the restriction point C (competence) but fails to allow progression in mid and late G1 (Cross et al., 1989; Denhardt et al., 1986; Pledger et al., 1977; Pledger et al., 1978). This period in early G1 was named competence. Following stimulation by PDGF, further progression in late G1 and S phase is achieved by stimulation with EGF or insulin (Leof et al., 1983; Yang and Pardee, 1986). However, in absence of essential amino acids cells arrest in mid-G1 at a restriction point named "V". The progression between points "C" and "V "defines the period called entry (Pardee, 1986) while the progression between point "V" and the mitogen-dependent restriction point (point "R") was called progression. Finally, the period beyond the mitogen-dependent restriction point and before the burst of DNA synthesis was named assembly (Pardee, 1989).

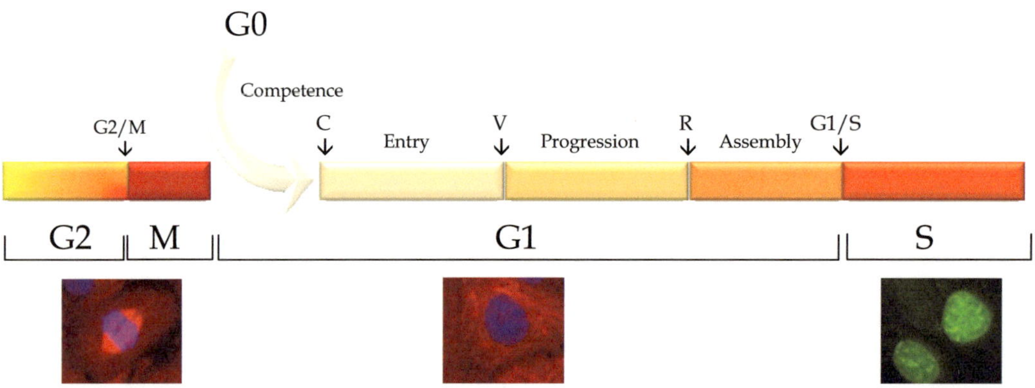

Fig. 2. Progression through the G1 phase is divided in several sub-phases. Photographs illustrate detection of cells in G2/M, G1 and S Phase : the cells in G2/M and G1 were stained with DAPI (DNA) and immuno-fluorescence detecting γ-tubulin while in S phase cells were incubated with BrdU to evidence DNA replication by indirect immunofluorescence. Four steps were identified during the G1 phase of the cell cycle: competence, entry, progression and assembly. Note that the convergence of molecular pathways in early G1 for cells entering G1 after completion of mitosis or re-entry in the cell cycle following stimulation by growth factors remains to be fully characterized in mammalian cells.

Similar studies were performed in other cell models such as mononuclear blood cells (Tushinski and Stanley, 1985) or hepatocytes (Loyer et al., 1996) leading to the same conclusion that G1 phase could be divided in sub-phases corresponding to major steps in the metabolic adaptation required for cells to initiate DNA replication and mitosis. From these data, soluble factors such as the PDGF that promote in early G1 were called priming factors while hormones and cytokines stimulating progression in late G1 and the G1/S transition were considered as mitogens or growth factors.

Following binding to their receptors on plasma membrane, priming and growth factors activate multiple phosphorylation events involving multiple protein kinases especially the MAPKinase pathways (Ruderman, 1993; Ussar and Voss, 2004). There are multiple cross-talks between these pathways but they ultimately control activation of transcription factors that sequentially trigger induction of cell cycle regulators such as the cyclins and Cdks (Talarmin et al., 1999). Cdks are nuclear effectors that play a pivotal role in orchestrating DNA replication, DNA repair, mitosis and centrosome duplication (Harrison et al., ; Muller et al., 2001; Ren et al., 2002). Because of the limited number of Cdk/cyclin complexes expressed in most mammalian cells in late G1 and at the G1/S transition, it was widely accepted until very recently that stimulation by growth factors triggered induction of D- and E--type cyclins in late G1, which associate with Cdk4/6 and Cdk2, respectively, to control entry into S phase. In this view of the cell cycle, by the time cells have reached late G1, the large diversity of growth factors and signaling pathways observed in early G1 is gone to leave the cells with ~four to six Cdk/cyclin complexes to regulate the entry into S phase. This view of the cell cycle has been partially revisited after the demonstration that Cdk2 knock-out mice were viable (Satyanarayana and Kaldis, 2009b; Sherr, 1994; Sherr and Roberts, 2004) and by the re-interpretation of data showing differences in the expression of Cdks and cyclins during G1 in different eukaryotic cells (Furukawa et al., 1990 ; Loyer et al., 1994). In the light of these recent data, it is tempting to ask the question whether additional combinations of Cdk/cyclin complexes can control the G1/S transition and progression in S phase and how such a diversity of complexes can activate the DNA replication machinery and centrosome duplication.

2.2 Expression and roles of Cyclin dependent kinases and cyclins during the G1 phase

Entry into and progression through the G1 phase of the cell cycle and the G1/S transition is associated with a sequential activation of Cdk/cyclin complexes upon the stimulation by priming and growth factors. The catalytic activities of these Cdk/cyclin complexes through the phosphorylation of "specific" protein substrates control the progression in G1 and commitment to DNA replication (Sherr, 1993), the chromosomal DNA replication (Araki, 2011) and centrosome duplication (Harrison et al., 2011). The identification of these substrates over the last 15 years has unveiled the crucial molecular mechanisms regulating the progression through G1 phase that need to be "unlocked" for the cell to proceed in S phase. In this section, we will briefly present the Cdk/cyclin complexes induced and activated during G1 phases and their phosphorylation substrates. Then, we will discuss how the differences in expression and/or activation of Cdk/cyclin complexes observed among mammalian cells may be compatible with the phosphorylation of the proteins controlling the initiation of DNA replication and centrosome duplication.

2.2.1 Sequential activation of Cdk/cyclin complexes during the cell cycle

For many years, the G0/G1 transition and progression in early G1 phase was thought to be associated with the induction of immediate-early and immediate delayed genes in a Cdk/cyclin independent manner. Following stimulation by priming factors a large set of immediate early genes is induced at a transcriptional level by pre-existing latent transcription factors such as NF-κB (FitzGerald et al., 1995). More recently Ren and Rollins made, however, a strong case that Cdk3/cyclin C complex could regulate the G0/G1 transition in human glioblastoma T98G cells (Ren and Rollins, 2004). The phosphorylation status of pocket protein family members including the retinoblastoma protein (pRb) and p130 changes throughout the cell cycle (DeCaprio et al., 1992). While cells leave quiescence to enter G1 this phosphorylation level varies and inactivation of pRb is sufficient to induce G0/G1 transition in quiescent cells (Canhoto et al., 2000). Based on these observations, Ren and Rollins postulated that hypophosphorylated or unphosphorylated pRb present in G0-arrested cells may be phosphorylated by Cdk/cyclin complexes to promote entry into G1 phase. They identified the Cdk3/cyclin C complex mediating pRb phosphorylation during G0/G1 transition (Ren and Rollins, 2004). Interestingly, cyclin C associated with Cdk8 (Tassan et al., 1995) plays a completely different role in transcriptional regulation through the phosphorylation of the C-terminal domain (CTD) of RNA polymerase II (Leclerc et al., 1996; Loyer et al., 2005; Rickert et al., 1999). This report associated for the first time a Cdk/cyclin complex with the G0/G1 transition (Figure 3).

This conclusion has not been generalized to a large panel of mammalian cell types in the past years. Indeed, many cells lack functional Cdk3 or express so little amounts that no conclusive data on the ubiquitous role of Cdk3/cyclin C complex at the G0/G1 boundary could be drawn. It was recently reported that in NIH3T3 cells, the absence of Cdk3 could be compensated by Cdk2 that interacts with cyclin C in early G1 (Hansen et al., 2009; Saxena et al., 2009). In this work, the authors did not investigate the phosphorylation of pRb by the Cdk2/cyclin C complex but rather showed that the transcription factor LSF (late simian virus 40 factor) (Kim et al., 1987) is phosphorylated by Cdk2 associated with cyclins C or E as well as Cdk3/cyclin C predominantly on serine 309. Phosphorylation of LSF on serine 291 by the MEK/extracellular signal-regulated kinase (ERK) signaling pathway upon stimulation by growth factors (Pagon et al., 2003; Ruderman, 1993; Volker et al., 1997) in mid-late G1 phase is essential for the G1/S transition since phospho(S291)-LSF controls the transcriptional activation of the thymidylate synthase (*Tyms*) (Powell et al., 2000). In contrast, phosphorylation of LSF on serine 309 in cells expressing Cdk3 inhibits LSF transactivation suggesting the required LSF shut-down in early G1 and its reactivation in late G1 mediated by Cdk/cyclin complex(es) and ERK, respectively (Hansen et al., 2009). This work appears important because it suggests functional redundancy of Cdk/cyclin complexes in early G1 and identifies LSF as the second known phosphorylation substrates of Cdk/cyclin complexes, in addition to pRb, during progression from quiescence to early G1 phase. There are too few reports describing the signaling pathways regulating the entry into G1 and early progression to draw the final conclusion that Cdk/cyclin complexes are crucial at this stage of the cell cycle but we can expect to learn more the molecular mechanisms regulating exit to quiescence in coming years.

In contrast, signaling pathways essential for the subsequent progression in late G1 are well documented and clearly involve the Cdk/cyclin complexes (Satyanarayana and Kaldis, 2009b). The transition from mid to late G1 phase is regulated by successive phosphorylation events of members of the pocket protein family including the retinoblastoma protein (pRb), p107, and p130 (DeCaprio et al., 1992). Cdk/cyclin complexes are responsible for the changes in pocket proteins phosphorylation status (Kato et al., 1993; Sherr, 1995). In mid-G1, the hypophosphorylated pRb binds to the transcription factor E2F family members thereby preventing active transcription of E2F-regulated genes. The negative regulation of E2F transcription factors mediated by pRb occurs through a conformation structure that prevents E2F's transactivation domain to be active and probably also by recruiting chromatin-modifying enzymes repressing transcription (Trimarchi and Lees, 2002). Upon stimulation by growth factors, D-type cyclins are up-regulated (Matsushime et al., 1991) and associate with Cdk4 and/or Cdk6 to form active complexes (Matsushime et al., 1992; Matsushime et al., 1994) that partially phosphorylate pRb and/or actively phosphorylate a fraction of pRb (Kato et al., 1993). In late G1, formation of Cdk2/cyclin E complex triggers additional phosphorylation of pRb to generate the hyperphosphorylated form of pRb (Figure 3) that looses the ability to negatively regulate the transactivation domain of E2F's factors (Lundberg and Weinberg, 1998). Consequently, the release of E2F proteins promote transcription of a large set of genes required for the progression in late G1 including Cdk2 and cyclin E (Fan and Bertino, 1997; Geng et al., 1996), S phase entry (DeGregori et al., 1995; Kowalik et al., 1995; Ren et al., 2002) and centrosome duplication (Harrison et al., 2011). In parallel, Cdk2 phosphorylates the Nuclear protein Ataxia-Telangiectasia implicated in the transcription of histones (Zhao et al., 2000) and the nucleophosmin/B23 regulating centrosome duplication (Okuda et al., 2000). At this stage of the cell cycle progression cells have committed to DNA replication and removal of growth factors (in culture cell systems) will not affect either the burst of DNA replication or the mitotic rate. Thus, turning on the E2F-dependent transcription coincides with the progression beyond the mitogen-dependent restriction point identified by Pardee and co-workers (Pardee, 1989) before the discovery of Cdk/cyclin complexes.

In eukaryotic cells, chromosomal DNA replication is ensured through periodic and tightly controlled assembly and disassembly of pre-replication complexes (pre-RC) loaded on DNA replication origins (Diffley, 2004; Fujita, 2006). In mid-late G1, the Origin Recognition Complex (ORC) containing several subunits associated to the proteins CDC6 and Cdt1 is responsible for loading a replicative helicase and the mini-chromosome maintenance (MCM) 2-7 subunits to form the pre-RC (Fujita, 2006). Interestingly, loading of the pre-RC components occurs in a low Cdk activity period (Wheeler et al., 2008) while at the onset of DNA synthesis the increasing Cdk-dependent kinase activities trigger the MCM complex to initiate replication and the degradation of Cdt1 to prevent reassembly of additional pre-RC (Katsuno et al., 2009; Lei and Tye, 2001; Thomson et al.). Recent data from our laboratory demonstrated that in quiescent hepatocytes, MCM7 is not expressed but its expression becomes detectable immediately after the mitogenic stimulation in mid-G1, almost concomitantly with the induction of cyclin D1 (Garnier et al., 2009) and prior the high Cdk-dependent kinase activity taking place in late G1 and early S phase. The induction of MCM7 and the formation of the pre-RC thus occur in a very narrow period of time since in S phase, ORC1 and Cdt1 are degraded through several mechanisms including the phosphorylation by Cdks and downstream ubiquitination by SCFSkp2 ubiquitin Ligase (Fujita, 2006; Fujita et al., 2002). These well documented mechanisms clearly point out the crucial role of Cdk/cyclin complexes in the regulation of pre-RC formation. Similarly, pre-RC are activated by phosphorylations involving the protein kinase Cdc7 and the Cdk2/cyclin E complex that trigger the recruitment of Cdc45 (Woo and Poon, 2003) a crucial docking factor for DNA helicase and polymerases. During S phase, the heterodimer Cdk2/cyclin A also contributes to DNA replication (Cardoso et al., 1993; Rosenblatt et al., 1992; Zindy et al., 1992) by phosphorylating components of the replication machinery including the Proliferating Cell Nuclear Antigen (PCNA) and DNA polymerases. The activity of Cdk2 is thus tightly associated with the entry into and progression through S phase (Figure 3). Following mitosis, daughter cells receive a single centrosome, which, like DNA, must duplicate prior mitosis. In early S phase, centriole duplication begins and by the late G2, two mature centrosomes have been generated to ensure proper chromosome segregation

(Harrison et al., 2011). Duplication of centrioles is in part regulated through the G1 phase Cdk/cyclin-dependent pRb pathway (Adon et al., 2010) and there is a large body of evidences for the Cdk2/cyclin E involvement in the activation by phosphorylation of crucial regulators of centriole duplication (Harrison et al., 2011).
The activity of Cdk1 associated with both A- and B-type cyclins is required for entry and progression through M phase in all eukaryotic cells (Doree and Hunt, 2002). The activity of the Cdk1/cyclin B complex, which was the first cyclin-dependent kinase activity detected in sea urchin and in *Xenopus* (Arion et al., 1988; Gautier et al., 1988), rapidly appeared to be a master regulator of the G2/M transition in all eukaryotic cells (Doree and Hunt, 2002) including in humans cells (Draetta and Beach, 1988). Recently, the Cdk11^{p58} protein kinase was also shown to be essential for mitosis (Hu et al., 2007; Petretti et al., 2006). In humans, the *Cell division control 2 Like* genes *Cdc2L1* and *Cdc2L2* encode two related protein kinases, denoted Cdk11B and A, respectively, which are expressed as two predominant protein isoforms designated by their apparent molecular weight of 110 and 58kDa for the Cdk11$^{p110A/B}$ and Cdk11$^{p58A/B}$ isoforms, respectively (Trembley et al., 2004). The CDK11^{p110} and CDK11^{p58} isoforms are produced from the same mRNAs through the use of an internal ribosome entry site (IRES) and two different AUG codons located in the coding sequence of the CDK11^{p110}A and B mRNAs. The CDK11^{p110} isoform thus contains the entire sequence of CDK11^{p58}, which includes the catalytic domain (Loyer et al., 2005). CDK11^{p110} protein is a nuclear protein present in two macromolecular complexes involved in the regulation of transcription and pre-RNA splicing. Expression of the large CDK11^{p110} isoform is ubiquitous and constant throughout the cell cycle while CDK11^{p58} expression is maximal during G2 and M phases of the cell cycle (Loyer et al., 2011; Loyer et al., 2008; Trembley et al., 2002). CDK11^{p58} is essential during mitosis for centrosome maturation and mitotic spindle formation, sister chromatid cohesion and cytokinesis (Hu et al., 2007; Petretti et al., 2006). Very recently, Franck & al., (Franck et al., 2011) showed that CDK11^{p58} is required for centriole duplication and that it could regulate centriole components such as the protein kinase Plk4 that mediates phosphorylation required for centriole duplication during the subsequent interphase. These data suggest that CDK11^{p58}-dependent kinase activity during mitosis would regulate mitotic events *per se* and downstream molecular pathways during the centriole duplication in S and G2 phases. The cyclin L's, encoded by the *CCNL1* and *CCNL2* genes, are the regulatory partners of CDK11^{p110} and CDK11^{p58} (Loyer et al., 2008) although it was not reported that CDK11^{p58} was associated to cyclin L's for its mitotic role. Nevertheless, CDK11^{p58} probably associated with L-type cyclins plays a pivotal role during mitosis (Figure 3).
Together, these data collected over more than 25 years have demonstrated that the sequential activation of Cdk/cyclin complexes is a hallmark of the cell cycle regulation.

2.2.2 Are Cdk/cyclin complexes functionally redundant to phosphorylate the retinoblastoma protein and components of the DNA replication machinery?

Because the kinase activities of Cdk2 and Cdk1 were mainly detected in G1/S and G2/M transitions respectively, they were thought to function independently at these two distinct periods without functional redundancy (Bashir and Pagano, 2005; Woo and Poon, 2003). This conclusion was reinforced by the experimental inactivation of Cdk1 and Cdk2 in human cell lines: enforced expression of kinase dead Cdk2 caused a G1 arrest while expression of kinase dead Cdk1 result in a G2/M arrest (van den Heuvel and Harlow, 1993). Similarly, cells expressing temperature-sensitive Cdk1 mutant arrest in G2 at the restrictive

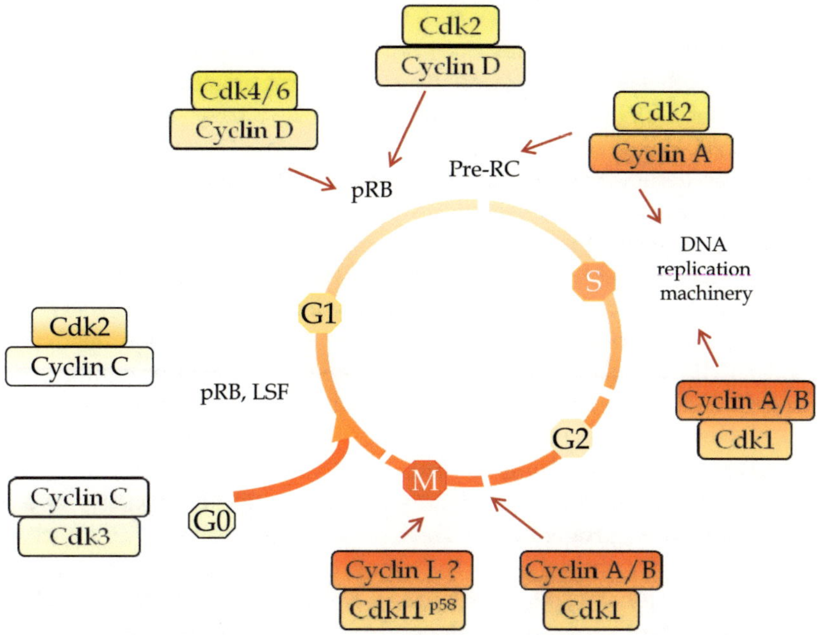

Fig. 3. Sequential activation of Cdk/cyclin complexes throughout the cell cycle.

temperature (Th'ng et al., 1990; Yasuda et al., 1991). This model of cell cycle control has first been challenged by the finding that some cancer cells proliferate despite Cdk2 inhibition (Tetsu and McCormick, 2003). Independently, the demonstration was brought that knock-out mice for Cdk2 as well as for E-type Cyclins are viable and that the cell cycle of cultured Cdk2-/- mouse embryonic fibroblasts (MEFs) did not show major alterations (Berthet et al., 2003; Ortega et al., 2003; Sherr and Roberts, 2004). In addition, in the hippocampus of Cdk2-/- mouse, the proliferation of granule neurons of the dentate gyrus that undergo continuous renewal throughout life, is not altered (Vandenbosch et al., 2007). Similarly, hematopoiesis is not affected in Cdk2 knockout mice (Berthet et al., 2007). These data indicated that Cdk2/Cyclin E complexes were dispensable for commitment to S phase and that other Cdk(s) could compensate for the loss of Cdk2. Along the same line, a Cdk1-dependent compensatory mechanism regulating S phase initiation and progression was also demonstrated in DT40 chicken cells lacking Cdk2 (Hochegger et al., 2007). Together, these data have led authors to propose a revised model of the cell cycle control in which Cdk1 compensates for Cdk2 ablation by controlling the G_1/S transition, initiation of DNA replication and centrosome duplication (Bashir and Pagano, 2005; Kaldis and Aleem, 2005).
Interestingly, it was recently demonstrated that both Cdk1 and Cdk2 were required for efficient DNA replication in *Xenopus* egg extracts (Krasinska et al., 2008) suggesting that, at least in some non-genetically modified cell types, Cdk1 could contribute to S phase initiation and/or DNA replication. In mammalian cells, the involvement of Cdk1 in S phase may have been underestimated mainly because the low levels of active Cdk1 compared to the high levels of Cdk2 during DNA replication suggested that Cdk2 was predominant over Cdk1 at this step of the cell cycle (Bashir and Pagano, 2005). In this emerging picture of the cell cycle regulation, these new data probably did not profoundly affect the roles that were initially attributed to the different Cdk/cyclin complexes but rather introduce the notion of redundancy and flexibility (Li et al., 2009b; Satyanarayana and Kaldis, 2009b).

Cdk/cyclin complexes are, at least in part, functionally redundant. Thus, interfering with the activity of one Cdk/cyclin complex does not systematically lead to cell cycle arrest and cell death. This hypothesis was verified by further investigating single and combined alterations in mice of Cdk4/6-Cyclin D, Cdk2-Cyclin E, $p27^{Kip1}$ and Rb (Li et al., 2009a; Malumbres et al., 2004; Satyanarayana and Kaldis, 2009b). These deletions did not affect early embryogenesis demonstrating multiple compensatory mechanisms and overlapping roles of these genes. Moreover, analysis of the cell cycle in MEFs derived from these knock-out mice evidenced compensatory mechanism between positive and negative regulators at the G_1/S transition and highlighted a complex network regulating the expression and activation of these cell cycle regulators in the progression from G_1 to S phase (Malumbres et al., 2009; Satyanarayana and Kaldis, 2009b). This important conclusion needs, however, to be softened since Cdk2 knockout mice exhibit altered self-renewal of neural progenitors in the adult subventricular zone of the brain (Jablonska et al., 2007). In this study, the authors showed that Cdk4 was able to compensate for the loss of Cdk2 during embryogenesis and during 2 weeks post-natal resulting in pRb inactivation. This compensatory pathway declines after a month leading to decreased self-renewal capacity and enhanced differentiation of neural progenitors. These data demonstrated that compensatory mechanisms for Cdk2 loss through the activation of other Cdk family members do not systematically occur in all cell types (Berthet and Kaldis, 2007). These molecular pathways can be silenced in some specific cell types depending upon the differentiation context.

The notion of redundancy between Cdks needs to be also modulated by the demonstration that knocking down certain Cdks in mouse is lethal for the embryos. For instance, $Cdk1^{-/-}$ mouse embryo's development is arrested at a very early stage (Santamaria et al., 2007) and knock-down of Cdk1 expression by shRNA in synchronized $Cdk2^{-/-}$ MEFs strongly reduced S phase entry (Aleem et al., 2005). Similarly, the $Cdk11^{p58}$ is essential for mitosis (Hu et al., 2007; Petretti et al., 2006) and the conventional knock-out of the Cdk11 gene in mouse is lethal as early as the blastocyst stage (Li et al., 2004) demonstrating that some Cdks have specific and essential functions that cannot be rescued by other Cdk family members. Nevertheless, in the experimental situations of genetic alterations of G1-associated Cdks and cyclins, Cdk1 is sufficient to drive the cell cycle in most cell types (Santamaria et al., 2007) illustrating the functional compensations among the Cdks. This conclusion based on models of genetic Cdk gene alterations and/or substitutions is also important to re-analyze some data that evidenced different patterns of cdk and cyclin expression in mammalian cells in absence of engineered genetic modifications. Indeed, both Cdk4 and Cdk6 can associate to Cyclins D1, D2 and D3 to form active complexes phosphorylating pRb (Bates et al., 1994; Kato and Sherr, 1993; Matsushime et al., 1994). However, these six complexes are rarely found expressed in a single cell type and are rather expressed differentially in normal or transformed cells (Alhejaily et al., 2011; Fiaschi-Taesch et al., 2010). In addition, while in cells actively proliferating Cdk1 is expressed constantly throughout the cell cycle, in cells proliferating after a cell cycle arrest in G0, such as lymphocytes and hepatocytes, Cdk1 is barely detectable in G1 but appears at the G1/S transition (Furukawa et al., 1990; Loyer et al., 1994). In fibroblast arrested in G0-like state by serum starvation, cdk1 appears only after the G1/S transition (Garnier et al., 2009) while in cells arrested in late G1 by a double thymidine block, Cdk1 is detected through the cell cycle with modest quantitative variations (Dulic et al., 1992).

The diversity of Cdk expression in G1 phase among mammalian cells may be explained in part by the fact that, in some experimental models, cells initiate the cell cycle from the quiescence in G0 while in others, cells enter G1 immediately after completion of mitosis without a cell cycle arrest in G0. However, these distinct patterns of expression of the Cdks especially during G1 phase may reflect a diversity of Cdk/cyclin-mediated pathways to promote the G1/S transition in absence of compensatory mechanisms generated by Cdk or cyclin gene invalidation. The diversity of Cdk/cyclin complexes expressed in G1 also raises the question of the phosphorylation events mediated by Cdks during interphase. Assuming that the phosphorylation of "specific" substrate proteins by Cdk/cyclin complexes during G1 and S phases such as pRb, LSF, pre-RC and DNA machinery components, is absolutely required for the cell cycle progression, the different combinations of Cdk and cyclin complexes expressed in interphase must all be capable of phosphorylating these substrates in order to promote cell cycle progression. To the best of our knowledge, detailed studies of all Cdk phosphorylation activities towards a large panel of candidate substrates have not been performed, however, several reports indicated that Cdk1 either associated to D- or A-type cyclins (Joshi et al., 2009; Santamaria et al., 2007) can indeed phsophorylate pRb and, thus, can compensate for the lack of Cdk4 or Cdk6 associated with G1 cyclins.

Recently, our view of the cell cycle regulation has significantly advanced towards a more complex and diversified picture. While in G2/M transition Cdk1/cyclin B complex remains a master regulator of the entry into mitosis, during G1 and in G1/S transition, differential expression of Cdk4, Cdk6 or Cdk2 and C- or D-type cyclins in various cell types obviously allows multiple options of Cdk/cyclin heterodimers that are capable of promoting S phase entry (Satyanarayana and Kaldis, 2009b). Even more surprising was the observation that genetic alterations of these G1/S regulator genes induce the recruitment of Cdk1 to promote S phase. Earlier in this chapter, we pointed out the striking contrast between the large diversity of mitogenic factors and proliferation signaling pathways opposed to the limited number of Cdk/cyclin complexes regulating the commitment to S phase. In the light of the recent findings on the diversity Cdk/cyclin complexes expressed at the G1/S transition in mammalian cells and their functional redundancy this opposition is no longer so evident. In contrast, the diversity of Cdk/cyclin complexes controlling the G1/S transition has emerged leading to the hypothesis that highly similar molecular pathways regulating cell cycle among mammalian cells only occur after the commitment to S phase.

3. Activation and involvement of Cdk1 during S phase in proliferating hepatocytes: synergy and redundancy between the protein kinases Cdk1 and Cdk2

The unique capacity of the liver to regenerate after tissue injury or resection has always fascinated biologists and makes the liver a unique model for studying mammalian adult organ regeneration. Centuries ago, the ancient Greeks recognized the liver regeneration potential in the myth of Prometheus (Fausto et al., 2006; Michalopoulos and DeFrances, 2005). The first "scientific" demonstration that the liver can restore its initial liver mass and its functional status within few days by a compensatory growth process was provided by using the experimental model of 2/3 hepatectomy in rats developed by Higgins and Anderson in 1931 (Fausto et al., 2006).

3.1 The rapid proliferating of differentiated hepatocytes allows the liver regeneration

In contrast to other regenerating tissue, the peculiar feature of the liver regeneration process is to involve massive proliferation of differentiated cells (Figure 4) in the remnant intact tissue. Hepatic progenitor cells are recruited only when intoxication alters the proliferation of mature cells for instance following administration of drugs targeting hepatocytes such as retrosine (Avril et al., 2004; Laconi et al., 1999).

After 2/3 hepatectomy, liver regeneration begins with a first synchronous wave of hepatocyte proliferation, followed by sequential proliferation waves of biliary, kupffer and endothelial cells (Fausto et al., 2006; Michalopoulos and DeFrances, 2005). Importantly, proliferation of mature hepatocyte occurs within the parenchyma in the vicinity of the portal triads and proceeds to the pericentral area close to the centolobular veins (Rabes et al., 1976) (Figure 4). Since the cell renewal is very low in the normal liver, the unique ability of differentiated cells to exit from quiescence after a tissue loss has aroused numerous studies to identify exogenous factors triggering the liver regeneration and regulators of hepatocyte cell cycle progression. Therefore, *in vivo* and *in vitro* models have been extensively studied for step by step identifications of the extracellular stimuli inducing cell cycle of mature hepatocytes and downstream signaling pathways. These models have also been used to investigate expression and activation of cdk/cyclin complexes throughout cell cycle progression (Fausto et al., 2006; Michalopoulos and DeFrances, 2005).

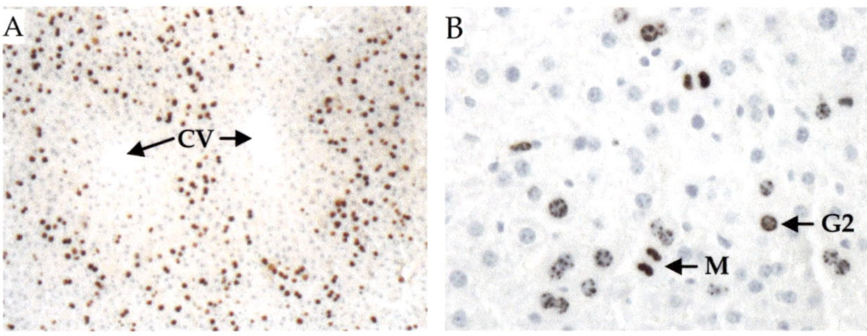

Fig. 4. Sections of mouse liver evidencing detection of DNA replication and G2 phase. Mice were hepatectomized, injected at 46 hours post-hepatectomy with BrdU and killed 2 hours later (at 48h). Livers were fixed for histological studies and detection of BrdU to visualize hepatocytes replicating DNA or phospho-histone H3 to detect cells in G2 and M phases.. A, this low magnification picture shows the detection of BrdU positive cells replicating DNA. It illustrates that replicating hepatocytes are initially localized in the vicinity of the portal vein while around centrolobular veins (CV) only few hepatocytes replicate DNA at 48h. B, a higher magnification picture shows nuclei of hepatocytes reaching G2 phase (detection of phosphor-histone H3 positive cells with punctuated nuclear signal : G2) and mitosis (M).

Using *in vivo* models, Molten and Bucher have shown that circulating growth factors present in the serum of hepatectomized rats induce hepatocyte replication in parabiosed non hepatectomized animals (Moolten and Bucher, 1967). Then using primary culture of rat hepatocytes, HGF, TGFα, and EGF have been identified as potent hepatocyte growth factors. However, the injection in rat of these growth factors does not induce massive hepatocyte DNA replication suggesting that normal hepatocytes *in vivo* are not able to respond to mitogenic signal without priming events allowing hepatocytes to become "sensitive" to growth factors. From different works, evidence was provided that the pro-inflammatory cytokines TNFα and IL-6 are the early stimulus during the liver regeneration allowing the exit of hepatocytes from quiescence (Cressman et al., 1996; Webber et al., 1998). Rapid induction of urokinase activity and urokinase receptor expression appeared within 5 min

followed within 30 min by a rapid activation of NFkB and STAT3. These transcription factors participate to the induction of a subset of genes called "immediate early genes" including c-fos and c-Jun leading to an increase in AP1 activity.
These events are followed by high levels of HGF in plasma around two hours after PH. This initiation phase controlled by pro-inflammatory cytokines thus results in the G0/G1 transition and early G1 progression allowing hepatocytes to become sensitive to growth factors and competent for commitment to DNA replication. Therefore, the complex regenerating process is now divided in three distinct phases: the initiation, proliferation and termination steps. In rat and, to a lesser extend, in mouse the first wave of hepatocyte proliferation following partial hepatectomy (PH) is synchronous. In both rat and mouse, within less than 15 minutes after the PH, hepatocytes exit quiescence and enter in G1-phase (Hsu et al., 1992). The timing of DNA replication and mitosis are however different between the two species. The peak of DNA synthesis is observed at 22-24h in rat followed by a peak of mitosis at 28-30h (Agell et al., 1994; Fabrikant, 1968; Grisham, 1962; Serratosa et al., 1988; Widmann and Fahimi, 1975). Seven days later, the liver has recovered its initial mass. In mouse, the progression in G1 phase of the cell cycle is slower and the peak of DNA and mitosis are delayed of approximately 20h highlighting differences of hepatocyte response between species.

3.2 Liver regeneration: a synchronized in vivo model of proliferation for cell cycle studies

During the 1990's, interest in hepatocyte cell cycle has increased because genes involved in the cell cycle control have been identified. This *in vivo* model of proliferation of non transformed cells was used for cell cycle studies since hepatocyte progression in the cell cycle is naturally synchronous with a long lasting G1-phase. Our group and others investigated Cdk2 and Cdk1 expression and activity as well as cyclin A, B, E and D1 expression during liver regeneration (Albrecht et al., 1993; Loyer et al., 1994; Lu et al., 1992; Zschemisch et al., 2006). Although Cdk2 is constantly expressed, Cdk1 is completely absent in resting hepatocytes and remains undetectable up to 20h after PH a time corresponding to late G1 phase and G1/S transition. Then, Cdk1 accumulates in S, G2 and M phase and both cyclin A/Cdk1 and cyclin B/Cdk1 complexes are formed. During S phase, Cdk2 associates with cyclin A. Additional experiments of kinase activity assays suggested that Cdk1 is active during both S and M phases while one peak of Cdk2 activity is detected in S phase only. At that time, these data contrasted with the dogma that Cdk1 is active only at the G2/M transition while Cdk2 would control G1/S transition. Our study raised the question of the significance of Cdk1 and Cdk2 expression during G1 phase and G1/S transition.
Unexpectedly, cyclins E and D1 are present in resting liver, which again contrasted with the admitted view of the mammalian cell cycle regulation with low D-type cyclin expression in early G1 and its dramatic induction at the mitogen-dependent restriction point in late G1 phase. In quiescent hepatocytes, Jaumot et *al.* (Jaumot et al., 1999) demonstrated that cyclin D3 and Cdk4 were localized in cytoplasm whereas cyclin D1 was nuclear. Low amounts of cyclin E are found in the cytoplasm (Pujol et al., 2000). Thirteen hours after PH cyclins D3 and Cdk4 are mostly located in the nucleus and significant amounts of cyclin D1/Cdk4 and cyclin D3/Cdk4 complexes are formed but remain inactive whereas at 24h they are fully activated. At 13 and 24h, cyclin E is detected in both cytoplasm and nuclei. Thereafter, the activity of Cdk4 decreases at 28h when cyclin D1 translocates to the nuclear matrix and the levels of cyclin D3 diminishes. Similarly, the inactivation of Cdk2 at 28h is associated with a

strong decrease in Cdk2 in the nuclear fraction and a decrease of cyclin E located in the nuclei. During this period, very low amounts of cyclin A are detected in the nuclear fraction at 13h after PH while following its strong induction in S phase, cyclin A is present in both cytoplasm and nuclei at 24 and 28h. Therefore, the specific nuclear localization of the complexes is associated with their activity in liver regeneration. The maximal activity of Cdk2 detected at 24h comes from cyclin E/Cdk2 and cyclin A/Cdk2 complexes whereas the activity at 28h is mainly attributable to the Cdk2/cyclin A heterodimer. However, the activity of Cdk2 rapidly decreases after the peak of DNA synthesis at 24h.

The presence of inactive cyclin D/Cdk4 complexes until 13h post PH and cyclin E/cdk2 at 28h has led authors to question the modulation of Cdk activity during rat liver regeneration. Indeed, reports indicated that Cdk inhibitors (Cdki's) are involved in modulating cell cycle progression following antagonist mitogenic and anti-mitogenic signals (Morgan, 1997; Sherr and Roberts, 1995). Two families of Cdki's were described: the Ink4 family ($p16^{Ink4a}$, $p15^{Ink4b}$, $p18^{Ink4c}$ and $p19^{Ink4d}$) which specifically bind Cdk4 and its homologue Cdk6 and the Cip/Kip family ($p21^{Cip}$, $p27^{Kip1}$, $p27^{Kip2}$) which bind and inhibit the activity of a wide range of Cdk/cyclin complexes including cyclin D/Cdk4/6, cyclin E/Cdk2 and cyclin A/Cdk2 (Sherr and Roberts, 1995). During liver regeneration in rat, Jaumot et *al*. (Jaumot et al., 1999) have observed that $p27^{Kip1}$ is associated with cyclin D/Cdk4 complexes when they are inactive. More precisely, Pujol et *al*. (Pujol et al., 2000) have evidenced that high amounts of $p27^{Kip1}$ bind to Cdk2/cyclin E complexes during the first 13h post-PH when the activity of Cdk2 is very low. At 24h, corresponding to the S phase, the amounts of $p27^{Kip1}$ associated to Cdk2/cyclin E decrease strongly while Cdk2 activity is maximal. Conversely, the amount of $p21^{Cip}$ bound to these complexes is low during the first 13h and subsequently increases. At 24h low levels of both inhibitors associated with the complexes are detected but increase in $p21^{Cip1}$ and $p27^{Kip1}$ proteins associated with Cdk2/cyclin A is observed at 28h after the peak of hepatocyte DNA synthesis. In hepatectomized mice, Albrecht et *al*., (Albrecht et al., 1997; Albrecht et al., 1998) obtained similar data and showed that expression of $p21^{Cip1}$ is induced during the pre-replicative phase and is maximal after the peak of hepatocyte DNA synthesis. In contrast, $p27^{Kip1}$ is present in quiescent liver and slightly induced after PH. Immuno-depletion experiments suggested that $p27^{Kip1}$ plays a role in down-regulating Cdk2 activity before and after the peak of DNA replication. Interestingly, study of liver regeneration in mice lacking $p21^{Cip1}$ evidenced a marked acceleration of hepatocyte progression into the cell cycle. DNA synthesis, up-regulation of cyclin A and PCNA, induction of cyclin D1- and Cdk2-associated kinase activities, and appearance of the hyperphosphorylated retinoblastoma protein (pRb) occur earlier in the $p21^{Cip1}$ knock-out mice. These results demonstrate the role of $p21^{Cip1}$ in the regulation of the hepatocyte progression through G1 phase *in vivo*.

Primary cultures of rat and mouse hepatocytes were also widely used to analyze hepatocyte cell cycle entry and progression through the G1 phase. It was clearly demonstrated that hepatocytes in culture undergo DNA replication when they were stimulated by growth factors alone (McGowan and Bucher, 1983; Sawada, 1989). Using this model of pure culture of hepatocytes, our group has shown that during cell isolation hepatocytes expressed immediate early proto-oncogenes like c-fos and c-myc suggesting a "spontaneous" G0/G1 transition following cell-cell interaction destruction (Etienne et al., 1988).

Then, Loyer et *al*., (Loyer et al., 1996) characterized different steps of G1 phase in hepatocytes. Confirmation that collagenase perfusion of the liver induces the G0/G1 transition of quiescent normal rat hepatocytes was provided and we showed that progression in late G1 triggers hepatocyte ability to respond to growth factor alone. Importantly, demonstration that hepatocytes are able to progress from an early G1 to a restriction point mitogen dependent (R point) located to mid-late G1 was shown. Indeed, in absence of growth factor and serum, hepatocytes are able to progress up to mid-late G1 phase as evidenced by the sequential over expression of c-fos, c-jun, c-myc, jun D and then c-Ki-ras and p53. In addition, low levels of cyclin D1 and D2 are observed while cyclin A and Cdk2 are not expressed. Moreover, the progression towards the G1/S is strictly dependent upon the stimulation by growth factor. Late addition of the EGF at day 2 and 3 of culture induces a sharp peak of DNA synthesis reflecting the high synchrony of the hepatocytes arrested at the R point. A lag phase between the R point and the onset of the DNA synthesis appeared to be approximately 18-20h. In this hepatocyte primary culture, Cdk2 mRNA is detectable throughout the G1 phase but significantly increased after the EGF stimulation. Cyclin A is detected at the entry of S phase and Cdk1 and Cdk2 dependent histone H1 kinase activity is mainly detected in S and M phases. Weak levels of cyclin E mRNA are found in unstimulated cultures but levels of this mRNA greatly increased after growth factor stimulation. Surprisingly, cyclin D3 mRNAs appear to accumulate in absence of EGF stimulation whereas a drastic increase in cyclin D1 expression accompanies the R point overcrossing. The cyclin D1 mRNA accumulation correlates with the R point onset and the cyclin D1 protein is detected 10-15h later. In accordance with these observations, accumulation of cyclin D1 is also detected when the hepatocytes are stimulated by HGF (Albrecht et al., 1995). Importantly, if progression beyond the restriction is delayed by late EGF stimulation, cyclin D1 induction is postponed accordingly demonstrating that cyclin D1 induction is essential for cell cycle progression at the mitogen-dependent restriction point.

The question arises whether this restriction point existed *in vivo*. Nicely, a growth factor dependency in mid-late G1 phase of proliferating hepatocytes *in vivo* was also evidenced (Talarmin et al., 1999). To reach that conclusion, we first analyzed the expression of cyclin D1 during liver regeneration and showed its induction at 12h post-hepatectomy, which is a time coinciding with the 2/3 of G1 progression as previously shown in primary culture of rat hepatocytes. We next isolated rat hepatocytes isolated 5, 7, 9, 12 or 15h after PH, and showed that only those isolated from 12-15h regenerating livers were able to replicate DNA without growth factor stimulation. Moreover, intravenous administration of a MEK inhibitor (PD98059) *in vivo*, before MEK activation at 10.5h post-PH was able to inhibit cyclin D1 mRNA accumulation and hepatocyte DNA replication demonstrating that MEK/ERK signaling pathway was involved in cyclin D1 induction and R point overcrossing. To the best of our knowledge, these data provide the unique evidence that the mitogen-dependent restriction point identified in cultured hepatocytes exists *in vivo* in whole organs and animals. These results were strengthened by Albrecht's observations showing that transient enforced expression of cyclin D1 in hepatocytes stimulates assembly of active cyclin D1/cdk4 complexes, robust hepatocyte proliferation and liver growth in rat liver (Nelsen et al., 2003). However, in this *in vivo* model, after several days, hepatocyte proliferation is inhibited despite the persistence of high levels of cyclin D1 and cyclin E, suggesting that anti-proliferative response related to marked up-regulation of $p21^{Cip1}$ represses cyclin D1/cdk4 and cyclin E/cdk2 dependent kinase actvities. More recently, using mice carrying a floxed *EGFR* allele to inactive the EGF receptor, Natarajan et al., (Natarajan et al., 2007) observed delayed liver regeneration characterized by defective G1/S phase entry, reduced cyclin D1 expression followed by moderate Cdk2 and Cdk1 expression. In parallel, these authors reported an increased mortality after PH associated to high levels of TNFα in the serum. They also suggested that soluble TNFα, which is a priming agent for hepatocytes, was produced at high levels by liver cells to compensate cell cycle arrest with a subsequent induction of cell death in absence of proliferation.

To evaluate the role of priming agents, another experimental *in vitro* model has been designed. For that purpose, we used a coculture model associating rat hepatocytes with rat liver epithelial cells (RLEC also called LEC for liver epithelial cells), in which heterotypic cell-cell contacts are restored and a spontaneous early production and deposition of extracellular matrix is observed (Clement et al., 1984; Corlu et al., 1991; Guguen-Guillouzo et al., 1983). This coculture model compared to the pure culture of hepatocytes (Figure 5) exhibits numerous advantages: adult hepatocytes remain highly differentiated for several weeks and are unable to proliferate under EGF or HGF stimulation alone as in liver tissue (Corlu et al., 1997; Fraslin et al., 1985). Therefore, based on the data obtained *in vivo*, we successfully designed a stimulation procedure allowing multiple hepatocyte division cycles without loss of differentiation (Serandour et al., 2005). In this coculture system, differentiated and quiescent hepatocytes are able to proliferate under co-stimulation with TNFα and EGF or HGF. Co-stimulation with TNFα and growth factors leads to proliferation of nearly all the hepatocyte population over a week. Peaks of DNA synthesis and mitotic activity occurred day 3 after stimulation. Both mono- and binuclear hepatocytes progressed up to mitosis and cytokinesis leading to significant expansion of hepatocyte colonies. Remarkably, these results are in accordance with *in vivo* experiments, in which co-injection of TNFα and growth factors induced hepatocyte proliferation (Webber et al., 1998). In contrast, TNFα alone does not act as complete mitogen in cocultures. Indeed, it induces DNA synthesis in less than 3% of hepatocytes as observed *in vivo* (Webber et al., 1998) and in long-term DMSO cultures (Iocca and Isom, 2003). In coculture, analysis of cell cycle proteins has revealed that growth factor alone such as EGF, induces cyclin D1 indicating that cells are sensitive to mitogen signal, override the R point in mid-late G1 but fail to reach the G1/S boundary. These observations diverged with Albrecht's results that showed that cyclin D1 expression *in vivo* or *in vitro* was sufficient to induce entry of these cells into S phase (Albrecht and Hansen, 1999; Nelsen et al., 2003). This discrepancy would be explained

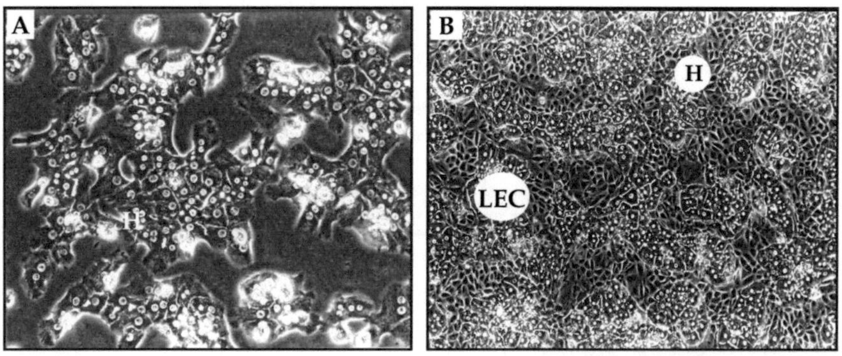

Fig. 5. Phase contrast photographs of A) pure culture of rat hepatocytes and B) co-culture of rat hepatocytes (H) and rat liver epithelial cells (LEC). Differentiated hepatocytes are characterized by a "dark" cytoplasm with one or two round nuclei with a single central nucleolus. In addition, hepatocytes in co-culture maintain a cubical shape and form colonies that remain viable for several weeks.

at least in part, by distinct experimental conditions, mainly the collagen gel system used *in vitro* and the level of cyclin D1 expressed. In contrast, when TNFα was associated with EGF, hepatocytes expressed both Cdk1 and Cdk2 and a progression into S phase was observed. From these data, we postulate that a late G1 checkpoint dependent on Cdk1, not yet described in hepatocyte cell cycle, may regulate entry into S phase independently from the Cdk2-mediated role at the G1/S transition.

3.3 Role of Cdk1 and Cdk2 in proliferating hepatocytes: synergy or redundancy

Most articles reporting data on liver regeneration focused on the G1 phase regulators but not on expression of Cdk1 during G1/S transition or S phase even if Cdk1 was observed *in vivo and in vitro* at this step by us and others (Albrecht et al., 1993; Loyer et al., 1994). Therefore, using *in vivo* and *in vitro* models, we have investigated the role of Cdk1 in normal adult hepatocytes. We have demonstrated that Cdk1 is expressed at high levels in S phase and that both Cdk1 and Cdk2, associated with cyclins A and/or B, are activated prior DNA replication in regenerating hepatocytes (Garnier et al., 2009). Assuming that Cdk1 and Cdk2 kinase activities towards the phosphorylation substrate histone H1 are identical, we provided evidence that Cdk1 activity is twice higher than Cdk2 activity during S phase in hepatocytes (Figure 6). Then, knock-down experiments of Cdk1 and/or Cdk2 were performed in isolated hepatocytes and human foreskin fibroblasts (HFFs) which differed in their ability to express high and low Cdk1 levels during S phase. Indeed, the levels of Cdk1 expression during S phase reached 80 and 15% of the expression levels during mitosis in hepatocytes and HFFs, respectively. Both siRNA-mediated repression of Cdk1 and Cdk2 significantly decreased DNA replication in hepatocytes. In contrast, in HFFs repression of Cdk2 significantly reduced the DNA synthesis while repression of Cdk1 had no effect on the rate of DNA replication but, as expected, reduced the mitotic index. Notably, in accordance with the Cdk1 and Cdk2 kinase activities during S phase in hepatocytes, the greatest decrease in DNA synthesis resulted from Cdk1 rather than Cdk2 silencing. In hepatocyte, the involvement of Cdk1 is evidenced in early S phase by showing that hepatocytes arrested after G1/S transition but prior to DNA replication by the iron chelator O-Trensox, express fully active Cdk1 and Cdk2. Moreover, the decrease in DNA replication after Cdk1 or Cdk2 silencing is not linked to a default in the formation of the pre-replication complex since Mcm7 nuclear localization and loading onto chromatin are not impaired. Therefore, Cdk1 may be involved in the origin firing events downstream the formation of replication complexes in hepatocytes, in agreement with a recent study showing that enforced expression of constitutively active Cdk1 mutant in HeLa cells results in abnormal origin firing and premature DNA replication in early S phase (Katsuno et al., 2009).

These data further support and extend the conclusion that Cdk1 compensates for Cdk2 gene ablation in genetically modified mice. Indeed, we showed for the first time the involvement of Cdk1 in S phase of normal and non-genetically modified mammalian cells. More precisely, both Cdk1 and Cdk2 play a critical role in hepatocyte cell cycle. Consistent with our observation, Satyanarayana et *al.*, (Satyanarayana et al., 2008) showed that the timing of S phase is not altered in regenerating livers of $Cdk2^{-/-}$ mice although the percentage of BrdU-positive cells slightly decreases compared to wild type. Interestingly, in $Cdk2^{-/-}$ $Cdk1^{+/cdk2k1}$ mice, in which a Cdk2 cDNA is knocked into the *Cdk1* locus, similar regenerative response and percentage of BrdU–positive cells are obtained compared to $Cdk2^{+/+}$ mice. These data indicated that Cdk2 expressed from the *Cdk1* locus is able to

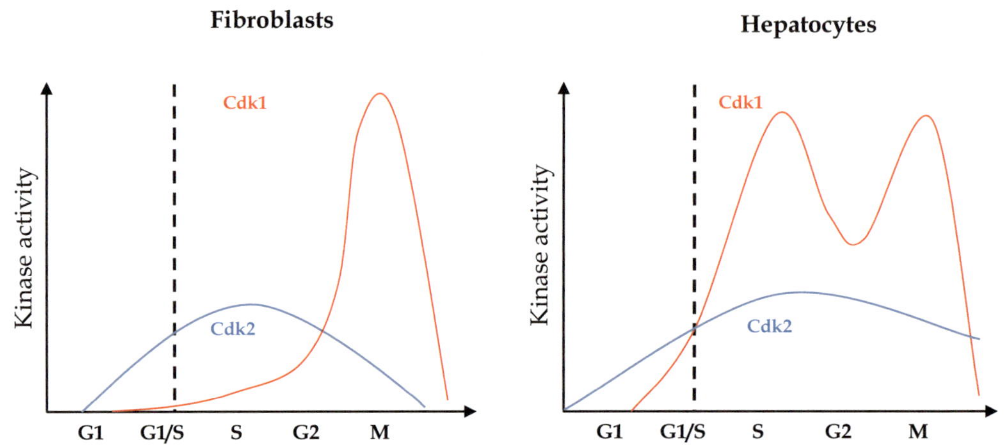

Fig. 6. Schematic representation of Cdk1 (red) and Cdk2 (blue) kinase activities in fibroblasts versus hepatocytes throughout the cell cycle. While in fibroblasts Cdk2 activity is dominant over Cdk1 at the G1/S transition and during S phase, both Cdk1 and Cdk2 are active in hepatocytes during S phase.

mimic the cell function of endogenous Cdk2 and restore normal regeneration process as well as that one copy of *Cdk1* is sufficient for a normal liver response after PH. Later, Hanse et *al.* (Hanse et al., 2009) showed that 42h after PH most hepatocytes enter S phase in wild-type mice whereas their number is diminished significantly in Cdk2$^{-/-}$ mice. In addition, hepatocytes isolated from livers of cdk2$^{-/-}$ mice respond to mitogenic stimulation but to a lower extent than hepatocytes coming from wild-type mice.

Altogether, these results strengthened the conclusion that physiological hepatocyte proliferation is dependent on both Cdk1 and Cdk2. While Cdk1/cyclin E complexes are not detected in normal hepatocytes, Cdk1, cyclins A and, unexpectedly, cyclin B1 are localized in the nucleus of replicating hepatocytes and form active complexes during S phase in regenerating hepatocytes. In addition, Cdk1 is active in all hepatocytes regardless of their ploidy status, excluding a peculiar regulation or role of Cdk1 related to the tetraploidy observed in half of adult hepatocytes in rat. Although the absolute requirement of cytosolic cyclin B1 during initiation of mitosis remains questioned, it has been postulated that relocating cyclin B1 to the nucleus in S phase might compromise entry into mitosis. This could explain why the accumulation of nuclear Cdk1/cyclin B1 complexes during DNA replication does not trigger premature mitosis in hepatocytes. Moreover, Phospho-Tyr15 Cdk1 found in replicating hepatocytes and known to be an inactive form of Cdk1 could also participate to this control. Indeed, recent reports showed that Tyr15 phosphorylation of Cdk1 is important to avoid premature entry into mitosis (Pomerening et al., 2008). Regulation of the ratio between pools of active and inactive Phospho-Tyr15 Cdk1 in hepatocytes might be essential to allow S phase initiation while preventing premature mitosis.

In absence of Cdk2, the induction of cyclin A is diminished consistent with the reduced proportion of hepatocyte in S phase, while Cdk1 is induced to higher levels than in control cells (Hanse et al., 2009). It is located in the nucleus at G1/S transition (Satyanarayana et al., 2008) and remained in the nucleus until the completion of mitosis. Cylin E/Cdk1, cyclin

A/Cdk1 and cylin B1/Cdk1 are successively activated. In this context, it is questioned whether p21^{Cip1} is able to arrest cells at G1/S transition in absence of Cdk2 after DNA damage and if cells are able to repair DNA and resume DNA replication. Indeed, Cdk2 is the primary target of the ATM/ATR, p53, p21 cascade (Bartek and Lukas, 2001). In Cdk2 knock-out mice, activation of p53– p21^{Cip1} pathway is not perturbed in the absence of Cdk2 and p21^{Cip1} can bind Cdk1. However, in Cdk2 knock-out mice DNA repair is delayed and partially impaired. Therefore, cells are more prone to lethal irradiation compared to wild-type although they display resumption of DNA replication in regenerating liver (Satyanarayana et al., 2008). The question of the involvement of Cdk2 in the induction of cyclin D1 has also been asked. Indeed, Albrecht's group has shown that infection with adenovirus leading to enforced expression of cyclin D1 in the liver triggers hepatocyte proliferation (Nelsen et al., 2001). In Cdk2$^{-/-}$ mice, they observed that this response is severely blunted leading to massive hepatocyte and animal death. This data highlights the critical role of Cdk2 in hepatocyte progression and survival after an acute mitogenic stimulation (Hanse et al., 2009). Altogether, these results could point out the emerging role of Cdk2 in proper DNA repair (Satyanarayana and Kaldis, 2009a) and how Cdk2 could be a sensor able to distinguish between moderate and extensive DNA damage to promote either survival or apoptosis.

4. Regulation of the Cdk1 expression and activation under the control of extracellular signals: involvement of extracellular remodeling and Cdk2 kinase activity

Although adult hepatocytes are quiescent and normally do not undergo cell division, they maintain the ability to proliferate in response to toxic injury and infection. Upon regenerative stimulus, 95% of the hepatocytes undergo cell division while maintaining their metabolic function and tissue architecture. This process involved a multitude of cellular processes including at early stage acute-phase reaction (Fausto et al., 2006), induction of pro-angiogenic signals (Ding et al.) and an important extracellular matrix (ECM) breakdown and remodeling (Kim et al., 1997) leading to local and transient changes in the liver architecture. Connective tissue is found around the portal triads whereas reticular fibers and small amounts of basement membrane are present between the sinusoid endothelial cells and the hepatocytes. In the portal areas, mainly type I, III and V collagens are found while type IV collagen, laminin, entactin and nidogen form the basement membrane along the sinusoids. Fibronectin is also present in the space of Disse (Clement et al., 1986).

Some proteins that are involved in the structural integrity of the liver are also required for normal regeneration. For example, deficiencies in connexin-32, a gap-junction protein (Temme et al., 2000) and keratin-8, an intermediate filament forming protein (Loranger et al., 1997) cause extended liver damage after partial hepatectomy. Connexin-32 is also required for normal mitosis by mediating cellular connections during cell division. Loss of certain proteases also results in prolonged liver injury. Mice lacking genes encoding the serine proteases urokinase-type plasminogen activator (uPA) and tissue-type plasminogen activator (tPA) exhibit delayed regeneration whereas the deficiency of the plasminogen inhibitors leads to accelerated liver regeneration (Roselli et al., 1998; Shimizu et al., 2001). Interestingly, injection or increased expression of collagenase in intact liver, associated with HGF or TGFα, induces hepatocyte proliferation, suggesting that ECM degradation may play a role in hepatocyte priming (Liu et al., 1994). Conversely, Issa et *al.* (Issa et al., 2003)

observed that failure in collagen-I degradation in mouse liver inhibits the hepatocyte proliferation response.
Spatial and temporal expression of protease occurs during liver regeneration. In rat, activation of plasminogen to plasmin begins within 15mim after PH and stays pronounced until 3-6h. Successive inductions of mRNA levels of the metalloproteinases (MMP)-9, MMP-2, MMP-13, MMP-14, MMP-24, which constitute a family of zinc-containing neutral proteinases involved in matrix remodeling in both normal and pathological processes, are observed in mouse. Moreover, in parallel, inhibitors of metalloproteinases (TIMP) -3, TIMP-4, TIMP-1 are also up-regulated. In particular, TIPM-1 expression appears just before DNA synthesis in rat and mouse models (Mohammed et al., 2005; Rudolph et al., 1999). After PH, its activation is linked to the hepatocyte cell cycle since experiments based on gain of TIMP-1 function in transgenic mice result in delayed cell cycle progression whereas loss of function in knout-out mice accelerates liver regeneration (Mohammed et al., 2005). Activation of pro-MMP9 in MMP-9 after PH, mediated by plasmin or by plasmin-activated MMP-3, is followed by activation of pro-MMP-2 in MMP-2 probably by the membrane-type 1 MMP. In regenerating liver 3h post-PH MMP-9 is located in the immediate periportal hepatocytes, then, its localization extends rapidly throughout the lobule before it decreases at 72h post-PH. In the meantime, MMP-2 expression enhances in the hepatocytes at 24 and 48h post-hepatectomy (Kim et al., 2000). Interestingly, migration of the MMP's staining pattern correlates with the gradual hepatocyte progression into the cell cycle from the periportal to the pericentral areas. This could be related to an important regulatory mechanism for controlling cell proliferation by the liberation of growth factors after ECM proteolysis. In accordance, mature HGF production is delayed by 12h in the $uPA^{-/-}$ mice along with a delayed DNA synthesis. Loss of uPA results in reduced plasmin levels responsible for activating MMP that in turn digest the ECM and allow release from ECM of activated growth factors like HGF (Schuppan et al., 1998). Deletion of the mouse gene *Timp3* results in the increase in TNF-α converting enzyme activity (TACE), constitutive release of TNFα and activation of TNFα-dependent signaling in the liver. In mice lacking *Timp3* gene, cyclin D1 and PCNA expression as well as hepatocyte division occur earlier than in wild-type mice with a shorter cell cycle time course. However, these mice succumbed of liver failure by a TNFα-signaling dependent cell death demonstrating also the importance of TIMP3 in controlling TNFα bioavailability (Mohammed et al., 2004).
Studies performed *in vitro* have shown that TNFα induces MMP-9 expression in mouse hepatocytes (Haruyama et al., 2000) and that MMP-9 transcription involves activation of NF-κB pathway (Mori et al., 2003). Cytokine-specific regulation of MMP/TIMP expression in hepatic stellate cells also suggests that the initial matrix breakdown following liver injury might be enhanced by TNFα, while diminished matrix degradation during chronic tissue injury might be due to the action of TGF-β1 through TIMP induction (Knittel et al., 1999). Together, these studies clearly demonstrated the importance in matrix remodeling to promote proliferation of adult hepatocytes. This conclusion is reinforced by the observation that normal rat hepatocytes plated on denatured collagen I are able to proliferate following stimulation by EGF while they do not respond to this growth factor when plated on collagen I gel (Hansen and Albrecht, 1999), collagen sandwich (De Smet et al., 2001) or matrigel (Nagaki et al., 2000). Cyclin D1 mRNA and protein expression as well as associated kinase activity are low on collagen gel relative to collagen film. Similar results are obtained when hepatocytes are spread on high fibronectin density (proliferation) or low fibronectin density (cell cycle arrest) coatings (Bhadriraju and Hansen, 2004). In this context, we asked the

question on how mitogen signals and extracellular matrix degradation are linked to promote cell cycle entry and progression of differentiated adult hepatocytes. For that purpose, the primary pure culture of hepatocytes did not appear as a pertinent model since hepatocytes progress regardless of priming factors in this model. In addition, we had previously shown that very low amounts of ECM were synthesized in pure culture. We therefore used quiescent adult rat hepatocytes in coculture with liver epithelial cells. Indeed, as mentioned above, hepatocytes in cocultures are stably differentiated for several weeks and capable of extracellular matrix deposition. This ECM located around the hepatocyte cords contains high amounts of type III, I collagens and fibronectin as *in vivo* (Clement et al., 1984). Moreover, cytoskeleton organization of hepatocytes is similar in coculture and *in vivo* i.e. beneath of the plasma membrane (Baffet et al., 1991; Corlu et al., 1991). Bile canaliculi structures present between the hepatocytes are also functional. Finally, in these *in vitro* conditions hepatocytes are unable to respond to growth factor alone as observed *in vivo* (Corlu et al., 1997).

Using this coculture system, we established new conditions allowing hepatocytes to undergo several proliferation waves (Figure 7) without loss of differentiation in presence of the priming cytokine, TNFα, and growth factors, HGF, EGF as *in vivo* (Serandour et al., 2005). For example, three days after TNFα/EGF or TNFα/HGF stimulation, 35% of hepatocytes divide whereas no DNA synthesis is observed in presence of HGF or EGF alone. Moreover, TNFα alone did not induce hepatocyte proliferation. However, hepatocytes gradually stop to synthesize DNA even under prolonged TNFα/EGF stimulation. Question is thus raised about the requirement of a cell cycle arrest following the first wave of divisions for inducing a second round of proliferation. When the cocktail TNFα/EGF is removed for few days before re-stimulation, induction of a new wave of DNA synthesis is obtained. This model of controlled induction of hepatocyte proliferation has been crucial to define whether the signaling mechanisms induced by TNFα could be linked to ECM remodeling (Figure 7). The quantification of ECM deposition detected using reticulin staining on cells stimulated by EGF alone, TNFα/EGF, or successively by EGF and then TNFα revealed several crucial data: 1) ECM is very abundant in both unstimulated and non proliferating EGF-treated cells, 2) in TNFα/EGF-treated cocultures, ECM deposition is very sparse and most fibers disappear within colonies of proliferating hepatocytes, 3) TNFα stimulation, before or after EGF exposure, induces ECM degradation, 4) during prolonged TNFα/EGF stimulation, DNA synthesis decreases concomitantly with new ECM deposition. In agreement with all these results, the phenanthroline, a specific inhibitor of MMP activities reduces the TNFα-mediated ECM degradation resulting in the decrease in DNA replication. This effect is reversible and after phenanthroline removal, DNA synthesis is completely restored. Among MMPs, MMP-9 expression by hepatocytes is induced by TNFα. Moreover, interferon-γ, described to inhibit TNFα-mediated MMP-9 expression via the Interferon Regulatory Factor-1 binding competition with NF-κB (Sanceau et al., 2002), prevents ECM remodeling and impairs DNA synthesis. Thus, ECM peri-cellular proteolysis controlled by TNFα via activation of the NF-κB pathway and induction of MMP-9 is necessary for S phase entry in hepatocytes. This ECM remodeling signal is also required for initiating any subsequent hepatocyte division wave in presence of mitogen (Serandour et al., 2005). These observations have been confirmed by Olle and coworkers using MMP-9$^{-/-}$ mice (Olle et al., 2006). Indeed, in these animals hepatic regenerative response is delayed compared with wild-type control animals. Moreover, they express significantly less HGF and TNFα at day 2

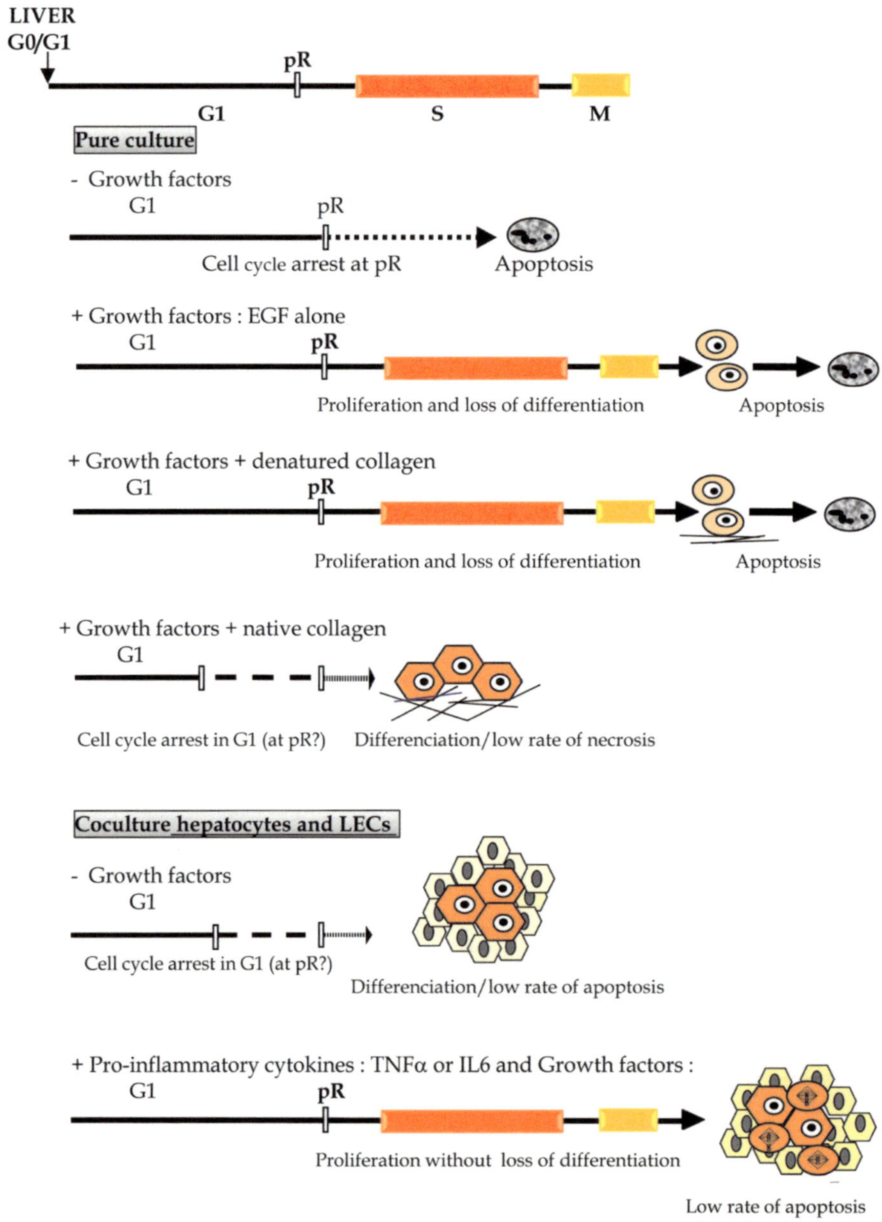

Fig. 7. Schematic representation of the commitment to cell death or proliferation in primary cultures of rat hepatocytes in different *in vitro* conditions. In pure culture, in absence of growth and survival factors, hepatocytes rapidly lose their differentiation and undergo apoptosis. In presence of growth factors they complete a single round of cell cycle before dying. When hepatocytes are maintained on complex bio-matrices (ex: matrigel and native collagens), they arrest in G1 and do not respond to growth factor stimulation. In co-culture, hepatocytes arrest in G1 unless a combination of pro-inflammatory cytokines and growth factors is added to the culture medium, which triggers a complete cell cycle without affecting differentiation and long-term survival.

post-PH corresponding to hepatocyte DNA synthesis in mice (Olle et al., 2006). In addition, in hepatoma cells, TNFα stimulates DNA replication by causing release of TGFα into the culture medium through the metalloproteinase disintegrin TACE. Then, TGFα activates EGFR and multiple downstream intracellular signaling cascades required for DNA replication (Argast et al., 2004).

Unexpectedly, experiments with successive addition of cytokine and growth factors as well as analysis of the expression of cell cycle regulation demonstrate that EGF alone promotes cell progression up to late G1. When we tested whether addition of TNFα before or after EGF stimulation might influence cell cycle progression, we observed that hepatocytes DNA synthesis is rapidly obtained in each situation. In addition, a pause of 2 days following EGF treatment does not affect hepatocyte responsiveness to TNFα, suggesting that these cells integrate a long-lasting mitogenic signal.

Using both pure culture of hepatocytes and the co-culture model, we compared expression of cell cycle markers to further investigate the molecular pathways involved in the progression in late G1 phase. In unstimulated co-cultures, cyclin D1 and Cdk2 are barely detectable (Figure 8). This pattern of expression, similar to that observed in unstimulated primary pure cultures of hepatocytes, suggestsed that they are blocked in G1 upstream the mitogen restriction point. Unexpectedly, although no BrdU-positive hepatocytes are detected in EGF-stimulated co-cultures, cyclin D1, Cdk4 and Cdk2 accumulate in this culture condition. Interestingly, even if Cdk2 was present no histone H1 kinase activity is detected (Figure 8). Therefore, EGF alone promotes the progression beyond the mitogen restriction point in late G1 although cells arrest before S phase.

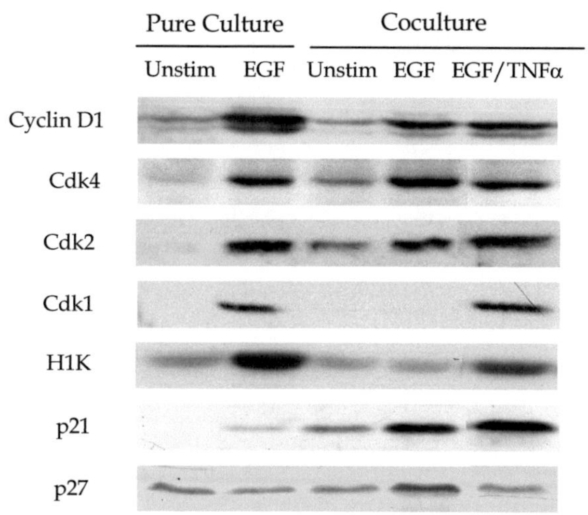

Fig. 8. Expression of Cdks, cyclins and Cdk's inhibitors in cultured rat hepatocytes. Cyclin D1, Cdk4, Cdk2, Cdk1 and the inhibitors $p21^{Cip1}$ and $p27^{Kip1}$ were analyzed by western blotting. In addition, kinase activities of Cdk1 and Cdk2 were measured using histone H1 as a substrate (H1K).

Our results could be linked to previous reports showing that cyclin E and Cdk2 are present in cells plated on collagen gel or film, but on collagen gel, hepatocytes do not proliferate and lack the Cdk2 activity (Hansen and Albrecht, 1999). In these conditions, $p27^{Kip1}$ protein levels are similar but higher amounts of p27^{Kip1} are associated with Cdk2 in cells plated on collagen gel than to those plated on collagen film. Similarly, p27^{Kip1} p21^{Cip1} are up-regulated in cell cultured on matrigel (Nagaki et al., 2000). In our co-culture condition, p27^{Kip1} p21^{Cip1} are also induced after EGF stimulation while in TNFα/EGF-stimulated co-cultures, expression levels of cyclin D1 and Cdk4 are strongly increased followed by up-regulation of Cdk1 and Cdk2. In contrast, p27^{Kip1} levels are reduced demonstrating that Cdk levels are up-regulated while Cdki's are repressed to favor cell cycle progression. Moreover, both Cdk2 and Cdk1 are active as evidenced by Histone H1 kinase activity. We therefore point out a new cell cycle control in late G1 associated with ECM deposition and overcome by TNFα addition that triggers ECM remodeling and induction of MMP9. Importantly, TNFα stimulation following EGF exposition induces the expression of Cdk1 and the activation of both Cdk2 and Cdk1 kinase activities. Altogether, our results show that induction of Cdk1, correlating with the hepatocyte S phase entry, requires remodeling of the extracellular matrix and induction of the metalloproteinase MMP9 by TNFα stimulation. They also suggest that catalytic activation of Cdk1 may be regulated by Cdk2 kinase activity. This led us to draw the conclusion that Cdk2 and Cdk1 would exhibit a sequential catalytic activation under the control of extracellular signals including cytokines, growth factors as well as extracellular matrix remodeling. TNFα–mediated ECM remodeling is necessary for Cdk2 activity, Cdk1 expression, G1/S transition and completion of the cell cycle of hepatocytes in co-cultures.

Several important questions remain unanswered. How does TNFα induce Cdk2 kinase activity? It could be hypothesized that low levels of p27^{Kip1} following TNFα stimulation favor activation of Cdk2/cyclin E and Cdk2/cyclin A kinase activities. In addition, the mechanism by which TNFα induces Cdk1 expression remains unclear. Does it involve a transcriptional regulation mediated by unidentified signaling pathways and transcription factors? Local remodeling of the ECM could lead to disruption of ECM-cell communications achieved by integrins. Through multiple protein-protein interactions and signaling events, they could activate various signaling cascades regulating transcriptional activities. For example, repression of Integrin-linked kinase (ILK), a cell-ECM-adhesion component implicated in cell–ECM signaling via the integrins, leads to enhanced cell proliferation and hepatomegaly (Gkretsi et al., 2008).

5. Conclusion

The peculiar biphasic pattern of Cdk1 activity during cell cycle of normal hepatocytes and the evenly active Cdk1 and Cdk2 during S phase contrasts with most mammalian cell types in which active Cdk2 is highly predominant over other Cdks in S phase. Indeed, in DT40 chicken cells expressing low levels of active Cdk1 in S phase, elimination of Cdk2 induced a Cdk1-dependent S phase but presence of a single Cdk2 allele rendered the S phase independent of Cdk1 suggesting that Cdk1 and Cdk2 are functionally exclusive at the level of kinase activity. However, in absence of Cdk2, Cdk1 can fully compensate for S phase function of Cdk2 but fails to compensate for Cdk2's DNA repair functions in mammalian cells. Because of its location and function, the liver which is a vital organ, is continuously exposed to a wide range of harmful substances, viral infections which alter the hepatic homeostasis by inducing changes in the balance between proliferation and apoptosis. Despite its efficient defense system, many agents are still able to produce liver damage. Thus, to overcome these damages, liver has to compensate tissue loss. A major feature of adult hepatocytes is their singular capacity to proliferate despite their high level of differentiation. This ability has been related to the low expression level of $p21^{CIP1}$ Cdk-inhibitors in adult liver and primary hepatocytes *in vitro*, which could explain their rapid exit from quiescence. Based on the data obtained by our laboratory and others, we hypothesize that those high levels of active Cdk1 and Cdk2 following G1/S transition could participate to cellular defense response following stress stimulus in controlling rapid DNA repair and synthesis. We also showed that Cdk1 expression and activation is correlated to ECM degradation via the involvement of the pro-inflammatory cytokine TNFα. We thus identified for the first time a new signaling pathway regulating Cdk1 expression at the G1/S transition upon stimulation by cytokines (Figure 8). It also further confirms the well-orchestrated regulation of liver regeneration via multiple extracellular signals and pathways.

6. Acknowledgement

The authors thank Dr Christiane Guillouzo for her guidance in the studies regarding the cell cycle regulation in hepatocytes. We also thank Drs Anne-Laure Serandour and Delphine Garnier for their involvement in some of the experiments described in this chapter and all the members of the team "Stress, Defences and Regeneration" from the laboratory Inserm UMR S-991. Our team is financially supported by federal funding through Inserm, CNRS and the University of Rennes1 and the European grant, Liv-ES, FP7 programme, Health F5-2008-223317.

7. References

Adon, A.M., X. Zeng, M.K. Harrison, S. Sannem, H. Kiyokawa, P. Kaldis, and H.I. Saavedra. 2010. Cdk2 and Cdk4 regulate the centrosome cycle and are critical mediators of centrosome amplification in p53-null cells. *Mol Cell Biol*. 30:694-710.

Agell, N., M.J. Pujol, A. Lopez-Girona, M. Bosch, J.L. Rosa, and O. Bachs. 1994. Calmodulin expression during rat liver regeneration. *Hepatology*. 20:1002-8.

Ajchenbaum, F., K. Ando, J.A. DeCaprio, and J.D. Griffin. 1993. Independent regulation of human D-type cyclin gene expression during G1 phase in primary human T lymphocytes. *J Biol Chem*. 268:4113-9.

Albrecht, J.H., and L.K. Hansen. 1999. Cyclin D1 promotes mitogen-independent cell cycle progression in hepatocytes. *Cell Growth Differ*. 10:397-404.

Albrecht, J.H., J.S. Hoffman, B.T. Kren, and C.J. Steer. 1993. Cyclin and cyclin-dependent kinase 1 mRNA expression in models of regenerating liver and human liver diseases. *Am J Physiol*. 265:G857-64.

Albrecht, J.H., A.H. Meyer, and M.Y. Hu. 1997. Regulation of cyclin-dependent kinase inhibitor p21(WAF1/Cip1/Sdi1) gene expression in hepatic regeneration. *Hepatology*. 25:557-63.

Albrecht, J.H., R.Y. Poon, C.L. Ahonen, B.M. Rieland, C. Deng, and G.S. Crary. 1998. Involvement of p21 and p27 in the regulation of CDK activity and cell cycle progression in the regenerating liver. *Oncogene*. 16:2141-50.

Aleem, E., C. Berthet, and P. Kaldis. 2004. Cdk2 as a master of S phase entry: fact or fake? *Cell Cycle*. 3:35-7.

Aleem, E., H. Kiyokawa, and P. Kaldis. 2005. Cdc2-cyclin E complexes regulate the G1/S phase transition. *Nat Cell Biol.* 7:831-6.

Alhejaily, A., B. Wood, C.J. Foster, P.L. Farmer, C.B. Gilks, J. Brettschneider, A.G. Day, H.E. Feilotter, T. Baetz, and D.P. Lebrun. 2011. Differential expression of cell-cycle regulatory proteins defines distinct classes of follicular lymphoma. *Hum Pathol.*

Araki, H. 2011. Cyclin-dependent kinase-dependent initiation of chromosomal DNA replication. *Curr Opin Cell Biol.* 22:766-71.

Argast, G.M., J.S. Campbell, J.T. Brooling, and N. Fausto. 2004. Epidermal growth factor receptor transactivation mediates tumor necrosis factor-induced hepatocyte replication. *J Biol Chem.* 279:34530-6.

Arion, D., L. Meijer, L. Brizuela, and D. Beach. 1988. cdc2 is a component of the M phase-specific histone H1 kinase: evidence for identity with MPF. *Cell.* 55:371-8.

Avril, A., V. Pichard, M.P. Bralet, and N. Ferry. 2004. Mature hepatocytes are the source of small hepatocyte-like progenitor cells in the retrorsine model of liver injury. *J Hepatol.* 41:737-43.

Baffet, G., P. Loyer, D. Glaise, A. Corlu, P.L. Etienne, and C. Guguen-Guillouzo. 1991. Distinct effects of cell-cell communication and corticosteroids on the synthesis and distribution of cytokeratins in cultured rat hepatocytes. *J Cell Sci.* 99 (Pt 3):609-15.

Bartek, J., and J. Lukas. 2001. Mammalian G1- and S-phase checkpoints in response to DNA damage. *Curr Opin Cell Biol.* 13:738-47.

Bashir, T., and M. Pagano. 2005. Cdk1: the dominant sibling of Cdk2. *Nat Cell Biol.* 7:779-81.

Bates, S., L. Bonetta, D. MacAllan, D. Parry, A. Holder, C. Dickson, and G. Peters. 1994. CDK6 (PLSTIRE) and CDK4 (PSK-J3) are a distinct subset of the cyclin-dependent kinases that associate with cyclin D1. *Oncogene.* 9:71-9.

Berthet, C., E. Aleem, V. Coppola, L. Tessarollo, and P. Kaldis. 2003. Cdk2 knockout mice are viable. *Curr Biol.* 13:1775-85.

Berthet, C., and P. Kaldis. 2007. Cell-specific responses to loss of cyclin-dependent kinases. *Oncogene.* 26:4469-77.

Berthet, C., M.C. Rodriguez-Galan, D.L. Hodge, J. Gooya, V. Pascal, H.A. Young, J. Keller, R. Bosselut, and P. Kaldis. 2007. Hematopoiesis and thymic apoptosis are not affected by the loss of Cdk2. *Mol Cell Biol.* 27:5079-89.

Bhadriraju, K., and L.K. Hansen. 2004. Extracellular matrix-dependent myosin dynamics during G1-S phase cell cycle progression in hepatocytes. *Exp Cell Res.* 300:259-71.

Canhoto, A.J., A. Chestukhin, L. Litovchick, and J.A. DeCaprio. 2000. Phosphorylation of the retinoblastoma-related protein p130 in growth-arrested cells. *Oncogene.* 19:5116-22.

Cardoso, M.C., H. Leonhardt, and B. Nadal-Ginard. 1993. Reversal of terminal differentiation and control of DNA replication: cyclin A and Cdk2 specifically localize at subnuclear sites of DNA replication. *Cell.* 74:979-92.

Clement, B., J.A. Grimaud, J.P. Campion, Y. Deugnier, and A. Guillouzo. 1986. Cell types involved in collagen and fibronectin production in normal and fibrotic human liver. *Hepatology.* 6:225-34.

Clement, B., C. Guguen-Guillouzo, J.P. Campion, D. Glaise, M. Bourel, and A. Guillouzo. 1984. Long-term co-cultures of adult human hepatocytes with rat liver epithelial cells: modulation of albumin secretion and accumulation of extracellular material. *Hepatology.* 4:373-80.

Coller, H.A., L. Sang, and J.M. Roberts. 2006. A new description of cellular quiescence. *PLoS Biol.* 4:e83.

Corlu, A., G. Ilyin, S. Cariou, I. Lamy, P. Loyer, and C. Guguen-Guillouzo. 1997. The coculture: a system for studying the regulation of liver differentiation/proliferation activity and its control. *Cell Biol Toxicol.* 13:235-42.

Corlu, A., B. Kneip, C. Lhadi, G. Leray, D. Glaise, G. Baffet, D. Bourel, and C. Guguen-Guillouzo. 1991. A plasma membrane protein is involved in cell contact-mediated regulation of tissue-specific genes in adult hepatocytes. *J Cell Biol.* 115:505-15.

Cressman, D.E., L.E. Greenbaum, R.A. DeAngelis, G. Ciliberto, E.E. Furth, V. Poli, and R. Taub. 1996. Liver failure and defective hepatocyte regeneration in interleukin-6-deficient mice. *Science.* 274:1379-83.

Cross, F., J. Roberts, and H. Weintraub. 1989. Simple and complex cell cycles. *Annu Rev Cell Biol.* 5:341-96.

De Smet, K., P. Loyer, D. Gilot, A. Vercruysse, V. Rogiers, and C. Guguen-Guillouzo. 2001. Effects of epidermal growth factor on CYP inducibility by xenobiotics, DNA replication, and caspase activations in collagen I gel sandwich cultures of rat hepatocytes. *Biochem Pharmacol.* 61:1293-303.

DeCaprio, J.A., Y. Furukawa, F. Ajchenbaum, J.D. Griffin, and D.M. Livingston. 1992. The retinoblastoma-susceptibility gene product becomes phosphorylated in multiple stages during cell cycle entry and progression. *Proc Natl Acad Sci U S A.* 89:1795-8.

DeGregori, J., T. Kowalik, and J.R. Nevins. 1995. Cellular targets for activation by the E2F1 transcription factor include DNA synthesis- and G1/S-regulatory genes. *Mol Cell Biol.* 15:4215-24.

Denhardt, D.T., D.R. Edwards, and C.L. Parfett. 1986. Gene expression during the mammalian cell cycle. *Biochim Biophys Acta.* 865:83-125.

Diffley, J.F. 2004. Regulation of early events in chromosome replication. *Curr Biol.* 14:R778-86.

Ding, B.S., D.J. Nolan, J.M. Butler, D. James, A.O. Babazadeh, Z. Rosenwaks, V. Mittal, H. Kobayashi, K. Shido, D. Lyden, T.N. Sato, S.Y. Rabbany, and S. Rafii. 2010. Inductive angiocrine signals from sinusoidal endothelium are required for liver regeneration. *Nature.* 468:310-5.

Doree, M., and T. Hunt. 2002. From Cdc2 to Cdk1: when did the cell cycle kinase join its cyclin partner? *J Cell Sci.* 115:2461-4.

Draetta, G., and D. Beach. 1988. Activation of cdc2 protein kinase during mitosis in human cells: cell cycle-dependent phosphorylation and subunit rearrangement. *Cell.* 54:17-26.

Dulic, V., E. Lees, and S.I. Reed. 1992. Association of human cyclin E with a periodic G1-S phase protein kinase. *Science.* 257:1958-61.

Etienne, P.L., G. Baffet, B. Desvergne, M. Boisnard-Rissel, D. Glaise, and C. Guguen-Guillouzo. 1988. Transient expression of c-fos and constant expression of c-myc in freshly isolated and cultured normal adult rat hepatocytes. *Oncogene Res.* 3:255-62.

Fabrikant, J.I. 1968. The kinetics of cellular proliferation in regenerating liver. *J Cell Biol.* 36:551-65.

Fan, J., and J.R. Bertino. 1997. Functional roles of E2F in cell cycle regulation. *Oncogene.* 14:1191-200.

Fausto, N., J.S. Campbell, and K.J. Riehle. 2006. Liver regeneration. *Hepatology.* 43:S45-53.

Fiaschi-Taesch, N.M., F. Salim, J. Kleinberger, R. Troxell, I. Cozar-Castellano, K. Selk, E. Cherok, K.K. Takane, D.K. Scott, and A.F. Stewart. 2010. Induction of human beta-cell proliferation and engraftment using a single G1/S regulatory molecule, cdk6. *Diabetes*. 59:1926-36.

FitzGerald, M.J., E.M. Webber, J.R. Donovan, and N. Fausto. 1995. Rapid DNA binding by nuclear factor kappa B in hepatocytes at the start of liver regeneration. *Cell Growth Differ*. 6:417-27.

Franck, N., E. Montembault, P. Rome, A. Pascal, J.Y. Cremet, and R. Giet. 2011. CDK11(p58) is required for centriole duplication and Plk4 recruitment to mitotic centrosomes. *PLoS One*. 6:e14600.

Fraslin, J.M., B. Kneip, S. Vaulont, D. Glaise, A. Munnich, and C. Guguen-Guillouzo. 1985. Dependence of hepatocyte-specific gene expression on cell-cell interactions in primary culture. *Embo J*. 4:2487-91.

Fujita, M. 2006. Cdt1 revisited: complex and tight regulation during the cell cycle and consequences of deregulation in mammalian cells. *Cell Div*. 1:22.

Fujita, M., Y. Ishimi, H. Nakamura, T. Kiyono, and T. Tsurumi. 2002. Nuclear organization of DNA replication initiation proteins in mammalian cells. *J Biol Chem*. 277:10354-61.

Furukawa, Y., H. Piwnica-Worms, T.J. Ernst, Y. Kanakura, and J.D. Griffin. 1990. cdc2 gene expression at the G1 to S transition in human T lymphocytes. *Science*. 250:805-8.

Garnier, D., P. Loyer, C. Ribault, C. Guguen-Guillouzo, and A. Corlu. 2009. Cyclin-dependent kinase 1 plays a critical role in DNA replication control during rat liver regeneration. *Hepatology*. 50:1946-56.

Gautier, J., C. Norbury, M. Lohka, P. Nurse, and J. Maller. 1988. Purified maturation-promoting factor contains the product of a Xenopus homolog of the fission yeast cell cycle control gene cdc2+. *Cell*. 54:433-9.

Geng, Y., E.N. Eaton, M. Picon, J.M. Roberts, A.S. Lundberg, A. Gifford, C. Sardet, and R.A. Weinberg. 1996. Regulation of cyclin E transcription by E2Fs and retinoblastoma protein. *Oncogene*. 12:1173-80.

Gkretsi, V., U. Apte, W.M. Mars, W.C. Bowen, J.H. Luo, Y. Yang, Y.P. Yu, A. Orr, R. St-Arnaud, S. Dedhar, K.H. Kaestner, C. Wu, and G.K. Michalopoulos. 2008. Liver-specific ablation of integrin-linked kinase in mice results in abnormal histology, enhanced cell proliferation, and hepatomegaly. *Hepatology*. 48:1932-41.

Grisham, J.W. 1962. A morphologic study of deoxyribonucleic acid synthesis and cell proliferation in regenerating rat liver; autoradiography with thymidine-H3. *Cancer Res*. 22:842-9.

Guguen-Guillouzo, C., B. Clement, G. Baffet, C. Beaumont, E. Morel-Chany, D. Glaise, and A. Guillouzo. 1983. Maintenance and reversibility of active albumin secretion by adult rat hepatocytes co-cultured with another liver epithelial cell type. *Exp Cell Res*. 143:47-54.

Hanse, E.A., C.J. Nelsen, M.M. Goggin, C.K. Anttila, L.K. Mullany, C. Berthet, P. Kaldis, G.S. Crary, R. Kuriyama, and J.H. Albrecht. 2009. Cdk2 plays a critical role in hepatocyte cell cycle progression and survival in the setting of cyclin D1 expression in vivo. *Cell Cycle*. 8:2802-9.

Hansen, L.K., and J.H. Albrecht. 1999. Regulation of the hepatocyte cell cycle by type I collagen matrix: role of cyclin D1. *J Cell Sci*. 112 (Pt 17):2971-81.

Hansen, U., L. Owens, and U.H. Saxena. 2009. Transcription factors LSF and E2Fs: tandem cyclists driving G0 to S? *Cell Cycle*. 8:2146-51.

Harrison, M.K., A.M. Adon, and H.I. Saavedra. 2011. The G1 phase Cdks regulate the centrosome cycle and mediate oncogene-dependent centrosome amplification. *Cell Div*. 6:2.

Haruyama, T., I. Ajioka, T. Akaike, and Y. Watanabe. 2000. Regulation and significance of hepatocyte-derived matrix metalloproteinases in liver remodeling. *Biochem Biophys Res Commun*. 272:681-6.

Hochegger, H., D. Dejsuphong, E. Sonoda, A. Saberi, E. Rajendra, J. Kirk, T. Hunt, and S. Takeda. 2007. An essential role for Cdk1 in S phase control is revealed via chemical genetics in vertebrate cells. *J Cell Biol*. 178:257-68.

Hsu, J.C., R. Bravo, and R. Taub. 1992. Interactions among LRF-1, JunB, c-Jun, and c-Fos define a regulatory program in the G1 phase of liver regeneration. *Mol Cell Biol*. 12:4654-65.

Hu, D., M. Valentine, V.J. Kidd, and J.M. Lahti. 2007. CDK11p58 is required for the maintenance of sister chromatid cohesion. *J Cell Sci*. 120:2424-34.

Iocca, H.A., and H.C. Isom. 2003. Tumor necrosis factor-alpha acts as a complete mitogen for primary rat hepatocytes. *Am J Pathol*. 163:465-76.

Issa, R., X. Zhou, N. Trim, H. Millward-Sadler, S. Krane, C. Benyon, and J. Iredale. 2003. Mutation in collagen-1 that confers resistance to the action of collagenase results in failure of recovery from CCl4-induced liver fibrosis, persistence of activated hepatic stellate cells, and diminished hepatocyte regeneration. *Faseb J*. 17:47-9.

Iyer, V.R., M.B. Eisen, D.T. Ross, G. Schuler, T. Moore, J.C. Lee, J.M. Trent, L.M. Staudt, J. Hudson, Jr., M.S. Boguski, D. Lashkari, D. Shalon, D. Botstein, and P.O. Brown. 1999. The transcriptional program in the response of human fibroblasts to serum. *Science*. 283:83-7.

Jablonska, B., A. Aguirre, R. Vandenbosch, S. Belachew, C. Berthet, P. Kaldis, and V. Gallo. 2007. Cdk2 is critical for proliferation and self-renewal of neural progenitor cells in the adult subventricular zone. *J Cell Biol*. 179:1231-45.

Jaumot, M., J.M. Estanyol, J. Serratosa, N. Agell, and O. Bachs. 1999. Activation of cdk4 and cdk2 during rat liver regeneration is associated with intranuclear rearrangements of cyclin-cdk complexes. *Hepatology*. 29:385-95.

Joshi, A.R., V. Jobanputra, K.M. Lele, and D.J. Wolgemuth. 2009. Distinct properties of cyclin-dependent kinase complexes containing cyclin A1 and cyclin A2. *Biochem Biophys Res Commun*. 378:595-9.

Kaldis, P., and E. Aleem. 2005. Cell cycle sibling rivalry: Cdc2 vs. Cdk2. *Cell Cycle*. 4:1491-4.

Kato, J., H. Matsushime, S.W. Hiebert, M.E. Ewen, and C.J. Sherr. 1993. Direct binding of cyclin D to the retinoblastoma gene product (pRb) and pRb phosphorylation by the cyclin D-dependent kinase CDK4. *Genes Dev*. 7:331-42.

Kato, J.Y., and C.J. Sherr. 1993. Inhibition of granulocyte differentiation by G1 cyclins D2 and D3 but not D1. *Proc Natl Acad Sci U S A*. 90:11513-7.

Katsuno, Y., A. Suzuki, K. Sugimura, K. Okumura, D.H. Zineldeen, M. Shimada, H. Niida, T. Mizuno, F. Hanaoka, and M. Nakanishi. 2009. Cyclin A-Cdk1 regulates the origin firing program in mammalian cells. *Proc Natl Acad Sci U S A*. 106:3184-9.

Kim, C.H., C. Heath, A. Bertuch, and U. Hansen. 1987. Specific stimulation of simian virus 40 late transcription in vitro by a cellular factor binding the simian virus 40 21-base-pair repeat promoter element. *Proc Natl Acad Sci U S A*. 84:6025-9.

Kim, T.H., W.M. Mars, D.B. Stolz, and G.K. Michalopoulos. 2000. Expression and activation of pro-MMP-2 and pro-MMP-9 during rat liver regeneration. *Hepatology*. 31:75-82.

Kim, T.H., W.M. Mars, D.B. Stolz, B.E. Petersen, and G.K. Michalopoulos. 1997. Extracellular matrix remodeling at the early stages of liver regeneration in the rat. *Hepatology*. 26:896-904.

Knittel, T., M. Mehde, D. Kobold, B. Saile, C. Dinter, and G. Ramadori. 1999. Expression patterns of matrix metalloproteinases and their inhibitors in parenchymal and non-parenchymal cells of rat liver: regulation by TNF-alpha and TGF-beta1. *J Hepatol*. 30:48-60.

Knockaert, M., P. Greengard, and L. Meijer. 2002. Pharmacological inhibitors of cyclin-dependent kinases. *Trends Pharmacol Sci*. 23:417-25.

Kowalik, T.F., J. DeGregori, J.K. Schwarz, and J.R. Nevins. 1995. E2F1 overexpression in quiescent fibroblasts leads to induction of cellular DNA synthesis and apoptosis. *J Virol*. 69:2491-500.

Krasinska, L., E. Besnard, E. Cot, C. Dohet, M. Mechali, J.M. Lemaitre, and D. Fisher. 2008. Cdk1 and Cdk2 activity levels determine the efficiency of replication origin firing in Xenopus. *Embo J*. 27:758-69.

Laconi, S., F. Curreli, S. Diana, D. Pasciu, G. De Filippo, D.S. Sarma, P. Pani, and E. Laconi. 1999. Liver regeneration in response to partial hepatectomy in rats treated with retrorsine: a kinetic study. *J Hepatol*. 31:1069-74.

Leclerc, V., J.P. Tassan, P.H. O'Farrell, E.A. Nigg, and P. Leopold. 1996. Drosophila Cdk8, a kinase partner of cyclin C that interacts with the large subunit of RNA polymerase II. *Mol Biol Cell*. 7:505-13.

Lei, M., and B.K. Tye. 2001. Initiating DNA synthesis: from recruiting to activating the MCM complex. *J Cell Sci*. 114:1447-54.

Leof, E.B., J.J. Van Wyk, E.J. O'Keefe, and W.J. Pledger. 1983. Epidermal growth factor (EGF) is required only during the traverse of early G1 in PDGF stimulated density-arrested BALB/c-3T3 cells. *Exp Cell Res*. 147:202-8.

Li, T., A. Inoue, J.M. Lahti, and V.J. Kidd. 2004. Failure to proliferate and mitotic arrest of CDK11(p110/p58)-null mutant mice at the blastocyst stage of embryonic cell development. *Mol Cell Biol*. 24:3188-97.

Li, W., S. Kotoshiba, C. Berthet, M.B. Hilton, and P. Kaldis. 2009a. Rb/Cdk2/Cdk4 triple mutant mice elicit an alternative mechanism for regulation of the G1/S transition. *Proc Natl Acad Sci U S A*. 106:486-91.

Li, W., S. Kotoshiba, and P. Kaldis. 2009b. Genetic mouse models to investigate cell cycle regulation. *Transgenic Res*. 18:491-8.

Liu, M.L., W.M. Mars, R. Zarnegar, and G.K. Michalopoulos. 1994. Collagenase pretreatment and the mitogenic effects of hepatocyte growth factor and transforming growth factor-alpha in adult rat liver. *Hepatology*. 19:1521-7.

Loranger, A., S. Duclos, A. Grenier, J. Price, M. Wilson-Heiner, H. Baribault, and N. Marceau. 1997. Simple epithelium keratins are required for maintenance of hepatocyte integrity. *Am J Pathol*. 151:1673-83.

Loyer, P., A. Busson, J.H. Trembley, J. Hyle, J. Grenet, W. Zhao, C. Ribault, T. Montier, V.J. Kidd, and J.M. Lahti. 2011. The RNA binding motif protein 15B (RBM15B/OTT3) is a functional competitor of serine-arginine (SR) proteins and antagonizes the positive effect of the CDK11p110-cyclin L2alpha complex on splicing. *J Biol Chem.* 286:147-59.

Loyer, P., D. Glaise, S. Cariou, G. Baffet, L. Meijer, and C. Guguen-Guillouzo. 1994. Expression and activation of cdks (1 and 2) and cyclins in the cell cycle progression during liver regeneration. *J Biol Chem.* 269:2491-500.

Loyer, P., G. Ilyin, S. Cariou, D. Glaise, A. Corlu, and C. Guguen-Guillouzo. 1996. Progression through G1 and S phases of adult rat hepatocytes. *Prog Cell Cycle Res.* 2:37-47.

Loyer, P., J.H. Trembley, J.A. Grenet, A. Busson, A. Corlu, W. Zhao, M. Kocak, V.J. Kidd, and J.M. Lahti. 2008. Characterization of cyclin L1 and L2 interactions with CDK11 and splicing factors: influence of cyclin L isoforms on splice site selection. *J Biol Chem.* 283:7721-32.

Loyer, P., J.H. Trembley, R. Katona, V.J. Kidd, and J.M. Lahti. 2005. Role of CDK/cyclin complexes in transcription and RNA splicing. *Cell Signal.* 17:1033-51.

Lu, X.P., K.S. Koch, D.J. Lew, V. Dulic, J. Pines, S.I. Reed, T. Hunter, and H.L. Leffert. 1992. Induction of cyclin mRNA and cyclin-associated histone H1 kinase during liver regeneration. *J Biol Chem.* 267:2841-4.

Lundberg, A.S., and R.A. Weinberg. 1998. Functional inactivation of the retinoblastoma protein requires sequential modification by at least two distinct cyclin-cdk complexes. *Mol Cell Biol.* 18:753-61.

Malumbres, M., and M. Barbacid. 2005. Mammalian cyclin-dependent kinases. *Trends Biochem Sci.* 30:630-41.

Malumbres, M., E. Harlow, T. Hunt, T. Hunter, J.M. Lahti, G. Manning, D.O. Morgan, L.H. Tsai, and D.J. Wolgemuth. 2009. Cyclin-dependent kinases: a family portrait. *Nat Cell Biol.* 11:1275-6.

Malumbres, M., R. Sotillo, D. Santamaria, J. Galan, A. Cerezo, S. Ortega, P. Dubus, and M. Barbacid. 2004. Mammalian cells cycle without the D-type cyclin-dependent kinases Cdk4 and Cdk6. *Cell.* 118:493-504.

Matsushime, H., M.E. Ewen, D.K. Strom, J.Y. Kato, S.K. Hanks, M.F. Roussel, and C.J. Sherr. 1992. Identification and properties of an atypical catalytic subunit (p34PSK-J3/cdk4) for mammalian D type G1 cyclins. *Cell.* 71:323-34.

Matsushime, H., D.E. Quelle, S.A. Shurtleff, M. Shibuya, C.J. Sherr, and J.Y. Kato. 1994. D-type cyclin-dependent kinase activity in mammalian cells. *Mol Cell Biol.* 14:2066-76.

Matsushime, H., M.F. Roussel, R.A. Ashmun, and C.J. Sherr. 1991. Colony-stimulating factor 1 regulates novel cyclins during the G1 phase of the cell cycle. *Cell.* 65:701-13.

McGowan, J.A., and N.L. Bucher. 1983. Pyruvate promotion of DNA synthesis in serum-free primary cultures of adult rat hepatocytes. *In Vitro.* 19:159-66.

Michalopoulos, G.K., and M. DeFrances. 2005. Liver regeneration. *Adv Biochem Eng Biotechnol.* 93:101-34.

Mohammed, F.F., C.J. Pennington, Z. Kassiri, J.S. Rubin, P.D. Soloway, U. Ruther, D.R. Edwards, and R. Khokha. 2005. Metalloproteinase inhibitor TIMP-1 affects hepatocyte cell cycle via HGF activation in murine liver regeneration. *Hepatology.* 41:857-67.

Mohammed, F.F., D.S. Smookler, S.E. Taylor, B. Fingleton, Z. Kassiri, O.H. Sanchez, J.L. English, L.M. Matrisian, B. Au, W.C. Yeh, and R. Khokha. 2004. Abnormal TNF activity in Timp3-/- mice leads to chronic hepatic inflammation and failure of liver regeneration. *Nat Genet*. 36:969-77.

Moolten, F.L., and N.L. Bucher. 1967. Regeneration of rat liver: transfer of humoral agent by cross circulation. *Science*. 158:272-4.

Morgan, D.O. 1997. Cyclin-dependent kinases: engines, clocks, and microprocessors. *Annu Rev Cell Dev Biol*. 13:261-91.

Mori, N., H. Sato, T. Hayashibara, M. Senba, R. Geleziunas, A. Wada, T. Hirayama, and N. Yamamoto. 2003. Helicobacter pylori induces matrix metalloproteinase-9 through activation of nuclear factor kappaB. *Gastroenterology*. 124:983-92.

Muller, H., A.P. Bracken, R. Vernell, M.C. Moroni, F. Christians, E. Grassilli, E. Prosperini, E. Vigo, J.D. Oliner, and K. Helin. 2001. E2Fs regulate the expression of genes involved in differentiation, development, proliferation, and apoptosis. *Genes Dev*. 15:267-85.

Nagaki, M., A. Sugiyama, T. Naiki, Y. Ohsawa, and H. Moriwaki. 2000. Control of cyclins, cyclin-dependent kinase inhibitors, p21 and p27, and cell cycle progression in rat hepatocytes by extracellular matrix. *J Hepatol*. 32:488-96.

Natarajan, A., B. Wagner, and M. Sibilia. 2007. The EGF receptor is required for efficient liver regeneration. *Proc Natl Acad Sci U S A*. 104:17081-6.

Nelsen, C.J., D.G. Rickheim, N.A. Timchenko, M.W. Stanley, and J.H. Albrecht. 2001. Transient expression of cyclin D1 is sufficient to promote hepatocyte replication and liver growth in vivo. *Cancer Res*. 61:8564-8.

Nelsen, C.J., D.G. Rickheim, M.M. Tucker, L.K. Hansen, and J.H. Albrecht. 2003. Evidence that cyclin D1 mediates both growth and proliferation downstream of TOR in hepatocytes. *J Biol Chem*. 278:3656-63.

Ninomiya-Tsuji, J., S. Nomoto, H. Yasuda, S.I. Reed, and K. Matsumoto. 1991. Cloning of a human cDNA encoding a CDC2-related kinase by complementation of a budding yeast cdc28 mutation. *Proc Natl Acad Sci U S A*. 88:9006-10.

Nurse, P. 2002. Cyclin dependent kinases and cell cycle control (nobel lecture). *Chembiochem*. 3:596-603.

Nurse, P., and P. Thuriaux. 1980. Regulatory genes controlling mitosis in the fission yeast Schizosaccharomyces pombe. *Genetics*. 96:627-37.

Okuda, M., H.F. Horn, P. Tarapore, Y. Tokuyama, A.G. Smulian, P.K. Chan, E.S. Knudsen, I.A. Hofmann, J.D. Snyder, K.E. Bove, and K. Fukasawa. 2000. Nucleophosmin/B23 is a target of CDK2/cyclin E in centrosome duplication. *Cell*. 103:127-40.

Olle, E.W., X. Ren, S.D. McClintock, R.L. Warner, M.P. Deogracias, K.J. Johnson, and L.M. Colletti. 2006. Matrix metalloproteinase-9 is an important factor in hepatic regeneration after partial hepatectomy in mice. *Hepatology*. 44:540-9.

Ortega, S., I. Prieto, J. Odajima, A. Martin, P. Dubus, R. Sotillo, J.L. Barbero, M. Malumbres, and M. Barbacid. 2003. Cyclin-dependent kinase 2 is essential for meiosis but not for mitotic cell division in mice. *Nat Genet*. 35:25-31.

Pagon, Z., J. Volker, G.M. Cooper, and U. Hansen. 2003. Mammalian transcription factor LSF is a target of ERK signaling. *J Cell Biochem*. 89:733-46.

Pardee, A.B. 1974. A restriction point for control of normal animal cell proliferation. *Proc Natl Acad Sci U S A*. 71:1286-90.

Pardee, A.B. 1986. Biochemical and molecular events regulating cell proliferation. *J Pathol*. 149:1-2.

Pardee, A.B. 1989. G1 events and regulation of cell proliferation. *Science*. 246:603-8.

Petretti, C., M. Savoian, E. Montembault, D.M. Glover, C. Prigent, and R. Giet. 2006. The PITSLRE/CDK11(p58) protein kinase promotes centrosome maturation and bipolar spindle formation. *EMBO Rep*.

Pledger, W.J., C.D. Stiles, H.N. Antoniades, and C.D. Scher. 1977. Induction of DNA synthesis in BALB/c 3T3 cells by serum components: reevaluation of the commitment process. *Proc Natl Acad Sci U S A*. 74:4481-5.

Pledger, W.J., C.D. Stiles, H.N. Antoniades, and C.D. Scher. 1978. An ordered sequence of events is required before BALB/c-3T3 cells become committed to DNA synthesis. *Proc Natl Acad Sci U S A*. 75:2839-43.

Pomerening, J.R., J.A. Ubersax, and J.E. Ferrell, Jr. 2008. Rapid cycling and precocious termination of G1 phase in cells expressing CDK1AF. *Mol Biol Cell*. 19:3426-41.

Powell, C.M., T.L. Rudge, Q. Zhu, L.F. Johnson, and U. Hansen. 2000. Inhibition of the mammalian transcription factor LSF induces S-phase-dependent apoptosis by downregulating thymidylate synthase expression. *Embo J*. 19:4665-75.

Pujol, M.J., M. Jaime, J. Serratosa, M. Jaumot, N. Agell, and O. Bachs. 2000. Differential association of p21Cip1 and p27Kip1 with cyclin E-CDK2 during rat liver regeneration. *J Hepatol*. 33:266-74.

Rabes, H.M., R. Wirsching, H.V. Tuczek, and G. Iseler. 1976. Analysis of cell cycle compartments of hepatocytes after partial hepatecomy. *Cell Tissue Kinet*. 9:517-32.

Reed, S.I. 1992. The role of p34 kinases in the G1 to S-phase transition. *Annu Rev Cell Biol*. 8:529-61.

Ren, B., H. Cam, Y. Takahashi, T. Volkert, J. Terragni, R.A. Young, and B.D. Dynlacht. 2002. E2F integrates cell cycle progression with DNA repair, replication, and G(2)/M checkpoints. *Genes Dev*. 16:245-56.

Ren, S., and B.J. Rollins. 2004. Cyclin C/cdk3 promotes Rb-dependent G0 exit. *Cell*. 117:239-51.

Rickert, P., J.L. Corden, and E. Lees. 1999. Cyclin C/CDK8 and cyclin H/CDK7/p36 are biochemically distinct CTD kinases. *Oncogene*. 18:1093-102.

Roselli, H.T., M. Su, K. Washington, D.M. Kerins, D.E. Vaughan, and W.E. Russell. 1998. Liver regeneration is transiently impaired in urokinase-deficient mice. *Am J Physiol*. 275:G1472-9.

Rosenblatt, J., Y. Gu, and D.O. Morgan. 1992. Human cyclin-dependent kinase 2 is activated during the S and G2 phases of the cell cycle and associates with cyclin A. *Proc Natl Acad Sci U S A*. 89:2824-8.

Ruderman, J.V. 1993. MAP kinase and the activation of quiescent cells. *Curr Opin Cell Biol*. 5:207-13.

Rudolph, K.L., C. Trautwein, S. Kubicka, T. Rakemann, M.J. Bahr, N. Sedlaczek, D. Schuppan, and M.P. Manns. 1999. Differential regulation of extracellular matrix synthesis during liver regeneration after partial hepatectomy in rats. *Hepatology*. 30:1159-66.

Sanceau, J., D.D. Boyd, M. Seiki, and B. Bauvois. 2002. Interferons inhibit tumor necrosis factor-alpha-mediated matrix metalloproteinase-9 activation via interferon regulatory factor-1 binding competition with NF-kappa B. *J Biol Chem*. 277:35766-75.

Sang, L., H.A. Coller, and J.M. Roberts. 2008. Control of the reversibility of cellular quiescence by the transcriptional repressor HES1. *Science*. 321:1095-100.

Santamaria, D., C. Barriere, A. Cerqueira, S. Hunt, C. Tardy, K. Newton, J.F. Caceres, P. Dubus, M. Malumbres, and M. Barbacid. 2007. Cdk1 is sufficient to drive the mammalian cell cycle. *Nature*. 448:811-5.

Satyanarayana, A., M.B. Hilton, and P. Kaldis. 2008. p21 Inhibits Cdk1 in the absence of Cdk2 to maintain the G1/S phase DNA damage checkpoint. *Mol Biol Cell*. 19:65-77.

Satyanarayana, A., and P. Kaldis. 2009a. A dual role of Cdk2 in DNA damage response. *Cell Div*. 4:9.

Satyanarayana, A., and P. Kaldis. 2009b. Mammalian cell-cycle regulation: several Cdks, numerous cyclins and diverse compensatory mechanisms. *Oncogene*. 28:2925-39.

Sawada, N. 1989. Hepatocytes from old rats retain responsiveness of c-myc expression to EGF in primary culture but do not enter S phase. *Exp Cell Res*. 181:584-8.

Saxena, U.H., C.M. Powell, J.K. Fecko, R. Cacioppo, H.S. Chou, G.M. Cooper, and U. Hansen. 2009. Phosphorylation by cyclin C/cyclin-dependent kinase 2 following mitogenic stimulation of murine fibroblasts inhibits transcriptional activity of LSF during G1 progression. *Mol Cell Biol*. 29:2335-45.

Schuppan, D., M. Schmid, R. Somasundaram, R. Ackermann, M. Ruehl, T. Nakamura, and E.O. Riecken. 1998. Collagens in the liver extracellular matrix bind hepatocyte growth factor. *Gastroenterology*. 114:139-52.

Serandour, A.L., P. Loyer, D. Garnier, B. Courselaud, N. Theret, D. Glaise, C. Guguen-Guillouzo, and A. Corlu. 2005. TNFalpha-mediated extracellular matrix remodeling is required for multiple division cycles in rat hepatocytes. *Hepatology*. 41:478-86.

Serratosa, J., J. Domingo, C. Enrich, and O. Bachs. 1988. Nuclear growth and chromatin relaxation-condensation cycle in hepatocytes during the proliferative activation of rat liver. *Virchows Arch B Cell Pathol Incl Mol Pathol*. 55:57-64.

Sherr, C.J. 1993. Mammalian G1 cyclins. *Cell*. 73:1059-65.

Sherr, C.J. 1994. G1 phase progression: cycling on cue. *Cell*. 79:551-5.

Sherr, C.J. 1995. Mammalian G1 cyclins and cell cycle progression. *Proc Assoc Am Physicians*. 107:181-6.

Sherr, C.J., and J.M. Roberts. 1995. Inhibitors of mammalian G1 cyclin-dependent kinases. *Genes Dev*. 9:1149-63.

Sherr, C.J., and J.M. Roberts. 2004. Living with or without cyclins and cyclin-dependent kinases. *Genes Dev*. 18:2699-711.

Shimizu, M., A. Hara, M. Okuno, H. Matsuno, K. Okada, S. Ueshima, O. Matsuo, M. Niwa, K. Akita, Y. Yamada, N. Yoshimi, T. Uematsu, S. Kojima, S.L. Friedman, H. Moriwaki, and H. Mori. 2001. Mechanism of retarded liver regeneration in plasminogen activator-deficient mice: impaired activation of hepatocyte growth factor after Fas-mediated massive hepatic apoptosis. *Hepatology*. 33:569-76.

Talarmin, H., C. Rescan, S. Cariou, D. Glaise, G. Zanninelli, M. Bilodeau, P. Loyer, C. Guguen-Guillouzo, and G. Baffet. 1999. The mitogen-activated protein kinase kinase/extracellular signal-regulated kinase cascade activation is a key signalling pathway involved in the regulation of G(1) phase progression in proliferating hepatocytes. *Mol Cell Biol*. 19:6003-11.

Tassan, J.P., M. Jaquenoud, P. Leopold, S.J. Schultz, and E.A. Nigg. 1995. Identification of human cyclin-dependent kinase 8, a putative protein kinase partner for cyclin C. *Proc Natl Acad Sci U S A*. 92:8871-5.

Temme, A., T. Ott, F. Dombrowski, and K. Willecke. 2000. The extent of synchronous initiation and termination of DNA synthesis in regenerating mouse liver is dependent on connexin32 expressing gap junctions. *J Hepatol*. 32:627-35.

Tetsu, O., and F. McCormick. 2003. Proliferation of cancer cells despite CDK2 inhibition. *Cancer Cell*. 3:233-45.

Th'ng, J.P., P.S. Wright, J. Hamaguchi, M.G. Lee, C.J. Norbury, P. Nurse, and E.M. Bradbury. 1990. The FT210 cell line is a mouse G2 phase mutant with a temperature-sensitive CDC2 gene product. *Cell*. 63:313-24.

Thomson, A.M., P.J. Gillespie, and J.J. Blow. 2010. Replication factory activation can be decoupled from the replication timing program by modulating Cdk levels. *J Cell Biol*. 188:209-21.

Trembley, J.H., D. Hu, L.C. Hsu, C.Y. Yeung, C. Slaughter, J.M. Lahti, and V.J. Kidd. 2002. PITSLRE p110 protein kinases associate with transcription complexes and affect their activity. *J Biol Chem*. 277:2589-96.

Trembley, J.H., P. Loyer, D. Hu, T. Li, J. Grenet, J.M. Lahti, and V.J. Kidd. 2004. Cyclin dependent kinase 11 in RNA transcription and splicing. *Prog Nucleic Acid Res Mol Biol*. 77:263-88.

Trimarchi, J.M., and J.A. Lees. 2002. Sibling rivalry in the E2F family. *Nat Rev Mol Cell Biol*. 3:11-20.

Tushinski, R.J., and E.R. Stanley. 1985. The regulation of mononuclear phagocyte entry into S phase by the colony stimulating factor CSF-1. *J Cell Physiol*. 122:221-8.

Ussar, S., and T. Voss. 2004. MEK1 and MEK2, different regulators of the G1/S transition. *J Biol Chem*. 279:43861-9.

van den Heuvel, S., and E. Harlow. 1993. Distinct roles for cyclin-dependent kinases in cell cycle control. *Science*. 262:2050-4.

Vandenbosch, R., L. Borgs, P. Beukelaers, A. Foidart, L. Nguyen, G. Moonen, C. Berthet, P. Kaldis, V. Gallo, S. Belachew, and B. Malgrange. 2007. CDK2 is dispensable for adult hippocampal neurogenesis. *Cell Cycle*. 6:3065-9.

Volker, J.L., L.E. Rameh, Q. Zhu, J. DeCaprio, and U. Hansen. 1997. Mitogenic stimulation of resting T cells causes rapid phosphorylation of the transcription factor LSF and increased DNA-binding activity. *Genes Dev*. 11:1435-46.

Webber, E.M., J. Bruix, R.H. Pierce, and N. Fausto. 1998. Tumor necrosis factor primes hepatocytes for DNA replication in the rat. *Hepatology*. 28:1226-34.

Wheeler, L.W., N.H. Lents, and J.J. Baldassare. 2008. Cyclin A-CDK activity during G1 phase impairs MCM chromatin loading and inhibits DNA synthesis in mammalian cells. *Cell Cycle*. 7:2179-88.

Widmann, J.J., and H.D. Fahimi. 1975. Proliferation of mononuclear phagocytes (Kupffer cells) and endothelial cells in regenerating rat liver. A light and electron microscopic cytochemical study. *Am J Pathol*. 80:349-66.

Woo, R.A., and R.Y. Poon. 2003. Cyclin-dependent kinases and S phase control in mammalian cells. *Cell Cycle*. 2:316-24.

Yang, H.C., and A.B. Pardee. 1986. Insulin-like growth factor I regulation of transcription and replicating enzyme induction necessary for DNA synthesis. *J Cell Physiol.* 127:410-6.

Yasuda, H., M. Kamijo, R. Honda, M. Nakamura, F. Hanaoka, and Y. Ohba. 1991. A point mutation in C-terminal region of cdc2 kinase causes a G2-phase arrest in a mouse temperature-sensitive FM3A cell mutant. *Cell Struct Funct.* 16:105-12.

Zhao, J., B.K. Kennedy, B.D. Lawrence, D.A. Barbie, A.G. Matera, J.A. Fletcher, and E. Harlow. 2000. NPAT links cyclin E-Cdk2 to the regulation of replication-dependent histone gene transcription. *Genes Dev.* 14:2283-97.

Zindy, F., E. Lamas, X. Chenivesse, J. Sobczak, J. Wang, D. Fesquet, B. Henglein, and C. Brechot. 1992. Cyclin A is required in S phase in normal epithelial cells. *Biochem Biophys Res Commun.* 182:1144-54.

Zschemisch, N.H., C. Liedtke, U. Dierssen, Y.A. Nevzorova, T. Wustefeld, J. Borlak, M.P. Manns, and C. Trautwein. 2006. Expression of a cyclin E1 isoform in mice is correlated with the quiescent cell cycle status of hepatocytes in vivo. *Hepatology.* 44:164-73.

24

Binding of Human MCM-BP with MCM2-7 Proteins

Ryoko Kon[1], Shunsuke Kusunoki[1], Naohito Nozaki[2] and Yukio Ishimi[1]
[1]*Ibaraki University, Mito, Ibaraki 351-8511,*
[2]*Kanagawa Dental College, Yokosuka, Kanagawa 238-8580*
Japan

1. Introduction

MCM2-7 proteins play essential roles in DNA replication in eukaryotic cells, probably by acting as a replicative DNA helicase that unwinds DNA duplexes at replication forks (Bell & Dutta, 2002; Forsburg, 2004; Masai et al., 2010). Several lines of evidences suggest that MCM2-7 hexameric complexes assembled on the replication origins are converted to an active form with the assistance of the CDC7, CDC45 and GINS complex (Moyer et al., 2006; Gambus et al., 2006). MCM-BP, which has been identified from human cells as a protein that binds to MCM6 and MCM7 proteins, has amino acids sequences homologous to MCM2-7 (Sakwe et al. 2007). The results in this report indicate that MCM-BP replaces MCM2 in MCM2-7 complex and it binds to a replication origin in HeLa cells, suggesting that the MCM complex containing the MCM-BP may play a role in the initiation of DNA replication. It has also been indicated that down-regulation of MCM-BP affects chromatin binding of MCM4. Recently it has been reported that *Arabidopsis thaliana* ETG1, which has been identified as an E2F target gene, is a homolog of MCM-BP (Takahashi et al., 2008). ETG1 protein is required for efficient DNA replication. Depletion of ETG1 results in inhibition of DNA replication and G2 arrest. Under these conditions, the G2 checkpoint system is induced. The report by Takahashi et al. (2010) indicates that ETG1 is involved in sister chromatid cohesion which is required for post-replicative homologous recombination repair. More recently, it has been reported that *Xenopus* MCM-BP regulates unloading of the MCM2-7 complex from chromatin in the late S phase by interacting with MCM7 (Nishiyama et al., 2011). These evidences suggest a possibility that MCM-BP may interact with the MCM2-7 complex at the replication forks to regulate the chromatin binding of the complex. Such interaction may be required for establishment of the cohesin complex at the forks.

Here we examined biochemical properties of human MCM-BP. First, we found that human MCM-BP can bind all the human MCM2-7 proteins when the MCM-BP and one of the MCM2-7 proteins are co-expressed in insect cells. However, the interaction of MCM-BP with MCM7 was mainly detected when all the MCM2-7 and MCM-BP were co-expressed at the same time. In HeLa cells, MCM-BP was mainly recovered in a Triton-soluble fraction, suggesting that it does not stably bind to chromatin. A small portion of MCM-BP in this fraction was bound to MCM4, MCM5, MCM6 and MCM7 proteins. These results suggest that MCM-BP is not a constituent of pre-RC and it exhibits its functions by interacting with

MCM7. The results are not inconsistent with the notion that MCM-BP may play a role in the dynamics of MCM complex at the forks.

2.1 Binding of human MCM-BP with MCM2-7

The human MCM-BP gene was synthesized from cDNA of HeLa cells by the RT-PCR method. The sequencing of the cloned gene indicates that an internal deletion of six nucleotides is present in comparison to the gene in Genebank (NM_002388). Thus two amino acids of Cys and Lys at amino acid no. 334 and 335 are deleted. This deleted portion is localized near the center of the protein where the Walker A and B motifs are located at amino acid no. 396-407 and 457-465, respectively. To examine the interaction of the MCM-BP and MCM2-7 proteins, Flag-tagged MCM-BP and one of MCM2-7 were co-expressed in High5 cells and the cell lysate was immuno-precipiated with anti-Flag antibody. We examined whether co-expressed MCM2-7 is co-precipiated with Flag-MCM-BP or not (Fig. 1). In all combinations, precipitation of expressed MCM-BP was confirmed, and all the co-expressed MCM2-7 proteins were co-precipitated. Since the amounts of MCM2-7 proteins present in the Triton-soluble fraction different, it is difficult to compare the strength of their interaction with MCM-BP in this system. However, the results suggest that the interaction between the MCM-BP and MCM2 is as strong as the interactions between the MCM-BP and MCM3-7 proteins. The interactions of MCM-BP with CDT1 and CDC6, which are MCM2-7 loaders, and with ORC2 and ORC4 were examined by using the same experimental system (Fig. 2). Only faint bands of CDT1 and ORC2 were detected in the fractions precipitated with MCM-BP, but co-precipitation with CDC6 and ORC4 were not detected. These results indicate that MCM-BP can specifically and directly interact with the MCM2-7 proteins. These results appear to be in contrast to the interaction of MCM7 with MCM2-6 proteins in that MCM7 mainly interacts with the MCM3 and MCM4 proteins (Numata et al., 2010). Such interaction of MCM7 is consistent with the placement of MCM2-7 proteins in the heterohexameric MCM2-7 complex (Yu et al., 2004).

To further examine the interaction of MCM-BP with the MCM2-7 proteins, all MCM2-7 proteins were co-expressed with MCM-BP in insect cells, and Flag-MCM-BP was precipitated with anti-Flag antibody. Proteins bound to the Sepharose beads were eluted with Flag peptide. In addition to MCM-BP, all the MCM2-7 proteins were detected in the eluted fractions, and the MCM7 protein was dominantly detected in silver-stained gel (Fig. 3). In glycerol gradient centrifugation of the eluted proteins, MCM-BP was mainly recovered in the fractions no. 7-13 (Fig. 4). Purified MCM-BP itself was recovered in fractions no. 9-13 (data not presented), suggesting a possibility that MCM-BP itself mainly forms a dimmer. MCM4/6/7 hexamer is recovered in fractions no. 3-6 under the same conditions. Both MCM-BP and MCM2-7 proteins were also detected in these fractions. Thus, it is assumed that MCM-BP may bind one to several molecules among the MCM2-7 proteins. Sedimentation profile supports the notion that MCM7 is mainly associated with MCM-BP. MCM-BP in the fraction no. 9 of the glycerol gradient was precipitated with anti-Flag antibody (Fig. 5). Although all the MCM2-7 proteins were hardly detected in unbound fractions, only MCM6 and MCM7 proteins were detected in elution fractions. Based on the finding that the direct interaction between MCM6 and MCM7 is not strong (Yu et al., 2004; Numata et al., 2010), all these results suggest that MCM-BP mainly interacts with MCM7 and also with MCM6.

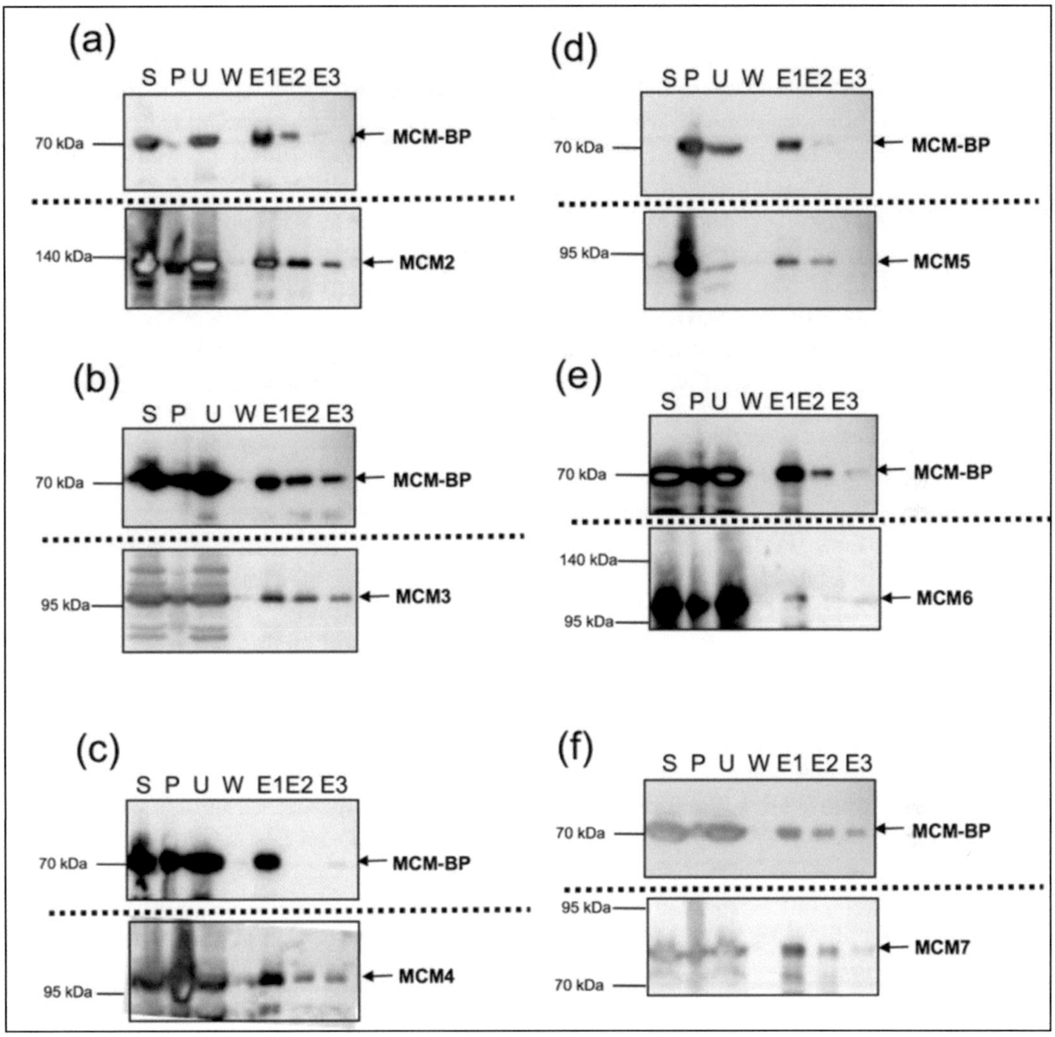
(a)
S P U W E1E2 E3
70 kDa
MCM-BP
140 kDa
MCM2
(b)
S P U W E1E2 E3
70 kDa
MCM-BP
95 kDa
MCM3
(c)
S P U W E1E2 E3
70 kDa
MCM-BP
95 kDa
MCM4
(d)
S P U W E1E2 E3
70 kDa
MCM-BP
95 kDa
MCM5
(e)
S P U W E1E2 E3
70 kDa
MCM-BP
140 kDa
MCM6
95 kDa
(f)
S P U W E1 E2 E3
70 kDa
MCM-BP
95 kDa
MCM7
70 kDa

(a-f) High5 cells (7x10^6 cells) were co-infected with the viruses expressing the MCM-BP protein (0.25 ml of viral stock solution) and MCM2-protein (a) (0.25 ml of viral stock solution), MCM3 (b), MCM4 (c), MCM5 (d), MCM6 (e) or MCM7 (f) for 2 days. The cells were suspended in a 500 μl of lysis buffer consisting of 10 mM Tris-HCl (pH 7.5), 130 mM NaCl, 1% Triton X-100, 10 mM NaF, 10 mM sodium phosphate buffer, 10 mM $Na_4P_2O_7$, and protease inhibitors (Pharmingen, BD, San Jose, CA). The mixture was incubated for 40 min on ice, and insoluble components were separated by centrifugation at 40,000 rpm (TLS55; Beckman, Fullerton, CA) for 40 min at 4°C. Supernatant of Triton-soluble (S) was recovered, and the precipitate was suspended with 100 μl of lysis buffer to obtain Triton-insoluble (P) fraction. The recovered supernatant (200 μl) was mixed for 1 h at 4°C with anti-Flag antibody (2.5 μg) and then protein G-Sepharose (20-30 μl) (Amersham Biosciences, Piscataway, NJ, USA) was added. The solution was mixed overnight at 4 °C. After spin, proteins unbound to the Sepharose beads were recovered (U). The beads were washed 10-12 times with 200 μl of phosphate-buffered saline (PBS) containing 0.1% Triton X-100, and supernatant after the final spin was recovered (W). The proteins bound to the beads were eluted three times with 20-30 μl of elution buffer (0.1 M glycine, pH 2.5 and 0.15 M NaCl) (E1, E2 and E3). These eluates were neutralized by adding 1/10 volume of 2 M Tris-HCl, pH 8.0. Proteins in the obtained fractions were separated by SDS-polyacrylamide gel electrophoresis. After the proteins in the gel were transferred to Immobilon-P transfer membrane (Millipore, Bedford, MA, USA), the membrane was incubated for 1 h at room temperature with a blocking buffer (EzBlock, ATTO, Tokyo, Japan) diluted by three-fold with TBS (50 mM Tris-HCl, pH7.9, 150 mM NaCl) plus 0.1% Triton X-100; it was then incubated overnight at 4 °C with 0.5-1 μg/ml of 1st antibodies in the diluted blocking buffer or culture supernatant of hybridoma cells producing anti-MCM-BP antibody (Nakaya et al., 2010). After washing the membrane with TBS containing Triton X-100, it was incubated for 2 h at 27°C with 2nd antibody conjugated with horseradish peroxidase (BioRad, Hercules, CA, USA). After washing, the membrane was incubated with SuperSignal West Pico Maximum Sensitivity Substrate (Pierce, Rockford, IL, USA), and chemiluminescent signals were detected by Light-Capture (ATTO). Anti-MCM2, -MCM3, and –MCM4 antibodies were prepared as reported (Nakaya et al., 2010). Anti-MCM5 (Santa Cruz, Bio, sc-165995), anti-MCM6 (Santa Cruz, Bio, sc-9843), anti-MCM7 (Santa Cruz Bio, sc-9966), and anti-Flag (Sigma, F-3165) antibodies were purchased. In the experiments (a-f), one filter was proved with anti-MCM-BP antibody (top) and the other was proved with anti-MCM2-7 antibodies (bottom). Due to over-loading, MCM2 bands in S and U fractions were not fully detected in (a). In (d), a band of MCM-BP in S fraction was hardly detected by unknown reason.

Fig. 1. Interaction of MCM-BP with MCM2-7 proteins

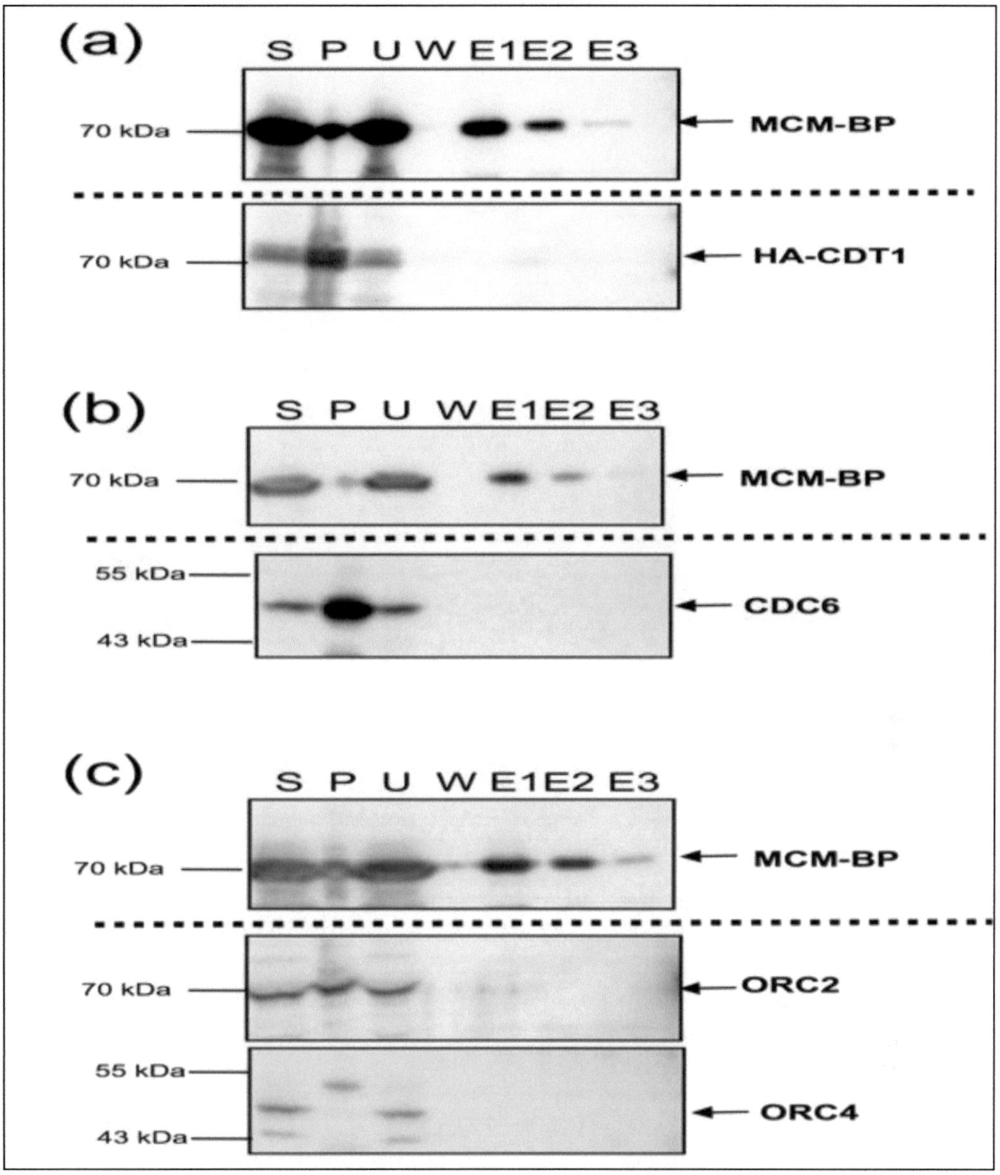

Human MCM-BP-Flag was co-expressed with human CDT1 (a), CDC6 (b) and ORC2 and 4 (c) in High5 cells and the cells were fractionated into Triton-soluble (S) and -insoluble (P) fractions. Proteins in the Triton-soluble fraction were immuno-precipitated with anti-Flag antibody. Unbound proteins (U) and those contained in the final wash (W) were recovered. In addition to the proteins eluted from the beads (E1, E2 and E3), proteins in other fractions were examined by immuno-blotting. In the experiments (a-c), one filter was proved with anti-MCM-BP antibody (top) and the other was proved with anti-HA(CDT1, Santa Cruz Bio. sc-7392), CDC6(Santa Cruz Bio. sc-8341), and ORC2, ORC4(Santa Cruz Bio. sc-20634) antibodies, (bottom).

Fig. 2. Interaction of MCM-BP with MCM loader proteins

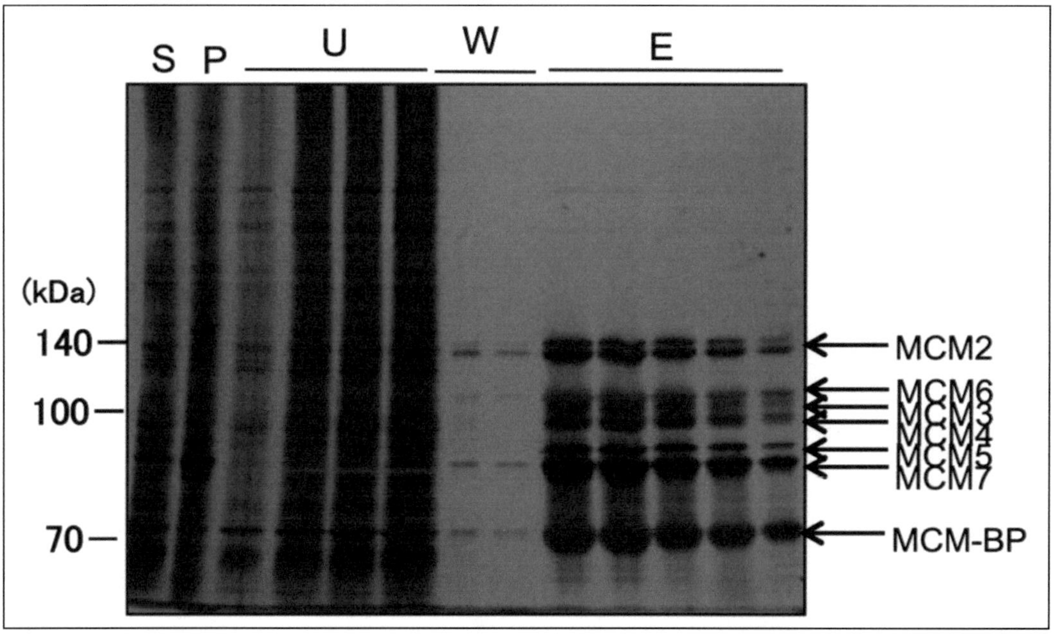

High5 cells (3x10[7] cells) were co-infected with recombinant baculoviruses producing Flag-MCM-BP (0.5 ml of stock solution), MCM2-MCM7(His) (0.5 ml), MCM3-MCM5(His) (1 ml) and MCM4(His)-MCM6 (0.5 ml). The infected cells (9x10[7] cell in total) were lysed with lysis buffer (4.5 ml) and fractionated into Triton-soluble (S) and -insoluble (P) fractions. Flag-MCM-BP in the Triton-soluble fraction was loaded onto a column of anti-Flag antibody beads (0.3 ml, Sigma, St. Louis, Missouri, USA)). Unbound proteins were collected (U). Supernatant after washing was recovered (W). Proteins bound to the beads were eluted by incubating with a buffer (50 mM Tris-HCl, pH 7.5, 0.15 M NaCl) containing Flag peptide (50 μg/ml, Sigma) (E). Proteins in these fractions were electrophoresed and they were stained with silver. Bands corresponding to MCM2-7 and MCM-BP proteins are indicated at the right.

Fig. 3. Preparation of MCM-BP-binding MCM2-7 proteins

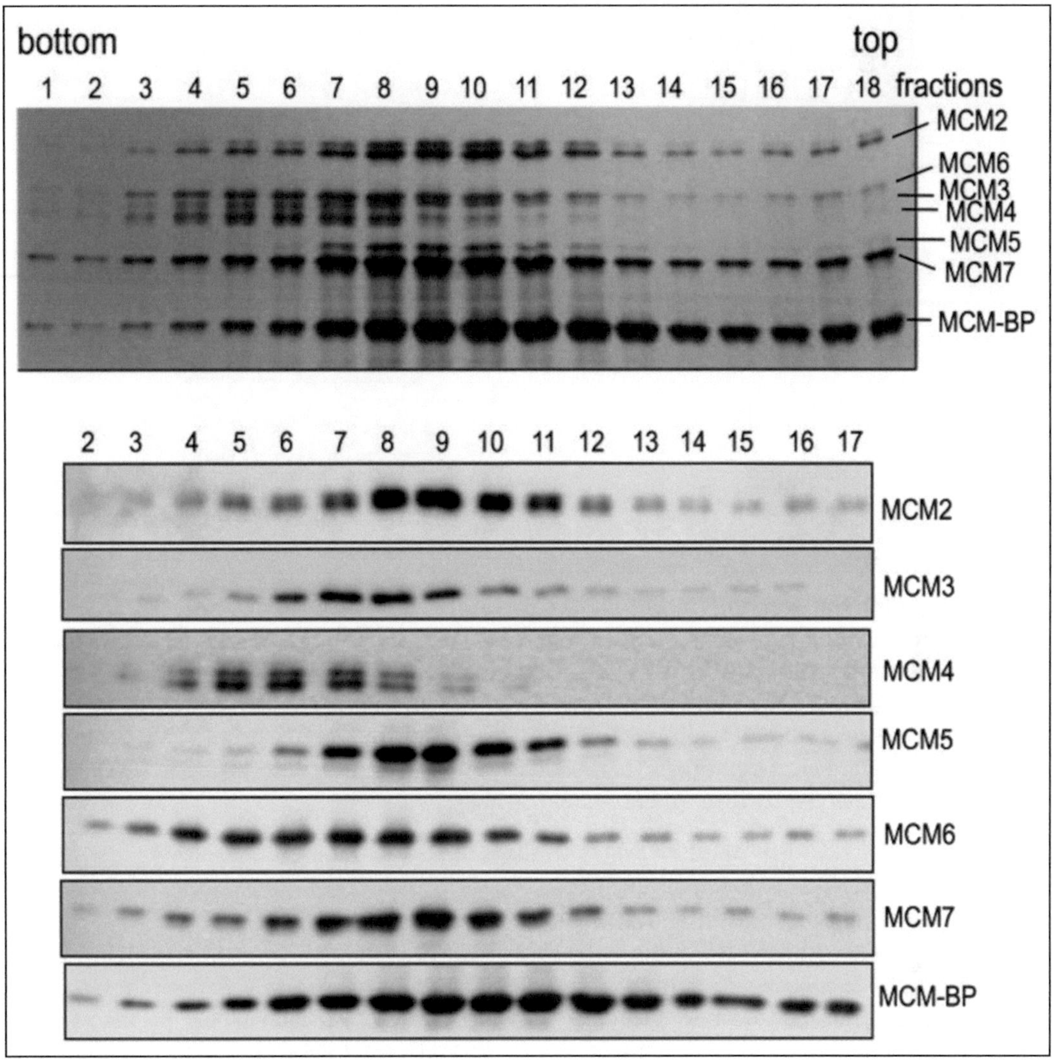

Proteins eluted from anti-Flag antibody column were fractionated by glycerol gradient centrifugation (Ishimi, 1997). Proteins were loaded onto a linear gradient of 15% to 30% glycerol and centrifuged at 36,000 rpm for 14 h in TLS55 rotor (Beckman). Aliquots of the obtained fractions (no. 1-18) were loaded on SDS-polyacrylamide gel. After electrophoresis, proteins were stained with silver (top). Positions of MCM2-7 and MCM-BP were indicated at the right. Proteins of MCM2-7 and MCM-BP in these fractions (no. 2-17) were detected by immuno-blotting using the specific antibodies (bottom). Two bands are detected for MCM4, which is probably due to degradation of the protein.

Fig. 4. Binding of MCM-BP with MCM2-7 proteins

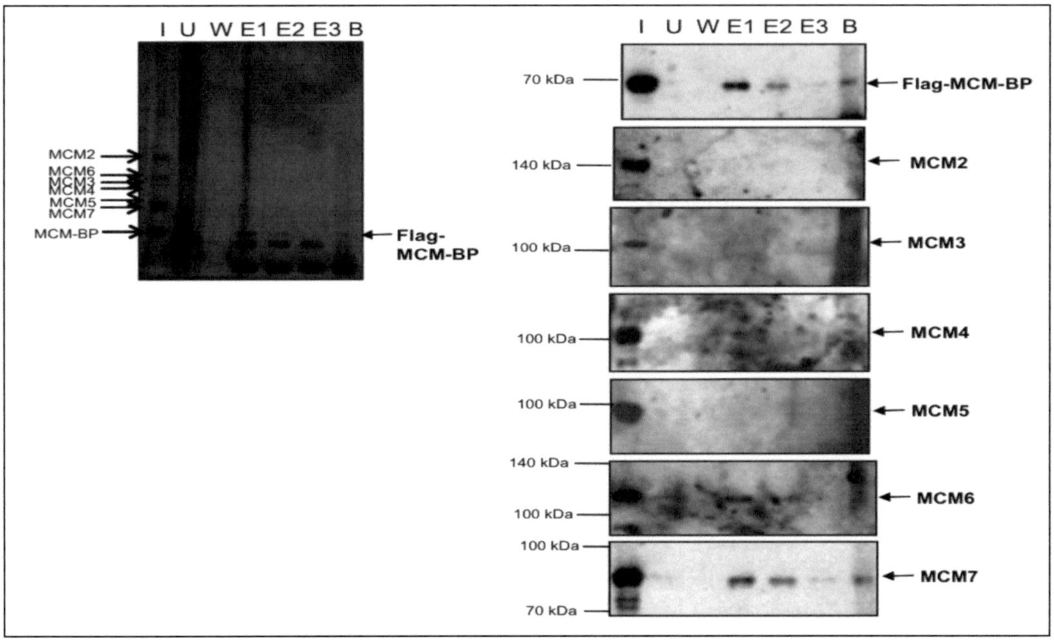

Proteins (I) in the fraction no. 9 in Fig. 4 were precipitated with anti-Flag antibody. After proteins unbound to the beads (U) and those in the supernatant of the final wash (W) were recovered, those bound to the beads were eluted three times by incubating with elution buffer (0.1 M glycine, pH 2.5 and 0.15 M NaCl) (E1, E2 and E3). Proteins remaining in the eluted beads were eluted by boiling in SDS-sample buffer for electrophoresis (B). Proteins in these fractions were electrophoresed and stained with silver (left), and MCM-BP and MCM2-7 were detected by immuno-blotting (right).

Fig. 5. Binding of MCM-BP with MCM6 and MCM7 proteins

2.2 Chromatin-binding of human MCM-BP

To examine whether MCM-BP binds with chromatin or not, logarithmically growing HeLa cells were lysed in a buffer containing Triton X-100 and 100 mM NaCl. After Triton-soluble nucleoplasmic and cytoplasmic proteins were recovered, nuclear DNA in the Triton-insoluble fraction was digested with DNase I. The DNase I-soluble fraction contained a small portion of histones, and DNase I-insoluble fraction contained a large portion of histones (Fig. 6). Proteins in these three fractions were examined by immuno-blotting. MCM4 protein distributed almost evenly into these three fractions. In contrast, MCM-BP was almost exclusively recovered into the Triton-soluble fraction and only a small portion of MCM-BP was detected in the DNase I-soluble chromatin fraction. When NaCl concentration in lysis buffer was increased to 200 mM, however, MCM-BP was not detected in the DNase I-soluble chromatin fraction, suggesting that a small portion of MCM-BP loosely associates with chromatin. To examine cellular localization of MCM-BP, logarithmically growing HeLa cells were stained with anti-MCM-BP antibody (Fig. 7A). The antibody almost exclusively stained nuclei, similarly to the antibody against MCM6. The intensities of the staining with anti-MCM-BP antibody appeared to be differ among cells. When the fluorescence of DAPI-staining and the anti-MCM-BP antibody staining was quantified, there was a weak correlation between these two intensities (Fig. 7A), suggesting that MCM-BP accumulates in nuclei from the G1 to G2 phases. A similar increase in the level of MCM6 protein during progression of cell cycle was detected. When proteins that do not stably bind to the nuclear structure including chromatin were extracted with a buffer containing Triton X-100, only half of the extracted cells strongly reacted with anti-MCM6 antibody (Fig. 7B). Probably this is due to the fact that the amounts of chromatin-bound MCM6 decrease during late S and G2 phases. In contrast, the fluorescence signal with anti-MCM-BP antibody was hardly detected in the Triton-extracted HeLa cells, and a small area in nuclei that may be nucleolus was faintly stained. These results, which are consistent with the immuno-blotting data, indicate that MCM-BP does not stably bind to chromatin during the cell cycle.

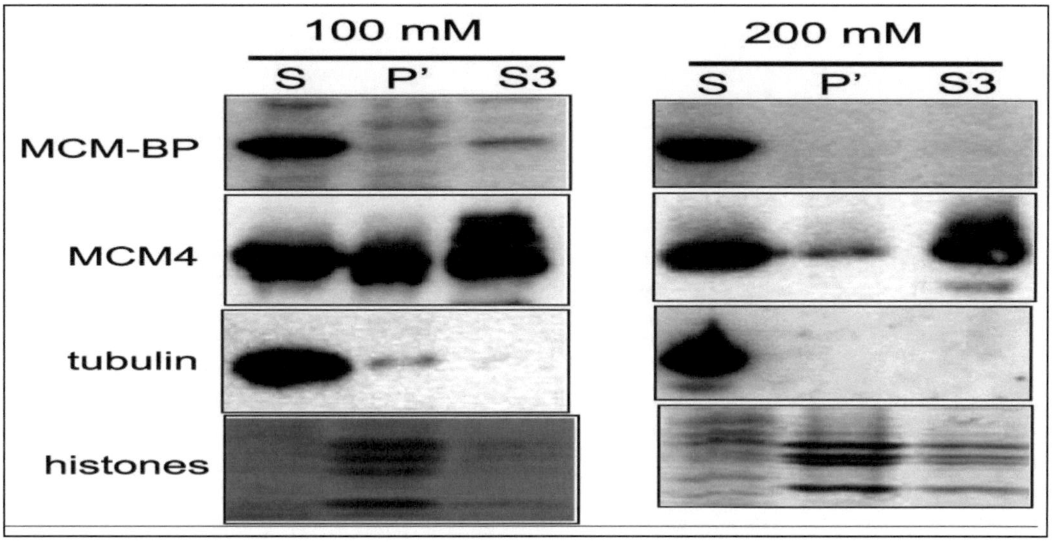

For biochemical fractionation of HeLa cells, the cells were lysed at 2 × 10^6 cells per 100 μl in modified CSK buffer (10 mM Pipes, pH 6.8, 100 mM NaCl, 1 mM $MgCl_2$ and 1 mM EGTA) containing 0.1% Triton X-100, 1 mM ATP, proteinase inhibitors (Pharmingen) (solution A) and placed on ice for 15 min. On the right, NaCl concentration in the lysis buffer was increased to 200 mM, as indicated at the top. The cell suspension was centrifuged (5,000 rpm for 5 min in a microcentrifuge), and its supernatant was saved (S). Recovered precipitate was suspended in solution A and centrifuged. The precipitate was suspended in a volume of solution A to yield 4 × 10^6 cells per 100 μl (P) and then incubated with DNase I (Takara, Tokyo, Japan) at 200 μg/ml at 30 °C for 15 min, and then soluble (S3) and insoluble (P') fractions were recovered after centrifugation. The insoluble materials (P') were suspended in a volume of solution A to yield 4 × 10^6 cells per 100 μl. The proteins in these fractions were electrophoresed and analyzed by immuno-blotting. MCM-BP, MCM4 and tubulin proteins in these fractions were analyzed. Distribution of histones was shown at the bottom.

Fig. 6. Chromatin-binding of MCM-BP

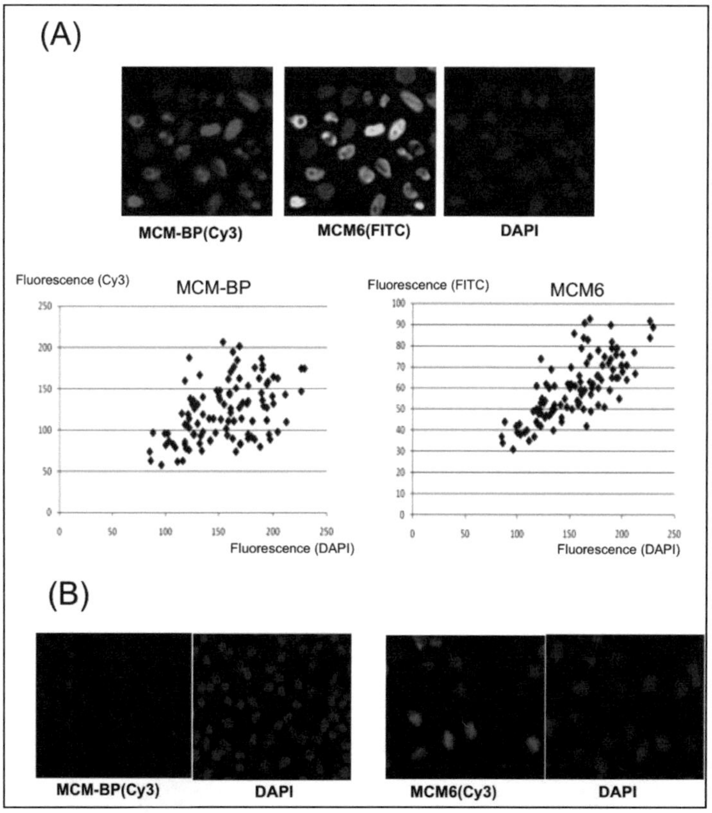

(A) Logarithmically growing HeLa cells were fixed by incubation with 4% paraformaldehyde in PBS for 5 min at room temperature, and then permeabilized and blocked by incubation with 0.1% Triton X-100, 0.02% SDS and 2% nonfat dried milk in PBS for 1 h at room temperature. The fixed cells were incubated at 4°C with anti-MCM-BP mouse antibody (culture supernatant of hybridoma cells) and anti-MCM6 goat antibody in the blocking solution. Cells were washed with the blocking solution and then incubated with Cy3-conjugated anti-mouse antibodies (Jackson Immuno-Research, West Grove, PA, USA) and FITC-conjugated anti-goat antibodies (Jackson Immuno-Research) for 1.5 h at 37°C in the blocking solution. Washed cells were stained with 2 μg/ml DAPI for 15 min at room temperature. After washing with PBS, cells were mounted in 90% glycerol and 10% PBS solution containing 1,4-diazabicyclo[2,2,2]-octane (DABCO, Sigma) (2.3%) and observed using fluorescence microscopy (BZ9000, KEYENCE, Japan). The levels of the fluorescence were measured (bottom). The values in each cell are plotted on a graph where DAPI fluorescence level is shown as a vertical line and Cy3 or FITC fluorescence level is horizontal line. (B) For extraction of chromatin-unbound proteins, HeLa cells were extracted by incubating with a buffer (10 mM PIPES, pH6.8, 0.1 M NaCl, 0.3 M sucrose, 3 mM $MgCl_2$ and 0.5 % Triton X-100) for 10 min at room temperature before fixation. After fixation, the extracted cells were stained with anti-MCM-BP antibody or with anti-MCM6 antibody. Fluorescence (Cy3) from the second antibody (Cy3-conjugated anti-mouse antibody and Cy3-conjugated anti-goat antibody) and from DAPI was detected.

Fig. 7. Cellular localization of MCM-BP

2.3 Binding of MCM-BP with MCM2-7 proteins in HeLa cells

Since it was found that MCM-BP was almost exclusively recovered in Triton-soluble fraction, we examined whether MCM-BP in the fraction binds with MCM2-7 proteins. It is known that considerable amounts of MCM2-7 were present in the nucleoplasm and they can be extracted with buffer containing Triton X-100. When MCM-BP in the Triton-soluble fraction was immuno-precipitated with the anti-MCM-BP antibody, MCM-BP was detected in the elution fractions (Fig. 8A). Among the MCM2-7 proteins, MCM4, MCM5, MCM6 and MCM7 were detected in the elution fractions. But MCM2 was not detected and MCM3 was only slightly detected in these fractions. Quantification of the data indicates that similar portions of MCM4-7 proteins were recovered in the elution fractions (Fig. 8B). As a control experiment, immuno-precipitation was performed in the absence of anti-MCM-BP antibody. Neither MCM-BP nor MCM2-7 was detected in the elution fractions.

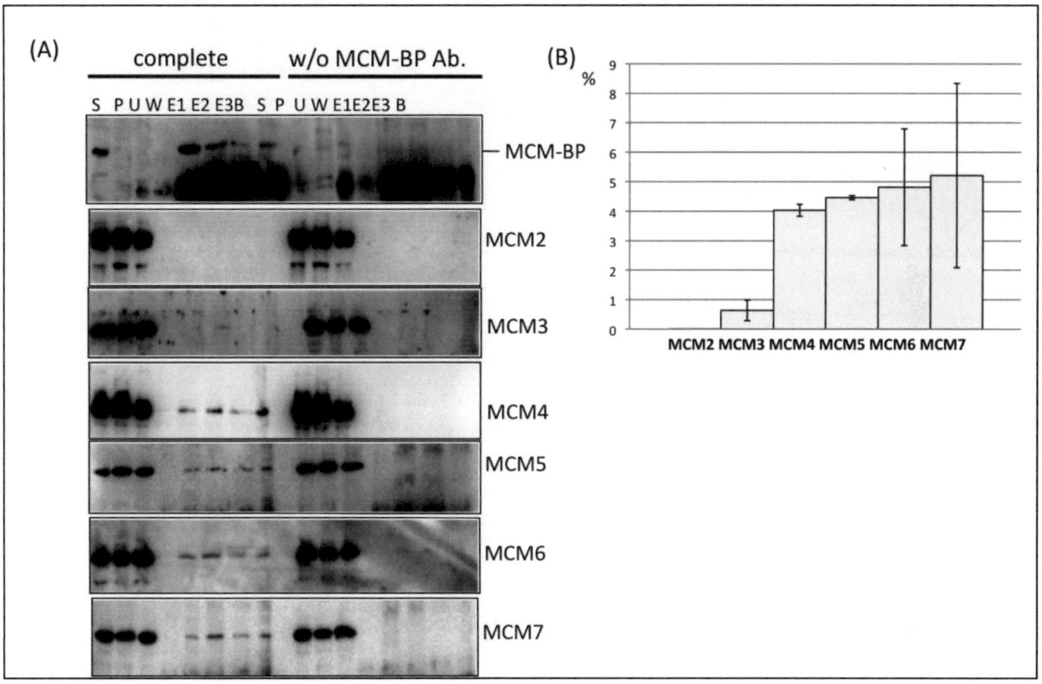

(A) (left) Logarithmically growing HeLa cells were lysed, and Triton-soluble (S) and -insoluble (P) fractions were obtained. MCM-BP in the Triton-soluble fraction was immuno-precipitated with anti-MCM-BP antibody bound to protein G beads. After proteins in the final wash were recovered (W), those bound to the beads were eluted three times by incubating with elution buffer (0.1 M glycine, pH 2.5 and 0.15 M NaCl) (E1, E2, and E3). Proteins bound to the beads after elution were eluted by boiling in SDS-sample buffer (B). MCM-BP and MCM2-7 proteins in these fractions were detected by immuno-blotting. (right) The same experiment was performed without addition of anti-MCM-BP antibody. (B) The levels of immuno-precipitated MCM2-7 proteins are shown with error bars by dividing the total chemiluminescence values detected in the E1-3 and B fractions by those in S and P fractions.

Fig. 8. Binding of MCM-BP with MCM2-7 proteins in HeLa cells

When proteins in the Triton-soluble fraction were fractionated by glycerol gradient centrifugation, all the MCM2-7 proteins were recovered at fraction no. 5-8 (Fig. 9). It is probable that the MCM2-7 hexameric complex is one of major components in these fractions. MCM-BP was mainly recovered at fraction no 10-14; the positions are comparable to those where MCM-BP purified from over-expressed insect cells is recovered (data not presented). Thus, it is suggested that MCM-BP is mainly present in a form free from MCM2-7 proteins in nucleoplasm and only a small portion of MCM-BP binds MCM4-7 proteins (Fig. 8).

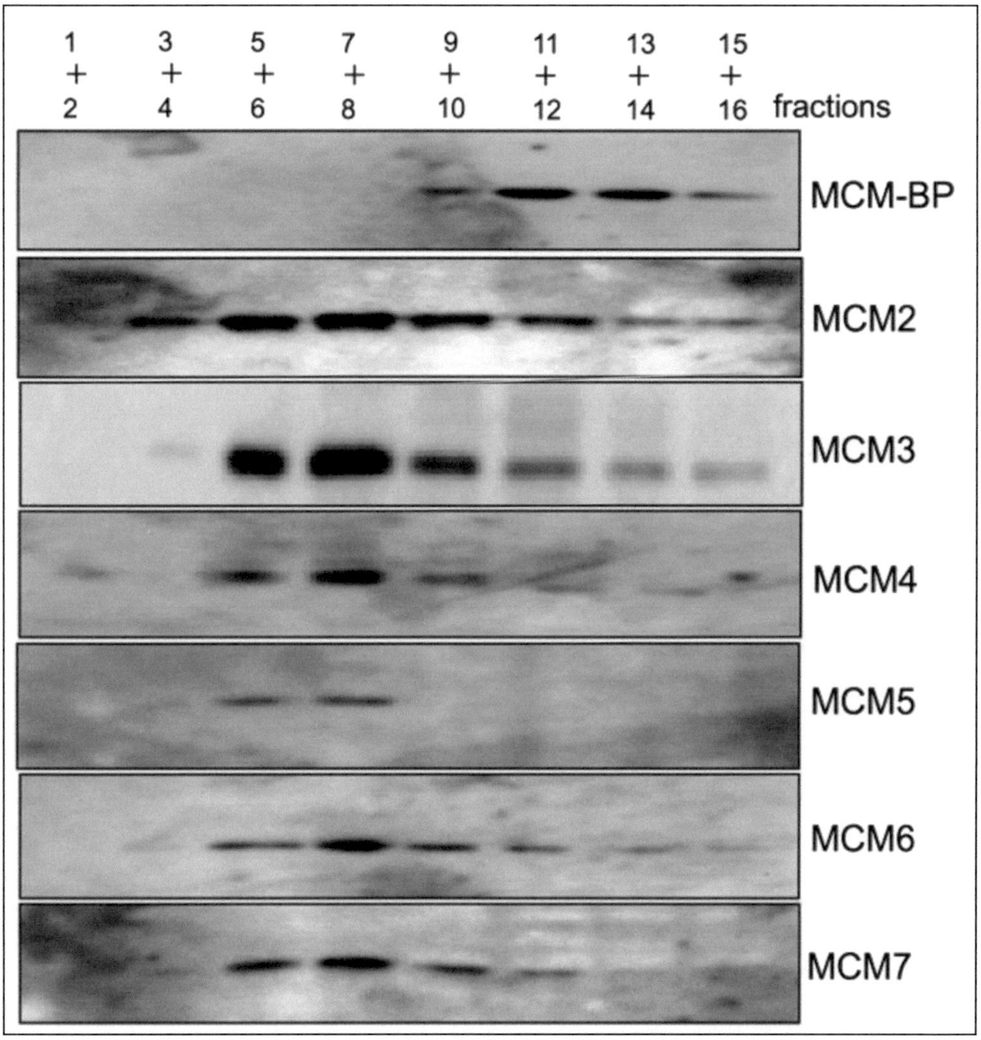

Proteins in the Triton-soluble fraction from HeLa cells were fractionated by glycerol gradient centrifugation (36,000 rpm for 14 h). After fractionation into 16 fractions, pairs of neighboring fractions were combined. Proteins in the combined fractions were concentrated and they were electrophoresed. MCM-BP and MCM2-7 were detected by immuno-blotting.

Fig. 9. MCM-BP does not stably bind to MCM2-7

3. Discussion

We presented data indicating that human MCM-BP can bind all of human MCM2-7 proteins when both are expressed in insect cells but it most strongly interacts with MCM7. It is possible that the central MCM domains are involved in the interaction of MCM-BP with MCM2-7 proteins. Consistently, it has been reported that *Xenopus* MCM-BP binds to the conserved MCM box in MCM7 (Nishiyama et al., 2011). In HeLa cells, endogenous MCM-BP protein was present in nuclei, and its amount increased during cell cycle. MCM-BP was almost exclusively recovered in a Triton-soluble fraction of HeLa cells and a small portion of MCM-BP in this fraction was bound with MCM4-7 proteins. As to chromatin binding of MCM-BP, a faint band was detected in DNase I-soluble chromatin fraction. When salt concentration in lysis buffer was increased from 100 mM to 200 mM, however, the MCM-BP band was not detected in the chromatin fraction. Under these conditions, MCM4 protein was still detected in the chromatin fraction. Thus, MCM-BP does not stably bind to DNA as MCM2-7 do in HeLa cells. These results suggest that MCM-BP, which is mainly present in nucleoplasm, plays a role in the S and G2 phases by interacting mainly with MCM7. We also found that the purified MCM-BP did not exhibit DNA helicase activity and did not show single-stranded DNA binding activity (data not presented). Consistent with the published results (Sakwe et al., 2007), MCM-BP did not significantly inhibit DNA helicase activity of the MCM4/6/7 hexamer (data not presented).

Recently, it has been reported that MCM-BP mainly interacts with MCM7 in *Xenopus* egg extracts (Nishiyama et al., 2011). It is suggested that MCM-BP plays a role in unloading of MCM2-7 complex from chromatin in late S phase. The results presented here are not inconsistent with the proposed function of MCM-BP. It has also been reported that MCM-BP is required for cohesion of replicated chromosomes in *Arabidopsis* and human cells (Takahashi et al., 2010). At the DNA replication forks, reorganization of cohesion complexes on chromosomes should occur, since they must encounter a large protein complex of DNA replication proteins that is required for replication fork progression (Uhlmann, 2009). The coordination of DNA replication fork movement and cohesion re-establishment may occur at the forks. Slowing down of MCM2-7 helicase movement or depletion of the MCM complex from the forks may be required for the cohesion re-establishment. It is possible that the interaction of MCM-BP with MCM7 is involved in the regulation of replication fork progression. Our data show that a small portion of MCM-BP binds with MCM4-7 proteins in nucleoplasm. These complexes may be generated from the interaction of MCM-BP and MCM proteins at the forks or on replicated DNA.

Recently, we comprehensively searched proteins that can interact with human RPA in insect cells (Nakatani et al., 2010). RPA plays an essential role in DNA replication by stabilizing the unwound single-stranded DNA region and assembling various replication proteins at the replication forks. In addition of MCM3-7, CDC45, TIPIN, Claspin and cyclin-dependent kinases, MCM-BP was found to interact with RPA among 30 proteins examined. This finding may support the role of MCM-BP in regulation of DNA replication fork movement. As mentioned above, it is probable that MCM helicase may be displaced from the replication forks or replicated DNA by active processes for regulation of DNA replication progression. Several factors could be involved in the displacement of MCM complex at the forks. Cyclin-dependent kinase that plays an essential role in preventing re-replication of DNA phosphorylates MCM4 during the S phase. MCM4 bound to chromatin is specifically phosphorylated with the kinase during the S phase, and MCM4 at G2 and M phases was highly phosphorylated with the kinase (Fujita et al., 1998). MCM4/6/7 DNA helicase activity was inhibited by the phosphorylation with CDK (Ishimi & Komamura-Kohno, 2001). MCM4 phosphorylation with CDK is stimulated under DNA replication checkpoint conditions (Ishimi et al., 2003). Thus MCM4 phosphorylation with CDK may be one of the reactions of the kinase to prevent re-replication of DNA. Consistently, the addition of excess cyclin-dependent kinase causes detachment of the MCM complex from chromatin to inhibit DNA replication in a replication system using *Xenopus* egg extracts (Hendrickson et al., 1996). Thus, it is possible that phosphorylation of MCM4 on chromatin may be involved in detachment of the MCM complex from the replication forks or DNA.

Here we showed biochemical characteristics of human MCM-BP. The MCM-BP has unique properties of binding capacity with MCM2-7 and high affinity to MCM7 in the experiments using insect cells and it shows weak chromatin-binding ability in HeLa cells. *In vitro* experimental system is required to evaluate the suggested role of MCM-BP at the replication forks.

4. Conclusion

Several lines of evidences suggest that an activated form of MCM2-7 complex functions as a replicative DNA helicase that unwinds duplex DNA at the replication forks. MCM-BP has been identified as a protein that binds to human MCM6 and 7 proteins (Sakwe et al., 2007). It has been suggested that MCM-BP bound to MCM3-7 proteins may play a role in the initiation of DNA replication. Recently, it has been shown that MCM-BP is required for the cohesion of replicated DNA (Takahashi et al., 2010), and it has been suggested that MCM-BP is involved in unloading of the MCM2-7 complex from chromatin at late S phase (Nishiyama et al., 2011). However, biochemical function of MCM-BP is not fully understood. Here, we examined the interaction of human MCM-BP with MCM2-7 in insect cells and in HeLa cells by immuno-precipitation. The results indicate that MCM-BP can bind all of MCM2-7 in insect cells, but it binds most with MCM7. In HeLa cells, MCM-BP was largely detected in a Triton-soluble fraction and only a small portion of MCM-BP was detected in chromatin fraction; the distribution is in contrast to that of MCM2-7. Immuno-precipitation experiment indicates that a small portion of MCM-BP in the Triton-soluble fraction is bound with MCM4, 5, 6 and 7 proteins. These results suggest that MCM-BP in nucleoplasm exhibits its function by interacting mainly with MCM7.

5. Acknowledgement

This study was supported by a grant-in-aid for scientific research from the Ministry of Education, Science, Sports and Culture of Japan.

6. References

Bell, S.P. & Dutta, A. (2002) DNA replication in eukaryotic cells. *Annu. Rev. Biochem.* 71, pp. 333-374.

Forsburg, S.L. (2004) Eukaryotic MCM proteins: Beyond replication initiation. *Microbiol. Mol. Biol. Rev.* 68, pp. 109-131.

Fujita, M., Yamada, C., Tsurumi, T., Hanaoka, F., Matsuzawa, K. & Inagaki, M. (1998) Cell cycle- and chromatin binding state-dependent phosphorylation of human MCM heterohexameric complexes. *J. Biol. Chem.* 273, pp. 17095-17101.

Gambus, A., Jones, R.C., Sanchez-Diaz, A., Kanemaki, M., van Deursen, F., Edmondson, R.D. & Labib, K. (2006) GINS maintains association of Cdc45 with MCM in replisome progression complexes at eukaryotic DNA replication forks. *Nat. Cell Biol.* 8, pp. 358-366.

Hendrickson, M., Madine, M., Dalton, S. & Gautier, J. (1996) Phosphorylation of MCM4 by cdc2 protein kinase inhibits the activity of the minichromosome maintenance complex. *Proc. Natl. Acad. Sci. USA* 93, pp. 12223-12228.

Ishimi, Y. (1997) A DNA helicase activity is associated with an MCM4, -6, and -7 protein complex. *J. Biol. Chem.* 272, pp. 24508-24513.

Ishimi, Y. & Komamura-Kohno, Y. (2001) Phosphorylation of MCM4 at specific sites by cyclin-dependent kinase leads to loss of Mcm4,6,7 helicase acivity. *J. Biol. Chem.* 276, pp. 34428-34433.

Ishimi, Y., Komamura-Kohno, Y., Kwon, H.-J., Yamada, K. & Nakanishi, M. (2003) Identification of MCM4 as a target of the DNA replication block checkpoint system. *J. Biol. Chem.* 278, pp. 24644-24650.

Masai, H., Matsumoto, S., You, Z., Yoshizawa-Sugata, N. & Oda, H. (2010) Eukaryotic chromosome DNA replication: where, when, and how? *Annu. Rev. Biochem.* 79, pp. 89-130.

Moyer S.E., Lewis P.W. & Botchan M.R. (2006) Isolation of the Cdc45-MCM2-7-GINS (CMG) complex, a candidate for the eukaryotic DNA replication fork helicase. *Proc. Natl. Acad. Sci. USA* 103, pp. 10236-10241.

Nakaya, R., Takaya, J., Onuki, T., Moritani, M., Nozaki, N. & Ishimi, Y. (2010) Identification of proteins that may directly interact with human RPA. *J. Biochem.* 148, pp. 539-547.

Nishiyama, A., Frappier, L. & Mechali, M. (2011) MCM-BP regulates unloading of the MCM2-7 helicase in late S phase. *Genes Dev.* 25, pp. 165-175.

Numata, Y., Ishihara, S., Hasegawa, N., Nozaki, N. & Ishimi, Y. (2010) Interaction of human MCM2-7 proteins with TIM, TIPIN and Rb. *J. Biochem.* 147, pp. 917-927.

Sakwe, A.M., Nguyen, T., Athanasopoulos, V., Shire, K. & Frappier, L. (2007) Identification and characterization of a novel component of the human minichromosome maintenance complex. *Mol. Cell. Biol.* 27, pp. 3044-3055.

Takahashi, N., Lammens, T., Boudolf, V., Maes, S., Yoshizumi, T., Jaeger, G.D., Witters, E., Inze, D. & Veylder, L.D. (2008) The DNA replication checkpoint aids survival of plants deficient in the novel replisome factor ETG1. *EMBO J.* 27, pp. 1840-1851.

Takahashi, N., Quimbaya, M., Schubert, V., Lammens, T., Vandepoele, K., Schbert, I., Matsui, M., Inze, D. Berx, G. & Veylder, L.D. (2010) The MCM-binding protein ETG1 aids sister chromatid cohesion required for postreplicative homologous recombination repair. *ProsGenet.* 6, e1000817.

Uhlmann, F. (2009) A matter of choice: the establishment of sister chromatid cohesion. *EMBO Rep.* 10, pp. 1095-1102.

Yu, Z., Feng, D. & Liang, C. (2004) Pairwise interactions of the six human MCM protein subunits. *J. Mol. Biol.* 340, pp. 1197-1206.

25

DNA Replication in Animal Systems Lacking Thioredoxin Reductase I

Edward E. Schmidt
Montana State University
United States of America

1. Introduction

Ribonucleotide reductase (RNR) activity is generally required to provide deoxyribonucleoside triphosphates (dNTPs or DNA-precursors) for DNA replication (Thelander and Reichard, 1979). This property has made both RNR and the pathways RNR depends upon important drug-targets. For example, the drug hydroxyurea is a specific inhibitor of RNR and has been used for many decades as an effective chemotherapeutic agent for certain cancers and viral diseases (Navarra and Preziosi, 1999; Wright et al., 1990; Yarbro, 1992). This chapter focuses on two critical pathways that lie upstream of RNR and are important for supporting RNR activity: namely, the glutathione (GSH) pathway and the thioredoxin (Trx) pathway. These pathways were first uncovered in bacterial systems roughly fifty years ago. In the ensuing half-century, the components and activities of these pathways have been intensely studied in bacterial, archaebacterial, and eukaryotic systems, both *in vivo* and *in vitro* (Holmgren, 1977; Holmgren, 1989). The GSH and Trx pathways, themselves, are ubiquitous in biology, yet various components of the pathways exhibit activities and, in some cases, evolutionary histories, that are particular to animal systems. Classic descriptive and biochemical studies laid the groundwork for understanding these pathways in animals; however, only in recent years have genetic systems been established in which the physiological activities of these pathways could be tested (Arner, 2009; Holmgren and Lu, 2010; Holmgren and Sengupta, 2010). Here I will overview the Trx and GSH pathways and their contributions to DNA replication. Particular attention will be paid to recent revelations on the activities and properties of these systems in animals that differ from those in other biological systems. Some recent advances have come from the development of mouse models bearing targeted "conditional" alleles of the gene encoding thioredoxin reductase I (TrxR1, also called Txnrd1 or TR1), which can be disrupted in a cell type- or developmental stage-specific manner. Whereas these models are yielding some exciting insights into the Trx and GSH systems in embryonic development, stress responses, toxicology, cancer, and other processes (Bondareva et al., 2007; Branco et al., 2011; Carvalho et al., 2008; Jakupoglu et al., 2005; Mandal et al., 2010; Rogers et al., 2004; Suvorova et al., 2009; Tipple et al., 2007; Zhang and Lu, 2007), the current treatise will emphasize the interplay of these pathways in supporting DNA replication in animal systems. The enormity of the body of literature on the Trx, GSH, and RNR systems precludes an exhaustive review of these materials, and it is my intention to cover these subjects in only a cursory manner to set the backdrop for understanding these systems in the context of DNA replication in animals. The reader is directed to more complete recent reviews on these subjects (Arner, 2009; Holmgren and Sengupta, 2010; Lu and Holmgren, 2009). I apologize in advance for my oversights and omissions related to the many important studies that have led to the current status of the field.

2. Thioredoxin reductase and glutathione reductase

Thioredoxin reductases (TrxRs) are enzymes that use electrons from NADPH + H^+ to restore the "active" reduced state of oxidized Trx (Fig. 1). Similarly, glutathione reductases (Gsrs) are enzymes that use electrons from NADPH + H^+ to convert oxidized glutathione disulfide (GSSG) into two molecules of reduced GSH (Arner and Holmgren, 2000; Holmgren, 1980; Holmgren, 2000). In both cases, electrons are typically exchanged as a "reductive currency" by altering the redox state of protein- or small molecule-sulfur residues. In combination, these two pathways provide reducing potential to countless reactions in cellular, sub-cellular and extracellular compartments, and constitute the predominant endogenous antioxidant system (Arner, 2009; Arner and Holmgren, 2006; Holmgren, 2000; Lillig and Holmgren, 2007; Nordberg and Arner, 2001). Trx and GSH serve as "electron-shuttles", transporting this reducing potential to various enzymes and reactions. Both systems participate in homeostatic antioxidant activities, for example by providing electrons to either the GSH-dependent glutathione peroxidases (Gpxs) or the Trx-dependent peroxiredoxins (Prxs) that each contribute to detoxification of reactive oxygen species in cells

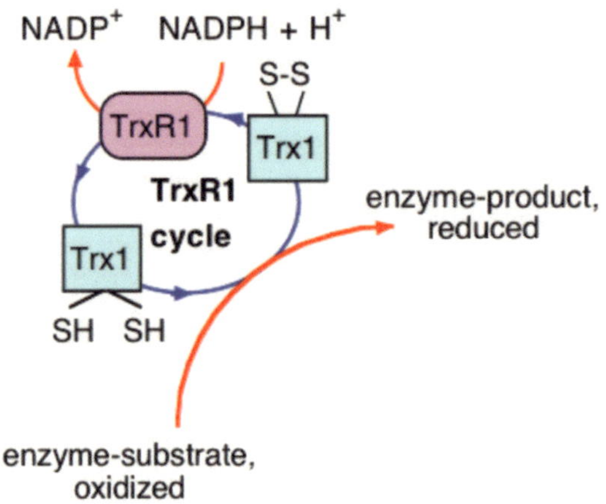

Fig. 1. Cytosolic thioredoxin reductase cycle. Reducing potential arrives at TrxR1 in the form of NADPH and a proton. TrxR1 reduces disulfide-form Trx1 (oxidized) to the dithiol-form. Trx1 is a small protein that can transport this reducing potential to locations throughout the cell; however it does not enter or exchange reducing potential with mitochondria. Reduced Trx1 is a major protein-disulfide reductase and the immediate source of electrons for many enzymatic reactions, including RNR, Prxs, 3′-phosphoadenylylsulfate (PAPS) reductase, methionine sulfoxide reductases, and others. This results in oxidation of Trx1 to the disulfide form, which then cycles back through TrxR1 (Arner, 2009; Holmgren and Bjornstedt, 1995).

(Arner and Holmgren, 2000; Berndt et al., 2007; Carmel-Harel and Storz, 2000; Holmgren, 2000). GSH can also reduce glutaredoxins (Grxs), which are small Trx-like proteins that further shuttle the electrons to various destinations, often but not always functioning analogous to Trxs (Fernandes and Holmgren, 2004; Holmgren, 1989; Holmgren, 2000; Holmgren et al., 2005; Meyer et al., 2009; Meyer et al., 2008). Although the Trx pathway and the GSH pathway are each most well known for somewhat different roles (Berndt et al., 2008; Carmel-Harel and Storz, 2000; Hayes and Pulford, 1995; Holmgren, 2000), there is enormous overlap between the two pathways and, for the most part, general physiological equivalence of the two pathways. Some evidence suggests the Trx pathway can respond to cellular damage by activating the cytoprotective Nrf2 stress-response pathway, which, in turn, induces expression of the genes encoding components of both the Trx and the GSH systems (Arner, 2009; Ishii and Yanagawa, 2007; Itoh et al., 1999; Nguyen et al., 2009; Suvorova et al., 2009). Generally, either the GSH or the Trx pathway can complement deficiencies in the other, resulting in a robust combined reductive system (Arner, 2009; Holmgren, 2000).

3. Activities and requirements of RNR

The role of RNR in replication is to provide dNTPs for synthesis of a duplicate genome by DNA polymerase during S phase of the cell cycle (Fig. 2). This pathway, in which DNA-precursors are made from endogenous RNA-precursors is termed the *de novo* biosynthesis pathway. Although salvage pathways can also provide a source of dNTPs using exogenous deoxyribonucleosides (Arner and Eriksson, 1995), sufficient exogenous sources of these substrates are rarely available. Thus, whereas salvage pathways might provide a sufficient source of DNA precursors for repair and perhaps for mitochondrial DNA replication, they generally will not support S phase genome replication (Iwasaki et al., 1997; Mathews and Song, 2007; Pontarin et al., 2007).

RNR functions by reductive conversion of generally abundant RNA precursors, in the form of ribonucleoside diphosphates (rNDPs), into deoxyribonucleoside diphosphates (dNDPs) (Holmgren et al., 1965; Reichard et al., 1961; Thelander and Reichard, 1979). The dNDPs are subsequently phosphorylated to the triphosphate state for use by DNA polymerase. In eukaryotes, although genomic replication is nuclear, RNR and dNTP biosynthesis occurs in the cytosol. dNTP pools in replicating cells are at a low steady-state concentration and are rapidly turned-over, indicating that the precursors are polymerized into DNA almost immediately upon their production (Rottgen and Rabes, 1989). Indeed, cellular DNA precursor pools, even during S phase, are typically only a small fraction of the concentration of RNA precursor pools (Rottgen and Rabes, 1989; Spyrou and Holmgren, 1996). Consistent with this, RNR shows tight product- and substrate-mediated allosteric regulation, in particular in response to local concentrations of dATP (Holmgren, 1981; Holmgren et al., 1965; Reichard et al., 2000). This feedback regulation is thought to be critical for maintaining replication fidelity and preserving genome-integrity. Thus, replication accuracy by DNA polymerase is optimal only within a narrow window of concentrations for each dNTP; treatments that skew normal dNTP pools have been shown to be either mutagenic or pro-apoptotic in different systems (Kunkel et al., 1982; Nicander and Reichard, 1983; Oliver et al., 1996).

Although three different classes of RNR enzymes are known to exist across the different biological kingdoms, all of these enzymes require a source of electrons and a metal co-factor, and all proceed by a reaction that involves a free radical intermediate (Atkin et al., 1973; Holmgren and Sengupta, 2010; Thelander and Reichard, 1979). Classes II and III are found only in a restricted subset of anaerobic or otherwise specialized microbes. These enzymes were discussed in detail in a recent review (Holmgren and Sengupta, 2010) and will not be considered further here. The most common class, class I, is found in eukaryotes and in most aerobic prokaryotes (Torrents et al., 2006). These enzymes are composed of two subunits: the B1 and B2 proteins in bacteria, or the functionally similar R1 and R2 proteins (also called M1 and M2) in eukaryotes (Brown et al., 1969; Thelander and Reichard, 1979). The B1 or R1 protein possesses the catalytic site for reduction of all four rNDPs, whereas the B2 or R2 subunit contains the protein-tyrosyl radical (Akerblom et al., 1981; Avval and Holmgren, 2009). Every cycle of nucleotide reduction results in generation of disulfide in the C-terminus of the B1 or R1 subunit, which must be reduced to a dithiol for the next reductive cycle (Avval and Holmgren, 2009).

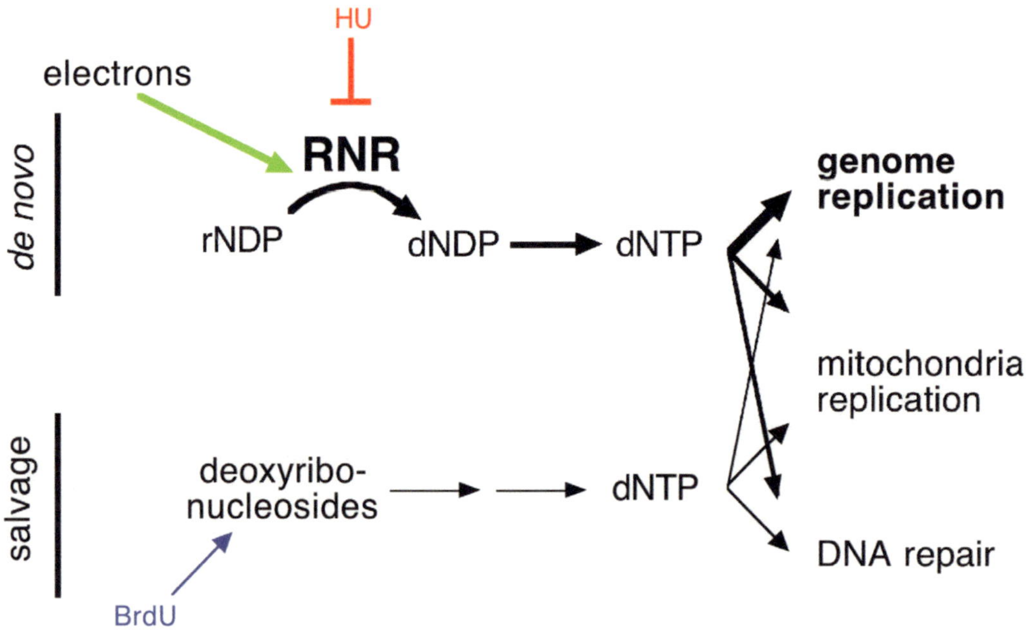

Fig. 2. Sources of DNA precursors. RNR is the key player on the *de novo* dNTP biosynthesis pathway, in which rNDPs are converted to dNDPs in eukaryotes and most prokaryotes. In addition to rNDPs, RNR requires a source of electrons as reducing potential (green arrow, see text). Arrow weight is diagrammatic of relative flux or activity of each step. The drug hydroxyurea (HU) scavenges the tyrosyl protein-free radical in RNR, thereby blocking RNR activity (red). Below is the salvage pathway, in which exogenous deoxyribonucleosides are assimilated by outer membrane transporters and kinased to form dNTPs. BrdU (blue) is incorporated via the salvage pathway, which, although it cannot generally support S phase replication (see text), does contribute sufficient DNA precursors to genome replication that BrdU will label all S phase (replicating) cells (Arner and Eriksson, 1995; Thelander and Reichard, 1979; Yarbro, 1992).

Mammalian cells have two distinct RNR enzymess that both share a common catalytic R1 subunit, but differ in their second subunit, with one isoform being S phase-specific and containing R2 protein and the other being expressed throughout the cell cycle as well as in post-replicative cells and having a distinct protein, p53R2, as the second subunit (Avval and Holmgren, 2009; Holmgren and Sengupta, 2010; Pontarin et al., 2007). The R1/R2 protein drives S phase genome replication; the R1/p53R2 protein is thought to play a major role in providing dNTPs for mitochondrial DNA replication and repair (Pontarin et al., 2007).

In addition to an obvious requirement for rNDPs, RNR requires a source of reducing potential or, more specifically, electrons, to restore the dithiol state of the B1 or R1 C-terminal disulfide after each catalytic cycle (Fig. 3) (Holmgren and Sengupta, 2010). The common distal source of this reducing potential is NADPH. In eubacteria, electrons can flow to RNR from NADPH by either a TrxR- or a Gsr-dependent route (Fernandes and Holmgren, 2004; Gleason and Holmgren, 1988; Holmgren, 1976; Holmgren, 1981; Holmgren, 1989; Laurent et al., 1964; Lillig and Holmgren, 2007). In the TrxR-dependent route, TrxR uses electrons from NADPH + H^+ to reduce oxidized (disulfide) Trx to the reduced (dithiol) form, while generating $NADP^+$ (Arner, 2009; Arner and Holmgren, 2000). Reduced Txn, then, can directly restore the active reduced state of RNR (Avval and Holmgren, 2009; Laurent et al., 1964). In the Gsr-dependent route, electrons extracted from NADPH + H^+ are used by Gsr to reduce oxidized di-glutathione (GSSG) to the reduced monomeric state (GSH), again yielding $NADP^+$ (Fernandes and Holmgren, 2004; Holmgren, 2000). Whereas GSH has numerous activities in cells (Fernandes and Holmgren, 2004), one of these is to restore oxidized (disulfide) Grxs to the reduced state (dithiol-Grx), which like reduced Trx, can restore the reduced active state of RNR (Avval and Holmgren, 2009; Holmgren, 1976; Holmgren, 1977; Holmgren, 1978; Holmgren, 1979; Luthman et al., 1979) (Fig. 3).

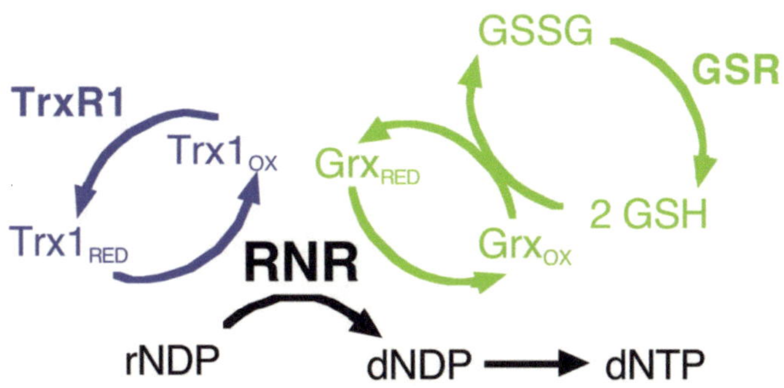

Fig. 3. Sources of electrons for RNR. Either the Trx cycle (blue) or the GSH cycle (green) can support reduction of ribonucleotides by RNR. The Trx cycle is summarized in Fig. 2. In the GSH cycle, Gsr uses reducing potential from NADPH to reduce one mole of oxidized di-glutathione (GSSG) to 2 moles of reduced glutathione (GSH). GSH has many roles in cells, one of which is to restore the reduced state of oxidized Grx. Reduced Grx, then, can serve as a proximal electron donor for RNR (Holmgren and Sengupta, 2010).

4. Contributions of the GSH and Trx pathways in supporting RNR

Although growth differences have not been reported between *E. coli* having only a GSH- or only a Trx-pathway (Holmgren, 1977; Holmgren, 1979), catalytically Grx is the most efficient electron donor for the reaction (Gon et al., 2006). By contrast, yeast and plants deficient in TrxRs show slow-growth phenotypes (Koc et al., 2006; Reichheld et al., 2007; Sweat and Wolpert, 2007), suggesting Gsr-dependent routes are poor at supporting DNA replication in these eukaryotes. It was anticipated that all eukaryotic systems might depend primarily on the Trx system to supply electrons to RNR for DNA replication. Consistent with this, mice homozygous for a spontaneous null mutation of the *gsr* gene showed no defects in growth or DNA replication (Rogers et al., 2004), and mice zygotically homozygous-null for either the *txn1* gene encoding cytosolic Trx1 (Matsui et al., 1996) or the *txnrd1* gene encoding cytosolic TrxR1 (Bondareva et al., 2007; Jakupoglu et al., 2005), are both embryonic-lethal. From these findings, it was inferred that, in mice under normal conditions, the GSH pathway may be superfluous for replication, yet the cytosolic Trx pathway is critical (Jakupoglu et al., 2005). However, since none of the studies on components of the cytosolic Trx systems directly showed that these mutations blocked DNA replication, *per se*, alternative explanations for embryonic lethality were not ruled out. Indeed, in reporting our study, we argued that the degree of cell proliferation seen prior to embryonic loss in TrxR1-deficient embryos was inconsistent with a block to proliferation, and instead suggested that the pre-resorption phenotype of TrxR1-deficient embryos was more consistent with an embryonic patterning defect (Bondareva et al., 2007)(see below).

5. Evolution of the TrxR protein families

GSH- and Trx-pathways are each ubiquitous in biology (Fig. 4). With the advent of organellar compartmentalization in early eukaryotes, it likely became important for cells to ensure an adequate level of activity for each pathway both in the cytosol as well as within the often relatively impervious confines of the organelles. For most components of these pathways in most eukaryotic systems, such as Grxs, Trxs, and TrxRs, separate genes arose by gene duplication that evolved to specialize, albeit to varying extents, in production of either cytosolic or mitochondrial isoforms of these enzymes (Gleason and Holmgren, 1981; Meyer et al., 2009; Meyer et al., 2008; Novoselov and Gladyshev, 2003; Sandalova et al., 2001; Taskov et al., 2005; Williams et al., 2000). For other components of these pathways, however, such as Gsr, cytosolic and mitochondrial functions are generally accomplished by expressing both cytosol- and mitochondria-targeted versions of the protein from a single gene. In an extreme example, the parasitic tapeworm *Echinococcus* has a single gene that issues the enzyme responsible for reduction of both Txr and GSSG in both the cytosol and the mitochondria (Bonilla et al., 2008) (see below).

Despite the ubiquity of these systems in the living world, TrxR enzymes underwent a striking evolutionary transition that sets it apart from other components in these systems (Zhong et al., 1998). Thus, whereas all Gsrs are homologous, all Grxs are homologous, and all Trxs are homologous, TrxRs are diphyletic, being represented by two distinct protein families (Arner, 2009; Arner and Holmgren, 2000; Sandalova et al., 2001). The more ancient family, here called the "*E. coli*-type TrxRs" for the species it was first described from (Moore et al., 1964), is found in all eubacteria, archaea, fungi, most protists, and most plants and algae (Fig. 4., shaded light blue). Metazoan animals universally share a distinct family of TrxR proteins ("metazoan-TrxRs"; shaded red in Fig. 4) (Arner, 2009; Arscott et al., 1997; Eckenroth et al., 2006; Novoselov and Gladyshev, 2003; Williams et al., 2000; Zhong et al., 1998).

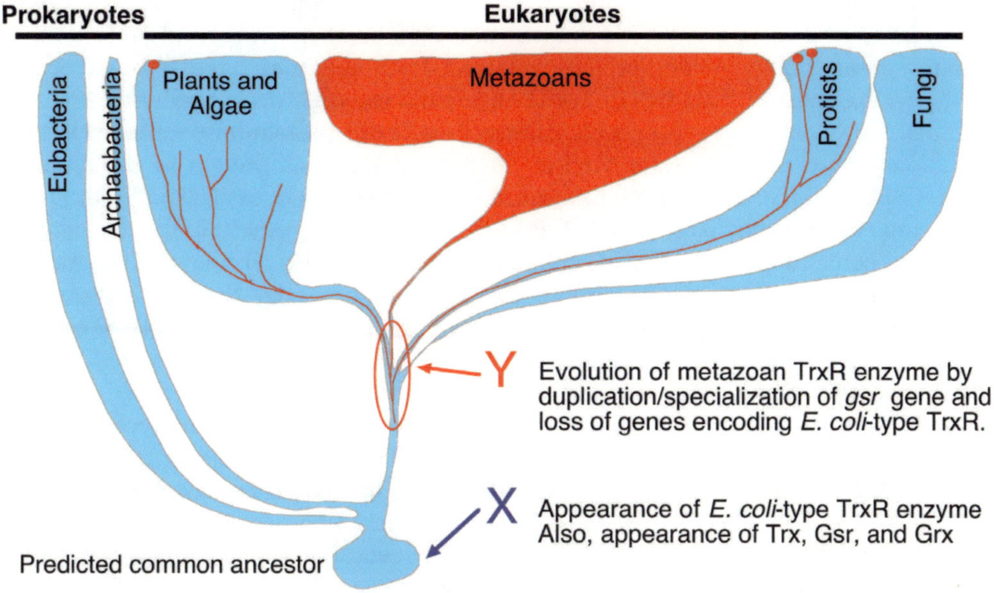

Fig. 4. Distribution of TrxR families in living kingdoms. *E. coli*-type TrxRs (blue) are found in most extant life forms, with the exception of metazoans (red), one green algae, and a few parasitic protists (red dots), which have metazoan-type TrxRs (Novoselov and Gladyshev, 2003). Thus, the metazoan-type TrxRs appeared before separation of ancestral metazoans onto a distinct lineage and was retained in a subset of plants and algae and in a subset of protists (Novoselov and Gladyshev, 2003) (fine red lines). See text for more details.

Evolution of the metazoan TrxR appears to have been brought about by extension of the C-terminal protein coding sequences of the *gsh* gene, leading to acquisition of the new C-terminal active site (Novoselov and Gladyshev, 2003). In this enzyme, the C-terminal active site, which directly reduces oxidized Trx, generally but not always contains the atypical 21st amino acid selenocysteine (Sec) translationally inserted in the penultimate position (Arner, 2009; Hondal and Ruggles, 2010; Lu and Holmgren, 2009). This overall design gives the impression of an enzyme that was built by "retrofitting" a new C-terminal active site onto an existing NADPH-dependent reductase (Schmidt and Davies, 2007), either by classical exon shuffling (Margulies and McCluskey, 1985) or by mutation of the stop codon and translational read-through into previously 3'-untranslated sequences (Novoselov and Gladyshev, 2003).

It is unclear why an ancestor to all extant metazoans eventually discarded its *E. coli*-type TrxRs, which presumably functioned adequately in its ancestors and continues to do so for nearly all contemporary non-metazoans within all biological kingdoms (Fig. 4). From the perspective of the nominal reaction catalyzed by TrxRs in either *E. coli* or mammalian systems, neither the distal source of electrons (NADPH) nor the substrate (oxidized Trx) differs. However, the *E. coli* and metazoan enzymes are not equivalent, and this evolutionary enzyme-exchange was unlikely to be selectively "neutral". Key differences between the two enzyme families are that the *E. coli*-type enzymes are smaller (~35 kDa) and highly specific for reduction of oxidized Trx, whereas metazoan TrxRs are larger proteins

(~55 kDa) that evolved from Gsr and are capable of reducing a broad range of substrates (Arner, 2009; Arscott et al., 1997; Holmgren and Bjornstedt, 1995; Lu and Holmgren, 2009; Williams et al., 2000). Although they evolved from Gsr and have a broad substrate specificity, the classical mammalian TrxR1 and TrxR2 enzymes do not reduce GSSG (Sun et al., 2001). However, the testis-specific mammalian TrxR3 protein, also called thioredoxin-glutathione reductase or TGR, as well as the Sec-lacking TrxR protein in *Drosophila*, does reduce GSSG (Gromer et al., 2003; Johansson et al., 2006; Sun et al., 2001; Sun et al., 2005), and in some lower metazoans such as *Echinococcus*, a single gene, within the metazoan TrxR family and containing Sec in its C-terminal active site, encodes all known Trx- and GSSG-reductase activities (Bonilla et al., 2008). One might hypothesize that, by exchanging the ancestral *E. coli*-type TrxR enzymes for the metazoan version, the evolutionary capacity of the lineage might have been potentiated; however since both enzymes will effectively reduce Trx, this model suggests the evolutionary advantage of the new enzyme for metazoans is related to other activities that differ between these enzyme types (Arner and Holmgren, 2000; Arner et al., 1996; Lothrop et al., 2009). Alternatively, one might imagine that, if an ancestral metazoan evolved a TGR enzyme that could replace both the ancestral TrxR and Gsr activities, as the *Echinococcus* version does, then perhaps the ancestral *E. coli*-type TrxR and the ancestral Gsr were simply and irrevocably lost as being redundant with the new bi-functional TGR enzyme, as seen in *Echinococcus*. Subsequent specialization could have led to a gene-duplication of TGR and loss of the C-terminal TrxR-specific domain in one of the duplicates, essentially reverting one copy of the gene to a classical Gsr protein that is still recognized as homologous to the ancestral version.

Interestingly, a few unicellular eukaryotes do contain "metazoan-type" TrxR enzymes (Novoselov and Gladyshev, 2003)(Fig. 4, red "dots" at top of "Plant and algae" and "Protist" branches of the tree). These include both a small number of protozoan parasites and a single known green alga (Holmgren and Lu, 2010; Novoselov and Gladyshev, 2003). In at least one case (the photosynthetic alga *Chlamydomonas*), both *E. coli*- type and metazoan-type TrxRs are found in the same genome (Novoselov and Gladyshev, 2003). Thus, there is a precedent for co-existence of both enzyme types in a single genome. One model to explain this odd disribution of the metazoan-type TrxR would be that these few non-metazoan species acquired the metazoan-type TrxR proteins by lateral gene transfer. Indeed, this hypothesis was raised previously when this isoform was discovered in members of genus *Plasmodium*, the malaria-causing parasites, and in other related protozoan parasites (Hirt et al., 2002; Rahlfs et al., 2002; Williams et al., 2000). Based both on the oddity of non-metazoans having this isoform and the intimate intracellular interaction between these intracellular protozoan parasites and both their vertebrate and invertebrate metazoan hosts, lateral gene transfer from host to parasite seemed a plausible model for the appearance of this unexpected isoform outside of metazoans. However, the subsequent discovery of a metazoan-type TrxR1 in *Chlamydomonas*, along with the absence of other signatures of lateral gene transfer between metazoans and the few single-cell eukaryotes that have this isoform, suggest lateral gene transfer is, in this case, an unlikely model (Novoselov and Gladyshev, 2003). Instead, the most parsimonious model of ancestry of the metazoan-type TrxRs is that the protein evolved only once by C-terminal extension of a copy of the *gsr* gene in a pre-metazoan ancestor; although lineages bearing this enzyme persisted to modern times in all metazoans as well as in a very small subset of algae and parasitic protozoa (Fig. 4, fine red lines) (Novoselov and Gladyshev, 2003).

6. Requirements of disulfide reductases for replication in rodent models

Early studies showed that some mammalian Grxs could reduce mammalian RNR *in vitro* (Luthman et al., 1979; Luthman and Holmgren, 1982), and that Trx generally did not co-localize to cells expressing the S phase-specific R1 subunit of RNR in rat tissues, suggesting that Trx is not the major physiological electron donor for RNR (Hansson et al., 1986). However experimentally, animal systems deficient in the Trx pathway were slow to appear. RNAi "knock-down" studies on mammalian cell cultures suggested replication was not impaired by ablation of TrxR1 (Yoo et al., 2006; Yoo et al., 2007); however questions of residual pre-formed TrxR1 protein in these systems lingered. The first studies on mouse knock-out models having homozygous zygotic disruption of the *txnrd1* gene, which encodes TrxR1, showed evidence of active and extensive proliferation prior to embryonic lethality (Bondareva et al., 2007; Jakupoglu et al., 2005). Because TrxR1-deficient embryos accumulated several thousand cells, it was unlikely that residual maternal TrxR1 had driven the replication cycles. More recently, by using conditional disruption of the *txnrd1* gene in mouse livers, my group has been able to provide a more detailed examination of the roles of TrxR1 for replication in animal cells (Rollins et al., 2010; Suvorova et al., 2009). During liver development and regeneration, normal mice and mice having TrxR1-deficient hepatocytes exhibit similar liver growth rates and similar levels of proliferative, S, and M phase hepatocytes. Regenerative thymidine incorporation is similar in normal and TrxR1-deficient livers, further indicating that DNA synthesis is unaffected (Rollins et al., 2010). The use of genetic chimeras in which a fluorescently marked subset of hepatocytes was TrxR1-deficient while others were not, revealed that the multigenerational contributions of both normal and Txnrd1-deficient hepatocytes to development and to liver regeneration were indistinguishable (Rollins et al., 2010). Thus, TrxR1 is truly superfluous for DNA replication and RNR activity in otherwise normal mouse hepatocytes.

Questions remain as to whether TrxR1-independent replication will prove to be a general phenomenon of mammalian cells or a peculiarity of hepatocytes. Both primary papers on mouse embryos lacking TrxR1 reported that it proved impossible to establish cultures of primary fibroblasts from mutant embryos; however it was not established whether this failure resulted from a block to replication or some other defect (Bondareva et al., 2007; Jakupoglu et al., 2005). As time passes, more and more cell types are being found to replicate in the absence of TrxR1. Recently, it was shown that lymphomas lacking TrxR1 can initiate and progress normally in mice (Mandal et al., 2010), adding another cell type to the list of cell types that can replicate in the absence of TrxR1. Also, in investigations using a fluorescent marker-tagged system in which both copies of the TrxR1 gene were disrupted in an arbitrary population of all cell types in fetal mice, my group assessed which, if any, cell types failed to contribute to the adult mouse two months later. No cell types could be identified that did not still contribute to the adult mouse under these conditions (CM Weisend and EE Schmidt, unpublished). Thus, whereas we cannot exclude the possibility that there could be some rare cell types in mice in which replication is critically dependent on TrxR1, our efforts to date have failed to pinpoint any such cell types.

Recently, a study was reported on disruption of TrxR1 in another metazoan, the nematode *C. elegans* (Stenvall et al., 2011). *C. elegans* has only a single TrxR protein, and this is the only Sec-containing protein in the worm genome (Stenvall et al., 2011). Surprisingly, although worms lacking TrxR1 show a molting defect due to an inability to reduce protein disulfides in the old cuticle to allow its removal, but like mouse livers lacking TrxR1 (Rollins et al., 2010; Suvorova et al., 2009), they show no evidence of oxidative stress or replicative insufficiency (Stenvall et al., 2011). Like in mice (Rollins et al., 2010), the source of electrons for RNR in worms remains unclear and will likely be an important subject for future investigation.

7. Alternative pathways of supplying electrons to RNR

Mammalian genomes contain three different genes encoding thioredoxin reductases. The *txnrd1* gene encodes TrxR1, the cytosolic enzyme; *txnrd2* encodes TrxR2 (also called Txnrd2 or TR3), the mitochondrial enzyme; and *txnrd3* encodes TrxR3 (also called Txnrd3, TGR, or TR2), a testis-specific cytosolic enzyme that can reduce either Trx1 or GSSG (Arner, 2009; Gerashchenko et al., 2010; Su et al., 2005). In most normal rodent tissues with the exception of testis, TrxR1 mRNA is about five-fold more abundant than TrxR2 mRNA, and TrxR3 mRNA is undetectable (Jurado et al., 2003). Previously, we have shown that neither TrxR2 mRNA nor TrxR3 mRNA are induced in TrxR1-deficient embryos (Bondareva et al., 2007) or livers (Suvorova et al., 2009), indicating that there is not an induction of the genes encoding either of the other known TrxRs that might compensate for ablation of TrxR1. However, it remained possible that normal levels of TrxR2 protein, though perhaps lower than normal levels of TrxR1 protein (see above), might be sufficient to compensate for loss of TrxR1 without an associated increase in mRNA levels. It is well established that the cytosolic and mitochondrial TrxR enzymes in *Arabidopsis* are cross-complementary. Thus, disruption of the gene encoding either of these *E. coli*-type TrxRs is compensated by a partial re-distribution of product from the other gene into the deficient sub-cellular compartment (Meyer et al., 2008; Reichheld et al., 2007; Sweat and Wolpert, 2007). To date, there is no *in vivo* evidence of similar cross-complementation occurring in mammalian systems. Nevertheless, several ESTs issued from the *txnrd2* gene but lacking the N-terminal mitochondrial transit signal have been reported from mammalian systems, which suggests the possibility that the *txnrd2* gene could yield cytosolic isoforms of TrxR2 (Turanov et al., 2006). Closer examination of this possibility will be important for determining whether cytosolic isoforms of TrxR2 participate in replication or homeostatic maintenance of mammalian cells lacking TrxR1.

Another system that might be compensating for loss of TrxR1 and supporting RNR activity and DNA replication in TrxR1-deficient hepatocytes is the GSH system. Neither livers nor embryos lacking TrxR1 exhibit compensatory induction of Gsr; however they do exhibit induction of mRNA encoding the modifier subunit of glutamate-cysteine ligase (Gclm), the rate limiting enzyme in GSH biosynthesis (Bondareva et al., 2007; Suvorova et al., 2009). A recent study showed that the GSH pathway, reconstituted entirely from recombinant or purified components (Gsr, GSH, and Grx), can effectively transfer electrons from NADPH to RNR and drive reduction of ribonucleoside diphosphates *in vitro* (Avval and Holmgren, 2009). In combination with the classical study showing that S-phase cells in normal rat tissues did not tend to exhibit Txr immunostaining (Hansson et al., 1986), there is a good possibility that the GSH system is supporting RNR activity in TrxR1-deficient hepatocytes (Holmgren and Sengupta, 2010); however other possibilities still exist, and all of these will need to be tested *in vivo*.

8. Considerations beyond supplying electrons to RNR

Decades of elegant studies on microbial and other non-metazoan systems revealed that, typically, if inhibition of disulfide reductases disrupted the supply of electrons to RNR, growth was abated; if not, growth was overtly normal (Gleason and Holmgren, 1988; Holmgren, 1985). In some cases, disruption of the Trx system was reported to yield intermediate growth phenotypes in non-metazoan eukaryotic systems (Koc et al., 2006; Meyer et al., 2009; Meyer et al., 2008; Reichheld et al., 2007; Sweat and Wolpert, 2007), apparently due to compromised output by RNR (Koc et al., 2006). Some studies on microbial models have shown that disruption of the Trx system can independently cause a disruption in homeostatic redox control or stress responses (Arner and Holmgren, 2000; Carmel-Harel et al., 2001; Carmel-Harel and Storz, 2000; Holmgren, 2000). Also, in mammalian systems, an intimate connection between intracellular signaling by the platelet-derived growth factor receptor (PDGFR), the T cell receptor, the epidermal growth factor receptor (EGFR), the tumor necrosis factor-α receptor (TNFAR), and likely other related phosphotyrosine receptors and Prxs has been established (Bae et al., 1997; Choi et al., 2005; Devadas et al., 2002; Kang et al., 1998; Rhee, 1999; Rhee et al., 2000), thereby indirectly linking the Trx pathway with physiological growth factor signaling. Thus, it is important to bear in mind that disruptions of cell physiology in response to perturbations in the Trx or GSH pathways, in particular in whole animals or other complex systems, is not necessarily indicative of a replicative block, and these distinctions can sometimes be difficult to tease apart experimentally.

A case in point is the as yet mechanistically uncertain causes of embryonic lethality in TrxR1-deficient mice (Bondareva et al., 2007; Jakupoglu et al., 2005). My group and that of Dr. Markus Conrad each generated independent and strategically distinct conditional-mutant alleles of the *txnrd1* gene that, in the zygotically homozygous-mutant state, result in embryonic lethality (Bondareva et al., 2007; Jakupoglu et al., 2005). In each case, the homozygous-mutant zygote proliferates to yield thousands of TrxR1-deficient cells prior to embryonic failure. Subsequently, using regulated disruption of these conditional alleles, mouse cells homozygous null for either allele have been shown to replicate vigorously (Mandal et al., 2010; Rollins et al., 2010), suggesting proliferation is normal in TrxR1-deficient cells. Why, then, do the mutant embryos die?

Although the reported details of embryonic progression differ between the two alleles, the system developed in my lab, with which I am most familiar, shows a phenotype that I believe lends clues to the answer. Despite the mutant embryos surviving and proliferating to embryonic day 8.5 (E8.5), the embryos become phenotypically abnormal much earlier (Bondareva et al., 2007). During post-blastocyst development, we detect no evidence of node formation, no development of primitive streak, and no differentiation of mesoderm (Bondareva et al., 2007). As a result, no body axis forms, normal patterning is not established, and the TrxR1-deficeint embryonic cells proliferate as a disorganized mass of primitive endoderm and ectoderm until, by E8.5, they have likely exceeded the volumetric constraints for survival without a functional (mesoderm-derived) cardiovascular and hematopoietic system. At this point, the embryo likely becomes necrotic and is simply resorbed by the mother (Bondareva et al., 2007). This phenotype is consistent with failure of early morphogen-signaling events. To date, we have not entirely ruled-out a possible proliferative defect in some unidentified early embryonic cell type as underlying embryonic lethality. Indeed, the recently reported metabolic eccentricities of mouse embryonic stem cells for replication (Wang et al., 2009) might suggest one rare but critical cell type that needs TrxR1 activity for full replicative potential, and whose perturbation might disrupt formation of node, primitive streak, and mesoderm. Further investigations will be required to test this possibility. However, the proliferative characteristics of the TrxR1-deficient mouse cells that have been studied to date disfavor this model (Mandal et al., 2010; Rollins et al., 2010). Conversely, the known interdependence of growth factor signaling on the Trx pathway (Choi et al., 2005; Rhee et al., 2005) is consistent with this embryonic phenotype. It is anticipated that these possibilities will be resolved in the very near future.

9. Summary and implications

Genome replication in most living systems is critically dependent on the activity of RNR. DNA synthesis is fairly rare in healthy adult mammals, being restricted to repair, mitochondrial renewal, and genome replication for a small subset of cells, including immune cells, germ cells, cells of the hair follicles, some intestinal epithelial cells, and a few others. However, certain diseases, such as cancers and some viral diseases, are critically dependent on DNA replication, and therefore are frequently combated with drugs that block this process. The key dependence of replication on RNR has made RNR an important drug-target for cancer and viral chemotherapies. Indeed, the classic chemotherapeutic drug HU directly inhibits RNR (Hatse et al., 1999; Lori and Lisziewicz, 1998; Newton, 2007; Romanelli et al., 1999; Szekeres et al., 1997; Yarbro, 1992), and various newer chemotherapeutics function similarly (Mayhew et al., 2002; Mayhew et al., 2005; Smart, 1995; Szekeres et al., 1994; Tsimberidou et al., 2002). Unfortunately, as with many chemotherapeutics, intra-host evolution of drug resistance by the diseased tissue is a common problem (Akerblom et al., 1981; Balzarini, 2000; Wright et al., 1990). The absolute dependency of RNR on a suitable electron-donor system has long suggested alternative mechanisms for blocking RNR activity, in particular in cases of HU resistance. Drugs that target either the Trx pathway, such as aurothioglucose, or the GSH pathway, such as buthionine sulfoxamine (BSO) have been developed and are well tolerated (Arner and Holmgren, 2000; Arner and Holmgren, 2006; Griffith and Meister, 1985; Lu et al., 2007; Williamson et al., 1982). Recent whole animal genetic studies reviewed here, however, suggest that in many if not all mammalian cells, either the GSH or the Trx pathway alone might be robust at supporting S phase RNR activity in the absence of the other. Thus, chemotherapeutic approaches to blocking DNA replication through disruption of disulfide reductase pathways will need to be cognizant of the potentially complete functional redundancy of the GSH and Trx pathways in animal systems, and sensitive to the various other physiological roles these pathways play in normal homeostatic and stress-response pathways.

10. References

Akerblom, L., Ehrenberg, A., Graslund, A., Lankinen, H., Reichard, P., and Thelander, L. (1981). Overproduction of the free radical of ribonucleotide reductase in hydroxyurea-resistant mouse fibroblast 3T6 cells. Proc Natl Acad Sci U S A *78*, 2159-2163.

Arner, E. S. (2009). Focus on mammalian thioredoxin reductases -- important selenoproteins with versatile functions. Biochim Biophys Acta.

Arner, E. S., and Eriksson, S. (1995). Mammalian deoxyribonucleoside kinases. Pharmacol Ther *67*, 155-186.

Arner, E. S., and Holmgren, A. (2000). Physiological functions of thioredoxin and thioredoxin reductase. Eur J Biochem *267*, 6102-6109.

Arner, E. S., and Holmgren, A. (2006). The thioredoxin system in cancer. Semin Cancer Biol *16*, 420-426.

Arner, E. S., Nordberg, J., and Holmgren, A. (1996). Efficient reduction of lipoamide and lipoic acid by mammalian thioredoxin reductase. Biochem Biophys Res Commun *225*, 268-274.

Arscott, L. D., Gromer, S., Schirmer, R. H., Becker, K., and Williams, C. H., Jr. (1997). The mechanism of thioredoxin reductase from human placenta is similar to the mechanisms of lipoamide dehydrogenase and glutathione reductase and is distinct from the mechanism of thioredoxin reductase from Escherichia coli. Proc Natl Acad Sci U S A *94*, 3621-3626.

Atkin, C. L., Thelander, L., Reichard, P., and Lang, G. (1973). Iron and free radical in ribonucleotide reductase. Exchange of iron and Mossbauer spectroscopy of the protein B2 subunit of the Escherichia coli enzyme. J Biol Chem *248*, 7464-7472.

Avval, F. Z., and Holmgren, A. (2009). Molecular mechanisms of thioredoxin and glutaredoxin as hydrogen donors for Mammalian s phase ribonucleotide reductase. J Biol Chem *284*, 8233-8240.

Bae, Y. S., Kang, S. W., Seo, M. S., Baines, I. C., Tekle, E., Chock, P. B., and Rhee, S. G. (1997). Epidermal growth factor (EGF)-induced generation of hydrogen peroxide. Role in EGF receptor-mediated tyrosine phosphorylation. J Biol Chem *272*, 217-221.

Balzarini, J. (2000). Effect of antimetabolite drugs of nucleotide metabolism on the anti-human immunodeficiency virus activity of nucleoside reverse transcriptase inhibitors. Pharmacol Ther *87*, 175-187.

Berndt, C., Lillig, C. H., and Holmgren, A. (2007). Thiol-based mechanisms of the thioredoxin and glutaredoxin systems: implications for diseases in the cardiovascular system. Am J Physiol Heart Circ Physiol *292*, H1227-1236.

Berndt, C., Lillig, C. H., and Holmgren, A. (2008). Thioredoxins and glutaredoxins as facilitators of protein folding. Biochim Biophys Acta *1783*, 641-650.

Bondareva, A. A., Capecchi, M. R., Iverson, S. V., Li, Y., Lopez, N. I., Lucas, O., Merrill, G. F., Prigge, J. R., Siders, A. M., Wakamiya, M., *et al.* (2007). Effects of thioredoxin reductase-1 deletion on embryogenesis and transcriptome. Free Radic Biol Med *43*, 911-923.

Bonilla, M., Denicola, A., Novoselov, S. V., Turanov, A. A., Protasio, A., Izmendi, D., Gladyshev, V. N., and Salinas, G. (2008). Platyhelminth mitochondrial and cytosolic redox homeostasis is controlled by a single thioredoxin glutathione reductase and dependent on selenium and glutathione. J Biol Chem *283*, 17898-17907.

Branco, V., Canario, J., Holmgren, A., and Carvalho, C. (2011). Inhibition of the thioredoxin system in the brain and liver of zebra-seabreams exposed to waterborne methylmercury. Toxicol Appl Pharmacol *251*, 95-103.

Brown, N. C., Canellakis, Z. N., Lundin, B., Reichard, P., and Thelander, L. (1969). Ribonucleoside diphosphate reductase. Purification of the two subunits, proteins B1 and B2. Eur J Biochem *9*, 561-573.

Carmel-Harel, O., Stearman, R., Gasch, A. P., Botstein, D., Brown, P. O., and Storz, G. (2001). Role of thioredoxin reductase in the Yap1p-dependent response to oxidative stress in Saccharomyces cerevisiae. Mol Microbiol *39*, 595-605.

Carmel-Harel, O., and Storz, G. (2000). Roles of the glutathione- and thioredoxin-dependent reduction systems in the Escherichia coli and saccharomyces cerevisiae responses to oxidative stress. Annu Rev Microbiol *54*, 439-461.

Carvalho, C. M., Chew, E. H., Hashemy, S. I., Lu, J., and Holmgren, A. (2008). Inhibition of the human thioredoxin system. A molecular mechanism of mercury toxicity. J Biol Chem *283*, 11913-11923.

Choi, M. H., Lee, I. K., Kim, G. W., Kim, B. U., Han, Y. H., Yu, D. Y., Park, H. S., Kim, K. Y., Lee, J. S., Choi, C., *et al.* (2005). Regulation of PDGF signalling and vascular remodelling by peroxiredoxin II. Nature *435*, 347-353.

Devadas, S., Zaritskaya, L., Rhee, S. G., Oberley, L., and Williams, M. S. (2002). Discrete generation of superoxide and hydrogen peroxide by T cell receptor stimulation: selective regulation of mitogen-activated protein kinase activation and fas ligand expression. J Exp Med *195*, 59-70.

Eckenroth, B., Harris, K., Turanov, A. A., Gladyshev, V. N., Raines, R. T., and Hondal, R. J. (2006). Semisynthesis and characterization of mammalian thioredoxin reductase. Biochemistry *45*, 5158-5170.

Fernandes, A. P., and Holmgren, A. (2004). Glutaredoxins: glutathione-dependent redox enzymes with functions far beyond a simple thioredoxin backup system. Antioxid Redox Signal *6*, 63-74.

Gerashchenko, M. V., Su, D., and Gladyshev, V. N. (2010). CUG start codon generates thioredoxin/glutathione reductase isoforms in mouse testes. J Biol Chem *285*, 4595-4602.

Gleason, F. K., and Holmgren, A. (1981). Isolation and characterization of thioredoxin from the cyanobacterium, Anabaena sp. J Biol Chem *256*, 8306-8309.

Gleason, F. K., and Holmgren, A. (1988). Thioredoxin and related proteins in procaryotes. FEMS Microbiol Rev *4*, 271-297.

Gon, S., Faulkner, M. J., and Beckwith, J. (2006). In vivo requirement for glutaredoxins and thioredoxins in the reduction of the ribonucleotide reductases of Escherichia coli. Antioxid Redox Signal *8*, 735-742.

Griffith, O. W., and Meister, A. (1985). Origin and turnover of mitochondrial glutathione. Proc Natl Acad Sci U S A *82*, 4668-4672.

Gromer, S., Johansson, L., Bauer, H., Arscott, L. D., Rauch, S., Ballou, D. P., Williams, C. H., Jr., Schirmer, R. H., and Arner, E. S. (2003). Active sites of thioredoxin reductases: why selenoproteins? Proc Natl Acad Sci U S A *100*, 12618-12623.

Hansson, H. A., Rozell, B., Stemme, S., Engstrom, Y., Thelander, L., and Holmgren, A. (1986). Different cellular distribution of thioredoxin and subunit M1 of ribonucleotide reductase in rat tissues. Exp Cell Res *163*, 363-369.

Hatse, S., De Clercq, E., and Balzarini, J. (1999). Role of antimetabolites of purine and pyrimidine nucleotide metabolism in tumor cell differentiation. Biochem Pharmacol *58*, 539-555.

Hayes, J. D., and Pulford, D. J. (1995). The glutathione S-transferase supergene family: regulation of GST and the contribution of the isoenzymes to cancer chemoprotection and drug resistance. Crit Rev Biochem Mol Biol *30*, 445-600.

Hirt, R. P., Muller, S., Embley, T. M., and Coombs, G. H. (2002). The diversity and evolution of thioredoxin reductase: new perspectives. Trends Parasitol *18*, 302-308.

Holmgren, A. (1976). Hydrogen donor system for Escherichia coli ribonucleoside-diphosphate reductase dependent upon glutathione. Proc Natl Acad Sci U S A *73*, 2275-2279.

Holmgren, A. (1977). The function of thioredoxin and glutathione in deoxyribonucleic acid synthesis. Biochem Soc Trans *5*, 611-612.

Holmgren, A. (1978). Glutathione-dependent enzyme reactions of the phage T4 ribonucleotide reductase system. J Biol Chem *253*, 7424-7430.

Holmgren, A. (1979). Glutathione-dependent synthesis of deoxyribonucleotides. Characterization of the enzymatic mechanism of Escherichia coli glutaredoxin. J Biol Chem *254*, 3672-3678.

Holmgren, A. (1980). Pyridine nucleotide - disulfide oxidoreductases. Experientia Suppl *36*, 149-180.

Holmgren, A. (1981). Regulation of ribonucleotide reductase. Curr Top Cell Regul *19*, 47-76.

Holmgren, A. (1985). Thioredoxin. Annu Rev Biochem *54*, 237-271.

Holmgren, A. (1989). Thioredoxin and glutaredoxin systems. J Biol Chem *264*, 13963-13966.

Holmgren, A. (2000). Antioxidant function of thioredoxin and glutaredoxin systems. Antioxid Redox Signal 2, 811-820.

Holmgren, A., and Bjornstedt, M. (1995). Thioredoxin and thioredoxin reductase. Methods Enzymol *252*, 199-208.

Holmgren, A., Johansson, C., Berndt, C., Lonn, M. E., Hudemann, C., and Lillig, C. H. (2005). Thiol redox control via thioredoxin and glutaredoxin systems. Biochem Soc Trans *33*, 1375-1377.

Holmgren, A., and Lu, J. (2010). Thioredoxin and thioredoxin reductase: current research with special reference to human disease. Biochem Biophys Res Commun *396*, 120-124.

Holmgren, A., Reichard, P., and Thelander, L. (1965). Enzymatic synthesis of deoxyribonucleotides, 8. The effects of ATP and dATP in the CDP reductase system from E. coli. Proc Natl Acad Sci U S A *54*, 830-836.

Holmgren, A., and Sengupta, R. (2010). The use of thiols by ribonucleotide reductase. Free Radic Biol Med *49*, 1617-1628.

Hondal, R. J., and Ruggles, E. L. (2010). Differing views of the role of selenium in thioredoxin reductase. Amino Acids.

Ishii, T., and Yanagawa, T. (2007). Stress-induced peroxiredoxins. Subcell Biochem *44*, 375-384.

Itoh, K., Ishii, T., Wakabayashi, N., and Yamamoto, M. (1999). Regulatory mechanisms of cellular response to oxidative stress. Free Radic Res *31*, 319-324.

Iwasaki, H., Huang, P., Keating, M. J., and Plunkett, W. (1997). Differential incorporation of ara-C, gemcitabine, and fludarabine into replicating and repairing DNA in proliferating human leukemia cells. Blood *90*, 270-278.

Jakupoglu, C., Przemeck, G. K., Schneider, M., Moreno, S. G., Mayr, N., Hatzopoulos, A. K., de Angelis, M. H., Wurst, W., Bornkamm, G. W., Brielmeier, M., and Conrad, M. (2005). Cytoplasmic thioredoxin reductase is essential for embryogenesis but dispensable for cardiac development. Mol Cell Biol *25*, 1980-1988.

Johansson, L., Arscott, L. D., Ballou, D. P., Williams, C. H., Jr., and Arner, E. S. (2006). Studies of an active site mutant of the selenoprotein thioredoxin reductase: the Ser-

Cys-Cys-Ser motif of the insect orthologue is not sufficient to replace the Cys-Sec dyad in the mammalian enzyme. Free Radic Biol Med *41*, 649-656.
Jurado, J., Prieto-Alamo, M. J., Madrid-Risquez, J., and Pueyo, C. (2003). Absolute gene expression patterns of thioredoxin and glutaredoxin redox systems in mouse. J Biol Chem *278*, 45546-45554.
Kang, S. W., Chae, H. Z., Seo, M. S., Kim, K., Baines, I. C., and Rhee, S. G. (1998). Mammalian peroxiredoxin isoforms can reduce hydrogen peroxide generated in response to growth factors and tumor necrosis factor-alpha. J Biol Chem *273*, 6297-6302.
Koc, A., Mathews, C. K., Wheeler, L. J., Gross, M. K., and Merrill, G. F. (2006). Thioredoxin is required for deoxyribonucleotide pool maintenance during S phase. J Biol Chem *281*, 15058-15063.
Kunkel, T. A., Silber, J. R., and Loeb, L. A. (1982). The mutagenic effect of deoxynucleotide substrate imbalances during DNA synthesis with mammalian DNA polymerases. Mutat Res *94*, 413-419.
Laurent, T. C., Moore, E. C., and Reichard, P. (1964). Enzymatic Synthesis Of Deoxyribonucleotides. Iv. Isolation And Characterization Of Thioredoxin, The Hydrogen Donor From Escherichia Coli B. J Biol Chem *239*, 3436-3444.
Lillig, C. H., and Holmgren, A. (2007). Thioredoxin and related molecules--from biology to health and disease. Antioxid Redox Signal *9*, 25-47.
Lori, F., and Lisziewicz, J. (1998). Hydroxyurea: mechanisms of HIV-1 inhibition. Antivir Ther *3 Suppl 4*, 25-33.
Lothrop, A. P., Ruggles, E. L., and Hondal, R. J. (2009). No selenium required: reactions catalyzed by mammalian thioredoxin reductase that are independent of a selenocysteine residue. Biochemistry *48*, 6213-6223.
Lu, J., Chew, E. H., and Holmgren, A. (2007). Targeting thioredoxin reductase is a basis for cancer therapy by arsenic trioxide. Proc Natl Acad Sci U S A *104*, 12288-12293.
Lu, J., and Holmgren, A. (2009). Selenoproteins. J Biol Chem *284*, 723-727.
Luthman, M., Eriksson, S., Holmgren, A., and Thelander, L. (1979). Glutathione-dependent hydrogen donor system for calf thymus ribonucleoside-diphosphate reductase. Proc Natl Acad Sci U S A *76*, 2158-2162.
Luthman, M., and Holmgren, A. (1982). Glutaredoxin from calf thymus. Purification to homogeneity. J Biol Chem *257*, 6686-6690.
Mandal, P. K., Schneider, M., Kolle, P., Kuhlencordt, P., Forster, H., Beck, H., Bornkamm, G. W., and Conrad, M. (2010). Loss of thioredoxin reductase 1 renders tumors highly susceptible to pharmacologic glutathione deprivation. Cancer Res *70*, 9505-9514.
Margulies, D. H., and McCluskey, J. (1985). Exon shuffling: new genes from old. Surv Immunol Res *4*, 146-159.
Mathews, C. K., and Song, S. (2007). Maintaining precursor pools for mitochondrial DNA replication. Faseb J *21*, 2294-2303.
Matsui, M., Oshima, M., Oshima, H., Takaku, K., Maruyama, T., Yodoi, J., and Taketo, M. M. (1996). Early embryonic lethality caused by targeted disruption of the mouse thioredoxin gene. Dev Biol *178*, 179-185.
Mayhew, C. N., Phillips, J. D., Cibull, M. L., Elford, H. L., and Gallicchio, V. S. (2002). Short-term treatment with novel ribonucleotide reductase inhibitors Trimidox and Didox

reverses late-stage murine retrovirus-induced lymphoproliferative disease with less bone marrow toxicity than hydroxyurea. Antivir Chem Chemother *13*, 305-314.

Mayhew, C. N., Sumpter, R., Inayat, M., Cibull, M., Phillips, J. D., Elford, H. L., and Gallicchio, V. S. (2005). Combination of inhibitors of lymphocyte activation (hydroxyurea, trimidox, and didox) and reverse transcriptase (didanosine) suppresses development of murine retrovirus-induced lymphoproliferative disease. Antiviral Res *65*, 13-22.

Meyer, Y., Buchanan, B. B., Vignols, F., and Reichheld, J. P. (2009). Thioredoxins and Glutaredoxins: Unifying Elements in Redox Biology. Annu Rev Genet.

Meyer, Y., Siala, W., Bashandy, T., Riondet, C., Vignols, F., and Reichheld, J. P. (2008). Glutaredoxins and thioredoxins in plants. Biochim Biophys Acta *1783*, 589-600.

Moore, E. C., Reichard, P., and Thelander, L. (1964). Enzymatic Synthesis Of Deoxyribonucleotides.V. Purification And Properties Of Thioredoxin Reductase From Escherichia Coli B. J Biol Chem *239*, 3445-3452.

Navarra, P., and Preziosi, P. (1999). Hydroxyurea: new insights on an old drug. Crit Rev Oncol Hematol *29*, 249-255.

Newton, H. B. (2007). Hydroxyurea chemotherapy in the treatment of meningiomas. Neurosurg Focus *23*, E11.

Nguyen, T., Nioi, P., and Pickett, C. B. (2009). The nrf2-antioxidant response element signaling pathway and its activation by oxidative stress. J Biol Chem *284*, 13291-13295.

Nicander, B., and Reichard, P. (1983). Dynamics of pyrimidine deoxynucleoside triphosphate pools in relationship to DNA synthesis in 3T6 mouse fibroblasts. Proc Natl Acad Sci U S A *80*, 1347-1351.

Nordberg, J., and Arner, E. S. (2001). Reactive oxygen species, antioxidants, and the mammalian thioredoxin system. Free Radic Biol Med *31*, 1287-1312.

Novoselov, S. V., and Gladyshev, V. N. (2003). Non-animal origin of animal thioredoxin reductases: implications for selenocysteine evolution and evolution of protein function through carboxy-terminal extensions. Protein Sci *12*, 372-378.

Oliver, F. J., Collins, M. K., and Lopez-Rivas, A. (1996). dNTP pools imbalance as a signal to initiate apoptosis. Experientia *52*, 995-1000.

Pontarin, G., Ferraro, P., Hakansson, P., Thelander, L., Reichard, P., and Bianchi, V. (2007). p53R2-dependent ribonucleotide reduction provides deoxyribonucleotides in quiescent human fibroblasts in the absence of induced DNA damage. J Biol Chem *282*, 16820-16828.

Rahlfs, S., Schirmer, R. H., and Becker, K. (2002). The thioredoxin system of Plasmodium falciparum and other parasites. Cell Mol Life Sci *59*, 1024-1041.

Reichard, P., Baldesten, A., and Rutberg, L. (1961). Formation of deoxycytidine phosphates from cytidine phosphates in extracts from Escherichia coli. J Biol Chem *236*, 1150-1157.

Reichard, P., Eliasson, R., Ingemarson, R., and Thelander, L. (2000). Cross-talk between the allosteric effector-binding sites in mouse ribonucleotide reductase. J Biol Chem *275*, 33021-33026.

Reichheld, J. P., Khafif, M., Riondet, C., Droux, M., Bonnard, G., and Meyer, Y. (2007). Inactivation of thioredoxin reductases reveals a complex interplay between thioredoxin and glutathione pathways in Arabidopsis development. Plant Cell *19*, 1851-1865.

Rhee, S. G. (1999). Redox signaling: hydrogen peroxide as intracellular messenger. Exp Mol Med *31*, 53-59.

Rhee, S. G., Bae, Y. S., Lee, S. R., and Kwon, J. (2000). Hydrogen peroxide: a key messenger that modulates protein phosphorylation through cysteine oxidation. Sci STKE *2000*, PE1.

Rhee, S. G., Kang, S. W., Jeong, W., Chang, T. S., Yang, K. S., and Woo, H. A. (2005). Intracellular messenger function of hydrogen peroxide and its regulation by peroxiredoxins. Curr Opin Cell Biol *17*, 183-189.

Rogers, L. K., Tamura, T., Rogers, B. J., Welty, S. E., Hansen, T. N., and Smith, C. V. (2004). Analyses of glutathione reductase hypomorphic mice indicate a genetic knockout. Toxicol Sci *82*, 367-373.

Rollins, M. F., van der Heide, D. M., Weisend, C. M., Kundert, J. A., Comstock, K. M., Suvorova, E. S., Capecchi, M. R., Merrill, G. F., and Schmidt, E. E. (2010). Hepatocytes lacking thioredoxin reductase 1 have normal replicative potential during development and regeneration. J Cell Sci *123*, 2402-2412.

Romanelli, F., Pomeroy, C., and Smith, K. M. (1999). Hydroxyurea to inhibit human immunodeficiency virus-1 replication. Pharmacotherapy *19*, 196-204.

Rottgen, V., and Rabes, H. M. (1989). Deoxyribonucleoside triphosphate pools in regenerating rat liver: effect of hydroxyurea and exogenous deoxypyrimidines. Biochim Biophys Acta *992*, 349-354.

Sandalova, T., Zhong, L., Lindqvist, Y., Holmgren, A., and Schneider, G. (2001). Three-dimensional structure of a mammalian thioredoxin reductase: implications for mechanism and evolution of a selenocysteine-dependent enzyme. Proc Natl Acad Sci U S A *98*, 9533-9538.

Schmidt, E. E., and Davies, C. J. (2007). The origins of polypeptide domains. Bioessays *29*, 262-270.

Smart, T. (1995). Beyond hydroxyurea. GMHC Treat Issues *9*, 5.

Spyrou, G., and Holmgren, A. (1996). Deoxyribonucleoside triphosphate pools and growth of glutathione-depleted 3T6 mouse fibroblasts. Biochem Biophys Res Commun *220*, 42-46.

Stenvall, J., Fierro-Gonzalez, J. C., Swoboda, P., Saamarthy, K., Cheng, Q., Cacho-Valadez, B., Arner, E. S., Persson, O. P., Miranda-Vizuete, A., and Tuck, S. (2011). Selenoprotein TRXR-1 and GSR-1 are essential for removal of old cuticle during molting in Caenorhabditis elegans. Proc Natl Acad Sci U S A *108*, 1064-1069.

Su, D., Novoselov, S. V., Sun, Q. A., Moustafa, M. E., Zhou, Y., Oko, R., Hatfield, D. L., and Gladyshev, V. N. (2005). Mammalian selenoprotein thioredoxin-glutathione reductase. Roles in disulfide bond formation and sperm maturation. J Biol Chem *280*, 26491-26498.

Sun, Q. A., Kirnarsky, L., Sherman, S., and Gladyshev, V. N. (2001). Selenoprotein oxidoreductase with specificity for thioredoxin and glutathione systems. Proc Natl Acad Sci U S A *98*, 3673-3678.

Sun, Q. A., Su, D., Novoselov, S. V., Carlson, B. A., Hatfield, D. L., and Gladyshev, V. N. (2005). Reaction mechanism and regulation of mammalian thioredoxin/glutathione reductase. Biochemistry *44*, 14528-14537.

Suvorova, E. S., Lucas, O., Weisend, C. M., Rollins, M. F., Merrill, G. F., Capecchi, M. R., and Schmidt, E. E. (2009). Cytoprotective Nrf2 pathway is induced in chronically txnrd 1-deficient hepatocytes. PLoS One *4*, e6158.

Sweat, T. A., and Wolpert, T. J. (2007). Thioredoxin h5 is required for victorin sensitivity mediated by a CC-NBS-LRR gene in Arabidopsis. Plant Cell *19*, 673-687.

Szekeres, T., Fritzer-Szekeres, M., and Elford, H. L. (1997). The enzyme ribonucleotide reductase: target for antitumor and anti-HIV therapy. Crit Rev Clin Lab Sci *34*, 503-528.

Szekeres, T., Gharehbaghi, K., Fritzer, M., Woody, M., Srivastava, A., van't Riet, B., Jayaram, H. N., and Elford, H. L. (1994). Biochemical and antitumor activity of trimidox, a new inhibitor of ribonucleotide reductase. Cancer Chemother Pharmacol *34*, 63-66.

Taskov, K., Chapple, C., Kryukov, G. V., Castellano, S., Lobanov, A. V., Korotkov, K. V., Guigo, R., and Gladyshev, V. N. (2005). Nematode selenoproteome: the use of the selenocysteine insertion system to decode one codon in an animal genome? Nucleic Acids Res *33*, 2227-2238.

Thelander, L., and Reichard, P. (1979). Reduction of ribonucleotides. Annu Rev Biochem *48*, 133-158.

Tipple, T. E., Welty, S. E., Rogers, L. K., Hansen, T. N., Choi, Y. E., Kehrer, J. P., and Smith, C. V. (2007). Thioredoxin-related mechanisms in hyperoxic lung injury in mice. Am J Respir Cell Mol Biol *37*, 405-413.

Torrents, E., Trevisiol, C., Rotte, C., Hellman, U., Martin, W., and Reichard, P. (2006). Euglena gracilis ribonucleotide reductase: the eukaryote class II enzyme and the possible antiquity of eukaryote B12 dependence. J Biol Chem *281*, 5604-5611.

Tsimberidou, A. M., Alvarado, Y., and Giles, F. J. (2002). Evolving role of ribonucleoside reductase inhibitors in hematologic malignancies. Expert Rev Anticancer Ther *2*, 437-448.

Turanov, A. A., Su, D., and Gladyshev, V. N. (2006). Characterization of alternative cytosolic forms and cellular targets of mouse mitochondrial thioredoxin reductase. J Biol Chem *281*, 22953-22963.

Wang, J., Alexander, P., Wu, L., Hammer, R., Cleaver, O., and McKnight, S. L. (2009). Dependence of mouse embryonic stem cells on threonine catabolism. Science *325*, 435-439.

Williams, C. H., Arscott, L. D., Muller, S., Lennon, B. W., Ludwig, M. L., Wang, P. F., Veine, D. M., Becker, K., and Schirmer, R. H. (2000). Thioredoxin reductase two modes of catalysis have evolved. Eur J Biochem *267*, 6110-6117.

Williamson, J. M., Boettcher, B., and Meister, A. (1982). Intracellular cysteine delivery system that protects against toxicity by promoting glutathione synthesis. Proc Natl Acad Sci U S A *79*, 6246-6249.

Wright, J. A., Chan, A. K., Choy, B. K., Hurta, R. A., McClarty, G. A., and Tagger, A. Y. (1990). Regulation and drug resistance mechanisms of mammalian ribonucleotide reductase, and the significance to DNA synthesis. Biochem Cell Biol *68*, 1364-1371.

Yarbro, J. W. (1992). Mechanism of action of hydroxyurea. Semin Oncol *19*, 1-10.

Yoo, M. H., Xu, X. M., Carlson, B. A., Gladyshev, V. N., and Hatfield, D. L. (2006). Thioredoxin reductase 1 deficiency reverses tumor phenotype and tumorigenicity of lung carcinoma cells. J Biol Chem *281*, 13005-13008.

Yoo, M. H., Xu, X. M., Carlson, B. A., Patterson, A. D., Gladyshev, V. N., and Hatfield, D. L. (2007). Targeting thioredoxin reductase 1 reduction in cancer cells inhibits self-sufficient growth and DNA replication. PLoS ONE *2*, e1112.

Zhang, J., and Lu, H. (2007). Ifosfamide induces acute renal failure via inhibition of the thioredoxin reductase activity. Free Radic Biol Med *43*, 1574-1583.

Zhong, L., Arner, E. S., Ljung, J., Aslund, F., and Holmgren, A. (1998). Rat and calf thioredoxin reductase are homologous to glutathione reductase with a carboxyl-terminal elongation containing a conserved catalytically active penultimate selenocysteine residue. J Biol Chem *273*, 8581-8591.

Part 6

Replication and Diseases

26

Prevalence of Reactivation of Hepatitis B Virus DNA Replication in Rheumatoid Arthritis Patients

Yukitomo Urata[1], Ryoko Uesato[2] and Dai Tanaka[2]
[1]*Department of Rheumatology Seihoku Chuo Hospital, Gosyogawara,*
[2]*Department of Orthopaedic Surgery, Seihoku Chuo Hospital, Gosyogawara,*
Japan

1. Introduction

Hepatitis B virus and rheumatoid arthritis

More than one-third of the worldwide population is infected with hepatitis B virus (HBV), and 350 million individuals have chronic HBV infection [1], with 75% of those living in the Southeast Asia and Western Pacific regions. HBV infection is a leading cause of cirrhosis and hepatocellular carcinoma (HCC) [2] and is estimated to be responsible for 500,000–700,000 deaths annually. Reactivation of hepatitis B in patients undergoing immunosuppressive therapy is a clinically important complication [3-5]. Hepatitis B reactivation can be transient and clinically silent but is often severe and results in acute hepatic failure.

Two clinical scenarios contribute to the reactivation of hepatitis B. The first occurs in patients with chronic hepatitis B. Fulminant HBV has been reported in hepatitis B surface antigen (HBsAg)-positive patients with rheumatoid arthritis (RA) taking tumor necrosis factor agents (TNFA) [6, 7].

Second, reactivation of hepatitis B occurs in patients with resolved hepatitis B. In these patients, low levels of HBV replication have been shown to persist in the liver and in peripheral blood mononuclear cells for decades [8-10], and reactivation occurs after transplantation, immunosuppressive therapy, and allogeneic and autologous hematopoietic stem-cell transplantation, with the reappearance of HBsAg [11-15]. Reactivation of hepatitis B can occur in RA patients with resolved hepatitis B who are on immunosuppressive therapy, including corticosteroids (CS), methotrexate (MTX) [16], and TNFA [17,18], and can result in fulminant or lethal hepatitis [4]. Optimal management practices for this group of patients are unclear [9].

We performed this study to determine the rate of reactivation of HBV DNA replication in RA patients with resolved hepatitis B.

2. Materials and methods

2.1 Patients and methods

In our departments, 516 patients who were treated for RA between January 2008 and August 2009 fulfilled the American College of Rheumatology 1987 revised criteria for RA.

All patients were evaluated for HBV markers, including HBsAg, anti-hepatitis B surface antibody (anti-HBs), and anti-hepatitis B core antibody (anti-HBc). HBV markers were detected using commercial enzyme immunoassays (HBsAg: ARCHITECT HBsAg QT, anti-HBs: ARCHITECT Anti-HBs, and anti-HBc: ARCHITECT Anti-HBc; Abbott Laboratories, Wiesbaden, Germany). If patients were HBsAg-positive or HBsAg-negative and anti-HBs- and/or anti-HBc-positive, HBV DNA levels were assessed. Sensitivity was 2 log copies/mL. When negative HBV DNA results were obtained, measurements were repeated every 3 months, and if HBV DNA became positive, measurements were repeated every month. Medications, including biologic agents, were generally not discontinued, irrespective of HBV DNA levels. All study protocols were approved by the ethics committees of the participating centers, and all patients provided written informed consent before enrolment.

2.2 Quantification of HBV DNA in blood by real-time PCR

HBV DNA levels were quantified using the automated COBAS TaqMan HBV Test version 2·0 (Roche, Basel, Switzerland). Samples were pretreated using the COBAS AmpliPrep System for amplification and quantification by real-time PCR and were analyzed using the COBAS TaqMan gene analyzer [19].

2.3 Statistical analysis

The Fisher's exact test, Student's *t*-test, and Mann–Whitney *U* test were used to compare baseline patient characteristics between subgroups. Two-tailed values of $p \leq 0.05$ were regarded as significant. Cox regression hazard analyses were used to separately investigate the influence of biologic agents, MTX, CS, and disease-modifying antirheumatic drugs (DMARDs) on reactivation of HBV DNA replication. To identify the relative important of these factors, we performed a stepwise forward elimination multiple logistic regression model. All analyses were performed using JMP version 8.0 software (JMP Japan, Tokyo, Japan).

3. Results

Background characteristics of the 516 patients are listed in Table 1. Seven patients were HBsAg-positive, while 157 were HBsAg-negative and anti-HBs- and/or anti-HBc-positive (30.4%). No resolved hepatitis B patients were positive for HBV DNA at baseline.
Subjects were followed for 18 months, and HBV DNA became positive (3.44 log copies/mL) in 13 of 157 patients (8.3%), whereas hepatic function remained normal in all cases (Table 1). Details of patients developing reactivation of HBV DNA replication are listed in Table 2; 1 patient developed reactivation of HBV DNA replication twice, 10 patients showed HBV DNA replication during biologic agent therapy [etanercept (ETN), n = 8; abatacept, n = 2; adalimumab, n = 1; infliximab, n = 1; tocilizumab, n = 1; and rituximab, n = 1], whereas 3 patient showed replication without biologic agent therapy. Types of DMARDs and immunosuppressants used for RA treatment during the study and numbers of patients being administered each pharmacotherapy are shown in Table 3. In 2 of the 13 patients, HBV DNA became negative without therapy. In 10 of the 13 patients, HBV DNA became negative with entecavir therapy (mean, 3.3 months). In the remaining 1 patient, after HBV DNA became positive, she suddenly died due to unknown causes.
Exploratory analysis was conducted on factors that were potentially associated with HBV replication development (Table 3). Among resolved hepatitis B patients who did and did not

Baseline demographic, clinical, and laboratory characteristics	HBV replication (+)	HBV replication (-)	*P* value
n	13	144	
Age, years (mean)	66.6 ± 10.7 (67.6)	64.9 ± 11.8 (66.2)	0.670
Female, n	8 (61.5%)	114 (77.9%)	0.505
RA duration, years	8.0 ± 7.7 (4.7)	7.6 ± 9.0 (4.0)	0.241
CRP, mg/dL	0.92 ± 2.46 (0.09)	1.04 ± 2.11 (0.20)	0.218
ESR, mm/h	26.0 ± 30.0 (13.0)	26.1 ± 26.8 (15.0)	0.476
IgM RF, IU/mL	46.2 ± 34.0 (49.3)	88.0 ± 151.2 (24.5)	0.791
AST, U/L	25.5 ± 6.5 (27.0)	27.9 ± 16.4 (23.0)	0.688
ALT, U/L	19.9 ± 6.8 (20.5)	26.0 ± 19.2 (19.0)	0.959
IgG, mg/dL	1454 ± 573 (1382)	1432 ± 450 (1358)	0.604
Neutrophil count	3326 ± 1567 (2722)	4462 ± 2302 (3868)	0.063
Lymphocyte count	1503 ± 425 (1431)	1732 ± 813 (1562)	0.323

Values are given as mean ± standard deviation (median)
RA, rheumatoid arthritis; *CRP*, C-reactive protein; *ESR*, erythrocyte sedimentation rate; *Ig*, immunoglobulin; *RF*, rheumatoid factor; *AST*, aspartate aminotransferase; *ALT*, alanine aminotransferase

Table 1. Comparison of hepatitis B virus (HBV) replication-positive and HBV replication-negative patients for baseline demographic, clinical, and laboratory characteristics

develop reactivation of HBV DNA replication, a significant difference was noted between the use of biologic agents (76.9% vs. 36.1%, respectively; p = 0.006), ETN (61.5% vs. 22.2%, respectively; p = 0.005), MTX (76.9% vs. 46.5%, respectively; p = 0.044), high-dose CS (15.4% vs. 1.4%; p = 0.035), and tacrolimus hydrate (30.8% vs. 5.6%; p = 0.010). Cox regression hazard analysis also revealed that biologic agent and ETN use can be as predictors for reactivation of HBV DNA replication. The hazard ratio (HR) for use of a biologic agent and etanercept was 10.9 (p = 0.008) and 6.9 (p = 0.001), respectively. Age at presentation, duration of RA, male gender, use of MTX and CS, dose of MTX and CS, levels of alanine aminotransferase and aspartate aminotransferase, immunoglobulin G level, neutrophil counts, and lymphoid cell counts were not associated with the reactivation of HBV DNA replication. The four variables extracted from the stepwise analysis were then entered as predictors of HBV DNA replication in a multivariate logistic regression model to determine their independent importance. The results of this model are shown in table 4. Predictive capacity was recognized for the use of tacrolimus hydrate only.

A recent study investigated 244 HBsAg-negative lymphoma patients receiving cytotoxic chemotherapy [13]. Reactivation of hepatitis B developed following therapy in 8 of these 244 patients (3.3%). Patients appeared to have a greater tendency to develop fulminant hepatic failure (3 of 8 patients, 37.5%). Direct DNA sequencing results confirmed that all 8 patients showed reactivation of hepatitis B from resolved hepatitis B. These patients were initially HBsAg-negative, and HBsAb- and/or HBcAb-positive, and serum liver enzyme levels were not elevated. At the time of hepatitis B reactivation, these patients became HBsAg positive. This change was associated with a more than 100-fold increase in serum HBV DNA levels, which occurred before the elevation of serum transaminases [13].

CD4+ T-helper cells may contribute to the control of HBV infection primarily by facilitating the induction and maintenance of HBV-specific cytotoxic T lymphocytes (CTL). MTX and

Case	Age (years)	RA disease duration (months)	Biologic agent	MTX (mg/week)	DMARDs	Prednisolone (mg/day)	HBV (log copies/ml)	Entecavir	Final status of HBV DNA	Time between emergence of HBV DNA and its disappearance (months)	ALT (U/L)
1	77	35	tocilizumab[a]	6	none	none	2.0	none	DNA negative	1	27
2	65	53	etanercept	none	none	2	5.0	yes	DNA negative	5	20
3	46	120	etanercept	8	tacrolimus 1 mg/day	none	3.7	yes	DNA negative	1	30
4	49	60	etanercept	none	bucillamine 200 mg/day	none	7.4	yes	DNA negative	18	20
5[b]	60	36	etanercept	none	leflunomide 10 mg/day	3mg	2.0	none	DNA negative	1	25
	61	48	adalimumab	2	tacrolimus 1mg/day	3mg	2.1	yes	DNA negative	1	25
6	75	18	etanercept	8	none	6	2.4	yes	DNA negative	2	26
7	74	19	none	7.5	none	5	3.0	yes	DNA negative	2	14
8	84	162	rituximab	7.5	tacrolimus 1mg/day	30	2.2	none			22
9	74	73	none	8	bucillamine 200 mg/day	4	2.1	yes	DNA negative	1	11
10	69	180	abatacept	8		2.5	7.8	yes	DNA positive		21
11	60	224	abatacept[c]	7.5			4.1	yes	DNA negative	1	13
12	66	317	etanercept		bucillamine 200 mg/day		2.2	yes	DNA negative	1	6
13	72	2		7.5		25	2.1	yes	DNA negative	1	18

RA, rheumatoid arthritis; *MTX*, methotrexate; *DMARDs*, disease-modifying antirheumatic drugs; *ALT*, alanine aminotransferase

[a]This patient sequentially received 3 biologic agents: infliximab, etanercept, and tocilizumab.

[b]This patient had HBV-DNA reactivation twice.

[c]This patient sequentially received 2 biologic agents: etanercept, and abatacept.

Table 2. Demographic, clinical, and laboratory characteristics of patients with HBV replication

Variables	Number of patients[a]		*P* value	HR (95% CI)
	HBV replication (+)	HBV replication (-)		
Total	13	144		
Biologic agent	10 (76.9%)	52 (36.1%)	0.006	2.1 (1.5–3.1)
Adalimumab	1 (7.7%)	8 (5.6%)	0.550	1.4 (0.2–10.2)
Etanercept	8 (61.5%)	32 (22.2%)	0.005	2.8 (1.6–4.7)
Infliximab	1 (7.7%)	17 (11.8%)	1.000	0.7 (0.1–4.5)
Tocilizumab	1 (7.7%)	7 (4.9%)	0.507	1.6 (0.2–11.9)
Abatacept	2 (15.4%)	3 (20.8%)	0.055	7.4 (1.4–40.3)
Rituximab	1 (7.7%)	0	0.08	
Methotrexate	10 (76.9%)	67 (46.5%)	0.044	1.7 (1.2–2.3)
mean dose	7.1 ± 1.9 mg/week	6.8 ± 1.9 mg/week	0.707	
Corticosteroids	6 (46.2%)	57 (39.6%)	0.770	1.2 (0.6–2.2)
mean dose	12.7 ± 15.6 mg/day	5.7 ± 5.0 mg/day	0.533	
High dose of corticosteroids (≥0.5mg $\cdot$kg^{-1} $\cdot$day^{-1})	2 (15.4%)	2 (1.4%)	0.035	11.1 (1.7–72.3)
Sulfasalazine	1 (7.7%)	36 (25.0%)	0.303	0.3 (0.0–2.1)
Bucillamine	3 (23.1%)	29 (20.1%)	0.729	1.1 (0.4–3.3)
Tacrolimus hydrate	4 (30.8%)	8 (5.6%)	0.010	5.5 (1.9–15.9)
Sodium aurothiomalate	1 (7.7%)	5 (3.5%)	0.410	2.2 (0.3–17.6)
Leflunomide	1 (7.7%)	2 (1.4%)	0.230	5.5 (0.5–57.1)
D-penicillamine	0	2 (1.4%)	1.000	
Actarit	0	1 (0.7%)	1.000	
Auranofin	0	7 (4.9%)	1.000	
Cyclosporine	0	1 (0.7%)	1.000	
Minocycline hydrochloride	0	2 (1.4%)	1.000	
Cyclophosphamide	0	1 (0.7%)	1.000	

[a]Values are given as the number of patients taking a drug; patients can take more than one drug and can switch to another biologic agent
HR, hazard ratio; *95% CI*, 95% confidence interval

Table 3. Number of patients using concomitant drugs related to rheumatoid arthritis during the study [comparing hepatitis B virus (HBV) replication-positive patients with HBV replication-negative patients]

	Odds Ratio (95% CI)	p value
Tacrolimus hydrate	11.1 (2.0-50.6)	0.0015
Sulfasalazine	0.3 (0.0-1.7)	0.2604
Abatacept	1.5 (0.1-17.4)	0.7726
immunoglobulin G	1.9 (0.0-160.3)	0.7572

95% CI, 95% confidence interval

Table 4. Logistic regression model predicting hepatitis B virus replication in rheumatoid arthritis patients

tacrolimus hydrate may inhibit the function of CTL that controls HBV proliferation, and trigger reactivation of HBV-DNA replication [20, 21]. CS has shown to have direct stimulatory effects on HBV replication, in addition to indirect effects mediated via generalized immune system suppression [4].

TNF is a proinflammatory cytokine that plays a key role in host responses to several types of infection and other stimuli [22]. Various observations have strongly implicated TNF in the pathogenesis of RA and ankylosing spondylitis (AS), and increased TNF production propagates rheumatoid synovitis, promotes osteoclast formation, and results in characteristic bone and joint destruction [23]. TNFA significantly affects the current treatment of RA and AS [24] but is associated with adverse reactions such as reactivation of tuberculosis [25]. Studies regarding the safety of TNFA with chronic viral infection are limited. Several theories exist regarding how TNF inhibitors reactivate hepatitis B. Elevated TNF levels are seen in both the serum and hepatocytes of patients with chronic hepatitis B [26], and are secreted by HBV-specific CTL [27]. TNF has biological activity and an amino acid sequence similar to lymphotoxin, which inhibits HBV replication [28]. Infected cells are also reported to be selectively killed by TNF [33]. TNF acts to suppress HBV DNA replication by reducing intracellular HBV transcription [29]. Animal studies have shown that TNF-knockout mice have defects in the proliferative capacity of HBV-specific CTL [30], suggesting that TNF plays a role in clearing or controlling HBV [30, 31]. Moreover, HBV-specific CTL inhibits HBV gene expression by secreting antiviral cytokines, such as interferon γ and TNF, and inducing apoptosis in HBV-infected hepatocytes [32, 33].

With increasing use of biologic agents such as TNFA, anti-IL-6 receptor, anti-CD20 [34], and anti-CD28, reactivation of HBV DNA replication in patients with resolved HBV will likely increase, particularly in endemic areas. Among patients who are scheduled to receive MTX, CS, tacrolimus hydrate, and biologic agents, patients who are HBsAg negative should be further screened for anti-HBc and anti-HBs.

4. Acknowledgments

We would like to thank the members of the Contract Research Organization for their assistance in collecting patient data.

Conflict of interest statement

None

5. References

[1] Lok AS, McMahon BJ. Chronic hepatitis B: update 2009. Hepatology 2009; 50: 61-2.
[2] Di Bisceglie AM. Hepatitis B and hepatocellular carcinoma. Hepatology 2009; 49: S56-60.
[3] Hoofnagle JH. Reactivation of hepatitis B. Hepatology 2009; 49 :S156-65.
[4] Calabrese LH, Zein NN, Vassilopoulos D. Hepatitis B virus (HBV) reactivation with immunosuppressive therapy in rheumatic diseases: assessment and preventive strategies. Ann Rheum Dis 2006; 65: 983-9.
[5] Zingarelli S, Airò P, Frassi M, Bazzani C, Scarsi M, Puoti M. Prophylaxis and therapy of HBV infection in 20 patients treated with disease modifying antirheumatic drugs or with biological agents for rheumatic diseases. Reumatismo 2008; 60: 22-7.
[6] Ostuni P, Botsios C, Punzi L, Sfriso P, Todesco S. Hepatitis B reactivation in a chronic hepatitis B surface antigen carrier with rheumatoid arthritis treated with infliximab and low dose methotrexate. Ann Rheum Dis 2003; 62: 686-7.
[7] Cansu DU, Kalifoglu T, Korkmaz C. Short-term course of chronic hepatitis B and C under treatment with etanercept associated with different disease modifying antirheumatic drugs without antiviral prophylaxis. J Rheumatol 2008; 35: 421-4.
[8] Zoulim F. New insight on hepatitis B virus persistence from the study of intrahepatic viral cccDNA. J Hepatol 2005; 42: 302-8.
[9] Rehermann B, Ferrari C, Pasquinelli C, Chisari FV. The hepatitis B virus persists for decades after patients' recovery from acute viral hepatitis despite active maintenance of a cytotoxic T-lymphocyte response. Nat Med 1996; 2: 1104-8.
[10] Yuki N, Nagaoka T, Yamashiro M, Mochizuki K, Kaneko A, Yamamoto K, Omura M, et al. Long-term histologic and virologic outcomes of acute self-limited hepatitis B. Hepatology 2003; 37: 1172-9.
[11] Yeo W, Johnson PJ. Diagnosis, prevention and management of hepatitis B virus reactivation during anticancer therapy. Hepatology 2006;43:209-20.
[12] Kitano K, Kobayashi H, Hanamura M, Furuta K, Ueno M, Rokuhara A, et al. Fulminant hepatitis after allogenic bone marrow transplantation caused by reactivation of hepatitis B virus with gene mutations in the core promoter region. Eur J Haematol 2006;77:255-8.
[13] Hui CK, Cheung WW, Zhang HY, Au WY, Yueng YH, Leung AY, et al. Kinetics and risk of de novo hepatitis B infection in HBsAg-negative patients undergoing cytotoxic chemotherapy. Gastroenterology 2006; 131: 59-68.
[14] Sera T, Hiasa Y, Michitaka K, Konishi I, Matsuura K, Tokumoto Y, et al. Anti-HBs-positive liver failure due to hepatitis B virus reactivation induced by rituximab. Intern Med 2006; 45: 721-4.
[15] Esteve M, Saro C, González-Huix F, Suarez F, Forné M, Viver JM. Chronic hepatitis B reactivation following infliximab therapy in Crohn's disease patients: need for primary prophylaxis. Gut 2004; 53: 1363-5
[16] Ito S, Nakazono K, Murasawa A, Mita Y, Hata K, Saito N, ea al. Development of fulminant hepatitis B (precore variant mutant type) after the discontinuation of low-dose methotrexate therapy in a rheumatoid arthritis patient. Arthritis Rheum 2001; 44: 339-42.
[17] Montiel PM, Solis JA, Chirinos JA, a Casis B, Sánchez F, Rodríguez S. Hepatitis B virus reactivation during therapy with etanercept in an HBsAg-negative and anti-HBs-positive patient. Liver Int 2008; 28: 718-20.

[18] Madonia S, Orlando A, Scimeca D, Olivo M, Rossi F, Cottone M. Occult hepatitis B and infliximab-induced HBV reactivation. Inflamm Bowel Dis 2007; 13: 508-9.
[19] Sasaki S, Sato S, Kano Y, Akaike A, Omura T, Sato T, et al. Validity of COBAS TaqMan HBV Test v2.0. Igaku to Yakugaku 2009; 61: 787-795 (in Japanese)
[20] Kuwano K, Arai S. The inhibitory effect of FK506 on cytotoxic T-lymphocyte killing. Immunol Lett. 1994; 43: 153-7.
[21] Strauss G, Osen W, Debatin KM. Induction of apoptosis and modulation of activation and effector function in T cells by immunosuppressive drugs. Clin Exp Immunol. 2002; 128: 255-66.
[22] Bradley JR. TNF-mediated inflammatory disease. J Pathol 2008; 214: 149-60
[23] Harris ED Jr. Rheumatoid arthritis. Pathophysiology and implications for therapy. N Engl J Med 1990; 322:1277-89.
[24] Gibbons LJ, Hyrich KL. Biologic therapy for rheumatoid arthritis: clinical efficacy and predictors of response. BioDrug 2009; 23: 111-24.
[25] Winthrop KL. Risk and prevention of tuberculosis and other serious opportunistic infections associated with the inhibition of tumor necrosis factor. Nat Clin Pract Rheumatol 2006; 2: 602-10.
[26] Daniels HM, Meager A, Eddleston AL, Alexander GJ, Williams R. Spontaneous production of tumour necrosis factor alpha and interleukin-1 beta during interferon-alpha treatment of chronic HBV infection. Lancet 1990; 335: 875-7.
[27] Fang JW, Shen WW, Meager A, Lau JY. Activation of the tumor necrosis factor-alpha system in the liver in chronic hepatitis B virus infection. Am J Gastroenterol 1996; 91: 748-53.
[28] Stoop JN, Woltman AM, Biesta PJ, Kusters JG, Kuipers EJ, Janssen HL, van der Molen RG. Tumor necrosis factor alpha inhibits the suppressive effect of regulatory T cells on the hepatitis B virus-specific immune response. Hepatology 2007; 46: 699-705.
[29] Wong GH, Goeddel DV. Tumour necrosis factors alpha and beta inhibit virus replication and synergize with interferons. Nature 1986; 323: 819-22.
[30] Kasahara S, Ando K, Saito K, Sekikawa K, Ito H, Ishikawa T, Ohnishi H, et al. Lack of tumor necrosis factor alpha induces impaired proliferation of hepatitis B virus-specific cytotoxic T lymphocytes. J Virol 2003; 77: 2469-76.
[31] Ganem D, Prince AM. Hepatitis B virus infection--natural history and clinical consequences. N Engl J Med 2004; 350: 1118-29.
[32] Guidotti LG, Ishikawa T, Hobbs MV, Matzke B, Schreiber R, Chisari FV. Intracellular inactivation of the hepatitis B virus by cytotoxic T lymphocytes. Immunity 1996; 4: 25-36.
[33] Marinos G, Naoumov NV, Rossol S, Torre F, Wong PY, Gallati H, Portmann B, et al. Tumor necrosis factor receptors in patients with chronic hepatitis B virus infection. Gastroenterology 1995; 108: 1453-63.
[34] Yeo W, Chan TC, Leung NW, Lam WY, Mo FK, Chu MT, Chan HL, et al · Hepatitis B virus reactivation in lymphoma patients with prior resolved hepatitis B undergoing anticancer therapy with or without rituximab. J Clin Oncol 2009; 27: 605-11.

27

Oncogenic Aspects of HPV Infections of the Female Genital Tract

Josko Zekan[1], Maja Sirotkovic-Skerlev[2] and Mihael Skerlev[3]
[1]*Department of Gynecologic Oncology, University Medical School, Zagreb,*
[2]*Department of Pathophysiology, University Medical School, Zagreb,*
[3]*Department of Dermatology and Venereology, University Medical School, Zagreb,*
Croatia

1. Introduction

Genital human papillomavirus (HPV) infection is a most common sexually transmitted infection among women (Muñoz et al., 2003). The immune system effectively repels most HPV infections, and is associated with strong localized cell mediated immune responses. However, approximately ten percent of individuals develop a persistent infection, with risk of development of high-grade precursor lesions and eventually invasive carcinoma (Stanley, 2006). The causal role of HPV in all cancers of the uterine cervix has been firmly established (zur Hausen, 1999; Walboomers et al., 1999; Bosch et al., 2008). Most cancers of the vulva and vagina are also induced by oncogenic HPV types. In precancerous lesions, most HPV genomes persist in an episomal state whereas, in many high-grade lesions and carcinomas, genomes are found integrated into the host chromosome. Two viral genes, E6 and E7, are invariably expressed in HPV-positive cancer cells. Their gene products are known to inactivate the major tumour suppressors, p53 and retinoblastoma protein (pRB), respectively. In addition, E6 oncoprotein is also capable to up regulate the expression of inhibitors of apoptosis, and E6 and E7 cooperate to effectively immortalise primary epithelial cells. Tumour formation is not an inevitable consequence of viral infection; it rather reflects the multi-step nature of oncogenesis where each step constitutes an independent (reversible or irreversible) genetic change that cumulatively contributes to deregulation of cell cycle, cell growth and survival.

2. Human papillomaviruses

Human papillomaviruses are a large family of small double-stranded DNA viruses which infect squamous epithelia (or cells with the potential for squamous maturation). Papillomaviruses are classified by genotype, and at present, about 130 types have been identified by sequences of the gene encoding the major capsid protein L1 (de Villiers et al.; 2004; Bravo et al., 2010, Van Doorslaer el al., 2011). HPVs can be classified into high or low-risk types depending upon their oncogenic potential. High-risk genotypes 16 and 18 are associated with 70% of cervical carcinoma (Muñoz et al., 2006), and about 80% HPV positive vulval and vaginal carcinoma (Madeleine et al., 1997; Daling et al., 2002; Hampl et al., 2006). Low-risk types 6 and 11 have been isolated in 90% of genital warts (Aubin et al., 2008).

2.1 HPV genome organization

Virus particles consist of about 7900 base-pairs (7.9 kbp) long circular DNA molecules wrapped into a protein shell. The HPV genome can be functionally divided into two regions: Upstream Regulatory Region (URR) and Open Reading Frames (ORFs). URR does not code for proteins but contains cis-elements required for the regulation of the gene expression, replication of the genome, and its packaging into virus particles. ORFs can be divided into the Early Region (E), necessary for the replication, cellular transformation and the control of viral transcription, and Late Region (L) that codes for the capsid proteins that comprises the outer coat of the virus (Figure 1).

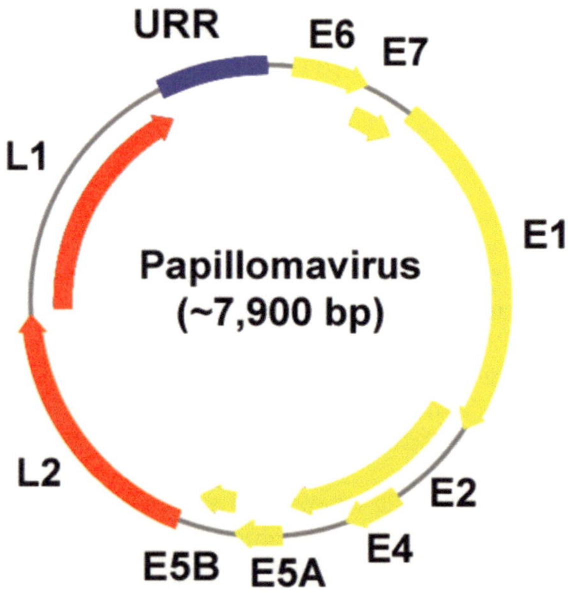

Fig. 1. Schematic presentation of the HPV genome. The non-coding region is the upstream regulatory region (URR). The open reading frames (ORFs) encode the early (E), and late (L) viral proteins. (Adapted from Muñoz et al., 2006).

Within the Early Regions (E) it is possible to distinguish different genes with specific functions. E1 and E2 genes have an important role in basal DNA replication. During viral persistence, the immune system keeps the infection in this state. E2 participates in the regulation of LCR (low-copy repeats) transcriptions, and decreases the expression of E6 and E7. The E4 gene codes for one family of small proteins involved in the transformation of the host cell by producing alterations of the mitotic signals and interacting with keratin. E5 decreases intercellular communication and isolates the transformed cells and interacts with the growth factor's receptors and encourages cellular proliferation. It also stimulates the expression of E6 and E7. E6 is oncogenic, stimulating the growth and transformation of the host cell by the inhibition of protein p53's normal tumour-suppressor function. E7 also acts as an oncogene, inducing cellular proliferation by inhibition of protein pRb. Within the Late Region (L), it is possible to distinguish the L1 gene, which codes for the major capsid protein and can form virus-like particles and L2, which codes for the minor capsid protein (Jones & Wells, 2006).

2.2 Natural history of genital HPV infection

Genital HPV infections are a very common sexually transmitted infection among women with a lifetime risk of 50-80% and have a peak prevalence between ages 18 and 30 (Koutsky, 1997). Most of these infections clear spontaneously. Seventy five per cent of infections clear within a year, and individuals with suboptimal immune responses may be at increased risk of persistent HPV infection and associated malignancy (Stanley, 2006). At present, in the female genital tract about 40 genotypes of HPV can be isolated; nevertheless only 15 types are usually associated with development of carcinoma. Genotypes 16 and 18 have been clearly shown to be predominant carcinogenic human viral agents, but in the majority of cases the presence of HPV alone is not sufficient for the development of neoplasm and different cofactors have been identified: tobacco, other sexually transmitted diseases (e.g. HIV), conditions of temporary immunodeficiency, alterations of hormonal status, beta-carotene deficiency, repeated local traumas, promiscuity and some modalities of sexual behaviour (Au, 2005; Cotton et al., 2007).

2.3 HPV life cycle

HPVs are perfectly adapted to their natural host tissue, the differentiating epithelial cells of skin or mucosa and exploit the cellular machinery for their own purposes. HPVs are undergoing a complete life cycle only in fully differentiated squamous epithelium. These viruses infect the basal cell layer where they establish their small double-stranded DNA genome, as a circular extra-chromosomal element or episome in the nucleus of infected cells. Following the entry into the suprabasal layer, the viral genome replicates and in the upper layers of epidermis complete viral particles are released (Doorbar, 2005). Existence of the viral genome in the infected cell is central to the life cycle of papillomaviruses and their associated pathologies. Maintenance of the viral genome requires the activity of E1 (the replicative helicase of papillomavirus) and E2, the two viral proteins necessary for replication of the HPV genome in conjunction with the host cell DNA replication machinery. As an initiator protein E1 acts both as a DNA binding protein to recognize the viral origin of DNA replication and subsequently as a helicase to unwind the origin and the DNA ahead of the replication fork. In lesions containing HPV episomes, the viral E2 protein directly represses early gene expression as part of a mechanism to regulate copy number. Integration of viral DNA usually disrupts E2 expression, leading to the deregulated expression of early viral genes, including E6 and E7. The expression of viral gene products is closely regulated as the infected basal cell migrates towards the epithelial surface. Genome amplification, which is necessary for the production of infectious virions, is prevented until the levels of viral replication proteins rise, and depends on the co-expression of several viral proteins. Viral persistence leads to clonal progression of the persistently infected epithelium. Events which are still not completely understood lead infected cells to malignant transformation. Tumour formation is not an inevitable consequence of viral infection; it rather reflects the multi-step nature of oncogenesis where each step constitutes an independent (reversible or irreversible) genetic change that cumulatively contributes to deregulation of cell cycle, cell growth and survival (Bosch et al., 2008).

3. HPV DNA replication

The papillomaviruses DNA replication is totally dependent upon the cellular DNA synthesis machinery. The problem for the virus is that the necessary cellular DNA polymerases and replication factors are only available in dividing cells. However, the virus replicates in non-dividing cells. To solve this problem, HPV encodes proteins that, in the context of the viral life cycle, reactivate cellular DNA synthesis in non-cycling cells, inhibit apoptosis, and delay the differentiation program of the infected keratinocyte, creating an environment permissive for viral DNA replication (Münger & Howley, 2002). The precise details by which this is achieved are not completely understood, but the relevant viral genes are E6 and E7. Rarely, by-product of high-risk HPV replication is the deregulation of growth control in the infected cell and the development of cancer (Swan et al., 1994; zur Hausen, 2002). The HPV episome is replicated by the viral E1 and E2 proteins together with the host DNA replication machinery. E1 acts both as a DNA binding protein to recognize the viral origin and subsequently as a helicase to unwind the DNA ahead of the replication. Structure-function studies have indicated that E1 is a modular protein comprised of a C-terminal enzymatic domain with ATPase/helicase activity, a replication origin DNA-binding domain located in the centre of the protein and the N-terminal regulatory domain. E1 binds to DNA with little sequence specificity. In vitro and in vivo, binding of E1 specifically to the origin is facilitated by its interaction with E2, a transcription/replication factor that binds with high affinity to sites in the viral origin. Assembly of a ternary complex between E1, E2 and the origin serves as a starting point for the assembly of a larger E1 complex that has unwinding activity, most likely a double hexamer necessary for bidirectional unwinding. E1 interacts with DNA replication factors, including the polymerase α-primase and the single-stranded binding protein RPA (Replication Protein A), to promote viral DNA replication (Thierry et al., 2004).

3.1 Inhibitors of HPV DNA replication

Interaction between the E2 protein and E1 helicase of human papillomaviruses is essential for the initiation of viral DNA replication. Research performed by Wang and colleagues (2004) led to the identification of the first small molecule inhibitors of HPV DNA replication. Characterization of their mechanism of action showed that this class of inhibitors binds to E2 and prevents its interaction with the E1 helicase. These inhibitors defined a previously unrecognized small-molecule binding pocket on E2. This class of inhibitors was found to antagonize specifically the E1-E2 interaction in vivo and to inhibit HPV DNA replication in transiently infected cells. These results highlighted for the first time the potential of the E1-E2 interaction as a small molecule antiviral target for the treatment of HPV infections (White et al., 2011). These inhibitors also provided a rare example of a class of small molecules that can antagonize a protein-protein interaction.

4. HPV-induced oncogenesis

The female genital tract, a continuum of squamous epithelium from the vulva to the cervix, is commonly infected by human papillomavirus. The outcome of HPV infection depends on the immune response, the viral genotype (low-risk or high-risk/oncogenic) and the site of infection (the cervical squamo-columnar junction is more susceptible to HPV disease). The key role of HPV in most cancers of the female lower genital tract has been firmly established biologically and epidemiologically (Herrero et al., 2000; Daling et al., 2002; Böhmer et al., 2003; Moscicki et al., 2006).

4.1 Malignant transformation of the lower genital tract

The cervical cancer is marked by a premalignant phase of various grades of cervical intraepithelial neoplasm (CIN) which is a genetically unstable lesion and is characterized by a spectrum of histological abnormalities. HPV viral integration into the host genomic DNA is associated with progressive genetic instability, and these events play a fundamental role in the progression from low-grade (CIN1) to high-grade (CIN2/3) lesions, and eventually to invasive cervical cancer (ICC). In longitudinal natural history studies, the time from the detection of high-risk HPV to the development of CIN3 is 3–5 years (Herrero et al., 2000), but the progression to ICC takes a further 10–20 years (Moscicki et al., 2006), and probably only 30–40% of CIN3 actually progress to invasive carcinoma (McCredie et al., 2008). Most cancers of the vulva and vagina in younger women are also induced by oncogenic HPV types (Madeleine et al., 1997; Hampl et al., 2006). These cancers are preceded by high-grade vulval intraepithelial neoplasia (VIN2/3) and vaginal intraepithelial neoplasia (VaIN2/3). Compared with cervical cancer, vulval and vaginal cancers develop less frequently.

4.2 Molecular basis of HPV-induced oncogenesis

The HPV DNA usually exists as extrachromosomal plasmid, mostly as a monomeric circular molecule in benign cervical precursor lesions. However, in cervical cancer cells the HPV DNA is integrated in the host genome. During HPV DNA integration, the viral genome breaks in the E1/E2 region. The break leads to the loss of the E2, which encodes proteins including one that inhibits the transcription of the E6 and E7 regions, resulting in increased expression of E6 and E7 oncogenic proteins (Moon et al., 2001). The proteins coded by these genes are multifunctional and interfere with important cell cycle regulatory proteins. Expression of viral oncogenes is tightly controlled in non-differentiated keratinocytes by at least two signalling cascades, one operative at the functional level and the other at the transcriptional level. Integration of the viral DNA could occur, resulting in increased expression of E6 and E7. Additionally, mutations or methylation of host DNA could occur that abrogate the transcriptional control of differentiation and viral gene expression; there is evidence for both of these mechanisms (Pett & Coleman, 2007; Kalantari et al., 2004). The oncoproteins E6 and E7 interact with many cellular proteins and change fundamental cellular functions like cell cycle regulation, telomere maintenance, susceptibility to apoptosis, intercellular adhesion and regulation of the immune response. These effects are in accordance with the essential changes in cell physiology that are acquired during tumour development and that have been proposed by Hanahan & Weinberg (2000). Evading the immune system surveillance has been recognized as an additional basic feature of malignant growth (Katz et al., 2008).

4.3 Regulation of the cell cycle

Maintenance of genetic integrity from one generation to the next requires the accurate replication of chromosomes during the S-phase and their faithful segregation during mitosis. The protein p53 (Figure 2) is know as the "genome's guardian" (Lane, 1992) and in the case of DNA damage, p53 can provoke the arrest of cellular division to assure the time necessary for DNA repair.

If damage can not be repaired, p53 is able to induce the programmed cellular death (apoptosis) and prevent the propagation of DNA damage in the subsequent generation of cells. The product of another tumour suppressor gene, pRb acts as a repressor of E2F transcription factor (Wu et al., 2000). E2F regulates various genes including those involved in the progression of the cell cycle (the G1-S transition). By binding E2F, pRb prevents the entry into the S phase, providing the time for checking genome integrity (Figure 3). Oncoproteins E6 and E7 cooperatively disrupt the functions of p53 and pRb, with profound changes in the cell cycle regulation (Vousden, 1993; Tungteakkhun & Duerksen-Hughes, 2008). Furthermore, E6 and E7 proteins can provoke directly DNA mutations of the host cell (Havre et al., 1995; Reznikoff et al., 1996; Moody & Laimins, 2010). As an aberration of virus infection, constant activity of the viral proteins E6 and E7 leads to increasing genomic instability, accumulation of gene mutations, further loss of cell-growth control and ultimately cancer (Münger et al., 1992; Ishiji, 2000).

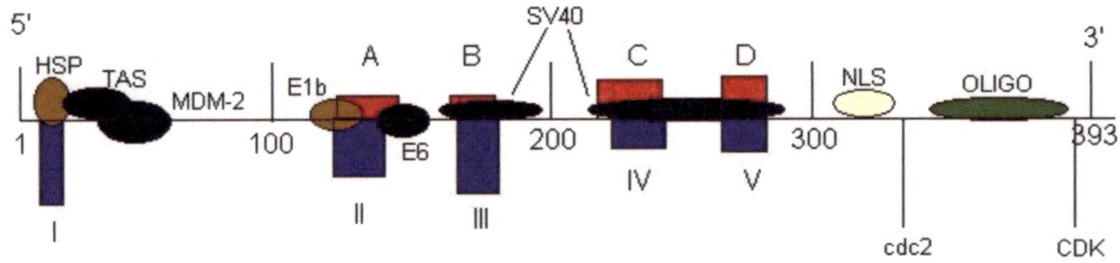

Fig. 2. Structural features of the p53 tumour suppressor gene. The transcription activation site (TAS), heat shock protein binding site (HSP), SV40 large T-antigen binding sites (SV40), adenovirus E1b and papillomavirus E6 binding sites, cellular Mdm2 binding site, nuclear localization signal (NLS), oligomerization domain (OLIGO) and phosphorylation sites (cdc2 and CDK) are indicated. The five evolutionarily conserved domains are labeled HCD I - V and the hot spot regions are HSR A-D (Adapted from Mietz et al., 1992).

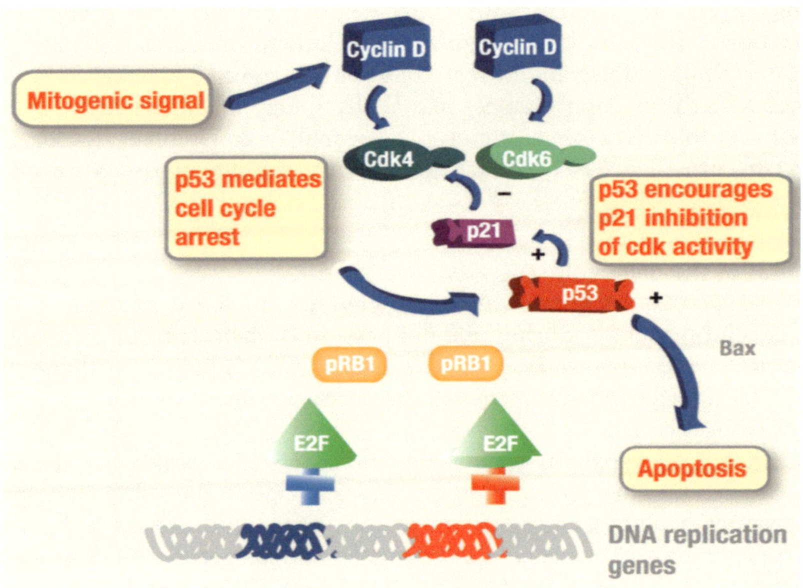

Fig. 3. Regulation of cell cycle: the role of p53 and pRb

4.3.1 Oncoprotein E6 functions

HPV 16 E6 is a 151 amino acid protein with two zinc finger domains. E6 is one of the primary oncogenes of the virus (Rapp & Chen, 1998; Fan & Chen, 2004). E6 together with E7 causes immortalization of cells and plays important roles in malignant transformation. Oncoprotein E6 interacts with numerous cellular proteins (Table 1).

Oncoprotein E6 functions	Investigators, year
Cell immortalization	Band et al., 1990
Binding of E6-AP results in degradation of p53	Tommasino et al., 2003
Antiapoptic effect	Thomas & Banks, 1998
Chromosomal destabilization	White et al., 1994
Foreign DNA integration	Kessis et al., 1996
Enhancement of DNA mutagenicity	Havre et al., 1995
Activation of telomerase	Klingelhutz et al., 1996
Blockade of interferon	Ronco et al., 1998
E2F-regulated mitotic genes	Thierry et al., 2004
E6 I/E6 II gene expression	Moodley et al., 2003

Table 1. Identified functions of the high-risk HPV oncoprotein E6

E6 targets p53 through recruitment of a cellular E3 ubiquitin ligase - E6 associated protein (E6AP). This trimeric complex leads to p53 degradation by ubiquitin-proteosomal pathway. Besides targeting it for degradation, E6 is capable of binding directly to p53, interfering with its DNA-binding activity (Lechner & Laimins, 1994). In addition, E6 protein blocks apoptosis, alters the transcription machinery and disturbs intercellular interactions, a crucial step towards malignancy. Another important target for E6 is the group of PDZ proteins (Wise-Draper & Wells, 2008). The name is related to the first three members identified: PSD-95 (a post-synaptic density signalling protein), Dlg (the *Drosophila* disc large protein) and ZO1 (the zonula occludens 1 protein with functional roles in epithelial polarity). Only high-risk E6 associates with PDZ proteins. These proteins play important role in cell signalling, cell adhesion and tight-junction integrity (Fanning & Anderson, 1999). Experimental evidence indicates that the interaction of E6 with PDZ proteins is necessary for development of epithelial hyperplasia (Nguyen, 2003).

4.3.2 Oncoprotein E7 functions

HPV 16 E7, a nuclear protein of 98 amino acids, has a casein kinase II phosphorylation site at serine residues 31 and 32 (Firzlaff et al., 1991). E7 interacts with various cellular proteins, most of which are important regulators of the cell cycle, especially the transition from the G1 to S phase (Table 2).

Oncoprotein E7 functions	Investigators, year
Cell immortalization	Münger & Phelps, 1993
Activation of cyclins E and A	Zerfass et al., 1995
Inhibition of pRb-related pocket proteins	Dyson et al., 1992
Induction of apoptosis	Puthenveettil et al., 1996
Inactivation of cyclin-dependent kinase inhibitors	Jones et al., 1997
Foreign DNA integration	Kessis et al., 1996
Enhancement of DNA mutagenicity	Reznikoff et al., 1996
Degradation of tyrosine kinase	Oda et al., 1999
Chromosomal abnormalities	Pett et al., 2004
E2F-regulated mitotic genes	Thierry et al., 2004

Table 2. Identified functions of the high-risk HPV oncoprotein E7

E7 proteins interact with the members of retinoblastoma protein family: pRb, p107 and p130 (also called "pocket proteins"). Most of the pRb functions are related to the repression of the E2F transcription factor. The E7 protein directly binds pRb and targets it for degradation through the ubiquitin-dependant pathway (Boyer et al., 1996). Suppression of Rb function by E7 results in the activation of E2F, and stimulation of the cell cycle progression (Dyson, 1998). E7 is also capable of direct interaction with E2F factors and chromatin modifiers such as histone deacetylases (HDACs), what additionally affects the expression of S phase genes (Hwang et al., 2002; Brehm et al., 1999). E7 protein interacts with cyclin dependent kinases (CDK) inhibitors like p21 and p27. While E6 inhibits p21 transcription by inactivating p53, E7 inhibits p21 functions by direct binding, thus contributing to sustained activity of CDK, such as CDK2. High-risk E7 also increases the expression of CDC25A phosphatase that promotes CDK2 activation (Nguyen et al., 2002). All these effects on cell proliferation are favourable for HPV life cycle and replication but they also contribute to the uncontrolled proliferation of infected cells. Besides disrupting cell cycle control, and allowing the cell division in the presence of DNA damage, E6 and E7 are capable of directly inducing DNA damage (Moody & Laimins, 2010). Thus, in HPV infected cells a deleterious combination could be present: increased DNA damage and impaired response to DNA damage.

4.4 Telomere maintenance

While normal cells have finite numbers of doublings before they become senescent ("Hayflick limit"), malignant cells acquire limitless replicative potential (Hanahan & Weinberg, 2000). The immortality of malignant cells is closely related with telomere maintenance (Shay & Bacchetti, 1997; Hanahan & Weinberg, 2000). The majority of malignant cells achieve telomere maintenance by up-regulation of telomerase, an enzyme that adds hexanucleotide repeats to the 3′ end of DNA strands in the telomere regions.

Telomerase is a ribonucleoprotein complex that contains three subunits: a catalytic subunit - human telomerase reverse transcriptase (hTERT), a RNA subunit and a protein subunit (dyskerin). The expression of hTERT is proportional to telomerase activity in the cells. It has been shown that high-risk E6 protein activates transcription of hTERT. E6 in complex with E6AP or alone interacts with Myc protein (Veldman et al, 2001; Howie et al., 2009). Heterodimer Myc/Max binds to the hTERT promoter and activates its transcription. E6 also affects other hTERT activators including Sp1 which binds to the hTERT promoter and histone acetyltransferases that increase histone acetylation at the hTERT promoter (Oh et al., 2001; James et al., 2006). E6 modulates activity of hTERT repressors as well. The HPV 16 E6/E6AP complex targets hTERT repressor X box-binding protein 1-91 (NFX1-91) for polyubiquitination and degradation. E6 affects binding of two other hTERT repressors - upstream stimulating factors 1 and 2 (USF1 and USF2). Additionally, E6 directly associates with NFX123 that increases hTERT activity by several mechanisms including those on transcriptional and post-translational level (Howie et al., 2009). A second mechanism of telomere maintenance is recombination-based and is termed alternative lengthening of telomeres (ALT) pathway. It has been suggested that the E7 protein affects telomere length through the ALT pathway (Spardy et al., 2008). Thus, a cooperative effect between E6 and E7 could be achieved regarding telomere maintenance and cell immortalization. The E7 effect could be important in early cancer development while E6 might play a role in later phases of oncogenesis (Moody & Laimins, 2010). This is in accordance with the observation that high levels of hTERT expression are found in advanced cervical lesions and invasive carcinomas (Zhang et al., 2004).

4.5 Evading apoptosis

HPV has developed numerous mechanisms that block host-mediated apoptosis. These mechanisms regulate the survival of infected cells thus facilitating the HPV replication cycle. Besides blocking p53 function in regulation of apoptosis, high-risk HPV proteins interact with both extrinsic and intrinsic apoptotic pathways. The extrinsic pathway is triggered by various extracellular signals that activate "death receptors", members of the tumour necrosis factor receptor (TNFR) family. After binding the ligand death receptors form trimers and associate with adaptor molecules and initiator caspases. The result is the formation of the death inducing signalling complex (DISC). DISC activates caspase 8 which cleaves downstream caspases in the apoptotic pathway leading to cell death. High-risk E6 protein interacts with all components of the DISC complex. E6 binds to the death receptor TNFR-1 and blocks its association with adapter molecules (Filippova et al., 2002). Furthermore, E6 can accelerate the degradation of some adapter molecules like FADD and the initiator caspase-8 (Garnett et al., 2006; Howie et al., 2009). The intrinsic apoptotic pathway is activated by various intracellular stressors (DNA damage, oxidative stress and others) and includes mitochondrial permeability transition. Then pro-apoptotic signals dominate changes in mitochondrial membrane are initiated with formation of pores and release of pro-apoptotic proteins. These proteins form an apoptotic signalling complex that results in cleavage of downstream caspases (like caspase-3 and caspase-7), leading to degradation of cellular components. The E6 protein interacts with intrinsic apoptotic pathway signalling by binding Bak, a pro-apoptotic member of Bcl-2 family. E6 binds Bak and induces its degradation through the ubiquitin-proteasome pathway (Thomas & Banks, 1998). The HPV E6 protein is also capable to up regulate the expression of inhibitors of apoptosis, such as survivin and the inhibitor of apoptosis protein 2 (IAP2). The studies of

HPV E7 in regulation of apoptosis obtained variable results; both, anti-apoptotic and pro-apoptotic effects have been found (Garnett & Duerksen-Hughes, 2006). HPV oncoproteins target a number of factors important for anoikis, a specific type of apoptosis that is induced by loss of cell adhesion or inappropriate cell adhesion (Valentijn et al., 2004; Chiarugi & Giannoni, 2008). High-risk HPV proteins bind or are associated with changes in expression levels of fibronectin, fibulin-1, focal adhesion kinase (FAK) and paxillin (Moody & Laimins, 2010). These interactions contribute to the capability of HPV infected cells to become resistant to anoikis and grow in the absence of anchorage to the extracellular matrix and their neighbouring cells. Anchorage independent growth is considered to be a hallmark of malignant phenotypes.

4.6 Escape from immune system surveillance

The major lines of defence against various pathogens are natural mechanical barriers, innate and adoptive immunity. Dendritic cells (DC) are highly specialized antigen presenting cells (APC) that play important roles in innate immunity and provide a link between innate and adoptive immunity. Toll-like receptors (TLR) located in the membrane or inside the DC recognize typical molecular motifs of various pathogens called pathogen-associated molecular patterns (PAMPS). Langerhans cells are main DC of the skin and mucosa, being important detectors at the site of HPV infection. Activated dendritic cells migrate to draining lymph nodes, mature during the migration to highly effective APC and present antigens to naïve T lymphocytes, thereby initiating cell-mediated responses. The activated effector (cytotoxic) cells target infected cells at the site of infection (Stanley, 2006). Indeed, in case of HPV infection in the majority of cases the virus is cleared by cell-mediated mechanisms that are clinically associated with complete remission. However, the time for clearance ranges from months to years suggesting a delay in immune response. Ten to twenty percent of infected persons do not manage to clear the HPV infection and they develop persistent infection that is associated with the risk of high-grade cervical lesions and invasive carcinoma (zur Hausen, 1996; Stanley, 2010). HPV has developed several mechanisms for evading the immune surveillance. The majority of these mechanisms contribute to evading of innate immunity that delays the adoptive immune response. Some of these mechanisms are related with the characteristics of the viral site of infection and some are related to the effects of viral oncoproteins. HPV does not have a lytic phase, and thereby does not cause cell injury that would initiate inflammation and/or immune response. There is no viraemic stage during HPV infection. Therefore both, locally and systemically there is no favourable situation for contact between HPV and the immune system. Hasan and colleagues (2007) have shown that high risk E6 and E7 proteins inhibit TLR9 transcription leading to impaired activation of the innate immune response. Additionally, high-risk proteins interact with interferon regulatory factors (IRF) required for the expression of type I interferons: E6 binds IRF-3 while E7 interacts with IRF-1 (Ronco et al., 1998; Park et al., 2000). Microarray analysis showed that high-risk proteins down-regulate the expression of IFN-inducible genes, including signal transducer and activator of transcription 1 (STAT1) (Chang & Laimins, 2000). One of the possible mechanisms that underlie this phenomenon is direct interaction of HPV 16 E7 with p48-the DNA binding component of the interferon-stimulated gene factor 3 (ISGF3) transcription complex, thus blocking the translocation of this complex to the nucleus (Barnard & McMillan, 1999). Furthermore, HPV proteins interact with the proximal components of interferon-inducible pathways. E6 binds and inhibits the function of tyrosin kinase (Tyk2), a component of the

JAK-STAT signalling pathway that mediates IFN cellular responses (Li et al., 1999). The activity of another interferon-inducible double-stranded RNA protein kinase (PKR) pathway is reduced by synergistic action of E6 and E7 (Hebner et al., 2006). Activated PKR-phosphorylates multiple products leading to various antiviral effects including the inhibition of translation. The reduced activity of this pathway results in the maintenance of viral protein synthesis. Furthermore, it has been shown that interferon induced growth arrest is dependent on p53 acetylation. Post-transcriptional modifications, like acetylation affect p53 stability and increases its transcriptional activity. Besides reducing p53 availability by targeting it for degradation, E6 interacts with p300/CBP that catalyzes acetylation of p53. E6 forms a complex with p300/CBP, thus preventing the acetylation of p53 (Hebner et al., 2007). This mechanism might contribute to the proliferation of HPV infected cells in the presence of interferon (Beglin et al., 2009).

5. Conclusions

Genital HPV infection is a most common sexually transmitted infection of viral origin among women. The association between persistent HPV infection and malignant transformation of the lower female genital tract is well established. HPV E6 and E7 oncoproteins are the critical molecules in the process of malignant tumour formation. Interacting with various cellular proteins, E6 and E7 influence fundamental cellular functions like cell cycle regulation, telomere maintenance, susceptibility to apoptosis, intercellular adhesion and regulation of immune responses. High-risk E6 and E7 cooperatively disrupt p53 and pRb functions with profound changes in the cell cycle regulation. Uncontrolled cell proliferation leads to increased risk of genetic instability; the generator of mutant phenotypes that will contribute to conferring other abnormalities and possible advantages for tumour growth. Furthermore, oncoproteins E6 and E7 are capable of directly provoking DNA damage. Usually, it takes decades for cancer to arise. Thus, cervical carcinogenesis is a multifactorial process involving genetic, environmental, hormonal and immunological factors in addition to HPV infection.

6. References

Au, WW. (2005). Life style, environmental and genetic susceptibility to cervical cancer. *Toxicology,* May 20, Vol.198, No.1-3, pp. 117-20, PMID: 15138035

Aubin, F.; Prétet, JL.; Jacquard, AC.; Saunier, M.; Carcopino, X.; Jaroud, F.; Pradat, P.; Soubeyrand, B.; Leocmach, Y.; Mougin, C. & Riethmuller, D. (2008). EDiTH Study Group. Human papillomavirus genotype distribution in external acuminata condylomata: a Large French National Study (EDiTH IV). *Clin Infect Dis,* Sep 1, Vol.47, No. 5, pp. 610-5, PMID: 18637758

Band, V.; Zajchowski, D.; Kulesa, V. & Sager, R. (1990). Human papilloma virus DNAs immortalize normal human mammary epithelial cells and reduce their growth factor requirements. *Proc Natl Acad Sci USA,* Jan, Vol.87, No.1, pp. 463-7, PMID: 2153303

Barnard,P. & McMillan, NA. (1999). The human papillomavirus E7 oncoprotein abrogates signaling mediated by interferon-alpha. *Virology,* Jul 5, Vol.259, No.2, pp. 305-13, PMID: 10388655

Beglin, M.; Melar-New, M. & Laimins, L. (2009). Human papillomaviruses and the interferon response. *J Interferon Cytokine Res*, Sep, Vol.29, No.9, pp. 629-35, PMID: 19715460

Böhmer, G.; van den Brule, AJ.; Brummer, O.; Meijer, CL. & Petry, KU. (2003). No confirmed case of human papillomavirus DNA-negative cervical intraepithelial neoplasia grade 3 or invasive primary cancer of the uterine cervix among 511 patients. *Am J Obstet Gynecol*, Jul, Vol.189, No.1, pp. 118-20, PMID: 12861148

Bosch, FX.; Burchell, AN.; Schiffman, M.; Giuliano, AR.; de Sanjose, S.; Bruni, L.; Tortolero-Luna, G.; Kjaer, SK. &Muñoz, N. (2008). Epidemiology and natural history of human papillomavirus infections and type-specific implications in cervical neoplasia. *Vaccine*, Aug 19, Vol.26, Suppl.10, K1-16, PMID: 18847553

Boyer, SN.; Wazer, DE. & Band, V. (1996). E7 protein of human papilloma virus-16 induces degradation of retinoblastoma protein through the ubiquitin-proteasome pathway. *Cancer Res*, Oct 15, Vol.56, No.20, pp. 4620-4, PMID: 8840974

Bravo, IG.; de Sanjosé, S. & Gottschling, M. (2010). The clinical importance of understanding the evolution of papillomaviruses. *Trends Microbiol*, Oct, Vol.18, No.10, pp. 432-8, PMID: 20739182

Brehm, A.; Nielsen, SJ.; Miska, EA.; McCance DJ.; Reid JL.; Bannister, AJ. & Kouzarides, T. (1999). The E7 oncoprotein associates with Mi2 and histone deacetylase activity to promote cell growth. *EMBO J*, May 4, Vol.18, No.9, pp. 2449-58, PMID: 10228159

Chang, YE. & Laimins, LA. (2000). Microarray analysis identifies interferon-inducible genes and Stat-1 as major transcriptional targets of human papillomavirus type 31. *J Virol*, May, Vol.74, No.9, pp. 4174-82, PMID: 10756030

Chiarugi P, & Giannoni E. (2008). Anoikis: a necessary death program for anchorage-dependent cells. *Biochem Pharmacol*, Dec 1, Vol.76, No.11, pp. 1352-64, PMID: 18708031

Cotton, SC.; Sharp, L.; Seth, R.; Masson, LF.; Little, J.; Cruickshank, ME.; Neal, K. & Waugh, N. (2007). TOMBOLA Group. Lifestyle and socio-demographic factors associated with high-risk HPV infection in UK women. *Br J Cancer*, Jul 2, Vol.97, No.1, pp. 133-9, PMID: 17519896

Daling, JR.; Madeleine, MM.; Schwartz, SM.; Shera, KA; Carter, JJ.; McKnight, B.; Porter, PL.; Galloway, DA.; McDougall, JK. & Tamimi, H. (2002). A population-based study of squamous cell vaginal cancer: HPV and cofactors. *Gynecol Oncol*, Feb, Vol.84, No.2, pp. 263-70, PMID: 11812085

de Villiers, EM.; Fauquet, C.; Broker TR.; Bernard HU. & zur Hausen H. (2004). Classification of papillomaviruses. *Virology*, Jun 20, Vol.324, No.1, pp. 17-27, PMID: 15183049

Doorbar, J. (2005). The papillomavirus life cycle. *J Clin Virol*, Mar, Vol.32, Suppl.1, S7-15, PMID: 15753007

Dyson, N. (1998). The regulation of E2F by pRB-family proteins. *Genes Dev*, Aug 1, Vol.12, No.15, pp. 2245-62, PMID: 9694791

Dyson, N.; Guida, P.; Münger, K. & Harlow E. (1992). Homologous sequences in adenovirus E1A and human papillomavirus E7 proteins mediate interaction with the same set of cellular proteins. *J Virol*, Dec, Vol.66, No.12, pp. 6893-902, PMID: 1331501

Fan, X. & Chen, JJ. (2004). Regulation of cell cycle progression and apoptosis by the papillomavirus E6 oncogene. *Crit Rev Eukaryot Gene Expr,* Vol.14, No.3, pp. 183-202, PMID: 15248815

Fanning, AS. & Anderson, JM. (1999). PDZ domains: fundamental building blocks in the organization of protein complexes at the plasma membrane. *J Clin Invest,* Mar, Vol.103, No.6, pp. 767-72, PMID: 10079096

Filippova, M.; Song, H.; Connolly, JL.; Dermody, TS. & Duerksen-Hughes, PJ. (2002). The human papillomavirus 16 E6 protein binds to tumor necrosis factor (TNF) R1 and protects cells from TNF-induced apoptosis. *J Biol Chem,* Jun 14, Vol.277, No.24, pp. 21730-9, PMID: 11934887.

Firzlaff, JM.; Lüscher, B. & Eisenman, RN. (1991). Negative charge at the casein kinase II phosphorylation site is important for transformation but not for Rb protein binding by the E7 protein of human papillomavirus type 16. *Proc Natl Acad Sci USA,* Jun 15, Vol.88, No.12, pp. 5187-91, PMID: 2052600

Garnett, TO. & Duerksen-Hughes, PJ. (2006). Modulation of apoptosis by human papillomavirus (HPV) oncoproteins. *Arch Virol,* Dec, Vol.151, No.12, pp. 2321-35, PMID: 16862386

Garnett, TO.; Filippova, M. & Duerksen-Hughes, PJ. (2006) Accelerated degradation of FADD and procaspase 8 in cells expressing human papilloma virus 16 E6 impairs TRAIL-mediated apoptosis. *Cell Death Differ,* Nov, Vol.13 No.11, pp. 1915-26. PMID: 16528386

Hampl, M.; Sarajuuri, H.; Wentzensen, N.; Bender, HG. & Kueppers, V. (2006). Effect of human papillomavirus vaccines on vulvar, vaginal, and anal intraepithelial lesions and vulvar cancer. *Obstet Gynecol,* Dec, Vol.108, No.6, pp. 1361-8, PMID: 17138767

Hanahan, D. & Weinberg, RA. (2000) The hallmarks of cancer. *Cell,* Jan 7, Vol.100, No.1, pp. 57-70, PMID: 10647931

Hasan, UA.; Bates, E.; Takeshita, F.; Biliato, A.; Accardi, R.; Bouvard, V.; Mansour, M.; Vincent, I.; Gissmann, L.; Iftner, T.; Sideri, M.; Stubenrauch, F. & Tommasino, M. (2007). TLR9 expression and function is abolished by the cervical cancer-associated human papillomavirus type 16. *J Immunol,* Mar 1, Vol.178, No.5, pp. 3186-97, PMID: 17312167

Havre, PA.; Yuan, J.; Hedrick, L.; Cho, KR. & Glazer, PM. (1995). p53 inactivation by HPV16 E6 results in increased mutagenesis in human cells. *Cancer Res,* Oct 1, Vol.55, No.19, pp. 4420-4, PMID: 7671255

Hebner, C.; Beglin, M. & Laimins, LA. (2007) Human papillomavirus E6 proteins mediate resistance to interferon-induced growth arrest through inhibition of p53 acetylation. *J Virol,* Dec, Vol.81, No.23, pp. 12740-7, PMID: 17898049

Hebner, CM.; Wilson, R.; Arder, J.; Bidder, M. & Laimins, LA. (2006). Human papillomaviruses target the double-stranded RNA protein kinase pathway. J Gen Virol, Nov, Vol.87, Pt 11, pp. 3183-93, PMID: 17030851

Herrero, R.; Hildesheim, A.; Bratti, C.; Sherman, ME.; Hutchinson, M.; Morales, J.; Balmaceda, I.; Greenberg, MD.; Alfaro, M.; Burk, RD.; Wacholder, S.; Plummer, M. & Schiffman, M. (2000). Population-based study of human papillomavirus infection and cervical neoplasia in rural Costa Rica. *J Natl Cancer Inst,* Mar 15, Vol.92, No.6, pp. 464-74, PMID: 10716964

Howie, HL.; Katzenellenbogen, RA. & Galloway, DA. (2009). Papillomavirus E6 proteins. *Virology,* Feb 20, Vol.384, No.2, pp. 324-34, PMID: 19081593

Hwang, SG.; Lee, D.; Kim, J.; Seo, T. & Choe, J. (2002). Human papillomavirus type 16 E7 binds to E2F1 and activates E2F1-driven transcription in a retinoblastoma protein-independent manner. *J Biol Chem,* Jan 25, Vol.277, No.4, pp. 2923-30, PMID: 11713253

Ishiji, T. (2000). Molecular mechanism of carcinogenesis by human papillomavirus-16. *J Dermatol,* Feb, Vol.27, No.2, pp. 73-86, PMID: 10721654

James, MA.; Lee, JH. & Klingelhutz, AJ. (2006). HPV16-E6 associated hTERT promoter acetylation is E6AP dependent, increased in later passage cells and enhanced by loss of p300. *Int J Cancer,* Oct 15, Vol.119, No.8, pp. 1878-85, PMID: 16708385

Jones, DL.; Alani, RM. & Münger K. (1997). The human papillomavirus E7 oncoprotein can uncouple cellular differentiation and proliferation in human keratinocytes by abrogating p21Cip1-mediated inhibition of cdk2. *Genes Dev,* Aug 15, Vol.11, No. 16, pp. 2101-11, PMID: 9284049

Jones, EE. & Wells, SI. (2006). Cervical cancer and human papillomaviruses: inactivation of retinoblastoma and other tumor suppressor pathways. *Curr Mol Med,* Nov, Vol.6, No.7, pp. 795-808, PMID: 17100604

Katz, JB.; Muller, AJ. & Prendergast, CG. (2008). Indoleamine 2,3-dioxygenase in T-cell tolerance and tumoral immune escape. *Immunol Rev,* Apr, Vol.222, pp. 206-21, PMID: 18364004

Kessis, TD.; Connolly, DC.; Hedrick, L. & Cho, KR. (1996). Expression of HPV16 E6 or E7 increases integration of foreign DNA. *Oncogene,* Jul 18, Vol.13, No.2, pp. 427-31, PMID: 8710383

Klingelhutz, AJ.; Foster, SA. & McDougall, JK. (1996). Telomerase activation by the E6 gene product of human papillomavirus type 16. *Nature,* Mar 7, Vol.380, No.6569, pp. 79-82, PMID: 8598912

Koutsky, L. (1997). Epidemiology of genital human papillomavirus infection. *Am J Med,* May 5, Vol.102, No.5A, pp. 3-8, PMID: 9217656

Lane, DP. (1992). Cancer. p53, guardian of the genome. *Nature,* Jul 2, Vol.358, No.6381, pp. 15-6, PMID: 1614522

Lechner, MS. & Laimins, LA. (1994). Inhibition of p53 DNA binding by human papillomavirus E6 proteins. *J Virol,* Jul, Vol.68, No.7, pp. 4262-73, PMID: 8207801

Li, S.; Labrecque, S.; Gauzzi, MC.; Cuddihy, AR.; Wong, AH.; Pellegrini, S.; Matlashewski, GJ. & Koromilas, AE. (1999) The human papilloma virus (HPV)-18 E6 oncoprotein physically associates with Tyk2 and impairs Jak-STAT activation by interferon-alpha. *Oncogene,* Oct 14, Vol.18, No.42, pp. 5727-37, PMID: 10523853

Madeleine, MM.; Daling, JR.; Carter, JJ.; Wipf, GC.; Schwartz, SM.; McKnight, B; Kurman, RJ.; Beckmann, AM.; Hagensee, ME. & Galloway, DA. (1997). Cofactors with human papillomavirus in a population-based study of vulvar cancer. *J Natl Cancer Inst,* Oct 15, Vol.89, No.20, pp. 1516-23, PMID: 9337348

McCredie, MR.; Sharples, KJ.; Paul, C.; Baranyai, J.; Medley, G.; Jones, RW. & Skegg, DC. (2008). Natural history of cervical neoplasia and risk of invasive cancer in women with cervical intraepithelial neoplasia 3: a retrospective cohort study. *Lancet Oncol,* May, Vol.9, No.5, pp. 425-34, PMID: 18407790

Mietz, JA.; Unger, T; Huibregtse, JM. & Howley, PM. (1992). The transcriptional transactivation function of wild-type p53 is inhibited by SV40 large T-antigen and by HPV-16 E6 oncoprotein. *EMBO J,* Dec, Vol.11, No.13, pp. 5013-20, PMID: 1464323

Moodley, M.; Sewart, S.; Herrington, CS.; Chetty, R.; Pegoraro, R. & Moodley, J. (2003). The interaction between steroid hormones, human papillomavirus type 16, E6 oncogene expression, and cervical cancer. *Int J Gynecol Cancer,* Nov-Dec, Vol.13, No.6, pp. 834-42, PMID: 14675321

Moody, CA. & Laimins, LA. (2010) Human papillomavirus oncoproteins: pathways to transformation. *Nat Rev Cancer,* Aug, Vol.10, No.8, pp. 550-60, PMID: 20592731

Moon, MS.; Lee, CJ.; Um, SJ.; Park, JS.; Yang, JM. & Hwang, ES. (2001). Effect of BPV1 E2-mediated inhibition of E6/E7 expression in HPV16-positive cervical carcinoma cells. *Gynecol Oncol,* Feb, Vol.80, No.2, pp. 168-75, PMID: 11161855

Moscicki, AB.; Schiffman, M.; Kjaer, S. & Villa, LL. (2006). Chapter 5: Updating the natural history of HPV and anogenital cancer. *Vaccine,* Aug 31, Vol.24, Suppl.3, S3/42-51, PMID: 16950017

Münger, K. & Howley, PM. (2002). Human papillomavirus immortalization and transformation functions. *Virus Res,* Nov, Vol.89, No.2, pp. 213-28, PMID: 12445661

Münger, K. & Phelps WC. (1993). The human papillomavirus E7 protein as a transforming and transactivating factor. *Biochim Biophys Acta,* May 25, Vol.1155, No.1, pp. 111-23, PMID: 8389201

Münger, K.; Scheffner, M.; Huibregtse, JM. & Howley PM. (1992). Interactions of HPV E6 and E7 oncoproteins with tumour suppressor gene products. *Cancer Surv,* Vol.12, pp. 197-217, PMID: 1322242

Muñoz, N.; Bosch, FX.; de Sanjosé, S.; Herrero, R.; Castellsagué, X.; Shah, KV.; Snijders, PJ. & Meijer, CJ. (2003). International Agency for Research on Cancer Multicenter Cervical Cancer Study Group. Epidemiologic classification of human papillomavirus types associated with cervical cancer. *N Engl J Med,* Feb 6, Vol.348, No.6, pp. 518-27, PMID: 12571259

Muñoz, N.; Castellsagué, X.; de González, AB. & Gissmann, L. (2006). Chapter 1: HPV in the etiology of human cancer. *Vaccine,* Aug 31, Vol.24, Suppl.3, S3/1-10, PMID: 16949995

Nguyen, DX.; Westbrook, TF. & McCance, DJ. (2002). Human papillomavirus type 16 E7 maintains elevated levels of the cdc25A tyrosine phosphatase during deregulation of cell cycle arrest. *J Virol,* Jan, Vol.76, No.2, pp. 619-32, PMID: 11752153

Nguyen, ML.; Nguyen, MM.; Lee, D.; Griep, AE. & Lambert, PF. (2003). The PDZ ligand domain of the human papillomavirus type 16 E6 protein is required for E6's induction of epithelial hyperplasia in vivo. *J Virol,* Jun, Vol.77, No.12, pp. 6957-64, PMID: 12768014

Oda, H.; Kumar, S. & Howley, PM. (1999). Regulation of the Src family tyrosine kinase Blk through E6AP-mediated ubiquitination. *Proc Natl Acad Sci USA,* Aug 17, Vol.96, No.17, pp. 9557-62, PMID: 10449731

Oh, ST.; Kyo, S. & Laimins, LA. (2001) Telomerase activation by human papillomavirus type 16 E6 protein: induction of human telomerase reverse transcriptase expression through Myc and GC-rich Sp1 binding sites. *J Virol,* Jun, Vol.75, No.12, pp. 5559-66, PMID: 11356963

Park, JS.; Kim, EJ.; Kwon, HJ.; Hwang, ES.; Namkoong, SE. & Um, SJ. (2000). Inactivation of interferon regulatory factor-1 tumor suppressor protein by HPV E7 oncoprotein. Implication for the E7-mediated immune evasion mechanism in cervical carcinogenesis. *J Biol Chem,* Mar 10, Vol.275, No.10, pp. 6764-9, PMID: 10702232

Pett, MR.; Alazawi, WO.; Roberts, I.; Dowen, S.; Smith, DI.; Stanley, MA. & Coleman N. (2004). Acquisition of high-level chromosomal instability is associated with integration of human papillomavirus type 16 in cervical keratinocytes. *Cancer Res,* Feb 15, Vol.64, No.4, pp. 1359-68, PMID: 14973079

Puthenveettil, JA.; Frederickson, SM. & Reznikoff, CA. (1996). Apoptosis in human papillomavirus 16 E7-, but not E6-immortalized human uroepithelial cells. *Oncogene,* Sep 19, Vol.13, No.6, pp. 1123-31, PMID: 8808685

Rapp, L. & Chen, JJ. (1998). The papillomavirus E6 proteins. *Biochim Biophys Acta,* Aug 19, Vol.1378, No.1, F1-19, PMID: 9739758

Reznikoff, CA.; Belair, CD., Yeager, TR.; Savelieva, E.; Blelloch, RH.; Puthenveettil, JA. & Cuthill, S. (1996). A molecular genetic model of human bladder cancer pathogenesis. *Semin Oncol,* Oct, Vol.23, No.5, pp. 571-84, PMID: 8893868

Ronco, LV.; Karpova, AY.; Vidal, M. & Howley, PM. (1998). Human papillomavirus 16 E6 oncoprotein binds to interferon regulatory factor-3 and inhibits its transcriptional activity. *Genes Dev,* Jul 1, Vol.12, No.13, pp. 2061-72, PMID: 9649509

Shay, JW. & Bacchetti, S. (1997). A survey of telomerase activity in human cancer. *Eur J Cancer,* Apr, Vol.33, No.5, pp. 787-91, PMID: 9282118

Spardy, N.; Duensing, A.; Hoskins, EE.; Wells, SI. & Duensing, S. (2008). HPV-16 E7 reveals a link between DNA replication stress, fanconi anemia D2 protein, and alternative lengthening of telomere-associated promyelocytic leukemia bodies. *Cancer Res,* Dec 1, Vol.68, No.23, pp. 9954-63, PMID: 19047177

Stanley, M. (2006). Immune responses to human papillomavirus. *Vaccine,* Mar 30, Vol.24, Suppl.1, S16-22, PMID: 16219398

Stanley, M. (2010). HPV - immune response to infection and vaccination. *Infect Agent Cancer,* Oct 20, Vol.5, No.19, PMID: 20961432

Swan, DC.; Vernon, SD. & Icenogle, JP. (1994). Cellular proteins involved in papillomavirus-induced transformation. *Arch Virol,* Vol.138, No.1-2, pp. 105-15, PMID: 7980001

Thierry, F.; Benotmane, MA.; Demeret, C.; Mori, M.; Teissier, S. & Desaintes, C. (2004). A genomic approach reveals a novel mitotic pathway in papillomavirus carcinogenesis. *Cancer Res,* Feb 1, Vol.64, No.3, pp. 895-903, PMID: 14871818

Thomas, M. & Banks, L. (1998). Inhibition of Bak-induced apoptosis by HPV-18 E6. *Oncogene,* 10, Vol.17, No.23, pp. 2943-54, PMID: 9881696

Tommasino, M.; Accardi, R.; Caldeira, S.; Dong, W.; Malanchi, I.; Smet, A. & Zehbe, I. (2003). The role of TP53 in Cervical carcinogenesis. *Hum Mutat,* Mar, Vol.21, No.3, pp. 307-12, PMID: 12619117

Tungteakkhun, SS. & Duerksen-Hughes, PJ. (2008). Cellular binding partners of the human papillomavirus E6 protein. *Arch Virol,* Vol.153, No.3, pp. 397-408, PMID: 18172569

Valentijn, AJ.; Zouq, N. & Gilmore, AP. (2004). Anoikis. *Biochem Soc Trans,* Jun, Vol. 32, Pt3, pp. 421-5, PMID: 15157151

Van Doorslaer, K.; Bernard, HU.; Chen, Z.; de Villiers, EM.; Hausen, HZ. & Burk, RD. (2011). Papillomaviruses: evolution, Linnaean taxonomy and current nomenclature. *Trends Microbiol,* Feb, Vol.19, No.2, pp. 49-50, PMID: 21144754

Veldman, T.; Horikawa, I.; Barrett, JC. & Schlegel, R. (2001) Transcriptional activation of the telomerase hTERT gene by human papillomavirus type 16 E6 oncoprotein. *J Virol,* May, Vol.75, No.9, pp. 4467-72, PMID: 11287602

Vousden, K. (1993). Interactions of human papillomavirus transforming proteins with the products of tumor suppressor genes. *FASEB J,* Jul, Vol.7, No.10, pp. 872-9, PMID: 8393818

Walboomers, JM.; Jacobs, MV.; Manos, MM.; Bosch, FX.; Kummer, JA.; Shah, KV.; Snijders, PJ.; Peto, J.; Meijer, CJ. & Muñoz N. (1999). Human papillomavirus is a necessary cause of invasive cervical cancer worldwide. *J Pathol,* Sep, Vol.189, No.1, pp. 12-9, PMID: 10451482

Wang, Y.; Coulombe, R.; Cameron, DR.; Thauvette, L.; Massariol, MJ.; Amon, LM.; Fink, D.; Titolo, S.; Welchner, E.; Yoakim, C.; Archambault, J. & White, PW. (2004). Crystal structure of the E2 transactivation domain of human papillomavirus type 11 bound to a protein interaction inhibitor. *J Biol Chem,* Feb 20, Vol.279, No.8, pp. 6976-85, PMID: 14634007

White, AE.; Livanos, EM. & Tlsty, TD. (1994). Differential disruption of genomic integrity and cell cycle regulation in normal human fibroblasts by the HPV oncoproteins. *Genes Dev,* Mar 15, Vol.8, No.6, pp. 666-77, PMID: 7926757

White, PW.; Faucher, AM. & Goudreau, N. (2011). Small molecule inhibitors of the human papillomavirus e1-e2 interaction. *Curr Top Microbiol Immunol,* Vol.348, pp. 61-88, PMID: 2067697

Wise-Draper, TM. & Wells, SI. (2008). Papillomavirus E6 and E7 proteins and their cellular targets. *Front Biosci,* Jan 1, Vol.13, pp. 1003-17, PMID: 17981607

Wu, L.; Goodwin, EC.; Naeger, LK.; Vigo, E.; Galaktionov, K.; Helin, K. & DiMaio, D. (2000). E2F-Rb complexes assemble and inhibit cdc25A transcription in cervical carcinoma cells following repression of human papillomavirus oncogene expression. *Mol Cell Biol,* Oct, Vol.20, No.19, pp. 7059-67, PMID: 10982822

Zerfass, K.; Schulze, A.; Spitkovsky, D.; Friedman, V.; Henglein, B. & Jansen-Dürr, P. (1995). Sequential activation of cyclin E and cyclin A gene expression by human papillomavirus type 16 E7 through sequences necessary for transformation. *J Virol,* Oct, Vol.69, No.10, pp. 6389-99, PMID: 7666540

Zhang, A.; Wang, J.; Zheng, B.; Fang, X.; Angström, T.; Liu, C.; Li, X.; Erlandsson, F.; Björkholm, M.; Nordenskjörd, M.; Gruber, A.; Wallin, KL. & Xu, D. (2004). Telomere attrition predominantly occurs in precursor lesions during in vivo carcinogenic process of the uterine cervix. *Oncogene*, Sep 23, Vol.23, No.44, pp, 7441-7, PMID: 15318175

zur Hausen H. (1996). Papillomavirus infections-a major cause of human cancers. *Biochim Biophys Acta,* Oct 9, Vol.1288, No.2, F55-78, PMID: 8876633

zur Hausen, H. (1999). Papillomaviruses in human cancers. *Proc Assoc Am Physicians,* Nov-Dec, Vol.111, No.6, pp. 581-7, PMID: 10591087

zur Hausen, H. (2002). Papillomaviruses and cancer: from basic studies to clinical application. *Nat Rev Cancer,* May, Vol.2, No.5, pp. 342-50, PMID: 12044010

28

The Role of E2 Proteins in Papillomavirus DNA Replication

Reet Kurg
Institute of Technology, University of Tartu
Estonia

1. Introduction

Papillomaviruses are small, nonenveloped, double-stranded DNA viruses, which infect a wide variety of vertebrate species and induce proliferative lesions in their host. The viruses are species-specific and to date, more than 150 different types of papillomaviruses have been identified; each virus infects a specific region of cutaneous or internal mucosal epithelium in its host (McLaughlin-Drubin and Münger, 2009). Papillomaviruses are widely spread in nature and in most cases, papillomavirus infections are cleared by the host immune system, however, sometimes papillomaviruses establish persistent infections. Papillomavirus classification is based on nucleotide sequence homology (de Villiers et al., 2004). Human papillomavirus (HPV) types that infect the genital epithelia belong to subgroup A (alpha-papillomaviruses), and are classified into high- or low-risk types, depending upon their oncogenic potential. Persistent infection with high-risk HPVs (HPV16, 18, 31, 33, 45) can lead to cervical cancer, the second most common cancer in women (Durst et al., 1983; zur Hausen, 2000). Low-risk HPVs, such as HPV6 and 11, can infect genital tract as well as oral sites where they are generally associated with benign papillomas. The second major group of HPVs, supergroup B, also known as beta-papillomaviruses, infect skin epithelia and may develop skin cancers at the site of HPV infection (McLaughlin-Drubin and Münger, 2009).

2. Papillomavirus life cycle

Papillomaviruses, with the help of only few genes, can achieve a complete replication cycle in the epidermal and mucosal keratinocytes. Most viral types are predominantly trophic for one or the other cell types, but certain genotypes can infect and persist in both. Papillomavirus virions enter the epithelial tissue through microwounds and infect a subset of basal cells, probably stem cells, at low copy number (Egawa, 2003). HPV virions migrate to the cell nucleus and establish their genomes as episomes. Next, the HPV early promoter is activated and the viral early proteins, E1 and E2, are transcribed, the synthesis of viral DNA is initiated and the copy number of viral episomes is raised up to 20-100 genomes per cell. During this amplification stage, rapid viral replication is required to quickly reach an optimal copy number. As basal cells divide, HPV genomes are replicated and distributed evenly between daughter cells in mitosis. This is a phase of episomal maintenance with minimal viral gene expression, viral replication proceeds at moderate level and is synchronized to cellular proliferation (De Geest et al., 1993). Papillomavirus persistence is set up through the maintenance of a constant copy number of extrachromosomal viral genomes in the nuclei of dividing host cells. The expression of late genes encoding the capsid proteins and virus assembly are tightly coupled to the differentiation of epithelial tissue (Longworth and Laimins, 2004). When the infected keratinocyte enters the differentiating compartment, exiting the cell cycle, the vegetative phase of the HPV life cycle leading to amplification of the viral genome is initiated. This phase includes amplification of viral copy number to at least 1000 copies per cell and expression of late transcripts encoding proteins for viral capsid. The viral DNA is packed into virions, which are released with dead cells after the infected cells reach the epithelial surface (for review, see Chow et al. 2010; Doorbar, 2005).

The dependence of papillomavirus life cycle on epithelial differentiation and difficulties in reproducing this process in cell culture has complicated the studies of papillomavirus replication. Short-term replication assays closely mimic the initial amplification phase of replication, while long-term replication assays mimic viral maintenance in undifferentiated basal cells. DNA amplification and virion assembly can be analyzed only in differentiating epithelial cells. The most extensively studied papillomavirus is bovine papillomavirus type-1 (BPV-1) because of its capacity to transform rodent cell lines in culture (Law et al., 1981). The mouse fibroblast cell line C127 transfected with the BPV1 genome maintaining the viral DNA as extrachromosomal plasmid with the constant copy number was historically the first model system for studying mechanisms of papillomavirus DNA replication. Our knowledge of initiation of papillomavirus DNA replication and maintenance of virus genomes has primarily derived from studies with BPV1. However, BPV-1 belongs to delta-papillomaviruses and is evolutionary distinct from the human papillomaviruses.

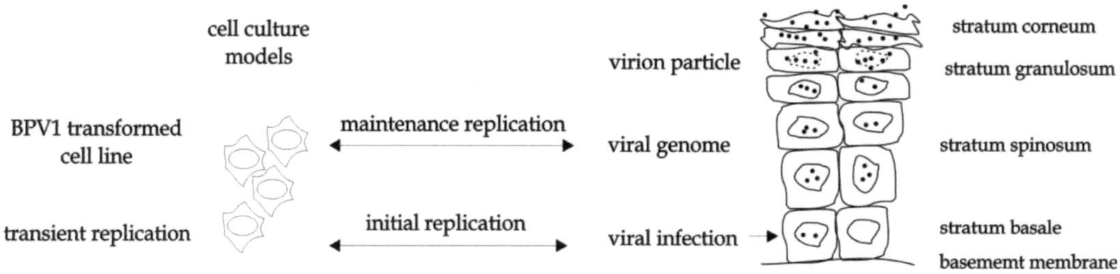

Fig. 1. Schematic representation of epithelia showing various differentiated layers and PV replication, and cell culture models mimicking papillomavirus DNA replication.

The limited availability of appropriate cell culture systems supporting HPV DNA replication has hampered research of HPV replication and regulatory pathways involved in these processes. Primary keratinocytes, transfected with circulized HPV genome, replicate HPV genomes at low copy number. Productive HPV replication needs culture systems where epithelial cells are able to differentiate. Adaptation of organotypic culture techniques, „raft“ culture systems, provide the basis for propagation of HPVs, although the yield of virions is very low (Dollard et al., 1992; McCance et al., 1988; Meyers et al., 1992). Introduction of adenovirus recombinants carrying the HPV genome flanked by loxP sites and Cre recombinase into PHK cells grown in raft cultures results in efficient establishment of cells harboring thousands of copies of the HPV18 genome. Virions obtained from these cultures efficiently infect PHKs at a multiplicity of infection (MOI) of <50, resulting in expression of spliced viral mRNAs (Wang et al., 2009a). However, organotypic culture of HPV-infected cells is not a very convenient system for long-term viral persistence and latency studies. Cell lines from mild dysplasia harboring episomal HPV genomes (W12 and CIN-612) have been very useful tools for studying stable episomal HPV replication, and also loss of episomes and integration of HPV into the host genome, a process accompanied by tumourigenesis (Pett and Coleman, 2007). At early passages in monolayer culture, the W12 cells retain HPV16 episomes at 100 to 200 copies per cell, but in long-term cultivation in the absence of feeder cells, the spontaneous loss of episomes and integration of HPV16 occurs (De Geest et al., 1993; Pett et al., 2004; Stanley et al., 1989). The genomes of both high- and low-risk alpha-papillomaviruses as well as cutaneous beta-papillomaviruses replicate in human osteosarcoma cell line U2OS, and are able to establish persistent replication in these cells. These cell lines might be a valuable and efficient tool for studying fundamental properties of HPV DNA replication, especially the long-term viral persistence, and for the development of inhibitors of HPV genome replication (Geimanen et al., 2011).

2.1 Papillomavirus genome

All papillomaviruses have a similar genomic organization. The papillomavirus genome of approximately 8000 base pairs in length contains a non-coding upstream regulatory region (URR), early (E) region of open reading frames (ORFs) and late (L) region of ORFs. The circular papillomavirus genome encodes roughly eight ORFs from a single DNA strand. The URR alone is 600-900 base pairs in length and contains the origin of replication and binding sites for transcription factors and enhancers (Fig. 2). All transcription takes place in the same direction (clockwise on the circular map) using multiple promoters. The E region and L region are both followed by a poly-A addition site. Within the virions, the papillomavirus genome is associated with cellular histones forming chromatin-like complexes.

Papillomavirus transcription is complex and involves the usage of different promoters, multiple splice patterns and differential production of mRNA species in different cells. In BPV1, seven different promoters, six of which being active in undifferentiated cells, have been identified (Ahola et al., 1987; Baker and Howley, 1987). In the high-risk HPV types, transcripts are initiated at two major viral promoters, one for early and the other for late transcripts. In contrast, early genes of low-risk HPVs are expressed from two independent promoters (Chow et al., 1987). The HPV early promoter (p105 in case of HPV18) is activated by binding of cellular transcription factors; however the factors that determine the cell specificity are still not fully understood. Among the main players involved in PV replication are the ubiquitous transcription factors Sp1 and AP1 (Gloss and Bernard, 1990; Hubert et al., 1999; Thierry, 2009; Thierry et al., 1992). In addition to the binding sites for the cellular transcription factors, the URR contains binding sites for the virally encoded E2 regulatory proteins and E1 helicase. Early region proteins, E6, E7, E1 and E2 are transcribed from the HPV early promoter active in basal, nonproductively infected cells and in transformed cells, and all four early proteins are translated from the same polycistronic mRNA (Hummel et al., 1992). E1 and E2 are directly involved in viral DNA replication; the other early proteins - oncoproteins E6 and E7 - support viral DNA amplification indirectly by inactivating major tumor suppressor proteins and activating signal transduction pathways (for review, see (McLaughlin-Drubin and Münger, 2009; Moody and Laimins, 2010).

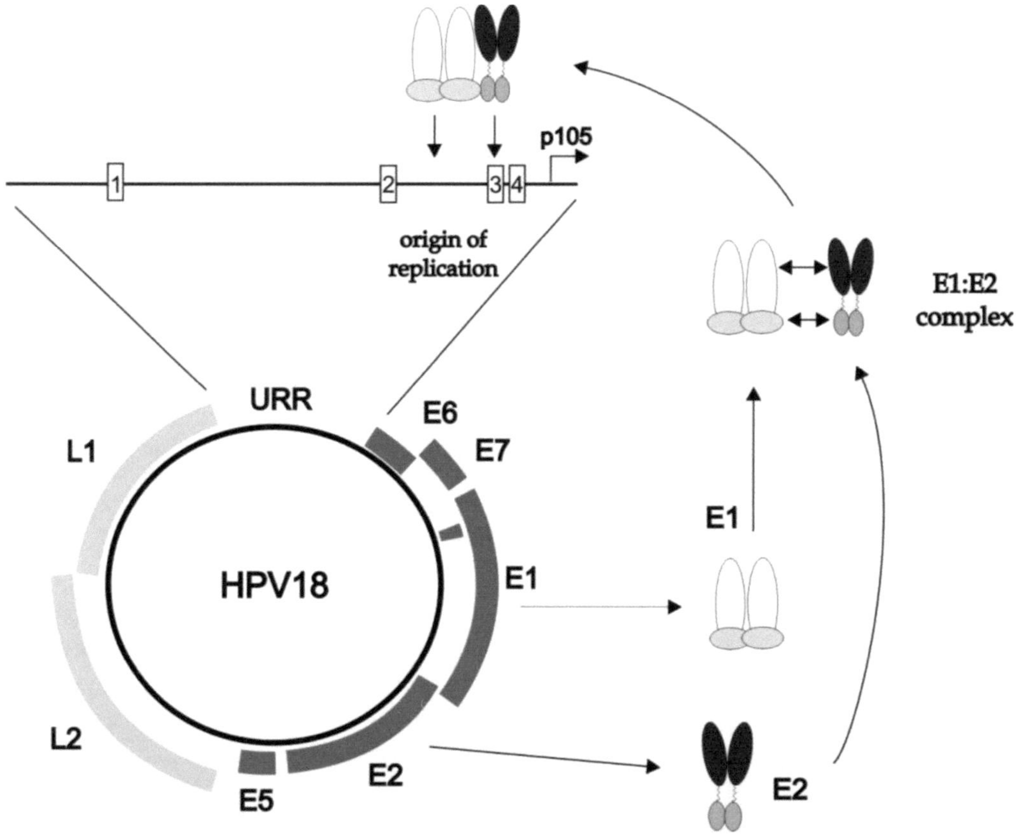

Fig. 2. Organization of the HPV18 circular genome showing the *cis*-sequences and viral proteins required for initiation of papillomavirus DNA replication. Open reading frames are indicated by dark grey (early region) and light grey (late region) boxes. The origin of replication, early promoter (p105) and E2 binding sites (boxes with numbers) are shown on the scheme of URR. Papillomavirus E1 and E2 proteins, transcribed from the early promoter, form a complex and bind cooperatively to their binding sites within the origin of replication locating in the URR.

3. Papillomavirus DNA replication

3.1 Initiation of replication

The double-stranded circular DNA replicates as a multi-copy extrachromosomal plasmid in the nucleus of infected cells. The replication of papillomavirus DNA is initiated from the origin of replication consisting of binding sites for E1 and E2 proteins (Del Vecchio et al., 1992; Ustav et al., 1993; Ustav et al., 1991). Transient, short-term replication requires the origin of replication *in cis* and the expression of viral E1 and E2 proteins, all other replication enzymes and proteins are supplied by the host cells (Remm et al., 1992; Ustav and Stenlund, 1991). Papillomavirus DNA replication is not cell-type specific, despite of high degrees of host and cell-type specificity for infection. The BPV1 genome can replicate and is maintained in murine C127 cells. HPV11 and HPV18 genomic DNA can replicate not only in its natural host cells, primary foreskin keratinocytes, but also in the human tongue squamous cell carcinoma cell line SCC4 and osteosarcoma cell line U2OS (Del Vecchio et al., 1992; Geimanen et al., 2011; Mungal et al., 1992). Transient replication of BPV1 and HPV origin-containing plasmids can take place in a number of mammalian cells if E1 and E2 proteins are provided from heterologous expression vectors (Chiang et al., 1992). HPV transcription exhibits stringent cell specificity and the lack of regulated gene expression of viral early proteins from HPV genomes could be the reason that restricts HPV genome replication to certain cell types. BPV1 DNA replication *in vitro* with purified proteins and cell extracts from murine, simian and human cells has been reconstituted showing that all cellular factors essential for papillomavirus DNA replication are provided by the host cell (Liu et al., 1995; Muller et al., 1994; Yang et al., 1991a). The cellular replication factors required for papillomavirus DNA replication include replication protein A (RPA), a single-stranded-DNA-binding protein, replication factor C (RFC), proliferating-cell nuclear antigen (PCNA) and DNA polymerase α–primase. It has been shown that E1 recruits Topo I to the papillomavirus replication fork and Topo I specifically stimulates the origin binding activity of papillomavirus E1 protein (Clower et al., 2006; Hu et al., 2006; Melendy et al., 1995; Park et al., 1994).

3.2 Origin of replication

The papillomavirus origin of replication consists of three E2 binding sites (E2BS), from which only one is absolutely required for replication, and an A/T-rich region containing an array of E1 protein binding sites (E1BS) (Remm et al., 1992; Ustav et al., 1991). The overall structure of BPV1 and HPV origins is conserved and various combinations of E1 and E2 proteins from different papillomaviruses can initiate DNA replication from several papillomavirus origins (Chiang et al., 1992; Del Vecchio et al., 1992; Kadaja et al., 2007). A relationship appears to exist between the affinity of the E2BS and the ability to function at a distance from the binding site for the E1 protein. A low-affinity site appears to be functional only when located close to the E1 binding site, while for function at greater distances higher affinities are required. In multimerized form, the high affinity E2BSs are able to function even when placed at a distance of one kilobase from the rest of the origin (Ustav et al., 1993). High-risk HPV genomes have been found integrated into host chromatin in tumors and cervix dysplasia biopsy specimens of patients (Dall et al., 2008; Kristiansen et al., 1994). Integration of the HPV genome is often accompanied by the disruption of E2 open reading frame and the loss of E2 activity, leading to enhanced expression of virus oncogenes E6 and E7. The HPV regulatory sequences are active in cervical cancer cells as expression of E7 promotes cell survival (Jiang and Milner, 2002). In patients, the HPV16 genome may exist at the same time in episomal as well as in an integrated form. Co-existence of the replicating episomal viral genome expressing the viral E2 protein, and integrated HPV with viral replication origin raises the question about the functionality of the integrated origins. Recent works have shown that expression of E1 and E2 proteins from expression vectors or from different HPV genomes can induce replication of the genomic integrated HPV origin. The replication forks initiated at the integrated HPV origins extend into the flanking regions of cellular DNA, and these amplified genomic sequences could be targets for the recombination and repair system. This suggests that replication induced from the papillomavirus integrated origin may induce genomic changes of the host cell (Kadaja et al., 2009; Kadaja et al., 2007).

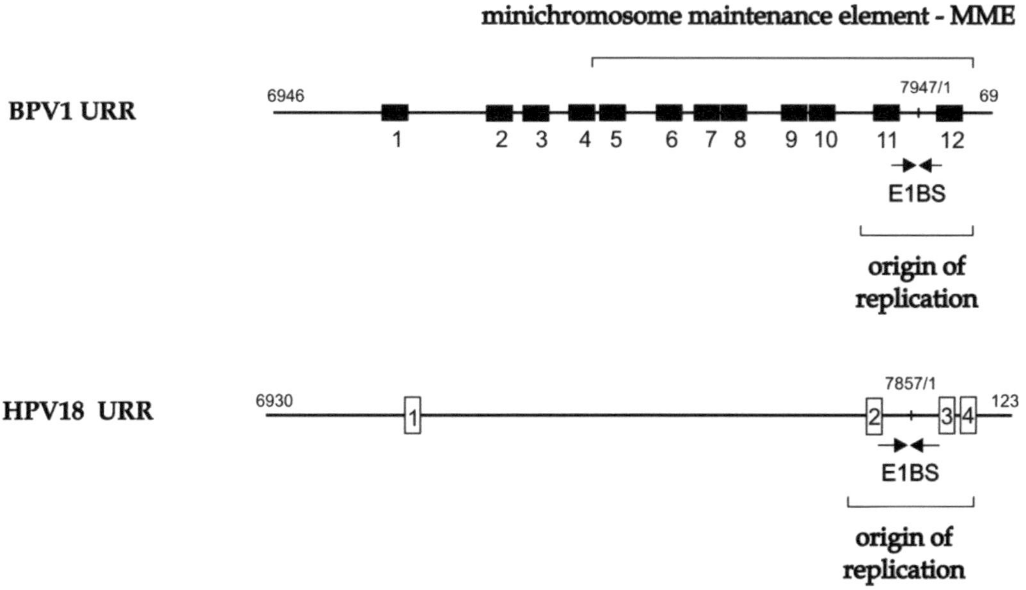

Fig. 3. Origin of replication of BPV1 and HPV18. E1 binding sites are depicted with arrows and E2 binding sites with boxes. The minimal origin of replication consisting of E1BS and E2BSs is shown for BPV1 and HPV18, and the minichromosome maintenance element MME, required for maintenance and segregation of viral DNA, for BPV1.

3.3 Assembly of the DNA replication initiation complex

E1 is an initiator protein of papillomavirus DNA replication. E1 is responsible for recognition of the replication origin, melting of the DNA at the origin as well as for subsequent unwinding of the double helix during progression of the replication fork. The viral E1 protein is an ATP-dependent helicase which binds as a dimer to pairs of its binding sites (Yang et al., 1993). The binding sites for the E1 replication helicase are short sequences, 5-6 base pairs in length, arranged as two pairs of inverted repeats (Chen and Stenlund, 1998; Chen and Stenlund, 2001). E1 has low sequence specificity and therefore it can initiate DNA replication in vitro, and from non-specific DNA sequences (Bonne-Andrea et al., 1995). Within the cells, the E1 and E2 proteins form a complex through multiple protein-protein interactions and bind cooperatively to adjacent binding sites in the origin of replication (Berg and Stenlund, 1997; Mohr et al., 1990). E1 by itself binds to the origin with low degree of sequence specificity, but in the presence of E2 the sequence specificity is increased (Sedman and Stenlund, 1995; Sedman et al., 1997). In this process, E2 functions transiently and "catalytically", providing sequence specificity for the formation of the E1-ori complex. In addition, E2 enhances E1 binding to DNA through the DNA-binding domain by inhibiting the non-specific DNA binding of the E1 helicase domain (Stenlund, 2003a). The E1-E2-ori complex is able to bind DNA with high specificity but lacks other biochemical activities. In the next step, additional E1 molecules are added by displacing E2 from the DNA-bound complex in an ATP-dependent manner (Sanders and Stenlund, 1998; Sanders and Stenlund, 2000). Two additional E1 molecules are recruited to the origin, which results in the formation of two E1 trimers on the ori, followed by formation of two hexamers in the presence of ATP. E1 hexameric complex has the DNA helicase activity which is able to unwind the DNA and initiate the papillomavirus DNA replication (Fouts et al., 1999; Schuck and Stenlund, 2005; Sedman and Stenlund, 1998).

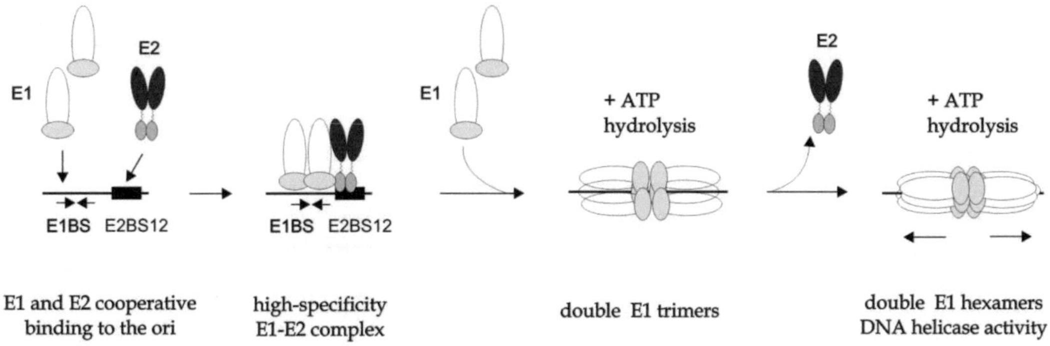

Fig. 4. Assembly of the replication initiation complex. The E1 and E2 proteins bind cooperatively to the origin of replication, which contains binding sites for both proteins (E1BS and E2BS). The resulting E1:E2 complex binds DNA with high affinity and specificity. In the next step, additional E1 molecules are recruited to the complex and E2 is displaced in the presence of ATP. ATP hydrolysis is also required for conversion of E1 complex into a double hexamer possessing DNA helicase activity (for review, see Stenlund, 2003b).

3.4 Stable maintenance replication

Papillomaviruses have the capacity to establish a persistent infection in mammalian epithelial cells. The BPV1-transformed C127 cells maintain the viral genome as a multicopy nuclear plasmid thus being a valuable tissue culture system for investigating the establishment and maintenance of papillomavirus genomic DNA. The studies with BPV1-C127 cells have revealed that during the maintenance of virus genomes BPV1 DNA is replicating by a conventional bi-directional (theta-type) replication mode throughout S phase of the cell cycle in a random-choice fashion (Gilbert and Cohen, 1987; Ravnan et al., 1992). Some molecules replicate once per cell cycle, some replicate more than once, and others do not replicate at all during a given cell cycle, resulting in statistically "once per cell cycle" replication of the viral DNA. Stable HPV DNA replication seems to be more complicated. This has been studied in human keratinocytes, where the HPV DNA is stably maintained at high copy number over several passages. HPV16 and HPV31 DNA can replicate randomly or in an ordered once-per-S-phase fashion depending on the cell line in which it is located. In W12 cells, which are derived from a natural cervical lesion, the HPV16 DNA replicates only once per S phase, but in another immortalized keratinocyte cell line, NIKS, it replicates randomly (Hoffmann et al., 2006). At later stages of the papillomavirus life cycle, there is a shift from the theta replication mode in the proliferating keratinocytes to the rolling-circle replication mode after the cells start to differentiate (Flores and Lambert, 1997).

Studies of subclones of BPV1-transformed C127 cells as well as U2OS cells maintaining HPV genomes have demonstrated cell to cell variation in the extent and state of genomic DNA. In addition to the monomeric form of genomic DNA, dimeric and sometimes higher oligomeric forms of BPV1 and mucosal and cutaneous HPV genomes are detected. Oligomeric forms of papillomavirus DNA are organized in a head-to-tail configuration and replication is initiated at only some of the origins (Geimanen et al., 2011; Schvartzman et al., 1990). In patient samples, HPV16 DNA, which is maintained in carcinoma cells as episome, is always multimeric, suggesting that oligomerization of HPV genomes is common during viral infections *in vivo* (Cullen et al., 1991; Kristiansen et al., 1994).

It is widely accepted that the E1 and E2 proteins are essential for long-term stable replication. However, some studies suggest that E1 is necessary to establish the viral genome as a nuclear plasmid, but is not required at the maintenance stage. The replication of the BPV1 genome containing temperature-sensitive mutation in the E1 gene was first initiated at the permissive temperature and then switched to the non-permissive temperature, where ts-E1 genomes were found to persist as nuclear plasmids for multiple cell generations (Kim and Lambert, 2002).

The functions of viral oncoproteins E6 and E7 are also essential for the maintenance of the extrachromosomal forms of HPV DNA (Thomas et al., 1999). Both E6 and E7 stimulate cell cycle progression and may create a cellular environment permissive to HPV maintenance and abrogate the checkpoints that would block the long-term retention of viral DNA (Garner-Hamrick et al., 2004). Oncogene expression in basal epithelial cells is shown to inhibit cellular differentiation thus promoting long-term persistence of HPV episomes (Hudson et al., 1990; Jones et al., 1997; Sherman and Schlegel, 1996). The E6 and E7 proteins of high-risk HPV types act as viral oncogenes. E6 binds the p53 tumor suppressor protein, which regulates the expression of proteins involved in cell cycle control, leading to degradation of p53 (Scheffner et al., 1990; Werness et al., 1990). Another important function of the high-risk E6 protein is the activation of telomerase in infected cells. High-risk HPV E6 has been shown to increase telomeric length by activating the catalytic subunit of the telomerase hTERT. This extends the life of epithelial cells containing HPV genomes (Oh et al, 2001; Stoppler et al., 1997). The function of the high-risk E7 protein is the binding and degradation of the RB family proteins, which are the major regulators of the cell cycle (Boyer et al., 1996; Schmitt et al., 1994). E7 interaction with histone deacetylases HDACs plays also an essential role in the viral life cycle, as cells harboring HPV genomes with mutations abolishing the E7-HDAC interaction display slower growth and a loss of episomal maintenance (Longworth and Laimins, 2004a). Integration of high-risk HPV into the host genome and loss of E2 expression leads to constitutive activation of the viral oncogenes. Reintroduction of E2 into HPV-associated cervical carcinoma cells, resulting in reactivation of p53 and pRB pathways, has shown to suppress cellular growth, because of cell cycle arrest in G1, apoptosis and senescence (Desaintes et al., 1997; Goodwin and DiMaio, 2000; Goodwin et al., 2000; Hwang et al., 1996; Thierry et al., 2004; Wells et al., 2000).

4. E2 as a viral regulatory protein

The proteins encoded by the papillomavirus E2 ORF play a crucial role in the viral life cycle and serve as major viral regulators of transcription, replication and segregation of the viral genome in the infected cells. The E2 protein is a modular protein consisting of three different structural as well as functional domains; the N-terminal transactivation domain (TAD) (aa 1-200), the C-terminal DNA-binding dimerization domain (DBD) (aa 310-410), and flexible unstructured "hinge region" which functions as a linker between the two domains. The carboxy-terminal DBD binds as a dimer to consensus sequence ACCN_6GGT (Androphy et al., 1987) and the N-terminal activation domain is required for the replication, transactivation and segregation function of the protein (Abroi et al., 2004; Bastien and McBride, 2000; McBride et al., 1989; Ustav and Stenlund, 1991). The three-dimensional structures of the C-terminal DBD and N-terminal transactivation domain of several E2 proteins have been reported revealing a tight dimer of the DBD bound to DNA and a L-shape structure of activation domain (Antson et al., 2000; Harris and Botchan, 1999; Hegde et al., 1992). The papillomavirus E2 proteins can function as activators or repressors of transcription depending on the concentration of proteins within the cell. At low concentrations, E2 activates, and at high concentrations, suppresses transcription from homologous and heterologous promoters containing E2 binding sites (Abroi et al., 1996; Schweiger et al., 2007). E2 has been demonstrated to be a transcriptional activator of early genes in BPV1 and a repressor of early genes in case of HPV16 (Soeda et al., 2006; Spalholz et al, 1985; Thierry and Yaniv, 1987).

E2 is a multifunctional protein. The transactivation domain of E2 is responsible for interactions with viral helicase E1 and with several cellular proteins. The transactivation and replication functions of E2 are separable by point-mutations in the N-terminal activation domain (Abroi et al., 1996; Brokaw et al., 1996; Ferguson and Botchan, 1996; Grossel et al., 1996). The X-ray crystal structures of a complex containing the activation domain of E2 and the helicase domain of E1, and the activation domain of E2 together with Brd4 have been solved and confirm that E2 interacts with E1 and Brd4 through different interaction surfaces (Abbate et al., 2004; Abbate et al., 2006). The cellular bromodomain protein Brd4 is the major cellular partner for E2, and interaction with Brd4 is crucial for both E2 transactivation and repression functions (Ilves et al., 2006; McPhillips et al., 2006; Schweiger et al., 2006). Brd4 is a component of the HPV11 E2 transcriptional silencing complex involved in repression of the E6/E7 promoter (Wu et al., 2006). Through the interaction of Brd4 and transactivation domain, E2 is associated with transcriptionally active cellular chromatin. This association is driving the E2-mediated tethering of viral genomes to host chromatin, and at the same time is retaining the viral genomes in transcriptionally active regions of the nucleus to escape silencing (Jang et al., 2009; Kurg et al., 2005). The transactivation domain mediates functional interactions with cellular transcription factors Sp1 and AP1, histone acetylase complexes containing CBP/p300 and pCAF, and with nucleosome assembly protein hNAP1 (Lee et al., 2002a; Lee et al., 2000; Li et al., 1991; Müller et al., 2002; Rehtanz et al., 2004; Thierry et al., 1992). E2-dependent activities are also modulated by interactions with Brm, a chromatin remodeling protein associated with SWI/SNF ATP-dependent chromatin remodeling complex, and with EP400, a component of the NuA4/TIP60 histone acetylase complex, and SMCX, also known as histone demethylase JARID1C , and Tax1BP1 (Kumar et al., 2007; Smith et al., 2010; Wang et al., 2009b).

E2 binds to the papillomavirus oncoproteins E6 and E7, leading to the modulation of their functions (Gammoh et al., 2006; Grm et al., 2005). E2 has activities that inhibit cell growth. High-risk, but not low-risk HPV E2 proteins can induce themselves growth arrest and apoptotic cell death in several HPV-negative carcinoma cell lines. Apoptosis can occur via a p53-dependent as well as independent pathways (Demeret et al., 2003; Parish et al., 2006b). E2 binds to the cellular protein p53. Expression of p53 can inhibit papillomavirus DNA replication and alter the transcriptional activity of E2 (Frattini et al., 1997; Lepik et al., 1998; Massimi et al., 1999). Interestingly, p53 inhibits the initial, amplificational replication, but not the stable, long-term replication of BPV1 (Ilves et al., 2003). E2 can modulate the activity of cellular proteins, like activators of the Anaphase Promoting Complex (APC) Cdh1 and Cdc20 inducing genomic instability (Bellanger et al., 2005). E2 is associated with transcriptionally active chromatin and as a transcription factor may directly regulate the expression of cellular genes. The HPV E2 proteins are reported to repress the hTERT promoter activity (Lee et al.,

2002b). HPV8 E2 protein suppresses β4-integrin expression and HPV16 E2 protein transcriptionally activates the promoter of a key cellular splicing factor SF2/ASF (Mole et al., 2009; Oldak et al., 2004). The expression of HPV8 E2 protein in transgenic mice can induce the formation of skin tumors through an unknown mechanism (Pfefferle et al., 2008).
The E2 proteins bind to inverted repeats with consensus sequence 5′ ACCGN$_4$CGGT, where N$_4$ represents a 4 bp central sequence (Li et al., 1989). Although the base pairs in the central spacer sequence are not in contact with the protein, they affect protein binding. The E2 DNA binding is accompanied by bending of DNA and depends on DNA flexibility (Hines et al., 1998). HPV E2 proteins bind with higher affinity to sites with A/T-rich central spacer while BPV1 E2 has no preference (Dell et al., 2003). E2 binding can be inhibited by CpG methylation of the E2 binding site (Kim et al., 2003; Thain et al., 1996). The BPV1 genome contains 17 E2 binding sites from which 12 sites are located within the URR region. In genital HPV genomes, there are four E2 binding sites with conserved sequences and positions. E2 remains associated with the BPV1 URR throughout the cell cycle including mitosis (Melanson and Androphy, 2009).

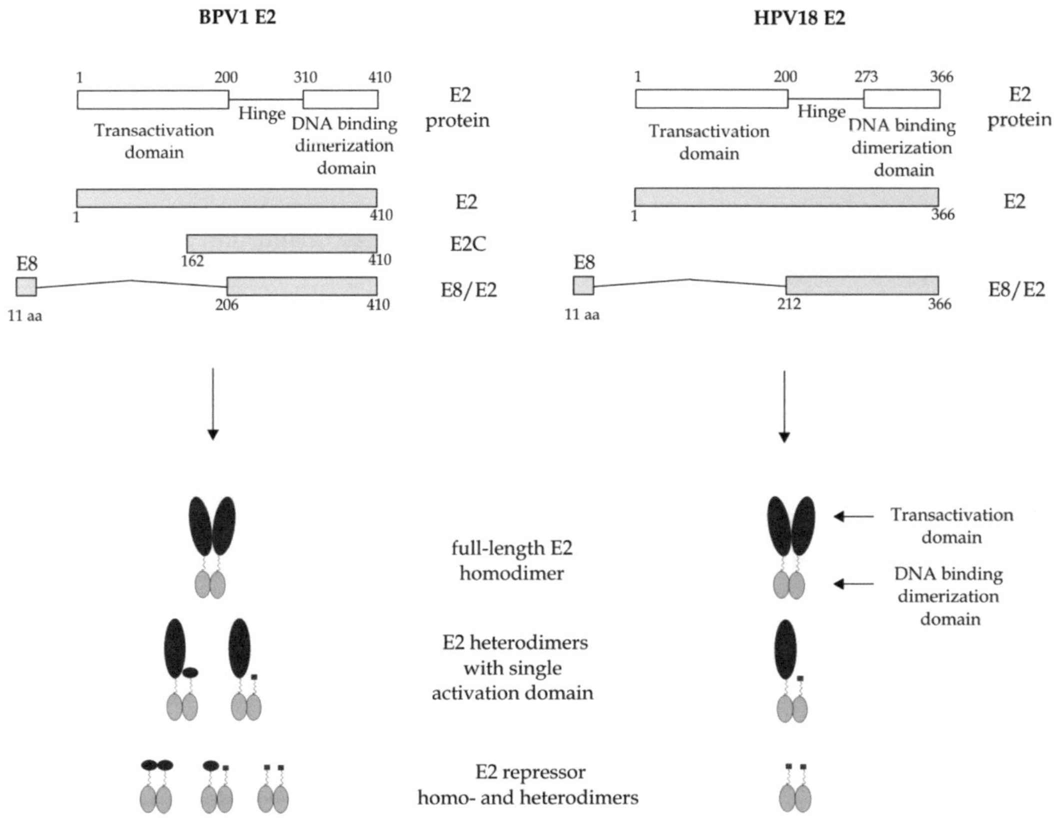

Fig. 5. Papillomavirus genomes encode multiple E2 proteins. In addition to the full-length E2 protein, BPV1 and HPV18 genomes encode truncated E2 proteins, which lack the activation domain and serve as repressors of replication and transcription. The full-length and truncated E2 proteins are able to form dimers through their common C-terminal DNA-binding-dimerization domain.

4.1 E2 repressors and heterodimers

In addition to the full-length E2 protein, the BPV-1 and mucosal HPV genomes encode truncated E2 proteins, which lack the activation domain, but maintain the DNA-binding-dimerization domain (DBD). For BPV1, mRNA for E2C is transcribed from a promoter internal to the open reading frame, and E8/E2 is created by splicing E8 ORF sequences to an acceptor located within the E2 ORF. The repressor proteins encoded by HPVs are similar to the BPV1 E8/E2 protein, since they contain a small conserved E8 ORF (HPV 11, 18, 31) or fragment of E1 ORF (HPV 11) fused to the C-terminus of E2. Transient over-expression assays have suggested that shorter E2 proteins act as negative regulators of E2 and function as repressors of transcription and replication (Chiang et al., 1991; Doorbar et al., 1990; Hubbert et al., 1988; Kurg et al., 2010; Lim et al., 1998; Stubenrauch et al., 2000). The shorter E2s antagonize the function of full-length E2 by competing for E2 DNA binding sites. In addition, the E8 of HPV 31 E8/E2 protein itself is a transcriptional repressor domain that functions independently of binding site competition inhibiting transcription and DNA replication by interacting with co-repressor molecules such as NCoR1/HDAC3, the histone methyltransferase SETDB1, and the TRIM28 protein (Ammermann et al., 2008; Powell et al., 2010).

The full-length and truncated E2 proteins are able to form dimers through their common C-terminal DNA-binding-dimerization domain (McBride et al., 1989). E2 heterodimers with single activation domain bind DNA sequence-specifically and serve as activators of transcription and replication in cell culture model systems (Kurg et al., 2006). E2 heterodimers can interact with viral helicase E1, and are able to recruit E1 to the origin of replication and activate the papillomavirus DNA replication in a cell-free system (Lim et al., 1998). Replacing the open reading frame of E2 with "single-chain" E2 in the context of BPV1 and HPV18 genome revealed that E2 heterodimer with single activation domain could support transient, but not long-term, replication in cell culture model systems (Kurg et al., 2009; Kurg et al., 2010). The full-length E2 protein is required for long-term papillomavirus DNA replication, the E2 heterodimer with single activation domain is crippled in this function. E2 requires two activation domains for interaction with Brd4, the cellular receptor for BPV1 E2 on mitotic chromosomes. Brd4 interacts efficiently with the BPV1 homodimer with two activation domains and with low affinity with the E2 heterodimer with single activation domain and with E2 mutants unable to form dimers between N-terminal activation domains (Cardenas-Mora et al., 2008; Kurg et al., 2006; You et al., 2004).

4.2 The role of E2 in initiation of DNA replication

The expression of E2 protein is required for initiation of papillomavirus DNA replication. The role of E2 in initiation of viral DNA replication is relatively well understood, E2 helps to recruit the viral helicase E1 to the viral replication origin by direct protein-protein and protein-DNA interactions as discussed above. The initiation step and interactions mediating the formation of the replication initiation complex are well studied and are conserved between BPV1 and alpha-papillomaviruses.

4.3 The role of E2 in stable maintenance

Segregation of papillomavirus genomic DNA is achieved through its attachment to mitotic host chromosomes during cell division. Non-covalent association of viral DNA with chromosomes is a general mechanism used by all papillomaviruses studied so far. This mechanism ensures that the replicated virus episomes are retained inside the nuclei of dividing host cells and faithfully partitioned to the daughter cells during mitosis (You, 2010).

Long-term replication and maintenance of BPV1 episomes requires the sequence of URR - the minichromosome maintenance element (MME) - consisting of at least six E2 binding sites and the minimal origin of replication as *cis*-elements. The plasmids containing BPV1 URR can be maintained as extrachromosomal elements in hamster CHO cells stably expressing the viral E1 and E2 proteins (Piirsoo et al., 1996). Extrachromosomal MME-containing plasmids containing ten oligomerized E2 binding sites segregate efficiently between daughter cells in the presence of E2 protein expressed from the same plasmid (Abroi et al., 2004; Silla et al., 2005). MME consisting of E2 binding sites and the E2 protein are responsible for anchoring of BPV1 genomes as well as URR reporter plasmids to host cell chromosomes (Ilves et al., 1999; Lehman and Botchan, 1998; Skiadopoulos and McBride, 1998). The functional organization of the HPV URR is significantly different from that of the BPV1. Alpha-papillomavirus genomes have four E2 binding sites in this region and only three of them are required for stable replication (Stubenrauch et al., 1998). The exact mechanism of segregation of HPV genomes is not yet known and needs further investigations.

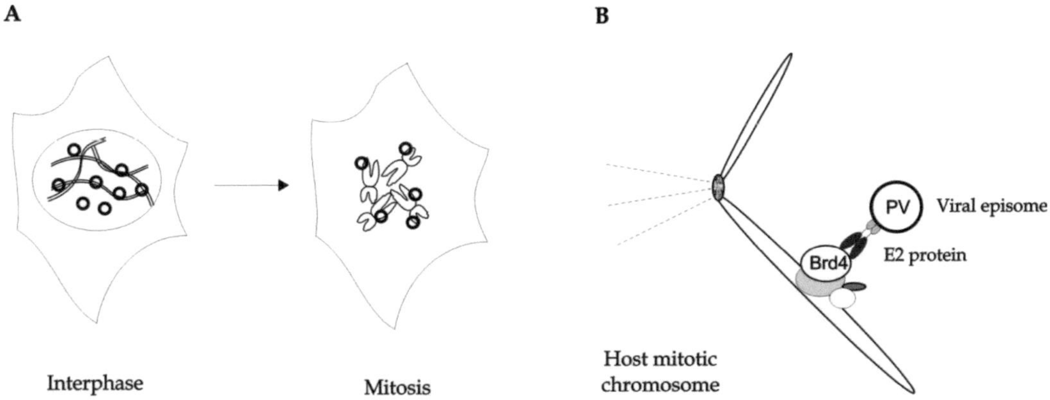

Fig. 6. Papillomaviruses establish persistent infection by maintaining viral genomes as episomes in host cell. (A) During mitosis, papillomavirus genomes are associated with cellular mitotic chromosomes. (B) For many papillomaviruses, association with mitotic chromosomes is mediated by the viral E2 protein and cellular bromodomain protein Brd4.

The role of E2 in long-term stable replication is not yet fully understood. The maintenance of papillomavirus genomes during latency is achieved by tethering viral genomes to host the mitotic apparatus in dividing cells. In this, BPV1 and HPVs may use different targets to achieve their goal. In BPV1, the activation domain of E2 is attached to chromosomes and the DNA-binding-dimerization domain tethers viral genomes to achieve their accurate segregation during mitosis. The point-mutations in the activation domain of E2, disrupting the transcription activity of E2, affect the chromatin attachment, suggesting that this activity is required for efficient segregation and maintenance of MME-containing plasmids (Abroi et al., 2004). The cellular receptor for BPV1 E2 on mitotic chromosomes is the bromodomain protein Brd4 (You et al., 2004). However, E2 proteins from different papillomaviruses interact with Brd4 with different affinities. E2 proteins of alpha-papillomaviruses interact with Brd4 weakly and do not co-localize with Brd4 on host mitotic chromosomes, suggesting that HPV E2 proteins may use different cellular targets for tethering virus genomes to host chromosomes (McPhillips et al., 2005; Oliveira et al., 2006). DNA helicase ChR1, a member of the mammalian cohesion complex, is a candidate partner for cellular receptor of HPV E2. ChlR1 and E2 co-localize at early stages of mitosis, however, during prometaphase, ChlR1 is localized to the spindle poles, suggesting that ChlR1 may help to load the papillomavirus E2 protein onto mitotic chromosomes during early mitosis (Parish et al., 2006a). HPV16 E2 co-localizes with TopBP1, a cellular protein involved in DNA damage response, on chromatin and centrosomes during late telophase, suggesting that TopBP1 could be the mitotic chromatin receptor for HPV16 E2 (Donaldson et al., 2007). On the other hand, E2 proteins of HPV11, HPV16 and HPV18 have been found to localize to centrosomes and mitotic spindles during cell division (Van Tine et al., 2004). MKlp2, mitotic kinesin-like protein 2, a kinesin-like motor protein of the central mitotic spindle, binds and co-localizes with papillomavirus E2 during mitosis (Yu et al., 2007). The beta-papillomavirus HPV8 E2 protein binds to the repeated ribosomal DNA loci that are found on the short arm of human acrocentric chromosomes. These speckles do not contain Brd4, the E2 protein co-localizes with UBF, the RNA polymerase I transcription factor (Poddar et al., 2009). A recent study using chimeric BPV1 E2 proteins has shown that attachment of the protein to chromatin is not sufficient for proper segregation. Successful partitioning of virus genomes during cell division is determined by effective formation of the segregation-competent complex which does not necessarily involve the Brd4 protein (Silla et al., 2010).

4.4 Regulation of replication by E2

The relative abundance of E2 proteins within the cell is an important factor regulating papillomavirus DNA replication. In BPV1-transformed cells, the relative ratio of E2 proteins is 1:5:1.5 for E2-E2C-E8/E2. The truncated E2 repressor proteins predominate in the steady state and the E2 heterodimers with single activation domain formed between the full-length and truncated E2 proteins are the preferential form for E2 (Kurg et al., 2006). The promoters for full-length E2 as well as for repressors are themselves controlled and differently regulated by E2, and furthermore, the ratio of the repressors to activators changes throughout the cell cycle. In G_1 cells, the repressors dominate, but in late S phase and G_2/M, the activator is present at about equal levels to that of the repressors. So, the level of E2 activators and repressors as well as E2 homo- and heterodimers is changing suggesting that the balance of different E2 proteins is a key event in the regulation of papillomavirus DNA replication (Szymanski and Stenlund, 1991; Yang et al., 1991b).

In papillomaviruses, there is a link between transcription and replication control, the protein that binds specifically to origin of replication also functions in control of transcription. BPV1 E2 protein levels are regulated by E2 itself and E2 activators and/or repressors have a positive or negative feedback to virus DNA replication. Initially the level of E2 activators is high to facilitate DNA amplification after infection, but later, the E2 expression is strictly controlled to avoid over-replication. Genetic studies have shown that the E8/E2 protein of HPV18, 31 and at least one of the BPV1 repressors are required for the long-term maintenance of virus episomes, demonstrating the important role of E2 repressors in the viral life cycle. Deletion of the E8 ORF results in robust initial replication of HPV genomes followed by rapid loss of virus episomes from dividing cells. The role of E2 repressors in the virus life cycle is to modulate the activity of full-length E2 protein by preventing the E2 binding to E2BS via binding site competition, and by acting as a repressor recruiting host co-

repressor molecules (Kurg et al., 2010; Lambert et al., 1990; Stubenrauch et al., 2000). However, the persistent replication and maintenance of virus genomes is not affected in E8 knock-out genomes of HPV16 and cotton-tail rabbit papillomavirus (CRPV), suggesting that E2 proteins of different papillomaviruses may regulate their expression and through this replication by different ways (Jeckel et al., 2003; Lace et al., 2008).
The efficiency of papillomavirus DNA replication is also controlled by the level of the E1 protein. E2 regulates E1 expression level through modulation of the activity of viral early promoters (Hubert and Laimins, 2002; Szymanski and Stenlund, 1991). However, it is still not clear to what extent HPV E2 proteins regulate HPV URRs. The HPV16 E2 protein does not repress HPV16 transcription when the URR is contained within an episomal HPV genome (Bechtold et al., 2003). Another group has shown that transcription activation function of the HPV31 E2 protein is not required for the viral life cycle (Stubenrauch et al., 1998). In addition to the transcriptional regulation by E2, the expression of E1 is regulated post-transcriptionally by mRNA splicing. In high-risk HPVs, E1 is translated by a discontinuous scanning mechanism and mRNA splicing within the E6 ORF is required for efficient expression of E1 (Hubert and Laimins, 2002)(Remm et al., 1999).

5. Conclusion

E2 is the master regulator of extrachromosomal replication of papillomaviruses. E2 regulates papillomavirus replication at multiple levels and through different mechanisms. First, E2 is essential for initiation of papillomavirus DNA replication. Second, E2 is required for long-term stable replication and is involved in maintenance and segregation of viral genomic DNA. Third, the abundance of E2 proteins and formation of homo- and heterodimers possessing different activities as well as the expression level of viral helicase E1 is regulated by E2. In addition to direct involvement in replication, E2 indirectly regulates papillomavirus replication through modulation of expression and activity of viral oncogenes E6 and E7, and the cellular environment.

6. Acknowledgment

I thank members of the Ustav lab for stimulating discussions and I am very grateful to Ivar Ilves for valuable comments. RK is supported by the Estonian Science Foundation (ETF7556) and by the European Regional Development Fund through the Center of Excellence in Chemical Biology.

7. References

Abbate, E. A., Berger, J. M., and Botchan, M. R. (2004). The X-ray structure of the papillomavirus helicase in complex with its molecular matchmaker E2. *Genes Dev* 18(16), 1981-1996.

Abbate, E. A., Voitenleitner, C., and Botchan, M. R. (2006). Structure of the papillomavirus DNA-tethering complex E2:Brd4 and a peptide that ablates HPV chromosomal association. *Mol Cell* 24(6), 877-889.

Abroi, A., Ilves, I., Kivi, S., and Ustav, M. (2004). Analysis of chromatin attachment and partitioning functions of the bovine papillomavirus type 1 E2 protein. *J.Virol.* 78, 2100-2113.

Abroi, A., Kurg, R., and Ustav, M. (1996). Transcriptional and replicational activation functions in the bovine papillomavirus type 1 E2 protein are encoded by different structural determinants. *J Virol* 70(9), 6169-6179.

Ahola, H., Stenlund, A., Moreno-Lopez, J., and Pettersson, U. (1987). Promoters and processing sites within the transforming region of bovine papillomavirus type 1. *J Virol* 61(7), 2240-2244.

Ammermann, I., Bruckner, M., Matthes, F., Iftner, T., and Stubenrauch, F. (2008). Inhibition of transcription and DNA replication by the papillomavirus E8-E2C protein is mediated by interaction with corepressor molecules. *J Virol* 82(11), 5127-5136.

Androphy, E., Lowy, D., and Schiller, J. (1987). Bovine papillomavirus E2 trans-activating gene product binds to specific sites in papillomavirus DNA. *Nature* 325(6099), 70-73.

Antson, A. A., Burns, J. E., Moroz, O. V., Scott, D. J., Sanders, C. M., Bronstein, I. B., Dodson, G. G., Wilson, K. S., and Maitland, N. J. (2000). Structure of the intact transactivation domain of the human papillomavirus E2 protein. *Nature* 403(6771), 805-809.

Baker, C., and Howley, P. (1987). Differential promoter utilization by the bovine papillomavirus in transformed cells and productively infected wart tissues. *EMBO J* 6(4), 1027-1035.

Bastien, N., and McBride, A. (2000). Interaction of the papillomavirus E2 protein with mitotic chromosomes. *Virology* 270, 124-134.

Bechtold, V., Beard, P., and Raj, K. (2003). Human papillomavirus type 16 E2 protein has no effect on transcription from episomal viral DNA. *J Virol* 77(3), 2021-2028.

Bellanger, S., Blachon, S., Mechali, F., Bonne-Andrea, C., and Thierry, F. (2005). High-risk but not low-risk HPV E2 proteins bind to the APC activators Cdh1 and Cdc20 and cause genomic instability. *Cell Cycle* 4(11), 1608-1615.

Berg, M., and Stenlund, A. (1997). Functional interactions between papillomavirus E1 and E2 proteins. *J Virol* 71(5), 3853-3863.

Bonne-Andrea, C., Santucci, S., and Clertant, P. (1995). Bovine papillomavirus E1 protein can, by itself, efficiently drive multiple rounds of DNA synthesis in vitro. *J Virol* 69(5), 3201-3205.

Boyer, S. N., Wazer, D. E., and Band, V. (1996). E7 protein of human papilloma virus-16 induces degradation of retinoblastoma protein through the ubiquitin-proteasome pathway. *Cancer Res* 56(20), 4620-4624.

Brokaw, J., Blanco, M., and McBride, A. (1996). Amino acids critical for the functions of the bovine papillomavirus type 1 E2 transactivator. *J Virol* 70(1), 23-29.

Cardenas-Mora, J., Spindler, J. E., Jang, M. K., and McBride, A. A. (2008). Dimerization of the papillomavirus E2 protein is required for efficient mitotic chromosome association and Brd4 binding. *J Virol* 82(15), 7298-7305.

Chen, G., and Stenlund, A. (1998). Characterization of the DNA-binding domain of the bovine papillomavirus replication initiator E1. *J Virol* 72(4), 2567-2576.

Chen, G., and Stenlund, A. (2001). The E1 initiator recognizes multiple overlapping sites in the papillomavirus origin of DNA replication. *J Virol* 75(1), 292-302.

Chiang, C., Broker, T., and Chow, L. (1991). An E1M--E2C fusion protein encoded by human papillomavirus type 11 is a sequence-specific transcription repressor. *J Virol* 65(6), 3317-3329.

Chiang, C., Ustav, M., Stenlund, A., Ho, T., Broker, T., and Chow, L. (1992). Viral E1 and E2 proteins support replication of homologous and heterologous papillomaviral origins. *Proc Natl Acad Sci U S A* 89(13), 5799-5803.

Chow, L., Nasseri, M., Wolinsky, S., and Broker, T. (1987). Human papillomavirus types 6 and 11 mRNAs from genital condylomata acuminata. *J Virol* 61(8), 2581-2588.

Chow, L. T., Broker, T. R., and Steinberg, B. M. (2010). The natural history of human papillomavirus infections of the mucosal epithelia. *Apmis* 118(6-7), 422-449.

Clower, R. V., Fisk, J. C., and Melendy, T. (2006). Papillomavirus E1 protein binds to and stimulates human topoisomerase I. *J Virol* 80(3), 1584-1587.

Cullen, A. P., Reid, R., Campion, M., and Lorincz, A. T. (1991). Analysis of the physical state of different human papillomavirus DNAs in intraepithelial and invasive cervical neoplasm. *J Virol* 65(2), 606-612.

Dall, K. L., Scarpini, C. G., Roberts, I., Winder, D. M., Stanley, M. A., Muralidhar, B., Herdman, M. T., Pett, M. R., and Coleman, N. (2008). Characterization of naturally occurring HPV16 integration sites isolated from cervical keratinocytes under noncompetitive conditions. *Cancer Res* 68(20), 8249-8259.

De Geest, K., Turyk, M. E., Hosken, M. I., Hudson, J. B., Laimins, L. A., and Wilbanks, G. D. (1993). Growth and differentiation of human papillomavirus type 31b positive human cervical cell lines. *Gynecol Oncol* 49(3), 303-310.

de Villiers, E. M., Fauquet, C., Broker, T. R., Bernard, H. U., and zur Hausen, H. (2004). Classification of papillomaviruses. *Virology* 324(1), 17-27.

Del Vecchio, A., Romanczuk, H., Howley, P., and Baker, C. (1992). Transient replication of human papillomavirus DNAs. *J Virol* 66(10), 5949-5958.

Dell, G., Wilkinson, K. W., Tranter, R., Parish, J., Leo Brady, R., and Gaston, K. (2003). Comparison of the structure and DNA-binding properties of the E2 proteins from an oncogenic and a non-oncogenic human papillomavirus. *J Mol Biol* 334(5), 979-991.

Demeret, C., Garcia-Carranca, A., and Thierry, F. (2003). Transcription-independent triggering of the extrinsic pathway of apoptosis by human papillomavirus 18 E2 protein. *Oncogene* 22(2), 168-175.

Desaintes, C., Demeret, C., Goyat, S., Yaniv, M., and Thierry, F. (1997). Expression of the papillomavirus E2 protein in HeLa cells leads to apoptosis. *EMBO J* 16(3), 504-514.

Dollard, S. C., Wilson, J. L., Demeter, L. M., Bonnez, W., Reichman, R. C., Broker, T. R., and Chow, L. T. (1992). Production of human papillomavirus and modulation of the infectious program in epithelial raft cultures. . *Genes Dev* 6(7), 1131-1142.

Donaldson, M. M., Boner, W., and Morgan, I. M. (2007). TopBP1 regulates human papillomavirus type 16 E2 interaction with chromatin. *J Virol* 81(8), 4338-4342.

Doorbar, J. (2005). The papillomavirus life cycle. *J Clin Virol* 32 Suppl 1, S7-15.

Doorbar, J., Parton, A., Hartley, K., Banks, L., Crook, T., Stanley, M., and Crawford, L. (1990). Detection of novel splicing patterns in a HPV16-containing keratinocyte cell line. *Virology* 178(1), 254-262.

Durst, M., Gissmann, L., Ikenberg, H., and zur Hausen, H. (1983). A papillomavirus DNA from a cervical carcinoma and its prevalence in cancer biopsy samples from different geographic regions. *Proc Natl Acad Sci U S A* 80(12), 3812-3815.

Egawa, K. (2003). Do human papillomaviruses target epidermal stem cells? *Dermatology* 207, 251-254.

Ferguson, M., and Botchan, M. (1996). Genetic analysis of the activation domain of bovine papillomavirus protein E2: its role in transcription and replication. *J Virol* 70(7), 4193-4199.

Flores, E. R., and Lambert, P. F. (1997). Evidence for a switch in the mode of human papillomavirus type 16 DNA replication during the viral life cycle. *J Virol* 71(10), 7167-7179.

Fouts, E. T., Yu, X., Egelman, E. H., and Botchan, M. R. (1999). Biochemical and electron microscopic image analysis of the hexameric E1 helicase. *J Biol Chem* 274(7), 4447-4458.

Frattini, M. G., Hurst, S. D., Lim, H. B., Swaminathan, S., and Laimins, L. A. (1997). Abrogation of a mitotic checkpoint by E2 proteins from oncogenic human papillomaviruses correlates with increased turnover of the p53 tumor suppressor protein. *Embo J* 16(2), 318-331.

Gammoh, N., Grm, H. S., Massimi, P., and Banks, L. (2006). Regulation of human papillomavirus type 16 E7 activity through direct protein interaction with the E2 transcriptional activator. *J Virol* 80(4), 1787-1797.

Garner-Hamrick, P. A., Fostel, J. M., Chien, W. M., Banerjee, N. S., Chow, L. T., Broker, T. R., and Fisher, C. (2004). Global effects of human papillomavirus type 18 E6/E7 in an organotypic keratinocyte culture system. *J Virol* 78(17), 9041-9050.

Geimanen, J., Isok-Paas, H., Pipitch, R., Salk, K., Laos, T., Orav, M., Reinson, T., Ustav, M., Jr., Ustav, M., and Ustav, E. (2011). Development of a cellular assay system to study the genome replication of high- and low-risk mucosal and cutaneous human papillomaviruses. *J Virol.*, in press.

Gilbert, D., and Cohen, S. (1987). Bovine papilloma virus plasmids replicate randomly in mouse fibroblasts throughout S phase of the cell cycle. *Cell* 50(1), 59-68.

Gloss, B., and Bernard, H. U. (1990). The E6/E7 promoter of human papillomavirus type 16 is activated in the absence of E2 proteins by a sequence-aberrant Sp1 distal element. *J Virol* 64(11), 5577-5584.

Goodwin, E. C., and DiMaio, D. (2000). Repression of human papillomavirus oncogenes in HeLa cervical carcinoma cells causes the orderly reactivation of dormant tumor suppressor pathways. *Proc Natl Acad Sci U S A* 97(23), 12513-12518.

Goodwin, E. C., Yang, E., Lee, C. J., Lee, H. W., DiMaio, D., and Hwang, E. S. (2000). Rapid induction of senescence in human cervical carcinoma cells. *Proc Natl Acad Sci U S A* 97(20), 10978-10983.

Grm, H. S., Massimi, P., Gammoh, N., and Banks, L. (2005). Crosstalk between the human papillomavirus E2 transcriptional activator and the E6 oncoprotein. *Oncogene* 24(33), 5149-5164.

Grossel, M., Sverdrup, F., Breiding, D., and Androphy, E. (1996). Transcriptional activation function is not required for stimulation of DNA replication by bovine papillomavirus type 1 E2. *J Virol* 70(10), 7264-7269.

Harris, S. F., and Botchan, M. R. (1999). Crystal structure of the human papillomavirus type 18 E2 activation domain. *Science* 284(5420), 1673-1677.

Hegde, R., Grossman, S., Laimins, L., and Sigler, P. (1992). Crystal structure at 1.7 A of the bovine papillomavirus-1 E2 DNA-binding domain bound to its DNA target [see comments]. *Nature* 359(6395), 505-512.

Hines, C., Meghoo, C., Shetty, S., Biburger, M., Brenowitz, M., and Hegde, R. (1998). DNA structure and flexibility in the sequence-specific binding of papillomavirus E2 proteins. *J Mol Biol* 276(4), 809-818.

Hoffmann, R., Hirt, B., Bechtold, V., Beard, P., and Raj, K. (2006). Different modes of human papillomavirus DNA replication during maintenance. *J Virol* 80(9), 4431-4439.

Hu, Y., Clower, R. V., and Melendy, T. (2006). Cellular topoisomerase I modulates origin binding by bovine papillomavirus type 1 E1. *J Virol* 80(9), 4363-4371.

Hubbert, N., Schiller, J., Lowy, D., and Androphy, E. (1988). Bovine papilloma virus-transformed cells contain multiple E2 proteins. *Proc Natl Acad Sci U S A* 85(16), 5864-5868.

Hubert, W. G., Kanaya, T., and Laimins, L. A. (1999). DNA replication of human papillomavirus type 31 is modulated by elements of the upstream regulatory region that lie 5' of the minimal origin. *J Virol* 73(3), 1835-1845.

Hubert, W. G., and Laimins, L. A. (2002). Human papillomavirus type 31 replication modes during the early phases of the viral life cycle depend on transcriptional and posttranscriptional regulation of E1 and E2 expression. *J Virol* 76(5), 2263-2273.

Hudson, J. B., Bedell, M. A., McCance, D. J., and Laiminis, L. A. (1990). Immortalization and altered differentiation of human keratinocytes in vitro by the E6 and E7 open reading frames of human papillomavirus type 18. *J Virol* 64(2), 519-526.

Hummel, M., Hudson, J. B., and Laimins, L. A. (1992). Differentiation-induced and constitutive transcription of human papillomavirus type 31b in cell lines containing viral episomes. *J Virol* 66(10), 6070-6080.

Hwang, E., Naeger, L., and DiMaio, D. (1996). Activation of the endogenous p53 growth inhibitory pathway in HeLa cervical carcinoma cells by expression of the bovine papillomavirus E2 gene. *Oncogene* 12(4), 795-803.

Ilves, I., Kadaja, M., and Ustav, M. (2003). Two separate replication modes of the bovine papillomavirus BPV1 origin of replication that have different sensitivity to p53. *Virus Res* 96(1-2), 75-84.

Ilves, I., Kivi, S., and Ustav, M. (1999). Long-term episomal maintenance of bovine papillomavirus type 1 plasmids is determined by attachment to host chromosomes, which Is mediated by the viral E2 protein and its binding sites. *J Virol* 73(5), 4404-4412.

Ilves, I., Maemets, K., Silla, T., Janikson, K., and Ustav, M. (2006). Brd4 is involved in multiple processes of the bovine papillomavirus type 1 life cycle. *J Virol* 80(7), 3660-3665.

Jang, M. K., Kwon, D., and McBride, A. A. (2009). Papillomavirus E2 proteins and the host BRD4 protein associate with transcriptionally active cellular chromatin. *J Virol* 83(6), 2592-2600.

Jeckel, S., Loetzsch, E., Huber, E., Stubenrauch, F., and Iftner, T. (2003). Identification of the E9/E2C cDNA and functional characterization of the gene product reveal a new repressor of transcription and replication in cottontail rabbit papillomavirus. *J Virol* 77(16), 8736-8744.

Jiang, M., and Milner, J. (2002). Selective silencing of viral gene expression in HPV-positive human cervical carcinoma cells treated with siRNA, a primer of RNA interference. *Oncogene* 21(39), 6041-6048.

Jones, D. L., Alani, R. M., and Munger, K. (1997). The human papillomavirus E7 oncoprotein can uncouple cellular differentiation and proliferation in human keratinocytes by abrogating p21Cip1-mediated inhibition of cdk2. *Genes Dev* 11(16), 2101-2111.

Kadaja, M., Isok-Paas, H., Laos, T., Ustav, E., and Ustav, M. (2009). Mechanism of genomic instability in cells infected with the high-risk human papillomaviruses. *PLoS Pathog* 5(4), e1000397.

Kadaja, M., Sumerina, A., Verst, T., Ojarand, M., Ustav, E., and Ustav, M. (2007). Genomic instability of the host cell induced by the human papillomavirus replication machinery. *Embo J* 26(8), 2180-2191.

Kim, K., Garner-Hamrick, P. A., Fisher, C., Lee, D., and Lambert, P. F. (2003). Methylation patterns of papillomavirus DNA, its influence on E2 function, and implications in viral infection. *J Virol* 77(23), 12450-12459.

Kim, K., and Lambert, P. (2002). E1 protein of bovine papillomavirus 1 is nor required for the maintenance of viral plasmid DNA replication. *Virology* 293, 10-14.

Kristiansen, E., Jenkins, A., and Holm, R. (1994). Coexistence of episomal and integrated HPV16 DNA in squamous cell carcinoma of the cervix. *J Clin Pathol* 47(3), 253-256.

Kumar, R. A., Naidu, S. R., Wang, X., Imbalzano, A. N., and Androphy, E. J. (2007). Interaction of papillomavirus E2 protein with the Brm chromatin remodeling complex leads to enhanced transcriptional activation. *J Virol* 81(5), 2213-2220.

Kurg, R., Sild, K., Ilves, A., Sepp, M., and Ustav, M. (2005). Association of bovine papillomavirus E2 protein with nuclear structures in vivo. *J Virol* 79(16), 10528-10539.

Kurg, R., Tekkel, H., Abroi, A., and Ustav, M. (2006). Characterization of the functional activities of the Bovine Papillomavirus type 1 E2 protein "single-chain" heterodimers. *J Virol* 80(22), 11218-11225.

Kurg, R., Uusen, P., Sepp, T., Sepp, M., Abroi, A., and Ustav, M. (2009). Bovine papillomavirus type 1 E2 protein heterodimer is functional in papillomavirus DNA replication in vivo. *Virology* 386(2), 353-359.

Kurg, R., Uusen, P., Vosa, L., and Ustav, M. (2010). Human papillomavirus E2 protein with single activation domain initiates HPV18 genome replication, but is not sufficient for long-term maintenance of virus genome. *Virology* 408(2), 159-166.

Lace, M. J., Anson, J. R., Thomas, G. S., Turek, L. P., and Haugen, T. H. (2008). The E8--E2 gene product of human papillomavirus type 16 represses early transcription and replication but is dispensable for viral plasmid persistence in keratinocytes. *J Virol* 82(21), 10841-10853.

Lambert, P., Monk, B., and Howley, P. (1990). Phenotypic analysis of bovine papillomavirus type 1 E2 repressor mutants. *J Virol* 64(2), 950-956.

Law, M., Lowy, D., Dvorezky, I., and Howley, P. (1981). Mouse cells transformed by bovine papillomavirus contain only extra-chromosomal viral DNA sequences. *PNAS* 78, 2727-2731.

Lee, D., Hwang, S., Kim, J., and Choe, J. (2002a). Functional interaction between p/CAF and human papillomavirus E2 protein. *J. Biol. Chem.* 277, 6483-6489.

Lee, D., Kim, H., Jeong, K., Shim, Y., Horikawa, I., Barrett, J., and Choe, J. (2002b). Human papillomavirus E2 down-regulates the human telomerase reverse transcriptase promoter. *J. Biol. Chem.* 277, 27748-27756.

Lee, D., Lee, B., Kim, J., Kim, D., and Choe, J. (2000). cAMP response element-binding protein-binding protein binds to human papillomavirus E2 protein and activates E2-dependent transcription. *J. Biol. Chem.* 275, 7045-7051.

Lehman, C. W., and Botchan, M. R. (1998). Segregation of viral plasmids depends on tethering to chromosomes and is regulated by phosphorylation. *Proc Natl Acad Sci U S A* 95(8), 4338-4343.

Lepik, D., Ilves, I., Kristjuhan, A., Maimets, T., and Ustav, M. (1998). p53 protein is a suppressor of papillomavirus DNA amplificational replication. *J Virol* 72(8), 6822-6831.

Li, R., Knight, J., Bream, G., Stenlund, A., and Botchan, M. (1989). Specific recognition nucleotides and their DNA context determine the affinity of E2 protein for 17 binding sites in the BPV-1 genome. *Genes Dev* 3(4), 510-526.

Li, R., Knight, J., Jackson, S., Tjian, R., and Botchan, M. (1991). Direct interaction between Sp1 and the BPV enhancer E2 protein mediates synergistic activation of transcription. *Cell* 65(3), 493-505.

Lim, D., Gossen, M., Lehman, C., and Botchan, M. (1998). Competition for DNA binding sites between the short and long forms of E2 dimers underlies repression in bovine papillomavirus type 1 DNA replication control. *J Virol* 72(3), 1931-1940.

Liu, J., Kuo, S., Broker, T., and Chow, L. (1995). The functions of human papillomavirus type 11 E1, E2, and E2C proteins in cell-free DNA replication. *J Biol Chem* 270(45), 27283-27291.

Longworth, M. S., and Laimins, L. A. (2004a). The binding of histone deacetylases and the integrity of zinc finger-like motifs of the E7 protein are essential for the life cycle of human papillomavirus type 31. *J Virol* 78(7), 3533-3541.

Longworth, M. S., and Laimins, L. A. (2004b). Pathogenesis of human papillomaviruses in differentiating epithelia. *Microbiol Mol Biol Rev* 68(2), 362-372.

Massimi, P., Pim, D., Bertoli, C., Bouvard, V., and Banks, L. (1999). Interaction between the HPV-16 E2 transcriptional activator and p53. *Oncogene* 18(54), 7748-7754.

McBride, A., Byrne, J., and Howley, P. (1989). E2 polypeptides encoded by bovine papillomavirus type 1 form dimers through the common carboxyl-terminal domain: transactivation is mediated by the conserved amino-terminal domain. *Proc Natl Acad Sci U S A* 86(2), 510-514.

McCance, D. J., Kopan, R., Fuchs, E., and Laimins, L. A. (1988). Human papillomavirus type 16 alters human epithelial cell differentiation in vitro. *Proc Natl Acad Sci U S A* 85(19), 7169-7173.

McLaughlin-Drubin, M., and Münger, K. (2009). Oncogenic activities of human papillomaviruses. *Virus Research* 143, 195-208.

McPhillips, M. G., Oliveira, J. G., Spindler, J. E., Mitra, R., and McBride, A. A. (2006). Brd4 is required for e2-mediated transcriptional activation but not genome partitioning of all papillomaviruses. *J Virol* 80(19), 9530-9543.

McPhillips, M. G., Ozato, K., and McBride, A. A. (2005). Interaction of bovine papillomavirus E2 protein with Brd4 stabilizes its association with chromatin. *J Virol* 79(14), 8920-8932.

Melanson, S. M., and Androphy, E. J. (2009). Topography of bovine papillomavirus E2 protein on the viral genome during the cell cycle. *Virology* 393(2), 258-264.

Melendy, T., Sedman, J., and Stenlund, A. (1995). Cellular factors required for papillomavirus DNA replication. *J Virol* 69(12), 7857-7867.

Meyers, C., Frattini, M. G., Hudson, J. B., and Laimins, L. A. (1992). Biosynthesis of human papillomavirus from a continuous cell line upon epithelial differentiation. *Science* 257(5072), 971-973.

Mohr, I., Clark, R., Sun, S., Androphy, E., MacPherson, P., and Botchan, M. (1990). Targeting the E1 replication protein to the papillomavirus origin of replication by complex formation with the E2 transactivator. *Science* 250(4988), 1694-1699.

Mole, S., Milligan, S., and Graham, S. (2009). Human papillomavirus type 16 E2 protein transcriptionally activates the promoter of a key cellular splicing factor, SF2/ASF *J Virol* 83(1), 357-367.

Moody, C., and Laimins, L. (2010). Human papillomavirus oncoproteins: pathways to transformation. *Nat Rev Cancer* 10, 550-560.

Muller, F., Seo, Y., and Hurwitz, J. (1994). Replication of bovine papillomavirus type 1 origin-containing DNA in crude extracts and with purified proteins. *J Biol Chem* 269(25), 17086-17094.

Mungal, S., Steinberg, B. M., and Taichman, L. B. (1992). Replication of plasmid-derived human papillomavirus type 11 DNA in cultured keratinocytes. *J Virol* 66(5), 3220-3224.

Müller, A., Ritzkowsky, A., and Steger, G. (2002). Cooperative activation of human papillomavirus type 8 gene expression by the E2 protein and the cellular coactivator p300. *J. Virol.* 76, 11042-11053.

Oh, S. T., Kyo, S., and Laimins, L. A. (2001). Telomerase activation by human papillomavirus type 16 E6 protein: induction of human telomerase reverse transcriptase expression through Myc and GC-rich Sp1 binding sites. *J Virol* 75(12), 5559-5566.

Oldak, M., Smola, H., Aumailley, M., Rivero, F., Pfister, H., and Smola-Hess, S. (2004). The human papillomavirus type 8 E2 protein suppresses beta4-integrin expression in primary human keratinocytes. *J Virol* 78(19), 10738-10746.

Oliveira, J. G., Colf, L. A., and McBride, A. A. (2006). Variations in the association of papillomavirus E2 proteins with mitotic chromosomes. *Proc Natl Acad Sci U S A* 103(4), 1047-1052.

Parish, J. L., Bean, A. M., Park, R. B., and Androphy, E. J. (2006a). ChlR1 is required for loading papillomavirus E2 onto mitotic chromosomes and viral genome maintenance. *Mol Cell* 24(6), 867-876.

Parish, J. L., Kowalczyk, A., Chen, H. T., Roeder, G. E., Sessions, R., Buckle, M., and Gaston, K. (2006b). E2 proteins from high- and low-risk human papillomavirus types differ in their ability to bind p53 and induce apoptotic cell death. *J Virol* 80(9), 4580-4590.

Park, P., Copeland, W., Yang, L., Wang, T., Botchan, M., and Mohr, I. (1994). The cellular DNA polymerase alpha-primase is required for papillomavirus DNA replication and associates with the viral E1 helicase. *Proc Natl Acad Sci U S A* 91(18), 8700-8704.

Pett, M. R., Alazawi, W. O., Roberts, I., Dowen, S., Smith, D. I., Stanley, M. A., and Coleman, N. (2004). Acquisition of high-level chromosomal instability is associated with integration of human papillomavirus type 16 in cervical keratinocytes. *Cancer Res* 64(4), 1359-1368.

Pett, M., and Coleman, N. (2007). Integration of high-risk human papillomavirus: a key event in cervical carcinogenesis? *J Pathol* 212, 356-367.

Pfefferle, R., Marcuzzi, G. P., Akgul, B., Kasper, H. U., Schulze, F., Haase, I., Wickenhauser, C., and Pfister, H. (2008). The human papillomavirus type 8 E2 protein induces skin tumors in transgenic mice. *J Invest Dermatol* 128(9), 2310-2315.

Piirsoo, M., Ustav, E., Mandel, T., Stenlund, A., and Ustav, M. (1996). Cis and trans requirements for stable episomal maintenance of the BPV-1 replicator. *EMBO J* 15(1), 1-11.

Poddar, A., Reed, S. C., McPhillips, M. G., Spindler, J. E., and McBride, A. A. (2009). The human papillomavirus type 8 E2 tethering protein targets the ribosomal DNA loci of host mitotic chromosomes. *J Virol* 83(2), 640-650.

Powell, M. L., Smith, J. A., Sowa, M. E., Harper, J. W., Iftner, T., Stubenrauch, F., and Howley, P. M. (2010). NCoR1 mediates papillomavirus E8;E2C transcriptional repression. *J Virol* 84(9), 4451-4460.

Ravnan, J., Gilbert, D., Ten Hagen, K., and Cohen, S. (1992). Random-choice replication of extrachromosomal bovine papillomavirus (BPV) molecules in heterogeneous, clonally derived BPV-infected cell lines. *J Virol* 66(12), 6946-6952.

Rehtanz, M., Schmidt, H., Warthorst, U., and Steger, G. (2004). Direct interaction between nucleosome assembly protein 1 and the papillomavirus E2 proteins involved in activation of transcription. *Mol.Cell.Biol.* 24, 2153-2168.

Remm, M., Brain, R., and Jenkins, J. (1992). The E2 binding sites determine the efficiency of replication for the origin of human papillomavirus type 18. *Nucleic Acids Res* 20(22), 6015-6021.

Remm, M., Remm, A., and Ustav, M. (1999). Human papillomavirus type 18 E1 protein is translated from polycistronic mRNA by a discontinuous scanning mechanism. *J Virol* 73(4), 3062-3070.

Sanders, C. M., and Stenlund, A. (1998). Recruitment and loading of the E1 initiator protein: an ATP-dependent process catalysed by a transcription factor. *Embo J* 17(23), 7044-7055.

Sanders, C. M., and Stenlund, A. (2000). Transcription factor-dependent loading of the E1 initiator reveals modular assembly of the papillomavirus origin melting complex. *J Biol Chem* 275(5), 3522-3534.

Scheffner, M., Werness, B. A., Huibregtse, J. M., Levine, A. J., and Howley, P. M. (1990). The E6 oncoprotein encoded by human papillomavirus types 16 and 18 promotes the degradation of p53. *Cell* 63(6), 1129-1136.

Schmitt, A., Harry, J. B., Rapp, B., Wettstein, F. O., and Iftner, T. (1994). Comparison of the properties of the E6 and E7 genes of low- and high-risk cutaneous papillomaviruses reveals strongly transforming and high Rb-binding activity for the E7 protein of the low-risk human papillomavirus type 1. *J Virol* 68(11), 7051-7059.

Schuck, S., and Stenlund, A. (2005). Assembly of a double hexameric helicase. *Mol Cell* 20(3), 377-89.

Schvartzman, J. B., Adolph, S., Martin-Parras, L., and Schildkraut, C. L. (1990). Evidence that replication initiates at only some of the potential origins in each oligomeric form of bovine papillomavirus type 1 DNA. *Mol Cell Biol* 10(6), 3078-3086.

Schweiger, M. R., Ottinger, M., You, J., and Howley, P. M. (2007). Brd4-independent transcriptional repression function of the papillomavirus e2 proteins. *J Virol* 81(18), 9612-9622.

Schweiger, M. R., You, J., and Howley, P. M. (2006). Bromodomain protein 4 mediates the papillomavirus E2 transcriptional activation function. *J Virol* 80(9), 4276-4285.

Sedman, J., and Stenlund, A. (1995). Co-operative interaction between the initiator E1 and the transcriptional activator E2 is required for replicator specific DNA replication of bovine papillomavirus in vivo and in vitro. *EMBO J* 14(24), 6218-6228.

Sedman, J., and Stenlund, A. (1998). The papillomavirus E1 protein forms a DNA-dependent hexameric complex with ATPase and DNA helicase activities. *J Virol* 72, 6893-6897.

Sedman, T., Sedman, J., and Stenlund, A. (1997). Binding of the E1 and E2 proteins to the origin of replication of bovine papillomavirus. *J Virol* 71(4), 2887-2896.

Sherman, L., and Schlegel, R. (1996). Serum- and calcium-induced differentiation of human keratinocytes is inhibited by the E6 oncoprotein of human papillomavirus type 16. *J Virol* 70(5), 3269-3279.

Silla, T., Haal, I., Geimanen, J., Janikson, K., Abroi, A., Ustav, E., and Ustav, M. (2005). Episomal maintenance of plasmids with hybrid origins in mouse cells. *J Virol* 79(24), 15277-15288.

Silla, T., Mannik, A., and Ustav, M. (2010). Effective formation of the segregation-competent complex determines successful partitioning of the bovine papillomavirus genome during cell division. *J Virol* 84(21), 11175-11188.

Skiadopoulos, M., and McBride, A. (1998). Bovine papillomavirus type 1 genomes and the E2 transactivator protein are closely associated with mitotic chromatin. *J Virol* 72(3), 2079-2088.

Smith, J. A., White, E. A., Sowa, M. E., Powell, M. L., Ottinger, M., Harper, J. W., and Howley, P. M. (2010). Genome-wide siRNA screen identifies SMCX, EP400, and

Brd4 as E2-dependent regulators of human papillomavirus oncogene expression. *Proc Natl Acad Sci U S A* 107(8), 3752-3757.

Soeda, E., Ferran, M. C., Baker, C. C., and McBride, A. A. (2006). Repression of HPV16 early region transcription by the E2 protein. *Virology* 351(1), 29-41.

Spalholz, B., Yang, Y., and Howley, P. (1985). Transactivation of a bovine papilloma virus transcriptional regulatory element by the E2 gene product. *Cell* 42(1), 183-191.

Szymanski, P., and Stenlund, A. (1991). Regulation of early gene expression from the bovine papillomavirus genome in transiently transfected C127 cells. *J Virol* 65(11), 5710-5720.

Stanley, M. A., Browne, H. M., Appleby, M., and Minson, A. C. (1989). Properties of a non-tumorigenic human cervical keratinocyte cell line. *Int J Cancer* 43(4), 672-676.

Stenlund, A. (2003a). E1 initiator DNA binding specificity is unmasked by selective inhibition of non-specific DNA binding. *Embo J* 22(4), 954-963.

Stenlund, A. (2003b). Initiation of DNA replication: lessons from viral initiator proteins. *Nature Reviews* 4, 777-785.

Stoppler, H., Hartmann, D. P., Sherman, L., and Schlegel, R. (1997). The human papillomavirus type 16 E6 and E7 oncoproteins dissociate cellular telomerase activity from the maintenance of telomere length. *J Biol Chem* 272(20), 13332-13337.

Stubenrauch, F., Colbert, A. M., and Laimins, L. A. (1998). Transactivation by the E2 protein of oncogenic human papillomavirus type 31 is not essential for early and late viral functions. *J Virol* 72(10), 8115-8123.

Stubenrauch, F., Hummel, M., Iftner, T., and Laimins, L. A. (2000). The E8E2C protein, a negative regulator of viral transcription and replication, is required for extrachromosomal maintenance of human papillomavirus type 31 in keratinocytes. *J Virol* 74(3), 1178-1186.

Stubenrauch, F., Lim, H. B., and Laimins, L. A. (1998). Differential requirements for conserved E2 binding sites in the life cycle of oncogenic human papillomavirus type 31. *J Virol* 72(2), 1071-1077.

zur Hausen, H. (2000). Papillomaviruses causing cancer: evasion from host-cell control in early events in carcinogenesis. *J Natl Cancer Inst* 92(9), 690-698.

Thain, A., Jenkins, O., Clarke, A., and Gaston, K. (1996). CpG methylation directly inhibits binding of the human papillomavirus type 16 E2 protein to specific DNA sequences. *J Virol* 70(10), 7233-7235.

Thierry, F. (2009). Transcriptional regulation of the papillomavirus oncogenes by cellular and viral transcription factors in cervical carcinoma. *Virology* 384(2), 375-379.

Thierry, F., Benotmane, M. A., Demeret, C., Mori, M., Teissier, S., and Desaintes, C. (2004). A genomic approach reveals a novel mitotic pathway in papillomavirus carcinogenesis. *Cancer Res* 64(3), 895-903.

Thierry, F., Spyrou, G., Yaniv, M., and Howley, P. (1992). Two AP1 sites binding JunB are essential for human papillomavirus type 18 transcription in keratinocytes. *J Virol* 66(6), 3740-3748.

Thierry, F., and Yaniv, M. (1987). The BPV1-E2 trans-acting protein can be either an activator or a repressor of the HPV18 regulatory region. *Embo J* 6(11), 3391-3397.

Thomas, J. T., Hubert, W. G., Ruesch, M. N., and Laimins, L. A. (1999). Human papillomavirus type 31 oncoproteins E6 and E7 are required for the maintenance of episomes during the viral life cycle in normal human keratinocytes. *Proc Natl Acad Sci U S A* 96(15), 8449-8454.

Ustav, E., Ustav, M., Szymanski, P., and Stenlund, A. (1993). The bovine papillomavirus origin of replication requires a binding site for the E2 transcriptional activator. *Proc Natl Acad Sci U S A* 90(3), 898-902.

Ustav, M., and Stenlund, A. (1991). Transient replication of BPV-1 requires two viral polypeptides encoded by the E1 and E2 open reading frames. *EMBO J* 10(2), 449-457.

Ustav, M., Ustav, E., Szymanski, P., and Stenlund, A. (1991). Identification of the origin of replication of bovine papillomavirus and characterization of the viral origin recognition factor E1. *EMBO J* 10(13), 4321-4329.

Van Tine, B., Dao, L., Wu, S.-Y., Sonbuchner, T., Lin, B., Zou, N., Chiang, C.-M., Broker, T., and Chow, L. (2004). Human papillomavirus (HPV) origin-binding protein associates with mitotic spindles to enable viral DNA partitioning. *PNAS* 101, 4030-4035.

Wang, H. K., Duffy, A. A., Broker, T. R., and Chow, L. T. (2009a). Robust production and passaging of infectious HPV in squamous epithelium of primary human keratinocytes. *Genes Dev* 23(2), 181-194.

Wang, X., Naidu, S. R., Sverdrup, F., and Androphy, E. J. (2009b). Tax1BP1 interacts with papillomavirus E2 and regulates E2-dependent transcription and stability. *J Virol* 83(5), 2274-2284.

Wells, S. I., Francis, D. A., Karpova, A. Y., Dowhanick, J. J., Benson, J. D., and Howley, P. M. (2000). Papillomavirus E2 induces senescence in HPV-positive cells via pRB- and p21(CIP)-dependent pathways. *Embo J* 19(21), 5762-5771.

Werness, B. A., Levine, A. J., and Howley, P. M. (1990). Association of human papillomavirus types 16 and 18 E6 proteins with p53. *Science* 248(4951), 76-79.

Wu, S. Y., Lee, A. Y., Hou, S. Y., Kemper, J. K., Erdjument-Bromage, H., Tempst, P., and Chiang, C. M. (2006). Brd4 links chromatin targeting to HPV transcriptional silencing. *Genes Dev* 20(17), 2383-2396.

Yang, L., Li, R., Mohr, I., Clark, R., and Botchan, M. (1991a). Activation of BPV-1 replication in vitro by the transcription factor E2. *Nature* 353(6345), 628-632.

Yang, L., Mohr, I., Fouts, E., Lim, D., Nohaile, M., and Botchan, M. (1993). The E1 protein of bovine papilloma virus 1 is an ATP-dependent DNA helicase. *Proc Natl Acad Sci U S A* 90(11), 5086-5090

Yang, L., Mohr, I., Li, R., Nottoli, T., Sun, S., and Botchan, M. (1991b). Transcription factor E2 regulates BPV-1 DNA replication in vitro by direct protein-protein interaction. *Cold Spring Harb Symp Quant Biol* 56, 335-346.

You, J. (2010). Papillomavirus interaction with cellular chromatin. *Biochim Biophys Acta* 1799(3-4), 192-199.

You, J., Croyle, J., Nishimura, A., Ozato, K., and Howley, P. (2004). Interaction of the bovine papillomavirus E2 protein with brd4 tethers the viral DNA to host mitotic chromosomes. *Cell* 117, 349-360.

Yu, T., Peng, Y. C., and Androphy, E. J. (2007). Mitotic kinesin-like protein 2 binds and colocalizes with papillomavirus E2 during mitosis. *J Virol* 81(4), 1736-1745.

29

Topoisomerase I and II Expression in Recurrent Colorectal Cancer Cells: A Dubious Matter

Panagiotis Gouveris, Elias Skopelitis and Nicolas Tsavaris
University of Athens, School of Medicine, Department of Pathophysiology, Athens Greece

1. Introduction

DNA topoisomerases are enzymes which alter and modify the topology of double-stranded DNA, without changing the sequence of the structural units of DNA, namely the nucleotides. They act by transiently breaking and then religating the DNA helix. Therefore, they unwind the double helix, relaxing the supercoiled DNA, and they allow DNA strands or double helices to pass through each other. Topoisomerases are essential for replication, transcription, translation and recombination of DNA because, relaxing the double helix, they facilitate the function of other enzymes, like DNA and RNA polymerases. Topoisomerases are the magicians of the DNA world, as they practically solve all the topological problems occurring during every aspect of DNA metabolism (Gupta et al., 1995; Pommier et al., 1998; Stewart et al, 1998; Champoux et al., 2001; Burden et al., 1998; Kellner et al., 2003; Wang et al., 2002).

The first topoisomerase discovered, in 1971, was *E. coli* topoisomerase I, originally known as ω protein (Wang, 1971). Next year there was the discovery of eukaryotic topoisomerase I in nuclei extract from secondary mouse-embryo cells (Champoux et al., 1972) In 1976, DNA gyrase (topoisomerse II) was purified from *Escherichia coli* cells (Gellert et al., 1976a). Topoisomerases have been categorized in two basic families, according to their structure and mechanism of action: type I topoisomerases and type II topoisomerases. Type I topoisomerases mediate transient breaks in one of the DNA strands. They are further classified in the subfamilies IA and IB. Type IA topoisomerases form a covalent intermediate with the 5′-phosphoryl end of DNA, while type IB topoisomerases form a covalent intermediate with the 3′-phosphoryl end of DNA (Champoux et al., 2001).

On the other hand, type II topoisomersases transiently cleave both of the two DNA strands. They are also further classified in the subfamilies IIA and IIB on the basis of differences in their protein structure. In human and higher eukaryotic organisms, three groups of topoisomerases have been described. The first group includes topoisomerase I and mitochondrial DNA topoisomerase, which are type IB enzymes. The second group includes topoisomerases IIα and IIβ, which are type II enzymes. The third group, which was later discovered, includes topoisomerases IIIα and IIIβ, which are type IA enzymes (Lodge et al., 2000; Kwan et al., 2001; Hanai et al., 1996). Topoisomerase IV has also been described, a bacterial type II topoisomerase (Kato et al., 1990). More recently, topoisomerase V has been described, which is a prokaryotic counterpart to the eukaryotic topoisomerase I (Slesarev et al., 1994).

Topoisomerase I is the well known Scl-70 antigen, against which high autoantibodies titters are developed in diffuse cutaneous systemic scleroderma (Shero et al., 1986; Guldner et al., 1986; Shero et al., 1987). Antibodies against topoisomerase IIα are detected in localized scleroderma (Takehara et al., 2005). Topoisomerases IIIα and IIIβ are possibly involved in the pathogenesis of Bloom, Werner and Rothmund-Thomson syndromes, which are associated with genetic instability (Kwan et al., 2001; Raynard et al., 2006).

Similar enzymes, as mentioned above, do exist in the prokaryotic cell (bacterial topoisomerases-gyrases) (Wang, 1971; Gellert et al., 1976a; Brown et al., 1979), and in viruses (e.g Vaccinia virus topoisomerase I) (Shaffer et al, 1987; Shuman, 1998). The clinical significance of bacterial gyrases is great, as they constitute targets for antibiotic drugs like novobiocin, nalidixic acid and new quinolones (Gellert et al., 1976b; Sugino et al., 1977; Smith, 1986; Maxwell, 1992).

Topoisomerase IIα and topoisomerase I are the best studied human topoisomerases, and constitute molecular targets for well known and widely used antineoplastic drugs (Pommier et al., 1998; Burden et al., 1998).

2. Topoisomerase I

Human DNA topoisomerase I is essential for vital cellular processes, namely DNA replication, transcription, translation, recombination and repair. It is a 91 kDa monomeric polypeptide which consists of 765 amino acids. It is encoded by a single copy gene which is located on chromosome 20q12-13.2 (Champoux et al., 2001). It catalyzes the relaxation of both positively and negatively supercoiled DNA, while bacterial topoisomerase I catalyzes the relaxation of negatively supercoiled DNA. Superhelix density for most natural DNA molecules ranges from -0.03 to -0.09 (Bauer et al., 1980). The negative sign means that DNA superhelices are left-handed. In other words, superhelices are derived from reverse winding of the helix. During the process of transcription, RNA polymerase follows the helical path along DNA double strand, having the tendency to generate positive supercoils in front of it and negative supercoils behind it. The accumulation of such supercoils could block the process of transcription, harming cell viability. Therefore, toposomerase I acts as a swivel to relieve the torsional strain caused by the generation of positive supercoils upstream and negative supercoils downstream of the moving RNA polymerase. It gives the solution, removing any undesirable supercoil (Liu et al., 1987; Wang et al., 1993).

During the process of replication, topoisomerase I has a similar function. There is a tendency of positive supercoils accumulation. Topoisomerase I relaxes the supercoils, relieving the torsional strain of the DNA molecule (Avemann et al., 1998; Hsiang et al., 1989). Topoisomerase I has also a role in the process of DNA recombination, DNA repair, and mitotic chromosome condensation (Pommier et al., 1998; Bullock et al., 1985; Wang et al., 1991; Shuman et al., 1989; Castano et al., 1996; Subramanian et al., 1998).

Topoisomerase I does not require ATP for its action, in contrast to topoisomerase II, which does need ATP (Wang et al., 1969). In the active centre of the enzyme there is the active site tyrosine (Tyr-723) of which the hydroxyl group performs a nucleophilic attack on the phosphodiesteric bond of one of the two DNA strands. The phosphodiesteric bond is broken now. The enzyme remains covalently attached to the 3′ end of the broken strand, creating a transient covalent complex, known as cleavable complex. The 5′ hydroxyl group of the broken strand remains free. The DNA molecule can now rotate around the intact strand. This rotation leads to the relaxation of the abovementioned positive and negative supercoils.

The whole process is completed as the exposed 5′ hydroxyl group performs a nucleophilic attack on the transient phosphotyrosine linkage. The active site tyrosin is detached from the 3′ end. The cleaved strand is resealed (Pommier et al., 1998; Sari et al., 2005).

In summary, topoisomrasre I unwinds and uncoils the DNA supercoiled double helix by transiently cleaving one of the two strands and allowing rotation over the other. In the end it reseals the cleaved strand.

Topoisomerase I is not essential for viability in yeast (Thrash et al., 1984; Uemura et al., 1984). On the contrary, it is essential for embryonic development in *Drosophila melanogaster* and mouse (Lee et al., 1993; Morham et al., 1996).

By contrast to topoisomerase II, topoisomerase I levels are not cycle-specific and remain relatively constant throughout the cell cycle (Heck et al., 1988). Topoisomerase I seems to be expressed in all cells, even those which do not divide. However, the enzyme levels are higher in cancer tissues, compared to the adjacent normal tissues. This fact renders topoisomerase I an attractive target for chemotherapy drugs (Bronstein et al., 1996; Husain et al., 1994).

Topoisomerase I catalytic activity was the first parameter of topoisomerase I evaluable in biomedical studies and it was detected in all normal tissues at a fairly constant level. Two more parameters were added in the investigational process: topoisomerase I immunoprotein levels, estimated by Western Blotting analysis, and topoisomerase I gene expression (toposomerase I mRNA), evaluated by Northern Blotting analysis. There seems to be a good correlation between topoisomerase expression and the catalytic activity of the enzyme (Bronstein et al., 1996; Husain et al., 1994). Using the abovementioned parameters and methods, elevated topoisoomerase I levels were detected in ovarian cancer, cervical cancer, colorectal cancer, prostate cancer, malignant melanoma, lymphoma (Bronstein et al., 1996; Husain et al., 1994; Van der Zee et al., 1991; Van der Zee et al., 1994; Perego et al., 1994; McLeod et al., 1994; Goldwasser et al., 1995; Guichard et al., 1999; Giovanella et al., 1989; Florell et al., 1996). On the other hand, there was no elevation in topoisomerase I levels detected in lung cancer, breast cancer, renal cancer, and rhabdomyosarcoma (Bronstein et al., 1996; Husain et al., 1994; McLeod et al., 1994). With regard to colorectal tumors, topoisomerase I levels have been found to demonstrate 5-35-fold increases in the cancer tissue, compared to the adjacent normal colonic mucosa (Bronstein et al., 1996; Husain et al., 1994). In 1997, a new evaluable parameter of topo I appeared in biomedical studies: topo I expression, evaluated by immunohistochemistry in paraffin embedded human tissues. Since then, topo I expression has been estimated in several neoplastic tissues. In fact, elevation of topo I was found in ovarian carcinomas (43% of tumors examined); colorectal carcinomas (ranging from 43% to 86% in different studies) ; testicular tumors (30-38% of seminomas, 30% of embryonal carcinomas, but 100% of teratomas and yolk sac tumours); urinary bladder carcinomas (77%); renal cell carcinomas (ranging from 36-100% according to histological grade); malignant melanomas (41,6%); gastric carcinomas (68%); sarcomas (13%); breast carcinomas (41%); oral dysplasias (79%) and squamous cell carcinomas (92%) (Holden et al., 1997; Boonsong et al., 2002; Staley et al., 1999; Paradiso et al., 2004; Monnin et al., 1999; Coleman et al., 2001; Coleman et al., 2000; Berney et al., 2002; Lynch et al., 2001; Gupta et al., 2000; Lynch et al., 1998; Hafian et al., 2004; Coleman et al., 2002). As far as topoisomerase I immunoreactivity in normal tissues is concerned, this appeared to be strongest in the germinal centres of the tonsil and in the lymphocytes of colonic mucosa, while it was also detected in the glandular colonic epithelium (Holden et al., 1997).

3. Topoisomerase II

Topoisomerase II is a ubiquitous enzyme which is essential for the viability of all eukaryotic organisms and plays a crucial role in literally every aspect of DNA metabolism and chromosome organization. In contrast to topoisomerase I, which is actually monomeric, topoisomerase II exists in two homologous but different isoforms, designated IIα and IIβ, which are closely related. The two isoforms share homology in the amino acid sequence (up to 70%), but they are encoded by separate genes. Topoisomerse IIα is the isoform originally described and characterized in mammalian species. It has a molecular mass of 170 kDa and is encoded by a gene which is located on chromosome 17q21-22. Topoisomerse IIβ has a molecular mass of 180 kDa and is encoded by a gene which is located on chromosome 3q24. Both of the proteins exist as homodimers (Burden et al., 1998; Kellner et al., 2003; Pommier et al., 2001; Jenkins et al., 1992; Austin et al., 1993).

Topoisomerase IIβ concentrations are relatively constant during the cell cycle. On the contrary, topoisomerase IIα levels are tightly associated with the proliferative state of the cell, and increase 2-3 fold during G_2/M phase. This increase takes place in rapidly proliferating tissues, while quiescent populations demonstrate low enzyme levels (Heck et al., 1988). Therefore, it is believed that the β isoform is responsible for the "housekeeping" functions of the enzyme, while the α isoform seems to be the type II enzyme which unlinks daughter chromosomes following replication. A small percentage of the total topoisomerase II pool in mammalian cells exists as α/β heterodimers (Biersack et al., 1996).

The enzymological characteristics of all eukaryotic type II appear to be similar. Each topoisomerase II monomer can be divided in three domains. The N-terminal domain, which includes the first 660 amino acids of the enzyme, is homologous to the B subunit of DNA gyrase and contains sequences for ATP binding. The central domain of the enzyme, which extends to amino acid 1200, is homologous to the A subunit of DNA gyrase and contains the active site tyrosine that forms the covalent bond with DNA during scission. The C-terminal domain of the enzyme varies from species to species and doesn't seem to have homology with DNA gyrase. The physiological function of this domain remains unclear. It possibly has a role in modulating the DNA cleavage/ligation reaction of the enzyme (Wang et al., 1996; Berger et al., 1998; Dickey et al., 2005).

Topoisomerase II works in a way similar to topoisomerase I, with the difference that it cleaves both strands of the nucleic acid substrate, allowing the passage of an intact double helix through the break. The enzyme Topoisomerase II is able to catalyze the relaxation of both positively and negatively supercoiled DNA. Its catalytic action begins with the simultaneous cleavage of both of the two DNA strands. The active site tyrosins (one for each monomer of the homodimer) covalently bind to the 5′ end of the broken strands and create the transient complex which is known as cleavable complex. Till this step, energy from ATP hydrolysis is not required. The protein dimer is stabilized with disulfide bridges that create a gate through which we have the passage of another intact double-stranded DNA helix. This passage takes place at the expense of ATP hydrolysis. The whole procedure is completed with the resealing of the cleaved double strand (Roca et al., 1994; Schultz et al., 1996; Lindsley et al., 1996).

As a result of this DNA passage mechanism, topoisomerase II is able not only to remove negative or positive DNA supercoils, but also to unlink intertwined pairs of newly replicated chromosomes. This extra feature of topoisomerase II is important for chromosome organization and segregation. Topoisomerase I doesn't share this feature (Roca et al., 1996).

As mentioned above, topoisomerase IIα levels are cell cycle-dependent, with maximum concentrations measured during the G2/M phase. That's why the percentage of positive of positive what? for topoisomerase IIα cells practically represents the percentage of dividing cells. Thus, several studies have displayed that topoisomerase IIα levels may act as a reliable marker of cell proliferation in tumors. Topoisomerase IIα has been used as a proliferation marker in several studies, including patients with colorectal cancer (Monnin et al., 1999; Holden et al., 1995; Nakopoulou et al., 2001; Gibbons et al., 1997).

Concerning normal tissues, topoisomerase IIα levels are higher in tissues with proliferating cells (eg. spermatocytes, germinal cells, and proliferative endometrium) references?. In contrast, no detectable topoismerase IIα was detected in terminally differentiated tissues, e.g cerebral cortex, skeletal muscle, and nerve (Bauman et al., 1997). Concerning neoplastic tissues, high levels of topoisomerase IIα are observed in biologically aggressive or rapidly proliferating tumors, like high-grade lymphomas or seminomas. Topoisomerase IIα is detectable in both the cell nucleus and cytoplasm. Topoisomerase IIβ is localized both in the nucleoli and the nucleoplasm. It is ubiquitously expressed in vivo and it is present in quiescent cell populations (Turley et al., 1997). Concerning normal colon mucosa, topoisomerase IIα is expressed only in the lower crypt zone. In adenomas, the topoisomerase IIα expression is expanded in the upper crypt region, while it is diffuse in carcinomas (Fogt et al., 1997).

Topoisomerase II constitutes the molecular target of a great number of antineoplastic drugs, which are widely used in cancer chemotherapy, including anthracyclins and epipodophyllotoxins. These drugs constitute substrates of the classic MDR proteins. It is interesting that topoisomerase II is implicated in a type of multiple drug resistance which is called atypical MDR. There is actually a type of multiple drug resistance only to anthracyclins and epipodophyllotoxins, not the vinca alkaloids and colchicine. This type has no relation with classical MDR (Borst et al, 1995). This atypical MDR is attributed to mutations associated with topoisomerase II. There are two basic types of such mutations:

1. Mutations which lead to low levels of the enzyme. Drugs targeting topoisomerase II stabilize the cleavable complexes between the enzyme and DNA, creating permanent breaks of the double strand. Reduced levels of topoisomerase II lead to reduced DNA strand breaks, therefore reduced drug activity (Zijlstra et al., 1990; Cole et al., 1991; Sullivan et al., 1987).
2. Mutations leading to a qualitatively modified topoisomerase II, less sensitive to the chemotherapy drugs (Beck et al., 1993; Glisson et al., 1987).

4. Topoisomerase I inhibitors

There are a lot of inhibiting topoisomerase I (Pommier et al., 1998; Wang et al., 1997). In clinical practice only camptothecin derivatives are used.

Camptothecin (CPT) is an alkaloid found in the wood and bark of the Chinese tree Camptotheca acuminata (Nyssaceae) (Wall et al., 1966). Wall and Perdue isolated CPT from Camptotheca acuminate during the '60s. CPT and its derivatives were also found in other plant families.

In the early phase-I and II clinical studies regarding CPT, the water soluble sodium salt NSC-100880 was used. Despite the antineoplastic activity, the studies were suspended due to unacceptable hematologic (myelosupression) and non hematologic (hemorrhagic cystitis) toxicity (Gottlieb et al., 1970; Muggia et al., 1972; Moertel et al., 1972; Gottlieb et al., 1972;

Schaeppi et al., 1974). Later, it was shown that the cytotoxic activity of camptothecin, that has pentacyclic structure, was attributed to its E-ring lactone. When the E-ring opens to form hydroxyacid, the drug becomes inactive. In water solutions the inactive open form is favored (Slichenmyer et al., 1993). On the other hand, the low water solubility of the drug was the main reason for its toxicity. Therefore, an effort began having to do with the synthesis of CPT derivatives that combine the maximum possible water solubility with the best cytotoxic activity. Semisynthetic water soluble derivatives were produced. The most important of them were topotecan (TPT) and irinotecan (CPT-11). These new drugs were developed with modification of the A-ring of the camptothecin molecule (Kerrigan et al., 2001).

Camptothecin derivatives act causing irreversible breaks on the DNA strands. They actually act stabilizing the cleavable complexes formed by topoisomerase I, which normally have short half life. This stabilization takes place bringing a guanine at the 5′ end of the cleaved DNA. While the stabilization is irreversible, it causes irreversible break of the double strand, when the replication fork meets a cleavable complex (Covey et al., 1989; Hsiang et al., 1989; Pommier et al., 1996; Jaxel et al., 1991). When topoisomerase I levels are higher, the cleavable complexes are more frequent, and the DNA strand breaks are more frequent, too. These breaks lead to the cell cycle arrest at S/G_2 phase, activation of apoptotic mechanisms and cell death (Hsiang et al., 1988). That's why camptothecin derivatives are cytotoxic in presence of active DNA replication or RNA transcription. Cells synchronized in S phase are 1000-fold more sensitive than in phases G_1 and $G_2/$ M. Despite the fact that topoisomerase levels remain stable during the cell cycle, camptothecin derivatives constitute cycle-specific drugs (Liu et al., 1983; D'Incalci et al., 1993).

The term "inhibitors" when we refer to topoisomerase I inhibitors is somewhat catachrestic. Camptothecin derivatives actually do not inhibit topoisomerase I but they use the enzyme function in order to transform the enzyme into a cell poison.

Irinotecan is bioactivated in liver by carboxylesterase to the active metabolite SN-38. SN-38 is 1000-fold more active (Slichenmyer et al., 1993). Both irinotecan and SN-38 are susceptible to pH - dependent reversible hydrolysis and transformation of the active closed ring (lactone) to the open form of hydroxyacid. Acidic pH favors the active form of closed ring. The open form not only lacks the ability of cleavable complexes stabilization, but also the ability of entrance into the cell via the cell membrane.

The active metabolite SN-38 is responsible not only for the antineoplastic activity of irinotecan, but also for the side-effects. Late diarrhea is the most important side effect and it often does not respond to common anti-diarrheic drugs. SN38 is further metabolized by the UDP-glucuronosyltransferase 1A1 (UGT1A1) enzyme to the inactive form SN38 glucuronide (SN38-Glu), which is excreted in the gastrointestinal lumen via bile. It is believed that intestinal bacteria produce β-glucuronidase, that hydrolizes SN38-Glu to the active form SN38. SN38 causes intestinal mucosa injury, that leads to late diarrhea. At the same time, the non-metabolized irinotecan constitutes a weak acetylcholinestarase inhibitor and may cause acute cholinergic symptoms, among which is the early diarrhea in some patients (Abigerges et al., 1994; Kehrer et al., 2001; Lokiec et al., 1995; Takasuna et al., 1996; Gupta et al., 1994).

Irinotecan received in 1996 and 1998 FDA approval for treatment of metastatic colorectal cancer after failure of treatment with fluorouracil. The importance of the drug was proved in two European randomized studies (Cunningham et al., 1998; Rougier et al., 1998). In 2000,

irinotecan received FDA approval for first line treatment in metastatic colorectal cancer, combined with fluorouracil/leucovorin (Saltz et al., 2000; Douillard et al., 2000).
Topotecan is the second camptothecin derivative. It is itself an active drug. A low percentage of the drug is metabolized by microsomal enzymes to N-demethyltopotecan, which is also an active metabolite. In contrast to irinotecan, which is metabolized in liver, topotecan is mainly excreted in urine. Topotecan received FDA approval as second line therapy in metastatic ovarian cancer (1996) and in SCLC (1998).

5. Topoisomerase II inhibitors

Topoisomerase II inhibitors are cytostatic drugs widely used in clinical practice since decades (Hande et al., 1998). According to their mechanism of action, they are divided in two broad categories. The first category includes DNA intercalators, which intercalate between the base pairs of DNA, disrupting DNA function. This category includes cytotoxic antibiotics like anthracyclines (eg. doxorubicin, epirubicin, mitoxantrone) and aminoacridines, among which amsacrine is the main drug (Bailly, 2000). The second category includes substances which do not act with an intercalation mechanism. Epipodophyllotoxins and some isoflavones, like genistein belong to this category. Genistein is included in soy, and it is possibly responsible for the low incidence of breast cancer, prostate cancer and colorectal cancer in Asian populations (Barnes et al., 1995; Stoll et al., 1997).
Quinolones, the well known family of broad spectrum antibiotic, are also topisomerase II inhibitors. They are the only group of drugs with activity against both eukaryotic topoisomerase IIα and its prokaryotic homologue, bacterial gyrase. Quinolones are not used as antineoplasic drugs, till now, but they include widely used antibiotics like ciprofloxacin and norfloxacin (Burden et al., 1998; Maxwell et al., 1992; Robinson et al., 1991; Robinson et al., 1992).
Epipodophyllotoxins were synthesized in an effort of amelioration of podophyllotoxin activity. Podophyllotoxin is a substance which constitutes extract of the plant *Podophyllum peltatum*, known by the American Indians for its emetical, cathartic, and anthelminthic activity (Mantle et al., 2000). Two semisynthetic glucosides were synthesized from podophyllotoxin: etoposide and tenoposide. Etoposide is produced with the attachment of podophyllotoxin to a glucopyranoside with a methyl group, while tenoposide is produced with the attachment of podophyllotoxin to a glucopyranoside with a thenyliden group. This simple modification causes an important change in the way of action of the drug. Therefore, while podophyllotoxin acts on microtubules that form mitotic spindle, etoposide and teniposide act as topoisomerase IIα inhibitors (Schilstra et al., 1989).
Etoposide and teniposide act on topoisomerase IIα, in a way similar to which irinotecan and topotecan act on topoisomerase I. They actually take advantage of the normal topoisomerase IIα action, in order to transform it into a cell poison. The whole process takes place during stabilization of DNA- topoisomerase IIα complexes, which induces double strand breaks (Burden et al., 1998). Cells in S and G_2 phases of the cell cycle are more sensitive to epipodophyllotoxins. However, in contrast to the camptothecins derivatives, which are characterized by high cycle specificity, DNA synthesis inhibition only partially affects epipodophyllotoxin induced cytotoxicity (Holm et al., 1989).
Etoposide is a widely used antineoplastic drug highly active in germ cell tumors, ovarian cancer, SCLC, NSCLC, non-Hodgkin lymphoma, acute leukemia, Ewing sarcoma, Kaposi sarcoma, neuroblastoma. Tenoposide is less used in clinical practice.

6. Original research

6.1. Pilot study

6.1.1 Materials and methods

6.1.1.1 Patients' characteristics - study and control groups

In the study we are describing in this chapter, a total of twenty-five patients were included. Those patients had colorectal cancer which had recurred following surgery and chemotherapy. Specifically, patients had undergone complete surgical resection of the primary tumour and subsequently were submitted to a 5-FU-based adjuvant chemotherapy regimen, postoperatively. Patients were followed-up until recurrence. When recurrences occurred, patients underwent a second surgical resection. Biopsy specimens from both surgical procedures for each patient were, therefore, collected, so that at the end of the study we evaluated two histological specimens from each patient: one from the primary tumour location (i.e. before the administration of 5-FU-based adjuvant chemotherapy) and a second one from the neoplastic tissue at the recurrence site (i.e. following the 5-FU-based chemotherapy regimen).
In order to be able to make comparisons we needed a control group, so we selected a group of twelve patients with colorectal cancer who underwent resection after initial diagnosis, but received no 5-FU-based adjuvant chemotherapy. Patients in the control group were age and gender mached and had also similar tumour characteristics with patients included in the main study group. For each patient in the control group two biopsy specimens were available for evaluation since they were submitted to surgery following recurrence.

6.1.1.2 Histologic evaluation - immunochemistry

For each biopsy specimen, the expression of topoismerase-I was quantified by means of standard three-step immunohistochemistry on paraffin embedded sections. For this purpose the Topogen Topo I Monoclonal Antibody (2012-3) was used; this is a monoclonal mouse antibody (IgG2b isotype). The epitope of the antibody has not been mapped. Normal human tonsil tissues served as positive control. Histological sections were examined by a single investigator with no previous knowledge of the clinical status of the examined specimen.
During histologic examination, immunostaining for topoisomerase I was graded according to the percentage of tumour cells with positive staining (- and ± for <5%, + for 5%-50% and ++ for 50% to 75%) and according to the intensity of staining (weakly positive, moderately positive, or strongly positive). Only specimens with strongly immunoreactive nuclei were considered as a positive biopsy for topoisomerase I; weak and moderate intensity of staining was considered as negative for the expression of topoisomerase I.

6.1.1.3 Statistical Analysis

Following this initial evaluation, the sections were examined in pairs (one section for the first surgery and one section for the second surgery for each patient) during the statistical analysis. For the latter, we used McNemar's paired chi-square test to assess the possible modification of the levels of topoisomerase I following chemotherapy with 5-FU. Fisher's exact test was performed in order to assess the possible relationship of the topoisomerase I increase with gender, Duke's stage, grade of differentiation and tumour localization. Mann-Whitney U-Test was performed in order to assess possible relationship between the age of patients and changes of topoisomerase I levels as well as to investigate possible correlations between the relapse free interval (RFI) and alteration of topoisomerase I levels.

6.1.2 Results

6.1.2.1 Topoisomerase I level increase

Patients were categorized into two groups according to the increase of topoisomerase I levels (Figure 1). Using McNemar's paired chi-square test, we found that malignant cells from the tumour recurrences were characterized by the presence of a statistically significant increase in the levels of topoisomerase I when compared to the cells from the primary tumours (2-sided p=0.01) (figure 1).

6.1.2.2 Correlation with tumour parameters and demographics

The raise in topoisomerase I levels observed in the previous section/Figure 1 did not demonstrate significant correlations with Duke's stage (Fisher's Exact Test p-value = 0.496), grade of differentiation (p value = 0.661), tumour localization (p value = 0.072), or patients' gender (p value = 0.434). On the other hand, a statistically significant relationship was observed between the age of patients and the increase in topoisomerase I levels (p = 0.011). Using Mann-Whitney U-Test, patients with an increase in topoisomerase I levels were found to be older in age (median=62.5 years) than patients without increase in topoisomerase I levels (median=50 years) (p = 0.038).
Moreover, patients with an increase in topoisomerase levels had a median relapse free interval (RFI) of 17.5 months, while patients without such increase had a median RFI of 16 months. This difference in the RFIs between the two groups was not statistically significant (p = 0.493).

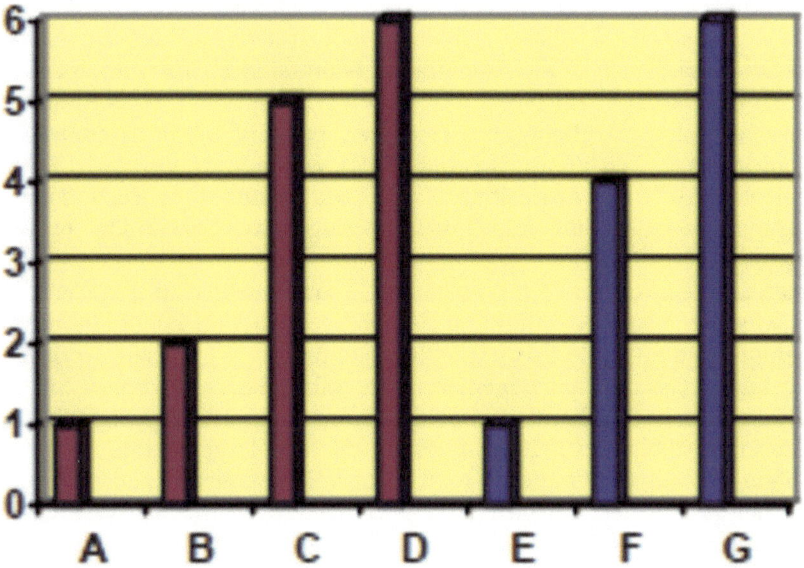

Y: 0-6 = Number of patients (n=25)
X: A (□ ▶++), B (+▶++), C (-▶+), D (□▶+): Group of increase (n=14)
E (+▶□), F (++▶++), G (+▶+): Group of non-increase (n=11)

Fig. 1. Distribution of the examined samples with regard to the combined expression of topoisomerase I (i.e at the tumour's first appearance and at its recurrence)

6.1.2.3 Comparison with control group

No statistically significant differences were found concerning topoisomerase I expression in malignant cells from the primary tumour between patients in the study and the control group.

6.1.2.4 Association with other morphologic characteristics

With regard to tumour-adjacent morphologically non-dysplastic mucosa, when colonic crypts were cut longitudinally, some topoisomerase I positive colonic cells were detectable in the proliferation zone (lower 1/3 of the colonic crypts). In totally normal colonic mucosa, obtained from tumour-free surgical margins, no such expression was detectable.

6.1.3 Discussion

In the current study, 13 out of the 25 patients with colorectal cancer (52%) stained positive for topoisomerase I (Figure 2). In respect with the percentage of tumour cells staining positive for topoisomerase I, 9 out of the 25 patients (36%) presented with 5% - 50% positive staining cells and 4 out of the 25 (16%) with >50% positive staining cells. These data are in line with Boonsong et al. (Boonsong et al., 2002), while Staley et al. (Staley et al., 1999) demonstrated a higher percentage (86%) of positive staining in samples of 29 patients.

Topoisomerase I immunoreactivity was confined to be present in the nucleus of all biopsy samples, a finding which is consistent with the role of topoisomerase I as a nuclear protein.

Importantly, we displayed a significant increase of topoisomerase I expression by means of immunohistochemistry in recurrences of the initial neoplasia, thus reinforcing the notion that topoisomerase I expression is likely to be part of the malignant cells' phenotype in recurrent colorectal carcinomas. This is in agreement with previous experiments (Ichikawa et al., 1999; Paradiso et al., 2004), which demonstrated a direct correlation between thymidylate synthase (TS) and topoisomerase I expression in tumours and hypothesized, similarly to TS (Leichman et al., 1997), that high topoisomerase I expression is related to a more aggressive biological phenotype. However, our finding is in contrast with other studies (Boonsong et al., 2002; Paradiso et al., 2004), which have postulated the absence of a role for topoisomerase I in the acquisition of a metastatic phenotype. Such disperse results in the literature may reflect an interlesion heterogeneity concerning topoisomerase I expression.

Since the increased expression of topoisomerase I immunostain in neoplastic tissues from recurrences was demonstrated following 5-FU-based adjuvant chemotherapy regimen, it would be tempting to attribute this particular alteration to 5-FU itself. Additionally, given the fact that high levels of topoisomerase I expression has been shown to correlate with sensitivity to camptothecin chemotherapy (Monnin et al., 1999), patients with advanced colorectal cancer are likely to benefit from topoisomerase I-targeted anticancer drug therapy. This also might explain why patients with metastatic colorectal cancer appear to benefit more when they are treated with a combination chemotherapy regimen. Of note, strong synergism between 5-FU and irinotecan (CTP-11) has been reported (Guichard et al., 1997, 1998) after sequential exposure to both agents, whereas additivity or antagonism has been reported only after simultaneous exposure. The above facts are suggestive that the mechanisms of interaction between these two drugs might be multifactorial and the specific schedule of administration represents a critical parameter of their chemotherapeutic efficacy. In fact, the combination of CTP-11 and 5-FU+leucovorin (LV) has been approved (Saltz et al., 2000, 2001; Vanhoefer et al., 2001) as reference first-line chemotherapy for

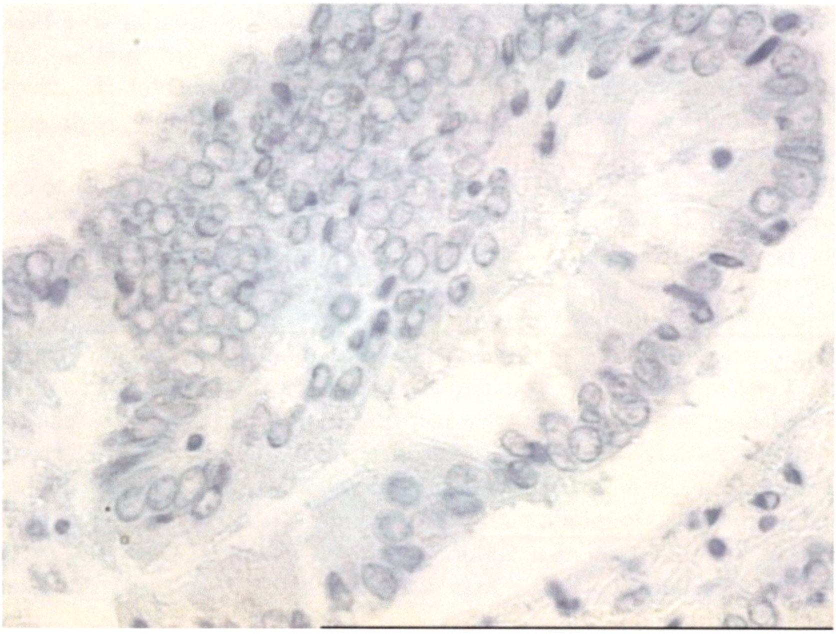

A

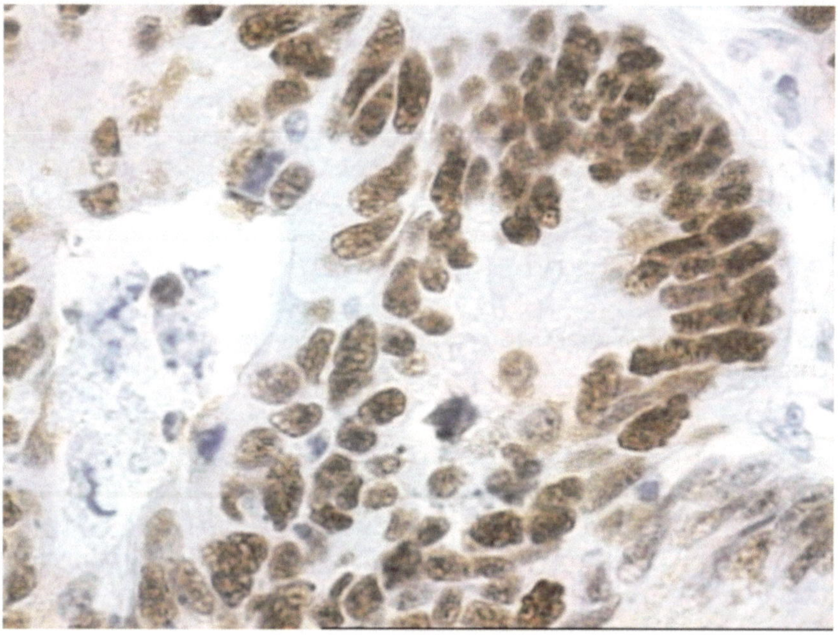

B

Fig. 2. (A) Absence of topoisomerase I staining in malignant cells of primary colorectal carcinoma (immunoperoxidase stain, x400) (B) Intense topoisomerase I reactivity, displaying a specific brown nuclear immunostaining, in malignant cells of the respective recurrence (immunoperoxidase stain, x400) patients with metastatic colorectal cancer, a regimen being superior to 5-FU+LV alone which has been demonstrated to offer consistently improved tumour control and prolonged survival, albeit, only approximately 40% of advanced colorectal cancer patients seem to be potentially responsive to the aforementioned combination regimen (Waters et al., 2001).

One method of increasing the above described percentage of responsiveness to combination chemotherapy is relied on the availability of biomarkers, capable for identifying patients who might potentially respond to topoisomerase I inhibitor-based chemotherapy. With regard to CPT-11 efficacy, in vitro data have suggested that topoisomerase I expression could be considered as an important cellular sensitivity determinant (Paradiso et al., 2004). In particular, decreased DNA topoisomerase I expression has been shown to correlate with camptothecin resistant cell lines (Sanghani et al., 2003), a finding being in agreement with Jansen et al. (Jansen et al., 1997), who conversely reported a positive correlation between CPT-11 sensitivity and increased topoisomerase I activity. Other indicators for topoisomerase I drug response of colorectal cancer cell lines, possibly include a high growth fraction and a functional apoptotic pathway (Hafian et al., 2004), while Saltz et al. (Saltz et al., 1998) have suggested an association between CPT-11 efficacy and topoisomerase expression in colorectal neoplastic tissue; the latter being a potential predictor of 5-FU resistance (Leichman et al., 1997).

Moreover, in our study, the percentage or intensity of increase of topoisomerase I protein expression in recurrences did not demonstrate any significant correlations with Duke's stage, grade of tumour differentiation, localization, and patients' gender. These data suggest that there might be no obvious benefit from evaluating histologicaly the tumour-cell sensitivity to topoisomerase I-targeted drugs; subsequently, such drugs appear to be effective across a various spectrum of pathologies, stage and gender. However, the aforementioned increase of topoisomerase I expression was correlated with age, a fact which might be suggestive that treatment with topoisomerase I inhibitors would be more beneficial in older colorectal cancer patients. Of note, these data should be interpreted with caution due to the limited number of evaluated patients.

6.2 Main research on topoisomerase I and II expression in colorectal cancer cells

6.2.1 Patients and methods

6.2.1.1 Patients

Forty patients with colorectal cancer that had recurred following surgery and adjuvant chemotherapy who underwent a second operation were included in this study. All had undergone surgical resection of the primary tumour and had received post-operatively 5-FU-based [5FU and Leucovorin (LV), Mayo Clinic regimen] adjuvant chemotherapy (Heidelberger et al., 1957). Patients' characteristics are described in Table 1.

6.2.1.2 Study plan

The first tumour tissue was collected from the primary tumour during the initial operation, before the administration of any adjuvant chemotherapy. The second tissue sample was obtained at the time of recurrence, during the second operation and following chemotherapy. Both tissue samples for each patient, were analyzed for the expression of both topoisomerase-I and topoisomerase-IIa proteins.

Patients (*n*)	40
Gender	
Men	25
Women	15
Median age at diagnosis (years)	58 (35–75)
Performance status (WHO), 0–1	40
Location of primary tumor	
Right colon	6
Left colon	28
Rectum	6
Stage (Dukes')	
B2	13
C	27
Relapse	
Local	17
Distant	23
Differentiation	
Well	2
Moderate	31
Poor	7
Disease-free survival (months)	18 (range, 6–79)

Table 1. Patients characteristics

6.2.1.3 Determination of topoisomerase-I and topoisomerase-IIα

The expression of topoisomerase-I and topoisomerase-II*a* was studied on paraffin embedded biopsy sections using a standard three-step immunohistochemistry approach. Topogen, an anti-topoisomerase-I monoclonal antibody (mAb) (2012-3) was applied. Topogen is a mouse mAb (IgG2b isotype); its epitope has not been mapped (Libutti et al., 2005; Gouveris et al., 2007; Lazaris, 2002). The primary mAb JH2.7 for topoisomerase-II*a* (Biocare Medical, CA, USA) is a mouse mAb (IgG1 isotype) that recognizes a 170-kDa protein, the epitope of which maps between aminoacid 854–1447 of topoisomerase-II*a* (Gouveris et al., 2007; Lazaris et al., 2002; Zorzos et al., 2003]. Counterstaining with hematoxylin was applied at the end of the classical immunohistochemistry procedure.

6.2.1.4 Positive and negative controls

For the expression of topoisomerase-I and -IIα, normal human tonsil tissue immunostaining served as positive control samples. Nonspecific, isotype-matched monoclonal antibodies worked well as substitute negative controls (Gouveris et al., 2007; Lazaris et al., 2002; Libutti et al., 2005; Zorzos et al., 2003).

First step: Sections were examined for quantified immunoreactivity by two independent investigators blinded to any relevant patient clinical data. They evaluated more than 1,000 malignant cells in consecutive sections of neoplastic tissue specimens. The numbers of positive cells were then expressed as a percentage of labeled tumour cells with respect to the total number of tumour cells that could be idendified. Immunostaining for topoisomerase-I and -II*a* was then graded according to the percentage of tumour cells staining positively (- and ± for <5%, + for 5-50% and ++ for 50 to 75% of cells with positive staining). A characterization was given additionally for the intensity of topoisomerase immunostaining (weakly positive, moderately positive, or strongly positive). To simplify the scoring, we graded them as 0 (negative cells), 1 (± and/or <5%), 2 (+ and/or 5-50%), 3 (++ and/or 50-75%). Then, the biopsy specimens were analysed as paired samples: one section from the first surgery and one section from the second surgery for each patient.
Second step: The percentages of immunoreactive malignant cells were calculated using an image analysis system with an appropriate software package [Sigma Scan Pro, Version 5.0 (SPSS Science, Erkrath, Germany)]. The ratio was calculated as a percentage of immunohistochemically positive neoplastic cells over the total number (stained and unstained) of neoplastic cells. The membrane, cytoplasmic or nuclear intensity of the specific immunohistochemical stain, was also assessed. All the positively stained cells were classified for the purpose of simplicity into two groups: weakly stained and strongly stained.
DNA ploidy of neoplastic cells was evaluated by image DNA flow-cytometry performed on Feulgen-stained sections. Images were acquired using a Zeiss Axiolab microscope (Carl Zeiss Jena GmbH, Jena, Germany) with a mechanical stage, fitted with a SONY-iris CCD video camera (SONY Corporation, Tokyo, Japan). The latter was connected to a Pentium II personal computer, which included the relevant software. Slides were examined at low power magnification (40x) to identify the areas with the highest cellularity. In each case, a total number of ≥200 Feulgen-stained nuclei was selected at high power magnification (400x) and stored as JPEG file [1,550 x 1,070 pixels, 16.7 million colors (24-bit)]. Then the images were converted to gray scale and the staining intensity of the Feulgen-stained nuclei was measured semi-automatically. A classification of the nuclei in pairs according to their staining intensity followed. Finally, a graphic presentation of the nuclei, demonstrating their distribution according to their DNA content, was also performed.

6.2.1.5 Statistical analysis

All analyses were performed with SPSS version 10.1 (Statistical Product and Service Solutions; SPSS Inc., Chicago, IL, USA). We used McNemar's paired Chi-square test to assess the possible alteration of the levels of topoisomerases after chemotherapy with 5-FU. Fisher's exact test was performed in order to assess the possible relationship of topoisomerase increase with gender, Dukes' stage, tumour grade and localization. Mann-Whitney *U* Test was performed to assess a possible relationship between patient age and alteration in topoisomerases levels.

6.2.2 Results

6.2.2.1 Patients

Forty patients were included in the present study. Of these, 25 were males and 15 were females. The median age was 58 years (range 35 - 75). All patients had a performance status

(PS) of 0 – 1. Tumour localization at the time of diagnosis was: right colon in six patients, left colon in 28 patients, and rectum in the remaining six patients. In respect with pathological classification, 13 patients had Dukes B2 tumours, and the remaining 27 had Dukes C tumours. With regard to differentiation, two patients had well differentiated tumours, 31 patients had moderately differentiated tumours and seven patients had poorly differentiated tumours. Of all forty patients, 17 relapsed locally and 23 manifested with distant metastases at the time of recurrence. Overall, the median relapse-free interval was 18 (range 6 – 79) months (Table 1). All patients who entered the trial were finally evaluable for analysis.

6.2.2.2 Ploidy

Out of the 40 primary tumours, 12 were highly aneuploid and the remaining 28 were moderately aneuploid. There was no association between the degree of DNA aneuploidy and the expression of any of the analyzed markers.

6.2.2.3 Topoisomerase I

Immunohistochemical analysis revealed that levels of topoisomerase-I expression were higher in malignant cells from tumour recurrences compared to cells from the primary tumours (2 sided paired Chi square test, P = 0.0001) (Table 2; Fig. 1). Topoisomerase-I expression was also decreased in grade 1 (P = 0.007) and increased in grade 3 tumours (2 sided Fischer's exact test, P = 0.003) (Table 2). By image analysis evaluation, a significant raise in malignant cells from the tumour recurrences could be recognised (2 sided paired Chi square test, P = 0.0001) (Table 3); low expression of topoisomerase-I was noticed in range 1–5 (P = 0.0001) and 26–30 (2 sided Fischer's exact test, P = 0.0143) (Table 3; Fig. 3). The increase in topoisomerase-I levels was not significantly correlated with gender, performance status (WHO), location of the primary tumour, Dukes' stage, grade of differentiation, and localization of relapse. There was a statistically significant correlation between the age of patients and the expression of topoisomerase-I (Mann–Whitney U Test, P = 0.011). Patients with an increased expression of topoisomerase-I levels were older in age (median=62.5 years) than patients without increased expression (median=50 years).

6.2.2.4 Topoisomerase IIα

Malignant cells from tumour recurrences showed a statistically significant increase of the levels of topoisomerase-II, compared to those of the primary tumours (2 sided paired Chi square test, P = 0.0001) (Table 2; Fig. 2). The topoisomerase-II levels were decreased in grade 3 lesions (2 sided Fischer's exact test, P = 0.0001) (Table 2; Fig. 4). In image analysis, a significant increase in malignant cells from tumour recurrences could be identified (2 sided Fischer's exact test, P = 0.0001) (Table 3); low expression of topoisomerase-II was noticed in the range of 16–20 (2 sided Fischer's exact test, P = 0.0143) (Table 3). Levels of topoisomerase-IIa expression were also higher in malignant cells from tumour recurrences compared to cells from primary tumours (Chi square test, P = 0.0001). There was a statistically significant positive correlation between the age of patients and increased levels of expression of topoisomerase-IIa (Mann–Whitney U Test, P = 0.011). The increase in topoisomerase-IIa levels did not demonstrate any significant correlation with gender, performance status (WHO), localization of primary tumour, Dukes' stage, tumour grade, and location of relapse, nor were such correlations found between the above parameters and the differences of topoisomerase-IIa levels in the primary tumours and relapses.

Examined parameters	Photo, microscopic evaluation			P
	Grade	First evaluation	Second evaluation	
Topoisomerase I	0	7	0	0.0117
	1	13	1	0.0007
	2	17	26	0.0722
	3	3	13	0.0103
Increased: 25, decreased: 0, no change: 15, $P = 0.0001$				
Topoisomerase IIa	0	0	0	1
	1	10	2	0.0252
	2	30	28	0.8027
	3	0	10	0.0010
Increased: 18, decreased: 0, no change: 22, $P = 0.0001$				

Table 2. Photomicroscopic evalution

6.2.3 Discussion

In our study, 33 out of 40 (83%) patients had biopsy samples obtained from colorectal cancer tissue that stained positive for topoisomerase (Table 2; Fig. 3). This finding is in close agreement with the results of a study by Staley et al. (Staley et al., 1999), who reported 86% of positive staining in a total of 29 samples, but in contrast with the results reported by Boonsong et al. (Boonsong et al., 2002), who demonstrated a lower percentage of cells expressing topoisomerase-I: 51% of the samples, including 24.4% with >50% positive tumour cells (Boonsong et al., 2002). Topoisomerase-I immunoreactivity in our study was confined to the nucleus in all samples, being consistent with the role of topoisomerase-I as a nuclear protein. For topoisomerase-II*a*, 21 out of the 40 samples (52%) of colorectal cancer tissue stained positive (Table 2; Fig. 4). Half of them, i.e. 10/40 (25%) presented only weak positive staining for topoisomerase IIα (grade 1), a finding confirmed by Image Analysis (Table 3). The above data are consistent with those reported by Burden and Osheroff (Burden et al., 1998).

In the present study, we reported a significant increase in topoisomerase-I and topoisomerase-II*a* expression in tissues from recurrent colorectal tumours, reinforcing the view that the expression of topoisomerases is likely part of the malignant-cell phenotype in colorectal carcinomas that relapse after initial treatment. This observation is in agreement with previous studies (Paradiso et al., 2004; Tsavaris et al., 2004), which demonstrated a direct correlation between thymidylate synthase (TS) and topoisomerase-I tumour expression and hypothesized, similar to TS (Ichikawa et al., 1999), that high topoisomerase-I expression is related to a more aggressive biological phenotype. Of note, increased topoisomerase-II*a* expression characterizes rapidly proliferating cells (Burden et al., 1998) and may represent a useful marker of aggressive tumour behavior (Leichman et al., 1997).

Since the increase of topoisomerase-I and -II*a* expression was demonstrated following 5-FU-based adjuvant chemotherapy therapy, it would be tempting to attribute this change to 5-FU itself. High levels of topoisomerase-I correlate with sensitivity to camptothecins (irinotecan and topotecan), as it has been shown in the litterature (Monnin et al., 1999), whereas high levels of topoisomerase-II*a* correlate with sensitivity to etoposide, a well-established topoisomerase-II*a*-targeting agent (Leichman et al., 1997). Thus, it would be reasonable to consider administering these agents sequentially in a regimen used for the treatment of colorectal cancer, i.e. 5-FU → irinotecan and 5-FU → etoposide.

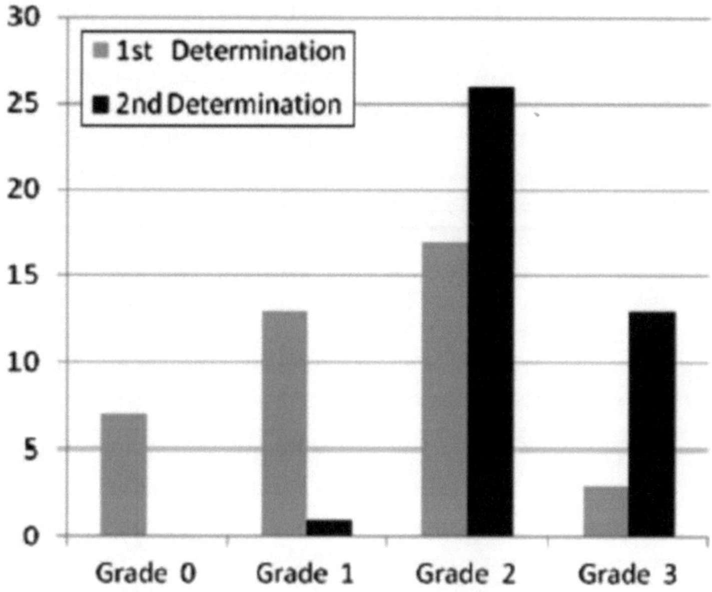

Fig. 1. Topoisomerase I (Topo-I) expression in relation to tumour grade according to immunohistochemical evaluation

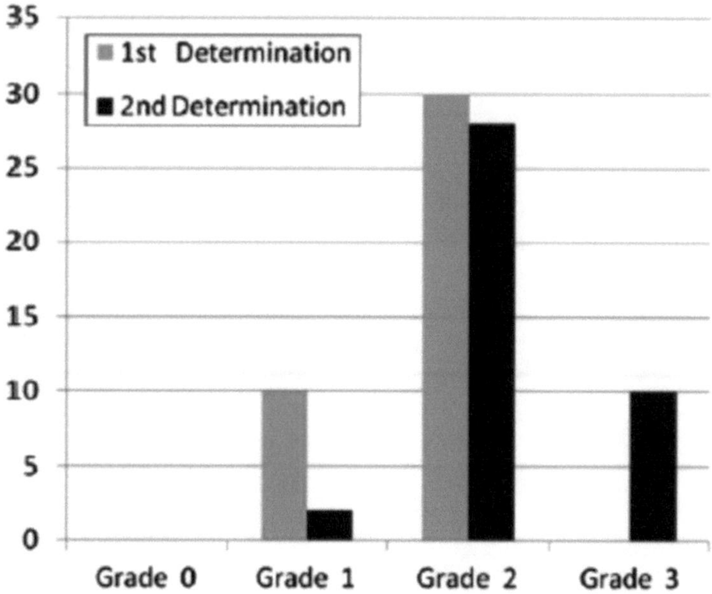

Fig. 2. Topoisomerase II*a* (Topo-II*a*) expression in relation to tumour grade according to immunohistochemical evaluation

Irinotecan (CPT-11) is a water soluble camptothecin derivative, which acts as a specific and potent inhibitor of topoisomerase-I (Hande et al., 1998). In a European-originated phase II study, irinotecan achieved response rates of 19% in chemotherapy-naive patients with colorectal cancer and 18% in chemotherapy pre-treated patients with advanced disease (Luzzio et al., 1995).

Irinotecan yielded response rates of 15–25% in colorectal cancer patients refractory to 5-FU-based treatments (Bognel et al., 1995; Conti & Saltz, 1994; Gennatas et al., 2006; Gupta et al., 1994; Pitot & O'Connell, 1994; Rothenberg & Burris, 1994; Tsavaris et al., 2003, 2007; Wilstermann et al., 2007), not dissimilar to those observed in first-line treatment of colorectal cancer patients (18–32%) (Mitry et al., 1998; Tsavaris NB et al., 2002; Van Custen & Peeters, 1998) and in contrast to the expected decreasing response rate from the application of irinotecan as a second-line treatment agent. Treating patients with irinotecan upon progression after chemotherapy with 5-FU+LV seems to be yielding more signiffcant results compared to the opposite sequence, based on our previous experience, where the best results with sequential monotherapies were obtained when 5-FU+LV was followed by irinotecan (5-FU/LV → CPT11) at disease progression or relapse (Gupta et al., 1994).

Range	First sample (no.)	Second sample (no.)	*P*	Range	First sample (no.)	Second sample (no.)	*P*
Topoisomerase I							
0	0	0	1	36–40	3	0	0.2405
1–5	21	1	0.0001	41–45	1	1	1.000
6–10	4	0	0.1156	46–50	1	1	1.000
11–15	2	4	0.6752	51–55	2	4	0.6752
16–20	3	5	0.7119	56–60	0	4	0.1156
21–25	2	3	1	61–65	0	5	0.0547
26–30	1	9	0.0143	66–70	0	0	
31–35	0	3	0.2405	71–80	0	0	
Topoisomerase IIa							
0	0	0	1	36–40	2	3	1
1–5	10	4	0.1395	41–45	5	1	0.2007
6–10	6	5	1	46–50	0	3	0.2405
11–15	5	2	0.4315	51–55	0	2	0.4937
16–20	9	1	0.0143	56–60	0	0	1
21–25	0	5	0.0547	61–65	0	1	1
26–30	3	3	1	66–70	0	2	0.4937
31–35	0	3	0.2405	71–80	0	5	0.0547

Total	First determination			Second determination			*P*
	Mean	Median	Range	Mean	Median	Range	
Topoisomerase I	13.875	4.5	1–54	35.375	29.5	4–65	0.0001
Topoisomerase IIa	16.775	15	1–45	34.575	31	2–79	0.0001

Table 3. Image analysis evalution (%)

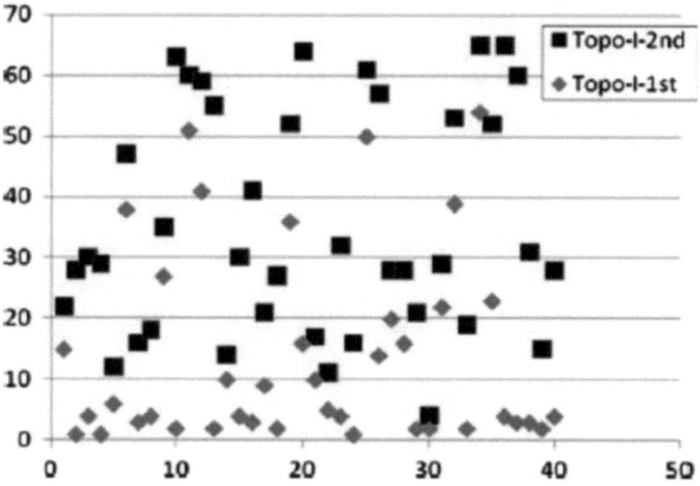

Fig. 3. Dispersion diagram of topoisomerase I (Topo-I) expression as assessed by immunohistochemistry (x axon are the number of cases analysed and the y axon represents the percentage of cells expressing topoisomerase I in first and recurrent tumour). It illustrates the increased levels of topoisomerase I in recurrences.

With regard to irinotecan efficacy, in vitro data suggest that topoisomerase-I expression could be regarded as an important cellular sensitivity determinant (Coleman et al., 2000). In particular, decreased DNA topoisomerase-I expression was correlated with camptothecin-resistant cell lines (Gouveris et al., 2007), while another study (Wilstermann et al., 2007) reported a positive correlation between irinotecan sensitivity and topoisomerae-I activity.

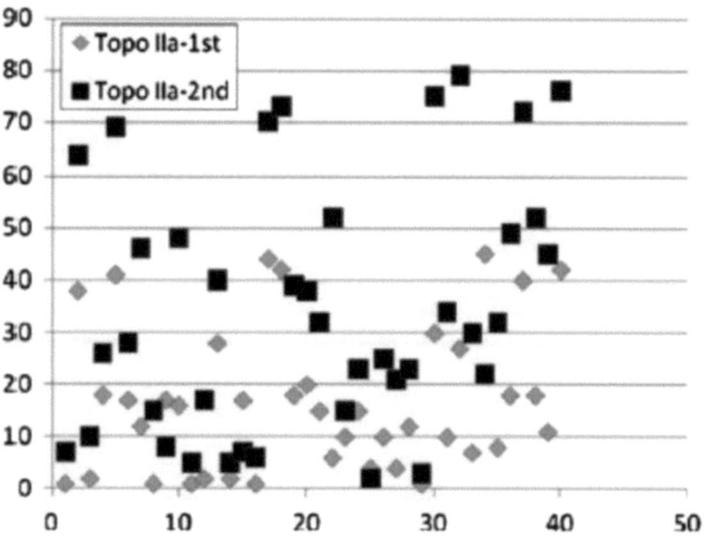

Fig. 4. Dispersion diagram of topoisomerase II*a* (Topo-II*a*) expression as assessed by immunohistochemistry (x axon are the number of cases analysed and the y axon represents the percentage of cells expressing topoisomerase II in first and recurrent tumour). It illustrates the increased levels of topoisomerase II in recurrences

Drugs that target topoisomerase-II, such as the epipodophylotoxins, etoposide (VP-16) and teniposide (VM-26) (Leichman et al., 1997) (VP-16), doxorubicin, and mitoxantrone, are among the most effective anticancer drugs still in clinical use. Especially, etoposide acts by destroying cells via inhibition of the ability of topoisomerase-II to ligate nucleic acids which are cleaved during the double-stranded DNA passage reaction (Bleiberg, 1998). Studies including previously untreated patients with advanced colorectal carcinoma evaluating the combination of etoposide with cisplatin or 5-FU demonstrated minimal activity in metastatic colorectal cancer (Boige et al., 1998; Passalacqua et al., 1991; Planting et al., 1996; Posner et al., 1990). There have been no clinical data supporting the in vitro synergy observed between these cytotoxic agents (Colucci et al., 1995; Zelkowitz et al., 1989). Other studies failed to prove any benefit with the combination of etoposide with 5-FU or cisplatin/carboplatin (Inaba et al., 1994). However, the combination of etoposide with 5-FU + LV had demonstrated some activity when administered as second-line treatment after failure of weekly 5-FU + LV in patients with metastatic colorectal cancer (Stuart et al., 1995; Tsavaris et al., 2002).

The results reported herein underscore the role of topoisomerases (topoisomerase-I and topoisomerase-II*a*) expression in colorectal cancer. It is believed that translational studies of molecular targets for currently applied cytotoxic and biological agents (like bevacizumab and cetuximab) might form the basis of shaping current and future drug combinations and of rationalizing the optimal chemotherapeutic drug schedule and sequence, which will eventually translate in improved tumour eradication and prolongation of survival.

This work is unique since it presents the first two of a series of studies that demonstrate an increase of topoisomerase expression following chemotherapy with 5FU. This may denote that such tumours are sensitized through 5FU chemotherapy regimens to topoisomerase inhibitors, providing a pathophysiologic mechanism to explain the described effectiveness of such agents in recurrent colorectal cancer after the first adjuvant chemotherapy.

7. References

Abigerges D, Armand JP, Chabot GG, Da Costa L, Fadel E, Cote C, Herait P, Gandia D. Irinotecan (CPT-11) high-dose escalation using intensive high-dose loperamide to control diarrhea. J Natl Cancer Inst. 1994 Mar 16;86(6):446-9.

Austin CA, Sng JH, Patel S, Fisher LM. Novel HeLa topoisomerase II is the II beta isoform: complete coding sequence and homology with other type II topoisomerases. Biochim Biophys Acta. 1993 Mar 20;1172(3):283-91.

Avemann K, Knippers R, Koller T, Sogo JM. Camptothecin, a specific inhibitor of type I DNA topoisomerase, induces DNA breakage at replication forks. Mol Cell Biol.1988 Aug;8(8):3026-34.

Bailly C. Topoisomerase I poisons and suppressors as anticancer drugs. Curr Med Chem. 2000 Jan;7(1):39-58. Review.

Barnes S, Peterson TG, Coward L. Rationale for the use of genistein-containing soy matrices in chemoprevention trials for breast and prostate cancer. J Cell Biochem Suppl. 1995;22:181-7.

Bauer WR, Crick FH, White JH. Supercoiled DNA. Sci Am. 1980 Jul;243(1):100-13.

Bauman ME, Holden JA, Brown KA, Harker WG, Perkins SL. Differential immunohistochemical staining for DNA topoisomerase II alpha and beta in human tissues and for DNA topoisomerase II beta in non-Hodgkin's lymphomas. Mod Pathol. 1997 Mar;10(3):168-75.

Beck WT, Danks MK, Wolverton JS, Kim R, Chen M. Drug resistance associated with altered DNA topoisomerase II. Adv Enzyme Regul. 1993;33:113-27. Review.

Berger JM. Type II DNA topoisomerases. Curr Opin Struct Biol. 1998 Feb;8(1):26-32. Review.

Berney DM, Shamash J, Gaffney J, Jordan S, Oliver RT. DNA topoisomerase I and II expression in drug resistant germ cell tumours. Br J Cancer. 2002 Sep 9;87(6):624-9.

Biersack H, Jensen S, Gromova I, Nielsen IS, Westergaard O, Andersen AH. Active heterodimers are formed from human DNA topoisomerase II alpha and II beta isoforms. Proc Natl Acad Sci U S A. 1996 Aug 6;93(16):8288-93.

Bleiberg H (1998) Continuing the fight against advanced colorectal cancer: new and future treatment options. Anticancer Drugs 9:18–28

Bognel C, Rekacewicz C, Mankarios H, Pignon JP, Elias D, Duvillard P, Prade M, Ducreux M, Kac J, Rougier P, Eschwège F, Lasser P (1995) Prognostic value of neural invasion in rectal carcinoma: a multivariate analysis on 339 patients with curative resection. Eur J Cancer 31A:894–898

Boige V, Raymond E, Armand JP (1998) Irinotecan: various administration schedules, study of drug combinations, phase I experience. Bull Cancer 26-32

Boonsong A, Curran S, McKay JA, Cassidy J, Murray GI, McLeod HL. Topoisomerase I protein expression in primary colorectal cancer and lymph node metastases. Hum Pathol. 2002 Nov;33(11):1114-9.

Bronstein IB, Vorobyev S, Timofeev A, Jolles CJ, Alder SL, Holden JA. Elevations of DNA topoisomerase I catalytic activity and immunoprotein in human malignancies. Oncol Res. 1996;8(1):17-25.

Brown PO, Peebles CL, Cozzarelli NR. A topoisomerase from Escherichia coli related to DNA gyrase. Proc Natl Acad Sci U S A. 1979 Dec;76(12):6110-4.

Bullock P, Champoux JJ, Botchan M. Association of crossover points with topoisomerase I cleavage sites: a model for nonhomologous recombination.Science. 985 Nov 22;230(4728):954-8.

Burden DA, Osheroff N: Mechanism of action of eukaryotic topoisomerase II and drugs targeted to the enzyme. Biochim Biophys Acta 1400:139-154, 1998.

Castano IB, Brzoska PM, Sadoff BU, Chen H, Christman MF. Mitotic chromosome condensation in the rDNA requires TRF4 and DNA topoisomerase I in Saccharomyces cerevisiae. Genes Dev. 1996 Oct 15;10(20):2564-76.

Champoux JJ, Dulbecco R. An activity from mammalian cells that untwists superhelical DNA--a possible swivel for DNA replication (polyoma-ethidium bromide-mouse-embryo cells-dye binding assay). Proc Natl Acad Sci U S A. 1972 Jan;69(1):143-6.

Champoux JJ. DNA topoisomerases: structure, function, and mechanism. Annu Rev Biochem 2001;70:369.

Cole SP, Chanda ER, Dicke FP, Gerlach JH, Mirski SE. Non-P-glycoprotein-mediated multidrug resistance in a small cell lung cancer cell line: evidence for decreased susceptibility to drug-induced DNA damage and reduced levels of topoisomerase II. Cancer Res. 1991 Jul 1;51(13):3345-52.

Coleman LW, Perkins SL, Bronstein IB, Holden JA (2000) Expression of DNA toposiomerase I and DNA topoisomerase IIalpha in testicular seminomas. Hum Pathol 31:728–733

Coleman LW, Bronstein IB, Holden JA. Immunohistochemical staining for DNA topoisomerase I, DNA topoisomerase II-alpha and p53 in gastric carcinomas. Anticancer Res. 2001 Mar-Apr;21(2A):1167-72.

Coleman LW, Rohr LR, Bronstein IB, Holden JA. Human DNA topoisomerase I: An anticancer drug target present in human sarcomas. Hum Pathol. 2002 Jun;33(6):599-607.

Colucci G, Maiello E, Giuliani F, Cifarelli RA, Giotta F (1995) Carboplatin and etoposide in previously treated colorectal cancer patients. Tumori 81:36–38

Conti JA, Saltz L (1994) Irinotecan is an active agent in untreated patients with metastatic colorectal cancer. Proc Am Soc Clin Oncol 13:195 (abstr)

Covey JM, Jaxel C, Kohn KW, Pommier Y. Protein-linked DNA strand breaks induced in mammalian cells by camptothecin, an inhibitor of topoisomerase I. Cancer Res. 1989 Sep 15;49(18):5016–5022.

Cunningham D, Pyrhonen S, James RD, Punt CJ, Hickish TF, Heikkila R, Johannesen TB, Starkhammar H, Topham CA, Awad L, Jacques C, Herait P. Randomised trial of irinotecan plus supportive care versus supportive care alone after fluorouracil failure for patients with metastatic colorectal cancer. Lancet. 1998 Oct 31;352(9138):1413-8.

Dickey JS, Osheroff N. Impact of the C-terminal domain of topoisomerase IIalpha on the DNA cleavage activity of the human enzyme. Biochemistry. 2005 Aug 30;44(34):11546-54.

D'Incalci M. DNA-topoisomerase inhibitors.Curr Opin Oncol. 1993 Nov;5(6):1023-8.

Douillard JY, Cunningham D, Roth AD, Navarro M, James RD, Karasek P, Jandik P, Iveson T, Carmichael J, Alakl M, Gruia G, Awad L, Rougier P: Irinotecan combined with fluorouracil compared with fluorouracil alone as first-line treatment for metastatic colorectal cancer: a multicentre randomised trial. Lancet 2000, 355:1041-1047.

Florell SR, Martinchick JF, Holden JA. Purification of DNA topoisomerase I from the spleen of a patient with non-Hodgkin's lymphoma. Anticancer Res. 1996 Nov-Dec;16(6B):3467-74.

Fogt F, Nikulasson ST, Holden JA, Alder SA, Hallgrimsson J, Jessup MJ, O'Brien MJ, Lavin PT, Goldman H. Topoisomerase II alpha expression in normal, inflammatory, and neoplastic conditions of the gastric and colonic mucosa. Mod Pathol. 1997 Apr;10(4):296-302.

Gellert M, Mizuuchi K, O'Dea MH, Nash HA. DNA gyrase: an enzyme that introduces superhelical turns into DNA. Proc Natl Acad Sci U S A. 1976 Nov;73(11):3872-6.

Gellert M, O'Dea MH, Itoh T, Tomizawa J. Novobiocin and coumermycin inhibit DNA supercoiling catalyzed by DNA gyrase. Proc Natl Acad Sci U S A. 1976 Dec;73(12):4474-8.

Gennatas C, Papaxoinis G, Michalaki V, Mouratidou D, Andreadis C, Tsavaris N, Paffiti A (2006) A prospective randomized study of irinotecan (CPT-11), leucovorin (LV) and 5-Xuorouracil (5FU) versus leucovorin and 5-Fluorouracil in patients with advanced colorectal carcinoma. J Chemother 18:538–544

Gibbons D, Fogt F, Kasznica J, Holden J, Nikulasson S. Comparison of topoisomerase II alpha and MIB-1 expression in uterine cervical squamous lesions. Mod Pathol. 1997 May;10(5):409-13.

Giovanella BC, Stehlin JS, Wall ME, Wani MC, Nicholas AW, Liu LF, Silber R, Potmesil M. DNA topoisomerase I-targeted chemotherapy of human colon cancer in xenografts. Science. 1989 Nov 24;246(4933):1046-8.

Glisson BS, Sullivan DM, Gupta R, Ross WE. Mediation of multi-drug resistance in a Chinese hamster ovary cell line by a mutant type II topoisomerase. NCI Monogr. 1987;(4):89-93.

Goldwasser F, Bae I, Valenti M, et al: Topoisomerase I–related parameters and camptothecin activity in the colon carcinoma cell lines from the National Cancer Institute and anticancer screen. Cancer Res 55:2116-2121, 1995.

Gottlieb JA, Guarino AM, Call JB, Oliverio VT, Block JB. Preliminary pharmacologic and clinical evaluation of camptothecin sodium (NSC-100880). Cancer Chemother Rep Part 1 1970; 54: 461-70.

Gottlieb JA, Luce JK: Treatment of malignant melanoma with camptothecin (NSC-100880). Cancer Chemother Rep 1972;56:103–105.

Gouveris P, Lazaris AC, Papathomas TG, Nonni A, Kyriakou V, Delladetsima J, Patsouris ES, Tsavaris N (2007) Topoisomerase I protein expression in primary colorectal cancer and recurrences after 5-FU-based adjuvant chemotherapy. J Cancer Res Clin Oncol 133:1011–1015

Guichard S, Cussac D, Hennebelle I, Bugat R, Canal P (1997) Sequence-dependent activity of the irinotecan-5FU combination in human colon-cancer model HT-29 in vitro and in vivo. Int J Cancer 73:729-734

Guichard S, Hennebelle I, Bugat R, Canal P (1998) Cellular interactions of 5- fluorouracil and the camptothecin analogue CPT-11 (irinotecan) in a human colorectal carcinoma cell line. Biochem Pharmacol 55:667-676

Guichard S, Terret C, Hennebelle I, Lochon I, Chevreau P, Fretigny E, Selves J, Chatelut E, Bugat R, Canal P. CPT-11 converting carboxylesterase and topoisomerase activities in tumour and normal colon and liver tissues. Br J Cancer. 1999 May; 80(3-4):364-70.

Guldner HH, Szostecki C, Vosberg HP, Lakomek HJ, Penner E, Bautz FA. Scl 70 autoantibodies from scleroderma patients recognize a 95 kDa protein identified as DNA topoisomerase I. Chromosoma. 1986;94(2):132-8.

Gupta D, Bronstein IB, Holden JA: Expression of DNA topoisomerase I in neoplasms of the kidney: Correlation with histological grade, proliferation, and patient survival. Hum Pathol 31:214-219, 2000.

Gupta E, Lestingi TM, Mick R, Ramirez J, Vokes EE, Ratain MJ. Metabolic fate of irinotecan in humans: correlation of glucuronidation with diarrhea. Cancer Res. 1994 Jul 15;54(14):3723-5.

Gupta M, Fujimori A, Pommier Y. Eukaryotic DNA topoisomerases I. Biochim Biophys Acta. 1995 May 17;1262(1):1-14.

Hafian H, Venteo L, Sukhanova A, Nabiev I, Lefevre B, Pluot M. Immunohistochemical study of DNA topoisomerase I, DNA topoisomerase II alpha, p53, and Ki-67 in oral preneoplastic lesions and oral squamous cell carcinomas. Hum Pathol. 2004 Jun;35(6):745-51.

Hanai R, Caron PR, Wang JC. Human TOP3: a single-copy gene encoding DNA topoisomerase III. Proc Natl Acad Sci U S A. 1996 Apr 16;93(8):3653-7.

Hande KR. Clinical applications of anticancer drugs targeted to topoisomerase II. Biochim Biophys Acta. 1998 Oct 1;1400(1-3):173-84.

Heck MM, Hittelman WN, Earnshaw WC. Differential expression of DNA topoisomerases I and II during the eukaryotic cell cycle. Proc Natl Acad Sci U S A. 1988 Feb;85(4):1086-90.

Heidelberger C, Chaudhuri NK, Danneberg P, Mooren D, Griesbach L, Duschinsky R, Schnitzer RJ, Pleven E, Scheiner J (1957) Fluorinated pyrimidines: a new class of tumor inhibitory compounds. Nature 179:663–666

Holden JA, Perkins SL, Snow GW, Kjeldsberg CR. Immunohistochemical staining for DNA topoisomerase II in non-Hodgkin's lymphomas. Am J Clin Pathol. 1995 Jul;104(1):54-9.

Holden JA, Rahn MP, Jolles CJ, Vorobyev SV, Bronstein IB. Immunohistochemical detection of DNA topoisomerase I in formalin fixed, paraffin wax embedded normal tissues and in ovarian carcinomas. Mol Pathol. 1997 Oct;50(5):247-53.

Holm C, Covey JM, Kerrigan D, Pommier Y. Differential requirement of DNA replication for the cytotoxicity of DNA topoisomerase I and II inhibitors in Chinese hamster DC3F cells. Cancer Res. 1989 Nov 15;49(22):6365-8.

Hsiang YH, Liu LF. Identification of mammalian DNA topoisomerase I as an intracellular target of the anticancer drug camptothecin. Cancer Res. 1988 Apr 1;48(7):1722-1726.

Hsiang YH, Lihou MG, Liu LF. Arrest of replication forks by drug-stabilized topoisomerase I-DNA cleavable complexes as a mechanism of cell killing by camptothecin. Cancer Res. 1989 Sep 15;49(18):5077-82.

Husain I, Mohler JL, Seigler HF, Besterman JM. Elevation of topoisomerase I messenger RNA, protein, and catalytic activity in human tumors: demonstration of tumor-type specificity and implications for cancer chemotherapy. Cancer Res. 1994 Jan 15;54(2):539-46.

Ichikawa W, Uetake H, Nihei Z, Mastuo K, Fujita H, Yamada Y (1999) Topoisomerase I (Topo-I) expression correlates to thymidylate synthase (TS) expression in colorectal cancer (CRC). Proc Am Soc Clin Oncol 18:946 (abstract)

Inaba M, Mitsuhashi J, Kawada S, Nakano H (1994) Different modes of cell-killing action between DNA topoisomerase I and II inhibitors revealed by kinetic analysis. Jpn J Cancer Res 85:187–193

Jansen WJ, Zwart B, Hulscher ST, Giaccone G, Pinedo HM, Boven E (1997) CPT-11 in human colon-cancer cell lines and xenografts: characterization of cellular sensitivity determinants. Int J Cancer 70:335–340

Jaxel C, Capranico G, Kerrigan D, Kohn KW, Pommier Y. Effect of local DNA sequence on topoisomerase I cleavage in the presence or absence of camptothecin. J Biol Chem. 1991 Oct 25;266(30):20418–20423.

Jenkins JR, Ayton P, Jones T, Davies SL, Simmons DL, Harris AL, Sheer D, Hickson ID. Isolation of cDNA clones encoding the beta isozyme of human DNA topoisomerase II and localisation of the gene to chromosome 3p24. Nucleic Acids Res. 1992 Nov 11;20(21):5587-92.

Kato J, Nishimura Y, Imamura R, Niki H, Hiraga S, Suzuki H. New topoisomerase essential for chromosome segregation in E. coli. Cell. 1990 Oct 19;63(2):393-404.

Kehrer DF, Sparreboom A, Verweij J, de Bruijn P, Nierop CA, van de Schraaf J, Ruijgrok EJ, de Jonge MJ. Modulation of irinotecan-induced diarrhea by cotreatment with neomycin in cancer patients. Clin Cancer Res. 2001 May;7(5):1136-41.

Kellner U, Sehested M, Jensen PB, et al. Culprit and victim—DNA topoisomerase II. Lancet Oncol 2003;3:235.

Kerrigan JE, Pilch DS. A structural model for the ternary cleavable complex formed between human topoisomerase I, DNA, and camptothecin. Biochemistry. 2001 Aug 21;40(33):9792-8.

Kwan KY, Wang JC. Mice lacking DNA topoisomerase IIIbeta develop to maturity but show a reduced mean lifespan.Proc Natl Acad Sci U S A. 2001 May 8;98(10):5717-21. Epub 2001 May 1.

Lazaris AC, Kavantzas NG, Zorzos HS, Tsavaris NV, Davaris PS (2002) Markers of drug resistance in relapsing colon cancer. J Cancer Res Clin Oncol 128:114–118

Lee MP, Brown SD, Chen A, Hsieh TS. DNA topoisomerase I is essential in Drosophila melanogaster. Proc Natl Acad Sci U S A. 1993 Jul 15;90(14):6656-60.

Leichman CG, Lenz HJ, Leichman L, Danenberg K, Baranda J, Groshen S, Boswell W, Metzger R, Tan M, Danenberg PV (1997) Quantitation of intratumoral thymidylate synthase expression predicts for disseminated colorectal cancer response and resistance to protracted-infusion fluorouracil and weekly leucovorin. J Clin Oncol 15:3223-3229

Libutti SK, Salz LB, Rustgi AK, Tepper JE (2005) Cancer of the colon. In: Devita VT, Hellman S, Rosenberg S (eds) Cancer: principles and practice of oncology, Chap 29, Sect 8. Lippincott Williams and Wilkins, Philadelphia

Lindsley JE. Intradimerically tethered DNA topoisomerase II is catalytically active in DNA transport. Proc Natl Acad Sci U S A. 1996 Apr 2;93(7):2975-80.

Liu, L. F. DNA topoisomerases: enzymes that catalyze the breaking and rejoining of DNA. CRC Critical Review of Biochemistry, 1983 15, pp. 1-24.

Liu LF, Wang JC. Supercoiling of the DNA template during transcription. Proc Natl Acad Sci U S A. 1987 Oct;84(20):7024-7.

Lodge AJ, Anderson JJ, Ng SW, Fenwick F, Steward M, Haugk B, Horne CH, Angus B. Expression of topoisomerase IIIalpha in normal and neoplastic tissues determined by immunohistochemistry using a novel monoclonal antibody. Br J Cancer. 2000 Aug;83(4):498-505.

Lokiec F, Canal P, Gay C, Chatelut E, Armand JP, Roche H, Bugat R, Goncalves E, Mathieu-Boue A. Pharmacokinetics of irinotecan and its metabolites in human blood, bile, and urine. Cancer Chemother Pharmacol. 1995;36(1):79-82.

Luzzio MJ, Besterman JM, Emerson DL, Evans MG, Lackey K, Leitner PL, McIntyre G, Morton B, Myers PL, Peel M, Sisco JM, Sternbach DD et al (1995) Synthesis and antitumor activity of novel water soluble derivatives of camptothecin as specific inhibitors of topoisomerase I. J Med Chem 38:395–401

Lynch BJ, Komaromy-Hiller G, Bronstein IB, Holden JA. Expression of DNA topoisomerase I, DNA topoisomerase II-alpha, and p53 in metastatic malignant melanoma. Hum Pathol. 1998 Nov;29(11):1240-5.

Lynch BJ, Bronstein IB, Holden JA: Elevations of DNA topoisomerase I in invasive carcinoma of the breast. Breast J 7:176-180, 2001.

Mantle D, Lennard TW, Pickering AT. Therapeutic applications of medicinal plants in the treatment of breast cancer: a review of their pharmacology, efficacy and tolerability.Adverse Drug React Toxicol Rev. 2000 Aug;19(3):223-40. Review.

Maxwell A. The molecular basis of quinolone action. J Antimicrob Chemother. 1992 Oct;30(4):409-14. Review.

McLeod HL, Douglas F, Oates M, Symonds RP, Prakash D, van der Zee AG, Kaye SB, Brown R, Keith WN. Topoisomerase I and II activity in human breast, cervix, lung and colon cancer. Int J Cancer. 1994 Dec 1;59(5):607-11.

Mitry E, Ducreux M, Rougier P (1998) Second-line irinotecan chemotherapy in the treatment of metastatic colorectal cancers: phase III trials. Bull Cancer 38-42

Moertel CG, Schutt AJ, Reitemeir RJ, et al: Phase II study of camptothecin (NSC-100880) in the treatment of advanced gastrointenstinal cancer. Cancer Chemother Rep 1972;56:95–101.

Monnin KA, Bronstein IB, Gaffney DK, Holden JA. Elevations of DNA topoisomerase I in transitional cell carcinoma of the urinary bladder: correlation with DNA topoisomerase II-alpha and p53 expression. Hum Pathol. 1999 Apr;30(4):384-91.

Morham SG, Kluckman KD, Voulomanos N, Smithies O. Targeted disruption of the mouse topoisomerase I gene by camptothecin selection. Mol Cell Biol. 1996 Dec;16(12):6804-9.

Muggia FM, Creaven PJ, Hansen HH, et al: Phase I clinical trial of weekly and daily treatment with camptothecin (NSC-100880): Correlation with preclinical studies. Cancer Chemother Rep 1972;56:515–521.

Nakopoulou L, Zervas A, Lazaris AC, Constantinides C, Stravodimos C, Davaris P, Dimopoulos C. Predictive value of topoisomerase II alpha immunostaining in urothelial bladder carcinoma. J Clin Pathol. 2001 Apr;54(4):309-13.

P. Borst and H.M. Pinedo. Drug Resistance. Oxford textbook of oncology, Oxford Press, 1995, Chapter 4.13.

Paradiso A, Xu J, Mangia A, Chiriatti A, Simone G, Zito A, Montemurro S, Giuliani F, Maiello E, Colucci G. Topoisomerase-I, thymidylate synthase primary tumour expression and clinical efficacy of 5-FU/CPT-11 chemotherapy in advanced colorectal cancer patients. Int J Cancer. 2004 Aug 20;111(2):252-8.

Passalacqua R, Bisagni G, Cocconi G, Boni C, Di Blasio B, Ceci G (1991) Cisplatin and etoposide in advanced colorectal carcinoma.Ann Oncol 2:687–688

Perego P, Capranico G, Supino R, et al: Topoisomerase I gene expression and cell sensitivity to camptothecin in human cell lines of different tumor types. Anticancer Drugs 5:645-649, 1994.

Pitot HC, O'Connell MJ (1994) A phase II trial of CPT-11 in patients with metastatic colorectal carcinoma: a North Central Cancer Treatment Group Study. Proc Am Soc Clin Oncol 13:197 (abstr)

Planting AS, van der Burg ME, van den Bent MJ, de Boer-Dennert M, Stoter G, Verweij J (1996) Phase II study of a short course of weekly high-dose cisplatin combined with long-term oral etoposide in metastatic colorectal cancer. Br J Cancer 73:1265–1267

Pommier Y. Eukaryotic DNA topoisomerase I: genome gate keeper and its intruders, camptothecins. Semin Oncol. 1996 23: 1-10.

Pommier Y, Pourquier P, Fan Y, Strumberg D. Mechanism of action of eukaryotic DNA topoisomerase I and drugs targeted to the enzyme. Biochim Biophys Acta. 1998 Oct 1;1400(1-3):83-105. Review.

Pommier YG, Goldwasser F, Strumberg D. Topoisomerase II inhibitors: epipodophyllotoxins, acridines, ellipticines, and bisdioxopiperazines. In: Chabner BA, Longo DL, eds., Cancer chemotherapy & biotherapy: principles and practice, 3rd ed. Philadelphia: Lippincott Williams & Wilkins, 2001:538.

Posner M, Slapak CA, Browne MJ, Clark JW, Curt G, Weitberg A, Calabresi P, Cummings FJ, Wiemann M, Urba S (1990) A phase I-II trial of continuous-infusion cisplatin, continuous-infusion 5-Fluorouracil, and VP-16 in colorectal cancer. Am J Clin Oncol 13:455–458

Raynard S, Bussen W, Sung P. A double holliday junction dissolvasome comprising BLM, topoisomerase IIIalpha, and BLAP75. J Biol Chem.2006 Apr 4.

Robinson MJ, Martin BA, Gootz TD, McGuirk PR, Moynihan M, Sutcliffe JA, Osheroff N. Effects of quinolone derivatives on eukaryotic topoisomerase II. A novel mechanism for enhancement of enzyme-mediated DNA cleavage. J Biol Chem. 1991 Aug 5;266(22):14585-92.

Robinson MJ, Martin BA, Gootz TD, McGuirk PR, Osheroff N. Effects of novel fluoroquinolones on the catalytic activities of eukaryotic topoisomerase II: Influence of the C-8 fluorine group. Antimicrob Agents Chemother. 1992 Apr;36(4):751-6.

Roca J, Wang JC. DNA transport by a type II DNA topoisomerase: evidence in favor of a two-gate mechanism. Cell. 1994 May 20;77(4):609-16.

Roca J, Wang JC. The probabilities of supercoil removal and decatenation by yeast DNA topoisomerase II. Genes Cells. 1996 Jan;1(1):17-27.

Rothenberg ML, Burris HA III (1994) Irinotecan as second line therapy for patients with 5-FU refractory colorectal cancer. Proc Am Soc Clin Oncol 13:198 (abstr)

Rougier P, Van Cutsem E, Bajetta E, Niederle N, Possinger K, Labianca R, Navarro M, Morant R, Bleiberg H, Wils J, Awad L, Herait P, Jacques C. Randomised trial of irinotecan versus fluorouracil by continuous infusion after fluorouracil failure in patients with metastatic colorectal cancer. Lancet. 1998 Oct 31;352(9138):1407-12.

Saltz L, Danenberg K, Paty P, Kelsen D, Salonga D, Park JM, Danemberg P (1998) High thymidylate synthase (TS) expression does not preclude activity of CTP-11 in colorectal cancer (CRC). Proc Am Soc Clin Oncol 17:991 (abstract)

Saltz LB, Cox JV, Blanke C, Rosen LS, Fehrenbacher L, Moore MJ, Maroun JA, Ackland SP, Locker PK, Pirotta N, Elfring GL, Miller LL. Irinotecan plus fluorouracil and leucovorin for metastatic colorectal cancer. Irinotecan Study Group. N Engl J Med. 2000 Sep 28;343(13):905-14.

Saltz LB, Douillard JY, Pirotta N, Alakl M, Gruia G, Awad L, Elfring GL, Locker PK, Miller LL (2001) Irinotecan plus fluorouracil/leucovorin for metastatic colorectal cancer: a new survival standard. Oncologist 6:81-91

Sanghani SP, Quinney SK, Fredenburg TB, Sun Z, Davis WI, Murry DJ, Cummings OW, Seitz DE, Bosron WF (2003) Carboxylesterases expressed in human colon tumor tissue and their role in CPT-11 hydrolysis. Clin Cancer Res 9:4983-4991

Sari L, Andricioaei I. Rotation of DNA around intact strand in human topoisomerase I implies distinct mechanisms for positive and negative supercoil relaxation. Nucleic Acids Res. 2005 Nov 27;33(20):6621-34.

Schaeppi V, Fleischman RW, Cooney DA: Toxicity of camptothecin (NSC-100880). Cancer Chemother Rep 1974;58: 25-36.

Schilstra MJ, Martin SR, Bayley PM. The effect of podophyllotoxin on microtubule dynamics. J Biol Chem. 1989 May 25;264(15):8827-34.

Schultz P, Olland S, Oudet P, Hancock R. Structure and conformational changes of DNA topoisomerase II visualized by electron microscopy. Proc Natl Acad Sci U S A. 1996 Jun 11;93(12):5936-40.

Shaffer R, Traktman P. Vaccinia virus encapsidates a novel topoisomerase with the properties of a eucaryotic type I enzyme. J Biol Chem. 1987 Jul 5;262(19):9309-15.

Shero JH, Bordwell B, Rothfield NF, Earnshaw WC. High titers of autoantibodies to topoisomerase I (Scl-70)in sera from scleroderma patients.Science.1986 Feb14;231(4739):737-40.

Shero JH, Bordwell B, Rothfield NF, Earnshaw WC. Antibodies to topoisomerase I in sera from patients with scleroderma. J Rheumatol Suppl. 1987 Jun;14 Suppl 13:138-40.

Shuman S. Vaccinia DNA topoisomerase I promotes illegitimate recombination in Escherichia coli. Proc Natl Acad Sci U S A. 1989 May;86(10):3489-93.

Shuman S. Vaccinia virus DNA topoisomerase: a model eukaryotic type IB enzyme. Biochim Biophys Acta. 1998 Oct 1;1400(1-3):321-37. Review.

Slesarev AI, Stetter KO, Lake JA, Gellert M, Krah R, Kozyavkin SA. DNA topoisomerase V is a relative of eukaryotic topoisomerase I from a hyperthermophilic prokaryote. Nature. 1993 Aug 19;364(6439):735-7.

Slichenmyer WJ, Rowinsky EK, Donehower RC, Kaufmann SH. The current status of camptothecin analogues as antitumor agents. J Natl Cancer Inst. 1993 Feb 17;85(4):271-91. Review.

Smith JT. [Mechanism of action of quinolones] Infection. 1986;14 Suppl 1:S3-15. German.

Staley BE, Samowitz WS, Bronstein IB, Holden JA (1999) Expression of DNA topoisomerase I and DNA topoisomerase II-αlpha in carcinoma of colon. Mod Pathol 12:356-361

Staley BE, Samowitz WS, Bronstein IB, Holden JA. Expression of DNA topoisomerase I and DNA topoisomerase II-α in carcinoma of colon. Mod Pathol 12:356-361, 1999.

Stewart L, Redinbo MR, Qiu X, Hol WG, Champoux JJ. A model for the mechanism of human topoisomerase I. Science. 1998 Mar 6;279(5356):1534-41.

Stoll BA. Eating to beat breast cancer: potential role for soy supplements. Ann Oncol. 1997 Mar;8(3):223-5.

Stuart K, Posner M, Campbell K, Huberman M (1995) Cisplatin and chronic oral etoposide as salvage therapy for advanced colorectal carcinoma. Am J Clin Oncol 18:300–302

Subramanian D, Rosenstein BS, Muller MT. Ultraviolet-induced DNA damage stimulates topoisomerase I-DNA complex formation in vivo: possible relationship with DNA repair. Cancer Res. 1998 Mar 1;58(5):976-84.

Sugino A, Peebles CL, Kreuzer KN, Cozzarelli NR. Mechanism of action of nalidixic acid: purification of Escherichia coli nalA gene product and its relationship to DNA gyrase and a novel nicking-closing enzyme. Proc Natl Acad Sci U S A. 1977 Nov;74(11):4767-71.

Sullivan DM, Chow KC, Glisson BS, Ross WE. Role of proliferation in determining sensitivity to topoisomerase II-active chemotherapy agents. NCI Monogr. 1987;(4):73-8.

Takasuna K, Hagiwara T, Hirohashi M, Kato M, Nomura M, Nagai E, Yokoi T, Kamataki T. Involvement of beta-glucuronidase in intestinal microflora in the intestinal toxicity of the antitumor camptothecin derivative irinotecan hydrochloride (CPT-11) in rats. Cancer Res. 1996 Aug 15;56(16):3752-7.

Takehara K, Sato S. Localized scleroderma is an autoimmune disorder. Rheumatology (Oxford). 2005 Mar;44(3):274-9. Epub 2004 Nov 23. Review. Erratum in: Rheumatology (Oxford). 2005 Apr;44(4):569.

Thrash C, Voelkel K, DiNardo S, Sternglanz R. Identification of Saccharomyces cerevisiae mutants deficient in DNA topoisomerase I activity. J Biol Chem. 1984 Feb 10;259(3):1375-7.

Tsavaris N, Kosmas C, Gennatas K, Vadiaka M, Skopelitis E, Xila V, Rokana S, Margaris E, Zografos G, Papastratis G, Kouraklis G (2002) Etoposide, leucovorin (LV) and 5-FLuorouracil (5-FU) in 5-FU + LV pre-treated patients with advanced colorectal cancer. J Chemother 14:406–411

Tsavaris N, Ziras N, Kosmas C, Giannakakis T, Gouveris P, Vadiaka M, Dimitrakopoulos A, Karadima D, Rokana S, Papalambros E, Papastratis G, Margaris H et al (2003) Two diVerent schedules of irinotecan (CPT-11) in patients with advanced colorectal carcinoma relapsing after a 5-Fluorouracil and leucovorin combination. A randomized study. Cancer Chemother Pharmacol 52:514–519

Tsavaris N, Kosmas C, Zorzos H, Lazaris A, Vadiaka M, Dimitrakopoulos A, Siakantaris MP, Rokana S, Papalambros E, Pangalis GA, Davaris P (2004) Breast cancer after curative chemotherapy in non-Hodgkin's lymphoma: examination of the role of drug resistance and retrospective comparison to the outcome of de novo breast cancer. Oncol Rep 11:899–903

Tsavaris N, Kosmas C, Skopelitis H, Papadoniou N, Polyzos A, Zografos G, Adoniou E, Gryniatsos J, Felekouras E, Zacharakis M, Sigala F, Bacoyiannis C et al (2007) Sequential administration of 5-Fluorouracil (5FU)/leucovorin (LV) followed by irinotecan (CPT-11) at relapse versus CPT-11 followed by 5-FU/LV in advanced colorectal carcinoma. A phase III randomized study. Chemotherapy 53:282–291

Tsavaris NB, Polyzos A, Gennatas K, Kosmas Ch, Vadiaka M, Dimitrakopoulos A, Macheras A, Papastratis G, Tsipras H, Margaris H, Papalambros E, Giannopoulos A et al (2002) Irinotecan (CPT-11) in patients with advanced colon carcinoma relapsing after 5-Fluorouracil-leucovorin combination. Chemotherapy 48:94–99

Turley H, Comley M, Houlbrook S, Nozaki N, Kikuchi A, Hickson ID, Gatter K, Harris AL. The distribution and expression and expression of the two isoforms of DNA topoisomerase II in normal and neoplastic human tissues. Br J Cancer. 1997;75(9):1340-6.

Uemura T, Yanagida M. Isolation of type I and II DNA topoisomerase mutants from fission yeast: single and double mutants show different phenotypes in cell growth and chromatin organization. EMBO J. 1984 Aug;3(8):1737-44.

Van Cutsem E, Peeters M (1998) Irinotecan monotherapy in the treatment of colorectal cancers: results of phase II trials. Bull Cancer 33-7

Van der Zee AG, Hollema H, de Jong S, Boonstra H, Gouw A, Willemse PH, Zijlstra JG, de Vries EG .P-glycoprotein Expression and DNA Topoisomerase I and II Activity in Benign Tumors of the Ovary and in Malignant Tumors of the Ovary, Before and After Platinum/Cyclophosphamide Chemotherapy. CancerRes. 1991, 51, 5915-5920.

Van der Zee AG, de Jong S, Keith WN, Hollema H, Boonstra H, de Vries EG. Quantitative and qualitative aspects of topoisomerase I and II alpha and beta in untreated and platinum/cyclophosphamide treated malignant ovarian tumors.CancerRes.1994 Feb1;54(3):749-55.

Vanhoefer U, Harstrick A, Achterrath W, Cao S, Seeber S, Rustum YM (2001) Irinotecan in the treatment of colorectal cancer: clinical overview. J Clin Oncol 19:1501-1518

Wall ME, Wani MC, Cook CE, Palmer KH, McPhail AT, Sim GA. Plant antitumor agents. I. The isolation and structure of camptothecin, a novel alkaloidal leukemia and tumor inhibitor from camptotheca acuminata. J Am Chem Soc 1966; 88: 3888-90.

Wang HK, Morris-Natschke SL, Lee KH. Recent advances in the discovery and development of topoisomerase inhibitors as antitumor agents. Med Res Rev. 1997 Jul;17(4):367-425. Review.

Wang HP, Rogler CE. Topoisomerase I-mediated integration of hepadnavirus DNA in vitro. J Virol. 1991 May;65(5):2381-92.

Wang JC. Cellular roles of DNA topoisomerases: a molecular perspective. Nat Rev Mol Cell Biol. 2002 Jun;3(6):430-40. Review.

Wang JC. Degree of superhelicity of covalently closed cyclic DNA's from Escherichia coli. J Mol Biol. 1969 Jul 28;43(2):263-72.

Wang JC. DNA topoisomerases.Annu Rev Biochem. 1996;65:635-92. Review.

Wang JC. Interaction between DNA and an Escherichia coli protein omega. J Mol Biol. 1971 Feb 14;55(3):523-33.

Wang, J. C. and Lynch, A. S., "Transcription and DNA supercoiling," Curr. Opin. in Genes and Dev. 3, 764-768 (1993).

Waters J, Cunningham D (2001) The changing face of chemotherapy in colorectal cancer. Br J Cancer 84:1-7

Wilstermann AM, Bender RP, Godfrey M, Choi S, Anklin C, Berkowitz DB, OsheroV N, Graves DE (2007) Topoisomerase II-drug interaction domains: identification of substituents on etoposide that interact with the enzyme. Biochemistry 46:8217–8225

Zelkowitz RS, Posner MR, Cummings F, Beitz J, Weitberg AB (1989) A phase I/II trial of 5-Fluorouracil and etoposide in metastatic colorectal carcinoma. Am J Clin Oncol 12:492–493

Zijlstra JG, de Jong S, de Vries EG, Mulder NH. Topoisomerases, new targets in cancer chemotherapy. Med Oncol Tumor Pharmacother. 1990;7(1):11-8. Review.

Zorzos HS, Lazaris AC, Korkolopoulou PA, Kavantzas NG, Tseleni-Balafouta S, Patsouris ES, Tsavaris NV, Davaris PS (2003) Multidrug resistance proteins and topoisomerase II alpha expression in colon cancer: association with metastatic potential. Pathology 35:315–318

30

Bacterial Genetics of Large Mammalian DNA Viruses: Bacterial Artificial Chromosomes as a Prerequisite for Efficiently Studying Viral DNA Replication and Functions

Felix Wussow[1,2], Tanja Spieckermann[1], Anne Brunnemann[1], Linda Hüske[1], Tuna Toptan[1,3] and Helmut Fickenscher[1]
[1]*Institute for Infection Medicine, Christian Albrecht University of Kiel and University Medical Center Schleswig-Holstein, Kiel,*
[2]*City of Hope Comprehensive Cancer Center and Beckman Research Institute, Translational Vaccine Research, Duarte, California,*
[3]*Cancer Virology Program, University of Pittsburgh Cancer Institute, Pittsburgh, Pennsylvania,*
[1]*Germany*
[2,3]*USA*

1. Introduction

Large DNA viruses such as herpesviruses and poxviruses constitute a group of highly relevant pathogens for animals and humans. Genetic and functional analysis of these viruses has been a constant research challenge mainly because of their large and complex genomes, which are difficult to access by standard molecular biology techniques. Homologous recombination is the major principle for the manipulation of such viral genomes. The simple site-directed integration of a selection marker gene into the viral DNA allowed for the first time the enrichment of recombinants in permissive eukaryotic cells (Mocarski et al., 1980; Smiley, 1980). Essential genomic sites including those involved in DNA replication cannot be efficiently investigated by this method, since mutants with such defects would not start to replicate and, thus, would not be generated. To some extent, amplicon constructs in the presence of a wild-type helper virus have been instrumental for functional studies, which were, however, hampered by the background of similar helper virus sequences. Such limitations were resolved by cloning entire virus genomes as cosmid libraries in *Escherichia (E.) coli* (van Zijl et al., 1988). The virus is reconstituted in permissive mammalian cells after cotransfection of overlapping viral cosmids. Essential genome sites involved in DNA replication can then eventually be identified by providing the missing function through *trans*-complementation. However, unwanted second-site mutations after recombination of the homologous overlapping sequences and the resulting spontaneous mutation possibilities at the overlapping stretches are considerable disadvantages, rendering this procedure rather unreliable.

The major methodological break-through was achieved by cloning entire herpesvirus genomes as infectious large plasmids, co-called bacterial artificial chromosomes (BACs) in *E. coli* (Messerle et al., 1997). This technology was first introduced for the murine cytomegalovirus genome and was subsequently applied to numerous other virus pathogens. This permitted the stable maintenance and the targeted mutagenesis of the virus genomes as single plasmids in *E. coli*. Afterwards, the transfer of the BAC DNA into virus-permissive eukaryotic cells allowed the reconstitution of the mutant virus representing a homogenous population. Initially, the selection marker and the BAC cassette remained obligatory after the manipulation of the genomes in *E. coli* and the virus reconstitution in eukaryotic cells, respectively. As an improvement, site-specific recombinase systems were applied for the excision of the BAC vector sequences, leaving behind only one recombinase recognition site. Also transposon mutagenesis was used for generating libraries of virus genomes saturated with single-site mutations. As the second break-through, manipulation techniques such as *en passant* mutagenesis enabled the seamless alteration of the BAC DNA in bacteria and, thus, the reconstitution of mutant progeny virus which was free of secondary mutations such as selection markers or recombinase recognition sites (Tischer et al., 2006). The third break-through was achieved, when all BAC vector sequences were deleted autonomically after transfection of restructured BACs into permissive eukaryotic cells, allowing the generation of virus progeny completely devoid of any operational sequences. This approach uses functional features of virus DNA replication in order to reconstitute the wild-type configuration at the previous BAC vector insertion site. In addition, methods were developed for the targeted transposition of the vector sequence within a BAC construct in order to optimize genomic vector design. Thus, BAC constructs of large mammalian DNA viruses have become crucial for functional studies, even of essential genes including that for viral DNA replication.

In this review, we summarize the development of viral BAC vectors and the bacterial genetics tools used. We discuss the advantages and disadvantages of different BAC vector strategies for herpes- and poxviruses, as well as the application potential for functional studies into DNA replication and other viral functions and the perspectives for future preventive and therapeutic strategies.

2. Generation of recombinant large DNA viruses

Herpesvirus genomes consist of 120-250 kb double-stranded (ds) linear DNA which is circularized after infection of the cell. They are composed of different unique and repetitive regions with densely packed or even overlapping open reading frames of approximately 70-220 genes. Poxvirus genomes are even larger. Whereas poxviruses replicate in the cytoplasm, the DNA replication of herpesviruses occurs in the nucleus. Functional studies in large DNA viruses require the precise generation of virus mutants; thus, accessory operational sequences and selection markers should be avoided in order to exclude unwanted side-effects which may hide or distort the effects mediated by the precise mutant position. The development of precise mutagenesis protocols has been a constant challenge in herpes- and poxvirology. Eight human herpesviruses are of major interest in this research field: herpes simplex virus 1 (HSV-1), herpes simplex virus 2 (HSV-2), varicella-zoster virus (VZV), Epstein-Barr virus (EBV), human cytomegalovirus (hCMV), human herpesvirus 6 (HHV-6), human herpesvirus 7 (HHV-7), and Kaposi's sarcoma-associated herpesvirus (KSHV). In addition, a series of animal herpesviruses have been subjected to recombinant mutagenesis. While all these herpesviruses are capable of persisting life-long in the human body, they can be reactivated and cause disease under specific conditions during primary infection or during reactivation. Among the poxviruses, the major interest lies in vaccinia viruses which are highly important tools for vaccine development.

2.1 Basic strategies for the manipulation of large viral genomes

The classical, pre-recombinant strategy for mutant generation was developed approximately forty years ago by the targeted phenotypic selection of chemically induced and randomly generated temperature-sensitive variants which are conditionally expressing specific virus proteins (Schaffer, 1975). This strategy was a pacemaker for virus research and allowed the temperature-dependent study of defined virus functions, including properties which are essential for virus replication. However, the precise definition of the respective mutation was demanding and unwanted second-site mutations were difficult to exclude.

The size of herpes- and poxviral genomes was by far too large in order to utilize naturally occurring unique endonuclease recognition sites for the precise manipulation of the viral DNA. The targeted mutagenesis of herpes- or poxviral genomes was successfully achieved by the integration of a selection marker flanked by viral DNA sequences including the desired genetic mutation by homologous recombination into the virus genome during virus replication in cultured permissive eukaryotic cells (Manning & Mocarski, 1988; Mocarski et al., 1980; Post & Roizman, 1981; Smiley, 1980; Spaete & Mocarski, 1987). Since the homologous recombination occurred as a rare event, the recombinants were difficult to isolate from a dominating amount of wild-type virus. This method did not yet allow the targeting of essential genes, since the strategy was dependent on active virus replication.

A considerable step forward was done by introducing the concept of virus reconstitution by cotransfection of overlapping genomic cosmid clones into permissive cells (Cohen & Seidel, 1993; Cunningham & Davison, 1993; Kemble et al., 1996; Tomkinson et al., 1993; van Zijl et al., 1988). For this purpose, virion DNA was prepared, degraded to fragment sizes of approximately 30-40 kb, and cloned in *E. coli* into cosmid vector libraries. Selected overlapping and complementing genomic cosmid DNA clones were then selected and transfected as sets of three to five cosmids into permissive cells in order to reconstitute infectious virus. The major advantage of the cosmid complementation method is the fact, that the cloned viral DNA can be manipulated precisely by molecular biology or bacterial genetic techniques. Moreover, the obtained virus progeny is free of cosmid vector sequences, although selection markers cannot be avoided in most cases. By providing essential functions *in trans* or by *trans*-complementing cell lines, even essential virus genes were analyzed using this method. The cosmid-complementation technique is limited in eukaryotic cells by illegitimate events of homologous recombination or unwanted second-site mutations which are difficult to exclude. The technique of cosmid complementation was instrumental for developing entire virus genomes in the form of viral BACs.

2.2 Bacterial artificial chromosomes of entire large viral genomes

BACs were established for studies in human and animal genetics. BACs are single-copy bacterial F-factor-derived plasmids of approximately 7.5 kb which carry an own origin of replication, encode own DNA replication factors (*e.g.*, repE), and an antibiotic resistance function (*e.g.*, against chloramphenicol). BACs can stably maintain DNA molecules of up to 300 kb in recombination-deficient *E. coli* strains (Shizuya et al., 1992). A frequently used BAC vector is pBeloBAC11. The F-plasmid based vector sequences are often designated "mini-F" fragments. The BAC copy number is strictly restricted to one or two copies per bacterial cell by regulatory elements (*e.g.,* parA & parB) of the mini-F vector. Thus, intermolecular homologous recombination events are largely excluded. However, repeated or duplicated sequences can still undergo homologous recombination (Shizuya et al., 1992). Bacteriophage P1-based vectors (PACs) are comparable to BACs. In contrast to BACs, yeast artificial chromosomes (YACs) can accommodate even larger inserts. However, YACs often have chimeric structures and sequence rearrangements (Ramsay, 1994; Schalkwyk et al., 1995). BACs show higher insert stability in *E. coli* in comparison to cosmid-based plasmids, which are restricted to DNA-fragment sizes of up to 50 kb (Kim et al., 1992). Therefore, BACs have become the vectors of choice for the cloning of large and complex genomes in *E. coli* (Ioannou et al., 1994; Shizuya et al., 1992). Moreover, BACs are instrumental in sequencing strategies, for functional genomics, and for the construction of gene targeting or gene therapy vectors (Copeland et al., 2001; Sparwasser & Eberl, 2007; Yang & Gong, 2005). For the application in cloning large DNA virus genomes, the BAC vector needs flanking virus homology regions of 300-500 bp for the precise targeting into the desired genomic region. Depending on the planned applications, accessory operational markers are included, such as genes for an autofluorescent protein, luciferase, or antibiotic resistance. Many strategies include flanking recognition sites (*e.g.,* loxP) for recombinases (*e.g.,* Cre) at the ends of the BAC insert sequence in order to allow the vector excision from recombinant progeny viruses.

Herpes- and also poxvirus BACs (Figure 1) can be constructed by inserting a mini-F vector into a specific site of a non-essential genomic region via homologous recombination of a linearized recombination construct during active virus replication in permissive eukaryotic cells after lipofection or electroporation. The recombination fragment may be cotransfected with virion DNA or the transfected culture may superinfected with wild-type virus after transfection. The transfer of the circular replication intermediates of recombinant progeny viruses or artificially created circular DNA is carried out into a RecA- *E. coli* strain, such as DH10B (Messerle et al., 1997). Alternatively, the BAC vector can be inserted into a non-essential region of a specific viral cosmid clone, in addition to the pre-existing cosmid vector fragment. After cotransfection of sets of three to five overlapping viral cosmids into permissive cells, the BAC vector-containing virus is reconstituted. Similarly, the circular replication intermediates are then transferred into *E. coli* (Saeki et al., 1998; Tischer et al., 2007). A detailed molecular analysis of the viral BACs is necessary in order to show genetic integrity. Importantly, viral BAC DNA can be prepared in large quantity and high quality in order to compensate for the inefficient transfection procedures into permissive eukaryotic cells. After retransfer of the viral BAC into permissive cells, the resulting recombinant virus is reconstituted and compared with wild-type virus for genome structure and replication properties. If possible, plaque purification is recommended in order to ensure a homogenous virus population. Selectable markers such as genes for autofluorescent proteins may be useful for the rapid identification of recombinant viruses. A detailed analysis is necessary since unwanted genotypic and phenotypic changes in viral BACs have been observed (Ali et al., 2009; Messerle et al., 1997). In viruses with particular large genomes, such as cytomegaloviruses, the 7.5 kb BAC vector insert may already lead to obvious retardation of viral replication (Yu et al., 2002).

After the initial cloning of murine cytomegalovirus (mCMV; Messerle et al., 1997), the genomes of many herpesviruses, some poxviruses, and some large RNA viruses were constructed as infectious viral BACs (Table 1; Adler et al., 2003; Britt, 2000; Brune et al., 1999,

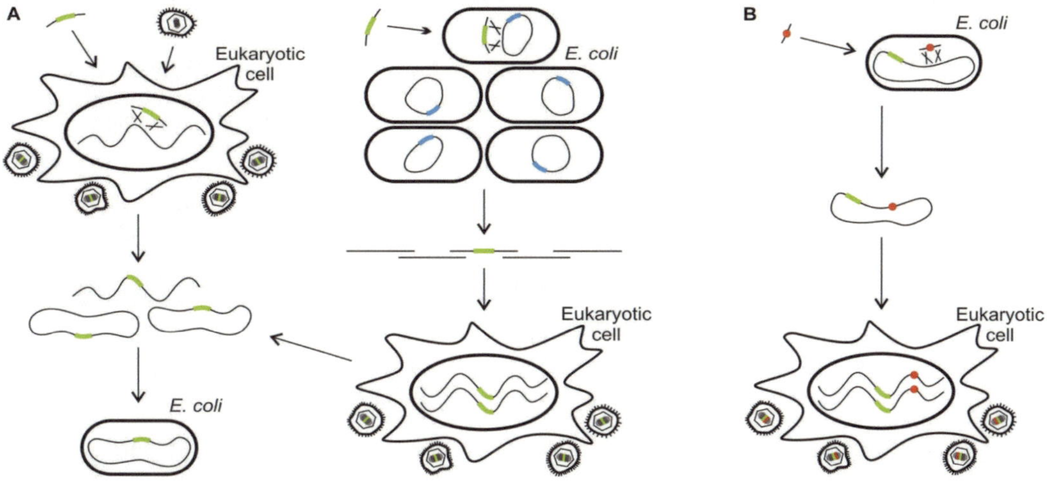

Fig. 1. Generation and mutagenesis of herpesvirus BACs. A) Cloning of a herpesviral genome as a bacterial artificial chromosome (BAC). A mini-F vector (green) is inserted into the viral DNA via homologous recombination (crossed lines) during virus replication in infected permissive eukaryotic cells. Circular replication intermediates are isolated and transferred into *E. coli* to establish an infectious viral BAC. Alternatively, the mini-F plasmid is first inserted into a viral cosmid (blue) DNA clone. Overlapping linear viral genome fragments from cosmid vectors are subsequently transfected into permissive cells. Circular DNA intermediates of recovered replicating virus are then isolated and transformed into *E. coli*. B) Herpesvirus BAC technology. The herpesviral BAC is maintained in *E. coli* and a mutation is introduced into the viral DNA by homologous recombination. The BAC is isolated and transfected into permissive eukaryotic cells, where mutant progeny is reconstituted (adapted from Felix Wussow, Ph.D. thesis, Christian Albrecht University of Kiel, 2009).

2000; Feederle et al., 2010; McGregor & Schleiss, 2001b; Wagner & Koszinowski, 2004; Wagner et al., 2002, 2004; Warden et al., 2011). Full-length viral DNA can be maintained and mutagenized in *E. coli* and delivered into permissive eukaryotic cells for virus reconstitution. Since poxviruses replicate in the cytoplasm, the initiation of viral transcription and DNA replication requires the presence of a related helper virus (Domi and Moss, 2002). Infectious homogenous progeny is recovered from mutated viral BAC-DNA in a defined manner without any further homologous recombination events to restore genome integrity, in contrast to virus reconstitution from overlapping cosmid fragments. Nevertheless, mini-F sequences in a non-essential genomic region can interfere with specific viral functions especially in further in vivo experiments. The complete removal of the mini-F vector by homologous recombination has been limited to laborious cotransfection experiments or to BAC constructs with restricted stability in bacteria (Strive et al., 2007; Wagner et al., 1999; Yu et al., 2002). Alternatively, the vector elements can be flanked by recognition sites for site-specific recombinases, which leave behind only one small recognition sequence (Adler et al., 2000, 2001; Chang & Barry, 2003; Smith & Enquist, 2000; Strive et al., 2006; Tanaka et al., 2003; Zhao et al., 2008).

Virus	Species	Abbr.	Major references
α-Herpesviruses			
- Simplexviruses			
Herpes simplex virus type 1	human	HSV-1	Horsburgh et al., 1999a, b; Nagel et al., 2008; Saeki et al., 1998; Stravropoulos & Strathdee, 1998; Tanaka et al., 2003
Herpes simplex virus type 2	human	HSV-2	Meseda et al., 2004
- Varicelloviruses			
Varicella-zoster virus	human	VZV	Nagaike et al., 2004; Tischer et al., 2007; Wussow et al., 2009; Yoshii et al., 2007; Zhang et al., 2007
Simian varicella virus	rhesus	SVV	Brazeau et al., 2011; Gray et al., 2011
Pseudorabies virus	porcine	PrV	Smith & Enquist, 1999
Bovine herpesvirus type 1	bovine	BHV-1	Mahony et al., 2002; Robinson et al., 2008
Equine herpesvirus type 1	equine	EHV-1	Rudolph & Osterrieder, 2002; Rudolph et al., 2002
Canine herpesvirus	canine	CHV	Strive et al., 2006
Feline herpesvirus type 1	feline	FHV-1	Costes et al., 2006; Tai et al., 2010
- Mardiviruses			
Marek's disease virus	turkey	MDV	Schumacher et al., 2000
Turkey herpesvirus	turkey	HVT	Baigent et al., 2006
β-Herpesviruses			
- Cytomegaloviruses			
Human cytomegalovirus	human	hCMV	Borst et al., 1999; Dulal et al., 2009; Hahn et al., 2002, 2003; Marchini et al., 2001; Murphy et al., 2003; Sinzger et al., 2008
Rhesus cytomegalovirus	rhesus	rhCMV	Chang & Barry, 2003
Murine cytomegalovirus	murine	mCMV	Messerle et al., 1997
Guinea pig cytomegalovirus	guinea pig	gpCMV	McGregor & Schleiss, 2001a
- Roseoloviruses			
Human herpesvirus 6	human	HHV-6	Borenstein & Frenkel, 2009
γ-Herpesviruses			
- Lymphocryptoviruses			
Epstein-Barr virus	human	EBV	Delecluse et al., 1998
- Rhadinoviruses			
Kaposi-Sarcoma associated herpesvirus	human	KSHV	Delecluse et al., 2001; Zhou et al., 2002
Rhesus rhadinovirus	rhesus	RRV	Estep et al., 2007
Murine γ-herpesvirus 68	murine	MHV-68	Adler et al., 2000; Song et al., 2005
Herpesvirus saimiri	saimiriine	HVS	White et al., 2003; Toptan et al., 2010
Alloherpesviruses			
Koi herpesvirus	carp	KHV	Costes et al., 2008
Poxviruses			
Vaccinia virus		VAC	Cottingham et al., 2008; Domi & Moss, 2002; Meissinger-Henschel et al., 2011
Cowpox virus	bovine	CPXV	Roth et al., 2011
Coronaviruses			
Transmissible gastroenteritis coronavirus	porcine	TGCV	Almazan et al., 2000
Severe acute respiratory syndrome coronavirus	human	SARS CoV	Almazan et al., 2006
Coronavirus OC43	human	OC43	St. Jean et al., 2006
Coronavirus NL63	human	NL63	Donaldson et al., 2008

Table 1. List of cloned viral bacterial artificial chromosomes with key references.

3. Manipulation of viral bacterial artificial chromosomes

The generation of a molecular viral BAC clone forms the prerequisite for efficient virus mutagenesis. The site-directed manipulation of single-copy plasmid DNA in *E. coli* by homologous recombination was established in several conditionally or transiently expressed forms. Alternatively, transposon mutagenesis can be used as a non-directed random method.

3.1 Site-directed mutagenesis of viral bacterial artificial chromosomes

Common techniques for the rapid and targeted DNA mutagenesis are based on Red recombination or RecET cloning encoded by prophages λ or Rac, respectively (Court et al., 2002; Lee et al., 2001; Murphy, 1998; Muyrers et al., 1999, 2001, 2004; Yu et al., 2000; Zhang et al., 1998). Recombination-mediated genetic engineering (termed "recombineering") via Red and RecET allows almost unlimited modifications of large BAC-cloned DNA sequences in *E. coli* and is widely used in functional genomics (Copeland et al., 2001; Muyrers et al., 2001; Narayanan et al. 1999; Sawitzke et al., 2007; Sharan et al., 2009; Thomason et al., 2007; Warming et al., 2005). The Red-recombination system from phage λ consists of the 5′-3′-exonuclease Exo and of the single-strand (ss) DNA-binding protein Beta. These proteins mediate the recombination between dsDNA ends and homologous target sequences on replicating DNA molecules in *E. coli* and are biologically responsible for the integration of λ phage DNA into the bacterial chromosome (Carter & Radding, 1971). Exo acts on dsDNA ends to generate 3′-ssDNA sticky ends (Little, 1967). Then, Beta recognizes the recessed ssDNA ends and anneals them to complementary ssDNA in preformed replication forks leading to their recombination with the homologous sequence (Kmiec & Holloman, 1981; Muniyappa & Radding, 1986). The Red genes are expressed together with the λ *gam* gene under a temperature-inducible promoter for the efficient induction and DNA manipulation in bacteria. Gam is a natural inhibitor of the *E. coli* RecBCD exonuclease, which rapidly degrades dsDNA invading into bacteria (Karu et al., 1975; Murphy, 1991, 1998, 2007; Yu et al., 2000).

While the Red recombination system is expressed, a linear DNA fragment with 40-50 bp homologous flanking regions is inserted into to the selected target sequence by Exo and Beta, whereas Gam blocks the RecBCD enzyme from degrading dsDNA ends. The Red system does not need the *E. coli* RecA protein, which is the main endogenous mediator of homologous recombination in *E. coli* (Murphy, 1998; Yu et al., 2000). Therefore, the Red recombination is useful for the easy manipulation of plasmids or bacterial chromosomes in a recA$^-$recombination-deficient *E. coli* background (*e.g.*, DY380-derived strains or GS1783) by linear products of the polymerase chain-reaction (PCR) that were generated with primers containing short homologous target sequences at their 5′-ends (Copeland et al., 2001; Oppenheim et al., 2004; Yu et al., 2000). The application of Red-mediated DNA mutagenesis for BAC mutagenesis was greatly simplified by expressing the *red* and *gam* genes from a defective prophage integrated in the *E. coli*-genome, when the culture temperature is increased from 32 to 42°C, without the need for additional expression plasmids. In comparison to the plasmid coexpression strategy, the λ prophage system is up to 100-fold more efficient in Red recombineering and the Red protein expression is more tightly controlled under the temperature-inducible promoter of the λ prophage (Lee et al., 2001; Yu et al., 2000). This more stringent control also reduces the risk for unwanted recombination during bacterial DNA replication. During the mutagenesis procedure, the mutation of interest is introduced into the target sequence together with an antibiotic resistance gene. The selection marker may be flanked by recombinase recognition sites in order to allow its secondary excision from the recombinants (Lee et al., 2001; Yu et al., 2000). The remaining single copy of a recombinase recognition site limits further repeated steps of the procedure and may also interfere with gene functions in tightly packed genomes. The site-directed mutagenesis may be used to delete further non-essential regions if the cloning capacity is limited in particularly large virus genomes. In addition, genetic elements of the BAC constructs can even be moved within the BAC by site-directed mutagenesis to optimized insertion positions (Wussow et al., 2009).

3.2 Two-step *en passant* mutagenesis

By the combination of homologous recombination steps, "traceless", "seamless", or "markerless" recombineering strategies were developed which allow the highly efficient mutagenesis of BAC DNA in *E. coli* without retaining any operational sequences (Sawitzke et al., 2007; Sharan et al., 2009; Thomason et al., 2007; Tischer et al., 2006, 2010a, b; Warming et al., 2005). The *en passant* procedure combines Red recombination with cleavage by the homing endonuclease I-SceI (Tischer et al., 2006, 2010a, b). The asymmetrical 18 bp I-SceI recognition site can be inserted into plasmid DNA and cleaved after induced expression of the homing enzyme. This highly sequence-specific restriction endonuclease produces dsDNA ends accessible for homologous recombination (Jamsai et al., 2003). For the *en passant* protocol, large oligonucleotide primers are designed which allow generation of a PCR product for the Red-mediated insertion of a selection marker together with an I-SceI recognition site flanked by a 50 bp direct sequence duplication. After selection of recombinants, a double-strand break is induced by I-SceI cleavage at the respective recognition site. This permits the seamless excision of the positive selection marker (psm) by a second Red-mediated homologous recombination event via short duplicated sequences. *En passant* mutagenesis can be used to generate single point-mutations, substitutions, deletions, or insertions, *e.g.*, of expression constructs, epitope tags, or autofluorescent fusion proteins (Figure 2). For the generation of single point mutations, a fragment including a psm and an I-SceI site is amplified with primers adding 60-80 bp extensions to the psm-I-SceI unit. The distal 40-50 bp of the primer sequences and of the resulting PCR fragments are homologous to the target site in the BAC. Additionally, 40-50 bp of the mutated target site are included into both primers in reverse complementary orientation. The psm fragment with the appropriate flanking sequence duplication and point mutation is inserted into the site of interest by the first Red recombination step. After induction of I-SceI cleavage, the psm is excised between the duplicated sequences and the markerless point mutation is generated by the second Red recombinetion step (Figure 2A). Similar procedures are used for large deletions. In this case, the PCR-primers for psm-I-SceI amplification carry 5'-extensions from the up- and downstream regions flanking the deletion area (Figure 2C). For the seamless insertion of large sequences by *en passant* mutagenesis, a cassette containing the psm and the I-SceI site and a 40-50 bp sequence duplication is PCR amplified. This PCR fragment is then inserted into a unique restriction endonuclease site of the cloned sequence of interest. The fragment is released from the plasmid by terminal restriction endonuclease sites and used for the precise insertion into the target region by Red recombination. In selected recombinants, the psm is seamlessly removed by the second *en passant* recombination of the 50 bp duplication of the inserted sequence of interest (Figure 2B).

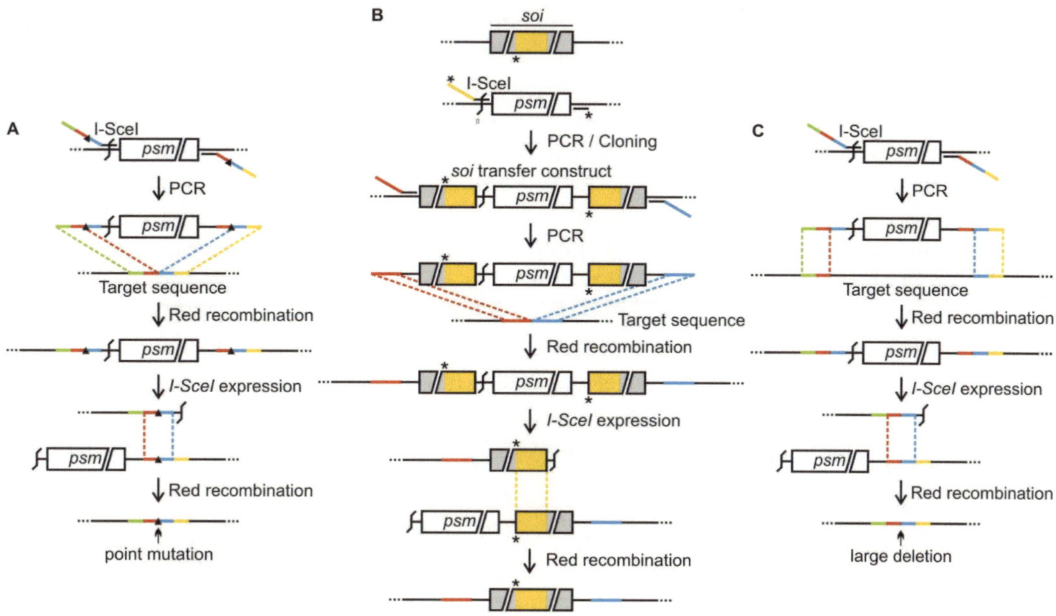

Fig. 2. *En passant* mutagenesis. A) Point mutation. A positive selection marker (psm) and an I-SceI site are PCR-amplified with primers carrying 60-80 bp homologous extensions (coloured elements). In both primers, 40-50 bp (red and blue) around the core sequence are reverse complementary and carry the mutation (triangles). The PCR product is inserted into the target site by Red recombination. After a double-strand break by I-SceI, the psm is excised by Red recombination of the duplication, resulting in the precise point mutation. B) Insertion of large sequences. The psm-I-SceI cassette is amplified using one primer with a 40-50 bp duplication (yellow) and inserted into a unique restriction site (*) of a cloned sequence of interest (soi). The soi transfer construct is then amplified using primers with 40-50 bp extensions (red and blue) and inserted into the target site by Red recombination. After I-SceI and red expression, the psm is deleted from soi by recombination of the short duplications. C) Large deletion. The psm-I-SceI element is amplified using primers with 5'-ends homologous to adjacent sequences from the deletion region (coloured). The soi is then deleted by Red recombination. The procedure follows the further steps as in panel A (adapted from Tischer et al., 2006; Felix Wussow, Ph.D. thesis, Christian Albrecht University of Kiel, 2009).

The well-established and highly versatile markerless manipulation techniques allow for the repetitive manipulation of the cloned genomes even within the direct or inverted viral repeat sequences. This unique feature makes the BAC technology especially useful to mutagenize elements involved in DNA replication or maturation, *e.g.*, the origin of DNA replication or DNA packaging signals, which are usually present in the repeat sequences or in the genomic termini of herpesviral genomes. Similarly, many DNA elements relevant for the establishment of latency and the reactivation from the latent state as well as for the integration of the viral DNA into the host genome are located in the viral repeats and can be efficiently studied by the BAC technology.

The *en passant* mutagenesis strategy can also be used for the seamless removal of the BAC-vector sequences from the viral genomes during virus reconstitution in eukaryotic cells

(Figure 3). Appropriately designed viruses will delete the mini-F element due to homologous recombination of duplications of viral genome fragments or due to intrinsic genome features. Such strategies were based on genomic duplications engineered in direct orientation at either site of the vector elements (Strive et al., 2007; Wagner et al., 1999). However, such BACs with direct duplications can apparently not be stably maintained in *E. coli* with the temperature-inducible Red expression cassette on a defective λ prophage integrate, since the mini-F vector will be lost presumably by homologous recombination between the duplicated viral sequences, even in the non-induced state. This has been overcome by providing the ET cloning functions from an additionally transfected plasmid for the efficient removal function after the mutagenesis procedure (Strive et al., 2007; Wagner et al., 1999), although recombineering mediated by plasmid-encoded functions is up to 100-fold less efficient than the integrated λ prophage system (Lee et al., 2001; Muyrers et al., 1999; Narayanan et al., 1999; Yu et al., 2000). In another λ-based self-excision system (Figure 3), the duplicated viral sequences flanking the mini-F integration site were inserted in inverse orientation. This arrangement allowed the stable maintenance of the BAC DNA in

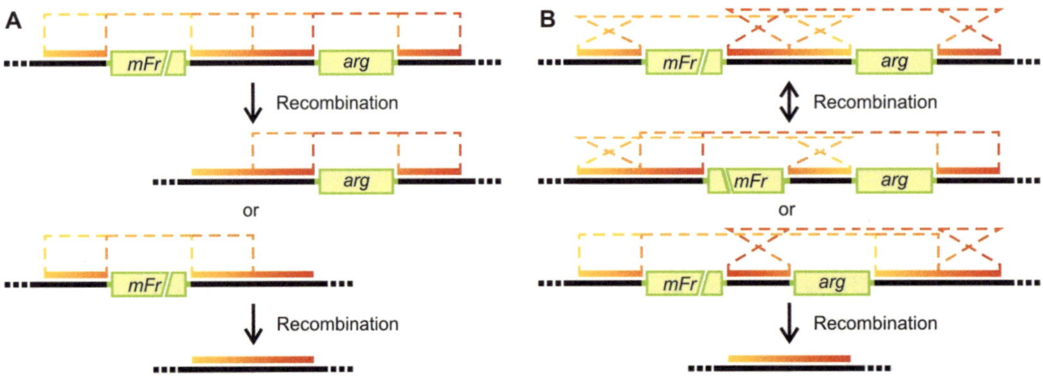

Fig. 3. Self-excision of BAC sequences by stabilized genomic duplication. A) BAC vector (green) self-excision from the viral DNA (black) by a forward genomic duplication (yellow to red gradient bars) inserted between the mini-F replicon (mFr) and the antibiotic resistance gene (arg). Two recombination events are necessary to release the mFr or the arg from the viral DNA. B) Self-excision of the BAC sequences from the viral DNA by a genomic duplication inserted in inverse orientation into the vector elements. Two successive events of recombination are required for the complete BAC vector excision from the viral DNA (adapted from Felix Wussow, Ph.D. thesis, Christian Albrecht University of Kiel, 2009).

E. coli, since two successive events of homologous recombination would be required for the deletion of the complete BAC sequences. BACs with these inverse viral duplications flanking the mini-F integration site within a viral direct S-repeat area did not lead to any detectable BAC instability in the recombineering *E. coli* strain GS1783 and allowed the efficient deletion of the vector moiety (Tischer et al., 2007).

Mini-F vector sequences containing inverse genomic duplications that were inserted into different essential viral replication genes also allow the efficient mini-F vector self-excision. Alternatively, certain repeat regions or terminal virus sequences are suitable under specific conditions for the autonomous vector excision (Tischer et al., 2007; Wussow et al., 2009; Zhou et al., 2010). Different genomic insertion sites for the mini-F vector were compared for the seamless reconstitution of recombinant virus. The most efficient variant pHJOFpac carried the mini-F vector insertion at the terminal genomic junction of VZV, which is an optimal vector integration site permitting the rapid and spontaneous generation of recombinant progeny devoid of any vector elements (Wussow et al., 2009). A similar integration site was described for rhesus rhadinovirus (RVV), from which the vector is also efficiently released (Zhou et al., 2010). Therefore, the terminal genomic junction might be in general an optimal integration site for the mini-F vector to construct other large linear viral DNA genomes as infectious BACs. In addition, the recombineering methodology even allows the transposition of genetic elements to defined new locations within the same BAC molecule (Wussow et al., 2009). Thus, the mini-F-transposition strategy eliminated the last hurdle to perform any imaginable kind of targeted seamless BAC modifications in *E. coli*. This is in general a valuable tool to reorganize or repair any other established BACs, *e.g.*, for the development of gene therapy or vaccine vectors or of specific targeting vectors for conditional knock-out mice.

3.3 Transposon mutagenesis of viral BACs

Alternatively, the random and non-directed approach of transposon mutagenesis was adapted for virus BAC mutagenesis (Brune et al., 1999; Smith & Enquist, 1999) and provides saturated libraries of diverse recombinant mutants. The random transposon mutagenesis was successfully performed for the large genomes of hCMV, mCMV, equine herpesvirus type 1 (EHV-1), and murine herpesvirus type 68 (MHV-68) (Bubeck et al., 2003; Hansen et al., 2006; Hobom et al., 2000; Song et al., 2005; Yu et al., 2003). Fortunately, the transposon insertion occurs preferentially into plasmid DNA in comparison to the bacterial genome. After transposon mutants have been tested for their functional phenotype, the respective genotype must be determined. This is accomplished using PCR primers which bind to the transposon insert and allow an easy genome-wide mapping and specific sequencing from the viral BAC genome. The major advantages of transposon mutagenesis are the unbiased random approach and the rapid generation of large BAC mutant libraries. However, this may be complicated by multiple insertions in the same BAC or by an uneven distribution of the insertion sites over the virus genome.

3.4 Functional mutagenesis of specific viral BACs

BAC generation and mutagenesis has been reported on numerous viruses (Table 1). HSV-1, the prototype genome of the herpesviruses in general, as well as of the α-herpesviruses and simplexviruses in particular, exists as BACs from different virus strains (Horsburgh et al., 1999a, b; Nagel et al., 2008; Saeki et al., 1998; Stavropoulos & Strathdee, 1998; Tanaka et al., 2003). Many BAC-based studies were performed on mutations in HSV-1 genes (*e.g.*, Boutell et al., 2002; Leege et al., 2009; O'Hara et al., 2010; Roberts et al., 2009; Tong & Stow, 2010). Also, HSV-2 is available as a viral BAC (Meseda et al., 2004). Several strains of the highly cell-associated varicellovirus prototype, VZV, were cloned as infectious BACs, the vaccine and parental OKA strains, as well as the wild-type isolate HJO (Nagaike et al., 2004; Tischer et al., 2007; Wussow et al., 2009; Yoshii et al., 2008; Zhang et al., 2007, 2008). A VZV BAC with a luciferase reporter gene allowed viral replication studies *in vivo* (Zhang et al., 2007, 2008). VZV was also subjected to saturating mutagenesis for determining essential genes for viral replication (Zhang et al., 2010). The genome of the closely related simian varicella virus (SVV) of rhesus monkeys has also been made available as a BAC (Brazeau et al., 2011; Gray et al., 2011). Pseudorabies virus (PrV) is another varicellovirus with highly important model function for herpesvirus biology. PrV was cloned as a BAC and used for pathogenesis studies *in vivo* (Smith & Enquist, 1999, 2000; Fuchs et al., 2009; Kopp et al., 2004]. Additional varicellovirus BACs of various animals have been studied *in vitro* and *in vivo*: Bovine herpesvirus type 1 (BHV-1; Gabev et al., 2009; Mahony et al., 2002; Robinson et al., 2008; Trapp et al., 2003), EHV-1 (Goodman et al., 2007; Rudolph & Osterrieder, 2002; Rudolph et al., 2002; Yao et al., 2003), canine herpesvirus (CHV; Strive et al., 2006), and feline herpesvirus type 1 (FHV-1; Costes et al., 2006; Richter et el., 2009; Tai et al., 2010). Moreover, BACs exist for the mardiviruses Marek's disease virus (MDV) and herpesvirus of turkeys (HVT) (Baigent et al., 2006; Petherbridge et al., 2003; Schumacher et al., 2000; Zhao et al., 2008). The particularly large BAC-cloned koi herpesvirus belongs to the alloherpesviruses and not to the typical α- to γ-herpesviruses (Costes et al., 2008, 2009).

The prototype for the β-herpesviruses, hCMV, has the largest genome among the human herpesviruses containing approximately 165 genes. Clinical hCMV isolates have larger genomes and replicate well in macrophages and endothelia cells, whereas the laboratory strains have undergone deletions and replicate efficiently only in fibroblasts (Dolan et al., 2004). Therefore, after the laboratory strain AD169, various laboratory strains and clinical isolates were cloned as infectious BACs in order to provide defined genetic conditions for functional studies (Borst et al., 1999; Dulal et al., 2009; Hahn et al., 2002, 2003; Marchini et al., 2001; Murphy et al., 2003; Sinzger et al., 2008). Many functional studies were performed with hCMV BACs (*e.g.*, Britt et al., 2004; Spaderna et al., 2005). Saturating random mutagenesis over the entire hCMV genome was performed by transposon insertion (Hobom et al., 2000; Yu et al., 2003). Moreover, the necessity for virus replication was determined for 162 individual hCMV genes (Dunn et al., 2003). mCMV as an important animal model for hCMV pathogenesis was the first herpesvirus genome to be cloned as an infectious BAC (Messerle et al., 1997) which has been used for *in vitro* and *in vivo* mCMV studies (*e.g.*, Wagner et al., 1999; Cicin-Sain et al., 2003, 2007; Menard et al., 2003; Schnee et al., 2006). BAC-clones have also been constructed for the genomes of rhesus CMV (rhCMV; Chang & Barry, 2003; Lilja et al., 2008; Rue et al., 2004) and guinea-pig CMV (gpCMV; Crumpler et al., 2009; McGregor & Schleiss, 2001a; Schleiss, 2008). The BAC of the human roseolovirus HHV-6 is still dependent on a helper virus infection (Borenstein & Frenkel, 2009; Borenstein et al., 2010).

The oncogenic γ-herpesvirus and lymphocryptovirus EBV (Delecluse et al., 1998) was one of the first cloned viral BACs and many studies have applied this technique, *e.g.*, on oncogene functions (Ahsan et al., 2005; Anderton et al., 2008; Chen et al., 2005; Kanda et al., 2004). The oncogenic rhadinovirus KSHV is hampered by its non-efficient replication in cell culture. Also for KSHV, several BACs were constructed and applied for functional analyses (Delecluse et al., 2001; Fan et al., 2006; Lu et al., 2010; Lukac et al., 2001; Luna et al., 2004; Majerciak et al., 2007; Xu et al., 2005, 2006; Yakushko et al., 2011 Zhou et al., 2002). Additionally, the major rhadinovirus animal model viruses were cloned in BACs, such as RRV (Estep et al., 2007; Zhou et al., 2010), MHV-68 (Adler et al., 2000; Pavlova et al., 2003), and herpesvirus saimiri (HVS; Calderwood et al., 2005; Toptan et al., 2010; White et al., 2003, 2007).

Besides the herpesviruses, BAC-cloning has been successfully applied for the poxvirus Vaccinia virus (Cottingham et al., 2008; Domi & Moss, 2002; Meissinger-Henschel et al., 2011) and cowpox virus (Roth et al., 2011). Moreover, this method was useful to generate full-length molecular clones of the large RNA genomes of different coronaviruses such as the porcine virus of transmissible gastroenteritis, the severe acute respiratory syndrome coronavirus and the human coronaviruses NL63 and OC43 (Almazan et al., 2000, 2006; Donaldson et al., 2008; St. Jean et al., 2006).

4. Conclusion

The viral DNA replication strategies were very well exploited for the generation of efficient BAC cloning, mutagenesis and reconstitution techniques. BAC cloning and recombineering strategies are essential for the efficient mutagenesis and analysis of herpesviral and poxviral gene functions and reduce problems due to unwanted mutations outside of the region of interest. In addition, only the existence of a cloned full-length genome guarantees the usage of defined genome structures, especially in variable virus genes. For example, the BAC-mediated expression of fusion proteins of viral factors with autofluorescent moieties can be used for analysing the expression and localization patterns of viral functions (*e.g.*, Antinone & Smith, 2006). The precise, seamless, and repetitive manipulation of repeat regions may facilitate the study of viral DNA elements involved in DNA replication, genome maturation, and packaging, as well as in latency, reactivation, and chromosomal integration.

Besides basic research, the BAC technology has its major translational applications in vector and vaccine development. In the case of viral vector design, the recombineering technique allows the easy deletion of useless non-essential regions or virulence genes from the viral vector genome (*e.g.*, Cicin-Sain et al., 2007). This may reduce unwanted side-effects and may increase the cloning potential for transgenes. Even large and complex multi-unit transgene cassettes can be inserted as well as novel conditional replication and expression control systems (*e.g.*, Glass et al., 2009). Such viral vectors include optimized transgene cassettes, the lack of genomic integration, and the advantage of physiologic infection routes. This may also comprise cell-type specific functions as for example in EBV or HVS vectors for B- or T-lymphocytes, respectively. Viral vectors may be constructed as efficiently replicating oncolytic agents (Kuroda et al., 2006; Marconi et al., 2009; Terada et al., 2006) or as packaging-cell dependent transduction vehicles (*e.g.*, Hettich et al., 2006).

The BAC technology has also provided new possibilities for vaccine development. For example, EHV-1 BAC-derived viruses were constructed for immunization against West Nile virus, bovine diarrhea virus or Venezuelan equine encephalitis virus (Rosas et al., 2007a, b, 2008). Especially for possible vaccination strategies for hCMV, the detailed analysis of the animal model viruses is important. In the case of mCMV and gpCMV, such BAC-based immunization strategies have shown promising results (Cicin-Sain et al., 2003, 2007; Crumpler et al., 2009; Redwood et al., 2005). In the rhesus monkey model, the viral inhibition mechanism for secondary rhCMV infections suggests respective strategies for hCMV vaccines (Hansen et al., 2010). Such observations may lead the way to novel recombinant human vaccines, for example by replication-deficient hCMV or HSV-1 (Schleiss et al., 2006; Suter et al., 1999).

Although the highly efficient modified vaccinia virus Ankara (MVA) has already been well established as a vaccine for the application in humans, the BAC strategy shows considerable advantage for optimizing novel vaccine generations (Cottingham et al., 2008; Domi & Moss, 2002; Meissinger-Henschel et al., 2011; Roth et al., 2011), especially since MVA and related poxviruses are also useful as transgene vectors for the efficient immunization against heterologous pathogens.

5. Acknowledgements

The scientific work underlying this manuscript was supported by the Deutsche Forschungs-gemeinschaft, the Excellence Cluster Inflammation at Interfaces, the Wilhelm Sander-Stiftung, and the Varicella-Zoster Virus Research Foundation. The authors thank Dr. Karsten Tischer for fruitful collaboration.

6. References

Adler, H.; Messerle, M.; Koszinowski, U.H. (2001). Virus reconstituted from infectious bacterial artificial chromosome (BAC)-cloned murine gammaherpesvirus 68 acquires wild-type properties in vivo only after excision of BAC vector sequences. *Journal of Virology*, Vol.75, No. X, 5692-5696

Adler, H.; Messerle, M.; Koszinowski, U.H. (2003). Cloning of herpesviral genomes as bacterial artificial chromosomes. *Reviews in Medical Virology*, Vol.13, No.12, 111-121

Adler, H.; Messerle, M.; Wagner, M.; Koszinowski, U.H. (2000). Cloning and mutagenesis of the murine gammaherpesvirus 68 genome as an infectious bacterial artificial chromosome. *Journal of Virology*, Vol.74, No.15, pp. 6964-6974

Ahsan, N.; Kanda, T.; Nagashima, K.; Takada, K. (2005). Epstein-Barr virus transforming protein LMP1 plays a critical role in virus production. *Journal of Virology*, Vol.79, No.7, pp. 4415-4424

Ali, A.K.; Saito, S.; Shibata, S.; Takada, K.; Kanda, T. (2009). Distinctive effects of the Epstein-Barr virus family of repeats on viral latent gene promoter activity and B-lymphocyte transformation. *Journal of Virology*, Vol.83, No.18, pp. 9163-9174

Almazan, F.; DeDiego, M.L.; Galan, C.; Escors, D.; Alvarez, E.; Ortego, J.; Sola, I.; Zuniga, S.; Alonso, S.; Moreno, J.L.; Nogales, A.; Capiscol, C.; Enjuanes, L. (2006). Construction of a severe acute respiratory syndrome coronavirus infectious cDNA clone and a replicon to study coronavirus RNA synthesis. *Journal of Virology*, Vol.80, No.21, 10900-10906

Almazan, F.; Gonzalez, J.M.; Penzes, Z.; Izeta, A.; Calvo, E.; Plana-Duran, J.; Enjuanes, L. (2000). Engineering the largest RNA virus genome as an infectious bacterial artificial chromosome. *Proceedings of the National Academy of Sciences of the United States of America*, Vol.97, No.10, 5516-5521

Anderton, E.; Yee, J.; Smith, P.; Crook, T.; White, R. E.; Allday, M.J. (2008). Two Epstein-Barr virus (EBV) oncoproteins cooperate to repress expression of the proapoptotic tumour suppressor Bim: clues to the pathogenesis of Burkitt's lymphoma. *Oncogene*, Vol.27, No.4, pp. 421-433

Antinone, S. E.; Smith, G.A. (2006). Two modes of herpesvirus trafficking in neurons: membrane acquisition directs motion. *Journal of Virology*, Vol.80, No.22, pp. 11235-11240

Baigent, S.J.; Petherbridge, L.J.; Smith, L.P.; Zhao, Y.; Chesters, P.M.; Nair, V.K. (2006). Herpesvirus of turkey reconstituted from bacterial artificial chromosome clones induces protection against Marek's disease. *Journal of General Virology*, Vol.87, No.4, pp. 769-776

Borenstein, R.; Frenkel, N. (2009) Cloning human herpesvirus 6A genome into bacterial artificial chromosomes and study of DNA replication intermediates. *Proceedings of the National Academy of Sciences of the United States of America,* Vol.106, No.45, pp. 19138-19143

Borenstein, R.; Zeigerman, H.; Frenkel, N. (2010). The DR1 and DR6 first exons of human herpesvirus 6A are not required for virus replication in culture and are deleted in virus stocks that replicate well in T-cell lines. *Journal of Virology,* Vol.84, No.6, pp. 2648-2656

Borst, E.M.; Hahn, G.; Koszinowski, U.H.; Messerle, M. (1999) Cloning of the human cytomegalovirus (HCMV) genome as an infectious bacterial artificial chromosome in Escherichia coli: a new approach for construction of HCMV mutants. *Journal of Virology,* Vol.73, No.10, pp. 8320-8329

Boutell, C.; Sadis, S.; Everett, R.D. (2002). Herpes simplex virus type 1 immediate-early protein ICP0 and its isolated RING finger domain act as ubiquitin E3 ligases in vitro. *Journal of Virology,* Vol.76, No.2, pp. 841-850

Brazeau, E; Wellish, M; Kaufer, B.B.; Tischer, B.K; Gray, W.; Zhou, F.; Osterrieder, N.; Hanlon, T.; Golive, A.; Hall, T.; Nair, S.; Owens, G. P.; Müller, N.H.; Cohrs, R.J.; Pugazhenthi, S.; Gilden, D.; Mahalingam, R. (2011) Simian varicella virus open reading frame 63/70 expression is required for efficient virus replication in culture. *Journal of Neurovirology,* (April 2011), published electronically ahead of print

Britt, W.J. (2000). Infectious clones of herpesviruses: a new approach for understanding viral gene function. *Trends in Microbiology,* Vol.8, No.6, pp. 262-265

Britt, W.J.; Jarvis, M.; Seo, J.Y.; Drummond, D.; Nelson, J. (2004). Rapid genetic engineering of human cytomegalovirus by using a lambda phage linear recombination system: demonstration that pp28 (UL99) is essential for production of infectious virus. *Journal of Virology,* Vol.78, No.1, pp. 539-543

Brune, W.; Menard, C.; Hobom, U.; Odenbreit, S.; Messerle, M.; Koszinowski, U.H. (1999). Rapid identification of essential and nonessential herpesvirus genes by direct transposon mutagenesis. *Nature Biotechnology,* Vol.17, No.4, pp. 360-364

Brune, W.; Messerle, M.; Koszinowski, U.H. (2000). Forward with BACs - new tools for herpesvirus genomics. *Trends in Genetics,* Vol.16, No.6, pp. 254-259

Bubeck, A.; Wagner, M.; Ruzsics, Z.; Lötzerich, M.; Iglesias, M.; Singh, I.R.; Koszinowski, U.H. (2004). Comprehensive mutational analysis of a herpesvirus gene in the viral genome context reveals a region essential for virus replication. *Journal of Virology,* Vol.78, No.15, pp. 8026-8035

Calderwood, M.; White, R.E.; Griffiths, R.A.; Whitehouse, A. (2005). Open reading frame 73 is required for herpesvirus saimiri A11-S4 episomal persistence. *Journal of General Virology,* Vol.86, No.10, pp. 2703-2708

Carter, D.M.; Radding, C.M. (1971). The role of exonuclease and beta protein of phage lambda in genetic recombination. II. Substrate specificity and the mode of action of lambda exonuclease. *Journal of Biological Chemistry,* Vol.246, No.8, pp. 2502-2512

Chang, W.L.; Barry, P.A. (2003). Cloning of the full-length rhesus cytomegalovirus genome as an infectious and self-excisable bacterial artificial chromosome for analysis of viral pathogenesis. *Journal of Virology,* Vol.77, No.9, pp. 5073-5083

Chen, A.; DiVisconte, M.; Jiang, X.; Quink, C.; Wang F. (2005). Epstein-Barr virus with the latent infection nuclear antigen 3B completely deleted is still competent for B-cell growth transformation in vitro. *Journal of Virology,* Vol. 79, No. 7, pp. 4506-4509

Cicin-Sain, L.; Brune, W.; Bubic, I.; Jonjic, S.; Koszinowski, U. H. (2003). Vaccination of mice with bacteria carrying a cloned herpesvirus genome reconstituted in vivo. *Journal of Virology,* Vol. 77, No. 15, pp. 8249-8255

Cicin-Sain, L.; Bubic, I.; Schnee, M.; Ruzsics, Z.M.; Mohr, C.; Jonjic, S.; Koszinowski, U.H. (2007). Targeted deletion of regions rich in immune-evasive genes from the cytomegalovirus genome as a novel vaccine strategy. *Journal of Virology,* Vol.81, No.24, pp. 13825-13834

Cohen, J.I.; Seidel, K.E. (1993). Generation of varicella-zoster virus (VZV) and viral mutants from cosmid DNAs: VZV thymidylate synthetase is not essential for replication in vitro. *Proceedings of the National Academy of Sciences of the United States of America,* Vol.90, No.15, pp. 7376-7380

Copeland, N.G.; Jenkins, N.A.; Court, D.L. (2001). Recombineering: a powerful new tool for mouse functional genomics. *Nature Reviews Genetics* Vol.2, No.10, 769-779

Costes, B.; Fournier, G.; Michel B.; Delforge, C.; Raj, V.S.; Dewals, B.; Gillet, L.; Drion, P.; Body, A.; Schynts, F.; Lieffrig, F.; Vanderplasschen, A. (2008). Cloning of the koi herpesvirus genome as an infectious bacterial artificial chromosome demonstrates that disruption of the thymidine kinase locus induces partial attenuation in Cyprinus carpio koi. *Journal of Virology,* Vol.82, No.10, pp. 4955-4964

Costes, B.; Thirion, M.; Dewals B.; Mast, J.; Ackermann, M.; Markine-Goriaynoff, N.; Gillet, L.; Vanderplasschen, A. (2006). Felid herpesvirus 1 glycoprotein G is a structural protein that mediates the binding of chemokines on the viral envelope. *Microbes and Infection,* Vol.8, No.11, pp. 2657-2667

Costes, B.; Raj, V. S.; Michel, B.; Fournier, G.; Thirion, M.; Gillet, L.; Mast, J.; Lieffrig, F.; Bremont, M.; Vanderplasschen, A. (2009). The major portal of entry of koi herpesvirus in cyprinus carpio is the skin. *Journal of Virology,* Vol.83, No.7, pp. 2819-2830

Cottingham, M.G.; Andersen, R.F.; Spencer, A.J.; Saurya, S.; Furze, J.; Hill, A.V.; Gilbert, S.C. (2008). Recombination-mediated genetic engineering of a bacterial artificial chromosome clone of modified vaccinia virus Ankara (MVA). PLoS One Vol.3, No.2, e1638

Court, D.L.; Sawitzke, J.A.; Thomason, L.A. (2002) Genetic engineering using homologous recombination. *Annual Reviews in Genetics,* Vol.35, pp. 361-388.

Crumpler, M.M.; Choi, K.Y.; McVoy, M.A.; Schleiss, M.R. (2009). A live guinea pig cytomegalovirus vaccine deleted of three putative immune evasion genes is highly atenuated but remains immunogenic in a vaccine/challenge model of congenital cytomegalovirus infection. *Vaccine,* Vol.27, No.31, pp. 4209-4218

Cunningham, C.; Davison, A. J. (1993). A cosmid-based system for constructing mutants of herpes simplex virus type 1. *Virology,* Vol. 197, No. 1, pp. 116-124

Delecluse, H.J.; Hilsendegen, T.; Pich, D.; Zeidler, R.; Hammerschmidt, W. (1998) Propagation and recovery of intact, infectious Epstein-Barr virus from prokaryotic to human cells. *Proceedings of the National Academy of Sciences of the United States of America,* Vol.95, No.14, pp. 8245-8250

Delecluse, H.J.; Kost, M.; Feederle, R.; Wilson, L.; Hammerschmidt, W. (2001). Spontaneous activation of the lytic cycle in cells infected with a recombinant Kaposi's sarcoma-associated virus. *Journal of Virology,* Vol.75, No.6, pp. 2921-2928

Dolan, A.; Cunningham, C.; Hector, R.D.; Hassan-Walker, A.F.; Lee, L.; Addison, C.; Dargan, D.J.; McGeoch, D.J.; Gatherer, D.; Emery, V.C.; Griffiths, P.D.; Sinzger, C.;

McSharry, B.P.; Wilkinson, G.W.; Davison,A.J. (2004). Genetic content of wild-type human cytomegalovirus. *Journal of General Virology,* Vol.85, No.5, pp. 1301-1312

Domi, A.; Moss, B. (2002). Cloning the vaccinia virus genome as a bacterial artificial chromosome in Escherichia coli and recovery of infectious virus in mammalian cells. *Proceedings of the National Academy of Sciences of the United States of America,* Vol.99, No.19, pp. 12415-12420

Donaldson, E.F.; Yount, B.; Sims, A.C.; Burkett, S.; Pickles, R.J.; Baric, R.S. (2008) Systematic assembly of a full-length infectious clone of human coronavirus NL63. Journal of Virology, Vol.82, No.23, pp. 11948-11957

Dulal, K.; Zhang, Z.; Zhu, H. (2009) Development of a gene capture method to rescue a large deletion mutant of human cytomegalovirus. *Journal of Virological Methods,* Vol.157, No.2, pp. 180-187

Dunn, W.; Chou, C.; Li, H.; Hai, R.; Patterson, D.; Stolc, V.; Zhu, H.; Liu, F. (2003). Functional profiling of a human cytomegalovirus genome. *Proceedings of the National Academy of Sciences of the United States of America,* Vol.100, No.2, pp. 14223-14228

Estep, R.D.; Powers, M.F.; Yen, B.K.; Li, H.; Wong, S.W. (2007). Construction of an infectious rhesus rhadinovirus bacterial artificial chromosome for the analysis of Kaposi's sarcoma-associated herpesvirus-related disease development. *Journal of Virology,* Vol.81, No.6, pp. 2957-2969

Fan, X.Z.; Li, X.; Zhou, F.; Gao, S.J.; Yuan, Y. (2006). Functional characterization of Kaposi's sarcoma-associated herpesvirus ORF45 by bacterial artificial chromosome-based mutagenesis. *Journal of Virology,* Vol.80, No.24, pp. 12187-12196

Feederle, R.; Bartlett, E.J.; Delecluse, H.J. (2010). Epstein-Barr virus genetics: talking about the BAC generation. *Herpesviridae,* Vol.1, No.1, 6.

Fuchs, W.; Klupp, B.G.; Granzow, H.; Leege, T.; Mettenleiter, T.C. (2009). Characterization of pseudorabies virus (PrV) cleavage-encapsidation proteins and functional complementation of PrV pUL32 by the homologous protein of herpes simplex virus type 1. *Journal of Virology,* Vol.83, No.8, pp. 3930-3943

Gabev, E.; Fraefel, C.; Ackermann, M.; Tobler, K. (2009). Cloning of bovine herpesvirus type 1 and type 5 as infectious bacterial artifical chromosomes. *BMC Research Notes,* Vol. 2, No. 209

Glass, M.; Busche, A.; Wagner, K.; Messerle, M.; Borst, E. M. (2009). Conditional and reversible disruption of essential herpesvirus proteins. *Nature Methods,* Vol. 6, No. 8, pp. 577-579

Goodman, L.B.; Loregian, A.; Perkins, G.A.; Nugent, J.; Buckles, E.L.; Mercorelli, B.; Kydd, J.H.; Palu, G.; Smith, K.C.; Osterrieder, N.; Davis-Poynter, N. (2007). A point mutation in a herpesvirus polymerase determines neuropathogenicity. *PLoS Pathogens,* Vol.3, No.11, pp. 1583-1592

Gray, W.L.; Zhou, F.; Noffke, J.; Tischer, K.B. (2011) Cloning the simian varicella virus genome in E. coli as an infectious bacterial artificial chromosome. *Archives of Virology,* (April 2011), published electronically ahead of print.

Hahn, G.; Khan, H.; Baldanti, F.; Koszinowski, U.H.; Revello, M.G.; Gerna, G. (2002) The human cytomegalovirus ribonucleotide reductase homolog UL45 is dispensable for growth in endothelial cells, as determined by a BAC-cloned clinical isolate of human cytomegalovirus with preserved wild-type characteristics. *Journal of Virology,* Vol.76, No.18, pp. 9551-9555

Hahn, G.; Rose, D.; Wagner, M.; Rhiel, S.; McVoy, M.A. (2003). Cloning of the genomes of human cytomegalovirus strains Toledo, Towne varRIT3, and Towne long as BACs and site-directed mutagenesis using a PCR-based technique. *Virology,* Vol.307, No.1, pp. 164-177

Hansen, K.; Napier, I.; Koen, M.; Bradford, S.; Messerle, M.; Bell, E.; Seshadri, L.; Stokes, H.W.; Birch, D.; Whalley, J.M. (2006). In vitro transposon mutagenesis of an equine herpesvirus 1 genome cloned as a bacterial artificial chromosome. *Archives of Virology,* Vol.151, No.12, pp. 2389-2405

Hansen, S.G.; Powers, C.J.; Richards, R.; Ventura,A.B.; Ford, J.C.; Siess, D.; Axthelm, M.K.; Nelson, J.A.; Jarvis, M.A.; Picker, L.J.; Früh, K. (2010). Evasion of CD8+ T cells is critical for superinfection by cytomegalovirus. *Science,* Vol.328, No.5974, pp. 102-106

Hettich, E.; Janz, A.; Zeidler, R.; Pich, D.; Hellebrand, E.; Weissflog, B.; Moosmann, A.; Hammerschmidt, W. (2006). Genetic design of an optimized packaging cell line for gene vectors transducing human B cells. *Gene Therapy,* Vol.13, No.10, pp. 844-856

Hobom, U.; Brune, W.; Messerle, M.; Hahn, G.; Koszinowski, U.H. (2000). Fast screening procedures for random transposon libraries of cloned herpesvirus genomes: mutational analysis of human cytomegalovirus envelope glycoprotein genes. *Journal of Virology,* Vol.74, No.17, pp. 7720-7729

Horsburgh, B.C.; Hubinette, M.M.; Qiang, D.; MacDonald, M.L.; Tufaro, F. (1999a). Allele replacement: an application that permits rapid manipulation of herpes simplex virus type 1 genomes. *Gene Therapy,* Vol.6, No.5, pp. 922-930

Horsburgh, B.C.; Hubinette, M.M.; Tufaro, F. (1999b). Genetic manipulation of herpes simplex virus using bacterial artificial chromosomes. *Methods of Enzymology,* Vol.306, pp. 337-352

Ioannou, P.A.; Amemiya, C.T.; Garnes, J.; Kroisel, P.M.; Shizuya, H.; Chen, C.; Batzer, M.A.; de Jong, P.J. (1994). A new bacteriophage P1-derived vector for the propagation of large human DNA fragments. *Nature Genetics,* Vol.6, No.1, pp. 84-89

Jamsai, D.; Orford, M.; Nefedov, M.; Fucharoen, S.; Williamson, R.; Ioannou, P.A. (2003). Targeted modification of a human beta-globin locus BAC clone using GET recombination and an I-SceI counterselection cassette. *Genomics,* Vol. 82, No.1, pp. 68-77

Kanda, T.; Yajima, M.; Ahsan, N.; Tanaka, M.; Takada K. (2004). Production of high-titer Epstein-Barr virus recombinants derived from Akata cells by using a bacterial artificial chromosome system. *Journal of Virology,* Vol.78, No.13, pp. 7004-7015

Karu, A.E.; Sakaki, Y.; Echols, H.; Linn, S. (1975). The gamma protein specified by bacteriophage gamma. Structure and inhibitory activity for the recBC enzyme of Escherichia coli. *Journal of Biological Chemistry,* Vol.250, No.18, pp. 7377-7387

Kemble, G.; Duke, G.; Winter, R.; Spaete, R. (1996). Defined large-scale alteration of the human cytomegalovirus genome constructed by cotransfection of overlapping cosmids. *Journal of Virology,* Vol.70, No.3, pp. 2044-2048

Kim, U.J.; Shizuya, H.; de Jong, P.J.; Birren, B.; Simon, M.I. (1992). Stable propagation of cosmid sized human DNA inserts in an F factor based vector. *Nucleic Acids Research,* Vol.20, No.5, pp. 1083-1085

Kmiec, E.; Holloman, W.K. (1981). Beta protein of bacteriophage lambda promotes renaturation of DNA. *Journal of Biological Chemistry,* Vol.256, No.24, pp. 12636-12639

Kopp, M.; Granzow, H.; Fuchs, W.; Klupp, B.; Mettenleiter T.C. (2004). Simultaneous deletion of pseudorabies virus tegument protein UL11 and glycoprotein M severely impairs secondary envelopment. *Journal of Virology,* Vol.78, No.6, pp. 3024-3034

Kuroda, T.; Martuza, R.L.; Todo, T.; Rabkin, S.D. (2006). Flipflop HSV-BAC: bacterial artificial chromosome based system for rapid generation of recombinant herpes simplex virus vectors using two independent site-specific recombinases. *BMC Biotechnology,* Vol.6, article No.40

Lee, E.C.; Yu, D.; Martinez, D.V.; Tessarollo, L.; Swing, D.A.; Court, D.L.; Jenkins, N.A.; Copeland, N.G. (2001). A highly efficient Escherichia coli-based chromosome engineering system adapted for recombinogenic targeting and subcloning of BAC DNA. *Genomics,* Vol.73, No.1, pp. 56-65

Leege, T.; Fuchs, W.; Granzow, H.; Kopp, M.; Klupp, B.G.; Mettenleiter, T.C. (2009). Effects of simultaneous deletion of pUL11 and glycoprotein M on virion maturation of herpes simplex virus type 1. *Journal of Virology,* Vol.83, No.2, pp. 896-907

Lilja, A.E.; Chang, W.L.; Barry, P.A.; Becerra, S.P.; Shenk, T.E. (2008). Functional genetic analysis of rhesus cytomegalovirus: Rh01 is an epithelial cell tropism factor. *Journal of Virology,* Vol.82, No.5, pp. 2170-2181

Little, J.W. (1967). An exonuclease induced by bacteriophage lambda. II. Nature of the enzymatic reaction. *Journal of Biological Chemistry,* Vol.242, No.4, pp. 679-686

Lu, F.; Stedman, W.; Yousef, M.; Renne, R.; Lieberman, P.M. (2010). Epigenetic regulation of Kaposi's sarcoma-associated herpesvirus latency by virus-encoded microRNAs that target Rta and the cellular Rbl2-DNMT pathway. *Journal of Virology,* Vol.84, No.6, pp. 2697-2706

Lukac, D.M.; Garibyan, L.; Kirshner, J.R.; Palmeri, D.; Ganem, D. (2001). DNA binding by Kaposi's sarcoma-associated herpesvirus lytic switch protein is necessary for transcriptional activation of two viral delayed early promoters. *Journal of Virology,* Vol.75, No.15, pp. 6786-6799

Luna, R. E.; Zhou, F.; Baghian, A.; Chouljenko, V.; Forghani, B.; Gao, S.J.; Kousoulas, K.G. (2004). Kaposi's sarcoma-associated herpesvirus glycoprotein K8.1 is dispensable for virus entry. *Journal of Virology,* Vol.78, No.12, pp. 6389-6398

Mahony, T.J.; McCarthy, F.M.; Gravel, J.L.; West, L.; Young, P.L. (2002). Construction and manipulation of an infectious clone of the bovine herpesvirus 1 genome maintained as a bacterial artificial chromosome. *Journal of Virology,* Vol.76, No.13, pp. 6660-6668

Majerciak, V.; Pripuzova, N.; McCoy, J.P.; Gao, S.J.; Zheng, Z.M. (2007). Targeted disruption of Kaposi's sarcoma-associated herpesvirus ORF57 in the viral genome is detrimenal for the expression of ORF59, K8α, and K8.1 and the production of infectious virus. *Journal of Virology,* Vol.81, No.3, pp. 1062-1071

Manning, W.C.; Mocarski, E.S. (1988). Insertional mutagenesis of the murine cytomegalovirus genome: one prominent alpha gene (ie2) is dispensable for growth. *Virology,* Vol.167, No.2, 477-484.

Marchini, A.; Liu, H.; Zhu, H. (2001) Human cytomegalovirus with IE-2 (UL122) deleted fails to express early lytic genes. *Journal of Virology,* Vol.75, No.4, pp. 1870-1878

Marconi, P.; Argnani, R.; Epstein, A.L.; Manservigi, R. (2009). HSV as a vector in vaccine development and gene therapy. *Advances in Experimental Medicine and Biology,* Vol. 655, pp. 118-144

McGregor, A.; Schleiss, M.R. (2001a). Molecular cloning of the guinea pig cytomegalovirus (GPCMV) genome as an infectious bacterial artificial chromosome (BAC) in Escherichia coli. *Molecular Genetics and Metabolism,* Vol.72, No.1, pp. 15-26

McGregor, A.; Schleiss M.R. (2001b). Recent advances in herpesvirus genetics using bacterial artificial chromosomes. *Molecular Genetics and Metabolism,* Vol.72, No.1, pp. 8-14

Meisinger-Henschel, C.; Späth, M.; Lukassen, S.; Wolferstätter, M.; Kachelriess, H.; Baur, K.; Dirmeier, U.; Wagner, M.; Chaplin, P.; Suter, M.; Hausmann, J. (2011) Introduction of the six major genomic deletions of modified vaccinia virus Ankara (MVA) into the parental vaccinia virus is not sufficient to reproduce an MVA-like phenotype in cell culture and in mice. Journal of Virology, Vol.84, No.19, pp. 9907-9919

Menard, C.; Wagner, M.; Ruzsics, Z.; Holak, K.; Brune, W.; Campbell, A.E.; Koszinowski, U.H. (2003). Role of murine cytomegalovirus US22 gene family members in replication in macrophages. *Journal of Virology,* Vol.77, No.10, pp. 5557-5570

Meseda, C.A.; Schmeisser, F.; Pedersen, R.; Woerner, A.; Weir, J.P. (2004). DNA immunization with a herpes simplex virus 2 bacterial artificial chromosome. *Virology,* Vol.318, No.1, pp. 420-428

Messerle, M.; Crnkovic, I.; Hammerschmidt, W.; Ziegler, H.; Koszinowski, U.H. (1997). Cloning and mutagenesis of a herpesvirus genome as an infectious bacterial artificial chromosome. *Proceedings of the National Academy of Sciences of the United States of America,* Vol.94, No.26, pp. 14759-14763

Mocarski, E.S.; Post, L.E.; Roizman, B. (1980). Molecular engineering of thc hcrpes simplex virus genome: insertion of a second L-S junction into the genome causes additional genome inversions. *Cell,* Vol.22, No.1, pp. 243-255

Muniyappa, K.; Radding, C.M. (1986). The homologous recombination system of phage lambda. Pairing activities of beta protein. *Journal of Biological Chemistry,* Vol.261, No.16, pp. 7472-7478

Murphy, E.; Yu, D.; Grimwood, J.; Schmutz, J.; Dickson, M.; Jarvis, M.A.; Hahn, G.; Nelson, J.A.; Myers, R.M.; Shenk, T.E. (2003) Coding potential of laboratory and clinical strains of human cytomegalovirus. *Proceedings of the National Academy of Sciences of the United States of America,* Vol.100, No.25, pp. 14976-14981

Murphy, K.C. (1991). Lambda Gam protein inhibits the helicase and chi-stimulated recombination activities of Escherichia coli RecBCD enzyme. *Journal of Bacteriology,* Vol.173, No.18, pp. 5808-5821

Murphy, K.C. (1998). Use of bacteriophage lambda recombination functions to promote gene replacement in Escherichia coli. *Journal of Bacteriology,* Vol.180, No.8, pp. 2063-2071

Murphy, K.C. (2007). The lambda Gam protein inhibits RecBCD binding to dsDNA ends. *Journal of Molecular Biology,* Vol.371, No.1, pp. 19-24

Muyrers, J.P.; Zhang, Y.; Benes, V.; Testa, G.; Rientjes, J.M.; Stewart, A.F. (2004). ET recombination: DNA engineering using homologous recombination in E. coli. *Methods in Molecular Biology,* Vol.256, pp. 107-121

Muyrers, J.P.; Zhang, Y.; Stewart, A.F. (2001). Techniques: Recombinogenic engineering - new options for cloning and manipulating DNA. *Trends in Biochemical Sciences,* Vol.26, No.5, pp. 325-331

Muyrers, J. P.; Zhang, Y.; Testa, G.; Stewart, A. F. (1999). Rapid modification of bacterial artificial chromosomes by ET-recombination. *Nucleic Acids Research,* Vol.27, No.6, 1555-1557

Nagaike, K.; Mori, Y.; Gomi, Y.; Yoshii, H.; Takahashi, M.; Wagner, M.; Koszinowski, U.; Yamanishi, K. (2004). Cloning of the varicella zoster virus genome as an infectious bacterial artificial chromosome in Escherichia coli. *Vaccine,* Vol.22, No.29-30, pp. 4069-4074

Nagel, C.H.; Döhner, K.; Fathollahy,M.; Strive, T.; Borst, E.M.; Messerle, M.; Sodeik, B. (2008) Nuclear egress and envelopment of herpes simplex virus capsids analyzed with dual-color fluorescence HSV1(17+). Journal of Virology, Vol.82, No.6, pp. 3109-3124

Narayanan, K.; Williamson, R.; Zhang, Y.; Stewart, A.F.; Ioannou, P.A. (1999). Efficient and precise engineering of a 200 kb beta-globin human/bacterial artificial chromosome in E. coli DH10B using an inducible homologous recombination system. *Gene Therapy,* Vol.6, No.3, pp. 442-447.

O'Hara, M.; Rixon, F.J.; Stow, N.D.; Murray, J.; Murphy, M.; Preston, V.G. (2010). Mutational analysis of the herpes simplex virus type 1 UL25 DNA packaging protein reveals regions that are important after the viral DNA has been packaged. *Journal of Virology,* Vol.84, No.9, pp. 4252-4263

Oppenheim, A.B.; Rattray, A.J.; Bubunenko, M.; Thomason, L.C.; Court, D.L. (2004). In vivo recombineering of bacteriophage lambda by PCR fragments and single-strand oligonucleotides. *Virology,* Vol.319, No.2, pp. 185-189

Pavlova, I.V.; Virgin IV, H.W.; Speck, S.H. (2003). Disruption of gammaherpesvirus 68 gene 50 demonstrates that Rta is essential for virus replication. *Journal of Virology,* Vol.77, No.10, pp. 5731-5739

Petherbridge, L.; Howes, K.; Baigent, S. J.; Sacco, M.A.; Evans, S.; Osterrieder, N.; Nair, V. (2003). Replication-competent bacterial artificial chromosomes of Marek's disease virus: novel tools for generation of molecularly defined herpesvirus vaccines. *Journal of Virology,* Vol.77, No.16, pp. 8712-8718

Post, L.E.; Roizman, B. (1981). A generalized technique for deletion of specific genes in large genomes: alpha gene 22 of herpes simplex virus 1 is not essential for growth. *Cell,* Vol.25, No.1, pp. 227-232

Ramsay, M. (1994). Yeast artificial chromosome cloning. Molecular Biotechnology, Vol.1, No.2, pp. 181-201.

Redwood, A.J.; Messerle, M.; Harvey, N.L.; Hardy, C.M.; Koszinowski, U.H.; Lawson, M.A.; Shellam, G.R. (2005). Use of a murine cytomegalovirus K181-derived bacterial artificial chromosome as a vaccine vector for immunocontraception. *Journal of Virology,* Vol.79, No.5, pp. 2998-3008

Richter, M.; Schudel, L.; Tobler, K.; Matheis, F.; Vögtlin, A.; Vanderplasschen, A.; Costes, B.; Spiess, B.; Ackermann, M. (2009). Clinical, virological, and immunological parameters associated with superinfection of latently with FeHV-1 infected cats. *Veterinary Microbiology,* Vol.138, No.3-4, pp. 205-216

Roberts, A.P.; Abaitua, F.; O'Hare, P.; McNab, D.; Rixon, F.J.; Pasdeloup, D. (2009). Differing roles of inner tegument proteins pUL36 and pUL37 during entry of herpes simplex virus type. *Journal of Virology,* Vol.83, No.1, pp. 105-116

Robinson, K.E.; Meers, J.; Gravel, J.L.; McCarthy, F.M.; Mahony, T.J. (2008). The essential and non-essential genes of bovine herpesvirus 1. *Journal of General Virology,* Vol.89, No.11, pp. 2851-2863

Rosas, C.T.; König, P.; Beer, M.; Dubovi, E.J.; Tischer, B.K.; Osterrieder, N. (2007a). Evaluation of the vaccine potential of an equine herpesvirus type 1 vector expressing bovine viral diarrhea virus structural proteins. *Journal of General Virology,* Vol.88, No.3, pp. 748-757

Rosas, C.T.; Paessler, S.; Ni, H.; Osterrieder, N. (2008). Protection of mice by equine herpesvirus type 1-based experimental vaccine against lethal Venezuelan equine encephalitis virus infection in the absence of neutralizing antibodies. *American Journal of Tropical Medicine and Hygiene,* Vol.78, No.1, pp. 83-92

Rosas, C.T.; Tischer, B.K.; Perkins, G.A.; Wagner, B.; Goodman, L.B.; Osterrieder, N. (2007b). Live-attenuated recombinant equine herpesvirus type 1 (EHV-1) induces a neutralizing antibody response against West Nile virus (WNV). *Virus Research,* Vol.125, No.1, pp. 69-78

Roth, S.J.; Höper, D.; Beer, M.; Feineis, S.; Tischer, B.K.; Osterrieder, N. (2011) Recovery of infectious virus from full-length cowpox virus (CPXV) DNA cloned as a bacterial artificial chromosome (BAC). *Veterinary Research,* Vol.42, No.1, 3

Rudolph, J.; O'Callaghan, D.; Osterrieder, N. (2002). Cloning of the genomes of equine herpesvirus type 1 (EHV-1) strains KyA and racL11 as bacterial artificial chromosomes (BAC). *Journal of Veterinary Medicine B,* Vol.49, No.1, pp. 31-36

Rudolph, J.; Osterrieder, N. (2002). Equine herpesvirus type 1 devoid of gM and gp2 is severely impaired in virus egress but not direct cell-to-cell spread. *Virology,* Vol.293, No.2, pp. 356-367

Rue, C. A.; Jarvis, M. A.; Knoche, A. J.; Meyers, H.L.; DeFilippis, V.R.; Hansen, S.G.; Wagner, M.; Früh, K.; Anders, D.G.; Wong, S.W.; Barry, P.A.; Nelson, J.A. (2004). A cyclooxygenase-2 homologue encoded by rhesus cytomegalovirus is a determinant for endothelial cell tropism. *Journal of Virology,* Vol.78, No.22, pp. 12529-12536

Saeki, Y.; Ichikawa, T.; Saeki, A.; Chiocca, E.A.; Tobler, K.; Ackermann, M.; Breakefield, X.O.; Fraefel, C. (1998). Herpes simplex virus type 1 DNA amplified as bacterial artificial chromosome in Escherichia coli: rescue of replication-competent virus progeny and packaging of amplicon vectors. *Human Gene Therapy,* Vol.9, No.18, pp. 2787-2794

Sawitzke, J.A.; Thomason, L.C.; Costantino, N.; Bubunenko, M.; Datta, S.; Court, D.L. (2007). Recombineering: in vivo genetic engineering in E. coli, S. enterica, and beyond. *Methods in Enzymology,* Vol.421, pp. 171-199

Schaffer, P.A. (1975). Temperature-sensitive mutants of herpesviruses. *Current Topics in Microbiology and Immunology,* Vol.70, pp. 51-100

Schalkwyk, L.C.; Francis, F.; Lehrach, H. (1995). Techniques in mammalian genome mapping. *Current Opinion in Biotechnology,* Vol.6, No.1, pp. 37-43

Schleiss, M.R. (2008). Comparison of vaccine strategies against congenital CMV infection in the guinea pig model. *Journal of Clinical Virology,* Vol.41, No.3, pp. 224-230

Schleiss, M.R.; Stroup, G.; Pogorzelski, K.; McGregor, A. (2006). Protection against congenital cytomegalovirus (CMV) disease, conferred by a replication-disabled, bacterial artificial chromosome (BAC)-based DNA vaccine. *Vaccine,* Vol.24, No.37–39, pp. 6175-6186

Schnee, M.; Ruzsics, Z.; Bubeck, A.; Koszinowski, U.H. (2006). Common and specific properties of herpesvirus UL34/UL31 protein family members revealed by protein complementation assay. *Journal of Virology,* Vol.80, No.23, pp. 11658-11666

Schumacher, D.; Tischer, B. K.; Fuchs, W.; Osterrieder, N. (2000). Reconstitution of Marek's disease virus serotype 1 (MDV-1) from DNA cloned as a bacterial artificial chromosome and characterization of a glycoprotein B-negative MDV-1 mutant. *Journal of Virology,* Vol.74, No.23, pp. 11088-11098

Sharan, S.K.; Thomason, L.C.; Kuznetsov, S.G.; Court, D.L. (2009). Recombineering: a homologous recombination-based method of genetic engineering. *Nature Protocols,* Vol.4, pp. 206-223.

Shizuya, H.; Birren, B.; Kim, U.J.; Mancino, V.; Slepak, T.; Tachiiri, Y.; Simon, M. (1992). Cloning and stable maintenance of 300-kilobase-pair fragments of human DNA in Escherichia coli using an F-factor-based vector. *Proceedings of the National Academy of Sciences of the United States of America,* Vol.89, No.18, pp. 8794-8797

Sinzger, C.; Hahn, G.; Digel, M.; Katona, R.; Sampaio, K.L.; Messerle, M.; Hengel, H.; Koszinowski, U.; Brune, W.; Adler, B. (2008) Cloning and sequencing of a highly productive, endotheliotropic virus strain derived from human cytomegalovirus TB40/E. *Journal of General Virology,* Vol.89, No.2, pp. 359-368

Smiley, J.R. (1980). Construction in vitro and rescue of a thymidine kinase-deficient deletion mutation of herpes simplex virus. *Nature,* Vol. 285, No.5763, pp. 333-335

Smith, G.A.; Enquist, L.W. (1999). Construction and transposon mutagenesis in Escherichia coli of a full-length infectious clone of pseudorabies virus, an alphaherpesvirus. *Journal of Virology,* Vol.73, No.8, pp. 6405-6414

Smith, G.A.; Enquist, L.W. (2000). A self-recombining bacterial artificial chromosome and its application for analysis of herpesvirus pathogenesis. *Proceedings of the National Academy of Sciences of the United States of America,* Vol.97, No.9, pp. 4873-4878

Song, M.J.; Hwang, S.; Wong, W.H.; Wu, T.T.; Lee, S.; Liao, H.I.; Sun, R. (2005). Identification of viral genes essential for replication of murine γ-herpesvirus 68 using signature-tagged mutagenesis. *Proceedings of the National Academy of Sciences of the United States of America,* Vol.102, No.10, pp. 3805-3810

Spaderna, S.; Kropff, B.; Ködel, Y.; Shen, S.; Coley, S.; Lu, S.; Britt, W.; Mach, M. (2005). Deletion of gpUL132, a structural component of human cytomegalovirus, results in impaired virus replication in fibroblasts. *Journal of Virology,* Vol.79, No.18, pp. 11837-11847

Spaete, R.R.; Mocarski, E.S. (1987). Insertion and deletion mutagenesis of the human cytomegalovirus genome. *Proceedings of the National Academy of Sciences of the United States of America,* Vol. 84, No.20, pp. 7213-7217

Sparwasser, T.; Eberl, G. (2007). BAC to immunology - bacterial artificial chromosome-mediated transgenesis for targeting of immune cells. *Immunology,* Vol.121, No.3, pp. 308-313

Stavropoulos, T.A.; Strathdee, C.A. (1998). An enhanced packaging system for helper-dependent herpes simplex virus vectors. *Journal of Virology,* Vol.72, No.9, pp. 7137-7143

St. Jean, J.R.; Desforges, M.; Almazan, F.; Jacomy, H.; Enjuanes, L.; Talbot, P.J. (2006) Recovery of a neurovirulent human coronavirus OC43 from an infectious cDNA clone. *Journal of Virology,* Vol.80, No.7, pp. 3670-3674

Strive, T.; Hardy, C.M.; French, N.; Wright, J.D.; Nagaraja, N.; Reubel, G.H. (2006). Development of canine herpesvirus based antifertility vaccines for foxes using bacterial artificial chromosomes. *Vaccine,* Vol. 24, No.7, pp. 980-988

Strive, T.; Hardy, C.M.; Wright, J.; Reubel, G.H. (2007). A virus vector based on canine herpesvirus for vaccine applications in canids. *Veterinary Microbiology,* Vol. 119, No.2-4, pp. 173-183

Suter, M.; Lew, A.M.; Grob, P.; Adema, G.J.; Ackermann, M.; Shortman, K.; Fraefel, C. (1999). BAC-VAC, a novel generation of (DNA) vaccines: a bacterial artificial chromosome (BAC) containing a replication-competent, packaging-defective virus genome induces protective immunity against herpes simplex virus 1. *Proceedings of the National Academy of Sciences of the United States of America,* Vol.96, No.22, pp. 12697-12702

Tai, S.H.; Niikura, M.; Cheng, H.H.; Kruger, J.M.; Wise, A.G.; Maes, R.K. (2010). Complete genomic sequence and an infectious BAC clone of feline herpesvirus-1 (FHV-1). *Virology,* Vol.401, No.2, pp. 215-227

Tanaka, M.; Kagawa, H.; Yamanashi, Y.; Sata, T.; Kawaguchi, Y. (2003). Construction of an excisable bacterial artificial chromosome containing a full-length infectious clone of herpes simplex virus type 1: viruses reconstituted from the clone exhibit wild-type properties in vitro and in vivo. *Journal of Virology,* Vol.77, No.2, 1382-1391.

Terada, K.; Wakimoto, H.; Tyminski, E.; Chiocca, E.A.; Saeki, Y. (2006). Development of a rapid method to generate multiple oncolytic HSV vectors and their in vivo evaluation using syngeneic mouse tumor models. *Gene Therapy,* Vol.13, No.8, pp. 705-714

Thomason, L.; Court, D.L.; Bubunenko, M.; Costantino, N.; Wilson, H.; Datta, S.; Oppenheim, A. (2007). Recombineering: genetic engineering in bacteria using homologous recombination. *Current Protocols in Molecular Biology,* Chapter 1, Unit 1.16.

Tischer, B.K.; Kaufer, B.B.; Sommer, M.; Wussow, F.; Arvin, A.M.; Osterrieder, N. (2007). A self-excisable infectious bacterial artificial chromosome clone of varicella-zoster virus allows analysis of the essential tegument protein encoded by ORF9. *Journal of Virology,* Vol.81, No.23, 13200-13208

Tischer, B.K.; Smith, G.; Osterrieder, N. (2010a). En passant Mutagenesis - A two step markerless Red recombination system. In: Braman, J., In Vitro Mutagenesis Protocols. Humana Press Inc., Tatowa, pp. 221-230.

Tischer, B.K.; Smith, G.A.; Osterrieder, N. (2010b). En passant mutagenesis: a two step markerless red recombination system. *Methods in Molecular Biology,* Vol.634, pp. 421-430

Tischer, B.K.; von Einem, J.; Kaufer, B.; Osterrieder, N. (2006). Two-step red-mediated recombination for versatile high-efficiency markerless DNA manipulation in Escherichia coli. *BioTechniques,* Vol.40, No.2, pp. 191-197

Tomkinson, B.; Robertson, E.; Yalamanchili, R.; Longnecker, R.; Kieff, E. (1993). Epstein-Barr virus recombinants from overlapping cosmid fragments. *Journal of Virology,* Vol.67, No.12, pp. 7298-7306

Tong, L.; Stow, N.D. (2010). Analysis of herpes simplex virus type 1 DNA packaging signal mutations in the context of the viral genome. *Journal of Virology,* Vol.84, No.1, pp. 321-329

Toptan, T; Ensser, A.; Fickenscher, H. (2010) Rhadinovirus vector-derived human telomerase reverse transcriptase expression in primary T cells. *Gene Therapy,* Vol.17, No.5, pp. 653-661

Trapp, S.; Osterrieder, N.; Keil, G.M.; Beer, M. (2003). Mutagenesis of a bovine herpesvirus type 1 genome cloned as an infectious bacterial artificial chromosome: analysis of glycoprotein E and G double deletion mutants. *Journal of General Virology,* Vol.84, No.2, pp. 301-306 van Zijl, M.; Quint, W.; Briaire, J.; de Rover, T.; Gielkens, A.; Berns, A. (1988). Regeneration of herpesviruses from molecularly cloned subgenomic fragments. *Journal of Virology*, Vol.62, No.6, 2191-2195

Wagner, M.; Jonjic, S.; Koszinowski, U.H.; Messerle, M. (1999). Systematic excision of vector sequences from the BAC-cloned herpesvirus genome during virus reconstitution. *Journal of Virology*, Vol.73, No.8, pp. 7056-7060

Wagner, M.; Koszinowski, U.H. (2004). Mutagenesis of viral BACs with linear PCR fragments (ET recombination). *Methods in Molecular Biology*, Vol.256, pp. 257-268

Wagner, M.; Ruzsics, Z.; Koszinowski, U.H. (2002). Herpesvirus genetics has come of age. *Trends in Microbiology*, Vol.10, No.7, pp. 318-324

Warden, C.; Tang, Q.; Zhu, H. (2011) Herpesvirus BACs: Past, present, and future. *Journal of Biomedicine and Biotechnology* Vol. 2011, Article ID 124595

Warming, S.; Costantino, N.; Court, D.L.; Jenkins, N.A.; Copeland, N.G. (2005). Simple and highly efficient BAC recombineering using galK selection. *Nucleic Acids Research*, Vol.33, No.4, article No.e36

White, R.E.; Calderwood, M.A.; Whitehouse, A. (2003). Generation and precise modification of a herpesvirus saimiri bacterial artificial chromosome demonstrates that the terminal repeats are required for both virus production and episomal persistence. *Journal of General Virology*, Vol.84, No.12, pp. 3393-3403

White, R.E.; Carline, L.; Allday, M.J. (2007). Mutagenesis of the herpesvirus saimiri terminal repeat region reveals important elements for virus production. *Journal of Virology*, Vol.81, No.12, pp. 6765-6770

Wussow, F.; Fickenscher, H.; Tischer, B.K. (2009). Red-mediated transposition and final reease of the mini-F vector of a cloned infectious herpesvirus genome. PLoS ONE, Vol.4, No.12, pp. 1-9, e8178

Xu, Y.; AuCoin, D.P.; Rodriguez Huete, A.; Cei, S.A.; Hanson, L.J.; Pari, G.S. (2005). A Kaposi's sarcoma-associated herpesvirus/human herpesvirus 8 ORF50 deletion mutant is defective for reactivation of latent virus and DNA replication. *Journal of Virology*, Vol.79, No.6, pp. 3479-3487

Xu, Y.; Rodriguez-Huete, A.; Pari, G.S. (2006). Evaluation of the lytic origins of replication of Kaposi's sarcoma-associated virus/human herpesvirus 8 in the context of the viral genome. *Journal of Virology*, Vol.80, No.19, pp. 9905-9909

Yakushko, Y.; Hackmann, C.; Günther, T.; Rückert, J.; Henke, M.; Koste, L.; Alkharsah, K.; Bohne, J.; Grundhoff, A.; Schulz, T.F.; Henke-Gendo, C. (2011). Kaposi's sarcoma-associated herpesvirus bacterial artificial chromosome contains a duplication of a long unique region fragment within the terminal repeat region. *Journal of Virology* (February 2011), published electronically ahead of print.

Yang, X.W.; Gong, S. (2005). An overview on the generation of BAC transgenic mice for neuroscience research. *Current Protocols in Neuroscience*, chapter 5.

Yao, H.; Osterrieder, N.; O'Callaghan, D.J. (2003). Generation and characterization of an EICP0 null mutant of equine herpesvirus 1. *Virus Research*, Vol.98, No.2, pp. 163-172

Yoshii, H.; Somboonthum, P.; Takahashi, M.; Yamanishi, K.; Mori, Y. (2007). Cloning of full length genome of varicella-zoster virus vaccine strain into a bacterial artificial chromosome and reconstitution of infectious virus. *Vaccine*, Vol.25, No.27, 5006-5012

Yu, D.; Ellis, H.M.; Lee, E.C.; Jenkins, N.A.; Copeland, N.G.; Court D.L. (2000). An efficient recombination system for chromosome engineering in Escherichia coli. *Proceedings of the National Academy of Sciences of the United States of America,* Vol.97, No.11, 5978-5983

Yu, D.; Silva, M.C.; Shenk, T. (2003). Functional map of human cytomegalovirus AD169 defined by global mutational analysis. *Proceedings of the National Academy of Sciences of the United States of America,* Vol.100, No.21, pp. 12396-12401

Yu, D.; Smith, G.A.; Enquist, L.W.; Shenk T. (2002). Construction of a self-excisable bacterial artificial chromosome containing the human cytomegalovirus genome and mutagenesis of the diploid TRL/IRL13 gene. *Journal of Virology,* Vol.76, No.5, pp. 2316-2328

Zhang, Y.; Buchholz, F.; Muyrers, J.P.; Stewart, A.F. (1998). A new logic for DNA engineering using recombination in Escherichia coli. *Nature Genetics,* Vol.20, No.2, 123-128

Zhang, Z.; Rowe, J.; Wang, W.; Sommer, M.; Arvin, A.; Moffat, J.; Zhu, H. (2007). Genetic analysis of varicella-zoster virus ORF0 to ORF4 by use of a novel luciferase bacterial artificial chromosome system. *Journal of Virology,* Vol.81, No.17, pp. 9024-9033

Zhang, Z.; Huang, Y.; Zhu, H. (2008). A highly efficient protocol of generating and analyzing VZV ORF deletion mutants based on a newly developed luciferase VZV BAC system. *Journal of Virological Methods,* Vol.148, No.1-2, pp. 197-204

Zhang, Z.; Selariu, A.; Warden, C.; Huang, G.; Huang, Y.; Zaccheus, O.; Cheng, T.; Xia, N.; Zhu, H. (2010). Genome-wide mutagenesis reveals that ORF7 is a novel VZV skin-tropic factor. *PLoS Pathogens,* Vol.6, No. e1000971

Zhao, Y.; Petherbridge, L.; Smith, L. P.; Baigent, S.; Nair, V. (2008). Self-excision of the BAC sequences from the recombinant Marek's disease virus genome increases replication and pathogenicity. *Virology Journal,* Vol.5, article No.19

Zhou, F.; Li, Q.; Wong, S.W.; Gao, S.J. (2010). Autoexcision of bacterial artificial chromosome facilitated by terminal repeat-mediated homologous recombination: a novel approach for generating traceless genetic mutants of herpesviruses. *Journal of Virology,* Vol.84, No.6, pp. 2871-2880

Zhou, F.C.; Zhang, Y.J.; Deng, J.H.; Wang, X.P.; Pan, H.Y.; Hettler, E.; Gao, S.J. (2002). Efficient infection by a recombinant Kaposi's sarcoma-associated herpesvirus cloned in a bacterial artificial chromosome: application for genetic analysis. *Journal of Virology,* Vol.76, No.12, pp. 6185-6196